THE HUGHSTON CLINIC
Sports Medicine Book

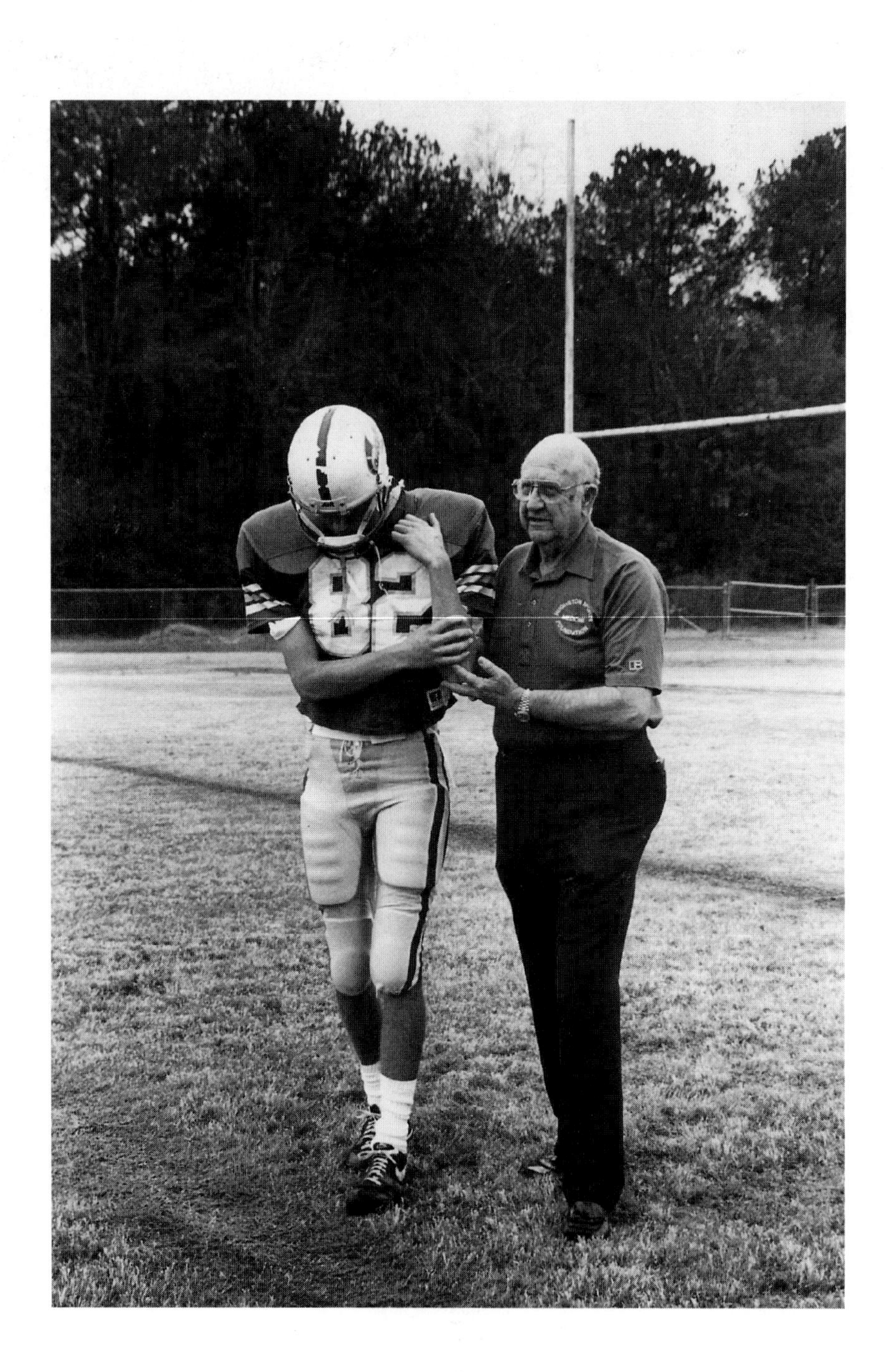

THE HUGHSTON CLINIC

Sports Medicine Book

Champ L. Baker, Jr., M.D., Editor-in-Chief

Fred Flandry, M.D., Section Editor

John M. Henderson, D.O., Section Editor

Hughston Sports Medicine Foundation, Inc.

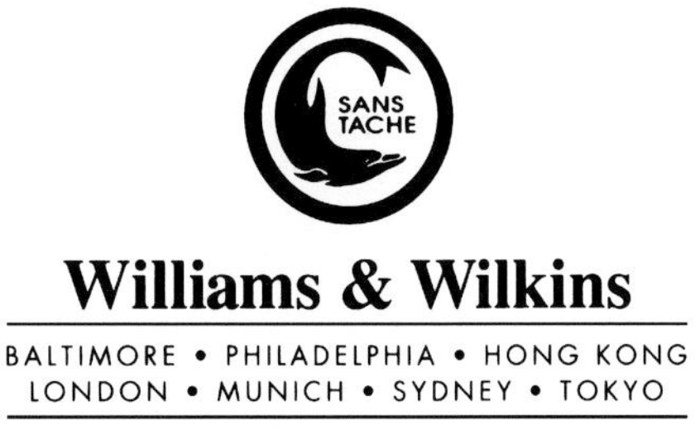

Williams & Wilkins

BALTIMORE • PHILADELPHIA • HONG KONG
LONDON • MUNICH • SYDNEY • TOKYO

A WAVERLY COMPANY

1995

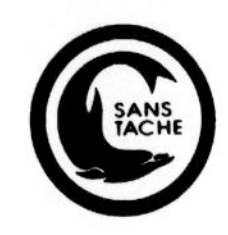

Executive Editor: Darlene B. Cooke
Developmental Editor: Sharon R. Zinner
Production Coordinator: Marette D. Magargle
Project Editor: Rebecca Krumm

Williams & Wilkins
Rose Tree Corporate Center, Building II
1400 Providence Rd., Suite 5025
Media, PA 19063-2043

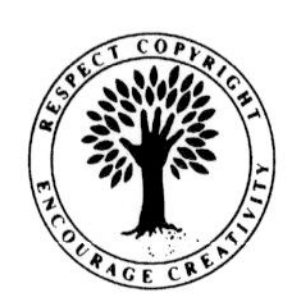

Accurate indications, adverse reactions, and dosage schedules for drugs are provided in this book, but it is possible they may change. The reader is urged to review the package information data of the manufacturers of the medications mentioned.

Printed in the United States of America

Library of Congress Cataloging in Publication Data
The Hughston Clinic sports medicine book / [edited by] Champ L. Baker.
p. cm.
"Hughston Sports Medicine Foundation, Inc."
Includes index.
ISBN 0-683-00397-6
1. Sports medicine. I. Baker, Champ L. II. Hughston Orthopaedic Clinic. III. Hughston Sports Medicine Foundation. IV. Title: Sports medicine book.
[DNLM: 1. Sports Medicine. 2. Athletic Injuries. QT 260 H8945 1995]
RC1210.H84 1995
617.1'027—dc20
DNLM/DLC
for Library of Congress 94-23442
CIP

The author and publishers have made every effort to trace the copyright holders for borrowed material. If they have inadvertently overlooked any, they will be pleased to make the necessary arrangements at the first opportunity.

95 96 97 98
1 2 3 4 5 6 7 8 9 10

To all past, present, and future residents and fellows at The Hughston Clinic and to Jack C. Hughston, M.D., our teacher, mentor, and friend.

FOREWORD

At long last. . . . We've been talking about producing a book on sports medicine for several years and have never gotten to first base. Congratulations to Champ Baker for taking the bull by the horns and organizing and forging ahead on this project. This thesis is now a reality.

Our roots go back to 1950, when we began to provide sideline "coverage" of high school football games in our community. Today, in 1995, in light of the flamboyant entrepreneurship that is sometimes seen in sports medicine, readers may find it hard to believe that, back then, our local medical community took a dim view of this activity and considered it unethical and indecent, even though this health service was provided at no charge. We persevered, however, and now we cover some 30 or 40 high schools in this region. High school athletics continues to be the most important area of organized sports, because at this level we are dealing with so many enthusiastic youngsters who may not have natural athletic ability. In addition, parents are often, understandably, over enthusiastic.

Over the 4 or 5 years after 1950, we met with county medical societies in the Georgia and Alabama area around Columbus, Georgia, to explain our experiences and the numerous advantages of medical coverage at athletic competitions. By 1959, this service had extended to nearly every community in the two-state area. The physicians interested in providing this coverage were a diverse group—internists, family practice physicians, pediatricians, even urologists and ophthalmologists, and a scattering of orthopedists.

The Board of Councilors of the Medical Association of Georgia became aware of the potential impact of these activities on the field of medicine as a whole and requested that we offer a postgraduate course for physicians, coaches, trainers, educators, and administrators involved in sports and sports medicine at the high school level. We put on the first course in 1960; it may have been the first one held in the United States. The leading neurosurgeon in the state, who long ago had given up going to medical meetings, observed that this was the most contributory and interesting meeting he had ever attended.

Luckily, it so happened that Sam Burke, then President of the National Federation of State High School Associations, lived in Thomaston, a town in central Georgia about 60 miles from Columbus. Although I did not know of him at the time, he turned out to be a stellar performer and a great force in the advancement of sports medicine in high schools throughout the United States. A considerable number of constructive advancements in sports medicine emanated from that initial postgraduate course. Sam Burke immediately made wearing mouthpieces mandatory for football players in the state of Georgia. The purpose of mouthpieces was to protect the teeth and decrease the incidence of concussions. The results were so dramatic that, the next year, he was instrumental in having the National Federation of State High School Associations institute this practice on a national basis. The health benefits (injury prevention) were obvious, and routine use of mouthpieces reduced the cost of medical treatment nationally by millions of dollars.

The National Athletic Trainers Association (NATA) was organized in 1950, and with Kenny Howard's association and interest we made a scientific presentation at their annual meeting in Miami, in 1955. There were about 50 members in attendance. Today, the attendees at annual meetings number in the thousands. Through the good work of Fred Hein of the American Medical Association (AMA) staff, NATA became an affiliate of the AMA in 1963. It was at about this time that NATA was becoming organized as an educational instrument for the trainers. We formed our first liaison with NATA in 1955, an association that continues today at their annual national meetings.

The AMA in 1959 organized a Committee on the Medical Aspects of Sports and began conducting scientific seminars at the AMA's annual clinical meetings. The Committee itself, composed of approximately 12 to 15 physicians, included representatives from various medical specialties: orthopedics, pediatrics, neurosugery, family practice, urology, and internal medicine. There were also three or four members from college infirmaries who had a special interest in various areas of sports medicine. In addition to the annual meetings, which usually attracted representatives from all sports-related societies, the Committee met at various times during the year to formulate policy, prepare instructional pamphlets, and propose recommendations for prevention of illness and injury. In these respects, the Committee worked closely with the National Federation of State High School Associations. Their achievements were many and important—to mention a few, elimination of "spearing," development of safety equipment, improvement of helmets and face masks, management of head injuries, and elimination of the crack-back block, resulting in an estimated 50% decrease in the incidences of knee injuries. Fred Hein was a great organizer and a moving force in the administration of this Committee.

The American Academy of Orthopaedic Surgeons (AAOS) established a Committee on Sports Medicine in 1965, for the intended purpose of education through postgraduate courses for the benefit of orthopedic surgeons. This was part of a general postgraduate approach found feasible by a 2-year experiment with a couple of postgraduate courses on general orthopedics and trauma held in Atlanta by AAOS. Because of my involvement with the Atlanta courses, as a member of the Education Committee, I was appointed Chairman of the newly formed Sports Medicine Committee. For the next 10 years we, the AAOS, conducted postgraduate courses on sports medicine in different areas throughout the United States on an annual basis.

Initially, faculty for these courses was quite limited, and their depth of knowledge was likewise limited in many areas. Thus, instructors had to be trained, and a new field for medical research emerged. For example, to learn more about the arm in throwing sports a physician who had some basic knowledge in this area was appointed and given 2 years to conduct research toward the end of developing meaningful information for a presentation. Situations such as this spurred research and organization of material in preparation for presentations. This process produced much of the knowledge we now regard almost as "given," without reflecting on the history of its development. Once presented, the ideas were quickly elaborated on by virtue of exchange between the faculty and the audience. I think it was these courses, and their tremendous educational benefits to so many interested and enthusiastic orthopedists, that led to the rapid expansion of knowledge and service in the field of sports medicine.

Many of the materials produced in these postgraduate courses needed to be published, but the subject matter was somewhat unusual and editorial boards of established orthopedic journals were not accustomed to such submissions. Thus, it became obvious to me that we were going to have to develop an outlet for much of this material. I began researching the feasibility of a journal on sports medicine in 1968. This finally developed into the initial publication of the *Journal of Sports Medicine* in 1972, which later became the *American Journal of Sports Medicine.* The journal is now a potent educational force in sports medicine and our present editor, Robert Leach, is striving to maximize its quality and volume. Competition always creates advancement; the established orthopedic journals saw the tremendous interest generated by the *American Journal of Sports Medicine* and began accepting and publishing similar reports related to sports medicine.

The avid participation in sports medicine postgraduate courses made us realize that an AAOS committee could not provide adequate representation for sports medicine. Thus, in 1970, we began developing plans for what became the American Orthopaedic Society for Sports Medicine (AOSSM). At its organizational meeting in Washington, D.C., during the Academy meeting of 1972, Don O'Donoghue was appointed chairman. The formation of the AOSSM and its subsequent status of an affiliate to the Academy met with considerable resistance; however, the Board of Directors of the Academy thought enough of the idea so that the resistance was finally overcome. As I best remember it at the moment, the driving forces that helped us accomplish this were Mason Hohl and John Hinchey. In the summer of 1975, the AOSSM held its first annual meeting in New Orleans, with much success and enthusiastic participation. As we all know, its growth has been great. I anticipated that, once we had this organization up and going, the Academy would dissolve the Committee on Sports Medicine in deference to the AOSSM, as an affiliate. I was wrong.

The American Board of Orthopaedic Surgery desired to explore whether the field of sports medicine should be included as a discipline of academic orthopedics. Thus, they requested that we function as an elective 1-year residency rotation with a university orthopedic training program. In 1968, Jack Wickstrom and Tulane University elected to establish this rotation, which is now in its 28th year. About 2 years thereafter, they recommended that we establish a fellowship in sports medicine, to complement the residency training, so that those not in the Tulane orthopedic residency program could have access to postgraduate sports medicine training after they completed their orthopedic residency, wherever they might be. It was odd, to me, at the time, that so many centers that promoted sports medicine were not enthusiastic about developing fellowships in that subspecialty. I am pleased to report that, today, around the country such fellowship programs are almost an institution, even to the extent that some regulatory mechanisms are developing.

Another advantage of the fellowships is that they offer opportunities for postgraduate training to orthopedists from outside the United States. It was this group of "foreign fellows" who trained with us that formed the nucleus of the International Society of the Knee.

One of us, Steve Hunter, instituted a fellowship in sports medicine as it is encountered in family practice, and there is now a sports medicine section in the American Academy of Family Physicians.

Many fine people—unselfish, hard working, and too numerous to be cited—have contributed to the recent development of sports medicine. My purpose in this Foreword is to offer a brief history of the involvement of The Hughston Clinic, in sports medicine—in the seminal research and as it is practiced today. The production of this book is one result. A few of the contributing authors who were not trained here have been close associates and friends. They have actively participated in the progress in sports medicine. I offer my congratulations to each of the authors for their stellar efforts and to Champ Baker for putting it all together.

Jack C. Hughston, M.D.
The Hughston Clinic
Columbus, Georgia.

PREFACE

The specialized field of treating athletes is not new. Herodicus of Selymbria, credited with being the father of sports medicine, practiced his craft more than 2000 years ago. As a medical and surgical subspecialty, sports medicine has gained credibility in the last decade, but the term *sports medicine* is, all too often, overused and abused. *Sports medicine* has many definitions. We at The Hughston Clinic believe that sports medicine involves education, treatment, and care, not just of the injury, but of the athlete. It involves understanding the sport and the climate of competition that motivates every athlete. Combining this understanding with a complete history and physical examination of the athlete enables the physician to reach a correct diagnosis and to determine the proper treatment, be it early rehabilitation and return to sport or surgical intervention, which might delay return to competition but might make it possible.

This philosophy of comprehensive care of the scholar athlete has been advocated at The Hughston Clinic since Dr. Jack Hughston founded the Clinic in 1949. In 1968, at the request of the American Board of Orthopaedic Surgery, the Clinic began training residents by offering a sports medicine rotation. A few years later, a year-long fellowship in sports medicine was established at the Clinic. These educational programs have continued, and past residents and fellows make up the Hughston Society, a cadre of orthopedic surgeons and primary care physicians who were trained in the Hughston Philosophy.

The Hughston Society includes orthopedic surgeons and physicians from other specialties, from the United States and abroad. The group is bound by a genuine concern for athletes and a desire to help them return to competition injury free in the shortest amount of time. We all know the importance of the preparticipation physical for discovering potential problems of athletes. We know the advantage of being on the sidelines during practice and competition and understanding the athlete and the sport as well as the mechanisms of injury. We also know the importance of preventive medicine. The art of the sports medicine physician is practiced on the field of competition and not in a laboratory or through expensive diagnostic imaging. The history of the injury—who, what, when, and how—is coupled with a complete examination to arrive at a clinical diagnosis.

The sports medicine physicians who have contributed to this book, both men and women, orthopedic surgeons and family physicians, have left The Hughston Clinic with knowledge they now share with others through seminars, presentations, and the written word. This book is a compilation of the thoughts and experiences of more than 100 members of the Hughston Society. It includes an administrative section that details some of the obligations of the team physician, the athletic trainer, and the physical therapist. The majority of the book covers clinical aspects of medical problems common in athletes and the injuries that may result from competitive play. This is not intended to be a surgical text but is to serve as a reminder for orthopedists who take care of teams and want information on treatment of common medical problems. For family physicians who serve as team physicians, this book gives more information on diagnosing and treating common injuries. The concept of a team approach to sports medicine is not new; it has been practiced at The Hughston Clinic for many years. The combined experiences of physicians from these two disciplines should help the reader care for injured athletes.

George McCluskey, a registered physical therapist and contributor to this book, is fond of saying, "As long as you have a mother and a child, you have sports medicine," This book is intended to help practitioners become more knowledgeable and better prepared to work in the realm that is truly sports medicine—the triangle of practitioner, parent, and child. Sports medicine is based on the physician's approach to athletes who have had an injury and are unsure what that injury means to them and their ability to participate in sports. The true sports medicine physician reassures, educates, and treats, to allow athletes to return to sports participation quickly, safely, and, more importantly, in good health.

ACKNOWLEDGMENTS

The task of editing this book was made easy by the expert guidance and assistance of Darlene Cooke, Sharon Zinner, and Rebecca Krumm at Williams & Wilkins. The majority of the work was done by Donna Tilton, who coordinated the efforts of more than 100 physicians throughout the United States and abroad and made each of their chapters readable and concise. When Donna went to work full-time for the *American Journal of Sports Medicine,* her position was ably assumed by Leslie Neistadt. I gratefully acknowledge the assistance of Carol Binns, senior medical writer at the Hughston Sports Medicine Foundation, who was a great source of guidance and wisdom. Thanks to Carolyn M. Capers, M.S.M.I., C.M.I., and Judy L. Barr, M.S.M.I, C.M.I., medical illustrators at the Hughston Sports Medicine Foundation, and Yvonne Ehrhart, medical photographer at the Hughston Sports Medicine Foundation, who have so beautifully illustrated this book. Most importantly, thank you to Dr. Jack C. Hughston, who inspired us all, and to the past and present residents and fellows and the staff at The Hughston Clinic, who have given counsel and advice on the production of this book.

CONTRIBUTORS

James R. Andrews, M.D.
Clinical Professor of Orthopaedics and Sports Medicine, University of Virginia Medical School
Charlottesville, Virginia
Clinical Professor, Department of Orthopaedic Surgery, University of Kentucky Medical Center
Lexington Kentucky
Orthopaedic Surgeon, Alabama Sports Medicine and Orthopaedic Center
Birmingham, Alabama

Richard L. Angelo, M.D.
Assistant Clinical Professor of Orthopaedics, University of Washington
Team Physician, UW Huskies
Washington Orthopaedics and Sports Medicine
Kirkland, Washington

Michael J. Axe, M.D.
Co-Director, All Sports Clinic of Delaware
Newark, Delaware

Champ L. Baker, Jr., M.D.
The Hughston Clinic, P.C.
Columbus, Georgia
Clinical Assistant Professor of Orthopaedics, Tulane University School of Medicine
New Orleans, Louisiana

Karl Lee Barkley II, M.D.
Family Practice, University Family Physicians
Charlotte, North Carolina
Team Physician, Davidson College
Davidson, North Carolina

Gene R. Barrett, M.D.
Mississippi Sports Medicine and Orthopaedic Center
Jackson, Mississippi

Major Kenneth B. Batts, D.O.
Director, Primary Care Sports Medicine, Family Practice Department, Tripler Army Medical Center
Honolulu, Hawaii

Paul W. Baumert, Jr., M.D.
Primary Care Sports Medicine, Kaiser Permanente
Overland Park, Kansas

Thomas N. Bernard, Jr., M.D.
Anderson, South Carolina

James L. Beskin, M.D.
Peachtree Orthopaedic Clinic, P.A.
Atlanta, Georgia
Assistant Clinical Professor of Orthopaedics, Tulane University School of Medicine
New Orleans, Louisiana

Kenneth M. Bielak, M.D.
Assistant Professor, Department of Family Medicine, Graduate School of Medicine, University of Tennessee Medical Center at Knoxville
Knoxville, Tennessee

Turner A. Blackburn, Jr., P.T., A.T.,C., M.Ed.
Cofounder and Director, Berkshire Institute of Orthopedic and Sports Physical Therapy, Inc.
Wyomissing, Pennsylvania
Adjunct Assistant Professor, Physical Therapy Program, University of Miami School of Medicine
Miami, Florida

James R. Bocell, Jr., M.D.
Clinical Professor, Department of Orthopaedic Surgery, Baylor College of Medicine
Houston, Texas

Thomas A. Boers, P.T., M.T.
Rehabilitation Services of Columbus
Columbus, Georgia

Mark R. Brinker, M.D.
Director of Orthopaedic Research, Department of Orthopaedic Surgery, University of Texas Medical School at Houston
Houston, Texas

Andrew A. Brooks, M.D.
Cedars-Sinai Medical Towers
Los Angeles, California

Douglas G. Browning, M.D., A.T.,C.
Assistant Professor in Family Medicine and Associate in Surgical Sciences-Orthopedics/Sports Medicine, Bowman Gray School of Medicine of Wake Forest University
Associate Team Physician, Wake Forest University
Winston-Salem, North Carolina

Michael E. Brunet, M.D.
Professor of Orthopaedic Surgery, Tulane University School of Medicine
New Orleans, Louisiana

Robert R. Burger, M.D.
Associate Director, Queen City Sports Medicine
Team Physician, Xavier University, The College of Mt. St. Joseph, Wilmington College
Volunteer Clinical Instructor, Department of Orthopaedic Surgery, University of Cincinnati
Cincinnati, Ohio

J. Kenneth Burkus, M.D.
The Hughston Clinic, P.C.
Columbus, Georgia

Peter D. Candelora, M.D.
Consulting Staff, Shriners Hospital
Tampa, Florida
Chairman, Department of Surgery, Northbay Hospital
New Port Richey, Florida

William G. Carson, Jr., M.D.
Clinical Assistant Professor of Orthopaedic Surgery, University of South Florida College of Medicine
Tampa, Florida

Peter M. Cimino, M.D.
Omaha Orthopedic Clinic & Sports Medicine, P.C.
Omaha, Nebraska

Massimo Cipolla, M.D.
Clinica Valle Giulia
Rome, Italy

Clark H. Cobb, M.D.
Faculty, Family Practice Residency Program, Co-Director, Primary Care Sports Medicine, Martin Army Hospital
Fort Benning, Georgia
Clinical Associate Professor of Family Practice, Uniformed Services University of the Health Sciences
Bethesda, Maryland

Mervyn J. Cross, MB., BS., M.D., F.R.A.C.S., F.A.Ortho A.
Crows Nest, New South Wales, Australia

Walton W. Curl, M.D.
Associate Professor of Orthopaedic Surgery, Bowman Gray School of Medicine of Wake Forest University
Director of Wake Forest University Sports Medicine Unit
Winston-Salem, North Carolina

Kenneth E. DeHaven, M.D.
Professor and Associate Chairman, Department of Orthopaedics, Director of Athletic Medicine, University of Rochester School of Medicine and Dentistry
Rochester, New York

R. Todd Dombroski, D.O.
Director of Primary Care Sports Medicine, Madigan Army Medical Center
Fort Lewis, Washington

Scott Dye, M.D.
Assistant Clinical Professor of Orthopaedic Surgery, University of California San Francisco
San Francisco, California

William Etchison, M.S.
Director of Industrial Relations and Wellness, Hughston Sports Medicine Foundation, Inc.
Columbus, Georgia

Fred Flandry, M.D., F.A.C.S.
The Hughston Clinic, P.C.
Chairman, Department of Surgery, and Chief, Section of Orthopaedic Surgery, The Medical Center Hospital
Columbus, Georgia
Clinical Associate Professor, Department of Orthopaedic Surgery, Tulane University School of Medicine
New Orleans, Louisiana
Adjunct Assistant Professor in Small Animal Surgery and Medicine, College of Veterinary Medicine, Auburn University
Auburn, Alabama

Robert S. Franco, M.D.
First Coast Medical Group
Medical Director, Riverside Hospital Sports Medicine Program
Chairman, Riverside Orthopaedic Foundation
Jacksonville, Florida

Vittorio Franco, M.D.
Clinica Valle Giulia
Rome, Italy

Hugh A. Frederick, M.D.
Associate Attending Physician, Orthopaedic Surgery, Baylor University Medical Center
Dallas, Texas

Gerard T. Gabel, M.D.
Assistant Professor, Department of Orthopaedic Surgery, Baylor College of Medicine
Houston, Texas

Angelo Galante, M.D.
Staff Physician, Athleticare and Health Care Plan
Team Physician, Buffalo Blizzard, Buffalo Stampede, and Canisius College Ice Hockey
Buffalo, New York

Sandra Gibney, M.D.
Family Practice Resident, Medical Center of Delaware
Newark, Delaware

Joe Gieck, Ed.D., A.T.,C., P.T.
Head Athletic Trainer, Professor, Curry School of Education
Associate Professor, Orthopaedics/Rehabilitation, University of Virginia
Charlottesville, Virginia

John M. Graham, Jr., M.D.
Orthopaedic Surgeon, Charleston Orthopaedics, P.A.
Team Physician, College of Charleston
Clinical Instructor, Medical University of South Carolina
Charleston, South Carolina

Brian Halpern, M.D.
Medical Director/Chairman of the Board, Sports Medicine New Jersey
Assistant Attending Physician, Sports Medicine Department, Hospital for Special Surgery
Assistant Attending Physician, New York Hospital, Cornell Medical Center
New York, New York
Clinical Assistant Professor, Sports Medicine, Robert Wood Johnson Medical School, University of Medicine and Dentistry of New Jersey
New Brunswick, New Jersey

James R. Harris, M.D.
Azalea Orthopedic and Sports Medicine Clinic
Tyler, Texas

David Harsha, M.D.
The Sports Medicine Institute of Indiana
Indiana Surgery Center
Indianapolis, Indiana

Jon M. Hay, M.Ed., A.T.,C.
Head Athletic Trainer, Georgia Southwestern College
Americus, Georgia

John M. Henderson, D.O.
Director, Primary Care Sports Medicine, The Hughston Clinic, P.C.
Columbus, Georgia

Jack H. Henry, M.D.
Clinical Professor of Orthopaedic Surgery, Columbia Presbyterian Medical Center
New York, New York

David L. Higgins, M.D.
Assistant Clinical Professor, Georgetown University School of Medicine
Washington, D.C.
Assistant Professor, Uniformed Services University of the Health Sciences
Bethesda, Maryland

Anne Hollister, M.D.
Adult Neuro Trauma Division, Rancho Los Amigos Medical Center
Downey, California

Kenny Howard, A.T.,C.
The Hughston Clinic, P.C.
Auburn, Alabama

Tanya L. Hrabal, M.D.
Emergency Room Physician
Jacksonville, Florida

Jack C. Hughston, M.D.
Chairman of the Board, The Hughston Clinic, P.C.
Columbus, Georgia
Professor Emeritus, Tulane University School of Medicine
New Orleans, Louisiana

Stephen C. Hunter, M.D.
The Hughston Clinic, P.C.
Columbus, Georgia

Mary Lloyd Ireland, M.D.
Assistant Professor, College of Medicine (Orthopaedics), Department of Family Practice, Orthopaedic Consultant to Sports Teams, University of Kentucky
Director, Kentucky Sports Medicine Clinic
Lexington, Kentucky
Orthopaedic Consultant to Sports Teams, Eastern Kentucky University
Richmond, Kentucky

Joseph G. Jacko, M.D.
Southwest Orthopedic Institute
Dallas, Texas

Kurt E. Jacobson, M.D., F.A.C.S.
The Hughston Clinic, P.C.
Columbus, Georgia

William D. Jones, P.T., C.S.C.S.
Human Performance and Rehabilitation Center
Columbus, Georgia

David M. Kahler, M.D.
Assistant Professor, Department of Orthopaedic Surgery, University of Virginia
Charlottesville, Virginia

Lee A. Kelley, M.D.
Peachtree Orthopaedic Clinic, P.A.
Atlanta, Georgia

Gary Keogh, M.D., M.R.C.G.P., D.A., M.L.C.O.M., M.R.O.
Pennington, New Jersey

David B. Keyes, M.D.
Clinical Assistant Professor of Orthopaedic Surgery, University of Miami
Active Staff, Baptist Hospital of Miami
Courtesy Staff, South Miami Hospital
Miami, Florida

Bernard G. Kirol, M.D.
Nalle Clinic
Charlotte, North Carolina

Daniel R. Kraeger, D.O., A.T.,C.
Medical Director, Southern Wisconsin Sports Medicine Center
Medical Director, Mercy Sports Medicine Center
Janesville, Wisconsin

Robert E. Leach, M.D.
Professor of Orthopaedic Surgery, Boston University Medical School
Editor, American Journal of Sports Medicine
Boston, Massachusetts

Mark J. Leski, M.D.
Associate Professor of Family Practice, Director of Sports Medicine, Department of Family and Preventative Medicine, University of South Carolina
Columbia, South Carolina

Steven D. Levin, M.D.
Midwest Sports Medicine and Orthopaedic Surgery
Elk Grove Village, Illinois

Stephen H. Liu, M.D.
Assistant Professor, Department of Orthopaedic Surgery, University of California, Los Angeles School of Medicine
Team Physician, UCLA Athletics
Los Angeles, California

Rene K. Marti, M.D.
Professor and Chairman, Orthopaedic Department, University of Amsterdam
Amsterdam, Netherlands
Chief Consultant, Klinik Gut
St. Moritz, Switzerland

David F. Martin, M.D.
Assistant Professor of Orthopaedic Surgery, Bowman Gray School of Medicine of Wake Forest University
Wake Forest University Sports Medicine Unit
Team Physician, Guilford College
Winston-Salem, North Carolina

Joseph A. Martino
Cumming, Georgia

George M. McCluskey, Jr., L.A.T., PT
Rehabilitation Services of Columbus, Inc.
Columbus, Georgia

George M. McCluskey III, M.D.
The Hughston Clinic, P.C.
Columbus, Georgia
Clinical Assistant Professor, Department of Orthopaedic Surgery, Tulane University School of Medicine
New Orleans, Louisiana

Leland C. McCluskey, M.D.
The Hughston Clinic, P.C.
Columbus, Georgia

Frank C. McCue III, M.D.
Alfred R. Shands Professor of Orthopaedic Surgery and Plastic Surgery of the Hand, Director, Division of Sports Medicine and Hand Surgery, Team Physician, Department of Athletics, University of Virginia
Charlottesville, Virginia

Craig C. McKirgan, D.O.
Orthopaedic Surgeon, Center for Orthopaedics and Sports Medicine
Team Orthopaedic Surgeon, Indiana University of Pennsylvania
Indiana, Pennsylvania

Thomas K. Miller, M.D.
Clinical Assistant Professor of Orthopaedic Surgery, University of Virginia, Roanoke Program
Roanoke Orthopaedic Center
Roanoke, Virginia

Michael A. Oberlander, M.D.
Coastal Orthopaedic and Sports Specialists
Director, Sports Medicine, Health and Fitness Institute
Concord, California

Dianne Bazor Olszak, P.T.
Birmingham, Alabama

Arnold R. Penix, M.D.
Cincinnati, Ohio

William W. Peterson, M.D.
Memorial Clinic
Olympia, Washington

Robert M. Poole, M.Ed., P.T., A.T.,C.
Director, Human Performance and Rehabilitation Center, Inc.
Atlanta, Georgia
Clinical Professor of Physical Therapy, North Georgia College
Dahlonega, Georgia

Julie A. Pryde, M.S., P.T., A.T.,C.
Coordinator, Health and Fitness Institute, Center for Sports Medicine
Instructor, Department of Physical Therapy, Samuel Merritt College
Consultant, Intercollegiate Athletics, Saint Mary's College of California
Walnut Creek, California

Giancarlo Puddu, M.D.
Professor of Orthopaedics, University of Roma "La Sapienza"
Rome, Italy

Reynold L. Rimoldi, M.D.
Las Vegas, Nevada

Lawrence D. Rink, M.D., F.A.C.C.
Clinical Professor of Medicine, Indiana University School of Medicine
Bloomington, Indiana

Lucien M. Rouse, Jr., M.D.
Assistant Professor, Department of Orthopaedics, Section of Athletic Medicine, University of Rochester School of Medicine and Dentistry
Rochester, New York

Carlton G. Savory, M.D.
The Hughston Clinic, P.C.
Columbus, Georgia

Todd A. Schmidt, M.D., F.A.C.S.
The Hughston Clinic, P.C.
Atlanta, Georgia

Alberto Selvanetti, M.D.
Clinica Valle Giulia
Rome, Italy

Robert M. Shalvoy, M.D.
Clinical Instructor in Orthopaedic Surgery, Brown University Program in Medicine
Director, Ortho Sports New England
Providence, Rhode Island

Herbert L. Silver, P.T., E.C.S.
Physical Therapist, Human Performance and Rehabilitation Center, Inc.
Atlanta, Georgia
Clinical Faculty, Department of Physical Therapy, North Georgia College
Dahlonega, Georgia

Patricia L. Skaggs, M.D.
The Hughston Clinic, P.C.
Auburn, Alabama

Robert S. Skerker, M.D.
The Rehabilitation Institute
Morristown Memorial Hospital
Morristown, New Jersey

Patrick A. Smith, M.D.
Team Physician, University of Missouri
Clinical Assistant Professor of Surgery, University of Missouri School of Medicine
Columbia, Missouri

Robert O'Neil Snoddy, Jr., M.D.
Suwanee, Georgia

Tarek O. Souryal, M.D.
Director, Texas Sports Medicine Group
Dallas, Texas

Gregory W. Stewart, M.D.
Assistant Professor, Section of Physical Medicine and Rehabilitation, Louisiana State University School of Medicine
Clinical Assistant Professor, Department of Orthopaedics, Tulane University
New Orleans, Louisiana

Laura Stokes, M.S.
Columbus, Georgia

Timothy B. Sutherland, M.D.
Alabama Sports Medicine and Orthopaedic Center
Birmingham, Alabama

William R. Sutton, M.D.
Wilmington, North Carolina

Suzanne Tanner, M.D.
Assistant Professor, Department of Orthopaedics and Pediatrics, University of Colorado Health Services Center
Denver, Colorado

Nancy J. Thompson, M.P.H., Ph.D.
Assistant Professor of Behavioral Science and Epidemiology, Rollins School of Public Health, Emory University
Atlanta, Georgia

Paula R. Tisdale, O.T.R.
Staff Therapist, Sundance Rehabilitation Center
Columbus, Georgia

David Tremaine, M.D.
Director, Foot and Ankle Center at Anderson Clinic
Arlington, Virginia
Clinical Assistant Professor of Surgery, Uniformed Services University of the Health Sciences
Bethesda, Maryland

Hugh S. Tullos, M.D.
Baylor College of Medicine
Houston, Texas

John Turba, M.D.
President, Queen City Sports Medicine and Rehabilitation
Cincinnati, Ohio

Tim L. Uhl, P.T.
Director of Physical Therapy, The Human Performance and Rehabilitation Center
Columbus, Georgia;
Adjunct Instructor of Clinical Physical Therapy, University of South Alabama
Mobile, Alabama

John Uribe, M.D.
Associate Professor, Chief, Sports Medicine Division, Department of Orthopaedics, University of Miami
Miami, Florida

Niek van Dijk, M.D.
University of Amsterdam
Amsterdam, Netherlands

J. William Van Manen, M.D.
Richmond, Virginia

Geoffrey Vaupel, M.D.
Medical Director, Institute for Sports Medicine, Davies Medical Center
San Francisco, California

W. Michael Walsh, M.D.
Clinical Associate Professor of Orthopaedic Surgery, University of Nebraska College of Medicine
Adjunct Graduate Associate Professor, School of Health, Physical Education and Recreation, Team Orthopaedist for all sports, University of Nebraska–Omaha
Omaha, Nebraska

Keith Webster, M.A., A.T.,C.
Director of Sports Relations, Hughston Sports Medicine Foundation, Inc.
Columbus, Georgia

Steven H. Weeden, B.A.
Medical Student, University of Texas Medical School at Houston
Houston, Texas

Barry L. White, P.T., M.S., E.C.S., R.E.P.T.
Physical Therapist, Clinical Electrophysiologic Specialist, Rehabilitation Services of Columbus
Columbus, Georgia

Franklin D. Wilson, M.D.
The Sports Medicine Institute of Indiana
Community Hospitals of Indianapolis Inc.
Assistant Professor of Orthopaedics, Indiana University Medical Center
Indianapolis, Indiana
Neutral Team Physician, National Football League

CONTENTS

I

ADMINISTRATIVE ASPECTS OF SPORTS MEDICINE

1 *Jack C. Hughston*

The Role of the Team Physician

The team physician is a person who is interested in using medical knowledge in an enjoyable, though serious, extra-curricular activity for the benefit of athletics and athletes. One's specific area of medical expertise or specialty does not really matter; we each have basic medical knowledge and can learn the fundamentals of emergency evaluation. Furthermore, a whole community of physicians is available to whom we can refer athletes for definitive treatment. The role of the team physician is to be supportive and unobtrusive, so the coach's attention can be directed to coaching without having to worry about an injured or sick player.

Being a team physician carries with it great responsibility. "It can be rewarding and at times demanding, inconvenient but entertaining, even obligatory but soul-satisfying" (Fig. 1–1).[1] Being a team physician is not something one can play at part-time or when it is convenient. The team physician should always be available to the athletes under his or her care. Athletes do not follow schedules for their injuries and must be treated in a timely fashion so that they can resume their athletic activities.

In the early 1950s, being a team physician was considered a community service that one performed without pay. Community physicians served one or more local high school athletic programs. In the 1960s physicians began being associated with college teams. This trend gradually gained momentum, and by 1980 most colleges had team physicians. Again, this coverage was performed by a physician in the local area on a volunteer basis.

For whatever reason, it was orthopedists who often functioned as the team physician at the high school level. Perhaps it was their strong interest in the musculoskeletal system, or perhaps because their training fit better "in the trenches" of athletic competition. As knowledge of athletic injuries and the importance of medical coverage grew, the family practice physician became an integral part of the college athletic health team. Today, there are postgraduate fellowships in sports medicine for primary care physicians.

Meanwhile, orthopedists moved into the arena of professional sports—an entirely different ballgame in many ways. The time commitments for traveling across the country, the long length of the playing season, and other factors often require financial remuneration for the team physician.

The coverage of college teams by physicians led to the association of two types of health care providers: the team physician and the athletic trainer. This association in turn has led to a more sophisticated sports medicine program. The role of the team physician has become one of support and cooperation with the athletic trainer, who is with the players daily and knows their personalities, their fatigue levels, and their idiosyncrasies. The trainer deals with their nutritional needs, their protective equipment, their weight training, and much more. The physicians interested in dealing with athletes have learned much from athletic trainers, and vice versa.

Physical therapists, another important part of the sports medicine team, help in the recovery of injured players. The team physician must see that this therapy is conducted at a site separate from the training room. Uninjured team members do not increase their mental toughness by being exposed to those working on recovery from injury. I have seen the adverse effects of such a program. Because the prepractice activities of the players require most of the attention of the trainer, the trainer cannot give full attention to players in a rehabilitation program. In this case, the athlete needing supervision of rehabilitation exercises suffers, and the vital role of the physical therapist becomes clear.

Today, the volunteer arrangement remains the most common one for team physicians and, in my view, is the most important contribution a physician can make to a

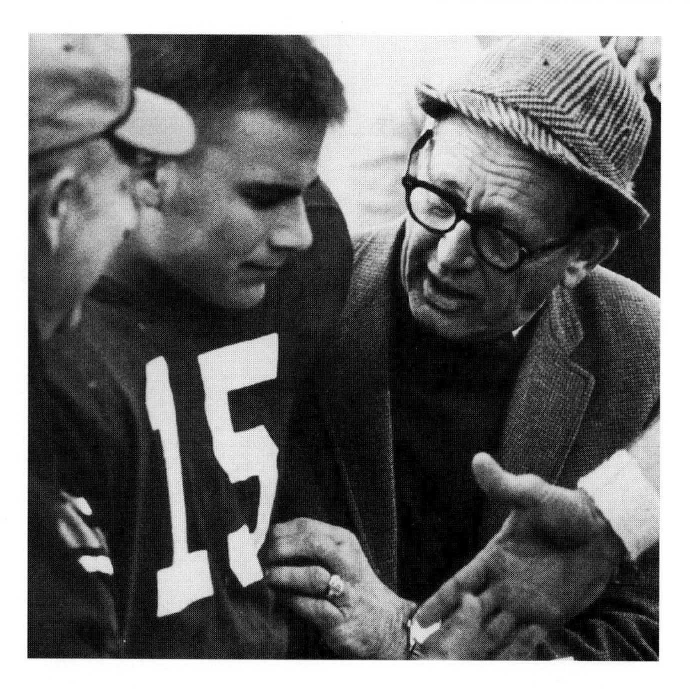

Fig. 1–1. Dr. Hughston on the sidelines caring for an injured player. Being a team physician "can be rewarding and at times demanding, inconvenient but entertaining, even obligatory, but soul-satisfying." (Committee on Sports Medicine: The Team Physician. Bulletin, The American Academy of Orthopaedic Surgeons. *20*:22, 1972.)

team. At the high school level in particular, the team physician helps in the evaluations that separate the athlete from the nonathletic person who wants to be an athlete. The preseason physical evaluation can identify individuals who would have difficulty competing. Further elimination may be necessary as training and the season progress. It is important to identify those who are not able to compete for their own protection, not just for the welfare of the team.

Most physicians acting as team physicians need to increase their knowledge of the requirements for each sport. This will help them better appreciate the demands placed on the athlete and help them evaluate the relationship of injury to performance. The physician should get to know the athletes' personalities, motivations, and tolerances for pain. Problems identified at the preseason physical evaluation can be corrected during preparticipation conditioning by having the athlete follow the physician's specific prescription to improve areas of noted physical deficit. The physician must remember that "all athletes cannot be All-American in the sports of their choice, and channeling them into other areas of participation is most important."[1]

Sideline etiquette is important for the team physician. Dress should be respectable and professional and the physician should stay in the background. Do not get into the coaches' area and block their movements. Go onto the field of play only when summoned. Trainers make the initial on-field examination, but they should know not to take the time to perform a complete knee examination on the field. The player should be taken off the field so the game can continue.

It is important for team physicians to be aware of the equipment needed for event coverage and to be sure it is available. In 1952, I remember having to find a two-by-four board in the Birmingham, Alabama, stadium to use as a splint for a lower limb. The player rode the train all the way back to Columbus, Georgia, splinted in this manner. Commercial splints were unheard of then, but after this incident I always kept some boxes of plaster of paris and bass wood splints on the sidelines.

The physician should always be prepared with basic equipment: the customary stethoscope, blood pressure apparatus, tongue depressors, flashlight, medications, suture sets for minor lacerations, and miscellaneous assistive devices. Splints of various types should be available on the sideline, along with such items as a stretcher, a spine board, fluids, ice, and oxygen, if possible. Today, an ambulance is often available at the game site. The physician should be aware of the resources available from the ambulance service. A clear plan of evacuation should be established so that no delay results if emergency equipment is needed. A working knowledge of cardiopulmonary resuscitation procedures is essential.

These are some of the highlights of the role of the team physician. Over the years, I have learned a great deal from the coaches, trainers, and others I have worked with. Availability, compassion, gentleness, and a true love of being helpful to those who are showing good sport are the hallmarks of a team physician.

REFERENCES

1. Committee on Sports Medicine: The Team Physician. Bulletin, The American Academy of Orthopaedic Surgeons *20*(3): 22, 1972.

2 *Kenny Howard*

The Role of the Athletic Trainer

The role of the athletic trainer is changing as these professionals gain more recognition in the area of sports medicine. Trainers are now employed in medical clinics and in industry. The role of the athletic trainer has evolved from the team water boy to masseur to the well-educated and respected professional of the present time. These advances have been made through hard work on the part of athletic trainers and with tremendous assistance from the medical profession.

Curricula designed for athletic training degrees are in place at many colleges and universities. This coursework includes the basic sciences; a core of studies about the human body, such as anatomy, physiology, kinesiology, and biomechanics; and the exercise sciences. Coursework also includes first aid, psychology, nutrition, personal and community health, and administrative topics such as budgeting and personnel management. Athletic injury prevention, diagnosis, treatment, and rehabilitation are also vital and required courses. In addition to the academic requirements, hands-on experience must be gained by working under the supervision of a certified athletic trainer for a total of 1600 hours. The prospective athletic trainer must also pass a certification test.

The administrative duties of an athletic trainer begin with responsibility for the facilities and materials. The supplies used in the training room must be ordered and stored, ready for use in preventing and treating athletic injuries. Administration of insurance programs and record keeping of the athletes' injuries are essential and must be coordinated with the medical staff. The athletic trainer also selects and manages assistant trainers and student trainers.

Once the facilities, supplies, and personnel are in place, the athletic trainer's main duty is to serve the athlete. Physical examinations for all athletes must be scheduled with the medical staff. The athletes with a problem requiring extra or special attention are referred to a medical specialist, and the athletic trainer makes sure that prescribed treatments are followed. The athletic trainer is responsible for the complete health of the athlete. As a health care professional, the athletic trainer must be accessible to the athlete when he or she is ill or injured and ensure that proper medical care is given. Periodic and thorough physical examinations are absolutely necessary to assure that no harm comes to the athlete from participating in a sport.

The results of medical examinations are reported to the coaching staff by the athletic trainer. Daily injury reports also take place throughout the season via staff meetings. The athletic trainer advises the coach regarding injured athletes. It is important that the athletic trainer have a thorough knowledge of the physical requirements of the athlete's chosen sport. The athletic trainer can thereby advise the coach as to which activity the athlete should participate in during practice if he or she has a limiting injury.

Athletic trainers can diagnose injuries, but this is done only in a supporting role to the physician when the injury is severe. By being present during each practice session and being observant and alert at all times, the athletic trainer can often see how and why an injury occurred, its mechanism, and its severity (Fig. 2–1). This information can be invaluable to a physician when taking the history of an injury and rendering a diagnosis. The athletic trainer's role at such times is to provide first aid to the athlete and information to the physician.

Rehabilitation of an athlete's injury is the responsibility of the athletic trainer, as is exercise for the rest of the body while the injury heals. It is important to maintain overall conditioning whenever possible.

Athletic trainers can treat injuries under the supervision of a physician. A trusting bond must be established between the trainer and the physician so that the athlete will benefit from the combined care of both individuals. This bond takes place when there is mutual respect and open communication.

While an athletic trainer must do many things, the most important responsibility is to be the advocate of

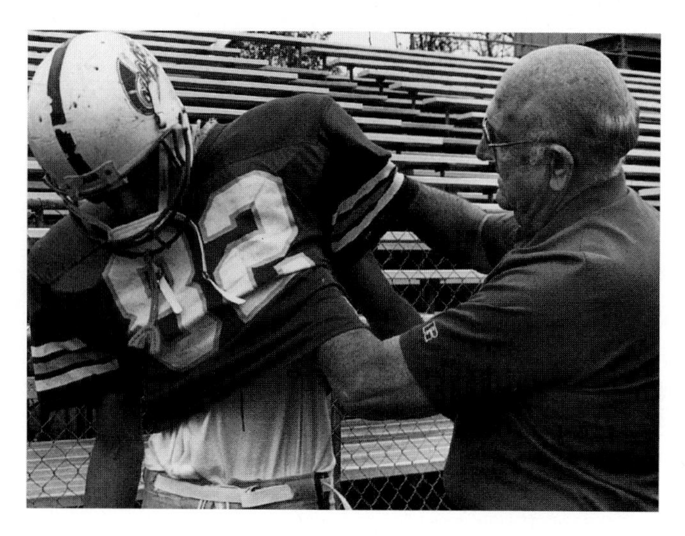

Fig. 2–1. The athletic trainer is usually present at practices and games to perform the initial examination when a player is injured.

the individual athlete. The athletic trainer should assist the athlete in becoming the best he or she can be in his or her chosen sport. Thus, the athletic trainer acts as an advocate between the athlete and the coaches, doctors, equipment custodian, and dieticians.

To become a successful advocate of the athlete, the athletic trainer must be familiar with the athlete's personality, work habits, pain tolerance, competitive spirit, friends (off as well as on the sports field), and relationship with the coach. An athletic trainer without these insights will miss the subtle changes that take place when something has interrupted the athlete's routine, such as trouble with a girlfriend or boyfriend, parents, roommate, or classwork.

The athletic trainer learns all of these things about an athlete by showing interest in the individual as a whole person—not just as an athlete. The athletic trainer becomes the athlete's friend, a trustworthy friend. Even as this friendship is present and growing, a athletic trainer must retain the respect of the athlete. It is most important that the injured athlete looks up and sees someone who he or she trusts and who is respected as a knowledgeable professional. An athletic trainer must understand what a devastating blow it is to the athlete to have a season-ending or career-ending injury.

An athletic trainer's primary responsibility is to the athlete. In accepting this responsibility the athletic trainer acts like a shadow, being with the athlete and observing behavior that affects the athlete's performance or health. Physicians and physical therapists cannot spend the majority of their time with the athletes because scheduled office appointments limit their flexibility.

The role of an athletic trainer is one of a trained health care professional who performs administrative duties, works to prevent injury, and aids in the treatment and rehabilitation of the athlete. Each of these can be taught from a book in a classroom, learned from an internship in a training room, or learned through trial and error on the job. But these skills do not complete the athletic trainer. The heart and soul of the dedicated athletic trainer must come first from a deep love of sports, a liking and understanding of young people who participate in sports, and a desire to help others feel well and be the best they can be in daily or sports activities. Athletic trainers must be willing to give a great deal of themselves in time and effort, but most athletic trainers will tell you it is not just a job but rather a way of life. Most athletic trainers also feel that they receive much more than they give.

If you can choose a person with heart and soul first and then give them the education, you will have the "ideal" athletic trainer.

3 *George M. McCluskey, Jr.*

The Role of the Physical Therapist in Rehabilitation

The word "rehabilitation" is a positive therapeutic word. It means restoration, or the process of returning something to its original status, as far as possible. It is a broad inclusive word. In the field of sports medicine, we use it to mean helping the athlete attain the highest possible skill in the shortest period of time after an injury or illness. Because they are highly motivated to return to sports, athletes are prime candidates for a well-organized and appropriately structured rehabilitation program after an injury or illness. Although physical therapists play an important role in caring for athletes at all levels of competition, the process should always be a team effort.

The physician serves as captain of the sports medicine team. But several health professionals also provide service in sports medicine rehabilitation: athletic trainer, physical therapist, occupational therapist, exercise physiologist, sports nutritionist, sports psychologist, nurse, and orthotist.

The athlete's level of competition and the environment in which he or she trains and competes usually determine the degree of sophistication of the medical coverage. In rural areas, recreational, high school, and small college athletes may have limited coverage and one health care professional will probably wear several hats. The primary care physician and the coach assigned to the training room may be required to provide all services. This does not mean that adequate care is not provided. It does mean that a good referral source or network is needed to meet the requirements of additional expertise. In areas that are fortunate enough to have an athletic trainer or physical therapist with special skills, such service is appreciated and respected.

Although physical therapists are trained to work with all types of patients, they have unique opportunities to acquire advanced skills in sports physical therapy. The Sports Physical Therapy Section of the American Physical Therapy Association has identified 11 competencies in the practice of sports physical therapy:

1. Organization and administration of a sports physical therapy service.
2. Administration of athletic evaluations.
3. Recognition and assessment of athletic related injuries.
4. Rendering of acute care.
5. Development and direction of conditioning programs.
6. Establishment of appropriate goals for athletes with respect to age, sex, skill level, and individual differences.
7. Nutritional counseling.
8. Recognition and recommendation related to environmental conditions.
9. Establishment of specific criteria for return to play.
10. Fabrication and fit of protective equipment.
11. Skill in taping, wrapping, and use of assistive supports.

A Specialty Board Examination determines competency in these areas. Therapists who pass this examination are recognized as Sports Clinical Specialists by The American Physical Therapy Association.

Rehabilitation for the athlete should be holistic in nature, using as many disciplines as is appropriate. Treatment plans should include not only the injured part but all aspects of training required for the athlete to return to play as quickly as possible without being vulnerable to re-injury. For example, an athlete recuperating from a shoulder injury should be on general strengthening and flexibility exercises as well as cardiovascular exercises to prevent deconditioning or detraining during the injury recovery period. This means that athletic trainers, physical therapists, and exercise physiologists could all be needed to treat injuries that occur in the athlete. It is possible that one member of the sports medicine team will attempt to provide all of the needs of the athlete even when other disciplines are available. The athlete is the loser in this situation. A defined network of specialists should be established and used as needed.

When dealing with college or professional athletes, or with high schools fortunate enough to have a certified athletic trainer, the athletic trainer continues to be the most visible health specialist in sports medicine. The athletic trainer has daily contact with all athletes, provides care when needed, and uses other specialists on a daily basis as indicated in the controlled training room environment or in the physical therapy clinic if one is conveniently located. In recreational and high-school athletics and in some professional sports (such as golf), the physical therapist should work with the attending physician to provide all services needed.

Physical therapists are trained to understand the pathologic damage and the kinesiologic mechanics of the injury (Fig. 3–1). They also understand the specific requirements of the sport involved and thus are uniquely qualified to design an appropriate rehabilitation program. The program should be designed to achieve the goals set forth by the attending physician. At the appropriate time in the recovery process, the program can be carried out under the direction of the athletic trainer in the training room, but the physical therapist should continue to monitor the athlete's progress. By working with the athletic trainer, the physical therapist can advance the program to meet the goals of the physician and the athlete.

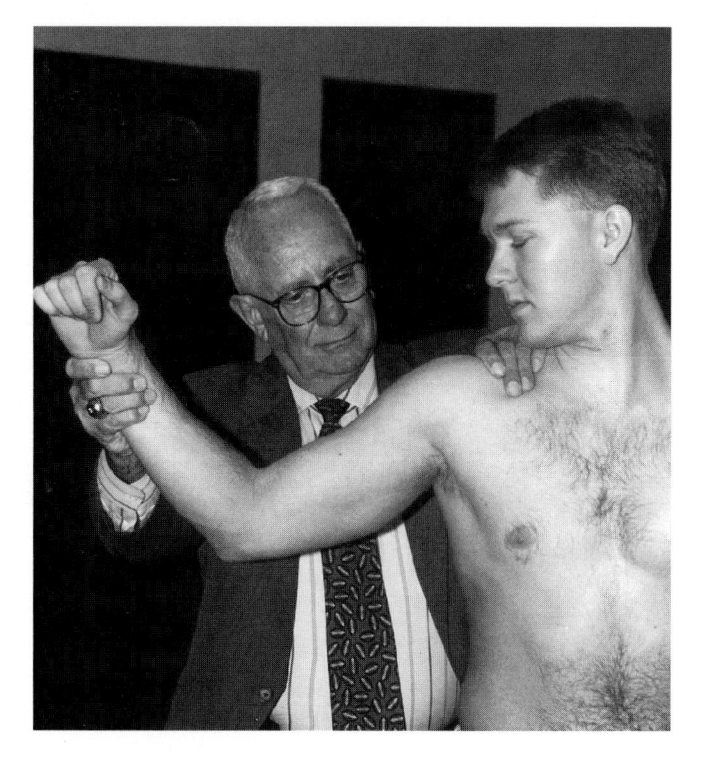

Fig. 3–1. The physical therapist has a thorough knowledge of the anatomic basis of the injury and designs a rehabilitation program to return the athlete to play as quickly as possible.

Athletes at all levels of competition should be educated about their injuries and instructed in the exercises required to return to play. If possible, they should be given the opportunity to carry out exercises at home or in other everyday settings rather than on daily visits to a physical therapy department. Of course, sometimes special equipment is required or the athlete needs special instruction or motivation to overcome a special problem during the recovery period. Athletes need to know why a specific exercise will help them, what to expect if they do that exercise, and what to expect if they do not follow instructions. They also need to know what *not* to do, because there are many myths about treating athletic injuries. The entire sports medicine team working together should maximize the athlete's potential to achieve the best possible results.

Many physical therapists are also certified athletic trainers. This combined expertise is excellent, but in some situations it can be a drawback. It is difficult for a physical therapist/athletic trainer to stay on the "cutting edge" of the physical therapy profession if he or she works as an athletic trainer day in and day out. Similarly, a physical therapist/athletic trainer who functions daily as a physical therapist, would find it difficult to stay on top of the athletic training profession.

Physical therapists who stay on the "cutting edge" are becoming more involved in verifying results of treatment procedures and in establishing new treatment protocols in pace with advances in sports medicine. The physical therapist should also be responsible for educating athletes, coaches, parents, peers, and the public. All professionals have a duty to update themselves, academically and technically, to better serve the community and general public as well as the athlete.

All specialists must respect one another and work together to provide the best care for athletes and all patients. Teamwork divides the task and doubles the success. Ken Blanchard, author of *The One Minute Manager* wrote, "No one of us is as smart as all of us." Working together always works best.

4 *Stephen C. Hunter*

Coverage of Games and Events

Physicians are present at most athletic events but are rarely seen or noticed until they appear at the side of an injured player along with the rest of the sports medicine team. This unobtrusive presence is ideal since the sport is for the players and spectators and should not be inhibited by an imposing medical professional.

Team physicians provide coverage at the professional, collegiate, high school, and recreational level, as well as at events for special athletes. At the organized professional level, the team physician often is contracted to attend team events and care for the individual team players. A physician may be present at recreational sports events as an interested spectator or a supportive parent. Organizers of events for special athletes usually seek physicians to cover their events because of the health risks of the participants.

An obligated team physician under contract is usually part of a well-organized sports medicine team that includes physicians, therapists, and athletic trainers. This group may include several physicians with subspecialty backgrounds, including primary care, orthopedics, physiatrics, and psychiatry, as well as podiatrists and chiropractors. The athletic trainer should direct the sports medicine team on the field and physicians and therapists should support the athletic trainer in this role.

High-school and recreational-level sporting events cannot afford a sophisticated sports medicine team, but they can still be effectively covered by a physician volunteer who works with the athletic trainer.

The athletic trainer should have primary responsibility for most of the medical equipment brought to the game (Table 4–1). The trainer's kit should include the supplies needed to repair equipment, treat minor injuries, and meet emergency needs. The team physician can inventory and suggest supplies for the trainer's kit, providing additional items needed to evaluate and treat potential emergencies during the sporting event. These items could include diagnostic instruments and the supplies for life support in emergency situations.

If an ambulance is present at the sporting event, the sports medicine team may not need to supply all the equipment for emergency use. The physician should check with the ambulance personnel regarding their supplies and their level of emergency-care training. The presence of a well-trained and supplied ambulance crew greatly enhances the capabilities of the sports medicine team on the sidelines.

The team physician should also be aware of the availability and capability of hospital and emergency-room support. If a problem arises at a game that requires transferring the patient, it is a comfort to know that such support is available.

Once on the field, the physician should contact the trainer and coaching staff to alert them to the medical team's presence. Any last-minute problems can be checked before the sports contest begins. From this point on, the sports event is for the players, coaches, and spectators. The medical team should remain inconspicuous, observing the contest from the sports medicine perspective and making themselves available when needed.

On the field, the athletic trainer remains the principal member of the sports medicine team, the person to whom the players and coaches will turn initially when injury and sports medicine problems arise. An injury or problem should be assessed first by the athletic trainer, who will be able to handle many of them alone, and who will call on the physician for help if needed. This practice will keep order in the delivery of sports medicine care and decrease anxiety in the athlete, coaches, and spectators.

If the physician is needed to care for an athletic injury on the field, he or she should continue to work closely with the athletic trainer and sports medicine team to

Table 4–1. Supplies That a Physician Should Have on Hand at Athletic Events

Tape supplies (variety of size and type of tape, prewrap, tape adherent, tape remover, etc.)
Scissors
Wound closures
Adhesive bandages (various sizes)
Gauze pads (sterile) and rolls
Elastic bandages (various sizes)
Gloves (sterile and nonsterile)
Slings
Crutches
Plastic bags for ice (make sure that ice is available)
Cryotherapy unit
Splints
Tongue depressors (sterile and nonsterile)
Bite stick
Hemostats
Penlight
Otoscope/ophthalmoscope
Suture kit including antiseptic cleanser (alcohol, Betadine, etc.), local anesthetic, syringes, and needles of various gauges. (Needles, syringes, and anesthetic must be kept in a secure place in the physician's kit.)
Thermometer
Scalpel handle and blades
Eye wash and saline for contact lens wearers
Pocket mirror
Dental kit
Antibiotic ointment and powder
Hydrogen peroxide
Cotton-tipped applicators (sterile)
Eye black
Cloth compression sleeves (compressionette, stockinette, etc.)
Bee sting kit, including epinephrine syringe
Paper bag (for hyperventilation)
Padding material (various sizes for protection of injuries incurred during practice or games)
Device to remove the facemask from a football helmet (e.g., bolt cutters, "trainer's angel," etc.)
Emergency information forms (one for each athlete)
An index card outlining an emergency plan with the following information: location of telephone, 911 service availability, availability of ambulance service, accessibility of the event site for the ambulance
Emergency equipment: mask and airway for CPR, stethoscope, blood pressure cuff
Emergency equipment (may be in conjunction with local ambulance service): spine board, stretcher, sand bags, rigid cervical collar, oxygen

This list is not intended to be all-inclusive. Add or delete items as they fit your particular needs. Items such as biomedical waste containers and disinfectant solutions used to prevent the spread of blood-borne pathogens should be included at your discretion. Quantities are determined by the number of athletes participating. Be sure to have other personnel available who are qualified to use emergency equipment. Review procedures about handling the football player who sustains a head or neck injury.

take advantage of their skills and provide optimum initial treatment to the injured athlete. Reliance on and support of the athletic trainer and sports medicine team is the key to successful care of an athletic team.

It is wise for the physician on the playing field to be able to contact additional support if necessary. Communication by cellular phone is sometimes available, but, if not, radio communications on the ambulance and line phones at the sports arena are usually available. The sports medicine team should identify the location and accessibility of such services before game time.

Serious injuries may require the presence of the physician on the field to treat life- and limb-threatening problems. She or he must be prepared to handle acute reactions to heat; head and spine injuries that present as neurologic emergencies; severe orthopedic injuries; and other medical emergencies, including cardiac and pulmonary distress. Fortunately these situations are uncommon, but they could be disastrous if the sports medicine team is inadequately trained and equipped.

More frequently, sports physicians must assess and treat routine injuries on the field. Triage and stabilization are the key factors. After diagnosing and assessing the extent of injury as well as possible on the field, the physician may be called on to determine a course of care. If the athletic trainer is uncomfortable returning an injured player to competition, he or she should ask the rest of the medical team for input. The decision should be based upon an assessment of the effect on the injured player and on the possibility of further injury to that player or others if they are treated and returned to the sports event. The team physician should be prepared to help make these decisions, as needed, on the sideline.

5 *Keith Webster*

Establishing a High School Sports Medicine Program

Every high school should have a well-thought-out program to provide care for its injured student athletes. The key people involved in establishing, running, and evaluating a sports medicine program include the school administrators, parents, team physician, and on-site program director.

School administrators must make the commitment to provide the best possible health care for their students who participate in extracurricular activities. Current economic, legal, and medical issues dictate that a comprehensive sports medicine program replace the all-too-common practice of only providing medical coverage at athletic events. While there is a high incidence of injury during actual contests, two-thirds of all injuries occur during daily practice sessions.[1] The school administration should name a team physician to provide the medical care and supervise the sports medicine program. After consulting the team physician, the school administrators should determine who will be the daily director. That person will answer to the school and work closely with the team physician in carrying out his or her duties. State laws regulating the practice of athletic training and allied health professions must be strictly adhered to.

Concerned parents and athletic booster club members are often the driving force behind getting a sports medicine program established at their school. One such group of parents won a legal battle in Washington, D.C. The result is a comprehensive sports-medicine program that includes a certified athletic trainer in each school in Washington, D.C. Booster clubs are also a great resource for fund-raising efforts to acquire facilities, equipment, and supplies needed to maintain such a program.

The team physician possesses unique qualities that allow him or her to work effectively with school administrators, coaches, athletic trainers, athletes, and their parents. They often give their time and service voluntarily and they spend a great deal of time on the playing fields with the athletes. The team physician, whether a general practitioner or orthopedic specialist, should be well-informed about the special demands and philosophies involved with sport medicine.

The key person whose presence on the "front lines" makes this program succeed is the on-site director. In addition to providing appropriate health care to injured athletes, he or she must possess the administrative skills necessary to conduct the program successfully. Frequently a member of an already overworked coaching staff is called on to assume the duties of the director with very little guidance. It is becoming increasingly clear that a coach cannot handle both jobs effectively. As a result, the team suffers and the athletes who become injured may not receive the attention they need. Coaches will continue to play an integral role in the sports medicine program, but the nationally certified athletic trainer who fulfills state regulatory requirements is best qualified to direct the program.

Athletic training is recognized as an allied health profession by the American Medical Association. Requirements for certification include a bachelor's degree with course work in health, human anatomy, exercise physiology, and other related courses. First aid and cardiopulmonary resuscitation certification or Emergency Medical Technician equivalency are also required. A practical experience requirement, which is evaluated through an oral/practical segment on the national certification test, makes the athletic trainer unique among allied health professionals. More than half of the states in the U.S. have laws regulating the practice of athletic training. The athletic trainer works under the

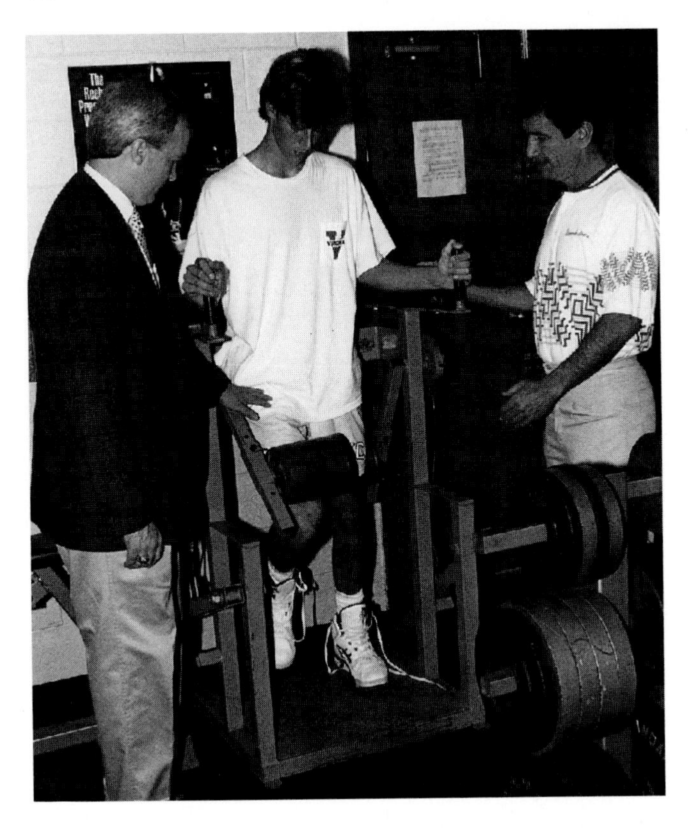

Fig. 5–1. The full-time athletic trainer works closely with athletes and coaches to rehabilitate an injury or guide a strengthening program.

direction and supervision of a physician and acts to extend the services of that physician. The athletic trainer also acts as a liaison between the medical community and the athletes, coaches, and parents.

The high-school athletic trainer who is hired on a full-time basis is in the best position to provide optimal sports healthcare (Fig. 5–1). These professionals can develop a comprehensive injury care program that includes the following:

1. Injury prevention strategies that can reduce potential liability. These strategies include ensuring a safe playing area, teaching athletes proper conditioning exercises, and preventing potentially fatal heat-related illnesses.
2. Proper, accurate assessment of the type and severity of injuries.
3. Appropriate first aid, including an emergency plan and treatment of injuries.
4. Determination of when and if the injured athlete can return to play.
5. Referrals of injured athletes to the appropriate medical professional or family's choice when indicated.
6. An effective rehabilitation program with the goal of returning the injured athlete to his or her sports activity as quickly as possible with minimal risk of reinjury.
7. Educational and counseling programs, such as in-service programs for coaches and seminars about health issues for athletes.

The athletic trainer is also uniquely qualified to administer the sports medicine program. He or she must keep accurate injury and treatment records, maintain a supply inventory, and operate within a budget. (In fact, centralizing the purchase of athletic training supplies alone is very cost effective.) The trainer also coordinates practice and event coverage and develops policy and procedure guidelines with school administrators. The athletic trainer must continually update the supervising physician as to the condition of the team's injured athletes. Together, the physician and the athletic trainer update or revise protocols as their relationship develops over time.

The athletic trainer can develop a network of medical specialists and allied health professionals in the region who can provide care to injured athletes who would benefit from their specialties. Members of the network will vary according to availability, but it is important to identify someone from each medical specialty so that a referral can be made quickly and appropriately when needed. Such a network will also enhance the team physician's effectiveness to the school.

Organizing preparticipation physical examinations is an important part of an athletic trainer's job. He or she can coordinate mass physicals with other schools to maximize the services of the medical community. In addition to basic general medical and orthopedic assessments, the athletic trainer may include strength and fitness stations, such as those that test flexibility, body fat, strength, power, and speed. These physical examinations can be followed up with exercise prescriptions to correct detected problems that might cause injuries.

School administrators should recognize that these components of the sports medicine team are necessary in every high school athletic program. The program should be directed by someone who has no additional teaching or coaching duties. The long-standing tradition of assigning a coach to perform athletic-training duties is fast becoming outdated and might even violate some state laws. Enlightened school boards and administrators understand that hiring an athletic trainer is cost effective. In addition to providing quality health care to student athletes, the investment of hiring an athletic trainer may be offset by reductions in school insurance, including both medical and liability coverage.

Another benefit of having a full-time athletic trainer in the high school is that he or she can provide instruction and guidance to students who develop an interest in pursuing a career in athletic training. For example, the trainer can teach athletic-training classes in a health occupations curriculum. Introducing high school students to athletic training can lead some to careers in sports medicine or allied health professions. Many young people have no role models in the health-care field. The athletic trainer, who bridges this gap, can introduce the student to new career possibilities.

Some high schools choose to hire the services of an athletic trainer through a clinic on a part-time or event-only basis. But an athletic trainer's effectiveness is somewhat diminished if he or she is not a full-time employee of the school or school system. Interaction with students during the school day is as important for the athletic trainer as it is for the coach and teacher. This interaction enables the athletic trainer to better understand students' personalities to better meet their health care needs. As a team physician, school administrator, coach, or concerned parent, determine your school athletes' health care needs and then strive to establish the best program to meet those needs. The National Athletic Trainers' Association office in Dallas is available for additional consultation to develop the best sports medicine program for your school.

REFERENCES

1. Powell, J.:636,000 injuries annually in high school football. Athletic Training *22*:19, 1987.

6 *Tarek Souryal*

Liability and Risk Management in Sports Medicine

Most public spirited physicians who look after high school teams are unaware of their precarious legal position.

—Dr. James Russell, 1962[1]

It is certainly a sign of the times that a medical book for team physicians contains a chapter such as this. Liability, malpractice, and negligence are words too often spoken in medicine these days. As health-care providers we must not only be aware of but also familiar with language and current trends in our profession. Liability and risk management play a significant role in the everyday practice of our profession. In this chapter, special consideration will be given to the legal language of liability. Current concepts and future trends in the field of sports medicine liability will also be discussed.

CASE REPORT

It was a typical Friday-night high school football game in an East Texas town. The squads were small. Early in the third quarter, a promising sophomore tight end dislocated his elbow on an end around play. The injury was obvious. Play was halted for nearly an hour. After 45 minutes of pain, chaos, and uncertainty, an ambulance took the boy and his family to a nearby hospital. Why did it take so long? Because no one had the key to the school building where the telephone was housed. The young man eventually recovered from this injury and returned to football the following year.

Who is at fault in this case? The coach? The principal? The grounds keeper? The doctor? Did the athlete or his parents know that football is a collision sport and that injuries are a part of the game? Knowing this, should the parents accept a delay in treatment? Did they sign a release? Is this a case of negligence?

As you proceed through this chapter you will become familiar with phrases and definitions that will help explain this case.

TORT LAW

There are two basic types of laws: *criminal,* in which the state has the authority to act, and *civil.* Civil law consists of *statutory law* and *common law.* Statutory law is legislated, and common law is a body of law that has accumulated over time, based on the decisions of the courts.

A tort is defined as "a private or civil wrong, other than a breach of contract, for which the court will provide a remedy in the form of an action for damages."[2] There are two types of torts: *statutory torts* and *common-law torts.* Defamation, product liability, fraud, and negligence are but a few types of tort actions. A tort action is not a criminal action. The courts, not the state, define the wrong and prescribe a remedy. Statutory torts in sports medicine involve workers' compensation, antitrust, and sexual and racial discrimination. Common-law torts in sports medicine usually involve negligence and product liability.

If a person feels that a wrong has been committed against him or her, that person can file a lawsuit. The person filing the lawsuit is called the *plaintiff,* and the alleged wrongdoer is the *defendant,* or *tort-feasor.* The majority of lawsuits filed in sports cases involve a claim of negligence, breach of contract (not a type of tort), defamation, or product liability. Several torts may be included in one lawsuit.

Three elements of every tort are duty, breach, and causation. To claim negligence, it must be proven to the courts that (1) a *duty* was established; (2) the duty was *breached;* and (3) as a result of this breach of duty harm did indeed occur, establishing *causation.* Then, and only then, can *damages* be awarded.

Liability is "a broad legal term." Simply stated, liability is assumption of responsibility. Risk management is limiting liability. In sports, risk management includes ensuring that equipment is maintained in good shape, proper emergency plans are made, and proper facilities are constructed.

Duty of Care

Society does not expect a person to act against his or her free will in a given situation unless that individual has an obligation to do so. This obligation to act is called *duty*. Duty is an important factor in any tort case. Without a duty to act, a person cannot be found at fault for not acting. The school administrators have a duty to the athlete to provide a safe place to play. The coaching staff have a duty to instruct the athlete in proper techniques for safe participation and to maintain the athlete in a state of good conditioning. The trainers have a duty to the athlete by advising the coaches in ways to minimize injuries and providing preliminary care to injured athletes. The physicians, however, do not have clearly outlined duties. Many donate their time to their local high schools in a spirit of community. But a person who chooses to do volunteer work must assume all the obligations associated with the role; thus the volunteer physician will find that the performance of these obligations will be judged in terms of the acceptable standard of care. Therefore, even on a voluntary basis a duty of care does exist. Some physicians are under contract to a professional team to provide complete medical care for their athletes. Under such a contractual agreement the duty is obvious. However, it can be argued that the duty is to the team, not to the athlete. In many cases where there are no clear-cut roles, the courts and attorneys must determine if a duty of care exists.

Some states have established guidelines to protect those who have no duty to act but choose to do so out of "the goodness of their own hearts." "Good samaritan" laws were established to protect those who act in an emergency situation but who are under no obligation to act. Not all states have good samaritan laws. The Texas good samaritan law is shown in Table 6–1. Specific exclusions pertain to the practice of medicine. Interpretation of such laws by the courts can be broad. Barring good samaritan action, one must still be able to prove that the defendant did have a duty to the plaintiff and that he or she failed to fulfill that duty in accordance with established standards.

Table 6–1. Texas Good Samaritan Law.

§ 74.001. Liability for Emergency Care

(a) A person who in good faith administers emergency care at the scene of an emergency or in a hospital is not liable in civil damages for an act performed during the emergency unless the act is wilfully or wantonly negligent.

(b) This section does not apply to care administered:

(1) for or in expectation of remuneration;

(2) by a person who was at the scene of the emergency because he or a person he represents as an agent was soliciting business or seeking to perform a service for remuneration;

(3) by a person who regularly administers care in a hospital emergency room; or

(4) by an admitting physician or a treating physician associated by the admitting physician of the patient bringing a health-care liability claim.

§ 74.002. Unlicensed Medical Personnel

Persons not licensed in the healing arts who in good faith administer emergency care as emergency medical service personnel are not liable in civil damages for an act performed in administering the care unless the act is wilfully or wantonly negligent. This section applies without regard to whether the care is provided for or in expectation of remuneration.

Texas Civil Practice and Remedies, Sections 74.001 and 74.002

Negligence

Negligence is defined as doing something that an ordinary prudent person would not have done under similar circumstances, or as failing to do something that an ordinary prudent person would have done in similar circumstances.[3] This concept applies to everyone under the law. School administrators, coaches, trainers, and doctors all have to abide by this definition or else risk a lawsuit. Another definition of negligence is failure to "live up to" an already established *standard of care*. In the past, the standard of care was established and limited to a given community. Today, the standard of care is established for much broader geographic areas. In the future, there might be a universal standard of care. Any action or treatment that falls outside the accepted standard of care can be termed negligence. It is society's responsibility to establish an acceptable standard of care and the courts' responsibility to define it. Attorneys on both sides of an issue must prove to the court that an action falls either within or without the standard of care. Proving negligence requires proof that the defendant had a duty to the claimant (plaintiff) and that this duty has been breached under established guidelines of standard-of-care doctrine.

For example, the standard of care in a given locale may be to provide ambulance service at all high school football games. If a school in this locale chooses not to have ambulance service, and if a serious injury occurs and ambulance service is delayed in providing necessary attention, that school is liable and may be sued for negligence.

Causation

After proving breach of duty, and in order to recover damages, the plaintiff's attorney must establish that the act resulted in physical harm, death, or economic or property damage.[4] That is, an injury must occur that is caused by the defendant's actions or inaction. This concept is called *causation*. If no injury results or there is no property or economic damage, the claim will be denied by the court. Causation can be difficult to prove in sports because of the doctrines of *assumption of risk* and *contributory negligence*.

Assumption of Risk and Contributory Negligence

Assumption of risk is the plaintiff's express or implied consent to encounter a known risk. Stated another way, the doctrine states that a party who voluntarily assumes a risk of harm arising from the conduct of another cannot recover damages if harm in fact results.[5] (Excluded from this doctrine are injuries arising out of bad faith and intentional or willful acts.[6]) A classic case that describes such an occurrence is the case of *Bourque* v. *Duplechin* in which a baserunner (Duplechin) went five feet off the basepath and ran full speed into the shortstop (Bourque) after he had already released the ball. This resulted in serious injury. The court stated that "Bourque did not assume the risk of Duplechin going out of his way to run into him at full speed. . . . A participant does not assume the risk of injury from fellow players acting in an unexpected or unsportsmanlike way with reckless lack of concern for others participating."[7]

Assumption of risk can be contractual, implied, or explicit. In some cases, the risk of the activity is so unreasonable that the mere participation is rendered contributory negligence (e.g., motorcycle stunt riders).[5]

Contributory negligence is conduct by the plaintiff that falls below the standard of care the law requires them to exercise for their own safety.[8] The same rules apply to this form of negligence as previously stated, that is, the defense must prove that the plaintiff had a duty of care to himself and that this duty was breached, resulting in an injury. In its original form, contributory negligence constituted a complete defense. Many states have now adopted a comparative form of contributory negligence that allows the plaintiff to recover a proportionate amount of damages for the resultant injury.[4]

LIABILITY FOR MEDICAL PERSONNEL

Coaches and Trainers

Coaches in charge of sports activities have a duty to exercise reasonable care for the protection of the athletes under their supervision. They must provide proper instruction, maintain a program of proper physical conditioning, and show diligence in delegating duty to competent personnel. The coach must also educate the athletes in the fundamental techniques of the game.[5] Liability cannot be proven if a coach fulfills these duties.

Problems arise when a coach oversteps the boundaries of what a prudent person should do or not do in a similar circumstance. The case of *Welch* v. *Dunsmuir Joint Union High School District* illustrates such a circumstance. This case involved a player with a known neck injury who was carried off the field by eight other players. Before being carried off the field, the player had full motor function, but as a result of the move he was rendered paraplegic. The coach was found negligent in ordering the injured player moved.[4] Another case in which a coach was found negligent occurred in Louisiana. In *Mogabgab* v. *Orleans Parish,* an athlete collapsed on the field from heat stroke. The coach waited two hours before obtaining medical help. The athlete later died.[7]

A coach has a difficult task in providing supervision and instruction to the athletes without being called on to be a paramedic. However, the courts do not expect much other than what a reasonable and prudent person would or would not do in a similar circumstance. It is very helpful for coaches and athletes to have certified athletic trainers on hand who, by training, are able to recognize urgent medical conditions. If trainers are not available, it may behoove the coaching staff to attend short educational seminars on medical conditions that they may encounter on the field. The team physician may be of great value in educating the coaching staff about some of the more common and urgent medical occurrences.

As allied health care professionals, athletic trainers and physical therapists are held to a higher standard of care than are coaches or lay people. However, the same principles apply as to negligence, i.e., the athletic trainer or physical therapist is expected to do as much as anyone with the same training would. The courts expect those who hold themselves to be sports medicine specialists, and therefore have expertise in the field, to uphold a higher standard of care and have basic skills equal to others who hold the same level.[8]

Physicians

Physicians are always aware of legal ramifications of their actions. Malpractice is a negative outcome that results from deviating from the accepted standard of care. In sports medicine, many physicians do not realize that they are not only expected to uphold the standard of care for the field of medicine, but are also held liable in other situations that do not necessarily involve medicine. Defamation, breach of contract, and the need to obtain consent are but a few of the issues sports physicians must contend with. A physician volunteering to take on the role of team physician must be aware that the courts view physicians as skilled professionals and hold them to a higher level of care than the general population. Those who call themselves sports medicine specialists are held to an even higher standard. A court may side against a sports medicine specialist in a given case simply because the standard of care is higher for a specialist than for a physician who does not specialize in sports medicine. The same case against a general practitioner might result in a different outcome. Self-proclaimed sports medicine specialists must be sure that they are indeed specially trained, because they will be held to the higher standard imposed on specialists.

When a physician takes on the task of team physician—whether for pay or simply out of goodness of heart—it means that he or she takes on a duty to provide service for all of the participating members of the team. This level of duty is no different than the duty they owe to their office patients. Medical decisions on the field are made without the benefits of proper equipment, radiographs, or examination positioning. At times, athletes are examined with their pads in place. These situations are compromising at best. Combine the disadvantage of working under such conditions with pressure from the players, the coach, the parents, and sometimes even the media, and the physician's liability increases. The sports medicine specialist should do everything possible to eliminate these outside influences and to establish a proper examination routine in order to treat the patients with the care and duty they deserve. Doing so also minimizes risk of mistakes on the part of the physician.

The team physician's function is to enhance safety and promptly initiate emergency medical care when an athlete is injured. To make sure that patients, athletes, families, and management are aware of the limitations of the team physician's role, it is best to circulate a written statement of your duties. This notification is most effective if it is circulated before the season begins.

It is not unusual for a team physician to cover an event in which all participants are under age. This situation places the physician in a precarious situation. Does he or she have proper informed consent for making nonemergency medical decisions? If so, did the physician fully explain to the athlete the nature, risks, benefits, and possible ramifications of his or her injury? Was the athlete able to respond in an intelligent manner? Are there pressures on the athlete to return to play too quickly? Is the physician at risk?

These concerns represent a new trend in sports medicine liability. The physician is at risk if it can be proved to the court that he or she failed to obtain proper consent from the athlete or the family.

It is important before an event to obtain a signed consent giving the supervisor or the coach permission to consult with a physician in case of an emergent or nonemergent injury; this procedure is especially important if the athletes are underage.

Speaking to any person other than the patient may be legal grounds for a defamation suit. This act is a breach in the confidentiality of the doctor-patient relationship, especially in the case of a professional athlete, who may lose income as a result. Such was the case in *Chuy* v. *Philadelphia Eagles football club,* in which it was found that the team physician disclosed erroneous medical information that caused the athlete emotional distress and financial loss. The athlete eventually was awarded damages.[8]

Another trend in sports medicine law is to file suit against a physician because of breach of contract. It can be argued that an assurance of outcome is a form of verbal contract, and if this outcome does not occur then the contract is breached. This type of suit falls under contract law and is governed by another set of standards. The physician should refrain from making guarantees or emphatic assurances.[4]

PHYSICAL EXAMINATIONS

The National Basketball Association holds yearly physical examinations for all incoming rookies. These examinations are very complete. They include echocardiograms, treadmill stress tests, hearing tests, vision tests, Cybex testing, radiographs, and magnetic resonance imaging scans. The purpose is to help detect a disease or defect that might harm the athlete during his career in professional basketball. Despite the thoroughness of these examinations, many medical problems still go undetected.

The NBA's thorough examination is an exception in sports. The typical preseason physical is usually provided by a family practitioner performing an examination that includes heart auscultation, hernia check, and vision check, as well as a cursory musculoskeletal evaluation. The courts have been evasive as to what constitutes a standard athletic physical examination. It is important to note that physical examinations for athletics are a serious matter and should be administered carefully.[9]

CONCLUSION

Risk management in sports medicine is not a phrase intended to help ward off attorneys. Before instituting a risk management protocol, one must be familiar with what the legal system considers liability. A knowledge of the language and definitions of liability and an awareness of the risks are essential for the sports medicine team.

In the case of the tight end in East Texas presented in the beginning of this chapter, the responsible personnel associated with it did indeed have a duty to provide prompt care. They collectively failed to fulfill that duty. Therefore, breach of duty did occur. However, because the outcome was uneventful and the young athlete regained full use of his arm and returned to sports, no harm resulted; thus there was no causation. The claim was denied.

The basic concepts of tort and liability have been in the law books for centuries. It is only recently that they have been introduced into the medical literature. Whether you realized it or not, you are acutely aware of and are currently practicing the principles of liability and risk management right now.

While no one can prevent all injuries, every effort can and should be made to reduce the total number that occur and to reduce their severity. Risk management is synonymous with safety in sports. The job of monitoring safety belongs to everyone involved with the sports activity. The school superintendent, the principal, the athletic director, the head coach, the trainer, the team physician, the parents, and the athletes themselves are all responsible. At the professional level, the owner, the general manager, the coach, the athletic trainer, the team physician, the player, and the player's agent also share the responsibility of risk management.

However, as one would expect, whenever so many people are involved in one action, conflicts of interest arise. As sports medicine physicians, we are not insurers of safety, but we should always strive to protect the athletes.

REFERENCES

1. Grieve, A.: *The Legal Aspects of Athletics.* Cranbury, NJ, A. S. Barnes and Co., 1969.
2. Black, H. C.: Black's Law Dictionary. 5th Ed. St. Paul, MN, West Publishing Co., 1979.
3. Schubert, G. W., Smith, R. K., Trentadue, J. C.: Sports Law. St. Paul, MN, West Publishing Co., 1986.

4. Waicukauski, R. J.: *Law and Amateur Sports.* Bloomington, IN, Indiana University Press, 1982.
5. Weistart, J. C., Lowell, C. H.: Law of Sports. Indianapolis, Bobbs-Merrill Co., 1979.
6. Jones, M. E.: *Current Issues in Professional Sports.* Durham, NH, Whittemore School of Business and Economics, University of New Hampshire, 1980.
7. Champion, W. T.: *Fundamentals of Sports Law.* New York, CBC Publishing, 1990.
8. Freedman, W.: *Professional Sports and Antitrust.* New York, Quorum Books, 1987.
9. King, J. H.: "The duty and standard of care for team physicians." *The Houston Law Review 18*:657, 1981.

7 *Daniel R. Kraeger*

Playing Surfaces in Sports

When many of us were playing sports in our youth, we used terms like "sandlot baseball" and "barnyard basketball." Playing surfaces have since become much more technical. Sports are played on many different surfaces, from wood to ice, blacktop to clay, and concrete to ground-up tires. Each surface has a different effect on the forces being applied to the body. Manufacturers make many claims regarding the benefits of one surface over another. However, except for natural grass and synthetic turf, there has been little published research regarding the effect these surfaces have on injuries.

Ideally, the playing surface would provide the cushioning and the shoe could be designed to provide the stability. Unfortunately it is often the other way around. The surfaces are so hard that the shoe is designed to provide cushioning, which then reduces the amount of stability it provides.

SYNTHETIC TURF VERSUS GRASS

Synthetic playing surfaces were first used in football in the late 1960s.[1] Some of the most common synthetic turfs are Astro Turf (Monsanto), Tartan Turf (3M Company, discontinued), Polyturf (U.S. Bilt-Rite, discontinued), Omniturf (Sportec), Polygrass (Adolff Co., West Germany), and Sporturf (All-Pro Athletic Surfaces). The initial claim by one manufacturer alleged that its synthetic turf offered reduced injury when compared with natural grass. Numerous researchers have tested these claims by comparing the number, severity, and type of injuries on synthetic turf versus natural grass. Unfortunately, more than 20 years later, the evidence is not conclusive. Whether less injuries occur on natural grass or synthetic turf depends on the study quoted and the type of synthetic turf studied.

Many factors are involved in a comparison of these surfaces for injury rates: whether the field is wet or dry, new or old; or the type of shoes worn. The Tartan Turf field appeared to have a higher injury rate when the field was wet. In contrast, in a study of Astro Turf injury rates were without exception significantly higher when the turf was dry than when wet.[2] Just as grass surface changes with wear, so do synthetic turfs. New Astro Turf fibers measure 1 cm in length and are upright. After three years of use these same fibers are 0.5 cm in height, and they are split and matted together.[3] These differences are important because the cleats on the athlete's shoes will not grip as well on the worn turf. Ultimately, this affects the athlete's skill and running and cutting ability. Appreciable differences in injury rates appear to exist not only among brands of synthetic turf but also among various types of turf coming from a single manufacturer.

Even a seemingly simple topic like running speed can lead to opposing conclusions depending on which study you read.[1,4]

INJURY RATES IN FOOTBALL: SYNTHETIC TURF VERSUS NATURAL GRASS

Although there is a benefit of increased fixation on the synthetic turf, the tradeoff is an increased risk of injury.[5] Some high school and college studies have shown that the differences between injury rates on synthetic turf and natural grass are statistically significant.[2,6] Adkison and colleagues found that injuries were more frequent on Astro Turf when compared with natural grass, while fewer injuries occurred on Tartan Turf compared with natural grass.[2] Martin and colleagues found the same results in intercollegiate tackle football.[7] There were 1.97 injuries per game on Astro Turf, 1.77 injuries per game on natural grass, and 1.41 injuries per game on Tartan Turf. In another comparison of injuries occurring to players on a collegiate team on natural grass (six seasons) and on Tartan Turf (six seasons), there were no significant differences in the *rate* of injuries, but there were in the *type* and *severity* of injuries. More serious sprains and torn ligaments occurred on the natural grass than on the Tartan Turf.[8]

The validity of such studies is questionable because change in coaching, training, equipment, practice, and game strategies may have affected the comparison of injuries that occurred before the team changed to playing on artificial turf with those that occurred after.[3] Also, not all studies find significant differences. In a four-season study of knee and ankle injuries occurring on natural grass and Astro Turf, there was very little difference between knee and ankle injuries occurring on either surface.[3]

Several studies have been done involving the National Football League. The earliest study (from 1969 to 1974) found many more major and minor injuries on all synthetic turf surfaces. The injury rates were highest when teams practiced on one type of surface and played on another.[9,10] The National Collegiate Athletic Association also found that all types of injuries were 50% more common on synthetic turf.[11] More recent studies have shown less discouraging results for synthetic turfs. Two recent studies found no significant differences between rates of injuries on natural grass versus synthetic turf.[12,13]

INJURIES MORE COMMON ON SYNTHETIC TURF

Prepatellar bursitis and olecranon bursitis are far more common on artificial surfaces than on grass.[14] Fortunately, padding can reduce the severity of these injuries and often prevent them. The term *turf toe,* meaning hyperextension of the metatarsal phalangeal joint, was coined because of the increased incidence of this injury on synthetic turf.[15]

Heat stroke, the second leading cause of death among American football players, is also more common among athletes playing on artificial surfaces. On hot days, athletes undergo a higher heat stress on the synthetic turf than on natural grass.[16] The air temperatures and mean radiant temperatures over synthetic turf have a persistent and slightly higher value than those temperatures over natural turf.[17,18] Although statistically significant, they represent a difference in the range of only 2°C (4°F) at the upper temperature levels.

Newer synthetic turfs have been and are being designed since the 1970s and 1980s, when much of the data on "turf" injuries were collected. These new synthetic turfs may be safer. Continued research should be done to assess these new products.

REFERENCES

1. Stanitski, C. L., McMaster, J. H., and Ferguson, R. J.: Synthetic turf and grass: A comparative study. J. Sports Med. *2*:22, 1974.
2. Adkison, J. W., Requa, R. K., and Garrick, J. G.: Injury rates in high school football. A comparison of synthetic surfaces and grass fields. Clin. Orthop. *99*:131, 1974.
3. Bowers, K. D., Jr.: Ankle and knee injuries at West Virginia University before and after Astro Turf. W. V. Med. J. *69*:1, 1973.
4. Krahenbuhl, G. S.: Speed of movement with varying footwear conditions. Res. Q. *45*:28, 1974.
5. Levy, I. M., Skovron, M. L., and Agel, J.: Living with artificial grass: A knowledge update. Part 1: Basic science. Am. J. Sports Med. *18*:406, 1990.
6. Alles, W. F., et al.: The National Athletic Injury/Illness Reporting System 3-year findings of high school and college football injuries. J. Orthop. Sports Phys. Ther. *1*:103, 1979.
7. Martin, G. L., Fuenning, S. I., Costello, D. F., and Inquanzo, J.: The 1970 intercollegiate tackle football injury surveillance report. Joint Commission on Competitive Safeguards and Medical Aspects of Sports, Lincoln, University of Nebraska, 1970.
8. Keene, J. S., Narechania, R. G., Sachtjen, K. M., and Clancy, W. G.: Tartan Turf on trial. Am. J. Sports Med. *8*:43, 1980.
9. Grippo: NFL Injury Study 1969–1972, Final Project Report (SRI-MSD 1961) Menlo Park, CA, Stanford Research Institute, 1973.
10. Stanford Research Institute: National Football League 1974 Injury Study. Menlo Park, CA, Stanford Research Institute, 1974.
11. Zemper, E.: Unpublished data, 1984.
12. Skovron, M. L., Levy, I. M., and Agel, J.: Living with artificial grass: A knowledge update. Part 2: Epidemiology. Am. J. Sports Med. *18*:510, 1990.
13. Powell, J. W., and Schootman, M.: A multivariate risk analysis of selected playing surfaces in the National Football League: 1980 to 1989. An epidemiologic study of knee injuries. Am. J. Sports Med. *20*:686, 1992.
14. Larson, R. L., and Osternig, L. R.: Traumatic bursitis and artificial turf. J. Sports Med. *2*:183, 1974.
15. Bowers, K. D., and Martin, R. B.: Turf-toe: A shoe-surface related football injury. Med. Sci. Sports *8*:81, 1976.
16. Buskirk, E. R., McLaughlin, E. R., and Loomis, J. L.: Microclimate over artificial turf. J. Health Phys. Edu. & Recreation, Nov. 1973. p. 29.
17. Kandelin, W. W., Krahenbuhl, G. S., and Schact, C. A.: Athletic field microclimates and heat stress. J. Safety Res. *8*:106, 1976.
18. Murphy, R. J.: Heat Illness. J. Sports Med. *1*:(4):26, 1973.

8 *Nancy J. Thompson*

Epidemiology of Injury

Epidemiology, the science of public health, is the study of the *distribution* and *determinants* of disease and disability in human populations.[1] Many persons outside the profession envision an epidemiologic study as one that describes in great detail where, when, and to whom an adverse health outcome occurs. This process, known as "descriptive epidemiology," is only the first stage of the science of epidemiology, the study of distribution. Of far more interest to most epidemiologists is "analytic epidemiology," the study of the "causes" or "determinants" of the adverse outcomes. Finding the cause of a health problem begins the process of identifying what groups are most likely to experience the problem and of intervening to prevent it.

Epidemiology has been applied to the study of sports injuries for at least three decades.[2,3] Numerous descriptive epidemiologic studies have been conducted, across sports and within sports, to identify what activities are most likely to result in injury and which athletes are most likely to be involved. In addition, analytic studies have been conducted to identify which sport factors, athlete factors, and environmental factors are most likely to cause or prevent a sports injury. As more attention has been focused on methodologic issues such as uniformly applying a definition of injury, consideration of the population at risk, representativeness of the study group, and randomization where appropriate, our knowledge base has grown.

DESCRIPTIVE EPIDEMIOLOGY

Because epidemiology is the science of public health, epidemiologic studies are designed to provide information that may be readily applied for the purpose of prevention. With this in mind, the epidemiologist generally classifies persons into categories and determines how many are injured and not injured in each category, so it will be apparent which categories most need intervention to reduce injuries. Because of the use of categorical (e.g., position played) and dichotomous (e.g., injured or not injured) data, the epidemiologist uses measures appropriate to these data: ratios, odds, proportions, and rates.

Ratios

Ratios are used to compare two numbers. In a study of 90 meniscal repairs, 68 were performed in conjunction with anterior cruciate ligament (ACL) reconstruction and 22 were isolated repairs.[4] Thus, the ratio of combined ACL and meniscal repairs to isolated meniscal repairs was 68 to 22, or 3.1 to 1. This ratio is generally written as 68:22 or 68/22 and reduced so that the number on the right is 1. When the two numbers being compared have no members in common (e.g., males to females), this is also known as the *odds* of being male to being female.

Proportions

Proportions, a particular type of ratio, are used when we compare a part of the whole to the whole. Using the example above, among the 90 meniscal repairs, 22 of 90 (22/90) were isolated repairs. Thus, 24.4% of the repairs were isolated ones. A proportion is usually expressed as a decimal or a percentage that, respectively, varies between 0 and 1 or 0% and 100%.

Rates

Rates are the most important measure in epidemiology because they measure probability, or risk, of the outcome among the persons to whom it might occur—those "at risk." Often, in clinical work, we see only persons to whom the injury occurs. This can give us a mistaken impression of the causes of the injury. For example, in a study of high school football players, 618 of 1228 (50%) football players with knee or ankle injuries wore shoes with short cleats whereas only 174 (14%) wore soccer shoes.[3,5] Looking only at the frequency of shoe type among the injured, one might conclude that shoes with short cleats are more dangerous than soccer shoes for playing football. However, out of the total of 7979 players studied, 4265 (53.5%) wore shoes with short cleats and only 937 (11.7%) wore soccer shoes. Thus, the rate of injuries among players wearing shoes with short cleats was 618/4265 (.145, or 14.5 per 100 players), whereas the rate among players wearing soccer shoes was 174/937 (.186, or 18.6 per 100 players). Soccer shoes were shown to be significantly more dangerous ($P<.05$) than shoes with short cleats when rates were considered.

Rates not only take into account the population at risk; they are also dynamic and specify a moment or period of time during which they were measured. *Prevalence* rates measure how many cases of a health problem are present in the population at a given point in time. For example, using prevalence we could determine how many high school students with ACL tears were in need of rehabilitation services in our community on January 1, 1994. The numerator of this rate includes both those who incurred an ACL tear on January 1 and those with a pre-existing ACL tear who were then still in need of supportive, rehabilitative, or other services. The denominator represents all high school students in the community who are at risk for an ACL tear. With chronic conditions or conditions of long duration, we are often most interested in prevalence.

Incidence rates measure how many new cases of the problem occur in individuals within a specified period of time. Using incidence rates, we could determine whether the likelihood of new ACL tears among high school students is increasing from year to year and, if so, whether factors such as changes in female sports participation might be associated. The numerator of the incidence rate would include all new ACL tears among high school students in the community. The denominator would include all youth at risk (i.e., all youth in the community who could still incur an ACL injury). Clearly, sports interventions such as rule and equipment changes cannot reduce the number of injuries that have already occurred (the prevalent cases). For this reason, incidence rates are important because they help us determine whether such interventions have reduced new occurrences.

ANALYTIC EPIDEMIOLOGY

Analytic epidemiology, as it applies to injury, includes evaluation of diagnostic and screening tests, observational studies to determine risk factors, and studies of the efficacy of interventions.

Evaluating Diagnostic and Screening Tests

Diagnostic and screening tests are evaluated in terms of their sensitivity, specificity, and yield (predictive value). The difference between a diagnostic test and a screening test is that when a patient has presented for diagnosis there are usually clinical data to support their being evaluated for a particular type of injury. In contrast, when a group of persons is screened they are usually asymptomatic. As a result, we expect to find more cases of the injury among persons presenting for diagnosis than among those who are being screened.

The *sensitivity* of a test assesses how well that test detects instances of the injury. Recently, Kalebo and coworkers assessed the diagnostic value of ultrasonography for partial ruptures of the Achilles tendon in 37 patients who underwent surgery for Achilles tendon disorders.[6] At surgery, the prevalence of partial ruptures was found to be 32 of the 37 (86%). Comparison of the results of presurgical ultrasonography to findings at surgery are shown in Table 8–1. Of 32 persons found at surgery to have partial tendon ruptures, ultrasonography had identified 30 of them. Thus, the test had a sensitivity of 30/32, or 94%.

The *specificity* of a test assesses how well that test rules out the injury among persons in whom it is not present. Using the same data from Kalebo's group, among the five persons found at surgery not to have partial tendon ruptures, ultrasonography had ruled out all of them. Thus, the specificity of the test was 5/5, or 100%.

In a similar study, Brenneke and Morgan assessed the diagnostic value of ultrasonography for rotator cuff tendon tears.[7] They studied 120 patients who were evaluated with preoperative ultrasonography of the rotator cuff tendon and subsequently underwent diagnostic arthroscopy. Eliminating the 19 patients found on ultrasound to have partial-thickness tears, the prevalence of full-thickness tears (by arthroscopy) was 36/101, or 36%. Their findings for ultrasound versus arthroscopy for full-thickness tears are shown in Table 8–2. Of the 36 persons found on arthroscopy to have full-thickness tears, all 36 were identified by ultrasound, a sensitivity of 36/36, or 100%. Of the 65 persons found not to have full-thickness tears on arthroscopy,

Table 8–1. Assessment of the Diagnostic Value of Ultrasonography for Partial Ruptures of the Achilles Tendon

	Surgery			
Ultrasonography	*Rupture*	*No Rupture*	*Total*	*Predictive Value*
Rupture	30	0	30	30/30
No Rupture	2	5	7	5/7
Total	32	5	37	

(Data from Kalebo, P., Allenmark, C., Peterson, L., and Sward, L.: Am. J. Sports Med. *20*:378, 1992.)

8

Table 8–2. Assessment of the Diagnostic Value of Ultrasonography for Detecting Rotator Cuff Tendon Tears

	Arthroscopy			
Ultrasonography	*Full Tear*	*Partial/No Tear*	*Total*	*Predictive Value*
Full Tear	36	6	42	36/42
Partial/No Tear	0	59	59	59/59
Total	36	65	101	

(Data from Brenneke S. L., and Morgan, C. J.: Am. J. Sports Med. *20*:287, 1992.)

59 were ruled out by ultrasonography, a specificity of 59/65, or 91%.

The yield of the test tells us how well we can predict the ultimate findings on the basis of the initial diagnostic or screening test. Yield is highly influenced by the prevalence of the condition in the population being tested.

Positive predictive value measures the likelihood that a person who tests "positive" on the diagnostic test will be positive by the criterion measure (surgery or arthroscopy). In the first example, where the prevalence of the disorder was 86% (see Table 8–1), the positive predictive value is 30/30 or 100%. In the second example, where the prevalence of the disorder was only 36% (see Table 8–2), the positive predictive value was 36/42, or 86%. In the first example, if the ultrasonography indicates there is a tendon rupture, then we may be certain that there is; in the second example we are less certain. When testing is performed for screening rather than diagnostic purposes, the prevalence is even lower, leading to a lower positive predictive value, (i.e., a greater proportion of *false*-positive results among all positive results).

Negative predictive value measures the likelihood that a person who tests "negative" on the diagnostic test will be negative on the criterion measure (surgery or arthroscopy). In the first example (see Table 8–1), the negative predictive value was 5/7, or 71%. In the second example (see Table 8–2), the negative predictive value was 59/59, or 100%. In this example, if ultrasonography indicates that a full tear is *not* present then we may be certain that there is none. In the first example, the sonogram might be negative when a tendon rupture was present.

Observational Studies to Determine Risk Factors

In epidemiology, when we study factors that contribute to risk (i.e., hazardous factors), we cannot use the typical randomized, blinded clinical trial because it is neither practical nor ethical to randomly expose persons to hazardous factors. For this reason, we rely on observational study methods. The two main types of observation studies are *cohort studies* and *case-control studies*. A cohort study of injury begins with a population at risk of the injury under study, eliminates those who are prevalent cases, and then subdivides the remaining participants into those who have been exposed to the factor of interest and those who have not. Both the exposed and the unexposed groups are then followed to determine their risk (or incidence rate) of injury. At the end of the follow-up period, the risks are compared using a ratio, the risk ratio.

In a recent cohort study of the injury risks associated with adult recreational fitness participation, Requa and associates followed 986 volunteers from fitness clubs and studios for a period of 3 months to determine the incidence of injury by activity.[8] Because participants varied in the number of activities and duration of participation, participant hours of exposure were used as the denominator for the incidence. Using a time loss definition of injury, there were 19 injuries for the activity "aerobic dance" (jazz, funk, etc.) and 1541 person hours of participation in this activity, yielding a 3-month incidence rate of 19/1541, or .0123:12.3 injuries per 1000 participant hours (Table 8–3). In contrast, there were 46 injuries for other aerobic dance activities and 12,059 person hours of participation, yielding a 3-month incidence rate of 46/12059, or .0038:3.8 injuries per 1000 participant hours. The risk ratio for jazz/funk as compared with other forms of aerobic dance was 12.3/3.8, or 3.2:1, indicating that the risk of injury was more than three times greater for jazz/funk than for other aerobic dance.

When the health event under study has a low incidence, it often is not feasible to conduct a cohort study, which involves following large numbers of persons for long periods that yield only a few injury events. Under these circumstances, a case-control study is more efficient. A *case-control* study begins with a representative sample of all cases of the injury under study. Then a second group, the controls, comprised of a representative sample of all persons without the injury under study, is also selected. Usually, one to four controls are selected for each case in the study. Both groups are then studied to determine their history of exposure to the risk factor under study and the odds of exposure to nonexposure are calculated. Finally, these odds are compared using an odds ratio.

In 1991, Mohtadi and coworkers conducted a case-control study of limitation of motion after ACL reconstruction.[9] In a series of 527 ACL reconstructions performed between 1983 and 1988, 37 cases were identified that required a manipulation under anesthesia because

Table 8–3. Cohort Study of Adult Recreational Fitness Participants

Activity	*Injuries*	*Exposure (Person Hours)*	*Incidence (per 1000)*	*Risk Ratio*
Aerobic dance (jazz/funk)	19	1,541	12.3	3.2
Aerobic dance (other)	46	12,059	3.8	1

(Data from Requa, R. K., DeAvilla, L. N., and Garrick, J. G.: Am. J. Sports Med. *21*:461, 1993.)

Table 8–4. Case-Control Study of Limitation of Motion Following ACL Reconstruction

Interval from Injury to Surgery (wk)	Limitation of Motion	
	Cases	Controls
<2	19	10
>2	18	27
Odds <2:>2	19/18	10/27
Odds Ratio	2.8	1

(Data from Mohtadi, N. G. H., Webster-Bogaert, S., and Fowler, P. J.: Am. J. Sports Med. *19*:620, 1991.)

of a flexion deformity of 10° or more, limitation of flexion to less than 120° as of 3 months after the surgery, or both. This gave a 5-year incidence of 37/527, or 7 per 100 reconstructions. An additional 37 persons (the controls) were randomly selected from among the remaining 490 persons who underwent ACL reconstruction. Among the cases, 19 had an interval from injury to surgery of less than 2 weeks and the remaining 18 had an interval of over 2 weeks, for odds of 19/18, or 1.1:1 (Table 8–4). Among the controls, 10 had an interval from injury to surgery of less than 2 weeks and the remaining 27 had a longer interval, odds of 10/27, or 0.4:1. The odds ratio for cases to controls was 1.1/0.4, or 2.8:1, suggesting that persons with limitation of motion were almost three times more likely to have had surgery shortly after their injury.

Studies of the Efficacy of Interventions

Interventions are designed to reduce the incidence of an adverse health problem and, so, are protective. According to current medical standards, surgical intervention must be selected on the basis of the state of the art and the surgeon's best clinical judgment. Consequently, it is not possible to study these interventions using a randomized design in which patients receive various procedures at random. Unfortunately, this approach is often extended to other interventions for which it is not only ethical but essential that we use study methods that include either randomization of subjects to receive and not to receive the intervention or comparison of the same subject with and without the intervention. Where acceptable, these designs are important because they ensure that the group that receives the intervention and the group that does not are comparable on all characteristics except the intervention. Then, if a difference is found between groups it can be attributed to the intervention.

Rosen and coworkers recently studied the efficacy of continuous passive motion (CPM) in the rehabilitation of ACL reconstruction using *randomization of subjects*.[10] Seventy-five patients undergoing arthroscopically assisted ACL reconstruction were randomly divided into three groups of 25 to assess the effects of (1) early active motion, (2) CPM, and (3) a combination of both. Knee motion was assessed at 1 week, 1 month, and then monthly until 6 months. After adjusting for the motion of the control knee, no differences were found among the three groups at any of these times. After 6 months, the rates of complications were 3/25 (12%) in the active motion group and 3/25 (12%) in the CPM group. Although the sample was large enough to detect differences in the continuous range of motion values, it should be noted that it was not sufficient to assess even a twofold difference in the rate of complications. Examples of other recent intervention studies conducted using a randomized design include a comparison of the effect of training using running, water running, or cycling on maximum oxygen consumption and 2-mile run performance, a comparison of development of lower leg strength and flexibility using the Strength Shoe versus the athlete's usual training shoes, and a comparison of basketball performance after imagery training alone versus imagery training combined with restricted environmental stimulation.[11–13]

Using a *repeated measures* design, Karlsson and Andreasson studied the effect on mechanical stability and reaction time of taping versus not taping the ankle in 20 patients with isolated unilateral ankle instability caused by supination trauma.[14] While there was no difference in instability, either in millimeters of anterior talar translation or degrees of talar tilt, between the taped and untaped conditions, the reaction time of the untaped ankle was significantly shortened ($P < .05$). Examples of other recent studies using the repeated measures design include a comparison of anterior compartment pressures in cross-country skiers who used the skating technique of skiing under two conditions: wearing the classic ski and wearing the skating ski.[15] In addition, Yack and colleagues compared alternating closed and open kinetic chain exercise in 11 volunteers with an ACL-deficient knee, and Highgenboten et al. compared oxygen consumption of four male runners when braced with each of four different commercially available braces.[16,17]

SUMMARY OF WHAT HAS BEEN ADEQUATELY STUDIED

Since the late 1980s we have made great advances in the descriptive epidemiology of sports injury. In large part, this is because of the greater attention paid to determining the population at risk.

Descriptive Studies

A number of authors have provided estimates of the incidence of injury in specific sports.[18–21] Still other authors have compared various sports using common methods to determine which are the most hazardous with respect to injury.[8,22–31] For all such studies in which American football was included, it has been found to have the highest risk. Garrick and Requa found that 81% of high school football players were injured during a single season, followed by 75% of wrestlers.[26] Similarly, McLain and Reynolds found that 61% of high school football players were injured during a single season, followed by girl gymnasts (46%) and wrestlers and boy gymnasts (40% each).[29] According to the NCAA Injury Surveillance System, the risk of injury in football games is 37.8 per 1000 athlete exposures.[32] Once again, this is followed by wrestling meets, which have a risk of 28.1 injuries per 1000 athlete exposures, and women's gymnastic meets, which have 24.6 injuries per 1000 athlete exposures. With respect to practice, women gymnasts had the highest risk of injury: 7.7 per 1000 athlete exposures. In several European studies that did not include American football, results were varied with regard to the highest-risk sport. In a study of 1818 school children in the Netherlands, basketball presented the greatest risk in physical education (99.8%) and in organized sports games (23 per 1000 game hours).[22] In a study of 31,620 inhabitants of a rural area in southwest Sweden, soccer was the highest-risk sport for both male and female athletes, with rates of 11.8 per 1000 and 3.5 per 1000, respectively.[24] In a study restricted to female college athletes in which soccer was not included, the highest risk (29.6% injured, 9.9% with disabling injuries) was in basketball.[28]

Within specific sports, descriptive studies have been conducted to determine who is most likely to be injured and during which activities.[5,19,21,27,32–42] Characteristics and activities of those at greatest risk vary from sport to sport. Furthermore, many such studies are limited because it is difficult and costly to assess the exact amount of exposure time for each athlete, let alone time spent in each activity during participation. In an extensive study at the college level, Cahill and Griffith actually monitored football player time on the field as well as exposure to specific activities.[43] They found that player risk was greatest during practice games: 59.37 injuries per 1000 player hours.

Many authors have studied frequency of injury to various body parts in specific sports.[18–21,24,28,34,40,41,44–45] According to Garrick and Requa, location of injury can be thought of as "sport specific" or "sport generic."[46] The physical demands of some sports create high frequencies of specific injuries that would not be present across all sports. It is overuse injuries, rather than acute injuries, that tend to be sport specific.

Rather than studying site of injury in a specific sport, some authors have studied the epidemiology across sports of injury to a particular site, such as the knee, foot and ankle, or cervical spine.[46–49] Garrick and Requa report that the majority of sports injuries occur to the lower extremity, injuries to the knee, ankle, and foot being most common.[46]

Another area that has been studied particularly well is risk in practice versus in competition. In all reported studies the greatest percentage of injuries occurs during practice. But when time spent in practice versus competition is taken into account, the risk during competition exceeds that during practice.[22,32,43,45] According to NCAA data on football, men's basketball, women's basketball, wrestling, ice hockey, men's gymnastics, and women's gymnastics, the risk ratios, comparing competition to practice, varied from 1.9:1 for men's basketball, to 9.5:1 for football.[32]

Other variables that have been studied well within a number of sports are injury by age and position played.[2,5,19,21,22,24,35,40,45,47,50,51] Within all sports, injury increased with age, which may be the result of increased levels of competition or greater intensity of play. Risk by position varies by sport.

Analytic Studies

Analytic studies have been conducted to identify factors that contribute to or protect against the likelihood of injury. These factors include types of equipment used, surfaces on which participation occurs, participant preparation, other physical characteristics of the participant, and psychological or emotional characteristics of the participant.[3,5,15,19,31,33,35,39–42,51–63] Among first-string high school football players, Thompson and Morris found psychological factors to be more predictive of injury than physical characteristics, perhaps because this is a generally fit and physically homogeneous group.[51] Psychological factors most studied have been personality characteristics, cognitive skills (e.g., reaction time or spatial skills), and life stress. Results on life stress as a risk factor for injury in contact sports have been most consistent.[63]

MAJOR ISSUES IN EPIDEMIOLOGIC STUDIES OF SPORTS INJURY

At present, the major issues to be addressed in the epidemiology of sports injury relate to the improvement of research methods. Of prime importance is the selection of a standard definition of injury. At present, injury definitions fall into two categories: medical attention and time loss. The benefit of a definition that requires medical attention is that the diagnosis is better, and serious injuries such as concussion that might not result in loss of time are identified. The benefit of a time loss definition is that medical attention is not equally available in urban and rural areas. Furthermore, many persons do not seek attention for injuries until long after the injury has occurred. At present, the most generally accepted definition is one that relies on a combination of time loss and medical attention.

A second research issue related to the injury itself is whether one is measuring a specific type of injury (e.g., knee injury) or whether one is collecting data on all injuries. In looking for injury mechanisms, study of a specific injury may be more fruitful because the mechanism of injury may vary by type; however, to identify a sufficient number of a particular type of injury, it may be necessary to study a much larger population than if all injuries were studied.

Another major issue, and one that can be very time consuming and expensive, is the monitoring of athlete exposures. For exposures such as practice versus game, one can obtain a good estimate of exposure time by knowing the length of each game and the number of players on the field, as well as the length of each practice and the number of players involved. However, when one is evaluating interventions such as knee or ankle braces, it is difficult to determine the number of hours during which each player was actually exposed to the brace. Similarly, for individual athletes, it is difficult to determine exactly how many hours were spent in practice or competition. For this reason, the role of individual factors in the risk of injury is very difficult to study.

Representativeness of the study group represents another research issue. While it is often most convenient to study the population of persons with knee or ankle injuries who present to a particular clinic or hospital for treatment, these cases are not representative of all cases. In the inner city teaching hospital, it is likely that persons with a history of timely and ongoing medical attention are under-represented. In addition, financial resources for medical attention may be related to financial resources for protective equipment, adequate diet, or other protective factors. For this reason, where possible, it is best to begin with a registry of "cases" representing the population. The same difficulty is present for the selection of clinic- or hospital-based controls. Once again, it is best to identify a population-based control group through random-digit telephone dialing or through recruitment at public areas such as shopping centers or malls.

A second problem of representativeness is the problem of "survivors." Often, researchers are tempted to survey persons who complete a race or who currently participate in aerobic dance to determine their lifetime prevalence of injury. Selection of such groups for study systematically excludes those who currently have injuries or who were injured severely enough to interrupt or end their participation in the sport. A far better research strategy is to identify the population of participants for a particular sport. This may be done through team rosters at the beginning of a season or through membership lists from sport organizations.

A final area important to consider is that of confounding variables. A confounding variable is one that is related to both the risk factor and the outcome being studied. For example, if we were to study the relationship between body weight and stress fractures in gymnastics, hours of practice might be a confounding variable. Certainly, hours of practice could influence body weight and could also lead to stress fractures. Thus, to determine the true relationship between body weight and stress fractures, hours of practice must be controlled in the analysis phase of the study or in the selection stage through the matching of cases and controls.

FUTURE DIRECTIONS

At present, the state of the descriptive epidemiology of sports injury is far in advance of analytic epidemiology. Future attention should be directed toward the development of more and better analytic studies to determine risk factors for injury. This must include the incorporation of a consistent definition of injury, selection of representative groups for study, adequate measures of exposure, and control for confounding variables. With this information, we will be able to develop intervention programs to reduce the risk of sports injuries among youth.

REFERENCES

1. MacMahon, B., and Pugh, T. F.: Epidemiology: Principles and Methods. Boston, Little, Brown, 1970.
2. Robey, J. M., Blyth, C. S., and Mueller, F. O.: Athletics injuries: Application of epidemiologic methods. JAMA *217*:184, 1971.
3. Mueller, F. O., and Blyth, C. S.: North Carolina high school football injury study: Equipment and prevention. J. Sports Med. *2*:1, 1974.
4. Cannon, W. D., and Vittori, J. M.: The incidence of healing in arthroscopic meniscal repairs in anterior cruciate ligament–reconstructed knees versus stable knees. Am. J. Sports Med. *20*:176, 1992.
5. Thompson, N. J., et al.: High school football injuries: Evaluation. Am. J. Sports Med. *16*(suppl):S97, 1988.
6. Kalebo, P., Allenmark, C., Peterson, L., and Sward, L.: Diagnostic value of ultrasonography in partial ruptures of the Achilles tendon. Am. J. Sports Med. *20*:378, 1992.
7. Brenneke, S. L., and Morgan, C. J.: Evaluation of ultrasonography as a diagnostic technique in the assessment of rotator cuff tendon tears. Am. J. Sports Med. *20*:287, 1992.
8. Requa, R. K., DeAvilla, L. N., and Garrick, J. G.: Injuries in recreational adult fitness activities. Am. J. Sports Med. *21*:461, 1993.
9. Mohtadi, N. G. H., Webster-Bogaert, S., and Fowler, P. J.: Limitation of motion following anterior cruciate ligament reconstruction. A case-control study. Am. J. Sports Med. *19*:620, 1991.
10. Rosen, M. A., Jackson, D. W., and Atwell, E. A.: The efficacy of continuous passive motion in the rehabilitation of anterior cruciate ligament reconstructions. Am. J. Sports Med. *20*:122, 1992.
11. Eyestone, E. D., Fellingham, G., George, J., and Fisher, A. G.: Effect of water running and cycling on maximum oxygen consumption and 2-mile run performance. Am. J. Sports Med. *21*:41, 1993.
12. Cook, S. D., et al.: Development of lower leg strength and flexibility with the strength shoe. Am. J. Sports Med. *21*:445, 1993.
13. Wagaman, J. D., Barabasz, A. F., and Barabasz, M.: Flotation rest and imagery in the improvement of collegiate basketball performance. Percept. Motor Skills *72*:119, 1991.
14. Karlsson, J., and Andreasson, G. O.: The effect of external ankle support in chronic lateral ankle joint instability: An electromyographic study. Am. J. Sports Med. *20*:257, 1992.
15. Lawson, S. K., Reid, D. C., and Wiley, J. P.: Anterior compartment pressures in cross-country skiers: A comparison of classic and skating skis. Am. J. Sports Med. *20*:750, 1992.
16. Yack, H. J., Collins, C. E., and Whieldon, T. J.: Comparison of closed and open kinetic chain exercise in the anterior cruciate ligament-deficient knee. Am. J. Sports Med. *21*:49, 1993.
17. Highgenboten, C. L., Jackson, A., Meske, N., and Smith, J.: The effects of knee brace wear on perceptual and metabolic variables during horizontal treadmill running. Am. J. Sports Med. *19*:639, 1991.
18. DeLee, J. C., and Farney, W. C.: Incidence of injury in Texas high school football. Am. J. Sports Med. *20*:575, 1992.
19. Engstrom, B., Johansson, C., and Tornkvist, H.: Soccer injuries among elite female players. Am. J. Sports Med. *19*:372, 1991.
20. Garrick, J. G., Gillien, D. M., and Whiteside, P.: The epidemiology of aerobic dance injuries. Am. J. Sports Med. *14*:67, 1986.
21. Lorish, T. R., Rizzo, T. D., Ilstrup, D. M., and Scott, S. G.: Injuries in adolescent and preadolescent boys at two large wrestling tournaments. Am. J. Sports Med. *20*:199, 1992.
22. Backx, F. J. G., Beijer, H. J. M., Bol, E., and Erich, W. B. M.: Injuries in high-risk persons and high-risk sports. Am. J. Sports Med. *19*:124, 1991.

23. Baxter-Jones, A., Maffulli, N., and Helms, P.: Low injury rates in elite athletes. Arch. Dis. Childhood *68*:130, 1993.
24. de Loes, M., and Goldie, I.: Incidence rate of injuries during sport activity and physical exercise in a rural Swedish municipality: Incidence rates in 17 sports. Int. J. Sports Med. *9*:461, 1988.
25. Gallagher, S. S., Finison, K., Guyer, B., and Goodenough, S.: The incidence of injuries among 87,000 Massachusetts children and adolescents: Results of the 1980–81 statewide childhood injury prevention program surveillance system. Am. J. Public Health *74*:1340, 1984.
26. Garrick, J. G., and Requa, R. K.: Injuries in high school sports. Pediatrics *61*:465, 1978.
27. Goldstein, J. D., Berger, P. E., Windler, G. E., and Jackson, D. W.: Spine injuries in gymnasts and swimmers. An epidemiologic investigation. Am. J. Sports Med. *19*:463, 1991.
28. Graham, G. P., and Bruce, P. J.: Survey of intercollegiate athletic injuries to women. Res. Q. *48*:217, 1977.
29. McLain, L. G., and Reynolds, S.: Sports injuries in a high school. Pediatrics *84*:446, 1989.
30. National Safety Council: Accident Facts. Itasca, IL, National Safety Council, 1987.
31. Watson, A. S.: Incidence and nature of sports injuries in Ireland. Analysis of four types of sport. Am. J. Sports Med. *21*:128, 1993.
32. National Collegiate Athletic Association: NCAA Injury Surveillance System: 1992–1993 Football. Overland Park, KS, NCAA, 1992.
33. Bouter, L. M., Knipschild, P. G., and Volovics, A.: Personal and environmental factors in relation to injury risk in downhill skiing. Int. J. Sports Med. *10*:298, 1989.
34. Halpern, B., et al.: High school football injuries: Identifying the risk factors. Am. J. Sports Med. *16*(1 suppl):S113, 1988.
35. Keller, C. S., Noyes, F. R., and Buncher, C. R.: The medical aspects of soccer injury epidemiology. Am. J. Sports Med. *16*(1 suppl):S105, 1988.
36. Krinsky, M. B., et al.: Incidence of lateral meniscus injury in professional basketball players. Am. J. Sports Med. *20*:17, 1992.
37. Kadel, N. J., Teitz, C. C., and Kronmal, R. A.: Stress fractures in ballet dancers. Am. J. Sports Med. *20*:445, 1992.
38. Laskowski, E. R., and Murtaugh, P. A.: Snow skiing injuries in physically disabled skiers. Am. J. Sports Med. *20*:553, 1992.
39. McAuley, E., et al.: Injuries in women's gymnastics: The state of the art. Am. J. Sports Med. *16*(1 suppl):S124, 1988.
40. Sim, F. H., Simonet, W. T., Melton, L. J., and Lehn, T. A.: Ice hockey injuries. Am. J. Sports Med. *16*(1 suppl):S86, 1988.
41. Taimela, S., et al.: Motor ability and personality with reference to soccer injuries. J. Sports Med. Phys. Fitness *30*:194, 1990.
42. Warren, B. L., and Davis, V.: Determining predictor variables for running-related pain. Physical Therapy *68*:647, 1988.
43. Cahill, B. R., and Griffith, E. H.: Exposure to injury in major college football: A preliminary report of data collection to determine injury exposure rates and activity risk factors. Am. J. Sports Med. *7*:183, 1979.
44. Andersson, G., Malmgren, S., and Ekstrand, J.: Occurrence of athletic injuries in voluntary participants in a 1-year extensive newspaper exercise campaign. Int. J. Sports Med. *7*:222, 1986.
45. Engstrom, B., Forssblad, M., Johansson, C., and Tornkvist, H.: Does a major knee injury definitely sideline an elite soccer player? Am. J. Sports Med. *18*:101, 1990.
46. Garrick, J. G., and Requa, R. K.: The epidemiology of foot and ankle injuries in sport. Clin. Sports Med. *7*:29, 1988.
47. Nielsen, A. B., and Yde, J.: Epidemiology of acute knee injuries: A prospective hospital investigation. J. Trauma *31*:1644, 1991.
48. Zarins, B., and Adams, M.: Knee injuries in sports. N. Engl. J. Med. *318*:950, 1988.
49. Torg, J. S.: Epidemiology, pathomechanics, and prevention of athletic injuries to the cervical spine. Med. Sci. Sports Exercise *17*:295, 1985.
50. Sutherland, G. W.: Fire on ice. Am. J. Sports Med. *4*:264, 1976.
51. Thompson, N. J., and Morris, R. D.: Predicting injury risk in high school football players: The role of psychological factors. Pediatr. Psychol. *19*:415, 1994.
52. Garrick, J. G., and Requa, R. K.: Prophylactic knee bracing. Am. J. Sports Med. *15*:S118, 1988.
53. Powell, J. W., and Schootman, M.: A multivariate risk analysis of selected playing surfaces in the National Football League: 1980–1989. An epidemiologic study of knee injuries. Am. J. Sports Med. *20*:686, 1992.
54. Skovron, M. L., Levy, I. M., and Agel, J.: Living with artificial grass: Knowledge update. Am. J. Sports Med. *18*:510, 1990.
55. Cahill, B. R., and Griffith, E. H.: Effect of preseason conditioning on the incidence and severity of high school football knee injuries. Am. J. Sports Med. *6*:180, 1978.
56. Garn, S. N., and Newton, R. A.: Kinesthetic awareness in subjects with multiple ankle sprains. Physical Therapy *68*:1667, 1988.
57. Giladi, M., Milgrom, C., Simkin, A., and Danon, Y.: Stress fractures. Identifiable risk factors. Am. J. Sports Med. *19*:647, 1991.
58. Bergandi, T. A.: Psychological variables relating to the incidence of athletic injury: A review of the literature. Int. J. Sport Psychol. *16*:141, 1985.
59. Bramwell, S. T., Masuda, M., Wagner, N. N., and Holmes, T. H.: Psychosocial factors in athletic injuries: Development and application of the social and athletic readjustment rating scale. J. Human Stress *1*:6, 1975.
60. Coddington, R. D., and Troxell, J. R.: The effect of emotional factors on football injury rates: A pilot study. J. Human Stress *6*:3, 1980.
61. Jackson, D. W., et al.: Injury prediction in the young athlete: A preliminary report. Am. J. Sports Med. *6*:6, 1978.
62. Kelley, M. J.: Psychological risk factors and sports injuries. J. Sports Med. Physical Fitness *30*:202, 1990.
63. Thompson, N. J., Curl, W. W., Maslanka, M., and Morris, R. D.: Psychological factors that predict injury: A review and integrating study. Under review.

II

MEDICAL ASPECTS OF SPORTS

9 *Robert O'Neil Snoddy, Jr.*

The Preparticipation Screening Examination

Almost anyone who has participated in organized sports can remember the ritual of the preseason physical examination. As it is performed today, the preparticipation screening examination is a great deal more sophisticated than simply listening to the heart and lungs and checking for a hernia.

The preparticipation screening examination serves many functions.[1] It can meet legal and insurance requirements related to athletic participation and can serve as a determination of the overall general health of the athlete. The examination may evaluate the athlete's level of physical conditioning, and it can assess the physical maturity of potential participants. Conditions that limit participation or that may be contraindications to participation can also be detected. The examination may detect conditions that may predispose to injury and allow for rehabilitation of these injuries before participation. The documented findings may serve as a baseline to use in determining when the injured athlete may return to play. Finally, the examination may afford an opportunity for health education.

One critical point to remember is that the athlete and the physician often view the event differently.[2] The athlete sees the evaluation as his or her "annual physical." The physician sees the examination as a screening tool. Athletes should be reminded that the preparticipation screening examination should not be considered a substitute for routine health care.

The legal requirements for the examination vary from state to state and with the level of athletic competition involved. When checking requirements with the appropriate authority, certain factors should be considered. The frequency of examinations is often specified, most commonly once a year. The authority may have a specific form that must be completed. If no form is specified, a standard form may be created (Fig. 9–1). The contents of the examination may be dictated to some degree, and there may be criteria for exclusion from participation. The athlete's parents may be required to sign documents authorizing emergency medical treatment before participation is allowed. The authority may even specify what types of health care providers can do the preparticipation screening examination.

Physicians doing preparticipation evaluations should keep in mind several other legal points. If the athlete is a minor, the parent must give permission for the examination. The findings of the examination should be carefully documented, and the recommendations for participation should be documented as well. While the physician's final opinion carries a great deal of weight, court rulings have generally held that the physician's recommendations on participation are not the final authority.[2] Ultimately, the decision on whether the athlete participates rests with the athlete or the athlete's parents.

Ideally, the preparticipation examinations should be scheduled several weeks before the season begins. This allows for correction or rehabilitation of many of the conditions that are detected. When the examination is scheduled, some documents, such as medical history or insurance forms, may be sent home with the athletes to be filled out before the event. The athletes should be instructed to come to the examination in loose-fitting shorts and tee shirt and to wear gym shoes.

There are two basic formats for the actual performance of the examination. These are the individual or office-based system, and the group or station system. Both systems have advantages and disadvantages. The office-based examination allows for more privacy, better availability of medical records, and a closer relationship between the examiner and the athlete. It also allows for

ATHLETIC EXAMINATION FORM

Name: ______ (Circle One) Sex: M · F Race: B · W · O

School Name: ______ Grade ____ Age: ____ Birthdate ______ Dominant Hand: R · L

Sport(s): ______ Position: ______

Exam Date: ___/___/___ (MONTH DAY YEAR)

CHECK OUT (DOCTOR'S INITIALS)			Conditions / Reasons
	PASS		
	FAIL		

Initial Exam ☐ Repeat Exam ☐

HISTORY

ILLNESS		MEDICATIONS	
ALLERGIES		INJURIES	
OPERATIONS		OTHER	
(Initial)			

HEIGHT / WEIGHT		PULSE	
BLOOD PRESSURE		DENTAL (Pass — Fail)	

MEDICAL

H.E.E.N.T.		SKIN	
HEART		LUNG	
ABDOMEN		OTHER	
(Initial)			

FLEXIBILITY

	L	R		L	R
HEELCORDS			HAMSTRINGS		
(Initial)			OTHER		

STRENGTH

	L	R		L	R
HIP FLEXOR (Pass - Fail)			THIGH GIRTH		
SHOULDER			OTHER		
(Initial)					

ORTHOPAEDICS

	L	R		L	R
SHOULDER			ANKLE		
ELBOW			FOOT		
HIP			SPINE		
KNEE			OTHER		
(Initial)					

FITNESS

			L	R
LATCH RUN		REACTION		
PULL UP or HANG TIME		GRIP STRENGTH		
REACH/JUMP		BODY FAT %		
MEDICINE BALL PUT				
		OTHER		

Fig. 9–1. The standard form for recording information from the preseason screening.

more comprehensive health care for the athlete in addition to meeting participation requirements. The drawbacks include higher cost, more time required, and increased demand for providers.

The group or station format is extremely time efficient and may reduce costs significantly. This form of examination also has the potential advantage of involving coaches, trainers, and other athletic personnel in the screening process. It is impersonal, however, and requires a great deal of coordination.

The most critical portion of the preparticipation screening examination is the medical history (Table 9–1). Studies have shown that 63 to 74% of athletes with potentially limiting conditions can be identified by an appropriately administered medical history. The athlete's parents should be included in this information-gathering process. When athletes and parents were allowed to fill out medical history forms independently, only 38% of the information reported matched. This finding suggests that sending the history questionnaires home with the athlete for completion with the parent's help before the examination date is advisable.[1]

Several subjects should be included in the screening history. The athlete should first be asked about his or her general health, medical illnesses, medications, allergies, and immunizations. Surgical history and the details of hospitalizations for any reason should be requested. A cardiovascular review of systems should be performed, including any history of heart disease, rheumatic fever, or hypertension. The athlete should be asked about any history of heart murmurs, even "innocent" ones. Probably the most critical events to ask about are episodes of exertional syncope, chest pain, and shortness of breath. The athlete should also be asked about a family history of cardiovascular disease and should be asked to list any musculoskeletal injuries sustained in the past and the present condition of the injured part. A history of neurologic injuries is important, particularly any injuries that resulted in concussion. The athlete should be asked about any previous heat or cold injuries. Finally, female athletes should be asked about their menstrual history and the possibility of pregnancy.

If the medical history is collected at the examination site, a standard report form can be completed by trained volunteers. It should be reviewed by the health care provider before the athlete receives clearance to participate. Computerized records of prior examinations are useful to keep track of previous findings. Athletes with documented normal examinations in the past may be allowed to provide abbreviated interval histories and undergo limited physical examinations.

The physical examination should begin with measurement of height and weight, resting pulse, and blood pressure, along with vision screening. If time permits, pulse rates can be collected after a standard amount of exercise such as running in place and after

Table 9–1. History Questions for Athletic Physicals

Illness
Are you currently seeing a doctor for a medical problem?
Have you ever had: Asthma or shortness of breath?
Allergies?
Bronchitis?
Epilepsy?
Hepatitis?
Mononucleosis?
Diabetes?
Heat illness or cramps?
Anemia?
Hernia?
High or low blood pressure?
Ulcer?
Tendency to bleed excessively?
Sickle cell disease or trait? [blacks only]
Do you tire easily?
Have you ever had chest pains or difficulty breathing, or passed out while exercising?
Do you have frequent or repeated backaches or strains?
Do you have frequent or repeated headaches?
Have you ever been told that you have a heart murmur, an irregular heartbeat, or any heart disease?
Have you ever been knocked out (unconscious)?
Have any members of your family had a "heart attack," "heart problems," or died before age 50?
Do you wear glasses or contact lenses?
Are you blind or partially blind in either eye?
Do you have any hearing problems?
Do you have any dentures or partials?
Do you smoke cigarettes or chew tobacco?
Males: Have you ever had a hydrocele?
Are you missing a testicle?
Females: Are you pregnant?
Do you have any menstrual disorders?
Medications
Are you taking any medications?
Are you allergic to any medications?
Injuries
Have you ever had a concussion, seizure, or convulsions?
Have you ever injured your: Neck?
Nose?
Throat?
Eyes or ears?
Head, arms or shoulders?
Knees, ankles or legs?
Chest or back?
Abdomen or stomach?
Operations
Have you *ever* had any surgery or operation?
Are you missing any organ (eye, kidney, lung, etc.)?
Please record any *yes* answers.

a standard recovery time. Dental screening may be included. This could be a formal screening examination by a dentist or a simple check for items such as braces or missing teeth. This portion of the examination could also include fitting for a mouthpiece if one is required for the sport.

The general physical examination should include inspection of the skin. The head, eyes, ears, nose, and throat should be examined as well as the heart, lungs, abdomen, and genitalia. It is important to perform the cardiac examination in a quiet location. The examiner should be able to remove the athlete's shirt and perform standing, sitting, and supine auscultation of the chest. The genital examination should include an assessment of the individual's physical maturity, such as Tanner staging.

A musculoskeletal screening examination should also be performed. The screening orthopaedic examination should include range of motion of the major joints and a screen for gross instability. Measurement of flexibility parameters is also useful. Laboratory screening such as urinalysis, hemoglobin measurement, or tuberculin tine test, is not recommended by the American Academy of Pediatrics, although certain tests may be required by state law or by the organization sanctioning the competition.[2] If any tests are required, arrangements must be made to have them done in advance or at the examination site, so the results are available to the health care provider who is responsible for reviewing the completed examination forms.

To provide even more information about the athlete, certain specialized tests may be included in the examination. Tests of flexibility such as sit and reach or popliteal angle for the hamstrings, knee hugs for the hip flexors, heel cord angle for the calf muscles, or range of motion for the shoulder girdle may alert trainers to problem areas. Simple tests of strength, including manual muscle testing, grip strength, push-ups, sit-ups, or isotonic weight lifts provide useful baseline values against which recovery from injury can be measured. Power can be tested by vertical jump and reach, stair climbing, medicine ball put, or by machinery. The athlete's speed can be assessed by a short sprint for time. Endurance can be measured by a 12-minute run or longer distance run for time. The athlete's body composition can be assessed by tape measure or caliper methods.

Once all of the information is collected, a health care provider should review all of the results with the athlete. This health care provider should be familiar with the demands placed on the athlete by the various sports. A simple scheme for classifying sports into demand categories based on level of potential impact and cardiovascular exertion is outlined in Table 9–2.[3]

After considering the health of the athlete and the sport, the health care provider should make specific recommendations for participation. Guidelines for participation in specific categories of sports for athletes with certain conditions have been published.[3]

The reviewer should limit the final disposition of the examination process to one of three recommendations. Most athletes should be found to pass the screening examination without restrictions. Some athletes may pass the examination subject to certain specified restrictions or conditions. Examples of such requirements might include a more extensive follow-up evaluation of a problem found during the screening, limitation of participation to certain sports or to positions within a sport, or use of additional protective equipment during participation. Finally, an athlete may fail the examination. As many as 15% of athletes may have a condition that requires further evaluation, but outright failure should be extremely rare.

If additional evaluation or rehabilitation is required for a problem uncovered during the screening, the ath-

Table 9–2. Classification of Sports

Contact/Collision	Softball
Boxing	Squash, handball
Field hockey	Volleyball
Football	**Moderately Strenuous Noncontact**
Ice hockey	Aerobic dancing
Lacrosse	Crew
Martial arts	Fencing
Rodeo	Field events:
Soccer	Discus
Wrestling	Javelin
Limited Contact/Impact	Shot put
Baseball	Running
Basketball	Swimming
Bicycling	Tennis
Diving	Track
Field events:	Weightlifting
High jump	**Strenuous Noncontact**
Pole vault	Badminton
Gymnastics	Curling
Horseback riding	Table tennis
Skating (ice or roller)	**Nonstrenuous Noncontact**
Skiing:	Archery
Cross country	Golf
Downhill	Riflery
Water	

(American Academy of Pediatrics: Recommendations for participation in competitive sports. Reproduced by permission of Pediatrics. *81*:737, 1988.)

lete should be restricted from participation until it is completed. If the athlete requires medication for participation, such as an inhaler for exercise-induced asthma, this should be noted as a condition of participation and the team should be notified to ensure that such medication is available.

Finally, it should be re-emphasized that the physician or other health care provider who reviews the results of the preparticipation screening examination is only making a recommendation concerning the athlete's participation. The right to make a final decision on whether to engage in athletics has been repeatedly recognized by the courts as resting with the athlete or with his or her parents.[2]

REFERENCES

1. Lombardo, J. A.: Preparticipation evaluation. *In* The Pediatric Athlete. Edited by J. A. Sullivan and W. A. Grana. Park Ridge, IL, American Academy of Orthopaedic Surgeons, 1988.
2. Feinstein, R. A., Soileau, E. J., and Daniel, W. A. Jr.: A national survey of preparticipation physical examination requirements. Physician Sportsmed. *16*(5):51, 1988.
3. American Academy of Pediatrics Committee on Sports Medicine: Recommendations for participation in competitive sports. Pediatrics, *81*:737, 1988.

10 *Paul W. Baumert, Jr.*

Preparticipation Evaluation: Disqualifying Conditions

Most, if not all, sports are associated with some risk. One of the primary objectives of the preparticipation evaluation is to detect conditions that may place the athlete or other participants at risk for injury. The preparticipation evaluation is not complete until a decision is made about the individual's ability to participate safely in a given sport. Clearance for activity is probably the most difficult, and the most important, decision that the physician can make as part of the preparticipation evaluation.

DETERMINING CLEARANCE

When a specific problem is found during the preparticipation evaluation that may limit the athlete's participation, the physician must consider several questions when determining the athlete's clearance.[1] First, one must determine if, because of the problem, the athlete or any other participant is at increased risk for injury. If the athlete could safely participate with treatment of the problem, such as medication, rehabilitation, bracing, or padding, the physician should determine if limited participation could be allowed while the treatment is being instituted. Finally, if clearance is denied for a particular activity, one should determine if there are any activities in which the athlete could safely participate. The physician should always strive to consider any alternatives that may allow the athlete some type of participation. It is also very important for the physician to explain any restrictions to the athlete, the parents or guardians, and the coach or athletic trainer whenever possible.

Guidelines

To help practitioners determine whether an athlete should be allowed to participate in a particular sport, the American Academy of Pediatrics' Committee on Sports Medicine has compiled a list of recommendations.[2] They classify three basic categories of sports activities—contact/collision, limited contact/impact, and noncontact—based on the intensity of exercise and the injury potential of the sport. The noncontact activities are further divided into strenuous, moderately strenuous, and nonstrenuous ones. The Committee's recommendations for sports participation, based on these categories, are listed in Table 10–1. These recommendations are not meant to be rigid and should be used only as a guide. It is imperative that the physician use his or her clinical judgment when interpreting these recommendations on an individual basis.

Types of Clearance

The type of clearance is best determined at the last station in the station screening evaluation (see Chapter 9) by a physician who is familiar with the demands of the activity, the limitations that result from various problems, and the American Academy of Pediatrics guidelines. Based on the findings in the preparticipation evaluation, one of three types of clearance may be recommended: (1) unrestricted clearance, (2) clearance with restrictions (following completion of evaluation or rehabilitation), or (3) no clearance or disqualification from a particular sport or classification. As one can see from Table 10–1, there are surprisingly few medical problems that actually limit athletic participation.

MEDICAL PROBLEMS

Atlantoaxial Instability

Athletes with documented atlantoaxial instability should not participate in any contact/collision or limited

Table 10–1. Recommendations for Participation in Competitive Sports

	Contact		*Noncontact*		
	Contact/Collision	*Limited Contact/Impact*	*Strenuous*	*Moderately Strenuous*	*Nonstrenuous*
Atlantoaxial instability	No	No	Yes*	Yes	Yes
Acute illness†					
Cardiovascular problems					
Carditis	No	No	No	No	No
Hypertension					
Mild	Yes	Yes	Yes	Yes	Yes
Moderate†					
Severe†					
Congenital heart disease‡					
Ocular disorders					
Absence or loss of function of one eye§					
Detached retina‖					
Inguinal hernia	Yes	Yes	Yes	Yes	Yes
Single kidney	No	Yes	Yes	Yes	Yes
Hepatomegaly	No	No	Yes	Yes	Yes
Musculoskeletal disorders†					
Neurologic problems					
History of serious head or spine trauma, repeated concussions, or craniotomy	†	†	Yes	Yes	Yes
Convulsive disorder					
Well-controlled	Yes	Yes	Yes	Yes	Yes
Poorly controlled	No	No	Yes¶	Yes	Yes**
Ovary					
Absence of one	Yes	Yes	Yes	Yes	Yes
Respiratory problems					
Pulmonary insufficiency	††	††	††	††	Yes
Asthma	Yes	Yes	Yes	Yes	Yes
Sickle cell trait	Yes	Yes	Yes	Yes	Yes
Boils, herpes, scabies	‡‡	‡‡	Yes	Yes	Yes
Splenomegaly	No	No	No	Yes	Yes
Absent or undescended testicle	Yes§§	Yes§§	Yes	Yes	Yes

*Swimming: no butterfly, breast stroke, or diving starts.
†Needs individual assessment.
‡Patients with mild forms can be allowed a full range of physical activities; patients with moderate or severe forms, or who are postoperative, should be evaluated by a cardiologist before athletics participation.
§Availability of eye guards approved by the American Society for Testing and Materials may allow competitor to participate in most sports, but this must be judged on an individual basis.
‖Consult ophthalmologist.
¶No swimming or weight lifting
**No archery or riflery.
††May be allowed to compete if oxygenation remains satisfactory during a graded stress test.
‡‡No gymnastics with mats, martial arts, wrestling, or contact sports until not contagious.
§§Certain sports may require protective cup.

(Reproduced with permission of Pediatrics–Vol 81. pg 738. Copyright 1988.)

contact/impact sports or sports that place too much repetitive flexion or extension stress on the cervical spine. In addition, if any neurologic signs or symptoms are present in an athlete who has atlantoaxial instability, any strenuous activity is contraindicated. Fortunately, the incidence of atlantoaxial instability in the general population is very low, but it can be as high as 10 to 20% in persons with Down syndrome.[3] Thus, it is recommended that all Down syndrome athletes have cervical spine radiographs as part of their preparticipation evaluation.

Acute Illness

There are a number of factors to consider when deciding whether an athlete with an acute illness should be withheld from sports participation. It has been shown that acute, febrile illnesses decrease muscle strength and performance.[4] Sports participation during an acute illness carries a risk of worsening the illness or transmitting it to others, an increased risk of dehydration or other thermoregulatory problems, and a risk of more serious complications of infection, such as myocarditis. Therefore, it is generally acceptable to limit athletic activity during a febrile illness. However, some athletes are so driven that they are afraid to miss a single workout, even when they are sick. A good rule of thumb is to perform a "neck check." If the athletes' symptoms are "above the neck," such as a stuffy or runny nose, sneezing, or a scratchy throat, they may proceed cautiously with their activity. If they have a fever, or "below the neck" symptoms, such as myalgias, a hacking cough, vomiting, or diarrhea, they should not be allowed to work out.

Cardiovascular Abnormalities

The guidelines for cardiovascular problems are based on the conditions that predispose the athlete to sudden cardiac death during activity or conditions that may be exacerbated by physical activity.

HYPERTENSION

The upper limit of normal blood pressure in young athletes is unknown. In addition to the question of what constitutes hypertension in children and adolescents is the issue of what level of hypertension should limit their participation in sports. The report of the Task Force on Blood Pressure Control in Children suggests using three consecutive blood pressure readings higher than the 95th percentile as the criteria for diagnosing hypertension in children and adolescents.[5] For children aged 10 to 12 years, the 95th percentile is approximately 125/80 mm Hg; for ages 13 to 15, it is approximately 135/85 mm Hg; and for those older than 15 years, adult standards are used (i.e., 140/90 mm Hg). Determining clearance for athletes diagnosed with hypertension requires individual assessment. The report of the 16th Bethesda Conference on Cardiovascular Abnormalities in the Athlete recommends that those with severe, uncontrolled hypertension according to adult standards (diastolic pressure higher than 115 mm Hg) or target organ involvement should not participate in competitive sports.[6] Those with controlled hypertension and no target organ disease may be allowed to compete in sports that make moderate to high dynamic and low static demands. Athletes with controlled hypertension but evidence of left ventricular hypertrophy or renal function impairment may participate in low-intensity activities such as bowling or golf.

CARDIAC MURMURS

Innocent cardiac murmurs—pulmonary flow murmur, Still's murmur, venous hum—are often found during the preparticipation evaluation. These benign functional murmurs do not preclude participation in sports. Mitral valve prolapse should not restrict an athlete from participation unless it is accompanied by a history of syncope, a family history of sudden death associated with mitral valve prolapse, chest pain or arrhythmias worsened by exercise, or moderate to severe mitral regurgitation. Any murmur that is questionable should be referred for further evaluation while clearance is deferred. Various maneuvers, such as deep inspiration, Valsalva's, and squat-to-stand, can be used to help differentiate benign murmurs from pathologic ones such as the murmur of hypertrophic cardiomyopathy.

HYPERTROPHIC CARDIOMYOPATHY

Hypertrophic cardiomyopathy is the most common cause of sudden death in young athletes. Athletes with hypertrophic cardiomyopathy should not participate in competitive sports if they have marked left ventricular hypertrophy or significant left ventricular outflow obstruction, arrhythmias, history of syncope, or a history of sudden death in relatives with hypertrophic cardiomyopathy.[1] Some athletes with hypertrophic cardiomyopathy may be allowed to participate in low-intensity activities if they are cleared by a cardiologist.

OTHER CARDIOVASCULAR ABNORMALITIES

A review of all cardiovascular abnormalities that may preclude athletic participation is beyond the scope of this discussion. Guidelines for clearance of athletes with arrhythmias or other cardiovascular abnormalities may be found in the report of the 16th Bethesda Conference on Cardiovascular Abnormalities in the Athlete.[6] The report is an excellent resource for any physician who is responsible for clearing athletes to participate in sports. If, after a complete evaluation has been performed by the athlete's personal physician there are any questions about the athlete's cardiovascular condition, referral to a cardiologist for a full evaluation is recommended.

Vision Impairment

It is difficult to define the level of vision impairment at which an individual should be considered functionally one-eyed for the purpose of clearance for sports participation. Many states require driver's license restrictions for persons whose best corrected vision in one eye is less than 20/50. Consequently, it is recommended that athletes with a best corrected visual acuity in one eye of less than 20/50 be considered functionally one-eyed and be prohibited from sports in which no eye protection can effectively be worn, such as boxing, wrestling, and full-contact karate. In other sports where there is high risk of eye injury, such as football, racquetball, and baseball, such athletes may be allowed to participate if they wear a lensed eye guard approved by the American Society for Testing and Materials. However, the ultimate decision of whether to allow a one-eyed athlete to participate should be made on an individual basis, and the potential risks and long-term serious consequences should be discussed with the athlete, his or her parents or guardians, coaches, and school administrators.

Inguinal Hernia

There is no reason to exclude athletes with asymptomatic inguinal hernias from participation in any activity. Symptomatic hernias may be affected by activity and should be evaluated on an individual basis.

Kidney Abnormalities

Although the incidence of renal trauma from athletics is relatively low,[7] and most forms of sports-related renal injury are mild, special consideration should be given to athletes with certain underlying kidney abnormalities. If an individual is found to have a solitary kidney, it should be determined whether the kidney is normal or abnormal. If it is abnormal (i.e., pelvic, iliac, or polycystic or shows evidence of hydronephrosis or ureteropelvic junction abnormality), the athlete should not participate in contact or collision sports. Athletes with a normal solitary kidney may be allowed to participate but should be advised of the risk involved in playing such sports and the long-term consequences—transplantation or dialysis—of losing a solitary functioning kidney.

Hepatomegaly and Splenomegaly

An enlarged liver or spleen that has surpassed the bony protection of the rib cage is at risk for injury in contact or collision sports, and participation in these sports should be restricted. Athletes with splenomegaly should also be restricted from strenuous noncontact sports, because splenic rupture has been known to occur after even mild trauma such as a simple Valsalva's maneuver.

Musculoskeletal Disorders

Musculoskeletal problems require individual assessment when determining clearance for participation. Before clearance is given, a thorough evaluation should be performed, which includes examination for swelling or other signs of inflammation, assessment of range of motion and strength compared to the uninjured side, and functional testing of the injured area. When evaluating fractures, one must consider the location, type, and risk of further damage in determining the athlete's clearance. Using a playing cast or splint to protect the fracture should always be considered. If, after a thorough evaluation, any question exists regarding clearance orthopedic consultation should be obtained.

Neurologic Disorders

Head injuries, burners or stingers, and seizure disorders are the most common types of neurologic problems encountered during the preparticipation evaluation. The most common head injury encountered is the cerebral concussion. Many classification schemes exist for grading the severity of concussion,[8–11] and, therefore, universally accepted guidelines for sports participation have not been established. The Colorado Medical Society Sports Medicine Committee has developed some basic guidelines for the management of concussion in sports, which can be readily used to help determine an athlete's clearance status.[11] History of a burner or stinger, more properly termed a nerve root or brachial plexus neurapraxia, should not limit an athlete from participation if it is completely asymptomatic and the physical examination findings are normal. A history of recurrent neurapraxia in a single season suggests a need for further evaluation. Athletes with a history of cervical spinal cord neurapraxia with transient quadriplegia should be fully evaluated. Those with well-controlled seizures should be allowed unrestricted clearance, provided that participation itself does not precipitate a seizure. Athletes with poorly controlled seizures should not participate in contact or any other potentially dangerous sports until they have gone seizure free at least 1 month and their medication(s) and neurologic findings are stable.

Gynecologic Disorders

Athletes with one ovary should not be restricted from sports participation. Competitors with signs or symptoms of any part of the female athlete triad (i.e., eating disorder, amenorrhea, and osteoporosis) may be cleared to participate after further evaluation.

Pulmonary Disorders

Asthma is not a contraindication to sports participation, provided appropriate medical treatment is given and symptoms are controlled. However, more significant pulmonary insufficiency may limit activity and usually requires a graded exercise test with oxygen saturation monitoring for clearance.

Sickle Cell Trait

Exercise performance usually is not impaired in persons with sickle cell trait, so restriction of activity is unnecessary. Persons with sickle cell disease and significant anemia usually are limited in their exercise capacity. Again, a graded stress test may be needed to further evaluate such persons who wish to participate in strenuous activity.

Dermatologic Disorders

The presence of an infectious dermatologic condition such as boils, herpes, impetigo, or scabies precludes participation in contact sports until the condition is no longer considered contagious. This is particularly important in sports for which mats are used, such as gymnastics, martial arts, and wrestling.

Testicular Disorders

Athletes with a single functioning testicle should be discouraged from participation in contact or collision sports. However, individuals may be allowed to participate if they clearly understand the risks and choose to participate using a protective cup that is approved by the American Society for Testing and Materials. Athletes found to have an undescended testicle should be referred for further evaluation.

Human Immunodeficiency Virus (HIV)

Clearing an HIV-infected person for athletic participation is very controversial. There is evidence that exercise may actually have a beneficial effect on the CD4 cell count[12]; however, allowing participation may place others at risk for contracting HIV. Although the risk of HIV transmission in sport is felt to be very low, no research is available that directly assesses this risk. As more data become available, specific recommendations about HIV and sports participation can be made.

LITERATURE REVIEW

Several large published studies have reported actual pass-fail rates for the preparticipation evaluation, as well as the most common conditions that result in an individual's failure to pass the preparticipation evaluation without restrictions.[13–17]

Clearance with Restrictions

The percentage of athletes who pass the preparticipation evaluation with restrictions varies from 3.4 to 13.5%, depending on the study. In the largest published study, Magnes and colleagues looked at the results of 10,540 preparticipation examinations and found that 10.2% of athletes were passed with restrictions.[17] The most common reason for clearing an athlete with restrictions was hypertension, which was diagnosed in 33.6% of the cases. The next most common conditions were eye abnormalities (13.5%) and musculoskeletal problems (12.2%).

No Clearance, or Disqualification

Only a very few persons are disqualified from participation as a result of findings of the preparticipation evaluation. Actual disqualification rates in the literature vary from 0.1 to 1.3%. In the study by Magnes' group, the disqualification rate was 0.4%, and the most common reason for disqualification was severe hypertension, which was found in 38% of those disqualified. Ophthalmic problems (principally loss of vision in one eye) were the next most common disqualifying condition (12%), followed by genitourinary tract abnormalities such as a single testicle or testicular mass (10%). Other reasons for disqualification included neurologic conditions (8%), recent mononucleosis with splenomegaly (4%), and musculoskeletal problems (4%).

SUMMARY

Clearance for activity is an important part of the preparticipation evaluation. The physician must be familiar with the available guidelines for participation but must rely on clinical judgment in interpreting these recommendations. Relatively few medical conditions actually restrict an athlete's participation; however, if restrictions are recommended, the physician must explain them fully to the athlete, the parents or guardians, and the appropriate coaches and trainers. One should always consider alternatives to disqualification so that the individual may experience the benefits of some form of participation. It is through genuine interest, thorough evaluation, and knowledgeable counseling, that the physician can positively influence the health care and safety of a local sports program.

REFERENCES

1. Bergfeld, J., et al.: Preparticipation Physical Evaluation Monograph. Kansas City, American Academy of Family Physicians, 1992.
2. American Academy of Pediatrics Committee on Sports Medicine: Recommendations for participation in competitive sports. Pediatrics *81*:737, 1988.
3. American Academy of Pediatrics Committee on Sports Medicine: Atlantoaxial instability in Down syndrome. Pediatrics *74*:152, 1984.
4. Eichner, E. R.: Infection, immunity, and exercise. Physician Sportsmed. *21*(1):125, 1993.
5. National Heart, Lung, and Blood Institute: Report of the Second Task Force on Blood Pressure Control in Children—1987. Pediatrics *79*:1, 1987.
6. Mitchell, J. H., Maron, B. J., and Epstein, S. E.: 16th Bethesda Conference: Cardiovascular abnormalities in the athlete: Recommendations regarding eligibility for competition. J. Am. Coll. Cardiol. *6*:1186, 1985.
7. Mandell, J., et al.: Sports-related genitourinary injuries in children. Clin. Sports Med. *1*:483, 1982.
8. Cantu, R. C.: Guidelines for return to contact sports after a cerebral concussion. Physician Sportsmed. *14*(10):75, 1986.
9. Gennarelli, T. A.: Cerebral concussion and diffuse brain injuries. *In* Athletic Injuries to the Head, Neck, and Face. 2nd Ed. Edited by J. S. Torg. St. Louis, C.V. Mosby, 1991.
10. Nelson, W. E., Jane, J. A., and Gieck, J. H.: Minor head injury in sports: A new system of classification and management. Physician Sportsmed. *12*(3):103, 1984.
11. Colorado Medical Society: Report of the Sports Medicine Committee: Guidelines for the Management of Concussion in Sports (revised). Denver, Colorado Medical Society, 1991.
12. Proceedings of the 5th International Conference on AIDS. Ottawa, Ontario, International Development Research Center, 1989, p. 337.
13. Linder, C. W., Durant, R. H., Seklecki, R. M., and Strong, W. B.: Preparticipation health screening of young athletes: Results of 1286 examinations. Am. J. Sports Med. *9*:187, 1981.
14. Goldberg, B., et al.: Pre-participation sports assessment—an objective evaluation. Pediatrics *66*:736, 1980.
15. Thompson, T. R., Andrish, J. T., and Bergfeld, J. A.: A prospective study of preparticipation sports examinations of 2670 young athletes: method and results. Cleve. Clinic Q. *49*:225, 1982.
16. Tennant, F. S. Jr., Sorensen, K., and Day, C. M.: Benefits of preparticipation sports examination. J. Family Pract. *13*:287, 1981.
17. Magnes, S. A., Henderson, J. M., and Hunter, S. C.: What conditions limit sports participation?: Experience with 10,540 athletes. Physician Sportsmed. *20*(5):143, 1992.

11 *Joseph G. Jacko*

Preparticipation Evaluation: Fitness Assessment

Although assessing fitness is considered a secondary objective of the preparticipation physical examination,[1] information from a fitness assessment may actually be of more benefit than is generally believed. Whereas the history, medical, and orthopedic examinations provide valuable information on health status, the fitness assessment provides information on human function or the impact of health on performance.

OBJECTIVES OF THE FITNESS ASSESSMENT

When discussing the objectives of the fitness assessment it is important to recognize that the results of fitness tests should be viewed as the means to an end, not as an end in itself. The objectives of the fitness assessment can be classified as primary or secondary.

Primary Objectives

The primary objectives of the fitness assessment are to minimize sports attrition due to injury and to improve athletic performance.[2] Although no conclusive proof has been offered, studies suggest (and it is generally accepted) that preseason conditioning programs can decrease the number of injuries.[3] Results from the fitness assessment can also identify weaknesses that may hinder athletic performance, such as deficiencies in strength, flexibility, endurance, or functional skills.

Secondary Objectives

The secondary objectives of the fitness assessment are to assess achievement of individual goals, help motivate athletes, provide an opportunity for wellness counseling, evaluate the success of a preseason conditioning program, and provide sport-specific athletic profiles.

When the fitness assessment is performed periodically, results can be used to verify the achievement of individual goals. Because results can be compared to established norms, and to one another, the fitness assessment may help to motivate athletes to reach their optimal level of fitness.

Results of the fitness assessment can be used to discuss health-related issues and provide an opportunity for wellness counseling. Results of body weight and body composition evaluation can be used to discuss the importance of proper nutrition and prevention of obesity. Results of flexibility and strength testing can be used to discuss prevention of low back pain and other common orthopedic problems. Results of cardiovascular or aerobic endurance testing can be used to discuss the relationship between activity level and risk for cardiac disease and the importance of maintaining an active lifestyle throughout adulthood.

Results also can be used to determine whether a preseason conditioning program is successful in achieving its goals. Weakness in the same area in many athletes may indicate a weakness in the program. Finally, information from the fitness assessment can be used to construct sport-specific profiles that may be helpful in matching athletes to sport, thus further minimizing injury risk and improving the likelihood for success. Sport-specific profiles also help explain the relationship between the demands of a sport and musculoskeletal adaptations that occur, providing further information on risk factors for injury.[4]

METHOD, TIMING, AND FREQUENCY

The advantages and disadvantages of performing the physical examination aspect of the preparticipation evaluation in the office setting, versus the station-screening format, were discussed in Chapter 9. Because of the need for space, equipment, and personnel, the fitness assessment invariably is best conducted in a station-screening format. The fitness assessment is best conducted at the time of the physical examination and to meet its primary objectives should be done at least 6 weeks before the start of the season. There is no consensus on how often a fitness assessment should be performed, but because of the rapid changes that can occur in developmental skills, strength, and flexibility secondary to growth and development of children and adolescents, it seems reasonable to perform a fitness assessment annually.

THE EVALUATION

The evaluation should include measurement of resting heart rate and blood pressure. The other major components are anthropometric characteristics and performance parameters or an abilities inventory. In deciding what parameters to test and how to test them, it is important to recognize that performance on a fitness assessment does not imply skill and skill does not ensure performance on the athletic field.[2,5] Psychological, emotional, and environmental factors are also important in determining athletic success. For purposes of the fitness assessment, it is not necessary to use the most elaborate, expensive equipment available. Tests and methods that are simple to perform, easy to measure, reproducible, and inexpensive should be considered.

In addition, I believe that the testing methods used must closely resemble the movements and activities actually used in competition. For example, throwing a medicine ball from the chest position (Fig. 11–1) more closely resembles the blocking technique of an offensive lineman than performance on a bench press and, so, may be a better indicator of strength and power. Likewise, a basketball player's performance on the vertical jump may be a better indicator of lower leg power than the maximum amount of weight he or she can toe raise or leg press.

Resting Heart Rate and Blood Pressure

The resting heart rate and blood pressure are indicators of cardiovascular health and current fitness level.

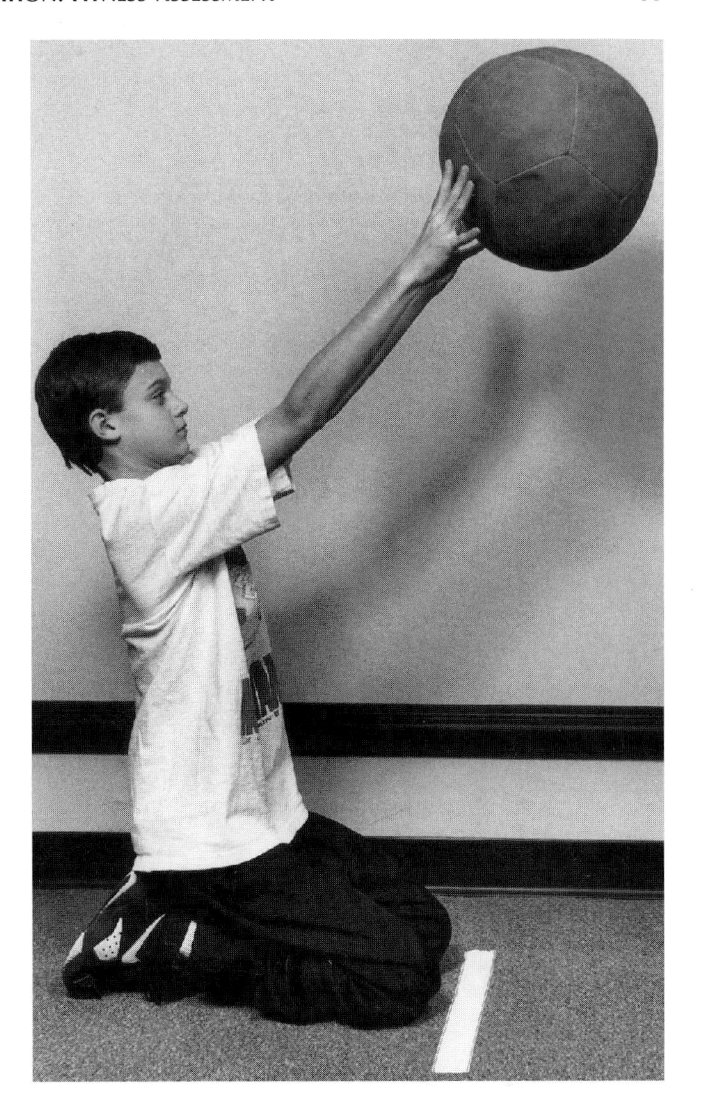

Fig. 11–1. The medicine ball throw measures an athlete's strength and power.

Anthropometric Characteristics

Height and weight are usually measured and when compared with standard growth charts may identify athletes who need further evaluation for possible growth abnormalities. Body composition is an indicator of general health and can be an important factor in determining success in certain sports, such as wrestling and gymnastics, for which a small proportion of body fat is desirable.

There are many methods for determining body composition. Height and weight measurements can be used to compute the body mass index by the following equation:

$$\frac{\text{WT (kg)}}{\text{HT}^2\text{ (cm)}} \times 10$$

Although useful for predicting obesity, the body mass index does not determine body composition. Skin fold measurements are perhaps the best overall method for determining body composition in a preparticipation fitness assessment. Skin fold measurements are easy, inexpensive, and, when performed by a skilled technician, reproducible and accurate.[6] Although underwater weighing is considered the most accurate test for determining body composition, it is time consuming, more expensive, and not readily available. Other methods of measurement use electrical impedance, photon absorptiometry, dual-energy x-ray absorptiometry, and magnetic resonance imaging. These, however, are too costly and impractical for preparticipation fitness assessment.

Abilities Inventory

By measuring various performance parameters, an athlete's functional or athletic ability can be determined. Where appropriate, tests for both upper and lower body determination should be done. Muscle strength, muscle endurance, and muscle power factor into the basic movements of athletics: running, jumping, lifting, and throwing. Although they are defined separately, they are closely related and therefore difficult to measure in isolation. Each varies in the force generated, velocity at which force is generated, and the number of repetitions involved. When the focus is on the maximum force generated, strength is the main component being tested. When the focus is on the force generated and the velocity at which it is generated, principally power is being tested. And when the focus is on the number of repetitions, principally endurance is being tested. For the purpose of this discussion, tests in which the number of repetitions is fewer than 25 are described as tests of muscle strength and tests in which the number of repetitions is greater than 25 are described as tests of muscle endurance.[7]

Also, note that muscle strength, muscle endurance, and muscle power can be tested and described in absolute or in relative terms. Absolute tests involve displacement of a known mass or use of loads identical for all athletes; relative tests involve displacement of one's own body weight or use of external loads in proportion to each athlete's maximum strength.

MUSCLE STRENGTH

Absolute strength generally refers to the ability to produce a maximum force in a one-time all-out effort, as in a bench press. Relative strength can be determined by counting repetitions in tests like pull-ups or dips, in which the maximum number of repetitions is fewer than 25.

MUSCLE ENDURANCE

Muscle endurance is the ability to perform work over an extended period without undue fatigue. Absolute endurance can be determined by performing tests that permit a weight to be lifted more than 25 repetitions. Relative endurance can be determined by performing tests involving the movement of body weight more than 25 repetitions, as in situps or leg lifts.

POWER

Power is the ability to exert force very rapidly (defined as $P = \text{Work}/\text{Time}$). Absolute power is the force in moving an external weight quickly and explosively, as in a medicine ball put or rapidly lifting an external load. Relative power is the force generated in moving body weight quickly and explosively, as in a vertical jump or standing broad jump.

FLEXIBILITY

Flexibility is the ability to move a joint through its normal maximal range of motion (Fig. 11–2). It is easily measured with a goniometer. Flexibility of the major muscle groups should be measured (quadriceps, hamstrings, calf, low back, and shoulder girdle muscles) as a part of the fitness assessment.

SPEED

Speed is the ability to move body mass over time. It is closely related to strength and power and difficult to isolate. Examples are the 40-yard or the 100-yard dash.

AEROBIC ENDURANCE

Aerobic endurance is the ability to exercise large muscle groups in a rhythmic fashion over a prolonged period of time. Examples include the 12-minute run or the 1.5 mile run.

ANAEROBIC ENDURANCE

Anaerobic endurance is the ability to move large muscle groups for at least 1 minute but generally not more than 2 minutes. These tests evaluate the muscle's short-

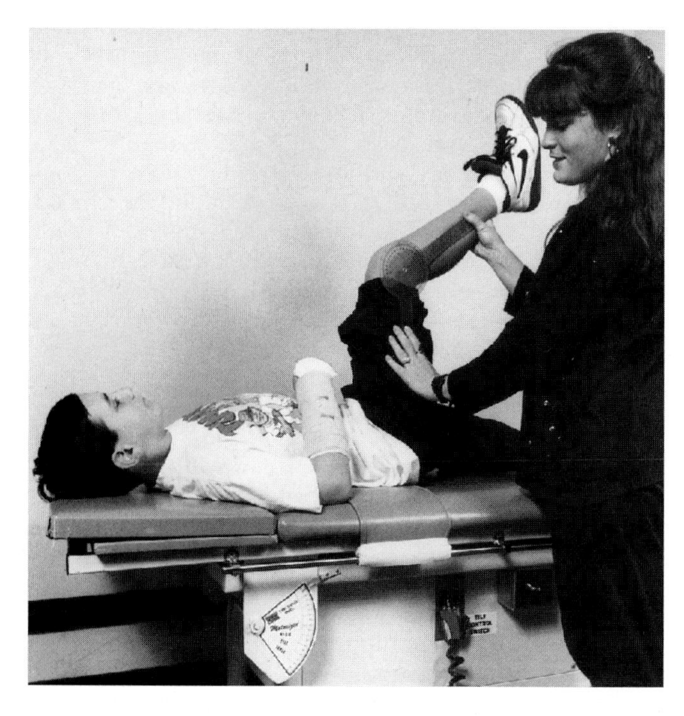

Fig. 11–2. Flexibility can be a determinant of athletic performance.

term energy supply. Examples are all-out running, swimming, or cycling for 1 or 2 minutes.

AGILITY

Agility is the combination of speed, power, and flexibility along with the ability to rapidly change directions. It can be measured by the time it takes to negotiate an obstacle course.

BALANCE

Balance is the coordinated neuromuscular response of the body to maintain a defined position of equilibrium in response to changing visual, tactile, or kinesthetic stimuli.[8] Dynamic balance can be determined by walking on a balance beam and static balance by the ability to maintain a "flamingo stance" (i.e., the athlete stands on one leg with the other leg flexed, externally rotated, and abducted at the hip).

REACTION TIME

Reaction time is the ability to respond to a stimulus. Common tests involve the ability to accomplish a hand or foot task in response to a visual stimulus. A simple test is to drop a yardstick through an athlete's open hand. The athlete grabs the yardstick after it is dropped. The distance the yardstick falls is an indication of the athlete's reaction time.

INTERPRETATION AND INTERVENTION

The results of the fitness assessment should be returned to the coaches, athletes, and parents in a timely fashion. This should include feedback on both team and individual performances in relation to standard norms and local peers. Recommendations should also be given to correct areas of weakness or deficiency.

In interpreting the results of the fitness assessment it is important to view each athlete's strengths and weaknesses in terms of the demands of each sport. In sports in which athletes must "control their bodies," relative tests that match the athlete against his own body weight may be more useful, whereas performance on absolute tests is more useful in evaluating athletes involved in sports and activities in which opposing players or objects must be moved (e.g., football lineman, shot putter, discus thrower).

In general, athletes with a smaller proportion of body fat perform better on tests of relative strength, relative endurance, and relative power. Athletes with a larger proportion of body fat, because they tend to also have greater absolute lean body mass, tend to perform better

Table 11–1. Most Important Components of Performance in Various Sports

Event or Position	*Absolute Strength*	*Relative Strength*	*Absolute Power*	*Relative Power*	*Aerobic Endurance*	*Anaerobic-Aerobic Endurance*	*Muscle Endurance*
Football							
Offensive back	X		X	X		X	
Defensive back	X		X	X		X	
Interior lineman	X		X	X		X	
Wide receiver				X		X	
Tight end	X		X	X		X	
Line backer	X		X	X		X	
Quarterback				X		X	
Baseball			X	X		X	X
Basketball				X	X	X	
Soccer				X	X	X	
Field hockey				X	X	X	
Wrestling	X	X	X	X	X	X	X
Fencing				X		X	X
Track: Running Events							
100 m				X		X	
200 m				X		X	
400 m						X	
800 m						X	
1 mile (1,500 m)					X		
2 miles					X		
5,000 m					X		
10,000 m					X		
Marathon					X		
Track: Field events							
Shot put			X	X			
Discus			X	X			
Hammer throw			X	X			
Pole vault				X			
High jump				X			
Long jump				X			

(Berger, R. A.: Applied Exercise Physiology. Philadelphia, Lea & Febiger, 1982, pp. 238–268.)

on tests of absolute strength, absolute endurance, and absolute power.

SPORTS PROFILING

A unique way to review the results of the fitness assessment and gain further insight into the significance of each performance parameter is to develop individual athletic profiles. When individual athletic profiles are compared to the specific demands of various sports (Table 11–1),[7] results from the fitness assessment can be better interpreted.

In addition, sports profiling can help explain the relationship between the demands of a sport and the musculoskeletal adaptions that occur.[4] An example is the increase in external rotation and the decrease in internal rotation of the dominant shoulder in athletes who participate in "overhead activities." Such information is useful for identifying athletes who may have strength and flexibility imbalances that may place them at an increased risk of injury.

Although there are many factors that determine athletic success and many risk factors for injury, sport profiling affords the physician a means of better counseling the athlete about sports participation, likelihood for success, and risk of injury, thus meeting the main objectives of the fitness assessment.

SUMMARY

Although frequently considered an optional part of the preparticipation evaluation, the fitness assessment can provide invaluable information describing the relationship between health, fitness, and athletic performance. When one considers the low yield of abnormalities detected during preparticipation physical examinations,[9,10] the fitness assessment can in fact provide more meaningful and useful information.

REFERENCES

1. Lombardo, J. A., et al.: Pre-Participation Physical Evaluation. Kansas City, MO. American Academy of Family Physicians, American Academy of Pediatrics, American Medical Society for Sports Medicine, American Orthopaedic Society for Sports Medicine and American Osteopathic Academy of Sports Medicine, 1992.
2. Henderson, J. M.: The preseason performance assessment. Exhibit at the American Academy of Orthopedic Surgeons 57th Annual Meeting. New Orleans, Feb 8–13, 1990.
3. Cahill, B. R., and Griffith, E. H.: Effect of preseason conditioning on the incidence and severity of high school football knee injuries. Am. J. Sports Med. *6*:180, 1978.
4. Kibler, W. B., Chandler, T. J., Uhl, T., and Maddux, R. E.: A musculoskeletal approach to the preparticipation physical examination. Preventing injury and improving performance. Am. J. Sports Med. *17*:525, 1989.
5. Foster, C.: Physiologic testing: Does it help the athlete? Physician Sportsmed. *17*(10):103, 1989.
6. Lohman, T. G., Roche, A. F., and Martorell, R. (eds.): Anthropometric Standardization Reference Manual. Champaign, IL, Human Kinetics Books, 1988.
7. Berger, R. A. Applied Exercise Physiology. Philadelphia, Lea & Febiger, 1982.
8. Nicholas, J. A.: Risk factors, sports medicine and the orthopedic system: An overview. J. Sports Med. *3*:243, 1975.
9. Risser, W. L., Hoffman, H. M., Bellah, G. G., and Green, L. W.: A cost-benefit analysis of preparticipation sports examinations of adolescent athletes. J. School Health *55*:270, 1985.
10. Runyan, D. K.: The preparticipation examination of young athletes: Defining the essentials. Clin. Pediatr. *22*:674, 1983.

12 *Clark H. Cobb, Tanya L. Hrabal, and Robert S. Skerker*

Environmental Injuries

Heat-Related Illnesses

Clark H. Cobb

Among the catastrophic causes of sudden death in athletes, heat stroke has the distinction of being almost totally preventable. Unfortunately, exertional heat injuries remain a common malady among athletes, laborers, and soldiers worldwide. A basic understanding of human thermoregulation, prompt recognition of clinical syndromes, and aggressive early intervention are necessary to minimize morbidity and mortality.

HUMAN THERMOREGULATION

The human body has available four means of transferring heat to the environment: conduction, convection, radiation, and evaporation. Conduction is the transfer of heat energy from warmer to cooler objects by direct contact. Convection implies heat loss to air and to water vapor molecules circulating around the body. Radiation is heat transfer by electromagnetic waves. Evaporation reflects heat loss via conversion of a liquid to a gas.

At rest, significant heat (perhaps 70% of the total) is lost via conduction, convection, and radiation.[1] With exertion most heat dissipation occurs at the skin surface, by evaporation of sweat. Each milliliter of evaporated sweat consumes about 0.6 kcal of heat.[2,3] Heat production in skeletal muscle rapidly increases while exercising; heat dissipation increases more slowly.[4]

Hubbard and Armstrong have proposed the "energy depletion model" to explain the devastating effects of excessive heat at the cellular level.[5] This model suggests that an exercise-induced thermal imbalance leads to an energy imbalance in the cells. Positive feedback via the sodium-potassium pump leads to increased membrane permeability, cellular energy depletion, and increased neurotransmitter activity that reduces heat tolerance and causes significant morbidity and mortality.

In humans, the hypothalamus is the primary regulator of heat transfer. In a reflex response to heated blood, the hypothalamus initiates the Benzinger reflex, which causes cutaneous blood vessels to dilate and eccrine sweat glands to produce sweat.[1] Blood is then cooled by transfer of heat to the environment, as mentioned above. The extent to which cardiac output can rise to meet the requirements of heat transfer is fixed by the maximum heart rate, the intravascular volume, and the achievable degree of renal and splanchnic vasoconstriction. Body temperature rises when heat is produced faster than it can be dissipated by these mechanisms. In certain circumstances, this imbalance may lead to a heat injury.

MINOR HEAT ILLNESSES

In addition to the more familiar cases of heat stroke and heat exhaustion frequently discussed, heat-related illnesses also include heat edema, heat tetany, miliaria rubra (prickly heat), heat syncope, and heat cramps (Table 12–1). Significant sunburn could also be considered a common heat-related injury.

Since heat-related illnesses lie along a spectrum whose divisions are somewhat arbitrary, it is understandable that similar signs and symptoms are common to a variety of these disorders. Common presenting symptoms include headache, vomiting, dizziness, gooseflesh, muscle cramps, chilling, fatigue, and apathy. Most patients with a heat-induced illness have at least some of these

Table 12–1. Characteristics of Minor Heat Illnesses

Heat edema:	Benign, self-limited swelling of the hands and feet, usually seen in the first few weeks of acclimatization and resolves with cooling, elevation of the affected part, and light compression when necessary. Diuretics should be avoided.
Heat tetany:	Carpopedal spasm (probably secondary to the normal hyperventilation seen with increased temperature)
Heat syncope:	Function of decreased vasomotor tone and venous pooling with exercise and elevated body temperature. Decreased hydration also contributes, but aggressive fluid replacement may not be required.
Miliaria rubra:	Maculopapular, erythematous rash on clothed parts of body when keratin plugs block sweat gland pores or when the glands themselves swell. Proper hygiene is usually sufficient treatment.
Heat cramps:	Cramps of heavily worked muscle groups (lower extremity and abdomen in particular) that appear to wander since the entire muscle is usually not affected. They are usually associated with a whole-body salt deficiency. Treatment often entails sodium replacement (0.1% oral saline solution or IV normal saline).

complaints, but some collapse suddenly without warning. Unusual findings on examination of these patients include hyperpyrexia, flushing, tachycardia, tachypnea, oliguria, hyperreflexia, mydriasis, hypotension, and dehydration. Altered mental status, seizures, or coma may be observed in more seriously affected victims.

The "Weak Link Rule" states that *any* heat injury in a military unit or among members of an athletic team or work group suggests that others are at risk for similar, or perhaps more dangerous, conditions. Precautions are therefore mandatory.[6]

HEAT EXHAUSTION AND HEAT STROKE

Historically, the label *heat exhaustion* has been applied to cases in which the patient's temperature did not exceed 102°F and no mental changes were present; however, nausea, vomiting, fainting, headache, cramping, and fatigue are considered commonplace.[7] Similarly, *heat stroke* was diagnosed when the patient's temperature was higher than 104°F, mental status was altered, and sweating was absent.[2,8,9] We now know that heat exhaustion and heat stroke may be indistinguishable on presentation, as the signs and symptoms of multiple organ system dysfunction seen with the latter may not become evident for hours or days.[6,7]

Any evidence of renal, neurologic, or hepatic injury during the first 24 hours should lead to the presumptive diagnosis of heat stroke.[6] It is vital to remember that a lower temperature *does not preclude* heat stroke.[9] Since heat stroke accounts for several hundred deaths annually in the United States,[7] intervention should err on the side of treating this more dangerous condition when confusion exists.[10]

Classic heat stroke, often seen during summer heat waves, typically affects poor, elderly, chronically ill, alcoholic, or obese persons. Exertional heat stroke is also more common in summer, but it is not uncommon in spring and fall. It is frequently seen in athletes, laborers, and military personnel, who often sweat profusely. Signs and symptoms may be similar in both cases; however, elderly patients who sustain heat stroke may present with dry skin whereas athletes who sustain exertional heat stroke may sweat profusely. The onset of illness may be more rapid in exertional cases. A number of factors increase a person's risk of heat injury (Table 12–2). A thorough history should uncover these clues.

Table 12–2. Predisposing Factors to Heat Illness

Endogenous	*Exogenous*
Age (extremes)	Increased temperature
Dehydration	Increased humidity
Obesity	No breeze
Exercise	No cloud cover
Hypokalemia	Inaccurate temperature information
Alcohol	
Mid-day overeating	
Heart disease	
Sweat gland problems	
Drugs*	
History of heat injury	
Sunburn	

*Drugs that either increase endogenous heat production (tricyclic antidepressants, amphetamines, LSD, PCP, cocaine, etc.) or those that impair heat dissipation (anticholinergics, antihistamines, diuretics, tricyclic antidepressants, β-blockers) are associated with increased risk.

Differential Diagnosis

In hot weather, the collapse of a previously healthy person during physical exertion implicates heat stroke unless another cause is obvious.[7,9] When a patient has a rectal temperature of 104°F or greater, cooling should begin as early as possible, regardless of the cause, with the intent to cool to a core temperature of 102°F within the first 30 to 60 minutes.[6,7] Nevertheless, other entities to be considered include meningitis, sepsis, malaria, influenza, thyroid storm, tickborne disease, and drug reaction.

Early Management

Since the severity of a heat injury is primarily a function of the severity and duration of hyperthermia, the value of prompt recognition, *rapid cooling,* and early transport to a medical facility cannot be overstated.[9,11] En route, oxygen should be administered, if available, since oxygenation may be hampered by pulmonary complications and metabolic demands are high.[9] Temperature should be monitored and intravenous access established. Glass or electric thermometers that do not register above 41°C (105.8°F) are inadequate,[10] so special thermometers are recommended. Heat-injury victims may *not* require aggressive administration of intravenous fluids,[12] and those who treat such patients should beware of overshoot hyponatremia and pulmonary edema that may follow overly vigorous fluid resuscitation.

Laboratory Abnormalities

A number of laboratory abnormalities are seen in patients who sustain a heat injury. Hyperventilation and elevated body temperature are associated with primary respiratory alkalosis. Metabolic acidosis often follows as a result of increased glycolysis and lactic acid accumulation.[9] Hypoglycemia or hyperglycemia may be seen. Hypokalemia is often seen early, and hyperkalemia may develop later (a factor in the electrocardiographic abnormalities so often recorded in these cases).[11] Sodium levels vary widely, depending to a significant degree on the patient's hydration status and the type of fluids used early in treatment. Low levels of phosphate, calcium, and magnesium are common.[11] Elevated liver function test results are consistent features, and the bilirubin value may be increased because of both hepatic dysfunction and hemolysis. White cell counts may be increased with hemoconcentration and catecholamine circulation, but a drop in platelets is usual (along with drops in Factors V and VIII). Hypoprothrombinemia and hypofibrinogenemia may lead to disseminated intravascular coagulation.[11] After prolonged endurance exercise, the creatine phosphokinase level may be extremely elevated (often over 20,000 IU,[10] but the transaminase level usually does not increase without associated heat injury. Transaminase, however, may not be significantly elevated until 24 to 48 hours after the initial insult, which means patients must be monitored at least that long.[9] Elevated levels of creatine phosphokinase and myoglobin are frequently observed with exertional heat stroke. Attributing such elevated levels to exertion or to heat injury may be challenging. The urine is usually concentrated and may contain ketones, protein, or myoglobin.[9]

Hospital Management

Strict attention to ABC management (airway, breathing, and circulation) is obviously the first priority.[10] The second should be *rapid* (0.15°C per minute) cooling to 102°F (39°C). The best method for this remains controversial, but it may be accomplished by immersion in iced or tap water, dousing the patient with water, applying ice packs, or spraying the patient with a cool mist after removing all restrictive clothing.[8–10,13,14] Immersion is probably the most rapid method, but obvious difficulties with cardiovascular monitoring, problems handling a submerged patient who may have a seizure or become incontinent, and the need for a ready supply of ice make it less than ideal. The spray and fan method is quick and easy and the preferred option in our hands.

Caregivers must beware of overshoot hypothermia or unmonitored rebound hyperthermia after cooling is complete.[11] Thermoregulory mechanisms function abnormally for at least several days in persons with severe heat injury. Baseline laboratory tests, chest radiographs, and electrocardiographs are advisable.

Complications

Nearly every organ system may be affected by hyperthermia. Because the brain is extremely sensitive to excess heat, a number of central nervous system disturbances are common, confusion, lethargy, depression, irritability, and delirium among them.[11] Seizures, cerebellar deficits, and coma may also occur from the associated decrease in perfusion, as well as microinfarcts.[9]

Transient conduction disturbances may be seen on electrocardiography,[11,13] reflecting widespread neuromuscular irritability. Cardiac output is low despite sinus tachycardia (low stroke volume and blood pressure from left ventricular dysfunction). These findings, as well as heart block and tachyarrhythmia, are especially prevalent in the cool-down period.[9] Continuous cardiac monitoring is therefore advisable. A Swan-Ganz catheter is clearly recommended when the circulatory status of the patient is uncertain.

The pulmonary system may be affected by increased pulmonary vascular resistance, pulmonary edema, adult respiratory distress syndrome, or disseminated intravascular coagulation. Aspiration pneumonia is not uncommon.[9,13] Azotemia may be either renal or prerenal. Acute renal failure may occur in as many as 25% of exertional heat stroke patients.[8–10] The liver is one of the most sensitive organs affected by excess heat: consistent elevations of liver function values are characteristic of heat stroke. Centrilobular necrosis with extensive cholestasis has been observed.[9]

Gastrointestinal dysfunction is common, often manifested by nausea, vomiting, and diarrhea that results from the gastroparesis and ileus frequently noted. Stress ulceration or frank hemorrhage may be seen in severe cases.[9,10]

Hemostasis is impaired by direct endothelial damage from the heat load, thermal activation of clotting factors, decreased production of clotting factors by an abnormally functioning liver, megakaryocyte damage in the bone marrow, and, finally, bone marrow suppression.[7,11]

Treatment

Prompt cooling and careful rehydration may correct the majority of early heat stroke complications. More aggressive management is obviously warranted for significant injuries. For acute renal failure, fluids, furosemide, and mannitol are generally sufficient; a lack of a diuretic response, anuria, uremia, or hyperkalemia may be indications for dialysis.[9] Congestive heart failure may signal a need for central monitoring and the use of dopamine in extreme cases (α-agonists should be avoided).[11] Dysrhythmias should be treated by established Advanced Cardiac Life Support (ACLS) protocols. Physical restraints should be avoided because of the risk of increased heat generation and further muscle injury in a combative patient.[8] Chemical sedation is preferable, and benzodiazepines are useful and safe. Similarly, diazepam (Valium) is recommended for controlling shivering or seizures. Some studies are assessing the benefit of phenytoin (Dilantin) as prophylaxis; others have looked at chlorpromazine hydrochloride (Thorazine) as a treatment for these common complications.[10] Unfortunately, Thorazine itself may impair thermoregulation.[9] Dantrolene, effective for both malignant hyperthermia and neuroleptic malignant syndrome, may have a secondary role in treating severe or refractory cases of heat stroke.[8,11]

There is no sound rationale for delayed cooling or the use of narcotics, steroids, antibiotics, dextran, or antipyretics.[6] Antipyretics are not effective against the elevated temperatures associated with heat-related illnesses. With these illnesses, the hypothalamic set point has not been reset upward as when fever is caused by infection.[8,13] Furthermore, commonly used antipyretics may have detrimental effects on injured hepatic, renal, or gastrointestinal organs.

Children and Heat Injury

Children may be at greater risk for heat-related injury for several reasons. Children gain heat more rapidly from the environment, sweat less effectively, produce more metabolic heat for a given work load, and become acclimatized more slowly than adults.[15] Children have a higher mass–surface area ratio and have a lower renal tubular filtration rate.[14] Moreover, children may lack the experience and judgment to perceive signs of impending heat injury.

Women and Heat Injury

Core temperature thresholds for all thermoregulating functions during exercise, heat, and cold exposure are increased during the luteal phase of the menstrual cycle. The mechanism of the increase in the hypothalamic set point is unknown. Thermoregulation may be somewhat compromised during prolonged exercise or heat exposure during the luteal phase.[16] Few differences exist, however, in the ability of men and women to become acclimatized to heat.[17]

Prognosis

Rapid reduction of body temperature, proper management of rehydration, control of seizures and other complications, and prompt evacuation to and management in an appropriate medical facility much improve chances for survival. Poorer prognostic indicators include an initial temperature higher than 106°F, longer duration of hyperthermia, coma lasting more than 2 hours (or persisting after temperature has returned to normal), oliguric renal failure, hyperkalemia, and aspartate aminotransferase (AST) levels over 1000 IU.[8,9] The LD_{50} of heat stroke appears to be 108°F.

Recurrence of Heat Stroke

A history of heat stroke seems to increase the chances of a subsequent episode. It is unclear whether there are inherent characteristics that predispose an individual to thermoregulatory dysfunction or whether this tendency is secondary to the initial heat-related episode.[14] We know that no measured variable consistently predicts recovery or acclimatization, that the rate of recovery is unique to each particular case (but may take up to a year), that all heat-injured patients are at higher risk for hyperthermia and hypothermia (those with lower V_{O_2}max levels are at greater risk), and that some victims sustain an elevated creatine phosphokinase value for 3 months. Nevertheless, only about 10% of heat stroke victims are rendered permanently heat intolerant (unable to acclimatize to heat).[6,18]

Postinjury Restrictions

Some modifications of a patient's activities are always prudent after any heat-related illness. Mild cases (no end-organ damage or dysfunction): The patient should avoid running, jumping, prolonged standing or walking, lifting more than 5 pounds, and strenuous exertion of any type. Exposure to adverse environmental conditions should be limited for 72 hours. No strenuous activity should be allowed if body weight drops 5% or more while training. Liberal intake of fluids and food should be encouraged.

Patients with severe injury (end-organ damage or significant laboratory abnormalities) should be treated as outlined above for 72 hours, then exercise at their own pace and distance in wet bulb–globe temperatures below 86°F for the next 90 days (Table 12–3). The wet bulb globe temperature is computed as follows:

$$(0.7 \times \text{wet bulb temperature}) + (0.2 \times \text{black globe temperature}) + (0.1 \times \text{shaded dry bulb temperature}).$$

The patient must be re-evaluated before resuming usual activities; this includes a thermoregulatory treadmill stress test to assess the ability to offload core heat.[19]

Prevention

CONDITIONING

Endurance training shares many characteristics with the human ability to adapt to heat stress. Training increases the sweat rate at a given temperature, lowers core temperature at given levels of physical stress, expands plasma volume, and decreases heat storage.[14] Intense interval training at more than 50% V_{O_2}max, even in a cool environment, improves heat tolerance more than mild to moderate exercise.[17] This is true if fluid balance is maintained and if factors that predispose to heat injury are avoided.

ACCLIMATIZATION

Heat acclimatization involves a complex of adaptations that include decreased heart rate, rectal temperature, and perceived exertion associated with increased plasma volume and sweat rate.[8,17] This reduces physiologic strain, improves an athlete's ability to exercise in a hot environment, and reduces the incidence of some forms of heat illness. Three to four hours of daily exposure to work and heat for 10 to 14 days allows for these changes.[9,17] Once a person is acclimatized, inactivity results in loss of these adaptations in a few days or weeks.[17]

Soldiers deployed to a hot environment or athletes arriving for competition in one on short notice arrive unacclimatized, regardless of their physical condition.[6] Furthermore, acclimatization *does not guarantee* that a soldier, athlete, or laborer will be immune to heat injury.

FLUID REPLACEMENT

Training and acclimatization do improve the body's ability to withstand a given heat load, but water requirements are not reduced by any form of conditioning.[6] Coaches and supervisors must understand this and the concept that thirst is a very poor indicator of hydration status. Humans are the only mammals that voluntarily dehydrate[20]: we do not fully replenish our losses through drinking and we do not experience thirst until we have lost about 2% of our body water content. The relatively "mild dehydration" of 2 to 3% decreases work capacity by 15 to 20%[21]; 4 to 5% losses may reduce capacity by 30%.[14] For every liter of water lost, rectal temperature increases by 0.3°C, cardiac output declines by 1 L per minute, and heart rate increases 8 beats per minute.[22]

Active persons may lose 2 L or more of water per hour through sweating, and the ideal goal would be to replenish this loss by drinking. Physical discomfort and intestinal absorption may be limiting factors, however. Drinking before, during, and after exercising or working in the heat is essential to maintain fluid balance.[23] Cool to cold fluids are absorbed best.

A reasonable recommendation is to consume 400 to 600 ml (13 to 20 ounces) of cold water or a 4- to 8% carbohydrate-electrolyte beverage 15 to 20 minutes before exercising. During exercise, 200 to 300 ml every 15 to 20 minutes is minimal replacement.[23] After the task is completed, an attempt should be made to restore at least 80% of the loss.[22] Exercises or work of more than 90 minutes' duration necessitates adequate replacement of water *and* carbohydrates and electrolytes.[23]

Water discipline must be involuntary. Once an athlete, soldier, or laborer is thirsty, his or her fluid status is already disturbed and the risk of heat injury is significant.[11] Nevertheless, military experience with cases of dilutional hyponatremia suggests that there is an upper limit to water consumption. Prolonged consumption of more than 2 L of plain water per hour may cause problems.

Table 12–3. Wet Bulb–Globe Temperature (WBGT) and Recommended Activity Levels

WBGT		
°C	*°F*	*Activity*
15.6	60	No precautions
19–21	66–70	No precautions as long as water, salt, and food are easily available
22–24	71–75	Postpone sports practice, avoid hiking
24	76	Lighter practice and work with rest breaks
27	80	No hiking or sports
28	82	Only necessary heavy exertion with caution
30	85	Cancel all exertion for unacclimatized persons; avoid sun exposure even at rest
31.5	88	Limited brief activity for acclimatized, fit persons only

(Yarbrough, B. E., Hubbard, R. W.: Heat related illness. *In* Management of Wilderness and Environmental Emergencies. 2nd Ed. Edited by P. S. Auerbach and E. C. Geehr. St. Louis, C. V. Mosby, 1989.)

TOOLS FOR PREVENTION

Several heat stress danger charts are available and a sling psychrometer is often used at high school or college events to measure temperature and humidity. The wet bulb–globe temperature (Table 12–3) is a heat index that is far more representative of heat stress than is ambient temperature. This index may be compared to published guidelines that indicate relative levels of heat stress risk and provide suggestions for activity modification. Scales for pre- and postexercise weighing also exist to help coaches and trainers recommend alterations in exertion.

Strategies also include uniform modifications, work-rest cycle changes, water discipline, spray cooling, and changing the time of practices to avoid the heat of the day. Also crucial is education of athletes, coaches, supervisors, and parents about acclimatization, fluid replacement, proper clothing, and early recognition and treatment of suspected heat-related illnesses. If these tools are properly used, heat injuries should be almost entirely preventable.

REFERENCES

1. Bracker, M. D.: Environmental and thermal injury. Clin. Sports Med. *11*:419, 1992.
2. Johnson, L. W.: Preventing heat stroke. Am. Family Physician *26*:1982.
3. Yarbrough, B. E., and Hubbard, R. W.: Heat-related illnesses. *In* Management of Wilderness and Environmental Emergencies. 2nd Ed. Edited by Auerbach, P. S., and Geehr, E. C. (eds): St. Louis, C. V. Mosby, 1989.

4. Young, A. J.: Energy substrate utilization during exercise in extreme environments. Exerc. Sports Sci. Rev. *18*:65, 1990.
5. Hubbard, R. W., and Armstrong, L. E.: Hyperthermia: New thoughts on an old problem. Physician Sportsmed. *17*(6):97, 1989.
6. US Army Research Institute of Environmental Medicine: Heat Illness: A Handbook for Medical Officers. US Army Technical Note 91–3. Natick, MA, 1991.
7. Tek, D., and Olshaker, J. S.: Heat illness. Emerg. Med. Clin. North Am. *10*:299, 1992.
8. Delaney, K. A.: Heatstroke: Underlying processes and lifesaving management. Postgrad. Med. *91*:379, 1992.
9. Shapiro, Y., Seidman, D. S.: Field and clinical observations of exertional heat stroke patients. Med. Sci. Sports Exerc. *22*:6, 1990.
10. Scott, J.: Heat-related illnesses: When are they a true emergency? Postgrad. Med. *85*:154, 1989.
11. Schwartz, M.: Recognition and management of heat stroke. Hosp. Phys. *26*:11, 1990.
12. Graham, B. S., Lichtenstein, M. J., Hinson, J. M., and Theil, G. B.: Nonexertional heatstroke: Physiologic management and cooling in 14 patients. Arch. Intern. Med. *146*:87, 1986.
13. Jacobson, S.: The ill effects of heat. Emerg. Med. *24*:313, 1992.
14. Squire, D. L.: Heat illness: Fluid and electrolyte issues for pediatric and adolescent athletes. Pediatr. Clin. North Am. *37*:5, 1990.
15. Nash, H. L.: Hyperthermia: Risks greater in children. Physician Sportsmed. *15*(2):29, 1987.
16. Stephenson, L. A., and Kolka, M. A.: Thermoregulation in women. Exerc. Sports Sci. Rev. *21*:231, 1993.
17. Armstrong, L. E., and Maresh, C. M.: The induction and decay of heat acclimatization in trained athletes. Sports Med. *12*:302, 1991.
18. Armstrong, L. E., De Luca, J. P., and Hubbard, R. W.: Time course of recovery and heat acclimation ability of prior exertional heatstroke patients. Med. Sci. Sports Exerc. *22*:36, 1990.
19. Epstein, Y.: Heat intolerance: Predisposing factor or residual injury? Med. Sci. Sports Exerc. *22*:29, 1990.
20. Noakes, T. D.: Fluid replacement during exercise. Exerc. Sports Sci. Rev. *21*:297, 1993.
21. Leski, M. J.: Thermoregulation and safe exercise in the heat. *In* Sports Medicine Secrets. Philadelphia, Hanley and Belfus, (in press).
22. Coyle, E. F., and Montain, S. J.: Benefits of fluid replacement with carbohydrate during exercise. Med. Sci. Sports Exerc. *24*:S324, 1992.
23. Millard-Stafford, M.: Fluid replacement during exercise in the heat; review and recommendations. Sports Med. *13*:223, 1992.

Cold Injuries

Tanya L. Hrabal

Humans must maintain their body temperature within a narrow range—75°F to 105°F (24°C to 40.5°C). Consistent temperature ranges must be maintained for optimal athletic performance. Cold affects the central nervous system, heart, lungs, and muscles. The *shell*—the skin, muscles, and extremities—are affected first; the result is decreased circulation to guard and protect the body's core temperature. This can result in weak, stiff muscles, delayed nerve conduction time, and decreased athletic performance.

Factors that predispose athletes to cold injury include inadequate or wet clothing, wind chill factor (Table 12–4), altitude, moisture content of air, and injury. Alcohol consumption, extremes of age, poor nutrition, fatigue, and medications can increase heat loss or impair judgment. Use of tobacco or constricting garments can diminish the peripheral blood supply and increase susceptibility to cold.

HYPOTHERMIA

Hypothermia, a problem for winter outdoor athletes, is defined as core body temperature below 95°F (35°C). Central nervous system and cardiovascular changes associated with hypothermia are the most serious ones. At body temperatures below 82.4°F to 86°F (28°C to 30°C), the heart's susceptibility to ventricular fibrillation increases and response to medical treatment decreases. Diminished blood flow and increased blood viscosity lead to impaired mentation and reduced ability to cooperate with rescuers.

Mild hypothermia—core temperature between 90°F and 95°F (32°C and 35°C)—produces changes in mentation. Such changes are the best indicator of the severity of hypothermia. Early signs of mental impairment are complaints of cold and loss of interest in activity. As hypother-

Table 12–4. Wind Chill Table*

Wind Speed (mph)	*Outside Air Temperature (°F)* 35	30	25	20	15	10	5	0	−5	−10	−15	−20	−25	−30	−35	−40	−45
	Equivalent Temperature (°F)																
5	32	27	22	16	11	6	0	−5	−10	−15	−21	−26	−31	−36	−42	−47	−52
10	22	16	10	3	−3	−9	−15	−22	−27	−34	−40	−46	−52	−58	−64	−71	−77
15	16	9	2	−5	−11	−18	−25	−31	−38	−45	−51	−58	−65	−72	−78	−85	−92
20	12	4	−3	−10	−17	−24	−31	−39	−46	−53	−60	−67	−74	−81	−88	−95	−103
25	8	1	−7	−15	−22	−29	−36	−44	−51	−59	−66	−74	−81	−88	−96	−103	−110
30	6	−2	−10	−18	−25	−33	−41	−49	−56	−64	−71	−79	−86	−93	−101	−109	−116
35	4	−4	−12	−20	−27	−35	−43	−52	−58	−67	−74	−82	−89	−97	−105	−113	−120
40	3	−5	−13	−21	−29	−37	−45	−53	−60	−69	−76	−84	−92	−100	−107	−115	−123
45	2	−6	−14	−22	−30	−38	−46	−54	−62	−70	−78	−85	−93	−102	−109	−117	−125

*Wind chill determination. To determine wind chill, find the ambient air temperature on the top line, then read down the column to the line that corresponds with the current wind speed. Example: When the air temperature is 10°F and the wind speed is 20 miles per hour, the rate of heat loss is equivalent to minus 24°F under calm conditions.

(From Medicine for the Outdoors by Paul Auerbach. Copyright © 1986 by Paul S. Auerbach, M.D. By permission of Little, Brown and Company.)

mia progresses, fine motor skills suffer, decision-making capabilities deteriorate, and the desire for sleep becomes strong. Motor function continues to deteriorate until the person is unable to walk. This is followed by an inability to be aroused. Physical examination reveals bradycardia, hypotension, muscle rigidity, and dilated pupils.

Early treatment

Treatment of mild hypothermia involves removing the victim from the cold environment to a warmer one. All wet clothing is removed after relocation. External heat sources should be placed in areas of high heat loss, like the neck, armpits, and groin. If external heat sources are not available, having another person lie next to the hypothermic one helps. If the patient is alert, oral hydration is given.

Severe hypothermia is defined by a core body temperature below 90°F (32°C). Rewarming patients in the field is still a controversial measure, because this shunts core blood to the periphery and results in dilatation of peripheral vessels, which returns blood rich in lactic acid to the core. Active external rewarming may precipitate a drop in core temperature, hypotension, and ventricular fibrillation. Other methods for rewarming include portable heat devices and humidified air for inhalation.

Evacuation of a severely hypothermic person to a treatment facility is a must. Physical exertion and rough handling are minimized to decrease chances of ventricular fibrillation. Before cardiopulmonary resuscitation is instituted, absence of pulse for 1 minute must be confirmed. Detection of a pulse may be difficult because of intense vasoconstriction, bradycardia, and shallow, irregular breaths. Poor outcome factors in hypothermic situations include body core temperatures less than 82°F (28°C) or equal to the ambient temperature, submersion for more than 50 minutes, an associated life-threatening injury, or elapsed time to definitive care of more than 4 hours.

FROSTBITE

Frostbite, the body's response to severe cold, is another injury sustained by athletes. Susceptible body parts include the nose, ears, feet, fingers, and penis. Frostbite occurs by direct freezing and vascular changes that produce ischemia. As tissue freezes, the crystals form within the cells and water is drawn out of them. Cell death occurs because of the resultant dehydration and electrolyte imbalance. Freezing produces vascular endothelial damage, resulting in fluid extravasation into tissue with accompanying erythrocyte sludge and thrombus formation in small vessels.

Superficial or first-degree frostbite results in white patches of frozen skin, but skin remains soft and resilient when depressed. Wounds usually heal without permanent sequelae. At times, it is difficult to distinguish superficial frostbite from the deep type until thawing is complete.

Second-degree frostbite results in bullus formation and edema within 24 hours after rewarming. The blisters usually dry within 7 to 10 days, leaving a hard black eschar that separates in 3 to 4 weeks, exposing delicate red skin.

Third- and fourth-degree frostbite produces "woody" frozen parts that remain cool and mottled after rewarming. Small, dark bullae form in a few days or weeks, (or, sometimes, not at all). Edema develops and resolves slowly. Loss of demarcation occurs over 3 to 6 weeks, followed by mummification and spontaneous amputation of dead tissue.

All frostbitten areas must be rewarmed only when there is no danger of refreezing. Patients may need heavy sedation as well as treatment for metabolic acidosis, hypoxia, and hypotension. Patients are kept in bed until edema subsides and blisters dry. Lamb's wool is applied between the toes to prevent maceration. Sterile escharotomy should be delayed until the eschar starts to separate. If necessary, tetanus immunization is updated. All nicotine products should be prohibited. Antibiotics are recommended. The patient starts gentle range of motion exercises as soon as possible.

Tendons and bones are relatively resistant to frostbite, whereas nerves, blood vessels, and muscles are not. Osteogenesis may occur in bones secondary to immobilization. Children may exhibit epiphyseal changes after severe frostbite. Other sequelae may include excessive sweating, causalgic-type pain, cold or cool extremities, persistent nail abnormalities, pigment changes, and scarring. Cold injuries render patients more susceptible to a second such injury (Table 12–5).

CHILBLAIN

Another cold-related athletic injury is chilblain, or pernio, which is caused by cool temperatures and high humidity. This neurocirculatory condition affects those who spend long periods outdoors in winter. Chilblain is rarely a problem, because the lesions are superficial and heal quickly. Symptoms include dermatitis, itching, skin ulcerations, and chronic inflammation. Trench foot results from prolonged exposure (more than 12 hours) of wet feet to temperatures of 32°F to 50°F (0°C to 10°C).

Table 12–5. Prognostic Signs for Recovery of Frostbitten Tissues After Thawing

Favorable	*Unfavorable*
Sensation to pinprick	Cold, cyanotic distal part
Normal color	Late appearance of small, dark bullae that do not extend across the affected part
Warm tissues	Absence of edema
Early appearance of large, clean bullae that extend across affected part	

PREVENTION

Cold injuries are prevented by protecting the body from heat loss and increasing heat production. Athletes who compete in cold weather must have a good nutritional base and physical conditioning, especially a broad aerobic base.

The principle of layering clothing is essential for outdoor sports. Several thin layers of clothing produces a still, warm layer of air next to the body that prevents overheating and associated excessive sweating and chilling. The best fabrics for cold weather sports are those that are good insulators *and* do not significantly lose that property when wet. Such fabrics include wool, wool-synthetic blends, polypropylene, and capeline. Cotton is not a good insulating fabric because of its poor insulating ability when wet. Pile garments and those containing down, Dacron, Hollofil, and Quallofil are also useful during exercise because of their thickness.

Wind protection is provided by wearing an outer jacket made from a windproof fabric such as GoreTex, nylon, or 60-40 cloth. The jacket should have a hood with a drawstring. Other special protection includes a face mask, balaclava, or ski-type neck warmer that may be pulled over the face. A cap to cover the head is useful, to prevent radiation losses. Ski goggles are worn to protect the eyes. Under cold conditions contact lenses can freeze to the eyeball. Feet and hands should be protected with polypropylene outerwear using GoreTex or nylon for extremely wet conditions.

Exercise during cold weather requires a longer warm-up period, to protect muscles, tendons, and ligaments. The warm-up should be done indoors, when possible. Common sense—and prompt medical attention in questionable situations—are key to safe activity in cold weather.

REFERENCES

1. Robinson, W.: Competing with the cold. Part II. Hypothermia. Physician Sportsmed. *20*(1):61, 1992.
2. Frey, C.: Frostbitten feet: Steps to treatment and prevention. Physician Sportsmed. *20*(1):67, 1992.
3. Robinson, W.: Competing with the cold: Part I. Frostbite. Physician Sportsmed. *19*(12):19, 1991.
4. Auerbach P. S., and Geehr, E. C. (eds.): Management of wilderness and environmental emergencies. 2nd Ed. St. Louis, C.V. Mosby, 1989.
5. Backer, M.: Environmental and thermal injuries. Clin. Sports Med. *11*:419, 1992.

Terrestrial Altitude Illness

Robert S. Skerker

Altitude is the vertical elevation of an object or land mass above sea level. Elevations above sea level are measured in units of distance, usually meters (m) or feet (ft) (3.28 m = 1 ft). Terrestrial elevations of 1500 to 3500 m (5000 to 11,500 ft) are considered *high altitude.* For example, Denver, Colorado, the "mile-high city," the Rocky Mountains, is at an elevation of 1610 m (5280 ft or 1 mile). In Colorado, every year, millions of people from areas of lower altitude ski at popular resorts with peak elevations of 2450 to 3500 m (8000 to 11,500 ft). The 1968 summer Olympics took place in Mexico City, whose altitude is 2300 m (7545 ft).

Terrestrial elevations of 3500 to 5500 m (11,480 to 18,000 ft) such as Pike's Peak at 4267 m (13,996 ft) are described as *very high altitude.* The lower barometric pressure causes physiologic sequelae, including a drop in arterial oxygen-hemoglobin saturation below 90%, as PaO_2 drops below 60 mm Hg. *Extreme altitudes* are those higher than 5500 m (18,000 ft), the most notable of which is Mt. Everest at 8848 m (29,028 ft). At these elevations, progressive deterioration of physiologic function occurs because of severe hypoxia, so that no permanent human habitation is possible. Ascents to the summit of Mt. Everest typically require oxygen equipment.

HIGH ALTITUDE ILLNESSES

The several illnesses or syndromes associated with exposure to high terrestrial altitudes can be grouped according to severity. The first group are those that are minor, rarely disabling, and not fatal. This group includes high-altitude systemic edema, high-altitude retinal hemorrhages, high-altitude flatus expulsion, ultraviolet keratitis (snow blindness), and altitude throat. The disabling but nonfatal illnesses of altitude include acute mountain sickness, chronic or subacute mountain sickness, and high-altitude deterioration.

Acute Mountain Sickness

Severe symptoms of acute mountain sickness rarely occur below 2440 m (8000 ft), and most people do not experience symptoms until 3050 to 3660 m (10,000 to 12,000 ft). Acute mountain sickness is the most common of all the altitude illnesses. Symptoms include headache, lassitude, anorexia, malaise, weakness, and dyspnea on exertion. Initially, urine output is diminished. Early after arrival at an area of unaccustomed high altitude, a feeling of warmth and flushing of the face may be noted for the first 24 to 48 hours. Tinnitus and vertiginous feelings may be present. Sleep, especially the first few nights after arrival at altitude, is difficult and marked by frequent periods of wakefulness and strange dreams.

Clinical signs of acute mountain sickness include tachypnea, tachycardia, Cheyne-Stokes respirations, and ataxia. Treatment of mild to moderate cases usually includes symptomatic relief using rest, light diet, fluids, and analgesics to relieve headache. Severe cases require descent from altitude, auxiliary oxygen, and pharmacologic therapy.

Honigman and coworkers recently published a survey that sampled participants at conventions in the Rocky

Mountain resort areas with altitudes between 1920 and 2960 m (6300 to 9700 ft).[1] Adequate survey responses were obtained from 3158 subjects aged 16 to 87 years. Twenty-five percent of travelers to moderate altitude met the case definition criteria (three or more symptoms) for acute mountain sickness, whereas 73% had at least one symptom. The majority (65%) developed symptoms within the first 12 hours after arrival at the higher altitude. Travelers from areas below 915 m (3000 ft) were more likely than those from higher elevations to develop symptoms (odds ratio 3.5:1). Visitors who had a history of episodes of acute mountain sickness developed symptoms 2.8 times more often than those who never experienced acute mountain sickness. Furthermore, those younger than 60 years were twice as likely to develop acute mountain sickness than older persons. Women, overweight persons, less physically fit ones, and those with underlying lung disease also had higher rates of acute mountain sickness.

PREVENTION

The best preventive measure is slow acclimatization by a 2- to 4-day sojourn at an intermediate altitude (1830 to 2440 m) and then gradual ascent to higher elevations.[2]

PHARMACOLOGIC PROPHYLAXIS

Acetazolamide (Diamox), a carbonic anhydrase inhibitor, can be taken in doses of 250 mg every 6 to 12 hours (or 500 mg per day of a sustained-release formulation) beginning 1 or 2 days before ascent and continuing at high altitude for 2 days or longer. For many, it prevents or blunts the severity of symptoms, but it is ineffective for a minority of high-altitude travelers.[3,4] Acetazolamide inhibits carbonic anhydrase and produces sodium bicarbonate diuresis.

Fluid retention is avoided and metabolic acidosis occurs as bicarbonate ions are excreted. This promotes compensatory hyperventilation (respiratory alkalosis) to normalize acid-base balance. The hyperventilation, in turn, increases alveolar oxygen partial pressure, which improves oxygen supply to the bloodstream and delivery to peripheral tissues, thus decreasing hypoxemia, especially during sleep. This helps ameliorate the symptoms of acute mountain sickness. The medication can cause dehydration because it is a mild diuretic, so high-altitude users should be warned to maintain hydration. Acetazolamide or Diamox can cause limb paresthesia and cause carbonated drinks to have a metallic taste because of buildup of carbonic anhydrase.

The synthetic glucocorticoid dexamethasone (Decadron), in doses of 4 mg every 6 hours, also offers prophylaxis against acute mountain sickness. A double-blind crossover trial of 16 men found that acute mountain sickness developed in 31% of those treated with Decadrone for 48 hours before and after rapid ascent to 4270 m (14,000 ft) and in 60% of those who took a placebo.[5] Another study at the same altitude found that acute mountain sickness occurred in 25% of 17 patients treated with Decadrone, 4 mg every 8 hours, 53% of 15 patients treated with acetazolamide, and 77% of 15 patients treated with placebo.[6] The combination of acetazolamide, 250 mg twice a day with dexamethasone, 4 mg four times a day for prophylaxis of acute mountain sickness was more effective than acetazolamide alone and much more effective than dexamethasone alone.[7]

The physiologic mechanism by which dexamethasone prevents acute mountain sickness is still unknown. It may work by reducing nausea and by producing euphoria. It may also work at the level of the endothelium to prevent vasodilatation, which could cause the symptoms of acute mountain sickness.[8]

TREATMENT

Initial treatment of acute mountain sickness is rapid descent to low altitude and administration of supplemental oxygen, especially during sleep. Acetazolamide has been used to treat symptoms of acute mountain sickness after onset, but no published trials demonstrate its efficacy. On the other hand, several published studies support the use of dexamethasone, 8 mg initially then 4 mg every 6 hours, for the treatment of acute mountain sickness symptoms.[9–11] Diamox should *not* be given to patients who are allergic to sulfa drugs.

High-Altitude Cerebral Edema

The symptoms of acute mountain sickness are probably related to increased intracranial pressure, and, thus, it is a neurologic disorder. Experienced physicians believe that acute mountain sickness progresses to high-altitude cerebral edema, although the distinction between the two is somewhat fuzzy. High-altitude cerebral edema is a life-threatening form of altitude illness that affects an estimated 1% of high-altitude travelers.[12] It usually occurs at altitudes above 3660 m (12,000 ft).

The clinical presentation is progressive neurologic signs and symptoms. Truncal ataxia, lassitude, and altered sensorium may progress to obtundity, stupor, and coma. Symptoms such as headache, nausea, and vomiting are often present, but not always.[13] Other symptoms may include paresthesia, diplopia, and vertigo. Focal neurologic deficits, including cranial nerve abnormalities, aphasia, and hemiparesis, may mimic stroke. Fundoscopic examination may reveal retinal hemorrhages and papilledema. The disease process may progress to unconsciousness within 12 hours but usually takes 1 to 3 days.[13]

Clinical evaluations have shown elevated cerebrospinal fluid pressure on lumbar puncture, cerebral edema on computed tomography of the head, and gross cerebral edema on necropsy.[14,15]

TREATMENT

Early recognition is the cornerstone of treatment, treatment being prevention of progression. Descent should begin immediately once symptoms are recognized. Also, if available, dexamethasone should be given, 4 to 8 mg IV, IM, or PO, followed by 4 mg every 6 hours. If supplemental oxygen is available it should be given. Seriously ill persons must be evacuated to a hospital where aggressive management, similar to that for other forms of cerebral edema, can be initiated. If high-altitude cerebral edema is caught early and managed with descent, steroids, and oxygen, the outcome is usually favorable.[13]

High-Altitude Pulmonary Edema

High-altitude pulmonary edema is a severe, potentially life-threatening form of high-altitude illness. It usually occurs within the first 2 to 4 days of ascent to altitudes higher than 2500 m (8,200 ft) and usually begins on the second night at altitude. Early warning signs include decreased exercise performance, tachypnea even at rest, fatigue, and weakness. Signs of acute mountain sickness, such as headache, anorexia, and lassitude, are also frequently present. Eventually, a dry cough develops, which proceeds to a productive cough. Cyanosis develops and audible congestion is noted. Progressive deterioration may ensue as severe hypoxemia produces mental changes, ataxia, and declining consciousness.[13,16]

On clinical examination, a low-grade fever is common; in severe cases patients are both tachycardiac and tachypneic. Unilateral or bilateral rales can be heard on auscultation. An electrocardiogram often reflects changes consistent with acute pulmonary hypertension and right-sided heart strain (i.e., right axis deviation, right bundle branch block, cor pulmonale, or right ventricular hypertrophy), and if Swan-Ganz catheterization is performed, mean pulmonary artery pressure and pulmonary vascular resistance are elevated in the face of low to normal capillary wedge pressure. Chest radiographic findings are consistent with noncardiogenic pulmonary edema. Arterial blood gas analysis usually shows severe hypoxia, hypocapnia, and acute respiratory alkalosis due to hyperventilation.

A subclinical form of high-altitude pulmonary edema was noted in 15% of climbers to the summit of Mt. Rainier (4390 m; 14,408 ft).[17] Clinically apparent high-altitude pulmonary edema has been described in 0.1% of vacationers who spent several nights above 2700 m (8850 ft) in a Colorado ski resort, and in 4.5% of a group of Himalayan trekkers above 4267 m (14,000 ft).[18,19]

PATHOPHYSIOLOGY

The trigger for high-altitude pulmonary edema is most certainly hypobaric hypoxia; however, the pathophysiology is not well understood. Several researchers hypothesize a neurogenic cause. Others believe that exaggerated pulmonary vasoconstriction occurs in some vascular beds and that other vascular beds with lower vascular resistance become overperfused, inducing increased vascular permeability and edema.[13,16] Bärtsch and colleagues studied the use of the calcium channel–blocking agent nifedipine as prophylaxis against high-altitude pulmonary edema.[20] Twenty-one subjects with a history of high-altitude pulmonary edema were randomly assigned to receive either slow-release nifedipine, 20 mg every 8 hours, or placebo while rapidly ascending from low altitude to 4559 m (14,954 ft) and during the next 72 hours. Seven of the eleven subjects (64%) who received placebo again developed high-altitude pulmonary edema, whereas only one of ten (10%) nifedipine-treated subjects did. This study supports the idea that high pulmonary pressure plays a role in high-altitude pulmonary edema, but, as Reeves and Schone pointed out,[21] there appear to be factors other than hypoxic vasoconstriction that cause pulmonary hypertension.

TREATMENT

As for all forms of altitude illness, treatment includes supplemental oxygen, 6 to 12 L per minute, and rapid descent to lower altitude. A recent review discusses hyperbaric treatment and expiratory positive airway pressure under field conditions when descent is not possible.[22] Severely affected persons should be hospitalized and cared for as if they had noncardiogenic pulmonary edema. It is reasonable to recommend nifedipine, 20 mg every 8 hours, for prophylaxis in susceptible persons and as a supplement to the treatment of high-altitude pulmonary edema in emergency situations.[21,23,24]

REFERENCES

1. Honigman, B., et al.: Acute mountain sickness in a general tourist population at moderate altitudes. Ann. Intern. Med. *118*:587, 1993.
2. High altitude sickness. Med. Lett. *30*:89, 1988.
3. Larson, E. B., Roach, R. C., Schoene, R. B., and Hornbein, T. F.: Acute mountain sickness and acetazolamide. J.A.M.A. *248*:328, 1982.
4. McIntosh, I. B., and Prescott, R. J.: Acetazolamide in prevention of acute mountain sickness. J. Int. Med. Res. *14*:285, 1986.
5. Rock, P. B., et al.: Effect of dexamethasone on symptoms of acute mountain sickness at Pikes Peak, Colorado. Aviat. Space Environ. Med. *58*:668, 1987.
6. Ellsworth, A. J., Larson, E. B., and Strickland, D.: A randomized trial of dexamethasone and acetazolamide for acute mountain sickness prophylaxis. Am. J. Med. *83*:1024, 1987.
7. Zell, S. C., and Goodman, P. H.: Acetazolamide and dexamethasone in the prevention of acute mountain sickness. West. J. Med. *148*:541, 1988.
8. Levine, B. D.: By what physiological mechanism is dexamethasone beneficial in the prevention of acute mountain sickness? J. Wilderness Med. *4*:106, 1993.
9. Ferrazzini, G., et al.: Successful treatment of acute mountain sickness with sesamethasone. Br. Med. J. *294*:1380, 1987.
10. Ferriera, P., and Grundy, P.: Dexamethasone in the treatment of acute mountain sickness. N. Engl. J. Med. *312*:1390, 1985.
11. Hacket, P. H., et al.: Dexamethasone for prevention and treatment of acute mountain sickness. Aviat. Space Environ. Med. *59*:950, 1988.
12. Tso, E.: High altitude illness. Emerg. Med. Clin. North Am. *10*:231, 1992.
13. Hackett, P. H., Roach, R. C., and Sutton, J. R.: High altitude medicine. *In* Management of Wilderness and Environmental Emergencies. 2nd Ed. Edited by P. S. Auerbach and E. C. Geehr. New York, Macmillan, 1989.
14. Dickinson, J. G.: High altitude cerebral edema: Cerebral acute mountain sickness. Semin. Respir. Med. *5*:151, 1983.
15. Dickinson, J. G., et al.: Altitude related deaths in seven trekkers in the Himalayas. Thorax *38*:646, 1983.
16. Rabold M: High altitude pulmonary edema, a collective review. Am. J. Emerg. Med. *7*:426, 1989.
17. Houston, C. S., and Dickinson, J.: Cerebral form of high altitude illness. Lancet *2*:758, 1975.
18. Hackett, P. H., Ronnie, D.: Rales, peripheral edema, retinal hemorrhages and AMS. Am. J. Med. *67*:214, 1979.

19. Hopewell, P. C., and Murray, J. F.: The adult respiratory distress syndrome. Ann. Rev. Med. *27*:343, 1976.
20. Bärtsch, P., et al.: Prevention of high altitude pulmonary edema by nifedipine. N. Engl. J. Med. *325*:1284, 1991.
21. Reeves, J. T., and Schone, R.B.: When lungs on mountains leak, studying pulmonary edema at high altitudes. N. Engl. J. Med. *325*:1306, 1991.
22. Bärtsch, P.: Treatment of high altitude diseases without drugs. Int. J. Sports Med. *13*:S71, 1992.
23. Jamieson, A., and Kerr, G. W.: Treatment of high-altitude pulmonary oedema. Lancet *340*:1468, 1992.
24. Oelz, O., et al.: Prevention and treatment of high altitude pulmonary edema by a calcium channel blocker. Int. J. Sports Med. *13*:S65, 1992.

13

Michael J. Axe and Sandra Gibney

Nutrition

In a quest for success, most athletes are willing to try almost any diet regimen or nutritional supplement. Unfortunately, these practices demonstrate the ignorance about sports nutrition often observed in coaches, trainers, and, most important, athletes, owing to the relative unavailability of objective information.

NUTRIENTS

Carbohydrates, proteins, fats, vitamins, minerals, and water are all nutrients. These absorbable components of food are necessary for energy, organ function, food utilization, and cell growth.

Micronutrients and Macronutrients

Vitamins and minerals are *micronutrients* and do not, themselves, provide energy. The *macronutrients*—carbohydrates, fat, and protein—do provide energy, but only when sufficient micronutrients are available to fuel the body's biochemical processes. Briefly stated, vitamins are organic substances necessary for life. They contain no calories and have no energy value of their own. With few exceptions, vitamins cannot be synthesized internally by the human body. Thus, they must be obtained (in minute quantities) in natural foods or from dietary supplements. A single vitamin deficiency can impair athletic performance. Although about 18 minerals are known to be required for body maintenance and regulatory functions, recommended dietary allowance (RDA) values have been established for only seven: calcium, iodine, iron, magnesium, phosphorus, selenium, and zinc.

The use of vitamin and mineral supplements has been a controversial issue in athletics. Many authorities claim that vitamin supplementation is unnecessary for athletes who consume a balanced diet (assuming that the increased energy needs are met by wise food choices). Unfortunately, many athletes do not eat a balanced diet: some are notorious "junk food junkies" whose intake rarely coincides with the criteria for a balanced diet.

Most important, the effect of these supplements on athletes' performance cannot be underestimated—whether that effect is attributable to placebo effect, psychologic effect, or actual deficiencies. Competitors at all levels have been reported to take supplements. Certainly, athletes whose vitamin intake is below the RDA guidelines benefit from supplements. Moreover, several studies have indicated that RDA levels for certain nutrients may be inadequate to meet the needs of athletes, or that athletes may improve their performance by ingesting particular nutrients in quantities that exceed the RDA. These specific nutrients include B vitamins, vitamin C, vitamin E, iron, supplemental protein, and supplemental carbohydrates.

Each athlete must be an "experiment of one" and determine the self-specific nutritional regimen that works for him or her. If there is a question of nutritional adequacy, a good-quality multivitamin-mineral supplement is recommended, to obviate deficiencies.

THE RDA AND THE U.S. RDA

The RDAs were established by the National Research Council of the National Academy of Sciences, an independent research organization based in Washington, D.C. The U.S. Food and Drug Administration (FDA) then adapted these requirements and called them the U.S. RDAs, which are the values found on food and supplement labels. The RDAs were established by the government to safeguard public health. It is important to realize that the RDAs are intended to address the needs of healthy persons, not those who are ill or are athletes.

The process of establishing RDAs is quite an involved and complicated one that is fraught with estimations and a less than ideal method for determining nutrient levels. Thus, people must be cautious in using these values as the "gold standard" for nutritional adequacy and athletic performance. Differences do exist between individuals; one such is their optimal levels of nutrients.

CARBOHYDRATES, PROTEIN, FAT, AND WATER—THE KEY PLAYERS

Carbohydrates

Carbohydrates are food components that are composed of *carb*on, *o*xygen, and *hydr*ogen. One or more basic sugar molecules bind together to form all carbohydrates. Sugar molecules that exist individually are called *monosaccharides;* in pairs they are called *disaccharides* and in chains of three or more, *polysaccharides.* All sugars are reduced to the simple sugar glucose, through digestion or conversion in the liver. Starch and glycogen are complex sugars that contain numerous glucose molecules. Once ingested, carbohydrates are first transported by the blood stream to the liver, where they are (1) converted to fat, (2) stored as glycogen, or (3) released into the bloodstream as glucose for transport to muscle and other tissues. Glycogen is the stored form of glucose found in liver and muscle. The glycogen stored in the liver can be converted to glucose and released into the bloodstream to meet the body's energy needs. Glycogen stored in the individual muscle fibers is available only for that muscle fiber.

A proper diet should contain 60 to 70% carbohydrates, the majority of these calories coming from starches (complex sugars). The remaining calories should be obtained from fat (15 to 20%) and protein (10 to 15%). Some carbohydrates tend to be inexpensive and readily available: breads, cakes, cereals, fruits, pancakes, pastas, potatoes, and baked beans. Candies, syrups, and pastries are generally considered simple carbohydrates and are less nutritionally sound food choices because they often lack other nutrients. Although most athletes who are training intensively recognize the importance of dietary carbohydrates, their diets often contain less than 40% carbohydrate (or 350 g per day). As a result, they feel chronically fatigued or "stale" during these periods. It is important to realize that, when a person's diet is rich in carbohydrates (550 to 650 g) the body requires less time to replenish the stored glycogen in exhausted muscles.

CARBOHYDRATE LOADING

Anyone who performs maximum-level exercise that is sustained longer than several seconds needs a readily available supply of glycogen. Ideally, before endurance activities or prolonged tournament-type activities, glycogen is stored at optimal levels, to prevent fatigue from fuel shortage. This is accomplished through carbohydrate loading. A minimum of 20 hours is generally required to totally replace depleted carbohydrate stores; however, during successive days of competition or intensive training, athletes should consume approximately 100 g of carbohydrates within 15 to 30 minutes after exercising. If this is followed by an additional 100 g of carbohydrates every 2 to 4 hours thereafter, needed glycogen stores will be replenished for the next day's competition. It appears the most simple way to accomplish this is to drink simple sugar drinks. Athletes are often thirsty, rather than hungry, after competitions and many prefer to consume carbohydrates in beverage form. This adds the benefit of rehydration of fluids lost during exercise.

Many studies have focused on the process of carbohydrate loading for athletes. Although carbohydrate diets may be beneficial for all athletes, the practice of carbohydrate loading to increase muscle glycogen stores to two to three times normal levels is more appropriate for those involved in repetitious, prolonged endurance-type events such as distance swimming, marathon running, tournament tennis, and cross-country skiing. Such athletes, who exercise constantly for more than 90 minutes, deplete their glycogen stores, and, when that happens, exhaustion sets in. The purpose and benefit of carbohydrate loading is to delay exhaustion by supersaturating the muscles with glycogen before the competition. Muscles begin to store this extra glycogen (load) only after heavy exercise that exhausts existing muscle stores. In general, it is recommended that all athletes increase their stores of carbohydrates before competition to provide optimal levels of available carbohydrate and glycogen.

COMPLEX CARBOHYDRATES

There are several reasons why it is more appropriate to eat complex carbohydrates, rather than simple carbohydrates, to replace glycogen stores and to maintain high glycogen levels in the muscles and liver:

1. Studies have shown that, within the first 24 hours, athletes who ingest simple carbohydrates store as much glycogen as those who use complex ones. On the second day, however, those who eat complex carbohydrate foods store *more* glycogen.
2. Complex carbohydrates tend to produce a less intense insulin response than simple carbohydrates, especially in sugar-sensitive persons. Some simple carbohydrates can cause a sharp rise in insulin production. The increase removes sugar too quickly into muscle, and the drop in blood sugar causes the athlete to feel light headed and lethargic.
3. Complex carbohydrate foods also include nutrients that are valuable to athletes, such as vitamins and minerals, whereas most simple carbohydrates do not contain these extra nutrients.

Protein

Protein, an organic substance, is the primary structural material of cells and tissues. In general, proteins are required for (1) maintenance and repair of body tissue; (2) manufacture of hemoglobin, which carries oxygen to the cells; (3) the formation of antibodies in the bloodstream to fight off infection and disease; and (4) production of enzymes and hormones that regulate body processes. It also supplies energy, when necessary.

Proteins are made of amino acids, building blocks that occur in various and complex combinations. Amino acids, in turn, are classified as either essential or nonessential. Eight of the twenty known amino acids are considered essential because they cannot be synthesized by the body at a rate sufficient to meet the needs for growth and maintenance and must therefore be provided in the diet. The other 12 amino acids can be synthesized by the body to build body proteins if sufficient nitrogen is available (Table 13–1). The question—or debate—for many years has been, How much protein should an athlete consume? Research has demonstrated that carbohydrates and fats are the principal sources of energy during exercise. However, recent research findings indicate that the need for dietary amino acids may increase as the result of regular exercise training. This increased protein need with exercise can occur directly, as a result of changes in amino acid metabolism, or indirectly, as a result of insufficient energy intake.

Traditionally, 0.8 g of protein per kilogram of body weight has been recommended, but these figures were based on observations of relatively sedentary persons. Many nutritionists currently recommend 1.2 to 2 g/kg/day of protein. Assuming the athlete's total energy intake is sufficient, this quantity of protein represents 12 to 15% of the energy intake in her or his mixed diet. There are two basic types of protein, complete proteins and incomplete proteins. Complete proteins provide the proper balance of the eight essential amino acids that build tissue and are found in foods of animal origin, such as meat, poultry, seafood, fish, milk, and cheese. Incomplete proteins lack certain essential amino acids although, when incomplete proteins are combined with small amounts of animal proteins, they become complete. Incomplete proteins are found in seeds, nuts, peas, grains, and beans.

BRANCHED-CHAIN AMINO ACIDS

Recent research has demonstrated that endurance athletes use higher levels of branched-chain amino acids, specifically leucine, isoleucine, and valine, as exercise fuel. Factors such as high-intensity exercise, prolonged exercise, endurance training, and decreased carbohydrate availability promote greater amino acid oxidation. These effects alter the rates of protein breakdown and synthesis and can lead to elevated dietary protein requirements. Also, muscle damage that results from endurance exercise and high-intensity exercise may cause additional dietary protein to be needed to ensure optimally rapid repair of muscle fibers. Branched-chain amino acids are naturally anabolic (muscle-building) supplements. They regulate how protein is used by the body and they play a unique role in protein metabolism within muscle.

While all of the amino acids can be broken down in the liver, branched-chain amino acids are oxidized in peripheral muscle as well. Branched-chain amino acids can be, in effect, the principal source of calories for human muscle. Intensive exercise produces rapid excretion of nitrogen, which causes a decrease in muscle protein synthesis. Branched-chain amino acids limit this decrease (anticatabolic). During strenuous exercise, stress on the muscle causes it to break down (catabolism). Branched-chain amino acids not only act to prevent this; they can actually reverse the process. They are, therefore, both anabolic and anticatabolic.

One-half of a healthy human's body weight is muscle and 15 to 20% of the muscle is branched-chain amino acids. A further consideration is that 50% of ingested branched-chain amino acids are available to muscles within 1 hour and 100% within 2 hours. Furthermore, branched-chain amino acids aid in glycogen production and help balance insulin secretion. They have statistically improved maintenance of high levels of performance and improved immune function. Although leucine can be consumed in readily available foods, the necessary volume, digestion times, and other factors prove limiting. Therefore, for optimal benefit, pharmaceutical-grade, crystalline, predigested capsule forms are recommended. While the U.S. RDA for leucine is 16 mg/kg body weight, this value was not formulated for athletes. Like many other (ergogenic) supplements, they are not intended to be used as calories but rather to promote muscle-building body processes.

Table 13–1. Amino Acids

Essential Amino Acids	*Nonessential Amino Acids*
Leucine	Alanine
Isoleucine	Arginine
Lysine	Asparagine
Methionine	Aspartic acid
Phenylalanine	Cystine
Threonine	Glutamic Acid
Tryptophan	Glutamine
Valine	Glycine
Histidine (for infants and children)	Ornithine
	Proline
	Serine

Fat

Fat is the most concentrated source of energy from food. It provides 9 calories per gram, whereas protein and carbohydrates provide just 4 calories per gram. Fats provide essential fatty acids, carry vitamins A, D, E, and K, and are part of the cell walls. Fats are a primary source of muscle energy at rest, and they can provide energy for latent endurance events. Fat is classified as either primarily saturated or primarily unsaturated. Saturated fats are found in animal fat, coconut oil, and palm oil. When eaten in large amounts, they are believed to predispose people to heart disease and atherosclerosis. Unsaturated fats, usually derived from plants, are liquid at room temperature. Examples are vegetable oils—peanut, soy, sunflower, corn—and fish oils.

During digestion, dietary fats are broken down into component parts called *fatty acids, monoglycerides,* and *glycerol.* Body cells can use fatty acids directly as an energy source; however, fatty acids that are not used as energy are stored in the body in the form of fat, as are unused carbohydrates and protein that is not converted to glycogen. Every person tends to have a genetic predisposition to sites of fat deposition. This fat can easily be measured by using a skin fold caliper or by more complicated methods, such as hydrostatic weighing.

Fat can serve as an energy source for athletes, but unfortunately it takes 20 to 30 minutes from the time exercise begins until fat can be available to contribute energy for exercise. Once more fat is being burned, through plasma and intramuscular triglyceride hydrolysis, less glycogen will be required to supply energy. There have been reports that highly trained marathon athletes, exercising at a pace of 70% of $\dot{V}O_2$max can derive as much as 75% of their total energy requirement from fat. Since glycogen stores are limited and fat stores abundant, fat can often serve athletes involved in endurance events; however, fat is a less efficient source of energy because greater amounts of oxygen are required to use it. Additionally, increased intensity of exercise often limits the degree to which fat can be used as an energy source. This case is an exception, in that, usually, activity at levels greater than 60% $\dot{V}O_2$max requires glycogen as an energy source, rather than stored fat.

Water

Water, by far the most abundant component of the human body, accounts for roughly 60% of body weight. This large reservoir furnishes an environment that is essential to the survival of tissues. Water is the main component of the cells, urine, sweat, and blood. When the body becomes dehydrated, cells become smaller and chemical reactions within the cell are impaired. Furthermore, cells are unable to use energy efficiently. Blood volume decreases, and less blood is available to transfer oxygen and nutrients throughout the body. The result is that the muscles become very weak and fatigued.

The most important function of water is to cool the body. As every athlete recognizes firsthand, exercise produces increases in body temperature. As a muscle contracts, the rate of heat production accelerates and the heat needs to be dissipated to avoid extreme elevations in body temperature (hyperthermia). Fortunately, such temperature elevations are avoided via the processes of radiation, convection, and most important, evaporation. The autonomic nervous system activates sweat glands to produce fluid secretions (perspiration). Without this process, the internal body temperature would accelerate rapidly—by almost 2°F every 5 to 7 minutes during moderate exercise. Note that, in cooler environmental temperatures, radiation and convection from the skin are the more important mechanisms of heat dispersal (across a large temperature gradient). When sweat evaporates from the skin and cools the body, the body loses large amounts of water. Fluid loss can be more than 2 L per hour. To prevent dehydration and improve performance, athletes must restore lost fluids and maintain an adequate level of hydration.

Why must athletes be concerned with hydration? Research has proven that humans lack the capacity to consume and retain fluids at a rate equivalent to that at which they are lost. This phenomenon is due, in part, to the fact that drinking plain water dilutes the blood. When a person drinks plain water, the blood becomes more diluted and urine production is stimulated. This fact is important because, when replacing fluid losses, one must consider replacing lost sodium to allow for appropriate rehydration to occur. Drinking pure water to rehydrate rapidly removes the thirst drive. The salt-dependent thirst drive needs to be maintained, and stimulation of urine production by dilution of plasma needs to be avoided. If fluid loss exceeds 3%, or approximately 5 pounds of body weight, both water and salt need to be replaced if rehydration is to be effective (Table 13–2).

As athletes become more conditioned and their physical fitness improves, several adaptations are made. The most significant of these is that physical training increases blood volume. This increase in blood volume then helps to ensure adequate cardiac function. Physical training also produces changes in sweat gland function: the body produces more dilute sweat, thus preserving sodium stores. While carbohydrate loading may be beneficial only to endurance athletes, fluid loading before events is recommended for all athletes. One of the most important points to realize is that an athlete cannot depend on a feeling of thirst as a *reliable indicator* of the need for fluid replacement.

Electrolyte Drinks

Choosing the appropriate "sports drink" for fluid replacement requires considering many factors. The major factor is how quickly the drink leaves the stomach. Gastric emptying rate is affected by the fluid's calorie content, volume load, osmolality, temperature, and

Table 13–2. How to Keep Your Body Hydrated

Never restrict fluids before or during an event.

Drink 2½ cups of fluid approximately 2 hours before competition and 1½ cups of fluid 15 minutes before competition.

During training and competition, drink fluids (5–8 oz.) every 15–20 minutes.

The fluid replacement beverage should contain some sodium and ideally 6–8% glucose or sucrose.

Avoid beverages that contain excessive caffeine or alcohol as they tend to increase urine production and exacerbate dehydration.

To establish adequate levels for rehydration, athletes should weigh in before and after exercise. As a guide, drink 2 cups of fluid for each pound of body weight lost during exercise.

hydrogen ion concentration (pH) as well as the metabolic state of the athlete (rest versus exercise), psychologic and emotional factors, and the ambient temperature. Among these, calorie content is the most critical variable. As the calorie content increases, the gastric emptying rate declines. Interestingly, isocaloric, isovolumic stomach contents of carbohydrates, fats, or proteins are emptied at equivalent rates.

After gastric emptying, intestinal absorption is the next critical factor, and fluid absorption in the small intestine is potentiated by the presence of glucose and sodium. They share a common membrane transport carrier across the epithelium of the small intestine. The carbohydrate type and content are also important. Glucose, glucose polymers, sucrose (table sugar), and a combination of glucose and fructose all equally stimulate food absorption, however, fructose is absorbed much less efficiently. In fact, concentrations greater than 10% fructose have been associated with gastrointestinal distress and osmotic diarrhea. Research indicates that beverages containing 6 to 8% glucose or sucrose are absorbed at rates comparable to that of plain water; however, unlike water, they provide performance-enhancing energy and nutrients without compromising cardiovascular or thermoregulatory function (i.e., blood volume or sweating mechanics). The performance-enhancing effects are attributed to muscle and liver glycogen sparing and improved plasma-glucose homeostasis.

The electrolyte content of fluids has been the focus of a nearly $1 billion industry. Beverages contain various concentrations of sodium, potassium, and chloride (Table 13–3). Losses less than 5 pounds can normally be replaced with plain water and a balanced diet. However, with heavy perspiration, ingestion of supplemental electrolytes during exercise in the form of carbohydrates and electrolyte beverages may potentiate glucose and fluid absorption. A little talked about, but equally important, consideration is palatability. Taste qualities of sports beverages can be enhanced by the addition of small amounts of electrolytes. Cool, slightly sweetened, and mildly lemon-lime–flavored fluids are preferred by exercisers and have been shown to promote voluntary consumption of larger volumes than does plain water or another fluid that is strong flavored and tends to "repeat," leaving an unpleasant aftertaste. Considering all factors, when exercising it is probably best to drink 5 to 8 ounces at 10- to 15-minute intervals of beverage containing 6 to 8% glucose and with an electrolyte concentration no greater than that of sweat.

Table 13–3. Comparison of Sports Beverages

Beverage	*Flavors*	*Carbohydrate Source*	*Calories (per 8 oz)*	*Sodium (mg/8 oz)*	*Potassium (mg/8 oz)*	*Other Vitamins, Minerals*
Breakthrough (Weider)	Tangerine, lemon	Glucose polymers, fructose polymers, maltodextrin	80	60	45	C, A, thiamine, riboflavin, niacin, iron, calcium, magnesium
Ultra Fuel (Twin Lab)	Lemon-lime, grape, fruit punch, orange	Glucose polymers, crystalline fructose	200	0	49.5	Magnesium, B_1, B_2, B_3, B_6, biotin, pantothenic acid, C
Carbo Force (American Body Building)	Strawberry, lemon-lime, cherry, orange	Glucose polymers, glucose, natural fructose	200	<17	49.5	C, A, thiamine, niacin, calcium, iron
Hydra Fuel (Twin Lab)	Fruit punch	Glucose, glucose polymers, fructose	66	25	49.5	Magnesium, chromium, C,
Carbo Power (Nature's Best)	Lemon-lime, lemonade, strawberry, watermelon	Maltodextrin, fructose	200	<17.5	50	C, B_1, B_2, niacin, folic acid, B_6, B_{12}
Powerade (Coca-Cola)	Lemon-lime	Glucose, sucrose	70	50	30	A, C, thiamine, riboflavin, niacin, calcium, iron
Gatorade (Stokely-Van Camp)	Lemon-lime, lemonade, fruit punch, orange, citrus cooler	Sucrose/glucose (powder), sucrose/glucose syrup solids (liquid)	50	110	25	Chloride, phosphorus
Cyberade (Cybergenics)	Lemon-lime	Fructose, dextrose	190	<7.5	49.5	C, A, thiamine, niacin, riboflavin, calcium, iron

TRAINING DIET

Recommendations of 60 to 70% carbohydrates, 15 to 20% fat, and 10 to 15% protein can be achieved without supplements by eating appropriately from the four basic food groups: milk group, meat group, fruit and vegetable group, and grain group. Both the age of the athlete and the level of activity must be considered when making recommendations. Diets can be divided into three types: the basic diet, training diet, and carbohydrate-loading diet (Table 13–4).

Precompetition meals pose a special problem. Too often, athletes concern themselves principally with the meal eaten immediately before the competition. They do not seem to realize that pre-event nutrition is a year-round task. By the time an athlete retires the night before competition, the stored glycogen already in place will be fuel for the next day's competition. What the athlete consumes on the day of the event does not affect the glycogen store as much as what was eaten 2 to 3 days before the actual competition. The following goals should be considered in planning a pre-event meal:

- Food intake should be voluminous enough to avoid feelings of hunger or weakness during the entire period of the competition.
- The diet plan should ensure that the stomach and upper bowel are empty at the time of competition.
- Food and fluid intake before and during prolonged competition should guarantee sufficient water. The immediate pre-event diet should include 2 to 3 glasses of some beverage, preferably water or diluted, low-sugar drinks.
- Precompetition diets should offer foods that minimize upset of the gastrointestinal tract. For example, fats and meats are generally digested slowly and may cause a feeling of fullness. Other categories of food to avoid may include gas-forming, greasy, and highly seasoned ones.
- The diet should include foods with which the athlete is familiar and is convinced provide optimal performance. In general, carbohydrates (bread, pasta, rice) should be the major constituent of the pregame meal, which should be taken 2 1/2 to 4 hours before competing. Carbohydrates are easy to digest and provide energy most quickly and efficiently. In addition, it is important that an athlete does not miss meals or eat a great deal shortly before competing.

Road Trips

The location of the competition may also pose a problem: It is difficult to sustain nutritionally balanced and sound eating habits on road trips or away from home anywhere. Difficulties include limited food budget, time constraints, restaurant availability, and unfamiliar foods. The key to effectively managing the situa-

Table 13–4. How to Select the Diet For You*

Food Groups	*Basic Diet*	*Training Diet*	*Carbohydrate-Loading Diet*
Appropriate for:	Athletes during off season Endurance athletes on the first 4 days of carbohydrate loading Anyone, as a weight loss diet	Athletes throughout the training season	Endurance athletes 3 days before competition
Recommended daily servings			
Milk: Milk, cheese, yogurt, cottage cheese, ice cream	Teenagers: ≥4 Adults: ≥2	Teenagers: ≥2 Adults: ≥4	Teenagers: 4–5 Adults: 2–3
Meats: Meat, fish, poultry, eggs, dry beans and peas, nuts	≥2	≥2	2–3
Fruits/vegetables: Fresh, frozen, canned, dried, and juiced fruits and vegetables; vitamin A, vitamin C	≥4	≥8	≥8
Grains: Cereals, breads, rolls, pastas, muffins, pancakes, grits; carbohydrates, thiamine, iron, niacin	≥4	≥8	≥12

*As an athlete you need about 50 nutrients for top performance. You can get these nutrients by including the recommended number of servings daily from each food group and by choosing a variety of foods from within each food group. The most important nutrient supplied by each food group is listed with each group. See Chapter 14 for serving sizes.

tion is, simply, to plan ahead. The Sports Science Exchange (Gatorade Sports Science Institute) provides information on menu items at fast-food restaurants that are readily available to meet the needs of traveling athletes so they can adhere to fundamental nutrition principles:

1. The serving guidelines from the four–food group pyramid are the framework for food selection.
2. Servings can be adjusted to meet energy needs with extra servings derived predominantly from the grains, fruits, and vegetables, not from the meat group.
3. The athlete must maintain a balance of 60% carbohydrates, 25% fat, and 15% protein.

Before the Event

In the last 15 to 30 minutes before exercising, it is probably best to avoid simple carbohydrates such as candy bars or simple sugars, especially for athletes susceptible to hyperglycemia. While the athlete remains inactive, the increased blood insulin level may have little effect. But once competition begins, the muscles become quite sensitive and the rapid influx of glycogen into muscle and the decrease in the blood sugar level will create a condition of fatigue and compromised performance.

Doubleheaders and tournament competition pose special problems. Playing back-to-back games can drain a player's energy (glycogen and fluid stores) and cause dehydration, especially in hot weather. The two most important considerations are fluid replacement and energy maintenance. Both goals can be accomplished by ingesting one of the various sports drinks. Formulated to enhance fluid replacement, they restore both fluid and carbohydrates. They can be drunk during competition as well as between and after contests. Some athletes feel the need for solid food between games, to offset hunger, emptiness, or weakness. Such persons can benefit from eating a candy bar or a "power bar." Power bars tend to be expensive, protein-rich, high-carbohydrate, low-fat foodstuffs that contain any of a variety of nutrients (vitamins/minerals).

Performance Supplements and Weight Gain Powders

To supplement is defined as to bring closer to the desired state. Research has shown that, when certain substances are taken at the appropriate times and in appropriate amounts, improved performance and increased body mass can be realized. Very often, supplements are expensive alternatives to good dietary consumption. Many athletes succumb to the advertisements of power improvement for every sport and for everyone. The "omnipotent" sports powder would be too expensive to be made commercially available, and since the optimal supplement would have to compensate for so much individual variability, it is unlikely that one will ever be formulated. Recent investigations have shown that protein needs are higher for endurance and strength athletes than for less active persons. While protein supplements are not *necessary*, some athletes find that protein powders help them to increase their protein consumption. Certain milk protein–based powders can be an effective means of increasing protein consumption without consuming a lot of fat. This is particularly true of dried milk. Athletes are encouraged to get their protein from dietary sources; however, some protein foods (e.g., fatty meats and whole milk cheese) are "rich" in fat.

In general, protein powders can enhance an athlete's dietary protein intake. In the past, these substances were commonly used by athletes who wanted to increase their muscle mass, usually body builders and weight lifters.

Powders ingested in the form of drinks can provide a highly assimilable, balanced mixture of amino acids, but it should be noted that it is important to use products that have additional co-factors and coenzymes that the body needs to use these amino acids and nutrient substances. It is also important to use high-quality multivitamins and mineral formulations designed for athletes, because these substances will assist the body generate maximum energy from foodstuffs, promote and enhance the immune system, and protect the body from deficiencies that are common in the diets of many players. The critical ingredients and features of some currently available commercial products are presented in Table 13–5.

Protein powders and weight gainers are formulated for convenience. They provide carbohydrates and protein and a complete spectrum of RDA vitamins and minerals. In essence, they are expensive vitamin-food complexes. They include Metabol and Protabalase. On the other hand, the currently publicized category of "Stuffs"—Real Strong Stuff, Hot Stuff, and Right Stuff—are great protein sources but lack carbohydrates and fat. They have essentially the same amount of protein as 6 to 7 ounces of meat. But the cost of Hot Stuff is equivalent to 4 to 5 pounds of good-quality steak. The common denominator of these products is that they are said to improve testosterone or growth hormone production. This is especially true of Orchic (testicle gland), Smilax, and Yohimbee Bark. While these ingredients may be used in a laboratory setting to produce testosterone, humans lack the enzyme system necessary to convert these sterols to steroids. Boron is worth mentioning, because this trace mineral is proposed to promote testosterone release, but the levels required would be toxic.

The weight gainers category of supplements is for people who do not have the opportunity to eat because of limited time or lack of a microwave or refrigerator. Other athletes at risk include those without the urge to eat (e.g., an athlete working construction in the summertime who loses his appetite because of the heat), those who were recently ill and therefore lost weight, or those who desire greater muscle mass. At a cost of approximately $20 to $40 per week, these products are expensive sources of calories (Table 13–6).

Table 13–5. Comparison of General Supplements

	Hot Stuff	*Metabolol II*	*Protabalase-EM*	*Right Stuff*
Manufacturer	National Health Products	Champion Nutrition	Cybergenics	Strength Systems USA Labs
Net weight per container	1 lb (454 g)	1 lb (454 g)	1.85 lb (840 g)	2.2 lb (998 g)
Ounces per serving	3.0 oz (86 g)	2.3 oz (66 g)	2.1 oz. (60 g)	2.5 oz. (70 g)
Servings per container	5.3	7	14	14
Cost per container*	$25.99	$17.99	$24.99	$36.98
Cost per serving	$4.90	$2.14	$1.78	$2.64
Cost per ounce	$1.62	$.93	$.96	$1.14
Cost per week	$34.30	$14.98	$13.44	$18.50
Calories per serving	320	260	220	200
Calories per ounce	106.7	130	110	80
Protein per serving (g)	60	20	16	50
Protein per ounce (g)	20	8.7	8	20
Carbohydrate per serving (g)	13	40gm	38	0
Carbohydrate per ounce (g)	4	17.4	19	0
Fat per serving (g)	2	2	2	0
Fat per ounce (g)	0.7	0.87	1	0
Nutrients per ounce				
Vitamins				
A (IU)		2500	1250	
B_1 (mg)		0.76	0.48	
B_2 (mg)		0.86	0.42	
B_6 (mg)		1.04	0.58	4
B_{12} (μg)		6	420	
C (mg)		30	30	10
D (IU)		200	90	
E (IU)		15.2	8.25	
Biotin (μg)			82.5	
Choline (mg)		150mg	0.050	
Folic Acid (μg)		200	100	
Inositol (mg)		150	25	
L-Carnitine (mg)	25	32.6	5	20
Niacin (mg)		10	41.5	
PABA				
Pantothenic acid (mg)		5	17.5	
Minerals				
Boron (mg)	1			1.2
Calcium (mg)		217.3	125	
Chromium (μg)	83	130.4	75	80
Copper (mg)		0.5	.5	
Iodine (mg)		23	12.5	
Iron (mg)		4.3	1	
Magnesium (mg)	83	173.9	62.5	80
Manganese (μg)		1.73	1000	
Molybdenum (μg)		43.4	25	
Phosphorus				
Potassium (mg)	66	240	150	79.2
Selenium (μg)		21.7	15	
Sodium				
Zinc (mg)	5	15	2.5	

*Cost data collected in Wilmington, DE, 1993.

SPECIAL PROBLEMS

Weight Control

Total food intake is measured in calories. Scientifically speaking, a calorie is the amount of heat required to raise the temperature of 1 kg of water 1°C. Nutritionally speaking, calories are the currency one must take in and save to gain weight or spend to lose weight. One pound of body weight contains about 3500 calories of energy. To gain a pound, one must take in and store that many calories over and above the daily need. Conversely, to lose a pound, one must burn or spend 3500 calories that are stored in the body. All carbohydrate, fat, and protein foods contain calories; water, minerals, and vitamins do not. Carbohydrates and protein contain 4 calories per gram whereas fat contains approximately 9 calories per gram.

Body weight is a function of genetics, diet, and the intensity and duration of sports training; however, the operable range of body fat varies with the demands of each sport. In most sports, fat contributes no strength, limits endurance and speed, and increases the likelihood of injury. Performance is also limited if there is an insufficient amount of body fat. One notices an

Table 13–6. Comparison of Weight Gain Formulations

	Gainer's Fuel 1000	*Infinity 1700*	*Mega Mass 2000*	*Perfect 1100*	*Weight Gainer 1850*
Manufacturer	Twin-Lab	Cybergenics	Weider	Nature's Best	Pro-Performance
Net weight per container	4.36 lb (1978 g)	3.15 lb (1431 g)	104 oz (2953 g)	7 lb (3171 g)	4 lb (1814 g)
Weight per serving	7 oz (197.4 g)	10.08 oz (285.7 g)	4.9 oz (140.6 g)	7.5 oz (214.5 g)	13.5 oz (383.4 g)
Servings per container	10	5	21	15	5
Cost per container*	$30.00	$29.00	$34.99	$37.00	$28.00
Cost per serving	$3.00	$5.80	$1.60	$2.46	$5.60
Cost per ounce	$0.42	$.57	$.32	$.33	$.41
Cost per week	$21.00	$40.60	$11.20	$16.52	$39.20
Calories per serving	700	1090	550	800	1500
Calories per ounce	100	109	110	106.7	111
Protein per serving (g)	30	40	27	35	50
Protein per ounce (g)	4.2	4	5.4	4.7	3.7
Carbohydrate per serving (g)	145	219	106	165	322
Carbohydrate per ounce (g)	20.7	22	21.2	22	238
Fat per serving (g)	<1	6	2	<1	<1
Fat per ounce (g)	<1	0.6	.4	<1	<1

*Cost data collected in Wilmington, DE, 1993.

increased number of musculotendinous injuries in athletes who have less than 5% or more than 15% body fat.

A certain amount of fat is essential to maintain a healthy body. The average male has 15 to 18% body fat and the average female, 25 to 28% body fat. A nutritionist or trainer can best measure body fat and help determine the ideal range. It is through monitoring percentage of body fat that reasonable guidelines can be offered for weight-dependent athletic competitions. It is recommended that growing athletes have no less than 7% body fat and for skeletally mature male athletes no less than 5%.

Athletes can safely lose 1 to 2 pounds of body fat per week, even when they are training. If they lose weight faster than 1 to 2 pounds a week, they can begin to break down muscle, and that harms their training performance. If a more rapid weight loss is desired, supplementation, in the form of amino acid complex, is recommended. Players should not restrict energy intake during growth periods; instead, they should be encouraged to maintain—or even increase—their weight.

To gain weight, energy output must be less than energy intake. Athletes must increase the calorie consumption over their expenditure. The goal is to increase lean body mass, and the diet must contain extra calories. There are several ways to increase the number of calories. One can eat larger portions at meals, eat more meals per day, snack between meals, or use one of several very expensive, high-calorie weight gain formulas. Further weight gain can be realized by substituting high-calorie foods for low-calorie ones, although one must remember that some high-calorie foods are nutrient poor. To supply the body with all the nutrients it needs, the following foods are found to be high in both calories and nutrients: nuts, dried fruit, milk and milkshake products, cheese, meat, pizza, and powdered weight gain products. A scale will serve to show how much weight is gained, but it is more important to determine percentage of body fat to be sure that gains are in lean body mass (muscle).

Anorexia Nervosa

Dietary practices of gymnasts and figure skaters often include poor nutrition habits that lead to reduced bone density and a factitious elevation of the percentage of body fat, reinforcing their self-perceived need to starve themselves. The American Psychiatric Association defines *anorexia nervosa* as the refusal to maintain a normal predicted body weight for height, intense fear of gaining weight or fat, a distorted body image, and amenorrhea. Most times, affected athletes are intelligent overachievers who demonstrate extreme discipline. They often have guilt associated with their family's total commitment to their achievement in their selected sport. Distinguishing features of anorexia have been offered by leaders in the field of nutrition disorders: aimless physical activity, poor or decreasing exercise performance, poor muscle development, flawed body image, body fat levels below normal range, electrolyte abnormalities, dry skin, cardiac arrhythmias, hirsutism, and leukocyte dysfunction. This disorder can be fatal, and, once recognized, requires a therapeutic plan involving the athlete, family members, and coaches.

Bulimia

While most wrestlers realize that precompetition weight loss can best be achieved through dieting and perspiration, others engage in the practice of purging. *Bulimia* is an act of excessive eating followed by a method of purging, either by vomiting or taking cathartics. Some authors report the prevalence of bulimia to be 20% for college students and 2 to 3% in the general population. Unfortunately, some wrestlers engage in this practice seasonally and some female athletes do it all the time to control their distorted body image.

Lactose (Milk) Intolerance

Many athletes, especially those of Mediterranean descent, lack the digestive enzyme lactase. When they ingest milk products, explosive diarrhea may result. This problem can be simply remedied by supplementing milk beverage or food products with the enzyme lactase in the form of tablets or powder. The purpose of this is to avoid calcium deficiency, since milk products are well known to be rich in calcium. If lactase tablets or powders are unsuccessful or inconvenient, calcium supplements are available in the form of calcium, chelated calcium, or calcium citrate. While known to be important to growing bones and functioning muscles, calcium deficiency was also recently recognized to be an underlying cause of hypertension.

Diabetes

Some coaches will have to recognize the signs and symptoms of insulin overload and hypoglycemia. They include confusion, weakness, unconsciousness, and convulsions. The athlete should always have ready access to sugar drinks and hard candies. Current recommendations for diabetic athletes center around control of daily insulin requirements through diet as opposed to adjusting the insulin for exercise and competition. In general, well-controlled, Type I, insulin-dependent diabetic athletes need not restrict physical activity. They must, however, regularly monitor their blood glucose level and maintain consistent eating habits and insulin injection schedules.

Hypertension

Many senior players and coaches have blood pressure problems and require daily medications. This is particularly true of players during the off season, but regular exercise and more controlled living standards during the season have often reduced the need for, or the amount of, such medication. Despite recommending controlled salt intake as part of the hypertension protocol, the same recommendations for electrolyte and fluid replacement are maintained.

SUGGESTED READINGS

MICRONUTRIENTS

Berning, J. R., and Steen, S. N. (eds.): Sports Nutrition for the 90s: The Health Professional's Handbook. Gaithersburg, MD, Aspen, 1991.

Keith, R. E.: Vitamins in sport and exercise. *In* Nutrition in Exercise and Sports. Edited by I. Wolinsky and J. F. Hickson, Jr. Boca Raton, FL, CRC, 1989.

CARBOHYDRATES/CARBOHYDRATE LOADING

Sherman, W., Costil, D. L., Fink, W. J., and Miller, J. M.: The effects of exercise and diet manipulation on muscle glycogen and its subsequent use during performance. Int. J. Sports Med. *2*:114, 1981.

Williams, M.: Nutrition in Fitness and Sport. 3rd Ed. Dubuque, IA, William C. Brown, 1992.

PROTEIN/BRANCHED-CHAIN AMINO ACIDS

Laritcheva, K. A., Yolavaya, N. I., Shubin, V. I., and Smirnov, D. V.: Study of energy expenditure and protein needs of top weightlifters. *In* Nutrition, Physical Fitness and Health. Edited by J. Parizkova, and V. A. Rogozkin. Baltimore, MD, University Park, 1978.

Walser, M.: Role of branched-chain keto acids in protein metabolism. Kidney Int. *38*:595, 1990.

FATS/TRIGLYCERIDES

Hegstead, D. M., et al. (eds.): Present Knowledge in Nutrition. 4th Ed. New York, Nutrition Foundation, 1976.

REHYDRATION/ELECTROLYTE DRINKS

Murray, R.: The effects of consuming carbohydrate-electrolyte beverages on gastric emptying and fluid absorption during and following exercise. Sports Med. *4*:322, 1987.

Owen, M. D., Kregel, K. C., Wall, P. T., and Gisolfi, C. V.: Effects of ingesting carbohydrate beverages during exercise in the heat. Med. Sci. Sports Exerc. *18*:568, 1986.

Pivornik, J. M.: Water and electrolytes during exercise. *In* Nutrition in Exercise and Sport. Edited by J. F. Hickson and I. Wolinsky. Boca Raton, FL, CRC, 1989.

TRAINING DIET/PRE-EVENT EATING

Coogan, A. R., and Coyle, E. F.: Effect of carbohydrate feedings during high intensity exercise. J. Appl. Physiol. *65*:1703, 1988.

Ivy, J. et al: Muscle glycogen synthesis after exercise: Effect of time of carbohydrate ingestion. J. Appl. Physiol. *64*:1480, 1988.

SUPPLEMENTS

Dubick, M.: Dietary supplements and health aids: A critical evaluation. III. Natural and miscellaneous products. J. Nutr. Educ. *14*:4, 1983.

Dubick, M., and Rucker, R. B.: Dietary supplements and health aids: A critical evaluation. I. Vitamins and minerals. J. Nutr. Educ. *15*:2, 1983.

WEIGHT CONTROL/WEIGHT LOSS

Brodie, D. A.: Techniques of measurement of body composition. Sports Med. *5*:11, 1988.

Lohman, T. G.: Body composition assessment in sports medicine. Sports Med. Digest *12*:1, 1990.

ANOREXIA/BULIMIA

Garkinel, P. E., and Garner, D. M.: Anorexia Nervosa: A Multidimensional Perspective. New York, Brunner/Mazel, 1982.
Story, M.: Nutrition management and dietary treatment of bulimia. J. Am. Diet. Assoc. *86*:517, 1986.

DIABETES

Franz, M.: Diabetes and Exercise; How to Get Started. Minneapolis, MN, Park Nicollete Medical Foundation, 1989.
Zinman, B., and Vranic, M.: Diabetes and exercise. Med. Clin. North Am. *69*:145, 1985.

14 *William Etchison*

Body Composition

Webster defines *obesity* as a condition characterized by excessive body fat. In Webster's definition, there is no reference to obesity as a condition characterized by excessive body *weight;* yet, the average person believes that obesity is determined by scale weight. The question then becomes, How do we determine excess fat, and what are optimal fat levels for nonathletes and athletes?

Fat is defined as adipose tissue that forms soft pads between various organs of the body and serves to smooth and round body contours and furnish a reserve supply of energy.[1] Fat is classified as either essential (physiologically necessary) or storage. Men need about 3% essential fat whereas women need about 10%. Sex-related fat deposits create the essential fat difference between men and women. Without the essential fat, health deteriorates. Fat is primarily found in the subcutaneous adipose tissue and the tissue surrounding the major organs of the body. Its function is explained in the aforementioned definition. The sum of essential fat and storage fat equals total body fat.[2]

For years, practitioners have determined weight parameters by scale weight, which equals the sum of fat, muscle, bone, and water. This was compared with height charts and size of body frame (small, medium, or large) to determine if a person was underweight or overweight. True ideal weight can be determined only by assessing how much of the body is composed of fat and how much is lean weight. When this is accomplished, the term *overweight* may not mean overfat and *underweight* may not mean underfat. Cases of extremes include a 314-pound football lineman who has 14% body fat compared with a petite, small-framed woman who has 30% body fat.

TECHNIQUES FOR MEASURING BODY FAT

Many of the techniques available for determining body fat are not practical for use by the average health-care practitioner. Some of the more exotic ways to determine body fat include chemical analysis of cadavers, helium dilution, radiographic analysis, K-40 (potassium) counting, total body water, and ultrasonography.[3] We will discuss three of the more commonly used techniques: (1) hydrostatic, or underwater weighing, a laboratory technique that requires special equipment, (2) bioimpedance, and (3) anthropometry, which is the use of skeletal diameters, circumferences, and skin folds. These techniques are used by exercise physiologists, health educators, athletic trainers, and various practitioners of sports medicine.

Hydrostatic Weighing

Hydrostatic weighing requires special equipment such as a large tank of water with a secured weighing cable suspended over the tank or a load cell system built into an underwater chair used for weight measurement.[3] The water must be chemically controlled, filtered, and heated for the health, safety, and comfort of the individual. This technique, generally confined to laboratory situations, is not cost effective and consumes a significant amount of time. If not performed carefully, hydrostatic weighing is subject to gross error.[3]

Hydrostatic weighing is based on the principle that fat is less dense than water and floats. Bone and muscle are more dense than water and sink. In other words, someone who has a large amount of body fat will float, or weigh less, in water than someone who has a large proportion of muscle tissue. To determine the percentage of body fat by hydrostatic weighing, it is necessary to know the individual's weight in the air (in kilograms), weight in water (in kilograms), density of the water at the temperature when the body is submerged, and the residual volume (volume of air left in the body after exhalation).[4]

$$\text{Body volume} = \frac{\text{Air weight} - \text{Water weight}}{\text{Water density}}$$

$$\text{Body density} = \frac{\text{Air weight}}{\text{Body volume} - \text{Residual volume}}$$

$$\text{Body fat \%} = 100 \times \left(\frac{4.570 - 4.142}{\text{Body density}}\right)$$

Bioimpedance

Thomas used bioelectric impedance to determine body composition in the 1960s and 1970s. A two-needle electrode technique was used to determine total body water and extracellular fluid. Patients resisted this technique because they did not want needles inserted into their muscles. Today's techniques use an electrode system that involves two electrodes placed on the back of the hand and wrist and two electrodes on the top of the foot at the tarsals and metatarsals.

Bioelectric impedance is based on the principle that free fatty mass has a much greater electrolyte content, and therefore far greater conductivity, than fatty tissue.[5] The estimation of body fat is based on this conduction principle. This can be a costly technique. Bioimpedance machines range in cost up to $5000 (Fig. 14–1). Accuracy could be affected by the subject's hydration status. There is evidence to indicate that, in young lean males, body fat percentage is overpredicted.[5]

Anthropometry

Anthropometry is the measurement of skin folds, skeletal diameter, and body girth.[3] Skin fold measurements require the use of hand-held calipers. Some of the more popular calipers are Skyndex (Caldwell Justice & Co., Inc, Fayetteville, Ark.), Lange (Cambridge Scientific Industries, Cambridge, Md.), and Harpenden (H. E. Morse Co., Holland, Mich.). Skyndex calipers are programmed to automatically calculate the percentage of fat. Lange and Harpenden calipers require the use of a nomogram, mathematical calculations, or estimated fat percentage tables based on the sum of various skin folds to determine fat (Tables 14–1 and 14–2) [2] If nomograms are used, the test populations must match the reference group.

Sites most commonly used to determine body fat are in the subscapular, triceps, axilla (armpit), chest, biceps, iliac crest, abdominal, and thigh areas (Fig. 14–2).[6] To perform this technique, the examiner grasps the skin firmly between the thumb and the index finger and pulls it slightly away from the muscle. The calipers are applied one-half inch below the pinch site, and the skin is measured in millimeters.[7]

In our health screening, we use the Skyndex caliper preprogrammed with the Jackson-Pollock formula. (There are several other formulas.) This formula requires the measurement of three sites on men: the chest is measured at a 45° angle between the lateral border of the pectoralis major and the armpit, the abdomen is measured vertically alongside the navel, and the thigh is measured vertically on the front of the thigh, halfway between the hip and the kneecap. Women's measurements are as follows: the triceps is measured vertically on the back of the arm halfway between the shoulder and the elbow, the iliac crest (suprailiac) is measured at a 45° angle on top of the crest in line with the armpit, and the thigh measurement is taken as for men.[7] If preprogrammed calipers are not available, the sum of the three sites is used (see Tables 14–1, 14–2).[1] Other measures of body fat include measuring skeletal diameters and body girth.

A simple field evaluation for predicting body fat for men without using calipers is this: The waist is measured at the navel and the wrist circumference just in front of

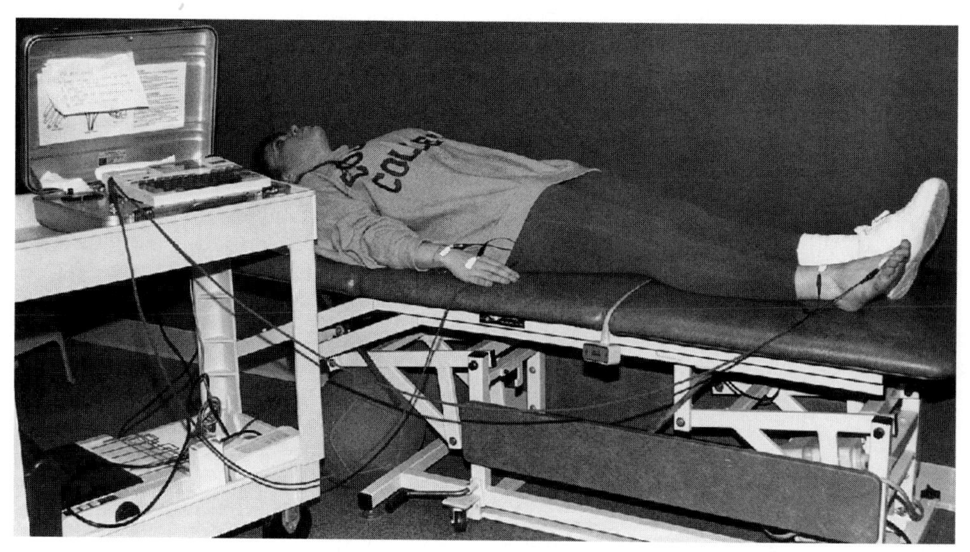

Fig. 14–1. Bioimpedance testing.

Table 14–1. Percent Fat Estimates for Women

Sum of 3 Skin Folds	*Age to the Last Year*								
	Under 22	*23 to 27*	*28 to 32*	*33 to 37*	*38 to 42*	*43 to 47*	*48 to 52*	*53 to 57*	*Over 58*
23-25	9.7	9.9	10.2	10.4	10.7	10.9	11.2	11.4	11.7
26-28	11.0	11.2	11.5	11.7	12.0	12.3	12.5	12.7	13.0
29-31	12.3	12.5	12.8	13.0	13.3	13.5	13.8	14.0	14.3
32-34	13.6	13.8	14.0	14.3	14.5	14.8	15.0	15.3	15.5
35-37	14.8	15.0	15.3	15.5	15.8	16.0	16.3	16.5	16.8
38-40	16.0	16.3	16.5	16.7	17.0	17.2	17.5	17.7	18.0
41-43	17.2	17.4	17.7	17.9	18.2	18.4	18.7	18.9	19.2
44-46	18.3	18.6	18.8	19.1	19.3	19.6	19.8	20.1	20.3
47-49	19.5	19.7	20.0	20.2	20.5	20.7	21.0	21.2	21.5
50-52	20.6	20.8	21.1	21.3	21.6	21.8	22.1	22.3	22.6
53-55	21.7	21.9	22.1	22.4	22.6	22.9	23.1	23.4	23.6
56-58	22.7	23.0	23.2	23.4	23.7	23.9	24.2	24.4	24.7
59-61	23.7	24.0	24.2	24.5	24.7	25.0	25.2	25.5	25.7
62-64	24.7	25.0	25.2	25.5	25.7	26.0	26.2	26.4	26.7
65-67	25.7	25.9	26.2	26.4	26.7	26.9	27.2	27.4	27.7
68-70	26.6	26.9	27.1	27.4	27.6	27.9	28.1	28.4	28.6
71-73	27.5	27.8	28.0	28.3	28.5	28.8	29.0	29.3	29.5
74-76	28.4	28.7	28.9	29.2	29.4	29.7	29.9	30.2	30.4
77-79	29.3	29.5	29.8	30.0	30.3	30.5	30.8	31.0	31.3
80-82	30.1	30.4	30.6	30.9	31.1	31.4	31.6	31.9	32.1
83-85	30.9	31.2	31.4	31.7	31.9	32.2	32.4	32.7	32.9
86-88	31.7	32.0	32.2	32.5	32.7	32.9	33.2	33.4	33.7
89-91	32.5	32.7	33.0	33.2	33.5	33.7	33.9	34.2	34.4
92-94	33.2	33.4	33.7	33.9	34.2	34.4	34.7	34.9	35.2
95-97	33.9	34.1	34.4	34.6	34.9	35.1	35.4	35.6	35.9
98-100	34.6	34.8	35.1	35.3	35.5	35.8	36.0	36.3	36.5
101-103	35.2	35.4	35.7	35.9	36.2	36.4	36.7	36.9	37.2
104-106	35.8	36.1	36.3	36.6	36.8	37.1	37.3	37.5	37.8
107-109	36.4	36.7	36.9	37.1	37.4	37.6	37.9	38.1	38.4
110-112	37.0	37.2	37.5	37.7	38.0	38.2	38.5	38.7	38.9
113-115	37.5	37.8	38.0	38.2	38.5	38.7	39.0	39.2	39.5
116-118	38.0	38.3	38.5	38.8	39.0	39.3	39.5	39.7	40.0
119-121	38.5	38.7	39.0	39.2	39.5	39.7	40.0	40.2	40.5
122-124	39.0	39.2	39.4	39.7	39.9	40.2	40.4	40.7	40.9
125-127	39.4	39.6	39.9	40.1	40.4	40.6	40.9	41.1	41.4
128-130	39.8	40.0	40.3	40.5	40.8	41.0	41.3	41.5	41.8

Body density calculated based on the generalized equation for predicting body density of women developed by A. S. Jackson, M. L. Pollock, and A. Ward. Medicine and Science in Sports and Exercise. *12*:175–182, 1980. Percent body fat determined from the calculated body density using the Siri formula. (Hoeger, W. W. K.: Lifetime Physical Fitness and Wellness. Englewood, CO, Morton, 1986.)

the wrist bones, where the wrist bends. The wrist measurement is subtracted from the waist measurement and the examiner refers to the conversion chart based on the Penrose-Nelson-Fisher equations.[8] For example, if the waist circumference is 32 inches and the wrist circumference is 7 inches, the difference would be 25 inches. If the person weighs 160 pounds, the chart shows he has about 11% body fat.[8] Interestingly, we compared the Penrose-Nelson-Fisher equation with actual skin fold measurements and were right on target, within 1% either way. Women's measurements for percentage of body fat take a little more effort on the part of the tester, who measures the hips at their maximum girth, the abdomen at the navel, and the height in inches. These measurements are then plugged into a computation table to find the constant value. The hip constant plus the abdominal constant minus the height gives the percentage of body fat (Table 14–3).[8]

LEVELS OF BODY FAT

The American College of Sports Medicine has set some recommended body fat levels for men and women.[3] As a general rule, 16 to 18% is acceptable for men of all ages and 22 to 26% for women. Once men exceed 22%, they should be on a weight loss program, and once women reach 30% or more, they should be working on weight loss. In studies done on the athletic population in Columbus, Ga., we found that girls 12 to 18 years old maintain 20% body fat. Boys maintain around 12% until they reach 18 years old, when the percentage drops to 10.4%.[9] Jacko and coworkers[10] did a study on all-star high school football players and found the following percentages of body fat: linemen, 17.4% (± 7.4%); tightends and linebackers, 11.9% (± 3.4%); offensive backs, 11.9% (± 6%); defensive backs and wide receivers, 8.8% (± 1.7%); and punters and place kickers,

Table 14–2. Percent Fat Estimates for Men Under 40

	Age to the Last Year							
Sum of 3 Skinfolds	*Under 19*	*20 to 22*	*23 to 25*	*26 to 28*	*29 to 31*	*32 to 34*	*35 to 37*	*38 to 40*
8-10	.9	1.3	1.6	2.0	2.3	2.7	3.0	3.3
11-13	1.9	2.3	2.6	3.0	3.3	3.7	4.0	4.3
14-16	2.9	3.3	3.6	3.9	4.3	4.6	5.0	5.3
17-19	3.9	4.2	4.6	4.9	5.3	5.6	6.0	6.3
20-22	4.8	5.2	5.5	5.9	6.2	6.6	6.9	7.3
23-25	5.8	6.2	6.5	6.8	7.2	7.5	7.9	8.2
26-28	6.8	7.1	7.5	7.8	8.1	8.5	8.8	9.2
29-31	7.7	8.0	8.4	8.7	9.1	9.4	9.8	10.1
32-34	8.6	9.0	9.3	9.7	10.0	10.4	10.7	11.1
35-37	9.5	9.9	10.2	10.6	10.9	11.3	11.6	12.0
38-40	10.5	10.8	11.2	11.5	11.8	12.2	12.5	12.9
41-43	11.4	11.7	12.1	12.4	12.7	13.1	13.4	13.8
44-46	12.2	12.6	12.9	13.3	13.6	14.0	14.3	14.7
47-49	13.1	13.5	13.8	14.2	14.5	14.9	15.2	15.5
50-52	14.0	14.3	14.7	15.0	15.4	15.7	16.1	16.4
53-55	14.8	15.2	15.5	15.9	16.2	16.6	16.9	17.3
56-58	15.7	16.0	16.4	16.7	17.1	17.4	17.8	18.1
59-61	16.5	16.9	17.2	17.6	17.9	18.3	18.6	19.0
62-64	17.4	17.7	18.1	18.4	18.8	19.1	19.4	19.8
65-67	18.2	18.5	18.9	19.2	19.6	19.9	20.3	20.6
68-70	19.0	19.3	19.7	20.0	20.4	20.7	21.1	21.4
71-73	19.8	20.1	20.5	20.8	21.2	21.5	21.9	22.2
74-76	20.6	20.9	21.3	21.6	22.0	22.2	22.7	23.0
77-79	21.4	21.7	22.1	22.4	22.8	23.1	23.4	23.8
80-82	22.1	22.5	22.8	23.2	23.5	23.9	24.2	24.6
83-85	22.9	23.2	23.6	23.9	24.3	24.6	25.0	25.3
86-88	23.6	24.0	24.3	24.7	25.0	25.4	25.7	26.1
89-91	24.4	24.7	25.1	25.4	25.8	26.1	26.5	26.8
92-94	25.1	25.5	25.8	26.2	26.5	26.9	27.2	27.5
95-97	25.8	26.2	26.5	26.9	27.2	27.6	27.9	28.3
98-100	26.6	26.9	27.3	27.6	27.9	28.3	28.6	29.0
101-103	27.3	27.6	28.0	28.3	28.6	29.0	29.3	29.7
104-106	27.9	28.3	28.6	29.0	29.3	29.7	30.0	30.4
107-109	28.6	29.0	29.3	29.7	30.0	30.4	30.7	31.1
110-112	29.3	29.6	30.0	30.3	30.7	31.0	31.4	31.7
113-115	30.0	30.3	30.7	31.0	31.3	31.7	32.0	32.4
116-118	30.6	31.0	31.3	31.6	32.0	32.3	32.7	33.0
119-121	31.3	31.6	32.0	32.3	32.6	33.0	33.3	33.7
122-124	31.9	32.2	32.6	32.9	33.3	33.6	34.0	34.3
125-127	32.5	32.9	33.2	33.5	33.9	34.2	34.6	34.9
128-130	33.1	33.5	33.8	34.2	34.5	34.9	35.2	35.5

Body density calculated based on the generalized equation for predicting body density of men developed by A. S. Jackson and M. L. Pollock. British Journal of Nutrition *40*:497–504, 1978. Percent body fat determined from the calculated body density using the Siri formula. (Hoeger, W. W. K.: Lifetime Physical Fitness and Wellness. Englewood, CO, Morton, 1986.)

12.1% (± 5.8%). The following percentage of body fat values seem to be ideal for high school football players: offensive and defensive linemen, 18 to 20%; linebackers, 12 to 14%; defensive backs, 9 to 11%; offensive backs, 10 to 12%; and quarterbacks, 14%.

WEIGHT LOSS AND WEIGHT GAIN

Ideal Weight

Ideal weight is based on the percentage of desired fat. The formula for determining ideal weight is as follows[6]:

Percent fat × Current weight = Fat weight

Current weight − Fat weight = Lean weight

Ideal weight = Lean weight / (1.00 − Ideal percentage fat)

For example, John has 16% body fat, weighs 180 pounds, and is a linebacker. His ideal fat level is 12%. To find the ideal weight for 12%, apply the previous formula:

16% × 180 = 29 pounds

180 − 29 = 151 pounds

Ideal weight = 151/(1 − 12%) = 151/.88 = 172 pounds

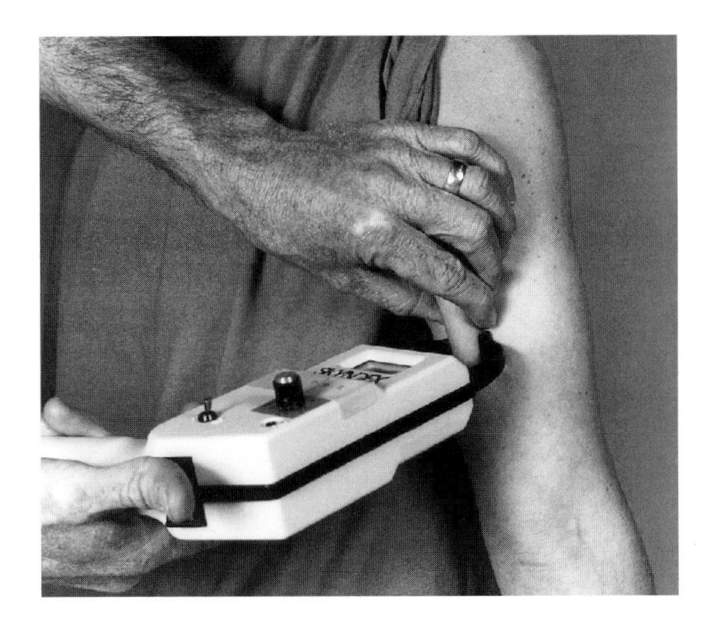

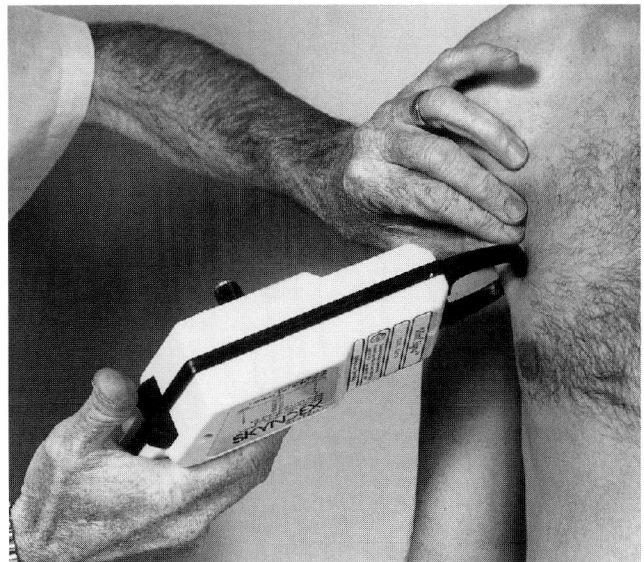

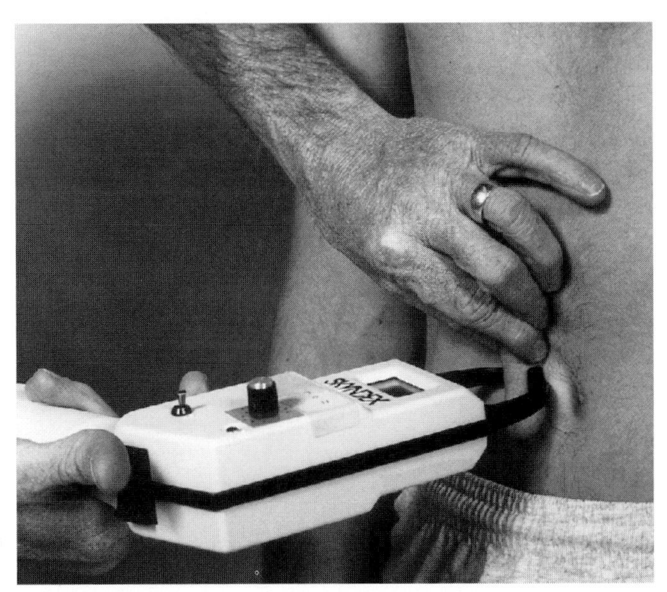

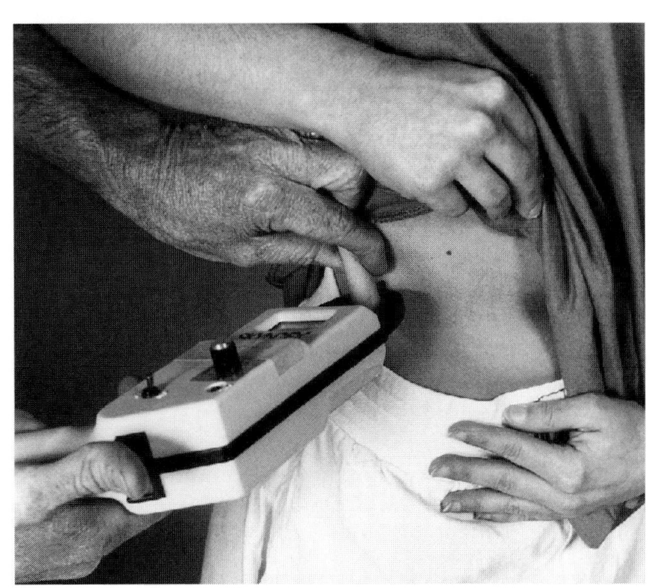

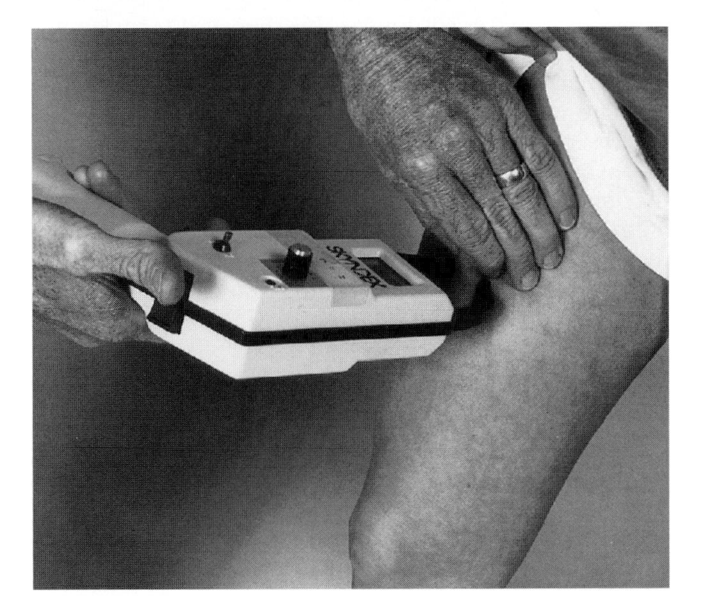

Fig. 14–2. Skin fold measurement sites. *(A)* Triceps: vertical fold on the upper arm over the triceps (midway between the shoulder and the elbow). *(B)* Chest: diagonal fold halfway between the anterior axillary line and the nipple. *(C)* Abdomen: Vertical fold about 1 inch from the navel. *(D)* Suprailium: diagonal fold above the crest of the ilium. *(E)* Thigh: vertical fold on the front of the thigh, midway between the hip and the knee.

Table 14–3. Conversion Constants to Predict Percent Body Fat for Women

Hips		Abdomen		Height	
In.	*Constant A*	*In.*	*Constant B*	*In.*	*Constant C*
30	33.48	20	14.22	55	33.52
31	34.87	21	14.93	56	34.13
32	36.27	22	15.64	57	34.74
33	37.67	23	16.35	58	35.35
34	39.06	24	17.06	59	35.96
35	40.46	25	17.78	60	36.57
36	41.86	26	18.49	61	37.18
37	43.25	27	19.20	62	37.79
38	44.65	28	19.91	63	38.40
39	46.05	29	20.62	64	39.01
40	47.44	30	21.33	65	39.62
41	48.84	31	22.04	66	40.23
42	50.24	32	22.75	67	40.84
43	51.64	33	23.46	68	41.45
44	53.03	34	24.18	69	42.06
45	54.43	35	24.89	70	42.67
46	55.83	36	25.60	71	43.28
47	57.22	37	26.31	72	43.89
48	58.62	38	27.02	73	44.50
49	60.02	39	27.73	74	45.11
50	61.42	40	28.44	75	45.72
51	62.81	41	29.15	76	46.32
52	64.21	42	29.87	77	46.93
53	65.61	43	30.58	78	47.54
54	67.00	44	31.29	79	48.15
55	68.40	45	32.00	80	48.76
56	69.80	46	32.71	81	49.37
57	71.19	47	33.42	82	49.98
58	72.59	48	34.13	83	50.59
59	73.99	49	34.84	84	51.20
60	75.39	50	35.56	85	51.81

(Fisher, A. G., and Conlee, R. K.: *The complete book of physical fitness,* Salt Lake City, Brigham Young University Press, 1979.)

The wave in weight loss today is counting fat grams. How many fat grams are required for John in the example above to maintain his ideal weight of 171 pounds? This is calculated as follows:

Ideal weight × 15 (15 calories per pound for active people) = 2,565 calories needed to maintain 171 pounds.

2,565 × 20% [recommended percentage of fat in diet] = 513 calories

513 ÷ 9 (9 calories/1 gram of fat) = 57 fat grams

Weight Gain

Many athletes are interested in gaining weight for contact sports. The key is to gain muscle and not fat. Therefore, increased eating of the proper food combined with weight training is the recommended mode. An ideal diet would be 65% carbohydrate, 15% protein, and 20% fat.[8] (Fats are more than twice as dense in calories as proteins and carbohydrates.) One gram of protein is equal to 4 calories, one gram of carbohydrate is 4 calories, and one gram of fat is 9 calories. So, fats are more than twice as calorie dense.

To gain 1 pound per week, you must consume 500 additional calories per day. (The calorie requirement of one pound of fat is 3500 calories, or 500 calories for 7 days.[11]) The average calorie requirement per pound of body weight based on activity patterns and sex is as follows[2]:

Men
- Sedentary 13.0
- Moderately physically active 15.0
- Very physically active 17.0

Women
- Sedentary 12.0
- Moderately physically active 13.5
- Very physically active 15.0

General nutrition guidelines are as follows[11]:

1. Keep a log of eating habits.
2. Do not skip meals.
3. Make nutritional food choices (i.e., choose foods from all the food groups)[12]:

   Milk and milk products 2–4 servings (serving = 1 cup) per day
   Fruits and vegetables 4–6 servings (serving = 1/2 cup) per day
   Breads and cereals 6–11 servings (serving = 1 slice or 1/2 cup of cereal) per day
   Meats 2–3 servings (serving = 1 ounce) per day

4. Eat three or more meals per day.
5. Eat high-calorie snacks between meals.
6. Eat complex carbohydrates.

Weight Loss

The fat thermostat theory is based on the principle that body fat is actually regulated in the brain by the hypothalamus. It is referred to as a kind of weight-regulating mechanism that actually chooses the amount of body fat it considers ideal for our needs and then works to protect it.[8] According to this theory, it turns on and off much as a thermostat would turn an air conditioner or furnace on and off. When we go on a very low-calorie diet we are sending a signal to our thermostat that it needs to protect our body. For example, if you have been overweight, your thermostat has become used to having that amount of body fat. If you go on an extremely low-calorie diet to lose weight, you generally become lethargic, tired, and irritable. These feelings occur because your regulating mechanism is very efficient. It is slowing your body function down to try and protect that body fat, which explains why it is very hard to starve yourself to death. The thermostat has a set point, and this set point is affected by what we eat and by our activity level. It will either conserve energy or waste energy.[8]

The danger of very low-calorie diets is that protein can be converted into sugar much more quickly than fat can. The body cannot utilize fat rapidly enough because it is such a long carbon chain compound, so it converts muscle tissue. Initially, some weight is lost but that eventually levels off, and the lost weight is mostly muscle. How can the fat thermostat be made to work properly? There are seven guidelines[8]:

1. Decrease fat consumption to 20% of total calories.
2. Reduce the refined carbohydrates or sugars in your diet (e.g., pies, cakes, candy, white flour, etc.).
3. Increase complex carbohydrates, such as whole grains, vegetables, and fruits.
4. Decrease consumption of calorie-containing fluids.
5. Drink adequate amounts of water.
6. Eat in harmony with one's weight-regulating mechanism.
7. Exercise aerobically.

To eat in harmony with the weight-regulating mechanism one must get in touch with eating drives. First, regular meals should be taken at least three times a day, and at one of those meals the diner should eat enough food to produce complete satiety.[8] To lose weight with an exercise program, it is necessary to exercise at least three times a week, and preferably five times at 60 to 70% of maximum heart rate for a minimum of 30 minutes. For maximum weight loss, at least 60 minutes of a continuous aerobic activity is recommended.[8] Aerobic activities include walking, jogging, swimming, hiking, bicycling, and aerobic dance (any large–muscle group activity).

Eating Disorders

One of the more common eating disorders, especially in young women, is anorexia nervosa. Anorexia nervosa is characterized by an overwhelming desire to get ever thinner. The person suffering from this disorder has an exaggerated fear of weight gain that harms her health. Coaches and trainers need to keep a close eye on these athletes, especially gymnasts and long-distance runners. They are typically intelligent, very self-disciplined, and from middle- and upper-class homes. Two common characteristics are a lack of self-confidence and low self-esteem. Signs of anorexia are excessive exercise, rapid weight loss, dry mottled reddish-purple skin, tiredness in workouts, dehydration, decreased sweating responses, brittle nails, hypotension, and Raynaud's phenomenon.[13]

Bulimia, another disorder of girls and young women, is characterized by ingestion of large quantities of food in a short period of time (bingeing) and then vomiting or taking laxatives (purging). This disorder often makes the individuals exhibit contempt for themselves. It is a very dangerous syndrome. Attempts to lose weight by severe diet restriction follow periods of binge eating. Persons with this problem are found to be frequent abusers of laxatives, alcohol, amphetamines, and sometimes cocaine. They have rapid fluctuations in weight. Fifty percent of anorexics become bulimic and 50% of bulimics become anorexic. Physical findings include hypokalemia, bradycardia, arrhythmias due to electrolyte imbalance, dehydration, bruising over the knuckles, dental caries, and fatigue.[13]

CONCLUSION

There are many ways to assess body composition, and although none is totally accurate, many are usable for the health-care practitioner or coach. The most important thing is to follow a generally accepted protocol and be consistent with it in the evaluation process.

REFERENCES

1. Dorland's Illustrated Medical Dictionary. 26th Ed. Philadelphia, W. B. Saunders, 1985.
2. Hoeger, W. W. K.: Lifetime Physical Fitness and Wellness. Englewood, CO, Morton, 1986.
3. American College of Sports Medicine Resource Manual for Guidelines for Exercise Testing and Prescription. Philadelphia, Lea & Febiger, 1988.
4. Brozek, J., et al.: Densitometric analysis of body composition: Revision of some quantitative assumptions. Ann. N.Y. Acad. Sci. *110*:113, 1963.
5. Body Composition Assessment in Youth and Adults. Report of the Sixth Ross Conference on Medial Research. Columbus, OH, Ross Laboratories, 1985.
6. Kirkendall, D. R., Gruber, J. J., and Johnson, R. F.: Measurement and Evaluation for Physical Educators. 2nd Ed. Champaign, IL, Human Kinetics Publishers, 1987.
7. Skyndex Instruction Manual. Fayetteville, AR, Caldwell Justice Co.
8. Remington, D., Fisher, G., and Parent, E.: How to Lower Your Fat Thermostat. Provo, UT, Vitality House International, 1983.
9. Hunt, J., Champion, W., and Broome, J. M.: Analysis of athletic fitness and medical history data of high school students in the Columbus, GA-Phenix City, AL area. Unpublished study.
10. Jacko, J. G., Henderson, J. M., Hunter, S. C., and Hunt, J. P.: Profiles of all-star high school football players. Unpublished study.
11. Knortz, K.: Weight gain and loss. APTA Sport Section Clinical Competencies. Columbus, GA, 1983.
12. Harris, R. J.: Personal communication.
13. Brendecke, P.: The female athlete: nonorthopaedic pathology, APTA Sport Section Clinical Competencies. San Diego, CA, 1983.

15 *Mary Lloyd Ireland and Craig C. McKirgan*

Performance-Enhancing Drugs: Ergogenic Aids

Humans have used many substances to enhance their athletic performance. As early as 200 to 300 A.D. Greek athletes and Nordic Berserkers ingested psychotropic mushrooms and herbs before competition and combat.[1] In the 19th century, caffeine, alcohol, nitroglycerin, ethyl ether, strychnine, and opium were commonly used by athletes.[2] In 1865, swimmers in a canal race in Amsterdam were charged with using ergogenic aids.[3] Cyclists used "speedballs" of heroine and cocaine in 1869.[4] In the late 19th century, a mixture of coca leaf extract and wine, called *vin Mariani* was used by French cyclists and a champion lacrosse team.[5] Amphetamines replaced other stimulants in the competitive arena in the 1940s and 1950s.[4]

In 1962, the International Olympic Committee (IOC) established a committee to control the use and abuse of drugs in athletics. In the 1968 Olympic games, ergogenic drugs were banned and drug testing began. The first person to be disqualified was Hans Gunnar Lijenvall, a Swedish pentathlete who took alcohol to steady his trigger finger.[6] In the late 1960s and early 1970s, there was an increase in the documentation of amphetamine abuse, especially in professional sports. The use of drugs in professional baseball was prohibited in 1971 by, then baseball commissioner, Bowie Kuhn.[7] During the 1980s, human growth hormone and human chorionic gonadotropin entered the world of ergogenic aids.[4] During the 1983 Pan-American Games in Caracas, Venezuela, 19 athletes, two from the United States, tested positive for banned substances. A number of other U.S. athletes returned home before competition and drug testing. In 1984, during the XXIII Olympiad in Los Angeles, four U.S. cyclists used blood doping and won four of the team's nine medals.

DRUGS IN SPORTS

The use of drugs falls into three general categories: therapeutic, performance enhancing, and recreational. Use of antibiotics for the treatment of an infection is an example of a therapeutic drug. The performance-enhancing drugs, or ergogenic aids, include drugs such as amphetamines and anabolic steroids (Table 15–1). Recreational drugs include alcohol, marijuana, and other mood-altering substances.

The term *ergogenic* comes from the Greek *ergon* (work) and *gennan* (to produce). Ergogenic aids increase work output. The American College of Sports Medicine's position statement in 1987 defined ergogenic aids as "physical, mechanical, nutritional, psychological, or pharmacological substances or treatments that either directly improve physiological variables associated with exercise performance or remove subjective restraints that may limit physiological capacity."[8]

The term *doping* originated in South Africa, where dope was the name of an alcoholic beverage used by the native population. According to the International Olympic Committee (IOC), doping is "the administration or use of any substance foreign to the body or any physiological substance taken in abnormal quantity or taken by an abnormal route of entry into the body with the sole intention of increasing in artificial and unfair manner . . . performance in competition. When necessity demands, medical treatment with any substance which, because of its nature, dosage or application, is able to boost the athlete's performance in competition in an artificial and unfair manner, this too is regarded by the IOC as doping."[9]

The IOC has divided the various types of drugs into doping *classes*. It should be noted that the doping

Table 15–1. Performance-Enhancing Drugs

Drug	*Mechanisms of Action*	*Enhancing Effects*	*Adverse Effects*
Amphetamines and sympathomimetics	Stimulate release of catecholamines from nerve cells; displace catecholamines from receptor sites, allowing an increased amount of catecholamines in the synaptic cleft; inhibit reuptake; act as catecholamine agonist; inhibit catecholamine breakdown	Increased alertness, increased self-confidence, elation, euphoria release of serum free fatty acids; decreased reaction time, appetite; fatigability, mood elevation	Central nervous system (CNS): Tremulousness, anxiety, insomnia, agitation, dizziness, irritability, headaches, psychosis, seizures, possible cerebrovascular accident (CVA) Cardiovascular (CV): Arrhythmias, hypertension, angina pectoris Gastrointestinal (GI): Nausea, vomiting, diarrhea, dry mouth, hyperthermia
Caffeine	Translocation of intracellular calcium; increase available cAMP; competitive antagonism of adenosine receptors; glycogen sparing by increasing free fatty acid availability	Decreased fatigue; increased concentration and alertness, endurance, muscle contractility, performance	CNS: Anxiety, nervousness, insomnia, delirium seizures, coma, death CV: Tachycardia, arrhythmias, hypertension Genitourinary (GU): Diuresis
Cocaine	Increased concentrations of dopaminergic and noradenergic transmitters at the neural synapse; blocks reuptake antagonism	Euphoria; sense of enhanced mental prowess	CNS: Addiction, CVA, seizures, visual changes, insomnia, confusion, delirium, paranoia, psychosis CV: Ventricular arrhythmia, angina pectoris, myocardial infarction, myocarditis, sudden death Other: Perforation of nasal septum, loss of smell, hyperthermia
Nicotine (tobacco)	Stimulation of CNS at low doses, depression of CNS (inhibition of catecholamine release) at high doses	CNS stimulation at low doses, decreased appetite, calming effect at high doses	CNS: Depression at high doses Respiratory (R): Chronic obstructive pulmonary disease, lung cancer CV: Hypertension, cornary artery disease Other: Periodontal disease
Beta blockers	Block beta receptors on end organs β_1: Heart, kidney, adipose tissue β_2: Liver, bronchi, and arteries	Relieving anxiety, decreased tremor and heart rate, improved hand-arm steadiness	CNS: Hallucinations, nightmares, insomnia, depression R: Increased airway resistance CV: Reduced blood pressure, congestive heart failure, retarded heart rate, atrioventricular block GI: Nausea, vomiting, diarrhea, constipation Other: Decreased endurance due to reduced $\dot{V}O_2$max; decreased muscle blood flow, O_2 uptake, and glucose concentration
Diuretics	*Types:* Osmotic diuresis; carbonic anhydrase inhibitor; increased concentration of Na^+ in urine; inhibition of electrolyte resorption; aldosterone antagonism	Weight reduction; dilution of drug concentration in urine	Dehydration, electrolyte imbalance, muscle cramps, orthostatic hypotension; decreased muscle strength, cardiac output, $\dot{V}O_2$max; poor temperature regulation
Blood doping and erythropoietin	Increased O_2 delivery to skeletal muscles via increased hemoglobin and hematocrit	Increased aerobic work; enhanced thermal regulation; increased cardiac output secondary to increased blood volume; increased buffering of lactic acid	Infection—viral (hepatitis or HIV) or bacterial Immune reactions: Fever, urticaria, hemolytic anemia, fatal transfusion reaction CV: Increased blood viscosity; decreased blood flow velocity; pulmonary emboli, deep venous thrombosis
Nutritional ergogenic aids: Amino acids, vitamin B_{15}, bee pollen, sodium, bicarbonate, baking powder, vitamins and minerals		Psychological benefit	Nutritional imbalance; vitaminosis; GI upset

definition is based on the banning of pharmacological *classes* of agents and not specific agents. The doping *method* refers to blood doping as well as other pharmacological, chemical, and physical manipulation of the urine. A third class of drugs that is subject to certain restrictions includes alcohol, marijuana, local anesthetics, corticosteroids, and beta blockers.[9] The doping classes are stimulants, narcotics, anabolic agents, diuretics, and peptide hormones and analogs.

STIMULANTS

Stimulants are the most commonly used ergogenic aid. The most common type is amphetamines (Table 15–2). Other stimulants include caffeine, nicotine, cocaine, crack cocaine, and over-the-counter sympathomimetic agents such as ephedrine. Stimulants have been most commonly used in events that require endurance, such as cycling, and in sports that require aggressiveness and explosive power.[4] The psychological effects of stimulants include enhanced alertness, increased ability to concentrate, decreased sensation of fatigue, mood elevation, and increased self-confidence and aggression. Stimulants also increase the musculoskeletal system's ability to improve muscle contractility and increase the release into the circulation of free fatty acids. Negative physiologic effects include anxiety, poor judgment, excessive aggressiveness, schizophrenia-like psychoses, increased heart rate, increased blood pressure, risk for cerebral vascular accident, cardiac arrhythmias, death, and interference with timing of technical skills.

Amphetamines

In the 1960s there was an increase in the use of amphetamines among American professional football players. In 1957, the American Medical Association condemned the use of amphetamines in athletics. A controlled substance act was passed by Congress in the 1970s that severely restricted the manufacturing of amphetamines and applied strict guidelines for their use.[10] The therapeutic uses of amphetamines have included the treatment of obesity, narcolepsy, minimal brain dysfunction (hyperkinesis), attention deficit disorder, depression, and severe menstrual cramps.[11,12]

Amphetamines, sympathomimetic agents, mimic the endogenous catecholamines epinephrine, norepinephrine, and dopamine.[13] Catecholamines stimulate the central and peripheral nervous system via the alpha and beta receptors. The stimulation of the central and peripheral nervous system by amphetamines is by an indirect method.[14] The cardiovascular effects of amphetamines include increased systolic and diastolic blood pressure, increased heart rate, and, with larger doses, reduced positive inotropic effect (via reflex action). Central nervous system effects of amphetamine use include stimulation of the medullary respiratory center, the spinal cord, and the reticuloendothelial system.[14] However, the most significant effect of amphetamines appears to be its psychological effects: increased alertness, decreased sense of fatigue, mood elevation, increased self-confidence, elation, and euphoria.

The ergogenic effects of amphetamines were the subject of a controlled study conducted by Smith and Beecher in 1959.[15] They evaluated swimmers, runners, and weight-throwing performers who were all trained athletes. Each subject was given a 14 mg/kg dose of amphetamine 2 to 3 hours before athletic performance. Better performance was noted in 93% of the swimmers, 73% of the runners, and 85% of the weight throwers. Although the percentage of increase in their respective fields ranged from a low of 0.5% for swimmers to a high of 4% difference for weight throwers, this difference may be significant for a high-class or world-class athlete. Other studies have shown that amphetamines do *not* produce a positive effect.[16] The psychological benefit from amphetamines appears to be the most significant one. The numerous side effects must be weighed against the known benefits.

The side effects of amphetamine use depend on dose and length of use. The adverse effects on the central nervous system include restlessness, insomnia, instability, agitation, confusion, paranoia, hallucinations, con-

Table 15–2. Amphetamines

Generic Name	*Trade Name*	*Street Name*
Amphetamine	Benzedrine	Uppers, bennies, peaches, greenies
Dextroamphetamine	Dexedrine	Dexies, oranges, greenies, orange heart caplets
Methamphetamine	Desoxynmethempex	Meth, crystal, whites, speed
Dextroamphetamine and amphetamine	Biphetamine	Footballs, black beauties

(Brill H., and Hirose, T.: The rise and fall of a methamphetamine epidemic: Japan 1945–55. Seminars in Psychiatry. *1*(2):179, 1969. Laties, V.G., and Weiss, B.: The amphetamine margin in sports. Fed. Proc. *40*:2689, 1981.)

vulsions, coma, and even death. Cardiovascular effects include headaches, chills, flushing, palpitations, angina, atrial or ventricular arrhythmias, hypertension, hypotension, bradycardia, tachycardia, cardiovascular collapse, necrotizing vasculitis, subarachnoid hemorrhage, and cerebral hemorrhage in doses as low as 20 mg. Gastrointestinal effects include gastrointestinal discomfort, weight loss, nausea, vomiting, abdominal pain, and decreased appetite. The sudden withdrawal from amphetamines, especially from long-term use, can result in chronic fatigue, lethargy, hypersomnia, hyperphagia, and depression.

Caffeine

Caffeine is one of the most commonly used drugs in the United States and Europe. Caffeine is a methylated xanthine similar to theophylline and theobromine.[12] Caffeine is found in the raw fruit of the coffee plant *(Coffea arabica)* as well as in 60 other species of plants, including tea leaves and coconuts. Today, caffeine is found principally in beverages such as coffee, tea, and soft drinks, and in some over-the-counter analgesics, cold medications, and antisomnolence drugs. The concentration of caffeine in an 8-ounce cup of coffee is roughly 100 to 150 mg. Tea has approximately 60 to 70 mg of caffeine per 8 ounce, cola drinks 40 to 60 mg in 12 ounce.[11,12]

Historically, caffeine was reported in France to cure smallpox, gout, and scurvy and in England to cure venereal disease and the common cold.[17] Today, the principal use of caffeine as an ergogenic aid is to increase endurance and increase alertness.[12] Some studies substantiate the hypothesis that the ingestion of caffeine may spare muscle glycogen use by mobilizing serum-free fatty acids.[18,19] The glycogen stores are then available for use later. There has also been evidence of an increase in muscle contractility associated with doses of caffeine.[20] Another primary effect of caffeine is its central nervous system stimulation, which may improve endurance, especially if an athlete is already fatigued. Studies of Vo_2max, an indicator of aerobic capacity, have shown no great effects after caffeine ingestion.

Because of conflicting reports about the ergogenic effects of caffeine, the IOC has changed its ban on caffeine and now allows it to be ingested in small amounts. The IOC banned the use of caffeine until 1972. At that time, any caffeine found in the urine was considered a banned substance. Just before the 1972 Olympics caffeine was removed from the banned list. This action reflected conflicting findings and the ubiquitous nature of caffeine. In the 1984 Olympic games in Los Angeles, the IOC returned caffeine to the "banned substance list," but only *restricted* the permissible level. Concentrations of caffeine greater than 15 μg/ml of urine were banned. In 1986, the IOC lowered the permissible caffeine level in the urine to less than 12 μg/ml.[9] The NCAA banned caffeine in urine concentrations greater than 15 μg/ml.[21] To reach a 12 μg/ml level, a person would have to drink six to eight cups of coffee over a short time and be tested within 2 or 3 hours.

The central nervous system effects of caffeine include anxiety, nervousness, insomnia, delirium, seizures, coma, and in larger doses, death. Withdrawal from long-term caffeine use can result in headaches, drowsiness, lethargy, rhinorrhea, irritability, nervousness, and depression. Cardiovascular side effects of increased caffeine ingestion include palpitations, hypertension, and arrhythmias (supraventricular and ventricular). Another complication is that the mild diuretic effect of caffeine could offset the performance-enhancing effect for endurance athletes.[13] Heat problems can occur with the reduced plasma volume and increased basal metabolic rate. Mild gastrointestinal irritation can also occur with excessive doses of caffeine.

Cocaine

Cocaine comes from the coca bush *(Erythroxylon coca)*, an indigenous plant in the Peruvian Andes. The coca leaf was originally chewed by the Incas. It was used for religious purposes and later became an abused drug. Its benefits were to fight off fatigue and suppress hunger.[13,22,23] Sigmund Freud also performed studies using cocaine on himself and felt exhilarated and at ease.[11,24] Cocaine was also used by Angelo Mariani, a Corsican chemist, who added it to wine *("vin Mariani")*, which was widely used by cyclists. In the United States, John Smythe Pemberton used cocaine in the original formula of Coca-Cola; however, it was removed from the formulation in 1903.[23] In 1986, cocaine caused the deaths of professional football player Don Rogers, of the Cleveland Browns, and amateur basketball player Len Bias, from the University of Maryland.[11]

Cocaine and crack cocaine use by athletes has been principally recreational rather than for ergogenic effect.[25,26] In the general population, one in every six high school seniors has admitted to trying cocaine, one in 18 students has tried crack cocaine, and nearly 40% of adults in their late 20s have used cocaine.[27] A study in 1985 showed that nearly 20% of professional baseball players and 75% of professional basketball players have used cocaine.[28] A 1986 National Football League (NFL) Players Association survey found that half of the respondents considered cocaine the most commonly abused drug in the NFL.[25]

The principal medical use for cocaine today is as an anesthetic. It is used principally in ear, nose, and throat procedures. The methods of use of cocaine include sniffing (snorting), smoking, chewing, and intravenous injection. The drug is usually snorted by illicit users.[11] Cocaine works primarily by blocking reuptake of neurotransmitters. The effects of cocaine are short lived. Since the exhilarating effects last only 5 to 15 minutes, it is not uncommon for users to take multiple doses during the day. Because of its short-lived action, cocaine is a poor ergogenic aid.[11] Unfortunately, cocaine is a very addictive drug. It is no longer considered "the safe drug." Side effects of cocaine include ulceration and perforations of the nasal septum, rhinitis, sinusitis, bronchitis, hyperthermia, agitation, restlessness, insomnia, anxiety, toxic psychoses, hallucinations, cardiac arrhythmias, sudden death, angina pectoris, myocardial infarction, and many others.

Nicotine

Nicotine, the addictive drug found in tobacco, has been used by humans for centuries. Tobacco can be smoked or used in smokeless forms. Smokeless tobacco can be further divided into loose leaf tobacco (chewing tobacco) and snuff. The use of smoking tobacco in the general population in the United States has been reported at approximately 31.5% of adult men and 25.7% of the adult women.[29] Nicotine use in the athlete population is principally by smokeless tobacco, usually by baseball players. It is hoped the current educational programs and rule changes will reduce the use of chewing tobacco during competition. It has been estimated that 34 to 39% of the U.S. professional baseball players in major and minor leagues use smokeless tobacco.[13,30]

Nicotine is a potent alkaloid that works on both the central and the peripheral nervous system. It also acts as both a depressant and a stimulant. The effect is dose dependent. At low doses, in the peripheral nervous system, stimulation occurs at the autonomic ganglia. At high doses, ganglionic depression occurs. Also at high doses, nicotine causes inhibition of catecholamine release from the adrenal medulla. In the central nervous system, norepinephrine and dopamine release occurs after nicotine administration. Tobacco appears to have paradoxical calming and stimulating effects because of the aforementioned dose-related effects of nicotine.[30]

The athlete uses nicotine for the stimulatory effect, calming effect, or appetite control.[12] The overwhelming side effects of the nicotine in tobacco far outweigh the benefits. The side effects of tobacco include pulmonary diseases, including various carcinomas; cardiovascular disease, including hypertension and coronary artery disease; gastrointestinal disease; and periodontal diseases, including leukoplakia and the risk of squamous cell carcinoma and others.

Although the benefits as an ergogenic aid to performance are small, the long-term risks of ill health far outweigh any possible benefit from nicotine. Nicotine is classed as a stimulant. It is not specifically listed in the IOC banned substance list. The rules of the NCAA and professional baseball are becoming more restrictive on the use of tobacco.

Sympathomimetics

Sympathomimetic amines are another group of agents that are principally stimulants. The sympathomimetics stimulate the sympathetic nervous system via α_1- or α_2- and β_1- or β_2-receptor stimulation. Examples of the sympathomimetic amines include phenylpropanolamine, ephedrine, and pseudoephedrine. These agents are commonly found in over-the-counter cold, decongestant, and asthma preparations (Table 15–3). The more selective the specific agent is for either alpha or beta stimulation, the more specific is the therapeutic benefit gained. For example, the β_2 agonists salbutamol and terbutaline are the only approved β_2 agonists for the treatment of asthma in the inhaled form.[9] Not only are these the only two β_2 agonists approved by the United States Olympic Committee (USOC) and IOC, but prior written notification of the use of these agents must be received by the USOC and the IOC.[9] Because of the ubiquitous nature of these agents in common cold remedies, appetite suppressants, and nasal decongestants, the use of sympathomimetic amines is common. Although there have been no specific studies that show an obvious ergogenic benefit for the sympathomimetics like ephedrine or phenylpropanolamine, the potential effects are still a concern.[31] The adverse cardiovascular effects include increased blood pressure (including life-threatening hypertensive episodes), cardiac arrhythmias, palpitations, and myocardial infarction. Central nervous system effects of these agents include nervousness, irritability, insomnia, dizziness, cephalgia, anorexia, agitation, confusion, paranoia, mania, hallucinations, stroke, cerebral vasculitis, and cerebral hemorrhage.

β-ADRENERGIC BLOCKING AGENTS

"Beta blockers" are therapeutic agents for hypertension, angina, and specific cardiac arrhythmias. Other

Table 15–3. USOC/IOC–Banned Cold and Asthma Preparations

Generic Name	*Example*
Ephedrine	Tedral, Bronkotabs, Rynatuss, Primatene, Bronkaid, Nyquil Nighttime Cold Medicine, herbal teas and medicines containing Ma Huang (Chinese Ephedra) and related compounds
Pseudoephedrine	Actifed, Afrin tablets, Afrinol, Co-Tylenol, Deconamine, Novafed, Sudafed, Chlor-Trimeton-DC, Drixoral and related compounds
Phenylephrine	Dristan, Neo-Synephrine, Sinex, and related compounds
Desoxyephedrine	Vicks inhaler and related compounds
Phenylpropanolamine	Alka-Seltzer Plus, Allerest, Contact Dexatrim, Dietac, Sine-Aid, Sine-Off Sinutab, Triaminic, Sucrets Cold Decongestant, and related compounds
Isoetharine HCl	Bronkosol, Bronkometer, Numotac, Dilabron, and related compounds
Isoproterenol	Isuprel, Norisodrine, Metihaler-ISO, and related compounds
Metaproterenol	Alupent, Metaprel, and related compounds
Methoxyphenamine	Ritalin, Orthoxicol cough syrup, and related compounds
Methylphenidate HCl	Ritalin and related compounds

(Gilman, A. G., Goodman, L. S., Rall, T. W., et al. (eds.): Goodman and Gilman's The Pharmacological Basis of Therapeutics. 7th ed. New York: Macmillan, 1985.)

uses for β blockers include the treatment of migraine headaches, essential tremors, overactivity, pheochromocytoma, thyroid toxicosis, and alcohol withdrawal. Beta blockers are agents that block β-adrenergic receptors on end organs. The β_1 receptors are found principally in heart, kidneys, and adipose tissue, and β_2 receptors in the liver, bronchi, and arteries. Beta-blocking agents, therefore, can be specific or nonspecific. Nonspecific agents block both the β_1 and β_2 receptor sites, whereas specific β blockers can block either the β_1 or the β_2 receptor sites. Although there is no pure β_1 or β_2 blocking without overlap, the agents principally affect either the β_1 or β_2 receptor sites.[13]

The most common β-blocking agent used has been propranolol (Inderal), a nonselective beta blocker.[32] Performance-enhancing effects of β blockers are relief of anxiety, decreased tremor, lower heart rate, a general calming effect, and improved hand-arm steadiness. Because of these potential ergogenic effects of using β blockers, the winter game sports of biathlon, bobsled, luge, and ski jumping, and summer game sports of archery, diving, equestrian, fencing, gymnastics, modern pentathlon, sailing, and shooting, have all been targeted by the IOC for β blocker abuse.[9] In events where shooting is involved, the athlete shoots between heartbeats, and β blockers provide the shooter more time to steady his aim between heartbeats.[33] Kruse and coworkers have shown a 13% improvement in pistol shooters using β blockers.[34]

Beta blockers decrease $\dot{V}O_2max$ by 15% or greater and decrease muscle blood flow, muscle oxygen uptake, and blood glucose concentrations. The adverse effects of beta blockers include increased airway resistance, nausea, vomiting, mild diarrhea, constipation, hallucinations, nightmares, insomnia, depression, shortened time to fatigue, decreased ability to perform endurance-type activities, hypotension, congestive heart failure, bradycardia, and atrioventricular block. Beta blockers are banned by the National Collegiate Athletic Association (NCAA), IOC, and USOC.

NARCOTICS

Pain can be controlled by narcotics or nonsteroidal anti-inflammatory agents. The latter are legal but should be declared by the tested athlete. The use of narcotic analgesics has been banned by the USOC and the IOC but is not restricted by the NCAA. Use of narcotics may mask symptoms of potentially severe injury or result in addiction, false feelings of invincibility, delusions of athletic prowess, and poor perception of dangerous situations that place the athlete and others at risk. No definitive studies have shown ergogenic effects for narcotics.

DIURETICS

Athletes use diuretics for two effects: rapid weight loss and urine dilution. In sports with weight categories, such as boxing, wrestling, judo, and equestrian, diuretic use is common. Weight loss potential using diuretics has been documented at 4.1% weight reduction over a 24-hour period. Reduction of the concentration of drugs in the urine with diuretics occurs because of more rapid excretion. Diuretics are banned by most governing bodies of athletic events.[9] Negative effects of diuretics are decreased $\dot{V}O_2max$, decreased work load to maximal exercise, and changes in blood lactate concentration.[34] Other adverse effects include dehydration, hypovolemia, muscle cramps, orthostatic hypotension, electrolyte imbalance, fatigue, and precipitation of gout.[13,34]

BLOOD DOPING AND ERYTHROPOIETIN

Blood Doping

Blood doping is also known as blood boosting, induced erythrocythemia, or blood packing. The definition of blood doping used by the USOC is "the administration of blood or related blood products, including erythropoietin, to an athlete other than for a legitimate medical treatment. This procedure may be preceded by the withdrawal of blood from the athlete, who continues to train in this blood-depleted state."[9] The use of blood doping goes back to the end of World War II, when attempts were made to enable pilots to avoid the adverse effects of high altitude.[35] In the athletic arena it was rumored that blood doping may have been used in 1972, during the Munich games, as well as in the 1976 Montreal games. In the 1984 summer Olympics in Los Angeles, seven U.S. cyclists (four gold medalists) admitted to using blood doping.[11]

The theory behind the use of blood doping is that it increases oxygen delivery to working muscles and increase the capacity for aerobic work, provided that oxygen delivery is the rate-limiting factor and cardiac output and blood distribution are not adversely affected by increased viscosity. Blood doping is also believed to enhance thermal regulation, buffer the inhibitory effect of lactic acid on skeletal muscles cells, and augment cardiac output secondary to increased blood volume and preload.[25] Results documented by Ekbloom demonstrated a maximum aerobic power increase of an average of 10%, and this lasted approximately 18 days after retransfusion.[36] Others have shown an increase in $\dot{V}O_2max$ by as much as 3.9 to 12.8% and an increase in endurance capacity from 2.5 to 35%.[8]

The actual technique for blood doping starts anywhere from 4 to 8 weeks before competition. Two units of blood are removed from the athlete and the athlete continues to train. The reinfusion takes approximately 1 to 2 hours and the best benefits are obtained within the next 24 hours to a week.[11,25]

Adverse effects of blood doping exist with either autologous or homologous blood transfusion techniques. Homologous transfusions carry the risk of infectious diseases such as hepatitis and AIDS.[35] Approximately 3% of all homologous blood transfusions cause immune reactions, including mild allergic reactions, fever, urticaria, and hemolytic transfusion reactions, which can be fatal.[11] Homologous and autologous blood transfusions carry the risks of elevated blood viscosity. Increased blood viscosity can lead to decreased cardiac output, decreased blood flow velocity, and decreased peripheral blood oxygen concentration, resulting in reduced aerobic capacity. Blood clots, deep venous thrombosis, and pulmonary emboli are also potential side effects. Most of these transfusion reactions of hyperviscosity are related to hematocrit values greater than 50 to 60%.[37]

Erythropoietin

Erythropoietin, in blood doping, is used primarily in the athletic population to increase the hematocrit of the athlete's blood. Erythropoietin is a hormone that is naturally produced in the human kidney. It stimulates bone marrow stem cells to differentiate into red blood cells. It has been shown to increase red blood cell mass as well as hemoglobin and hematocrit.[38] Presently, erythropoietin is genetically engineered using recombinant gene technology.[39] The effects of long-term recombinant erythropoietin administration on healthy persons has not been determined, but stroke and renal failure are known complications.

Knowing the results of blood-doping studies and the effects of erythropoietin, it would then appear that erythropoietin could be used as an ergogenic aid. Erythropoietin and blood doping are indetectable by present testing methods. Erythropoietin and blood doping are both banned by the NCAA, the USOC, and the IOC.[9,21]

NUTRITIONAL ERGOGENIC AIDS

History documents use of such ergogenic aids as honey, bee pollen, wheat germ oil, and other natural substances.[40] *Nutrients* are proteins, fats, carbohydrates, and vitamins and minerals. These nutrients provide energy, maintain growth and development of the tissues, and regulate metabolic enzymatic processes. The scientific literature is equivocal about the uses of various nutritional supplements and foods as ergogenic aids. Some nutritional ergogenic aids like teas and herbal medications may actually contain stimulants detectable in the urine and subsequently disqualify an athlete. This has, however, not prohibited commercial entities from using various data to support their beliefs.

Amino Acids

The amino acids arginine and ornithine have been marketed as agents that increase muscle development, decrease body fat, and increase human growth hormone levels.[41] L-Tryptophan has been touted as being able to raise growth hormone levels, enhance performance, and relieve depression and insomnia.[42]

The possible adverse consequences of using amino acids and protein powders include dehydration, gout, calcium loss, and increased urea production.[40] There is no overwhelming evidence that protein powders or amino acids in supplemental form provide any benefit over those of a balanced adequate diet.

Vitamin B_{15}

Vitamin B_{15} (pangamic acid), though not a true vitamin, has been theorized to enhance aerobic endurance performance by improving oxidative metabolism by enzyme stimulation of succinate dehydrogenase and cytochrome oxidase. The evidence to date does not support vitamin B_{15} as an ergogenic aid.[40]

Bee Pollen

Bee pollen, a mixture of microspores from flowers and nectar from the beehive, has historically been considered an ergogenic aid. Some believe that it may help the athlete recover faster during workouts. Available scientific evidence does not support bee pollen as a true ergogenic aid.[40]

Soda Doping

The use of sodium bicarbonate or baking soda to increase the normal alkaline reserve of the body has been termed soda doping or buffer boosting.[35,40] In theory, fatigue may be reduced. By increasing pH by soda loading, lactic acid production may be reduced.

This would be most beneficial for athletes who use anaerobic metabolism, such as sprinters, as opposed to aerobic metabolism, such as endurance athletes. A decrease in subjective fatigue ratings and perceived exertion during exercise has been reported. Complications of soda doping are principally gastrointestinal, like gastrointestinal upset and diarrhea.

General Nutrition

The best advice is sound nutrition in all phases: training phase, performance, and recovery. Unlike pharmacologic ergogenic aids, no one specific nutritional source has been shown to enhance performance.

CONCLUSION

"Higher, faster, stronger." Although these are the words of the Olympic motto, they by no means reflect or condone achieving these goals by *any* means, including ergogenic aids. The use of ergogenic aids is evident at all levels of competition, including high school, college, and international competition. Our roles as health care givers to athletes is one of education, support, and providing quality health care and safety. Although not paramount in the minds of present-day athletes, "The important thing in the Olympic games is not to win but to take part; the important thing in life is not the triumph but the struggle. The essential thing is not to have conquered but to have fought well," as stated in 1908 by the founder of the modern Olympic games, Baron Pierre D. de Coubertin. This spirit should be the goal.

REFERENCES

1. Prokop, L.: The struggle against doping and its history. Physical Fitness *10*:45, 1970.
2. Hollyhock, M.: The application of drugs to modify human performance. Br. J. Sports Med. *4*:119, 1969.
3. Thomason, H.: Drugs and the athlete. *In* Science and Sporting Performance: Management or Manipulations? Edited by B. Davies and G. Thomas. Oxford, Clarendon Press, 1982.
4. Anstiss, T. J.: Uses and abuses of drugs in sport: The athlete's view. *In* Medicine, Sport and the Law. Edited by S. D. W. Payne. Oxford, Blackwell Scientific Publications, 1990.
5. Murray, T. H.: The Coercive Power of Drugs in Sport. The Hastings Center Report. New York, 1983, pp. 24.
6. Wood, C., et al.: The drug busters. Maclean's, February, 1988, p. 123.
7. Cooter, G. R.: Amphetamine use, physical activity and sport. J. Drug Issues Summer, 323, 1980.
8. American College of Sports Medicine: Position on blood doping as an ergogenic aid. Med. Sci. Sports Exerc. *19*:540, 1987.
9. United States Olympic Committee Drug and Education and Doping Control Program: Guide to Banned Medications. 1993.
10. Ryan, A. J.: Use of amphetamines in athletics. J.A.M.A. *170*:152, 1959.
11. Wadler, G. I., and Hainline, B.: Drugs and the Athlete. Philadelphia, F. A. Davis, 1989.
12. Lombardo, J. A.: Stimulants. *In* Drugs and Performance in Sports. Edited by R. H. Strauss. Philadelphia, W. B. Saunders, 1987.
13. Gilman, A. G., Goodman, L. S., Rall, T. W., et al. (eds.): Goodman and Gilman's The Pharmacological Basis of Therapeutics. 7th ed. New York, Macmillan, 1985.
14. Cooper, J. R., Bloom, F. E., and Roth, R. H.: The biochemical basis of neuropharmacology. 5th Ed. New York, Oxford University Press, 1986.
15. Smith, G. M., and Beecher, H. R.: Amphetamine sulfate and athletic performance: 1. Objective effects. J.A.M.A. *170*:542, 1959.
16. Haldi, J., and Wynn, W.: Action of drugs on the efficiency of swimmers. Res. Q. *17*:96, 1946.
17. Goulart, F. S.: The Caffeine Book—A User's and Abuser's Guide. New York, Dodd, Mead, 1984.
18. Costill, D. L., Dalsky, G. P., and Fink, W. J.: Effects of caffeine ingestions on metabolism and exercise performance. Med. Sci. Sports *10*:155, 1978.
19. Toner, M. M., et al.: Metabolic and cardiovascular responses to exercise with caffeine. Ergonomics *25*:1175, 1982.
20. Lopes, J. M., et al.: Effect of caffeine on skeletal muscle function before and after fatigue. J. Appl. Physiol. *54*:1303, 1983.
21. The 1993–94 NCAA Drug Testing Education Programs. Overland Park, KS, NCAA Publishing, 1993.
22. Kunkel, D. B.: Cocaine then and now. Part I. Its history, medical botany and use. Emerg. Med. *18*:113, 1986.
23. Van Dyke, C., and Gyck, R.: Cocaine. Scientific Am. *246*:128, 1982.
24. Freud, S.: On the general effect of cocaine. *In* Cocaine Papers. Edited by R. Byck. New York, Stonehill Publishing, 1974.
25. Smith, D. A., and Perry, P. J.: The efficacy of ergogenic agents in athletic competition. Part II: Other performance-enhancing agents. Ann. Pharmacother. *26*:653, 1992.
26. Wagner, J. C.: Enhancement of athletic performance with drugs: An overview. Sports Med. *12*:250, 1991.
27. Johnston, L., and Bachman, J.: The Monitoring the Future Study. Institute for Social Research, The University of Michigan, 1987.
28. Boswell, T.: Drug case puts game into reality. Virginia-Pilot and Ledger-Star, Sept. 22, 1985.
29. Fielding, J. E.: Smoking and women: tragedy of the majority. N. Engl. J. Med. *317*:1343, 1987.
30. Lombardo, J. A.: Stimulants and athletic performance: Part 2. Cocaine and nicotine. Physician Sportsmed. *14*:85, 1986.
31. Martin, W. R., et al.: Physiologic, subjective, and behavioral effects of amphetamine, methamphetamine, ephedrine, phenmetrazine and methylphenidate in man. Clin. Pharmacol. Ther. *12*:245, 1971.
32. Haupt, H. A.: Ergogenic aids. *In* Sports Medicine: The School-Age Athlete. Edited by B. Reider. Philadelphia, W. B. Saunders Co., 1991.
33. Rogers, C.: Shooters aim to score with beta-blockers. Physician Sportsmed. *12*:35, 1984.
34. Kruse, P., et al.: β-blockade used in precision sports: Effect on pistol shooting performance. J. Appl. Physiol. *61*:417, 1986.
35. Caldwell, J. E., Ahonen, E., and Nousiainen, U.: Differential effects of sauna-, diuretic-, and exercise-induced hypohydration. J. Appl. Physiol., *57*:1018, 1984.
36. Williams, M. H.: Drugs and sport performance. *In* Sports Medicine. 2nd Ed. Edited by A. J. Ryan and F. L. Allman, Jr. San Diego, Academic Press, 1989.
37. Ekbloom, B.: Blood doping, oxygen breathing and altitude training. *In* Drugs and Performance in Sports. Edited by R. H. Strauss. Philadelphia, W. B. Saunders Co., 1987.
38. Gledhill, N., Blood doping and related issues: A brief review. Med. Sci. Sports Exerc. *14*:183, 1982.
39. Eschbach, J. W., et al.: Correction of the anemia of end-stage renal disease with recombinant human erythropoietin. Results of a combined phase I and II clinical trial. N. Engl. J. Med., *316*:73, 1987.
40. Flaharty, K. K., Grimm, A. M., and Vlasses, P. H.: Epoetin human recombinant erythropoietin. Clin. Pharm. *8*:769, 1989.
41. Williams, M. H.: Ergogenic aids. *In* Sports Nutrition for the 90s: The Health Professional's Handbook. Edited by J. R. Berning and S. N. Steen. Gaithersburg, MD, Aspen, 1991.
42. Slavin, J. L., Lanners, G., and Engstrom, M.: Amino acid supplements: Beneficial or risky? Physician Sportsmed. *16*(3):221, 1988.
43. Muller, E. E., et al.: A slight effect of L-tryptophan on growth hormone release in normal human subjects. J. Clin. Endocrinol. Metabol. *39*:1, 1974.

SOURCES OF ADDITIONAL INFORMATION

National Collegiate Athletic Association (NCAA)
6201 College Boulevard
Overland Park, KS 66211-2422
(913) 339-1906

National Federation of State High School Association
11724 Plaza Circle
Kansas City, MO 64195
(816) 464-5400

United States Olympic Committee Drug Control Hotline
1750 East Boulder Street
Colorado Springs, CO 80909
(800) 233-0393

16

Suzanne Tanner

Anabolic Steroids and Human Growth Hormone

Weekly news reports attest that the use of drugs, such as anabolic steroids and growth hormone, is not restricted to Olympic and professional athletes. A great problem facing sports today is drug abuse by high school, collegiate, and recreational athletes who hope to gain an edge over other competitors. Health-care providers may play an important role in tempering an athlete's desire to become a champion athlete by any means with education on potentially irreparable harm from anabolic steroids and growth hormone.[1]

ANABOLIC-ANDROGENIC STEROIDS

Pharmacology

Anabolic-androgenic steroids (AAS) are synthetic derivatives of testosterone, the male sex hormone. Although they are commonly referred to as "anabolic steroids," no pure tissue-building agent has been isolated. All these compounds also have androgenic (masculinizing) properties.[2]

Anabolic-androgenic steroids increase cellular protein synthesis.[3] They may enhance rapid recovery from strenuous workouts, perhaps via inhibition of the catabolic effect of glucocorticoids.[3] Aggression in AAS users might be enhanced by neurologic changes directly rather than by a placebo effect alone.[3]

Anabolic-androgenic steroids may be taken orally or by injection. Taken orally, testosterone has poor efficacy because of liver degradation.[2] Adding a 17-alpha alkyl group or administering AAS by injection prevents first-pass metabolism and enhances efficacy.[2]

Legitimate Uses

Therapeutic uses of AAS include treatment of certain anemias, hereditary angioedema, some cases of breast cancer, male hypogonadism, and possibly osteoporosis.[4] Doses of AAS used by athletes may far exceed therapeutic doses.[5]

History of Use

The first "athlete" to use testosterone may have been a gelding named Holloway, in 1942. His trotting speed improved after implantation of testosterone pellets and several months of training.[6] It is alleged that German soldiers took steroids during World War II to enhance aggressiveness, but Yesalis and coworkers point out that this is not documented and is unlikely, since the Nazis were opposed to organism-altering drugs.[6]

West Coast American body builders may have experimented with testosterone preparations in the late 1940s and early 1950s.[6] Successful Soviet weight lifters probably used AAS in the early 1950s.[6] By the mid 1960s, AAS use was reported in Olympic track and field athletes, and AAS use appeared to escalate among National Football League players in the 1970s and 1980s.[6]

Motives for Use

Athletes in a variety of sports use AAS to enhance strength and performance. AAS use may be most prevalent in the "strength sports," such as weight lifting, body building, football, wrestling, and certain track and field events.[7] Some swimmers and cyclists believe AAS enhances recovery from strenuous workouts. Increased aggressiveness is a benefit claimed by some football players.[8] Many males use AAS merely to improve their appearance (Fig. 16–1).

Epidemiology of Use

A 1988 national survey revealed that 6.6% of 12th graders reported that they used or had used steroids.[8] A more recent (1992) survey of 6930 high school students in Denver revealed that 4% of male students and 1.3% of female students used or had used AAS.[9] Windsor and Dumitru found a higher prevalence of AAS use among male athletes in affluent schools (10.2%) than in poorer schools (2.8%).[10] High school students' knowledge of the risks of AAS is poor. Many students (30%) in the Denver study did not know steroids could stunt growth, 28% did not know that cardiac disease is a risk, and 25% of students did not realize that AAS could cause liver tumors.[9]

The greatest users of AAS among college athletes appear to be football players. Anderson found that 10% of university football players reported AAS use in 1991.[11] Swimming, track and field, and basketball were associated with lower rates of use. One fourth of athletes started using AAS before college.[12]

Efficacy

A comprehensive review of 25 studies addressing the effects of AAS on strength supports the American College of Sports Medicine conclusion that AAS can increase lean body mass and strength when combined with proper diet and high-intensity training.[12,13] The American College of Sports Medicine also points out that AASs are not effective in increasing aerobic capacity.[13]

Risks

As shown in Table 16–1, AAS may adversely affect multiple physiologic systems. Most adverse effects appear to be reversible, but this has not been rigorously studied.[2] Permanent risks include alopecia, gynecomastia, and premature closure of epiphyseal growth plates in adoles-

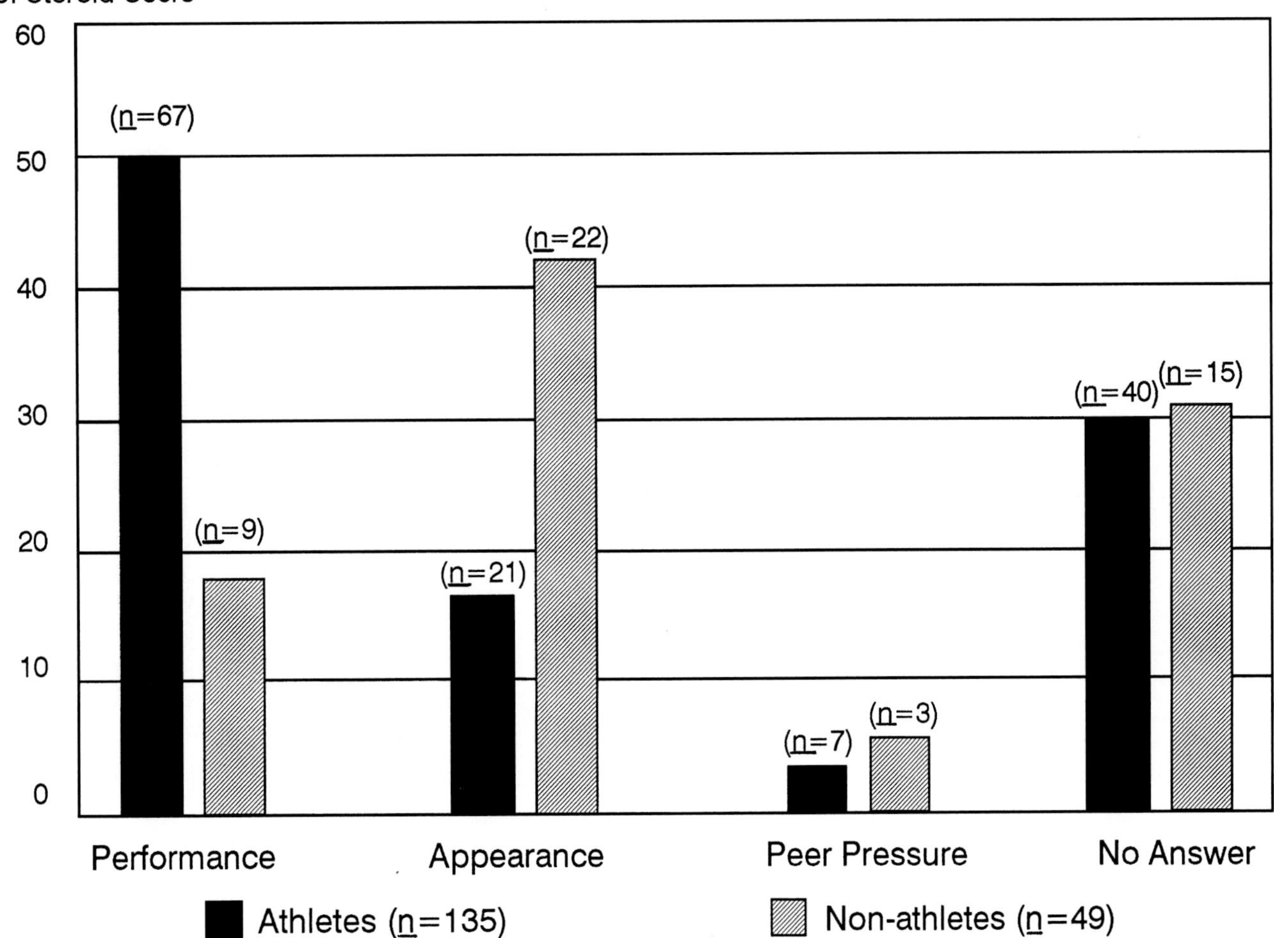

Fig. 16–1. Motives for steroid use. (From Tanner, S. M., Miller, D. W., and Alongi, C.: Unpublished study, 1993.)

Table 16–1. Adverse Effects Associated with Anabolic-Androgenic Steroids

Skin:	Oily skin, folliculitis, cystic acne, hirsutism, striae, alopecia
Breasts:	Gynecomastia
Cardiovascular:	Hypertension,* decreased serum high-density lipoprotein, increased levels of other serum lipids, atherosclerotic coronary artery disease, cardiomyopathy, myocardial infarction, thrombotic stroke
Liver:	Altered liver enzymes, cholestatic jaundice, peliosis hepatitis,† hepatic adenoma, hepatocellular carcinoma, hepatic angiosarcoma
Gastrointestinal:	Iliopsoas hypertrophy with small bowel obstruction
Renal:	Wilms' tumor
Metabolic:	Hyperinsulinemia, impaired glucose tolerance
Immune function:	Uncertain effects
Reproductive function:	Testicular atrophy, decreased spermatogenesis, sterility, altered libido, symptomatic prostatic hypertrophy, prostatic carcinoma
Musculoskeletal:	Tendon rupture
Fluid balance:	Edema
Psychological:	Fluctuating moods, aggressiveness ("roid rage"), depression, psychosis, addiction
Infections from shared needles:	Human immunodeficiency virus, hepatitis
Virilizing effects in females:	Hirsutism, hoarse voice, breast atrophy, clitoral hypertrophy, amenorrhea
Stunted growth:	In adolescents, permanent short stature due to premature closure of epiphyses

*Not a well-established effect of AAS

†Peliosis hepatis is a potentially life-threatening hepatic lesion characterized by blood-filled cysts.

(Catlin, D. H., Hatton C. K.: Use and abuse of anabolic and other drugs for athletic enhancement. Adv. Intern. Med. *36*:399, 1991. Friedl, K. E.: Effects on anabolic steroids on physical health. In Anabolic Steroids in Sport and Exercise. Edited by C. E. Yesalis. Champaign, IL., Human Kinetics Publishers, 1993.)

cents.[2] Deaths among AAS users have been attributed to liver tumors and sudden cardiac death.[5]

If an athlete exhibits a rapid increase in muscularity and acne, and excessive aggressiveness, a team physician should suspect the possibility of AAS use.

Sources

The main source of AAS for athletes is the illicit market. The Interagency Task Force on Anabolic Steroids (1991) contends that one third of the drugs are smuggled into the United States from foreign countries, a third are manufactured in the United States and diverted to the illegal market, and a third are manufactured in clandestine laboratories. Probably fewer than 10% of athletes obtain AAS by prescription.[14]

To restrict availability, the Federal Anti-Drug Abuse Act of 1988 "prohibits distribution of anabolic steroids" for "any use in humans other than the treatment of disease . . ." and outlines penalties, including imprisonment.[14] Anabolic-androgenic steroids became a controlled substance in 1990.[15] Violation of state and federal provisions by physicians may lead to loss of license and incarceration.[7]

Concurrent Use of Other Drugs

Body builders and athletes using AAS may also take tamoxifen to prevent gynecomastia,[5] growth hormone (GH), thyroid hormone, and diuretics. Some of these compounds may enhance the adverse effects of AAS.[5]

Methods of Decreasing Steroid Abuse

It is unlikely that drug testing alone will be an effective deterrent to AAS use. The high cost of drug testing prohibits widespread implementation. Education may help dissuade athletes from using AAS. Junior high school may be the appropriate level to start education, since AAS use often starts before age 16.[8] Educators' credibility may be enhanced by presenting balanced information about the potential benefits of AAS, health risks, and ethical concerns. Scare tactics—presenting only the detrimental effects of AAS—have proven ineffective.[16]

More difficult challenges are changing the attitude among athletes that it is acceptable to win at any cost and the values that place such a premium on appearance.

If a team physician suspects an athlete of using AAS, he or she may present the athlete with alternatives, including nutritional guidance and supervision in a weight-training program. Evidence of side effects, such as decreased high-density lipoprotein or abnormal liver function tests, may help dissuade an athlete from using AAS. During withdrawal from AAS, psychological counseling and referral to an endocrinologist for possible hormone replacement therapy may be warranted.

GROWTH HORMONE

Compared with abuse of anabolic steroids, abuse of GH is a new phenomenon. Popularity of GH supplementation stems from hopes that it will increase strength and height yet escape detection by drug tests. Increased availability of growth hormone may be a problem because of the recent technologic advances that allow production of human growth hormone (hGH) from recombinant DNA.

Mechanism of Action

Growth hormone is a polypeptide secreted by the anterior pituitary gland. Its most important function is to stimulate somatic growth.[17] By stimulating fatty acid oxidation, it may spare protein for anabolic pathways.[17]

History of Growth Hormone

Since the 1950s, GH has been used as replacement therapy for children with a deficiency of endogenous hormone.[18] Initially, it was extracted from pituitary glands of cadavers. In 1985, this extraction was stopped because of discovery of viral contamination.[1] A slow virus was implicated in several cases of Creutzfeldt-Jakob disease, a fatal encephalopathy.[4,19] The potential supply of hGH abruptly increased in 1984 with the development of methods to produce it via recombinant DNA technology.

Pharmacology

Supplemental GH must be administered by injection because the gastrointestinal tract destroys most of the hormone.[1] Development of a GH "drug test" is difficult because GH is a natural compound and has a half-life of only 15 minutes to 1 hour, and because very little is eliminated in the urine.

Efficacy

Although administration of GH is known to increase height in GH-deficient children and may boost the growth rate in some short children who are not GH deficient, it is not known if supplemental GH accelerates growth or increases final height in other children.[20,21]

Administration of GH to animals may increase muscle size and performance of atrophied muscle, but the ability of GH to increase strength and performance of normal human muscles is unknown.[17] The fact that muscles of persons with acromegaly are large, but weak, suggests that GH administration may not increase strength in normal human muscles.[2] Also, enhancement of muscle bulk may be caused by an increase in connective tissue but not of contractile fibers.[17]

In one study in humans, 8 mg hGH was given each week for 6 weeks to well-trained exercising adults. (Production of endogenous GH has been estimated at 0.4 to 1.0 mg/day in adult males.[17]) The subjects' body fat decreased and fat-free weight increased; athletic performance was not evaluated.[22] No other published reports present evidence that GH supplementation improves performance.[17]

Anecdotal reports yield inconsistent findings on the efficacy of GH in reducing body fat, increasing muscle bulk, and enhancing strength.[17]

Adverse Effects

Adverse effects of hGH in athletes can be predicted from complications of endogenous growth hormone hypersecretion,[4] although most adverse effects in athletes have not been studied directly. Hypersecretion of GH by the pituitary gland leads to gigantism, with increased linear growth in prepubertal children. After closure of epiphyseal growth plates, hypersecretion of GH leads to acromegaly.[2,17] Acromegaly is irreversible and develops insidiously (Table 16–2). The myopathy of acromegaly is unusual; although muscles appear large, they are weak and exercise tolerance is poor.[17] The life span is reduced by acromegaly. Mortality is 50% by age 50 years and 89% by 60 years.[17]

Other potential problems with GH supplementation include decreased high-density lipoprotein cholesterol, transmission of viruses, and formation of antibodies. In one study, six body builders who self-administered anabolic steroids plus hGH for 6 weeks developed significantly decreased levels of HDL cholesterol.[23] Transmission of hepatitis virus and human immunodeficiency virus may occur if needles used for injection of GH are shared. Exogenous GH administration may lead to antibodies, which neutralize exogenous GH—and perhaps endogenous GH. This could lead to permanent GH deficiency.[17]

Abuse by Athletes

Abuse of GH is probably limited by its high cost and limited availability. Although the Food and Drug Administration and other agencies are attempting to curb illegal distribution of GH, some may still reach the illegal market. There is also risk of foreign product introduction.[1] Illegal suppliers may substitute other preparations for this still scarce substance, including animal extracts of unlikely efficacy and steroids.[1] The incidence of GH abuse by athletes is unknown. Five percent of 224 male adolescents surveyed at several suburban high schools reported past or present use of GH.[24] Such a high prevalence of abuse is questionable, however, since the authors could not confirm that adolescents *were* using GH, the population studied was small,

Table 16–2. Complications of Acromegaly

Soft tissue and bone thickening
Hypothyroidism
Hyperlipidemia
Hypertension
Atherosclerotic heart disease
Cardiomyopathy
Congestive heart disease
Diabetes mellitus
Hypercalciuria
Hypogonadism
Impotence
Peripheral nerve compression
Osteoarthrosis

and the students exhibited poor knowledge about GH, suggesting that perhaps they were unable to identify it for purchase.

Few physicians admit to prescribing GH to athletes. One physician, however, in 1983 reported he had for years prescribed hGH for hundreds of athletes and body builders.[1]

Alternative Compounds

Athletes may try to increase endogenous GH release by taking amino acids, clonidine, levodopa, propranolol, or vasopressin and by exercising.[17] The efficacy of these compounds is unknown. Intermittent, high-intensity exercise produces higher levels of GH than does continuous exercise.[17]

CONCLUSION

While AASs may help an athlete increase strength, they deserve the title "bitter pill," because of their multiple, serious side effects. Although the efficacy of GH, in terms of gaining a height and strength advantage, is unproven, athletic abuse may be a growing problem as its availability increases and athletes try to maximize their performance by any means while beating drug tests.

REFERENCES

1. White, G. L., et al.: Preventing growth hormone abuse: an emerging health concern. Health Education Aug./Sept.:4, 1989.
2. Catlin, D. H., and Hatton C. K.: Use and abuse of anabolic and other drugs for athletic enhancement. Advances in Internal Medicine. *36*:399, 1991.
3. Lombardo, J.: The efficacy and mechanisms of action and anabolic steroids. *In* Anabolic Steroids in Sport and Exercise. Edited by C. E. Yesalis. Champaign, IL, Human Kinetics Publishers, 1993.
4. Council on Scientific Affairs, AMA: Drug abuse in athletes: Anabolic steroids and human growth hormone. J.A.M.A. *259*:1703, 1988.
5. Friedl, K. E.: Effects of anabolic steroids on physical health. *In* Anabolic Steroids in Sport and Exercise. Edited by C. E. Yesalis. Champaign, IL, Human Kinetics Publishers, 1993.
6. Yesalis, C. E., Courson, S. P., and Wright, J.: History of anabolic steroid use in sport and exercise. *In* Anabolic Steroids in Sport and Exercise. Edited by C. E. Yesalis. Champaign, IL, Human Kinetics Publishers, 1993.
7. Hallagan, J. D., Hallagan, L. F., and Snyder, M. B.: Sounding board: Anabolic-androgenic steroid use by athletes. N. Engl. J. Med. *321*:1042, 1989.
8. Buckley, W. E., et al.: Estimated prevalence of anabolic steroid use among male high school seniors. J.A.M.A. *260*:3441, 1988.
9. Tanner, S. M., Miller, D. W., and Alongi, C.: Unpublished study, 1993.
10. Windsor, R., and Dumitru, D.: Prevalence of anabolic steroid use by male and female adolescents. Med. Sci. Sports Exerc. *21*:494, 1989.
11. Anderson, W. A., et al.: A national survey of alcohol and drug use by college athletes. Physician Sportsmed. *19*(2):91, 1991.
12. Haupt, H. A., and Rovere, G. D.: Anabolic steroids: A review of the literature. Am. J. Sports Med. *12*:469, 1984.
13. American College of Sports Medicine: Position stand on the use of anabolic-androgenic steroids in sports. Med. Sci. Sports Exerc. *19*:534, 1987.
14. Interagency Task Force on Anabolic Steroids (1991, January). Washington, DC. U.S. Department of Health and Human Services, Public Health Service, 1991.
15. Yesalis, C. E., and Wright, J.: Societal alternatives. *In* Anabolic Steroids in Sport and Exercise. Edited by C. E. Yesalis. Champaign, IL, Human Kinetics Publishers, 1993.
16. Goldberg, L., et al.: Anabolic steroid education and adolescents: Do scare tactics work? Pediatrics *87*:283, 1991.
17. Macintyre, J. G.: Growth hormone and athletes. Sports Med. *4*:129, 1987.
18. Ilkos, D., Luft, R., and Gemzell, C. A.: The effect of human growth hormone in man. Lancet *1*:720, 1958.
19. Underwood, L. E.: Degenerative neurologic disease in patients formerly treated with human growth hormone. J. Pediatr. *107*:10, 1985.
20. Underwood, L. E.: Report of conference on uses and possible abuses of biosynthetic human growth hormone. N. Engl. J. Med. *311*:606, 1984.
21. VanVliet, G., et al.: Growth hormone treatment for short stature. N. Engl. J. Med. *309*:1016, 1983.
22. Crist, D. M., et al.: Body composition response to exogenous GH during training in highly conditioned adults. J. Appl. Physiol. *65*:579, 1988.
23. Zuliani, U., et al.: Effects of anabolic steroids, testosterone, and HGH on blood lipids and echocardiographic parameters in body builders. Int. J. Sports Med. *10*:62, 1989.
24. Rickert, V. I., et al.: Human growth hormone: A new substance of abuse among adolescents? Clin. Pediatr. *31*:723, 1992.

17 Karl Lee Barkley II

Child and Adolescent Athletes

It has often been said, in one way or another, that children and adolescents are not "little adults." This certainly is true when comparing young athletes to adult ones. There are many similarities between the two groups, but some of the differences must be highlighted to afford a better understanding of the medical and orthopedic concerns of young competitors.

It is estimated that, in the United States, 20 million sports participants between the ages of 8 and 16 years are involved in nonscholastic sports and community-sponsored programs. Additionally, 20 million adolescents are involved in recreational or unstructured physical activities. Seven million are estimated to participate in high school athletics—in at least 32 boys' and 27 girls' sports.[1]

Children and adolescents exercise for various reasons: (1) to have fun (probably the most important), (2) to socialize and be with friends, (3) to attain self-confidence and personal satisfaction, (4) to further life goals (in the case of adolescents), and (5) to become physically fit. The last one is perhaps the most important reason why *adults* exercise and the least important motive for children and adolescents.[1,2]

GROWTH AND DEVELOPMENT

Understanding the difference between pediatric and adult athletes requires a brief review of growth and physiology as it pertains to athletics. Specific medical conditions and injuries can better be reviewed against this background.

Boys and girls grow at approximately the same rate during childhood. Boys are born slightly bigger, grow slightly more during the first year, and sustain this "lead" throughout the prepubertal stage. Average growth per year is about 5 cm of height and 2.5 kg of weight for both genders. The maximum growth spurt occurs earlier in girls (age 12 to 13 years) than in boys (age 14 to 15 years). Men are taller overall because of this longer period of preadolescent growth and the fact that their maximum growth period tends to last longer as well.[2,3] There is an increase in body weight for both groups; boys experience a greater increase in lean body mass than postadolescent girls, who on average have about two thirds the amount of muscle and twice as much body fat as their male peers.[2]

Physiologic capabilities are important to understand in the pediatric and adolescent age groups. The physiologic term VO_2max is used to describe the greatest amount of oxygen that an exercising subject can consume and process during a progressively increasing exercise test. Exercise physiologists use this term to represent a person's fitness or aerobic capacity. The VO_2max/kg of the preadolescent child is often very close to adult levels. This age group is already at maximum efficiency regardless of training status. At puberty, unless a training effect is maintained, VO_2max declines. Adolescents, unlike their prepubescent counterparts, are able to increase their VO_2max with regular training. This suggests that improving skill proficiency is the main benefit of exercise for prepubescent children.[1,4] Long conditioning sessions do not increase aerobic capacity and should be discouraged in this age group because they may predispose to overuse injuries.

Preparticipation physical examinations are required in some form for all aspiring pediatric athletes who participate in organized school athletics and in many recreational leagues. These evaluations often include assessing the physical maturity of the child. There are still some unresolved questions about the use of Tanner's staging guidelines for assessing and making decisions for play.

Tanner's stages are used to assess secondary sex characteristics, as a way of judging the physical maturity of boys and girls. This sexual maturation scale or rating was developed in 1962 and further refined in 1969. There has recently been some controversy about its suitability for determining whether pediatric and adolescent athletes are approved for sports participation. Currently, the debate centers on whether physically immature athletes are at greater risk for injury in competition with physically mature athletes, especially in contact and collision sports. The recently published monograph entitled Preparticipation Physical Evaluation is a joint project of several groups.[5] It outlines the controversy but does not take a stand. The risks are largely theoretical; no current research supports excluding an athlete from participation on the basis of an immature rating on the Tanner scale. Until better prospective studies are available, the Tanner scale should not be used routinely to make participation decisions, although, common sense dictates some counseling of athletes and their parents about the theoretical risks of competition with bigger or stronger competitors.

MEDICAL CONCERNS OF CHILD AND ADOLESCENT ATHLETES

Causes of sudden death in the pediatric age group usually involve some sort of congenital condition as opposed to coronary artery disease, which is the most common cause of sudden death in exercising persons older than 35 years. Common features of the adolescent sudden death victim include male gender, participation in a variety of sports (football, basketball), and junior high or high school age. The incident usually occurs on the playing field or just after a period of exertion. The most common cause of sudden death in this age group is hypertrophic obstructive cardiomyopathy. In one study this was the cause of 48% of sudden deaths.[6]

Screening for possible cardiac conditions must concentrate on a history of syncope during exercise or family history of sudden death at a young age. A physical examination of the young athlete may reveal a heart murmur, but one third of normal athletes have a murmur. Echocardiography is considered the diagnostic test of choice, but it should not be ordered without obtaining an electrocardiogram first. If an athlete has a normal electrocardiogram or findings of the athletic heart syndrome (sinus bradycardia, etc.), most often reassurance is called for rather than further workup.

There is currently no test that can be applied on a broad basis to detect potentially lethal conditions in young athletes. The best current methods involve a complete cardiac history and physical as part of a routine preparticipation physical examination by a qualified health professional. The examination should include cardiac auscultation, blood pressure and heart rate measurement, pulses, and body habitus assessment for Marfanoid features (associated with risk of sudden death from aortic rupture). Echocardiography is the test of choice to exclude structural abnormalities, but it has not been cost effective when applied for screening. Exercise and rest electrocardiography can play a role when history indicates. Serum lipids should be assessed in a younger athlete with a significant family history of premature coronary artery disease.

There is truly no substitute for the history and physical examination when assessing for risk of sudden death. Historical "red flags" include chest pain on exertion, syncope, exercise-related syncope, presyncope or lightheadedness, known congenital or acquired cardiovascular disease, fatigue with light exercise, and suspicious family history.

Infectious disease often affects the younger population and may affect an athlete's ability to participate. Mononucleosis is a well-known condition associated with adolescents. Epstein-Barr virus is the agent of this acute, self-limiting, lymphoproliferative disease with autoimmune features. A 3- to 5-day prodrome of malaise, fatigue, anorexia, headache, and myalgia heralds the onset. The classic triad consists of pharyngitis (usually incapacitating), lymphadenopathy in the posterior cervical chain, and fever. The spleen is palpable in 50 to 70% by the second week.[7] It is this splenomegaly that concerns most practitioners when making the decision to send an athlete back to play. Splenic rupture is rare (prevalence 0.1 to 0.2% of all cases).[7] Many ruptures are spontaneous, occurring without trauma.

The athlete with mononucleosis may return to easy activity after 3 weeks, as long as the spleen is not painful or enlarged, the athlete is afebrile, and symptoms and laboratory abnormalities are resolved. Full return can be granted in 1 month for noncontact sports. The physician should consider ultrasound measurement of the spleen when in doubt about resumption of a contact sport. It is better to err on the side of keeping such athletes out too long than sending them back too early.[7,8]

Unlike mononucleosis, which is relatively easy to recognize in young athletes, exercise-induced asthma or bronchospasm is often overlooked. Clinical features usually appear after 5 to 8 minutes of intensive exercise or hyperpnea. There are the usual obvious symptoms, such as wheezing, chest tightness, or pain, and sometimes not so obvious symptoms such as cough, a feeling of being out of shape, or a lack of energy. The criterion for diagnosis is a 10 to 15% decline in forced expiratory volume or peak expiratory flow rate following exercise at 80 to 90% of predicted maximum heart rate for 6 to 8 minutes.[9] If the clinical history suggests the diagnosis, a trial of a β_2 agonist inhaler 15 to 30 minutes before competition or practice can be considered.

Recognition of eating disorders in adolescent athletes is difficult and they are often overlooked. Sports that promote a lean body image or where leanness is equated with optimal performance are higher-risk sports for athletes with eating disorders. This includes sports such as gymnastics, figure skating, distance running, swimming, and diving. Girls experience the highest number of eating disorders (9:1 ratio of girls to boys), and young adolescent girls are especially vulnerable. Anorexia nervosa and bulimia are the two most common eating disorders. Warning signs include solitary eating, trips to the restroom after eating (for the purposes of purging), preoccupation with weight, mood swings, rapid weight fluctuations, and self-statements that do not accurately reflect the true body image (e.g., "I'm so fat" from an obviously lean cross-country runner). Treatment of these disorders is difficult but it depends first on recognition by the practitioner. Usually treatment is carried out in a multispecialty approach employing physician, psychologist, coach, and nutritionist to execute a treatment plan and intervention.[10]

Another type of abnormal eating is seen in sports that have weight classifications such as wrestling, boxing, weight lifting, and martial arts sports. Unhealthy techniques used to "cut weight" include fasting, and dehydration through sweating, purging, and use of diuretics or laxatives. In these type of sports, boys outnumber girls. Counseling of the athlete by the physician or an available nutritionist is helpful, as is educating coaches in safe weight loss techniques.

ORTHOPEDIC CONCERNS OF CHILD AND ADOLESCENT ATHLETES

Pediatric and adolescent athletes sustain many of the same overuse injuries, such as Achilles tendinitis, plantar fasciitis, and patellar tendinitis, that mature adults incur. Of special concern in child athletes are the epiphyseal and apophyseal areas of the immature skeleton, which are subject to injury and repetitive stress during sports competition. Young athletes may sustain a different set of sports injuries related to these growing areas of the skeleton.

Children and adolescents have at both ends of long bones growth areas, or epiphyses. These areas "close" at an average bone age of 14.5 years for girls and 16.5 years for boys. An important fact to note is that these areas are the weakest part of the bone. The ligaments are 300% stronger than the physeal area in a Tanner Stage 3 child (period of maximum growth). It is this weak area that is prone to injury in active children and adolescents.[11]

The Salter and Harris classification of growth plate injuries is commonly used to describe these injuries (Fig. 17–1). The Salter I injury is a nondisplaced fracture. The radiograph often appears normal, and this can cause the examining practitioner to miss the diagnosis. The diagnosis should be based on clinical findings of point tenderness over the physeal area.

Treatment of epiphyseal injuries usually consists of immobilization and gradual return to play. Referral to an orthopedist or management by a primary care physician who is comfortable casting fractures is recommended. Types II through IV have been described in various orthopedic texts and should be recognized radiographically and referred for treatment. Generally, Types I and II have excellent prognoses for prompt healing and no residual problems or growth disturbance. Types III and IV require open reduction and internal fixation and have a more guarded prognosis. Type V can go unrecognized and has the potential to lead to major growth disturbances. The patient with this type of injury should be followed for potential growth disturbances until growth stops, and the family should be advised of the potential complications.[12]

The growing athlete who presents with a chief complaint of "sprain" should be examined carefully to exclude epiphyseal injury. The "sprained ankle" in this age group may represent a distal fibular physeal fracture, and the "sprained knee" may represent a Salter injury of the distal femur or proximal tibia. In this area of the knee stress radiographic views are helpful. In a 12-year-old pitcher the repeated stress of throwing can lead to Little League shoulder, a fracture of the physis of the proximal humerus. This condition is often caused by repetitive throwing but can be associated with just one throw.[16] The distal radial physis can be injured by trauma or repetitive stress as well. The term *gymnast's wrist* has often been applied. Figure 17–2 highlights some potential areas of epiphyseal and apophyseal injury.

The apophysis is an area where major tendons attach via an interfacing layer of physeal cartilage. These areas are prone to avulsion or overuse stress. The areas where avulsions most often occur are around the hip and pelvis area (see Fig. 17–2). The sartorius can be pulled off the anterosuperior iliac spine. With this injury, point tenderness over the anterosuperior iliac spine is noted. The physician asks the patient to place the foot of the affected limb on the opposite knee and flex the affected hip against resistance. As this motion is performed, the physician observes for pain. The rectus femoris attaches to the anteroinferior iliac spine. If an avulsion injury occurs at this insertion, point tenderness should be present, and passive flexion of the knee with the hip extended should produce pain. The hamstrings attach to the ischial tuberosity and can be avulsed by sudden effort. This injury can be diagnosed by having the athlete flex at the hip with the knee extended; a positive finding is pain in the area of the ischial tuberosity. The iliopsoas attaches to the lesser trochanter, and pain elicited by medially rotating the thigh with the knee and hip flexed at 90° indicates avulsion of the tendon attachment. Avulsions from the posterior iliac crest are rare.

Management of apophyseal avulsion is usually conservative and includes rest, immobilization, anti-inflammatory medications, and time. Some avulsions may be reattached if the avulsed tendon attachment is significantly displaced. One author has suggested greater than 15 mm as a guide to consider surgery, at least in the ischial tuberosity avulsion.[13] Occasionally, an avulsion of the mid–iliac crest apophysis can occur, but more than likely this would be an overuse apophysitis of characteristically insidious onset.

Other conditions about the hip include osteitis pubis, which is not confined to the adolescent athlete but may be more predominant in the adolescent distance runner or soccer player. With osteitis pubis, pain is noted about the symphysis pubis and is made worse with activity. An adductor strain can sometimes mimic osteitis pubis, as can a stress fracture of the pubic ramus, which is sometimes seen in female distance runners. Radionuclide bone scan findings can be positive with both stress fractures and osteitis pubis, but they may help differentiate the two if necessary. Management of osteitis pubis is conservative (the usual measures), but occasionally bed

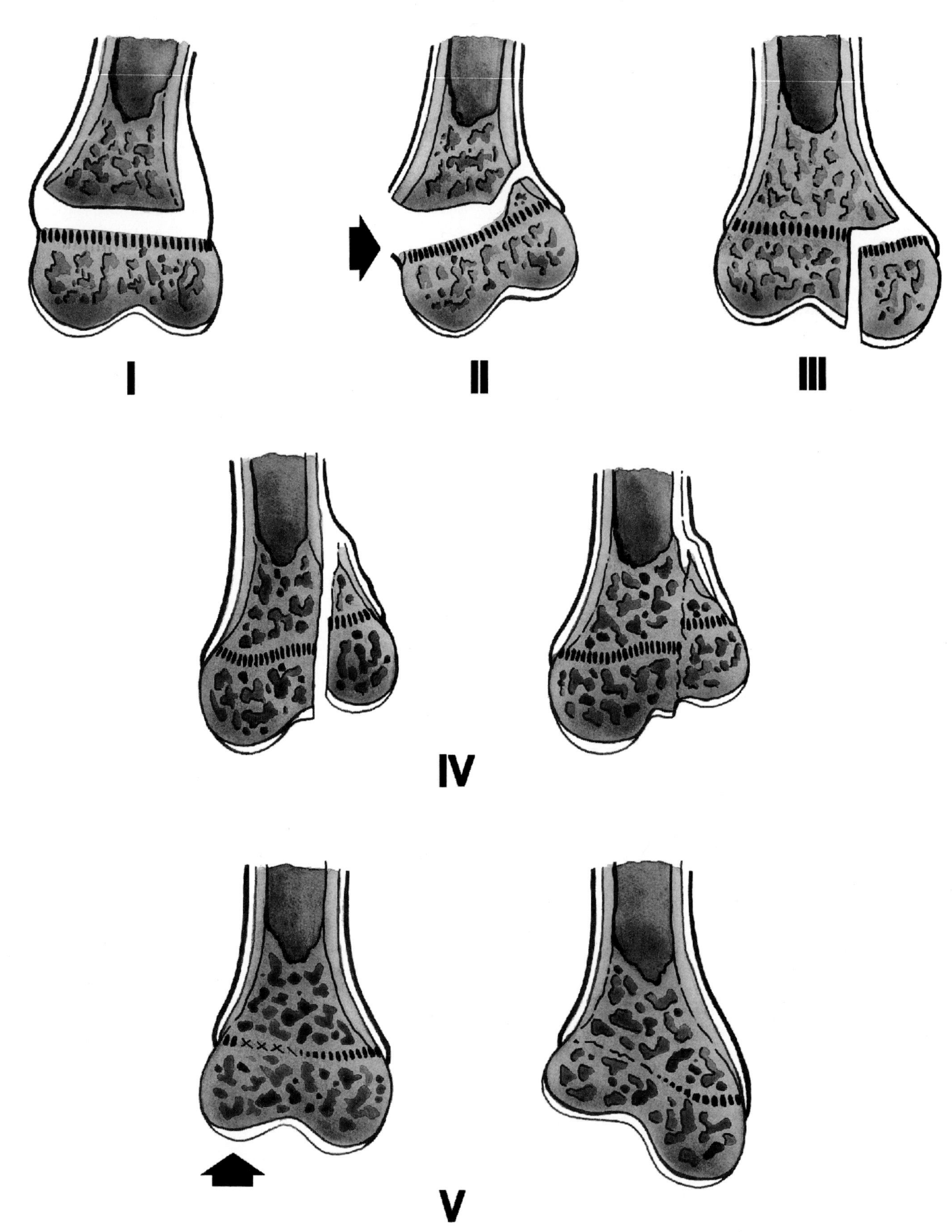

Fig. 17–1. Salter-Harris classification of epiphyseal injury: Type I, nondisplaced fracture; Type II, fracture through most of the plate that involves part of the metaphysis; Type III, fracture along the growth plate and into the joint through the epiphysis; Type IV, intra-articular fracture involving the epiphysis, the growth plate, and the metaphysis; Type V, crushed growth plate.

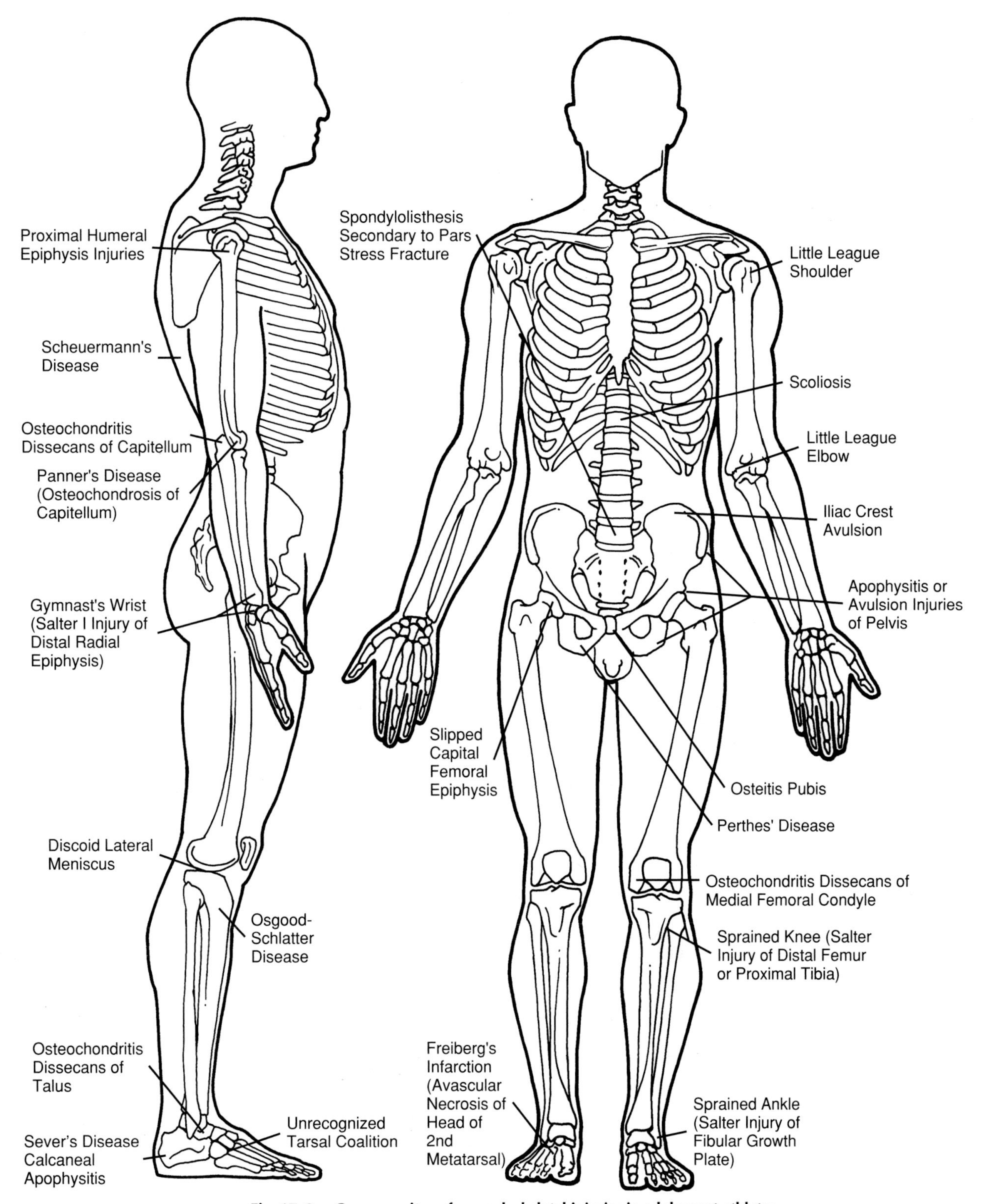

Fig. 17–2. Common sites of musculoskeletal injuries in adolescent athletes.

rest may be required, followed by gradual return to ambulation with crutches.[14]

One important condition about the hip that may develop in an adolescent or child athlete is slipped capital femoral epiphysis. This can occur abruptly (5 to 10% of cases) or gradually (90%). The baseball player who slides into base and experiences sudden pain or the basketball player who gradually develops pain during the course of the season may both represent the same entity. The patient is usually a 9- to 17-year old male who is taller and heavier than average.[15] Clinically, the patient may present with a limp and pain. Physical examination reveals the pathognomonic external rotation of the hip as it is moved into flexion. It is always wise to keep in mind the diagnosis of slipped capital femoral epiphysis when an adolescent has unexplained knee pain.

For the sake of completeness, Perthes' disease should be considered as a potential diagnosis in the younger age group (5- to 9-year-olds and occasionally 10- to 12-year-olds). This is an avascular necrosis of the femoral head of unknown cause. Symptoms may be indistinguishable from transient synovitis on first presentation. Although Perthes' disease is not typically associated with sports, youngsters who play sports are not excluded either. Another avascular necrosis with considerably better prognosis is Freiberg's infarction, avascular necrosis of the metatarsal head, usually the second one. Pain, swelling, and limp are all symptoms of Freiberg's infarction. Radiographs reveal some sclerosis, irregularity, and even collapse of the metatarsal head (several weeks after the onset of pain). Usually, restriction of activity, and possibly casting, is necessary, but the condition is often self-limited.[15]

Another category of injury seen in children and adolescents is osteochondritis dissecans, which can occur at the knee, ankle, or elbow. This group of conditions shares the common feature of "the separation of an abnormal ossification area within the epiphysis covered by articular cartilage."[16] The most common site is the knee—or, more specifically, the medial femoral condyle (75%). Repeated trauma to the flexed knee may predispose the athlete to this condition. Osteochondritis dissecans is more common in boys than in girls, and the clinical presentation may include poorly localized pain, effusion, locking, and giving way. Referral to an orthopedist is generally recommended since the unstable fragment may need pinning. Osteochondritis dissecans of the ankle involves the superomedial or superolateral aspect of the talus and must be distinguished from an acute fracture associated with ankle sprains. Adolescents present with general aching and swelling of insidious onset or with a "recurrent sprain."

The elbow joint of young pitchers (and gymnasts) is subject to osteochondritis dissecans at the capitellum. Restriction of activity is necessary and may last up to a year. This condition should not be confused with Little League elbow, a term that has been used to describe 12 different entities about the elbow but was originally applied to avulsion of the medial ossification center at the elbow in an adolescent throwing athlete. Splinting and rest may suffice for this entity, but a complete separation may require surgery.[17]

Panner's disease, or osteochondrosis of the capitellum, is yet another separate entity not to be confused with osteochondritis dissecans. It, too, is thought to be associated with the valgus stress placed on the lateral elbow of young pitchers. Pain and inability to extend the elbow are noted, and radiographs reveal fragmentation of the capitellum. A sling or splint may be necessary; the athlete returns gradually to movement as symptoms allow. The athlete may need to switch to a sport that does not involve throwing or weight bearing.[16]

Perhaps one of the most common sports injuries is Osgood-Schlatter disease, which sounds very ominous but in reality is seldom associated with complications. The tibial tubercle apophysis becomes inflamed, swollen, and painful to the touch. The pain is often worse with activities such as running and jumping and is most common in 11- to 14-year-old boys. Treatment usually includes rest, activity as tolerated, anti-inflammatory medications, ice, and stretching. Similarly, Sever's disease, the heel's version of apophysitis, causes pain over the posterolateral aspect of the os calcis. The same type of conservative treatment measures are helpful.

Back pain in a child or adolescent can be caused by many of the same things that cause it in adults, but there are several specific ones to note. Certainly, scoliosis should be sought on the preparticipation physical examination, and students who exhibit it should be referred, if necessary. Kyphosis, or roundback, comes in two forms: the postural variety and Scheuermann's disease. The second type is more common in boys and by definition has structural vertebral changes, including greater than 5° wedging at two consecutive vertebrae. End plate irregularities and loss of disc space are often noted. The postural variety is usually painless, as opposed to Scheuermann's disease, with which the patient complains of localized back pain.[15] Treatment can include observation, extension exercises, and even bracing. In some cases surgery may be necessary.

Another cause of back pain in weight lifting or power athletes or those who often hyperextend the back (gymnasts) is spondylolysis, with or without spondylolisthesis. The pars interarticularis of the posterior vertebral arch can become weakened with repetitive stresses and can fracture. This event can be associated with pain alone, but it is sometimes accompanied by forward slippage of one vertebra on another (spondylolisthesis), which can also be associated with pain. The slippage may be the result of either a congenital pars defect or stress-related changes. Having the patient hyperextend the spine while standing on one leg often reproduces the pain in either spondylolysis or spondylolisthesis. Conservative measures, such as rest and possibly a back brace, may suffice for a pars stress fracture. Patients with spondylolisthesis should be followed on a regular basis with standing lateral radiographs. Progression may mean that stabilization is warranted.

Two final conditions that can be added to the list of pediatric and adolescent orthopedic concerns are tarsal coalition and discoid meniscus. Tarsal coalition is marked by two or more tarsal bones that are joined by a bony bar or fibrocartilaginous bridge. Although this condition is congenital, most cases do not become symptomatic until adolescence, when the patient may present with a painful and rigid flat foot sometimes associated with spasm of the peroneal muscles. Referral is indicated, and probably surgical intervention.

Discoid lateral meniscus is thought to be a normal meniscus with abnormal attachments to the periphery of the joint. There is an abnormal shape and thickness to this meniscal tissue. Often a popping or snapping sensation is present, and a small mass may be noticed at the lateral joint line. Excision may be required to prevent further degenerative changes.[18,19]

REFERENCES

1. McKeag, D.: Adolescents and exercise. J. Adolesc. Healthcare *7*:121S, 1986.
2. Smith, R. E., Smoll, F.L., and Smith, N. J.: Parents' Complete Guide to Youth Sports. Costa Mesa, CA, HDL Publishing, 1989.
3. Fujii, C. M., and Felice, M. E.: Physical growth and development: Current concepts. Adolesc. Med. Primary Care *14*:1, 1987.
4. Dyment, P. G.: Sports Medicine: Health Care for Young Athletes. Elk Grove, IL, American Academy of Pediatrics, 1991.
5. Preparticipation Physical Evaluation (Monograph). A joint publication of AAFP, AAP, AMMSM, AOSSM, and AOASM. Kansas City, MO. 1992.
6. Maron, B. J., et al.: Sudden death in young athletes. Circulation *62*:218, 1980.
7. Maki, D. G., and Reich, R. M.: Infectious mononucleosis in the athlete: Diagnosis, complications and management. Am. J. Sports Med. *10*:162, 1982.
8. Haines, J. D.: When to resume sports after infectious mononucleosis: How soon is safe? Postgrad. Med. *81*:331, 1987.
9. Katz, R. M.: Coping with exercise-induced asthma in sports. Physician Sportsmed. *15*(7):100, 1987.
10. Murphy, S. M.: Effects of Competition on the Athlete: Psychological Issues to be Encountered in Sport. Presentation at ACSM Team Physician Course, Part III. March, 1991.
11. Ehrlich, M. G., et al.: Sports injuries in children and the clumsy child. Pediatr. Clin. North Am. *39*:443, 1992.
12. Mayer, P. J.: Lower limb injuries in childhood and adolescence. *In* Pediatric and Adolescent Sports Medicine. Edited by L. J. Micheli. Boston, Little, Brown & Co., 1984.
13. Weiker, G.: Apophyseal avulsion, osteitis pubis, hip pointer, and others. Presentation at ACSM Team Physician Course, Part III. March 1991.
14. Micheli, L. J.: Injuries to the hip and pelvis. *In* The Pediatric Athlete. Edited by J. A. Sullivan and W. A. Grana. Park Ridge, IL, American Academy of Orthopaedic Surgeons, 1990.
15. DeRosa, G. P.: Orthopedic conditions. *In* Textbook of Adolescent Medicine. Edited by E. R. McAnarney, et al. Philadelphia, W.B. Saunders, 1992.
16. Garrick, J. G.: Sports injuries and the osteochondroses. *In* Textbook of Adolescent Medicine. Edited by E. R. McAnarney, et al. Philadelphia, W. B. Saunders, 1992.
17. Hunter, S. C.: Little Leaguer's elbow. *In* Injuries to the Throwing Arm. US Olympic Sports Medicine Council. Edited by B. Zarins, J. Andrews, and W. Carson. Philadelphia, W.B. Saunders, 1985.
18. Watts, H. G.: The bones and joints: Orthopedic problems. *In* Nelson Textbook of Pediatrics. 13th Ed. Edited by R. E. Behrman, and V. C. Vaughan III. Philadelphia, W. B. Saunders, 1987.
19. Grana, W. G.: Injuries to the knee. *In* The Pediatric Athlete. Edited by J. A. Sullivan and W. A. Grana. Park Ridge, IL, American Academy of Orthopaedic Surgeons. 1990.

18 *Patricia L. Skaggs*

The Pregnant Athlete

Understandably, active women are interested in continuing exercise throughout pregnancy. Over the last several decades, studies have more clearly defined the interrelationship of pregnancy and exercise. In 1985, the American College of Obstetricians and Gynecologists responded to an increased demand for information by developing and publishing guidelines for exercise during pregnancy.[1] The medical literature now supports well-documented conclusions regarding the effects of exercise on mother and fetus.

PHYSIOLOGIC RESPONSES TO EXERCISE

Despite significant biomechanical, physiologic, endocrine, and metabolic alterations in pregnancy, response to exercise is similar to that of nonpregnant athletes. Some responses to exercise, while they represent advantageous adaptations for the mother, may potentiate deleterious effects on the fetus.

Hemodynamic Response

During pregnancy, women's cardiac output increases 30 to 50% above the normal level during the first trimester. The heart rate is increased throughout the gestation period, but the increased myocardial oxygen requirements generally have little negative effect unless some underlying condition is also present. This increase in heart rate limits the maximum work capacity of women during pregnancy, by limiting the incremental change in output available with exercise.

The immediate response to exercise stress is increased cardiac output and oxygen consumption; relative tachycardia occurs later. A similar response is seen in pregnant exercisers.[2–6] Throughout pregnancy, cardiac output is higher at all levels of exercise than it is in nonpregnant control subjects. It is not clear whether the entire magnitude of the change can be attributed to higher resting values or whether this represents an augmented exercise-induced increase.

Blood volume is also increased in pregnant women as a response to circulating estrogen and because of the increased demands of the large arteriovenous shunt created by the placenta.[7] It is tempting to attribute increased cardiac output to the increased uterine blood flow, but the fact that maximum cardiac output occurs early in pregnancy suggests another mechanism. The major mechanism of increased cardiac output is cardiac enlargement: both left ventricular distension and muscle hypertrophy. In late pregnancy, posture dominates the control of cardiac output, because of its influence on venous return. When the woman is upright, the uterus is situated anteriorly; when she lies supine, the uterus rests posteriorly, compressing the inferior vena cava to the extent that cardiac filling is compromised. Decreased cardiac output of 22% in the supine position has been reported.[7]

The greater increase in plasma volume than in red blood cell mass leads to a decreased hematocrit value in pregnancy. A decrease in mean arterial pressure occurs early in pregnancy and rises toward nonpregnant values at term. Most reports indicate that maternal arterial blood pressure response during exercise is not affected by pregnancy,[3,6,8,9] but conflicting findings have been reported.[7]

The hemoconcentration seen during exercise is familiar to exercise physiologists and occurs in active pregnant patients as well. Plasma volume can decrease 17% with exercise in nonpregnant women. This change occurs rapidly and no further decrease is observed after 3 minutes' exercise; recovery occurs within 10 minutes after exercise stops. This hemoconcentration ensures adequate oxygen delivery capability during exercise despite altered blood flow distribution.

Uterine blood flow increases dramatically with gestational age, approaching 1 L/min in resting women near term. Uterine blood flow is controlled by sympathetic stimulation and by vascular resistance changes due to circulating catecholamines and hormones. There is evidence that pregnancy blunts the vascular response to the autonomic nervous system.[10] This would explain the common finding of decreased severity of Raynaud's phenomenon during pregnancy.

The exercise-induced redistribution of cardiac output away from splanchnic vessels and to skin and exercising muscles in the nonpregnant female suggests decreased uterine blood flow with exercise during pregnancy. Studies in sheep have demonstrated a fall in uterine blood flow of up to 35% with maternal exercise.[4,11] Other animal data reveal that uterine flow is inversely related to the intensity and duration of exercise.[4] In contrast, human studies suggest maintenance of uterine flow with exercise.[6]

Even in a setting of altered perfusion, several compensatory responses occur to prevent fetal hypoxia. A downward shift in the oxygen dissociation curve permits increased oxygen extraction and increased oxygen content differential across the umbilical circulation.[11] Some researchers attribute a greater role in maintaining oxygen delivery to the hemo-concentration that occurs with exercise.[4] Preferential shunting of blood within the uterus itself further contributes to stable placental VO_2 during exercise.[7,12]

Respiratory Response

Respiratory rate increases with exercise, and in pregnant women, it accelerates more than in nonpregnant ones.[13,14] The increased minute volume and tidal volume seen in pregnant women at rest increase further during exercise and at a higher rate for a given workload than in nonpregnant exercisers.[7,13] Artal and colleagues showed that pregnant women were not able to obtain the VO_2max level observed in nonpregnant controls.[15] Significantly lower ventilatory equivalent during moderate exercise suggests increased ventilatory efficiency, perhaps owing to the respiratory alkalosis of pregnancy. At maximal exercise intensity, this respiratory alkalosis may not be able to compensate for developing metabolic lactic acidosis. This inability to exercise anaerobically is a protective mechanism to avoid hypoxia or carbohydrate depletion.

Oxygen delivery to the fetus is enhanced by small but significant changes in maternal erythrocyte 2,3-diphosphoglycerate that counteract the Bohr effect of the alkalosis, shifting the oxygen dissociation curve back to the right and facilitating oxygen release to the fetus.

Other authors contend that respiratory ventilation does not limit exercise capacity in pregnant women unless they have an underlying pulmonary disease.[7] During both cycling and treadmill exercises, VO_2max was unaffected by pregnancy in subjects who served as their own controls.[16] Because of the progressive increase in basal oxygen consumption with gestation, the oxygen reserve available for exercise tended to decrease in pregnancy, but the degree was significant only with weight-bearing exercises or in late gestation.

COMMON MUSCULOSKELETAL PROBLEMS

The most obvious musculoskeletal change in pregnancy is the exaggerated lumbar lordosis that develops as the uterus grows anteriorly. A pelvic organ until 12 weeks' gestation, the uterus enlarges, increasing its weight by 1.5 to 2 pounds and its area by more than 150%. Dynamic adjustment in posture is achieved by increasing lumbar lordosis and cervical flexion, described by Shakespeare as "the proud posture." Enlarging breasts, with an average weight of 500 g, also add to the altered mechanical forces on the vertebral column and the shifted center of gravity. Increasing maternal weight stresses the musculoskeletal system. The total average gain of 25 to 30 pounds is comprised of fetus (7.5 pounds), amniotic fluid (2 pounds), placenta (1.5 to 2 pounds), uterus (1.5 to 2 pounds), breasts (1 pound), and the rest is increased total body water.

Hormonally mediated changes in the connective tissue of pregnant women occur early: relaxin (derived from the ovary) and estrogen induce softening of ligamentous cartilage. The resulting relaxation across the joints leads to increased joint mobility and, therefore, instability. These adaptations permit widening of the pelvis to allow fetal transit at birth.

Back Pain

Low back pain is estimated to occur in 50% of pregnant women. The asymptomatic group cannot be distinguished by age, weight gain, baby weight, or gravidity or parity. Although most reported onset of pain in the fifth to seventh month, the number of back complaints actually decreased beyond the seventh month. Fast and colleagues did record a significant racial distinction: more Caucasians in the back pain group and more Hispanics in the asymptomatic group.[17] The high incidence of low back pain was attributed to lordotic posture, effects of relaxin on ligamentous laxity, and the resultant pelvic insufficiency, as well as direct pressure on neural elements by the gravid uterus or herniated disc.

The pathologic role of lordotic posture is debated in the literature. Many authors support Fast and colleagues, who identify lordosis as a major contributor to low back pain in pregnancy. A review of women in primitive societies found zero incidence of low back pain among these women, who assume a stance of hip flexion with straight lumbar spine, again supporting the role of lordosis in producing low back pain.[18]

It is postulated that relaxin, which is involved in the remodeling of collagen, may directly affect the intervertebral joint and result in greater vulnerability to a given degree of lordotic stress.

Herniated discs remain uncommon during pregnancy. In a review of over 48,000 deliveries the incidence of herniated lumbar disc was found to be one per 10,000,[19] no greater than that in the general population. Although acute herniation during pregnancy is rare, previous vaginal delivery has been identified as a predisposing factor to later lumbar disc herniation.[20] As many as 50% of pregnant patients do not complain of low back pain. These patients may benefit from better overall fitness or trunk musculature, and they may be better able to tolerate altered load distribution.

The treatment of low back pain is similar in both pregnant and nonpregnant patients. The mechanics of daily activity must be optimized, and exercises must be aimed at improving strength, endurance, and control of trunk muscles learned. The lengthened abdominal muscles may be less effective in preventing anterior pelvic tilt in pregnant patients; hamstring strength becomes relatively more important in gravid patients. Flexion exercises should be prescribed with caution owing to the laxity of the pregnant woman's joints. Some investigators have found trochanter belts and lumbosacral corsets effective in decreasing pain.[21]

The sacroiliac joint becomes vulnerable to stress during pregnancy. In the nongravid female, ligaments that stabilize the joint limit virtually all movement. Relaxin-induced ligamentous laxity allows the sacroiliac joint to gradually stretch, accommodating the passage of the fetal head through the pelvic outlet at delivery. Weakening of the central fibrous tissue in the rectus abdominis leads to diastasis in approximately 30% of all pregnant patients. Abdominal exercise can cause further separation.

Idiopathic scoliosis does not progress beyond skeletal maturity in most females. Pregnancy has no effect on the degree of spinal curvature despite the presence of relaxin and altered spinal mechanics. In the few reported scoliosis patients whose deformity progressed throughout adulthood, the rate of curvature seems to be unaffected by pregnancy as well.[23] Pregnancy outcomes are unaffected by the presence of scoliosis.

Hand and Wrist Pain

Hand and wrist pain is the second most common orthopedic complaint of pregnant patients. Median nerve compression develops in approximately 20% of pregnant women, leading to typical symptoms of carpal tunnel syndrome.[22] Symptoms are bilateral in as many as two thirds of patients.[23] As in nonpregnant women, positive Tinel's and Phelan's signs with decreased sensation characterize the clinical examination. Delayed nerve conduction or thenar muscular atrophy is rare. The predilection for this syndrome in pregnancy may have a hormonal basis because the incidence of carpal tunnel syndrome is also increased by taking oral contraceptives. A reported 59% incidence of edema predisposes to this and other nerve compression syndromes.[22] Additionally, relaxation of the transverse carpal ligament may compress the median nerve by decreasing the height of the carpal tunnel. There is no association with excess weight gain or maternal age.[23]

Splinting and injection are mainstays of therapy. Symptoms generally resolve by 3 months post partum, but recurrence with subsequent pregnancies is common.

Pregnancy-associated fluid retention may also contribute to compression of the posterior tibial nerve, causing tarsal tunnel syndrome, or on the extensor pollicis brevis and abductor pollicis longus tendons, resulting in stenosing (or De Quervain's) tenosynovitis. The ulnar nerve is also subject to compression at two sites: (1) Guyon's canal at the wrist and (2) posterior to the medial epicondyle at the elbow.

Lower Extremity Problems

Not surprisingly, complaints of patellofemoral dysfunction increase in pregnant women. Indeed, it is the mechanics of the female pelvis, with increased Q angle and increased femoral torsion, that produces lateral vectors about the knee during flexion and extension. The increased weight and decreased activity of pregnancy may exacerbate this problem. Therapy is generally conservative and nonoperative. Weight loss cannot be recommended during pregnancy.

Recurrent leg cramps are a particularly bothersome symptom during pregnancy, and they affect 15 to 30% of women.[23] The cause of these often severe nocturnal cramps is unknown, but it has frequently been postulated to be a calcium or magnesium deficiency. Serum levels of these minerals are not different in pregnant and nonpregnant populations, but a negative calcium balance has been reported in the gravid population because of the large fetal requirement.[23] Oral administration of 1 g elemental calcium resulted in a significant decrease in severity and incidence of cramps in one study.[23] No significant side effects of this treatment were observed in the mother or the fetus. Other authors believe cramps represent mechanical pain resulting from chronic distension of the fascia in these patients and lower extremity venous pooling.[24] Lactic acid accumulation has also been postulated as a cause. The negative calcium balance suggests the possibility of a "pregnancy osteomalacia." However, no evidence of delayed bone healing in pregnancy has been confirmed.

The frequency of fractures in exercising pregnant women is not increased over that in the general population.[24] The diagnosis of fracture in this population becomes problematic because of the known teratogenic effects of radiation exposure, especially exposure in the first trimester. Every attempt should be made to reduce fetal exposure to radiation and to delay that exposure beyond the embryonic period of gestation.

Hip pain in pregnant women is generally related to mechanical back complaints; however, the possibility of osteonecrosis of the femoral head must be considered. Symptoms of osteonecrosis are vague: unilateral hip, thigh, and pelvis or groin pain are often attributed to fatigue. A high index of suspicion must be maintained to diagnose and treat this condition and to avoid the potential for femoral neck fracture. Investigators who reported seven cases of pregnancy-related osteonecrosis of the femoral head postulated that higher adrenocortical activity during pregnancy, aggravated by the stress of maternal weight gain, is responsible.[25] Radiographic findings are typical: lucency and possibly segmental collapse. Treatment includes avoidance of full weight bearing. Orthopedic follow-up with these patients is important, but spontaneous resolutions of symptoms and reconstitution of the skeleton is the rule by 4 to 6 months post partum. In cases complicated by stress fracture, surgical intervention may be required.

A history of pelvic fracture deserves special mention. Although there may be no exercise intolerance, permanent pelvic deformity may lead to cephalopelvic disproportion and be a contraindication to vaginal delivery. Examples of such deformities include central fracture-dislocation of the hip, which results in medial protrusion of the acetabulum and femoral head, or cephalad displacement of the hemi-pelvis seen in Malgaigne-type fracture dislocations.

Rheumatoid arthritis that results in synovial proliferation and inflammation affects women of child-bearing age. Interestingly, pregnancy frequently ameliorates both the acute symptoms and the progression of the disease. A protein found to be markedly elevated in pregnancy is now believed to be responsible for rheumatoid arthritis remissions.[21] Pregnancy α-glycoprotein is known to suppress monocyte activity. Still unexplained is that remission generally lasts 6 weeks post partum. Almost 70% of rheumatoid arthritis patients experience improvement during pregnancy. Symptoms recur later in more than 90%.[22]

METABOLISM

The metabolism of pregnancy has parallels with the increased metabolism and increased glucose use during exercise (Table 18–1). "Accelerated starvation" appears in pregnant females, even with short-term fasting, because of the glucose and amino acids used by the fetus.[8] This phenomenon predicts differences in energy metabolism in exercising pregnant women.

Late in pregnancy a fall in blood glucose is seen with even short-term exercise.[9,26,27] Glucose production can lag behind the accelerated glucose use. It is unclear whether this represents a detrimental effect.

Plasma lactate levels are generally similar in both pregnant and nonpregnant exercisers,[4,27,28] but concentrations are higher in pregnant women after more intensive exercise.[7,29]

As lactate and glucose are actively metabolized by the placenta and fetus, the physiologic impact of increased fetal and maternal levels is difficult to assess. A theoretical risk exists that the hypoglycemic response to endurance exercise and pregnancy would be additive. As noted, there are inconsistencies in the literature. A reviewer suggests that the specifics of the exercise itself, as well as individual maternal variables, can determine the glucose response to exercise during pregnancy.[26]

Table 18–1. Changes in Physiologic Parameters During Pregnancy

Parameter	*Change (%)*
Cardiovascular system	
Cardiac output	↑ (20–40)
Heart rate	↑ (0–20)
Stroke volume	↑ (25)
Arterial pressure:	
Systolic	↓ (5)
Diastolic	↓ (5)
Systemic vascular resistance	↓ (20–30)
Pulmonary vascular resistance	↓ (34)
Heart volume	↑ (12)
Pulmonary capillary wedge pressure	None
Blood volume	↑ (55)
Peripheral blood flow	↑ (600)
Hematocrit	
Respiratory system	
Tidal volume	↑ (30–40)
Respiratory rate	None
Expiratory reserve	↓ (40)
Residual volume	↓ (40)
Functional residual capacity	↓ (25)
Vital capacity	None
Minute volume	↑ (40–50)
Arterial P_{CO_2}	None
Blood pH	↑ to slight ↓
Renal system	
Renal plasma flow	↑ (25–50)
Glomerular filtration rate	↑ (50)
Metabolism and others	
Fibrinogen	↑ (50)
Platelets	↑ (33)
Free thyroxine and tri-iodothyronine	None
Plasma insulin	↑
Plasma glucagon	↑
Insulin resistance	↑ (80)
Cholesterol	↑ (100)
Triglycerides	↑ (300)
Free fatty acids	↑ (60)
Serum electrolytes	None
Nitrogen stores	↑
Oxygen consumption	↑ (15–20)

THERMOREGULATION

The profound thermoregulatory effects of the reproductive cycle suggest an interaction between the endocrine and thermoregulatory systems. Progesterone acts to reset the thermoregulatory control center, elevating the maternal temperature by at least 0.3°F. The elevated core temperature occurs early, peaks in midpregnancy, and may actually decline late in gestation. In addition, temperature is elevated because of the higher metabolic rate in pregnancy.

Exercise of sufficient intensity can induce heat stress. The temperature response to exercise is similar in both pregnant and nonpregnant women.[29] Sweat production does not change in the gravid state.[29]

At rest, the fetal temperature averages 0.5°C higher than maternal temperature. The main determinant of fetal temperature is maternal temperature, with changes in fetal metabolism and uterine blood flow having lesser effects.

The increased plasma volume in pregnancy helps to maintain optimal feto-maternal heat transfer and dissipation. However, the maximum increase in plasma volume occurs after the period of greatest vulnerability during fetal development.

In an animal model, treadmill exercise to exhaustion resulted in a 1.5°C elevation in core temperature.[11] Lotgering also observed a hyperthermic response in pregnant ewes.[16] Fetal temperature remained elevated for one hour postexercise, but despite decreased uterine blood flow and decreased Po_2 by 30%, no fetal distress was noted. McMurray and Katz concluded that no evidence for significant fetal effects was found in animal studies in which core temperature elevations did not exceed 1.5°C.[30] In human subjects, Clapp observed an improved efficiency of heat dissipation in late pregnancy similar to that seen with athletic training and heat acclimation.[26]

In a small study of trained runners who were observed in a climate-controlled environment, no change in thermoregulatory response was seen throughout pregnancy.[29] A pattern of early transient decrease in temperature was noted to be of greater magnitude in late pregnancy. It was felt that, owing to decreased vascular tone and increased peripheral pooling, cooler blood was mobilized with the onset of exercise, leading to the observed drop in core temperature. The increased plasma volume of pregnancy was thought to be responsible for optimizing uterine blood flow and heat dissipation in the setting of exercise-induced hemoconcentration and sweating.

Concern regarding hyperthermia in humans arises from literature in mammalian pregnancies strongly suggesting the teratogenicity of heat exposure. The central nervous system is most frequently and severely affected. Although direct evidence of fetal well-being is difficult to obtain, it appears moderate exercise does not pose a great risk of hyperthermia in humans.

Risks for markedly elevated core temperature and potentially detrimental fetal effects include maternal dehydration, prolonged vigorous exercise, decreased heat diffusion capacity (as with hot ambient temperature or humidity), poor maternal conditioning, and preexisting uteroplacental insufficiency. There may also be some risks of hyperthermia during the fetus' most vulnerable time of organogenesis in women who continue vigorous workouts before learning of the pregnancy.

FETAL RESPONSE TO EXERCISE

A discussion of response to exercise in the pregnant woman must focus on potential effects on the fetus. The relationship between the fetus and the mother is essentially a parasitic one: the fetus is wholly dependent on the mother for its development.

Normal exercise-induced changes in the mother may result in deleterious effects on the fetus. Of particular concern are the possibility of fetal hypoxemia due to decreased uterine blood flow, teratogenesis secondary to hyperthermia, and the metabolic changes of the "accelerated starvation" seen with high energy demands. Research in this area is problematic because of the obvious ethical constraints on study design. The conclusions from animal studies are difficult to extrapolate to human experience. Human studies have focused on indirect evidence of fetal well-being with noninvasive measurements of fetal heart rate and respiratory patterns as well as outcome studies.

Human studies offer indirect evidence of fetal tolerance during maternal exercise. An increased fetal heart rate is noted in response to moderate exercise (61 to 73% of maximum) in trained pregnant women,[31] and during exercise in both trained women and controls without deleterious effects on fetal outcome[32]; no rate greater than 100 bpm was observed. Rates in excess of 180 bpm were recorded in 60% of subjects after jogging without increased risk of poor fetal outcome.[27] More recent studies have reported fetal bradycardia during maternal exercise.[7] Fetal heart rate decreased within 30 to 60 seconds of the beginning of cycle exercise in 100% of trained subjects in one study.[33] Recovery occurred immediately on cessation of exercise, even in the presence of maternal lactic acidemia, suggesting fetal well-being.

DRUG USE

Drug use during pregnancy carries special risks. Prescription medicine is usually taken under direct supervision of a physician. Pregnant women may not, however, be aware of the detrimental effects of over-the-counter medications, assuming them to be safe because of their availability.

The health risks of cigarette smoking are well known. Infants of smoking mothers weigh an average of 200 g less at birth than those born to nonsmokers.[34] The reduction in birth weight is directly related to the degree of smoking. The level of maternal smoking is also correlated with the incidence of preterm delivery, placenta previa, abruptio placentae, premature rupture of membranes, and perinatal mortality. Nicotine has a direct vasoconstrictive effect; plus, inhaled carboxy-hemoglobin reduces the oxygen-carrying capacity of the blood.

The deleterious effects of alcohol have been increasingly demonstrated. The structure most sensitive to the effects of prenatal alcohol is the developing brain. The FDA recommends limiting consumption to less than 2 drinks per day; however, significant developmental effects have been documented in babies exposed to lesser amounts. The occurrence of fetal alcohol syndrome correlates with preconception maternal alcohol intake. Of particular relevance for exercising mothers is the transfer of ibuprofen and its metabolites across the placental barrier. Persistent pulmonary hypertension in the newborn is the most serious potential consequence of ibuprofen use.

Aspirin can lead to platelet dysfunction and decreased Factor VII, leading to hemorrhagic problems in the nursery, including periorbital purpura and encephalohematoma.

RISKS AND BENEFITS

The pregnancy-induced physiological alterations outlined in this chapter are not invariably disadvantageous to the exercising athlete. Indeed, the physiologic response to training has many parallels in the response to pregnancy.

A wealth of pregnancy outcome studies provide compelling evidence of the benign nature of the physiologic alterations to exercise. No effects on gestational age, birth weight, one minute Apgar score, or length of labor were noted in a group of women participating in aerobics, swimming, or walking.[35] More than 300 women involved in endurance exercise had no increased obstetrical complications or fetal morbidity, despite significantly less weight gain, shorter gestation, and decreased infant weight.[14] Trained joggers have a low incidence of maternal and fetal complications.[27,28] No correlation was found between the total number of miles run or miles run in just the third trimester, and either birth weight or gestational age. In a classic study, Zaharieva reported on pregnancy outcomes of Olympic athletes.[36] Without specifying training schedules, she noted "normal" pregnancy in 70.4% of cases, with minor complaints of nausea, anorexia, or vomiting constituting the remainder. A shortened second stage of labor was noted; however, there was no difference in infant birth weights. Interestingly, the Olympic athletes delivered more boys (63%) than girls in this small study. Only primigravidas experienced shortened labor in a study of recreational athletes; no difference was noted in multiparous patients.[37] No correlation was seen between the number of medications used during labor and previous training activity.

A recent meta-analytic review included data on more than 2000 exercising pregnant women.[38] For the variables of maternal weight gain, infant birth weight, length of gestation, length of labor, and Apgar scores, women who exercised during their pregnancy did not differ from sedentary women. Exercise duration and intensity averaged 43 minutes daily, 3 times per week, at heart rates up to 144 beats per minute, exceeding the published recommendations of the American College of Obstetricians and Gynecologists (ACOG). Meta-analysis of studies involving pregnant females who complied with these guidelines and those who exceeded them revealed no difference in pregnancy outcome between the two groups.

Despite generally good pregnancy outcomes, exercise does pose *potential* risks for both the pregnant woman and her unborn child. Of greatest theoretical concern are the effects of hyperthermia and fetal hypoxia.

Hyperthermia can be associated with unfavorable blood flow redistribution, increased oxygen requirements, and congenital central nervous system defects. The risk is greatest early in pregnancy and in the setting of maternal dehydration, prolonged or intensive exercise, and high ambient temperature and humidity.

Fetal hypoxia can occur either as a direct effect of redistributed circulation during exercise, or secondary to maternal hyperventilation, acidosis, or uteroplacental insufficiency.

The metabolic demands of exercise may further compromise the maternal stores of iron and sodium. Later in pregnancy, musculoskeletal adaptations may predispose the gravid exerciser to injury. Premature labor risks may be increased by high circulating catecholamines during exercise.

In an otherwise uncomplicated pregnancy, these risks appear to be minimal when precautions are followed. Exercise intensity and duration should be modified as pregnancy progresses; consideration should be given to switching from weight-bearing to non–weight-bearing activity in the last trimesters. Exercise in the supine position is to be avoided after the first trimester. Activity requiring coordination and balance should be modified as the gravid uterus shifts the center of gravity.

Specific exercise recommendations must come from the patient's physician. Updated guidelines have recently been published by the ACOG.[39]

Restrictions on exercise may be necessary during a complicated pregnancy. Maternal conditions that may contraindicate exercise include cardiopulmonary disease, hypertension, diabetes, severe anemia, poor prior conditioning, fever, uterine bleeding, and high risk of premature labor because of incompetent cervix or history of premature delivery. Fetal placental contraindications to exercise may include intrauterine growth retardation, decreased fetal movement, breech presentation, and multiple gestation.

REFERENCES

1. American College of Obstetricians & Gynecologists (ACOG). Technical Bulletin on Exercise in Pregnancy. Washington, D.C., 1985.
2. Artal, R., et al.: Exercise in pregnancy. Am. J. Obstet. Gynecol. *140:*123, 1981.
3. Fierobe, T., et al.: Sport and pregnancy—A review of the literature. J. Gynecol. Obstet. Biol. Reprod. *19:*375, 1990.
4. Lotgering, F. K., Gilbert, R. D., and Longo, L. D.: Exercise responses in pregnant sheep: blood gases, temperatures, and fetal cardiovascular system. J. Appl. Physiol. *55:*834, 1983.
5. Morton, M. J., et al.: Exercise dynamics in late gestation: Effects of physical training. Am. J. Obstet. Gynecol. *152:*91, 1985.
6. Sady, S. P., et al.: Cardiovascular response to cycle exercise during and after pregnancy. J. Appl. Physiol. *66:*336, 1989.
7. Lotgering, F. K.: Pregnancy In Women and Exercise: Physiology and Sports Medicine. Edited by M. Shangold and G. Mirkin. Philadelphia, F. A. Davis Co., 1988.
8. Gorski, J.: Exercise during pregnancy: maternal and fetal responses. A brief review. Med. Sci. Sports Exerc. *17:*407, 1985.
9. Platt, L. D., et al.: Exercise in pregnancy and fetal responses. Am. J. Obstet. Gynecol. *146:*587, 1983.
10. Quilligan, E. J.: Maternal physiology. *In* Obstetrics and Gynecology. 4th Ed. Edited by D. Danforth. Philadelphia, Harper & Row, 1982.
11. Clapp, J. F., III: Acute exercise stress in the pregnant ewe. Am. J. Obstet. Gynecol. *136:*489, 1980.
12. Huch, R., and Erkkola, R.: Pregnancy and exercise—exercise and pregnancy. A short review. Br. J. Obstet. Gynaecol. *97:*208, 1990.
13. Artal, R., et al.: Pulmonary responses to exercise in pregnancy. *In* Exercise in Pregnancy. Edited by R. Artal and R. Wiswell. Baltimore, Williams & Wilkins, 1986.
14. Clapp, J. F., III., and Dickstein, S.: Endurance exercise and pregnancy outcome. Med. Sci. Sports Exerc. *16:*556, 1984.
15. Artal, R., Wiswell, R., Romem, Y., and Dorey, F.: Pulmonary responses to exercise in pregnancy. Am. J. Obstet. Gynecol. *154:*378, 1986.
16. Lotgering, F. K. et al.: Maximal aerobic exercise in pregnant women: Heart rate, O_2 consumption, CO_2 Production and ventilation. J. Appl. Physiol. *70:*1016, 1991.
17. Fast, A., et al.: Low-back pain in pregnancy. Spine *12:*368, 1987.

18. Fahrni, W. H.: Conservative treatment of lumbar disc degeneration: Our primary responsibility. Orthop. Clin. North Am. *6:*93, 1975.
19. LaBan, M. M., Perrin J. C. S., and Latimer, F. R.: Pregnancy and the Herniated Lumbar Disc. Arch. Phys. Med. Rehabil. *64:*319, 1983.
20. Kelsey, J. L., Grenberg, R. A., Hardy, R. J., Johnson, M. F.: Pregnancy and the syndrome of herniated lumbar intervertebral disc: An epidemiologic study. Yale J. Biol. Med. *48:*361, 1975.
21. Heckman, J. D.: Managing musculoskeletal problems in pregnancy. J. Musculoskel. Med. 7(9):17, 1990.
22. Friedman, M. J.: Orthopaedic Problems in Pregnancy. *In* Exercise in Pregnancy. Edited by R. Artal and R. Wiswell. Baltimore, Williams & Wilkins, 1986.
23. Heckman, J. D.: Managing musculoskeletal problems in pregnancy. J. Musculoskel. Med. 7(8):29, 1990.
24. Artal, R., Friedman, M. J., and McNitt-Gray, J. L.: Orthopedic problems in pregnancy. Physician Sportsmed. *18*(9):93, 1990.
25. Bealieu, J. G., Razzano, C. D., and Levine, R. B.: Transient osteoporosis of the hip in pregnancy. Clin. Orthop. *115:*165, 1976.
26. Clapp, J. F., III, Wesley, M., and Sleamaker, R. H.: Thermoregulatory and metabolic responses to jogging prior to and during pregnancy. Med. Sci. Sports Exerc. *19:*124, 1987.
27. Hauth, J. C., Gilstrap, L. C., III, and Widmer, K.: Fetal heart rate reactivity before and after maternal jogging during the third trimester. Am. J. Obstet. Gynecol. *142:*545, 1982.
28. Jarrett, J. C., II, and Spellacy, W. N.: Jogging during pregnancy: an improved outcome? Obstet. Gynecol. *61:*705, 1983.
29. Jones, R. L., Botti, J. J., Anderson, W. M., and Bennett, N. L.: Thermoregulation during aerobic exercise in pregnancy. Obstet. Gynecol. *65:*340, 1985.
30. McMurray, R. G. and Katz, V. L.: Thermoregulation in pregnancy: Implications for exercise. Sports Medicine *10:*146, 1990.
31. Collings, C., and Curet, L. B.: Fetal heart rate response to maternal exercise. Am. J. Obstet. Gynecol. *151:*498, 1985.
32. Collings, C. A., Curet, L. B., Mullin, J. P.: Maternal and fetal responses to a maternal aerobic exercise program. Am. J. Obstet. Gynecol. *145:*702, 1983.
33. Jovanovic, L., Kessler, A., and Peterson, C. M.: Human Maternal and fetal responses to graded exercise. J. Appl. Physiol. *58:*1719, 1985.
34. Giacoia, G., and Sumner, Y.: Drugs and the Perinatal Patient. *In* Neonatology. Edited by G. B. Avery. Philadelphia, J.B. Lippincott Co., 1975.
35. Work, J.: Study: Exercise okay in normal pregnancy. Physician Sportsmed. *15*(7):51, 1987.
36. Zaharieva, E.: Olympic participation by women: Effects on pregnancy and childbirth. J.A.M.A. *221:*992, 1972.
37. Kulpa, P. J., White, B. M., and Visscher, R.: Aerobic exercise in pregnancy. Am. J. Obstet. Gynecol. *156:*1395, 1987.
38. Lokey, E. A., Tran, Z. V., Wells, C. L., Myers, B. C., and Tran, A. C.: Effects of physical exercise on pregnancy outcomes: A meta-analytic review. Med. Sci. Sports Exerc. *23:*1234, 1991.
39. American College of Obstetricians and Gynecologists. Exercise during pregnancy and the postpartum period. ACOG Technical Bulletin 189. Washington, D.C. 1994.

19 *Robert E. Leach*

The Older Athlete

In a sports medicine practice of 25 years ago, the assumption was that most patients would be in the 15- to 25-year age range, that high school- and college-aged athletes would be the majority of the patients seen by a sports medicine practitioner. Year by year, but particularly during the past decade, sports medicine doctors have been seeing more and more patients in the older "masters athlete" category.

Masters, junior veterans, veterans, and *seniors* are all terms used to define older athletes. I will use the generic term *masters athletes,* meaning athletic people in the 40- to 85-years age group. Many readers may ask, Are there enough masters athletes to warrant writing specifically about them? The answer is a definite *Yes.* A variety of sports have local and national competitions for masters athletes, including cycling, track and field, tennis, swimming, skiing, squash, hockey, soccer, rowing, basketball, baseball, and undoubtedly others of which I am less aware. Not only are there a variety of sports for masters athletes to practice and compete in, but the number of people who are engaging in these sports is rapidly increasing, both at the competitive and the recreational level.

Older people do many athletic activities, such as hiking, climbing, cross-country skiing, and water skiing, for recreation. People who engage in these recreational sports as youngsters often continue most of them in later life. The gradual aging of the population, combined with a sense of staying in good health and the appearance of more leisure time, has enabled the masters athlete group to grow rapidly.[1] Early retirement and the financial security enjoyed by many older Americans have added to an older athletic population. There is also a sense that staying athletic contributes to good health, and even happiness.

Another question is, Do masters athletes present specific problems different from those of the high school, college, and younger adult athletes? Again, the answer is *Yes.* As the masters athlete grows older yet continues to be active in competitive or recreational sport, he or she faces new problems and conditions that may require the help and advice of a sports-oriented physician.[1] Most of these problems are not as acute as those that occur in the younger athletes; however, even masters athletes can suffer a fracture while skiing or rupture an Achilles tendon while playing squash. Many of the conditions that affect masters athletes become chronic and may affect both the working and leisure life of these active people. Some injuries may interfere with activities of daily living and with the maintenance of good health. In some ways, the conditions that affect masters athletes may prove more crucial to their general well-being than those that affect younger athletes.

COMPONENTS OF ATHLETIC PERFORMANCE

I am going to consider some of the components of athletic activity that all athletes draw on and see how these specifically relate to masters athletes. Endurance, strength, power, flexibility, agility, quickness, and coordination are all elements that we should consider for people who are active in athletics. Does the process of aging affect these elements, and, if so, what can we as physicians advise to help masters athletes perform over the long term?

Endurance

Endurance is a component of most athletic competitions. Many factors affect endurance, most of them within the control of the individual athlete. Genetically, some people seem endowed with certain internal characteristics, such as a high Vo_2max, that allow them to be one step ahead of the general populace. However, we know that, by training, most healthy people can gradually build and enhance endurance, and that this is one component of athletic activity that can be sustained long into the masters athlete years. Certain factors determine the masters athlete's ability to build endurance.[2] For instance, people who were active and had high cardiovascular endurance when they were young have a much easier time maintaining or rebuilding this endurance at a later age. People who have never been in shape find it more difficult to build cardiovascular endurance once they are older. There appears to be some "memory" in the body that allows people to retrain at an older age more easily than to train for the first time.

There is some gradual loss of the Vo_2max with aging, but studies have demonstrated conclusively that this loss can be reduced substantially by maintaining a training program.[2] By playing sports, rowing, jogging, cross-country skiing, biking, and using machines such as the Stair Master, we should be able to maintain our endurance virtually throughout our lifetime.

Illness is a factor for masters athletes that we rarely have to think about in younger athletes. As we move into the super seniors or super masters category, it becomes more of a worry. People who have any heart, lung, or major organ problem find it more difficult to train and maintain endurance. This means that people who had a previous illness, who suspect an illness, or who have a family history of cardiovascular problems must consult with their physician before undertaking any serious athletic training.

There is recent evidence that people can add to their longevity and general health by staying in good cardiovascular condition. The flip side of this question is that perhaps people who enjoy good health and who would be expected to have a long life may be the ones who choose to participate in sports. However, the evidence seems to point to cardiovascular conditioning as a significant factor in longevity.

Strength

Strength is another element of athletic activity that seems to apply to most sports. As we age, most people do gradually become weaker in both the upper and lower extremities. For years, this was accepted as an inevitable process of aging, but recent work shows that this may not be the case. What we have often attributed to aging may be due to decreased activity.[3,4] We need to exercise and to continue to use our major motor muscle groups to maintain strength. Athletic people who have continued to do resistance exercises or who have continued to be active in their sports maintain muscle strength at much higher levels than those who do not. Interestingly, those who have previously been strong or have done resistance training seem to have some type of internal muscle memory recall that allows them to gain strength in their older age more easily than those who have never done resistance training before. Studies performed on nonathletic people show that people, even in their late 80s, can increase the muscle strength of a motor group such as the quadriceps.[5] This has enabled such patients to walk faster, get out of a chair more easily, and have better balance as the result of increased strength.

Most masters athletes' objective should be to develop sport-specific strength. There is no need to "bulk up." The idea is to maintain or gain strength in those muscle groups that are most important for the sport or other activity the person is performing. With resistance exercises, the usual rule is to start at lower resistance than one would use at a younger age. I would advise a gradual increase in repetitions and, when a comfort level is reached at a particular resistance, one can then progress to further resistance if he or she wants (Fig. 19–1). All that the masters athlete should be thinking of doing is maintaining or gaining that strength essential to perform the sport at a good level. It appears that people with more strength may be less injury prone because they are able to use the muscle strength to protect themselves. For instance, in skiing, strong thigh muscles may afford better control of the skis, which could help avoid a potentially injurious fall.

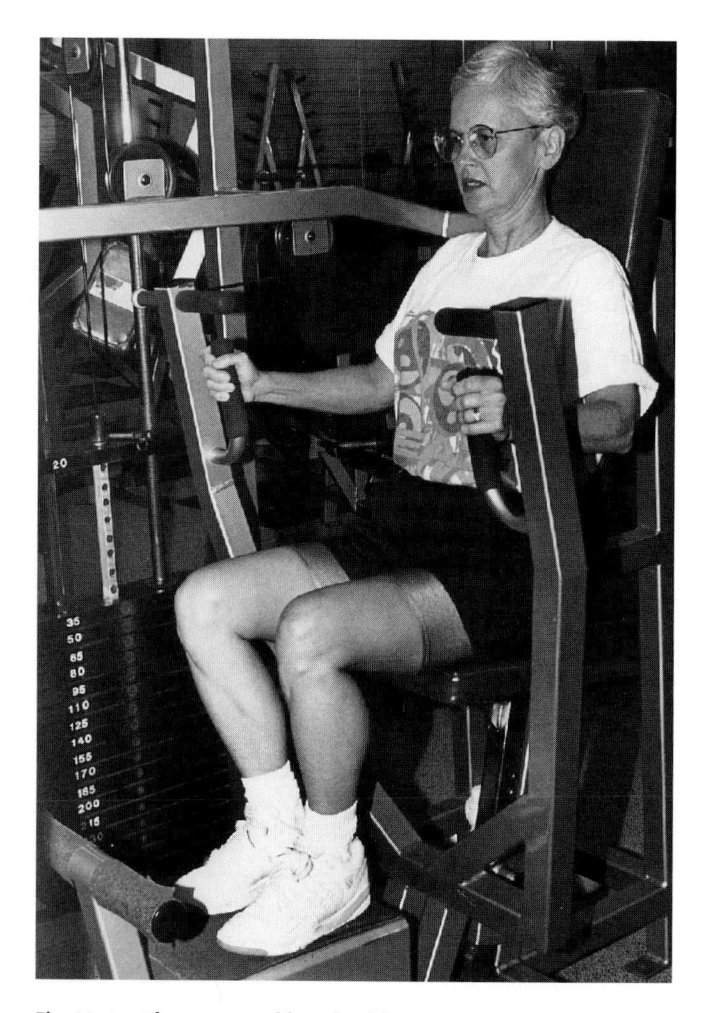

Fig. 19–1. The masters athlete should start resistance training at a lower level than younger athletes and then increase the number of repetitions.

Some older (and even younger) athletes worry about the possibility of becoming "muscle bound." This is an out of date term that describes a person who becomes very strong and loses flexibility, which it was thought would render him unable to perform athletics well. All that one has to do is to maintain a full range of motion in the involved joints. There is no reason to have decreased flexibility just because one is gradually getting stronger. I would advise any masters athlete pursuing a weight training program, particularly for the first time or if there is any question of cardiovascular disease, to get a check-up from his or her physician. Problems with the heart, particularly hypertension, may indicate the need for modification—or perhaps, even more rarely, a complete ban—of resistance exercises, but most physicians feel that moderate strength training can be done by people of any age.

Power

Power, important in most sports, is a function of both strength and time. The quicker a given measure of strength is delivered, the more power exists. Masters athletes can do quite well with regard to strength, and this is half of the equation for power.[3] There *is* a definite loss of quickness associated with aging. This is more evident in the lower extremities than in the upper ones. If we maintain strength and continue to be active in sports that require quickness, we should maintain power better than those who do not exercise or work out. We will not, however, usually be at the level of younger people. It is of interest to note that certain athletes seem to have maintained power well into their forties. Examples such as Nolan Ryan in baseball and Al Oerter in the discus throw come immediately to mind. Both men trained intensively, leading us to believe that even power can be maintained at a higher level than we had once thought.

Flexibility

So far, masters athletes have been seen to do reasonably well with regard to the elements of athletic performance, but in the next area to consider, flexibility, there is a definite loss as we age.[6] There are genetic differences between people, and women are generally more flexible than men. With age and accumulated injuries or inactivity, there is a gradual loss of flexibility in both joint motion and in certain muscle-tendon units. Research points out that, if people do nonballistic stretching exercises and follow a faithful regimen, they can maintain much of their flexibility.[4,7] Even those who have lost flexibility can regain some of what has been lost.

For masters athletes, the tendo Achilles complex, the thigh adductors, the hamstrings, the back, the neck, and the shoulder all tend to lose flexibility. All of these areas are important in athletic activity. There are well-known stretching exercises for each of these areas and a 7- to 10-minute period each day would go a long way toward maintaining flexibility and helping to decrease many of the common and chronic muscle-tendon strains seen in older athletes. Loss of flexibility in certain joints may limit an athlete's ability to generate power. For instance, if the shoulder cannot go through a full range of motion, the arc of motion that normally goes into producing the tennis serve is reduced. Thus, racket speed and the eventual speed of the ball are reduced.

Speed

Every competitive masters athlete, and probably most recreational athletes, become aware that, with age they lose quickness and speed. I define *quickness* as the time needed to take the first two steps or the first motion with the hands; whereas *speed* is associated with how long it takes to go 10 to 50 yards. We lose some of both of these elements as we age.[8,9] Generally, people who were quick or speedy as children are usually those who are quick or speedy as adults, and they seem to maintain the same relationship with their peers as masters athletes, if they do not become injured. Even though we lose speed and quickness, the masters athletes usually have learned a great deal about the sport, so that they can compensate by knowing where they should be at a given time in a particular sport.

Both of these elements, quickness and speed, seem to have a strong genetic component. Other athletes and coaches are usually well aware of the people who have these abilities when they start athletics, and it is unusual to hear about someone who was slow at age 16 and suddenly becomes the fastest person on the team at a later age. Endurance plays a role in maintaining quickness and speed, because as one becomes tired it is obviously impossible to maintain the other elements of athletic competition. We seem to lose quickness more slowly in the upper extremities than in the lower ones. People in their 70s seem to maintain good hand speed, which augurs well for people playing sports such as squash and tennis.

Coordination

One area important in athletic performance, and in which I have seen a change in thinking, concerns coordination. Many people in their 40s, 50s, and perhaps even their 60s seem remarkably well-coordinated, though, we know that, with age, there is loss of nerve tissue. There is usually a gradual decrease in nerve conduction velocity and decreased reaction time.[8] However, the rate of aging is highly individual. Also, there is evidence that inactivity exaggerates the negative aspects.

It does appear that, in many people in their 50s through the 70s, coordination and hand-eye control do disappear. What we are probably seeing is a combination of effects: decreased endurance, decreased strength, and decreased activity or practice of a particular skill.[2] With practice of repetitive patterns, much coordination can be maintained unless other physical disabilities interfere.

Agility, coordination, and balance are all elements of athletic participation and also are very important in life. Most people think these elements are present in masters athletes in their 40s and 50s, but there is a general feeling that athletes in their 60s and 70s gradually lose them. In all probability, what observers are noticing is a combination of decreasing levels of other elements of athletic competition. Many previously active people stop doing a lot of the activities that they did or start doing them less often. They then appear to lose the easy facility for performing a particular athletic maneuver, and it looks as if they have lost their coordination. The same could be said for agility. Certainly, as we grow older, agility is lost, but fatigue and decreased endurance play a role in this for masters athletes. From my personal observation of many masters athletes, it appears that carrying out certain athletic patterns, maintaining an active life style, and maintaining the other elements of athletic performance allow one to keep coordination, agility, and balance at much higher levels. This is very important, particularly for avoiding injury. A more athletic population may be less at risk for the trivial stumbles and falls that have led to severe injuries in older people.

INJURY AND ILLNESS

Injury and illness must be considerations in masters athletes. As we age, chronic health conditions such as diabetes, heart problems, cancer, osteoarthritis, and osteoporosis all have to be considered. Masters athletes may have to deal with these factors on a long-term basis, and the advice of the physician will be critical to being able to continue to compete and enjoy athletic activity. Acute injuries are less common in masters athletes than in younger ones, but muscle and muscle-tendon injuries are very common.[9,10] We see many muscle strains in older athletes, probably because of the relative lack of flexibility and the fact that most people do not work very hard on maintaining flexibility. Masters athletes play sports at a lower level, in terms of strength and power, than do young athletes, and that is probably what causes muscle strains—as opposed to complete ruptures or disruptions—to occur. Gradual degeneration in tendons such as the rotator cuff tendons or the Achilles may lead to ruptures of either of these muscle-tendon units.

We often see many more of what may be termed "wear-and-tear" disorders, those that result from years of athletic endeavor and the stresses induced by it. Back problems, which are ubiquitous in the population overall, may gradually increase in the masters athlete group because of long-term stresses on the back. In the shoulder, adhesive capsulitis is a more common diagnosis in masters athletes than in the younger age group. The same can be said for tears of the muscle belly of the gastrocnemius.

Another problem for masters athletes relates to previous injuries, particularly those that may have occurred in early years. For example, a tear of a medial meniscus at age 20 that resulted in a meniscectomy will cause increased forces on the medial articular cartilage and eventual deterioration of the joint.[11] At age 48, this may be a minor problem, but 10 years later it could threaten athletic performance. The meniscus presents a problem after age 40 because it loses much of its resilient inner structure.[3,12] Posterior horn cleavage tears are common. Repairs usually are not possible, and partial meniscectomy is the rule. This takes care of the early problem, but for some reason the underlying articular cartilage seems more prone to degeneration, even with later meniscectomy.[13] The masters' knee requires some decreased activity, good quadriceps strength, perhaps nonsteroidal anti-inflammatory drugs, and, sometimes, judicious surgery to keep the athlete going.

More important than a mere listing of the conditions that are seen more commonly in the masters athlete is how to deal with them. It may not be possible to completely cure a condition of a masters athlete as we would expect to do in a 25-year-old. The physician's objective should be to try to decrease pain and increase function, which would allow the masters athlete to enjoy athletic activity. He or she may have to learn to moderate their activity and not to play their sports every day. They may find that taking nonsteroidal anti-inflammatory drugs allows them to play relatively pain free, and, with judicious advice from the physician, they may find that medication allows them to increase playing time. One must balance the effects of the increased playing time with the pleasure derived from it. We see many more supportive braces such as neoprene sleeves or counterforce braces in masters athletes than in younger athletes, and, again, judicious use of such external supports may allow the athlete to play in comparative comfort.

Muscle soreness is common in athletes aged 40 and over. Sometimes this is due to a sudden increase in activity. Younger athletes playing sports seem to be able to use their general muscular and cardiovascular conditioning and go from one sport to another without significant muscle soreness. With age, some of the resiliency is gone, and each sport seems to require some training of the involved muscles to avoid soreness after the athletic activity.

Some older athletes who engage in vigorous physical activity find that muscle soreness is the biggest problem for a day or two after the activity. For others who are more used to physical activity it may not be soreness but simply a drop-off in performance or the vigor with which one can perform on the second or third day after a very active day. This must be taken into account when masters athletes are going to compete, or even when they go into intensive training for a particular performance. To put it bluntly, we do not seem at age 50, to have the ability to bounce back the way we once did at 20, and this must be considered, particularly when competing.

Another problem for the over-40 group is night cramps after muscle activity. Many people playing sports have had the unpleasant experience of cramping while playing sports, but even more common is waking up at night with a hamstring, calf, or foot cramp.[14] We do not yet know the exact causes of muscle cramps, although we understand that heat, dehydration, and intense physical activity all play a role. Some people never have muscle cramps, whereas others have a pattern of cramping during activity or later at night. Even well-conditioned athletes can have muscle cramps after activity. Some athletes are able to forestall the appearance of night cramps by taking quinine before they go to sleep. Once a muscle cramp sets in, gentle stretching of the involved area or even light massage of the muscle usually breaks the cramp. Relaxation is an important component of any treatment, although it is very hard to achieve when the pain is acute, as it often is with muscle cramps.

The mind set of older athletes is often different from that of younger ones. They have been through the process of being hurt, having treatment, or playing injured. The sport that they are playing is very important to them, but for different reasons than when they were 20 years old. Often, masters athletes seek advice from physicians but do not want to be told, "Don't play." They understand treatment plans and, in many instances, faithfully carry out the plan, but the vicissitudes of earning a living and caring for a family may interfere with any therapeutic plan. On the positive side, masters athletes realize how much they have invested in their activity and try hard to resume it.

Physicians must remember that sometimes small losses of muscle mass or joint motion make it difficult for a person to perform a sport. Rehabilitation and maintenance therapy are critical for masters athletes. A small loss of function or motion each decade makes a great deal of difference in a person's ability to enjoy a sport in their 60s. If people do not maintain their muscle mass, they may not be able to enjoy taking a hike, going for a swim, or skiing later in life. As a result of injury, there may be gradual deterioration of the previous health status, which relates not only to maintaining fitness but to maintaining good health.

With age come differences in body tissues such as bones, tendons and muscles that are measurable—and, to some extent, inevitable—though a number of them are partially within our control. Many of the changes that we thought were due to age are in fact due to disuse, at least in part. Those of us who stay active and pay attention to the elements that enhance athletic performance will probably continue to play sports longer and also to enjoy better health. The doctor's role in this is to help masters athletes reach these goals.

REFERENCES

1. Legwold, G.: Masters competitors age little in ten years. Physician Sportsmed. *10*(10):27, 1982.
2. Astrand, P. O.: Exercise physiology of the mature athlete. *In* Sports Medicine for the Mature Athlete. Edited by J. R. Sutton and R. M. Brock. Indianapolis, Benchmark Press, 1986.
3. Green, H. J.: Characteristics of aging human skeletal muscles. *In* Sports Medicine for the Mature Athlete. Edited by J. R. Sutton and R. M. Brock. Indianapolis, Benchmark Press, 1986.
4. Menard D., and Stanish W. D.: The aging athlete. Am. J. Sports Med. *17*:187, 1989.
5. Fiatarone, M. A., et al.: High-intensity strength training in nonagenarians. J.A.M.A. *263*:3029, 1990.
6. Vailas, A. C., Pedrini, V. A., Pedrini-Mille, A., and Holloszy, J. D.: Patellar tendon matrix changes associated with aging and voluntary exercise. J. Appl. Physiol. *58*:1572, 1985.
7. Taylor, D. C., Dalton, J. D., Seaber, A. V., and Garrett, W. E.: Viscoelastic properties of muscle-tendon units. The biomechanical effects of stretching. Am. J. Sports Med. *18*:300, 1990.
8. Larsson, L., Grimby, G., and Karlsson, J.: Muscle strength and speed of movement in relation to age and muscle morphology. J. Appl. Physiol. *46*:451, 1979.
9. DeHaven, K. E., and Lintner, D. M.: Athletic injuries: Comparison by age, sport, and gender. Am. J. Sports Med. *14*:218, 1986.
10. Kannus, P., Niittymäki, S., Järvinen, M., and Letho, M.: Sports injuries in elderly athletes: A three-year prospective, controlled study. Age Aging *18*:263, 1989.
11. Jackson, R. W.: The masters knee—past, present, and future. *In* Sports Medicine for the Mature Athlete. Edited by J. R. Sutton and R. M. Brock. Indianapolis, Benchmark Press Inc., 1986.
12. Jackson, R. W., and Rouse, D. W.: The results of partial arthroscopic meniscectomy in patients over 40 years of age. J. Bone Joint Surg. *64B*:481, 1982.
13. Litchman, H. M., Silver, C. M., and Simon, S. D.: Injuries to the medial meniscus in the aging patient. J.A.M.A. *196*:178, 1966.
14. Benda, C.: Outwitting muscle cramps—is it possible? Physician Sportsmed. *17*(9):173, 1989.

20

Kenneth M. Bielak

The Handicapped Athlete

A growing arena for team physicians is the care (and management) of handicapped athletes. Over the last few decades there has been an explosion of interest in sports and recreation for athletes who are disabled, either physically or mentally. This is due partly to the pioneering efforts of individuals who overcame the obstacles of a disability and showed the rest of the world that "they belonged." More recently, federal legislation has mandated equal access and equal opportunity for persons with handicaps, including access to physical education and sports.

The boundaries of man's imagination and determination are limitless; blind and disabled athletes ski down and climb up mountains, wheelchair marathon racers break new records in endurance, paraplegic weight lifters bench press over 600 pounds, and severely retarded teenagers sprint a 50-yard dash to the thunderous applause of thousands of spectators.

The value of sport for the disabled lies in fun of movement, joy and pleasure of competition, and the satisfaction of being able to realize normal and healthy desires.[1] Studies show that disabled athletes have higher self-esteem, are better educated, and express more satisfaction and happiness with life than disabled "nonathletes."[2] The more a disabled athlete can accomplish, the greater is the feeling of belonging and the self-esteem.[3] It is important for all who participate in the care and management of disabled athletes to remember that the ultimate goal of all athletes, be they abled, disabled, or impaired, is to be part of the overall team, developing skills, achieving goals, meeting new challenges, and building self-esteem while enjoying themselves.

WHAT IS *DISABLED?*

The term *handicapped* is an umbrella term that encompasses those who are crippled, disabled, or mentally retarded. Physical disability is defined by the presence of amputation, blindness, cerebral palsy, dwarfism, spinal cord injury, hemiplegia, spina bifida, and *les autres. Les autres* (literally, "the others") is the official term, in the United States and world competitions, for locomotor conditions not included in other organizations (e.g., osteogenesis imperfecta, arthritis, muscular dystrophy, and multiple sclerosis).[4] There are numerous supporting organizations for people with each of these disabilities. Athletes with mental retardation are served exclusively by the Special Olympics International organization. Participants must have an IQ score of 70 or below and be at least 8 years old.

THE SPECIAL OLYMPICS

In the late 1960s, the Joseph P. Kennedy, Jr. Foundation, under the direction of Eunice Kennedy Shriver, established the Special Olympics as a means of promoting exercise and participation in sport by persons with mental retardation. According to their mission statement, year-round sports training is promoted in the spirit of courage, joy, and sharing. Annual local, state, and international competitions are arranged for an estimated 2 million participants in more than 126 countries.

The following age classes are used for individual sports at the Special Olympics (slight differences are noted in team sports): youth, ages 8 to 10 years; junior, 12 to 15 years; senior, 16 to 21 years; masters, 22 to 29 years; senior masters, more than 30 years; and open-age group. The average age of Special Olympic athletes is 23 years. The athletic competition loosely follows the structure of the Olympic games for summer and winter venues. In the summer, athletes can compete in softball, track and field, equestrian events, roller skating, soccer or football, volleyball, bocce, cycling, power lifting, table tennis, team handball, tennis, and golf events. The winter games include cross-country and Alpine skiing, skating, basketball, gymnastics, and bowling.

Athletic injury patterns for athletes with mental retardation are very similar to those for athletes without this impediment.[5–7] The most common injuries involve soft tissue, strained muscles, heat-related problems, and dehydration. Robson tallied the number and types of medical problems encountered among 1512 competitors at the 1989 United Kingdom Special Olympics Games and found joint injuries were most frequent (36%), followed by syncope and heat exhaustion (11%), strains (7%), and upper respiratory tract infections (5%).[8]

Mental retardation typically is associated with other physical and medical disorders. Robson reported the conditions encountered at the pregame medical examination of the 1512 competitors (Table 20–1). Only seven convulsions occurred during the competition. Other preparticipation screening studies of Special Olympics athletes have found visual acuity worse than 20/30 (40%), heart murmurs (5%), deficient flexibility of the lower extremities (31%), clonus (12%), and spasticity (8%).[9]

Reichow and colleagues performed vision testing on athletes at the 1991 Special Olympics International Games and found that 10 to 15% of athletes had some type of visual performance deficit. Other medical problems can be encountered, such as hypoglycemic reactions in diabetic athletes. Easy fatigue, tachycardia, and changes in mental status are the first signs of potential trouble. The two most common problems encountered are Down syndrome and seizure disorder.

Table 20–1. Conditions Encountered at the Pregame Medical Examination of 1512 Competitors (942 Male, 570 Female) at the U.K. Special Olympics, 1989

Condition	Number
Down syndrome	417
Confirmed atlantoaxial subluxation (AAS) by radiograph	(24)
Confirmed negative for AAS by radiograph	(312)
No radiographs available	(81)
Epilepsy, receiving treatment	167
Epilepsy, history but not currently taking medication	72
Congenital cardiac lesions, mostly septal defects	88
Cerebral palsy	33
Asthma	24
Hypothyroidism	22
Hemiparesis	11
Severe vision impairment	11
Diabetes mellitus	10
Hydrocephalus	9
Ataxia	7
Microcephaly	6
Paraplegia	5
Hepatitis B carrier	4
Phenylketonuria	3
Colostomy	1
Seto's syndrome	1
Celiac disease	1
Hydronephrosis	1
Oxycephaly	1
Hypertension	1
Congenital absence of all four limbs	1

(Robson, H.E.: Br. J. Sports Med. *24*:225, 1990.)

Down Syndrome

There are special concerns for athletes with Down syndrome. As many as 50% of moderately to severely mentally retarded people have Down syndrome.[10] Several major disorders are associated with Down syndrome, including atlantoaxial instability and other orthopedic conditions such as metatarsus primus varus, patellar instability, pes planus, and slipped capital femoral epiphysis.[11] These conditions can affect proper shoe fitting and can be associated with Achilles tendinitis, patellofemoral pain syndrome, posterior tibial tendinitis, and other complications of overpronation.[12] Furthermore, 40 to 60% of Down syndrome patients have congenital heart disorders such as heart murmur, ventricular septal defect, and endocardial cushion defects.[4,13] Persons with these more serious heart conditions should be evaluated by a cardiologist and take a graded exercise test to determine their functional capacity so a physician can prescribe a safe level of activity.[14] McCormick found that athletes with Down syndrome had 3.2 times more medical problems than other Special Olympics athletes.[6] For these reasons, athletes with Down syndrome should be monitored closely.

Some 12 to 18% of people with Down syndrome have atlantoaxial instability,[15,16] excessive play between the C1 and C2 vertebrae. Because of the weak supporting muscles and ligaments of this area, any stress, such as an axial load, flexion, or excessive torque from a collision or contact could damage the spinal cord. Since 1983, it has been required that athletes with Down syndrome be evaluated for this disorder. In Canada, the condition is diagnosed if either a fixed or mobile translation gap of 0.5 to 1.0 cm is seen between the first and second cervical vertebrae on lateral flexion or extension views.[17] The American Academy of Pediatrics released a position paper in 1984 that defined atlantoaxial instability as the condition of the distance between the odontoid process of the axis and the anterior arch of the atlas being more than 4.5 mm.[18] Affected persons are not allowed to participate in any collision sports or venues that could involve trauma to the head and neck. Specifically, they are prohibited from participating in diving, gymnastics, butterfly stroke, soccer, high jump, pentathlon, and horseback riding.[19]

Neurologic manifestations of atlantoaxial instability include fatigue with walking, gait disturbance, imbalance, and incoordination, with spasticity, hyper-reflexia, and toe extensor reflexes developing later on. In addition, torticollis and neck pain should suggest this disorder and prompt immediate evaluation.[18] Before 1984, only 24 cases of cord compression were reported in patients with Down syndrome.[20] Nonetheless, when the complication does occur, the treatment of choice is posterior stabilization and fusion.

Seizure Disorders

Seizure disorders occur in 14 to 46% of mentally retarded persons.[21,22] Chaperones, coaches, trainers, and physicians should be prepared to handle seizure episodes in these athletes and monitor medication needs and schedules. The team physician should be prepared to treat a prolonged seizure. Hyperventilation is known to lead to seizures; thus, in swimming events the lifeguard should be strong enough to pull the heaviest swimmer out of the water.[23] At high altitudes, the decreased oxygen tension and subsequent hyperventilation, as well as fatigue, may lower the seizure threshold.[9]

DISABLED ATHLETES

Common sense dictates that, if there is a will, there is a way. Many disabled athletes had to overcome numerous roadblocks to develop their skills and show everyone else that they, too, can enjoy sport, competition, and training. The unofficial United States Census Bureau report of 1990 estimated that 12.6 million people (8% of Americans from age 16 to 64) have some type of mobility limitation. Legislation has provided the basis for protection of the rights of the handicapped with the Rehabilitation Act of 1973, which mandated equal opportunity for comparable participation in physical education classes.[24] The courts have established handicapped athletes' right to access to every sporting venue where able-bodied athletes participate. Beyond athleticism, the Americans with Disabilities Act of 1990 mandated that public places be accessible to the disabled, which was a progressive step toward affording all people equal access.

History of Organized Athletics for Disabled Persons

The first wheelchair sports ventures were introduced in England in the 1940s and spread to the United States by 1952. By the 1960s, formal venues for competitive games were organized with the first Paralympics and the first Wheelchair Olympics in Rome following the 1960 Olympics. The Paralympics included archery, track and field, basketball, bocce, cycling, fencing, goalball, judo, shooting, soccer, swimming, table tennis, volleyball, and weight lifting.[25] In 1976, the Olympiad for the Physically Disabled (blind, amputee, paralyzed) in Toronto attracted more than 1500 athletes from 38 countries.[26] In 1984, demonstration events for disabled athletes for the first time were held with the Olympic Games in Sarajevo and Los Angeles.

Over the last few years the number of organizations that support and organize games for individuals with "handicaps" has increased. The competitions for the National Wheelchair Athletic Association include archery, table tennis, swimming, track and field, weight lifting, slalom races, and marathon racing.[27] More people are realizing the benefits of physical exercise and participation in sport for the disabled, and opportunities will continue to increase. The appendix provides a list of resources.

For competition to be fair among participants, elaborate schemes are devised that separate athletes by ability. For example, the 12 categories for amputees are made up of combinations of conditions: loss of one or both legs, loss of leg above or below the knee, loss of one or both arms, and loss of arm above or below the elbow.[25] For the athlete with a spinal cord injury, there are six categories of participation, based on level of the spinal lesion and the extent of injury (Table 20–2).

Table 20–2. Classification System for Wheelchair Athletes

Classification	*Description*
I	Most disabled athletes fit this category
IA	C6 or higher lesion or equivalent with an active wrist extensor but only fair/poor triceps extensors
IB	Good/normal triceps, functional wrist flexors and extensors, but no intrinsic muscle power
IC	Good/normal triceps, functional finger flexors and extensors, but no intrinsic muscle power
II	High thoracic paraplegia with no abdominal muscle power
III	Midthoracic paraplegia or equivalent with some functioning upper abdominal muscles
IV	Good abdominal muscle power but no hip musculature except weak quadriceps
V	Fair or greater quadriceps
VI*	For swimmers only: ability to push off wall with lower extremities
The National Wheelchair Basketball Association†	
Class 1	Equivalent to T7 paraplegia or above
Class 2	T8–L2 with significant loss of hip and thigh function
Class 3	All other disabilities, higher functioning

*There is a point system for lower extremity muscle power and sensation to help differentiate between Class III and VI.[26,27]

†A player is assigned value points equal to his class number, so no more than a total of 12 player points may be on the floor at one time.

(For an updated classification system see Curtis, K. A.: Sport-specific functional classification for wheelchair athletes. Sports 'n Spokes, 17(2):45, 1991.)

Profile of Wheelchair Athletes

In a survey of 210 wheelchair participants conducted by Curtis and coworkers in 1985, 65% of athletes had spinal cord injuries, 12% had once had poliomyelitis, 9% had congenital disorders, 3% were amputees, and 10% had neuromuscular and musculoskeletal disorders.[28] The largest percentage of athletes were involved in track (79%), basketball (71%), swimming (61%), field events (60%), and road racing (57%). Athletes with disabilities have essentially the same injury risks as able-bodied athletes.[29]

The wheelchair athlete is more likely to injure the upper extremity (shoulder), and Nichols and coworkers described "wheelchair user's shoulder" in 50% of spinally paralyzed patients who propel themselves using a wheelchair.[30] The five highest-risk sports for wheelchair athletes, in descending order of risk, are track, basketball, road racing, tennis, and field events.[10]

Ferrara found 57% of injuries to elite wheelchair athletes were minor, causing loss of less than 7 days' practice, whereas 32% were major injuries (more than 22 days of practice lost).[31] The upper extremity (shoulder and wrist) was involved in 58%, the lower extremity in 22%, the head and spine in 18%, and illness in 2%. The type of injuries that Ferrara found in his year-long survey of elite wheelchair athletes were strain (48%), abrasion (22%), contusion (10%), blisters (6%), fracture (6%), sprain (4%), laceration (2%), and illness (2%).

The most common mechanisms of injury were falls as the result of direct impact with another chair or other objects (49%) and repetitive stress and overuse (35%).[31] Ferrara found that wheelchair athletes had the same type and frequency of injury as athletes without a disability; however, he also found that the time lost was greater for the disabled ones. He explains that this may be the result of the delayed healing process associated with the spinal cord injury or more conservative rehabilitation. Conversely, in a review of the 1976 Olympiad for Disabled Athletes in Toronto, Jackson and Fredrickson found that disabled athletes were slightly more vulnerable to stress and fatigue.[26]

Soft tissue injuries, blisters, lacerations, decubitus ulcers, and joint disorders were the most commonly reported injuries in a survey of wheelchair athletes by Curtis and Dillon in 1985.[28] More than 70% of all reported injuries in that survey occurred during wheelchair track (26%), road racing (22%), and basketball (24%). Decubitus ulcers and temperature regulation disorders were noted as particular risks for athletes with spinal cord injuries. The very low-risk sports include pool, bowling, archery, slalom, and table tennis. Injuries occurred more frequently in untrained handicapped athletes who started exercising too vigorously, as they do in all athletes.[32]

Injury prevention techniques for wheelchair athletes include static stretching, progressive warm-up periods, padding bony exposed extremities and push rims to prevent blisters and lacerations, building calluses, and wearing gloves.[10,28,33,34] Because pressure sores are a major cause of concern in this population, special effort needs to be made for systematic and regular monitoring coupled with adequate cushioning and ventilation. Early warning signs include areas of redness and blistering. Recurrent urinary tract infections and bowel dysfunction can be dealt with in a systematic manner.

Hoeberigs and coworkers found that five of eight new injuries in an elite wheelchair marathon were related to spills.[32] Problems were relatively more frequent in athletes with paraplegia and polio-related disabilities. Downhill portions of courses are particularly risky because speeds can reach 30 to 35 miles per hour.[35] Proper control of crowds and road conditions are essential to ensure safety.

Thermoregulatory problems occur more often in athletes with high spinal cord lesions, because of sympathetic dysreflexia. Autonomic dysreflexia can raise the blood pressure dangerously high, as the result of an injury or irritation below the level of the spinal cord injury.[9] If wheelchair athletes have symptoms of flushing, tachycardia, headache, or spasticity and pain of unknown origin they should rest at least 24 hours before continuing training.[34]

Hypothermia becomes a high-risk factor for endurance wheelchair athletes because they lack muscle mass, which prevents adequate shivering to generate heat. Prevention is the most important issue to consider, and it may be accomplished with attention to adequate clothing that provides both insulation and a wind barrier and can be "layered," as conditions require (Fig. 20–1). For these athletes it is vitally important to strip off wet clothes and replace them with dry ones and to provide adequate hydration.[10] Hyperthermia can be a critical risk, since sweating may be deficient below the level of the spinal cord injury and may not allow for adequate evaporative cooling in hot environments. Increased hydration (more than 1 L per hour), lighter clothing that allows more evaporation, and spraying the extremities with water are techniques used to prevent hyperthermia.[10,35]

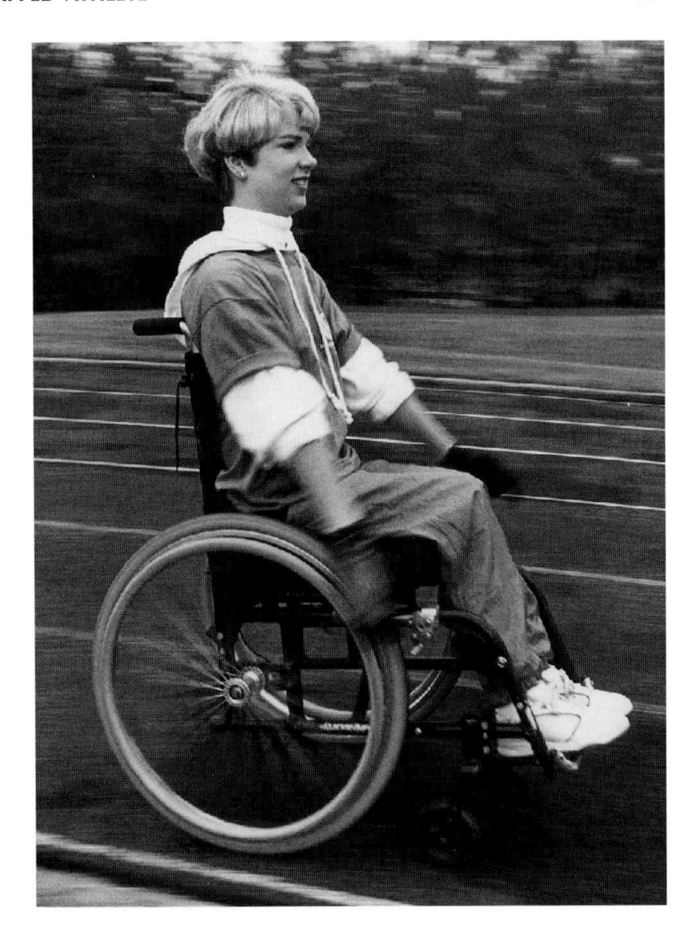

Fig. 20–1. Hyperthermia is a great risk for wheelchair athletes. Adequate clothing that provides both insulation and a wind barrier should be worn and layered as needed.

Athletes involved in a greater number of sporting venues reported a higher number of injuries, and it was noted that increasing the number of training hours per week corresponded to a greater number of reported injuries.[28]

Skiing for Disabled Athletes

Approximately 3 of every 1000 Americans are blind, but there is very little literature on blind athletes. For competition, divisions are made according to available sight: partial or total loss of vision. The most common injury to blind athletes is trauma to the lower extremity, since that is the part of the body that most closely interacts with the environment. Trips, falls, and unseen obstacles affect the lower extremity first. The Blind Outdoor Leisure Development is a nonprofit corporation dedicated to helping blind persons enjoy the outdoors. Skiing has become a popular pursuit with the adaptation of a "guide," who directs the skier by verbal cues. The blind skier must be able to heed the command "Sit down!" on a moment's notice, to avoid potential injury from obstacles.[9]

There has been somewhat more written on the highly visible sport of skiing for athletes with a disability. Studies have shown no significant differences in overall injury rates between able-bodied and physically disabled skiers.[36,37] The overall rate of skier injury per 1000 skier days in the able-bodied population has been reported as 2.8 to 3.5.[36,38] For disabled skiers, the rate was 2.0 to 3.7.[36,37] Laskowski found that disabled skiers have fewer fractures and lacerations but more abrasions and bruises than able-bodied skiers.[36] McCormick found that 70% of disabled skiers had never been injured.[37] Knee injuries were the most common, followed by fractures of the leg and back, contusions, lacerations, and sprains of the upper extremities. Hazards related to injury were equally blamed on ski conditions and equipment. The outrigger, a small ski attached to the poles, has been found to be an additional hazard if it is not properly released from the body during a fall. Rates of injury increase toward the end of the ski day, probably because of fatigue and deteriorating light and snow conditions.

To understand potential areas of injury and concern, the attending physician should become familiar with the wide range of adaptive equipment available for disabled athletes, such as outrigger skis, flip skis, canting wedges, ski bras, toe spreaders, sit skis, and monoskis.[39] The role of the team physician for disabled athletes is similar to that in any other athletic venue—to ensure the health and welfare of participants and spectators. The desire of disabled athletes to push themselves to the limit is a common problem. A balance must be struck that allows for this expression but in a safe, reasonable manner.

The attending physician should emphasize the prevention of injuries by ensuring safe environmental conditions. When warranted, the physician should be able to advise athletes and coaches about the potential dangers of dehydration, heat prostration, hypothermia, and cold exposure, and how to prevent them. Ample space should be allowed for accommodating large numbers of athletes and spectators who need a place to rest or who are overcome by the effects of extreme heat or cold. As many team physicians can attest, there are probably just as many injuries at an event from the population of spectators as among the participants.

There must be a plan, and sufficient organization, to treat a variety of illnesses and injuries, and procedures must be established to transfer athletes to the hospital if necessary. The physician must also be aware that a disability can mask an injury. For example, Corcoran reported a paraplegic basketball player who fell off his wheelchair in competition and resumed play, not realizing until hours later when swelling occurred that he had fractured his femur.[35]

LIABILITY ISSUES

Since the courts have granted disabled athletes equal opportunity to participate in competition, it has placed the responsibility on the team physician to determine what is allowable and safe. As with athletes who have only one of a pair of organs, the decision for participation should involve the athlete, coaches, and parents after full disclosure by the physician of the inherent risks and potential outcomes.[40] In most states, a team physician is protected under the Good Samaritan laws when providing volunteer first aid on site at sporting venues. Additional liability may fall on a physician who clears an athlete with a known condition for participation. So far, courts have intervened on behalf of athletes seeking not to be restricted, and there are no reported cases of physicians being sued by a disabled or handicapped athlete who was a participant in athletic contests.

REFERENCES

1. Klapwijk, A.: The multiple benefits of sports for the disabled. Int. Dis. Studies *9*:87, 1987.
2. Valliant, P. M., Bezzubyk, I., Daley, L., and Asu, M. E.: Psychological impact of sport on disabled athletes. Psychol. Rep. *56*:923, 1985.
3. Levy, A. M.: The disabled athlete: An approach. NJ Med. *88*:647, 1991.
4. Sherrill, C., et al.: Self-concepts of disabled youth athletes. Percept. Motor Skills *70*:1093, 1990.
5. Birrer, R. B.: The Special Olympics: An injury overview. Physician Sportsmed. *12*(4):95, 1984.
6. McCormick, D. P., Nieburg, V., and Risser, W. L.: Injury and illness surveillance at local Special Olympic games. Br. J. Sports Med. *24*:221, 1990.
7. Mangus, B. C., and French, R.: Wanted: Athletic trainers for Special Olympic athletes. Athlet. Training *20*:204, 1985.
8. Robson, H. E.: The Special Olympic Games for mentally handicapped—United Kingdom 1989. Br. J. Sports Med. *24*:225, 1990.
9. Hudson, P. B.: Preparticipation screening of Special Olympics athletes. Physician Sportsmed. *16*(4):97, 1988.
10. Bloomquist, L. E.: Injuries to athletes with physical disabilities: Prevention implications. Physician Sportsmed. *14*(9):96, 1986.
11. Diamond, L. S., Lynne, D., and Sigman, B.: Orthopedic disorders in patients with Down's syndrome. Orthop. Clin. North Am. *12*:57, 1981.
12. Tanji, J. L.: The preparticipation exam. Special concerns for the Special Olympics. Physician Sportsmed. *19*(7):61, 1991.
13. Park, S. C., et al.: Down's syndrome with congenital heart malformation. Am. J. Dis. Child. *131*:29, 1977.
14. Starek, P. J.: Athletic performance in children with cardiovascular problems. Physician Sportsmed. *10*(2):78, 1982.
15. Cooke, R. E.: Atlantoaxial instability in individuals with Down's syndrome. Adapted Phys. Activity Q. *1*:194, 1984.
16. Cope, R., and Olson, S.: Abnormalities of the cervical spine in Down's syndrome: Diagnosis, risks, and review of the literature, with particular reference to the Special Olympics. South. Med. J. *80*:33, 1987.
17. Sullivan, J. D.: Down's syndrome and the Canadian Special Olympics. Can. Med. Assoc. J. *132*:1004, 1985.
18. Committee on Sports Medicine, American Academy of Pediatrics: Atlantoaxial instability in Down syndrome. Pediatrics *74*:152, 1984.
19. Low, L. J., and Sherrill, C.: Sports medicine concerns in Special Olympics. Palaestra, 1988, p. 56

20. Pueschel, S. M., et al.: Symptomatic atlantoaxial subluxation in persons with Down syndrome. J. Pediatr. Orthop. *4*:682, 1984.
21. Rubin, I. L.: Health care needs of adults with mental retardation. Mental Retardation *25*:201, 1987.
22. Nelsen, R. P., and Crocker, A. C.: The medical care of mentally retarded persons in public residential facilities. N. Engl. J. Med. *299*:1039, 1978.
23. McCormick, D. P.: The preparticipation sports examination in Special Olympic athletes. Texas Med. *84*:39, 1988.
24. PL 93–112. The Rehabilitation Act. 1973.
25. Hamel, R.: Getting into the game. New opportunities for athletes with disabilities. Physician Sportsmed. *20*(11):121, 1992.
26. Jackson, R. W., and Fredrickson, A.: Sports for the physically disabled: The 1976 Olympiad (Toronto). Am. J. Sports Med. *7*:293, 1979.
27. Clark, M. W.: Competitive sports for the disabled. Am. J. Sports Med. *8*:366, 1980.
28. Curtis, K. A., and Dillon, D. A.: Survey of wheelchair athletic injuries: Common patterns and prevention. Paraplegia *23*:170, 1985.
29. Ferrara, M. S., et al.: The injury experience of the competitive athlete with a disability: Prevention implications. Med. Sci. Sports Exerc. *24*:184, 1992.
30. Nichols, P. J. R., Norman, P. A., and Ennis, J. R.: Wheelchair user's shoulder: Shoulder pain in patients with spinal cord lesions. Scand. J. Rehabil. Med. *11*:29, 1979.
31. Ferrara, M. S.: Injuries to elite wheelchair athletes. Paraplegia *28*:335, 1990.
32. Hoeberigs, J. H., Debets-Eggen, H. B. L., and Debets, P. M. L.: Sports medical experiences from the International Flower Marathon for disabled wheelers. Am. J. Sports Med. *18*:418, 1990.
33. Madorsky, J. G. B., and Curtis, K. A.: Wheelchair sports medicine. Am. J. Sports Med. *12*:128, 1984.
34. Nilsen, R., Nygaard, P., and Bjorholt, P. G.: Complications that may occur in those with spinal cord injuries, who participate in sport. Paraplegia *23*:152, 1985.
35. Corcoran, P. J., et al.: Sports medicine and the physiology of wheelchair marathon racing. Orthop. Clin. North Am. *11*:697, 1980.
36. Laskowski, E. R., and Murtaugh, P. A.: Snow skiing injuries in physically disabled skiers. Am. J. Sports Med. *20*:553, 1992.
37. McCormick, D. P.: Injuries in handicapped Alpine ski racers. Physician Sportsmed. *13*(12):93, 1985.
38. Jafflin, B.: An epidemiologic study of ski injuries: Vail, Colorado. Mt. Sinai J. Med. *48*:353, 1981.
39. Laskowski, E. R.: Snow skiing for the physically disabled. Mayo Clin. Proc. *66*:160, 1991.
40. Wichmann, S., and Martin, D. R.: Single-organ patients. Balancing sports with safety. Physician Sportsmed. *20*(2):176, 1992.

RESOURCES: Addresses and Phone Numbers of Prominent Organizations

National Handicapped Sports
1145 19th St. NW
Suite 717
Washington, DC 20036
(202) 393-7505

National Handicapped Sports
451 Hungerford Dr.
Suite 100
Rockville, MD 20850
(301) 217-0960

US Cerebral Palsy Association
34518 Warren Rd.
Suite 264
Westland, MI 48185
(313) 425-8961

US Quad Rugby Association
1037 Cragmore Dr.
Fort Collins, CO 80521
(303) 484-7395

US Wheelchair Racquet-Sports Association
1941 Viento Verano Dr.
Diamond Bar, CA 91765
(714) 861-7312

Special Olympics International
1350 New York Ave. NW
Washington, DC 20005

National Wheelchair Athletic Association
3593 E. Fountain Blvd.
Suite L-1
Colorado Springs, CO 80910
(719) 574-1150

National Wheelchair Softball Association
1616 Todd Ct.
Hastings, MN 55033
(612) 437-1792

North American Riding for the Handicapped Association
Box 33150
Denver, CO 80233
(800) 369-7433

US Association for Blind Athletes
33 N. Institute
Colorado Springs, CO 80903
(719) 630-0422

American Blind Bowling Association
411 Sheriff St.
Mercer, PA 16137
(412) 662-5748

American Blind Skiing Foundation
610 S. William St.
Mount Prospect, IL 60056
(708) 255-1739

Handicapped Scuba Association
7172 W. Stanford Ave.
Littleton, CO 80123
(303) 933-4864

International Wheelchair Road Racers Club
30 Myano Ln.
Stamford, CT 06902
(203) 325-1429

National Amputee Golf Association
Box 1228
Amherst, NH 03031
(800) 633-6242

National Association of Wheelchair Tennis
940 Calle Amanacer
Suite B
San Clemente, CA 92672
(714) 361-6811

Winter Park Handicap Ski Program
P.O. Box 36
Winter Park, CO 80482
(303) 726-5514

Blind Outdoor Leisure Development, Inc.
0714 Meadows Rd.
P.O. Box 5429
Snowmass Village, CO 81615

21 *Joseph G. Jacko*

Head Injuries

All physicians who care for athletes should have a working knowledge of head trauma—of recognition, evaluation, treatment, and prevention. They should also be aware of associated injuries and complications that may follow head trauma. Head injuries occur in all sports, and each sport carries certain risks. Although head injuries in boxing and football have received the most attention, they commonly occur in other sports associated with high-risk maneuvers or activities, such as horseback riding, swimming, diving, gymnastics, ice hockey, martial arts, cycling, rugby, and skydiving.

PATHOPHYSIOLOGY

The scalp, skull, meninges, and cerebrospinal fluid (CSF) form a multilayered barrier that protects the brain from injury. Despite this protection, injuries to the brain still occur, and they can be discussed in terms of the mechanisms of injury, forces applied, and stresses generated. The skull and brain are generally injured in one of two ways. In one, an object strikes the resting but movable head, causing maximal brain injury beneath the point of impact *(coup injury)*. In the other, the moving head strikes a nonmoving object, usually producing maximal brain injury on the side opposite the site of impact *(contrecoup injury)*. These two mechanisms produce two types of forces that are applied to the brain.

Brain injury results from rotational (angular) or translational (linear) forces. These two forces generate distinct stresses; the three most important when discussing brain injury are compressive, tensile, and shearing stresses. Rotational forces produce shearing stresses on the nerve fibers, commonly leading to loss of consciousness. Conversely, translational forces more commonly produce compressive stresses that lead to skull fracture, intracranial hematoma, and cerebral contusion rather than unconsciousness.[1]

The brain tolerates compressive stress better than tensile or shearing stress. In part, this is related to the semisolid composition of the brain, which is not very compressible, and to the presence of the CSF, which helps absorb and distribute compressive forces uniformly. Shearing stress, however, is applied parallel to the surface of the brain; thus, the CSF does not totally prevent shearing stresses from being imparted to the brain.

The degree of brain injury is related to the position and motion of the head at the time of impact. For example, a baseball player hit by a pitched ball may suffer focal damage to the brain (translational force, compressive stress), but a gymnast who falls backward from a balance beam may suffer more diffuse brain injury (rotational force, shearing stress).

CLASSIFICATION OF HEAD INJURIES

Head injuries can be classified as *focal* or *diffuse* brain injuries. (Some authors classify them as either severe or minor; however, concussion, the mildest of head injuries, may not be so benign, so it is probably best to avoid the word *minor* when discussing head injuries.)

Focal brain injuries include cerebral contusions, intracerebral hematomas, epidural hematomas, and subdural hematomas (Fig. 21–1). These result from translational forces. Diffuse brain injuries include the concussion and diffuse axonal injury. Rotational force is the primary mechanism involved in diffuse brain injuries and is associated with global disruption of neurologic function. Diffuse brain injuries usually are not associated with focal or macroscopically visible brain lesions.

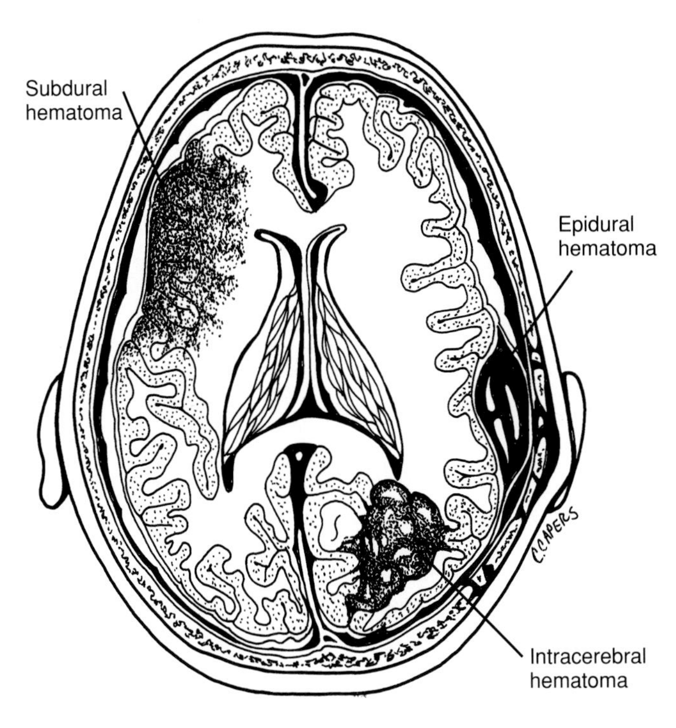

Fig. 21-1. Types of focal brain injury: subdural hematoma, hemorrhage in the subdural space between the dura and arachnoid membrane; epidural hematoma, accumulation of blood in the epidural space owing to damage to the middle meningeal artery; and intracerebral hematoma, hemorrhage into the cerebrum.

Focal Brain Injuries

CEREBRAL CONTUSION

Cerebral contusion is an ill-defined area of small hemorrhages, necrosis, and edema that occurs most often from an acceleration-deceleration (translational) force, such as that produced when an athlete's head strikes the ground. This causes the typical contrecoup lesion, which results in local loss of brain function as well as the creation of a mass effect compressing adjacent brain tissue.

INTRACEREBRAL HEMATOMA

Intracerebral hematomas occur deep within the brain and often result from a force applied to the head over a small area. Symptoms are determined by the size and location of the hematoma. Because of brain parenchymal injury, there is usually some decrease in the level of consciousness. Those who remain conscious complain of severe persistent headaches and amnesia. Evaluation with computed tomography (CT) or magnetic resonance imaging (MRI) is necessary.

EPIDURAL HEMATOMA

An epidural hematoma most often results from a tear of the middle meningeal artery in association with a temporal skull fracture. Of the focal head injuries, it is the most potentially life threatening, and death results from the mass effect of the rapidly expanding hematoma, which causes brain herniation. The mortality and morbidity rates associated with epidural hematoma are quite high, even with early recognition and treatment.

The classic presentation of an epidural hematoma is loss of consciousness at the time of injury followed by a lucid period of variable length. Rapid deterioration, characterized by severe headache and decreasing level of consciousness follows, and coma and death sometimes occur in a matter of only 15 to 30 minutes. This classic picture, however, occurs in only 12 to 33% of the patients.[2] Therefore, absence of the classic presentation cannot be relied on to exclude the diagnosis. Because injury to the brain itself usually is not significant, complete neurologic recovery is possible if the hematoma is recognized promptly and treated by surgical evacuation. Athletes suspected of having an epidural hematoma should be evaluated by CT or MRI.

SUBDURAL HEMATOMA

Subdural hematomas occur when the bridging veins between the brain and the dura are torn or when injury results in laceration of the brain parenchyma. Generally, less primary parenchymal injury occurs in subdural hematomas occurring in sports than from vehicular accidents because less force is involved.

Athletes may or may not be briefly lucid, and the need for neurosurgical evaluation is usually obvious because patients rendered unconscious at the time of injury generally remain so. The bleeding and associated swelling create an enlarging mass that may lead to nausea, vomiting, seizures, and hemiparesis. Depending on the location, a subdural hematoma may lead to uncal herniation compressing the brain stem and cranial nerves. Herniation should be suspected if ipsilateral ocular ptosis or pupillary dilatation develops.

Once an acute subdural hematoma has developed, rapid evacuation of the hematoma best decreases the chance of serious complications and death associated with this injury. Mortality rates for subdural hematoma are as high as 70%, and only 11% of patients can return to work.[3] Because some brain parenchymal injury usually occurs, the possibility of returning to contact sports is extremely small. In some patients a subdural hematoma develops, not immediately but more slowly, over 1 to 3 days. This is the result of slow bleeding and is generally associated with less parenchymal injury. In these subacute cases, the initial head injury is often assumed to have been insignificant. Symptoms range from generalized headache and dizziness to confusion, memory loss, and personality changes. A high index of suspicion must be maintained if an athlete is not steadily improving. If such symptoms persist, further evaluation with CT or MRI is indicated.

Diffuse Brain Injuries

CONCUSSIONS

Of all head injuries, concussion is the most common—and sometimes the most difficult to recognize.

Thus the potential for missed diagnosis and mismanagement is great.

It is estimated that, in football alone, more than 250,000 concussions, and an average of eight deaths, occur owing to head injury every year.[4,5] Twenty percent of high school football players suffer a concussion each year, and the chance of suffering a second concussion while playing football is four times greater than the chance of sustaining a first concussion.[6]

There is no universally accepted definition of concussion. In this discussion, however, concussion is defined "as a traumatically induced alteration in mental status."[7] Therefore, concussion can occur without loss of consciousness. The hallmarks of concussion are confusion and amnesia. These symptoms, as well as the presence or absence of consciousness, were described using an animal model created by Ommaya and Gennarelli.[1] Their findings indicate that confusion and amnesia occur when the shearing stress affects only the cortical and diencephalic structures. Loss of consciousness does not occur unless the shearing stress also reaches the reticular activating system.

There are many classification systems for grading the severity of concussions.[8,9] Some are based on the duration of unconsciousness, others on the duration of posttraumatic amnesia, and others on a combination of both. The Colorado Medical Society Sports Medicine Committee has developed a simple and practical grading system (Table 21–1) along with guidelines for the management (Table 21–2) of concussions based on the presence or absence of the three clinical findings already discussed: confusion, amnesia, and loss of consciousness.[10] These guidelines are not absolute and are no substitute for the sound clinical judgment of the examining physician.

Although most patients appear to recover uneventfully, a concussion is not a "benign" injury. Neuropsychologic deficits may exist despite normal neurologic findings. The ability to process information is reduced, and the effects are cumulative.[11] Twenty-five percent of athletes with three mild head injuries, 33% of those with four mild head injuries, and 40% of those with five mild head injuries showed persistent abnormalities on neuropsychologic testing 6 months after injury.[9] In addition, intracranial lesions are sometimes detected on CT and MRI.[12] Recently, there was a case report of a high school football player who died after developing severe brain swelling after a second mild head injury and another of a high school football player who developed a subdural hematoma after two mild concussions.[2,7,13] Sequelae of concussions such as postconcussion syndrome and second-impact syndrome will be discussed later.

DIFFUSE AXONAL INJURY

Diffuse axonal injuries represent more severe brain dysfunction and result from structural disruption of axons in the white matter of the cerebral hemispheres and brain stem. Prolonged traumatic coma occurs, with loss of consciousness generally lasting several hours. Because of axonal disruption, residual neurologic, psychologic, or personality deficits often result.

Table 21–1. Grading Scale for Concussions

Grade	*Symptoms*
Grade I (mild)	Confusion No amnesia No loss of consciousness
Grade II (moderate)	Confusion Amnesia No loss of consciousness
Grade III (severe)	Loss of consciousness

(Adapted from Colorado Medical Society: Report of the Sports Medicine Committee: Guidelines for the management of concussion in sports (revised). Denver: Colorado Medical Society, 1991.)

Table 21–2. Guidelines for Return to Play After Concussion

Grade	*First Concussion*	*Second Concussion*	*Third Concussion*
Grade I (mild)	May return to play when asymptomatic for at least 20 min	Terminate contest/ practice; may return to play if asymptomatic for at least 1 week	Terminate season; may return to play in 3 months if asymptomatic
Grade II (moderate)	Terminate contest/ practice; may return to play when asymptomatic for 1 week	Consider terminating season, but may return to play if asymptomatic for 1 month	Terminate season; may return to play next season if asymptomatic
Grade III (severe)	Terminate contest/practice and transport to hospital; may return to play 1 month after two consecutive asymptomatic weeks; conditioning allowed after 1 asymptomatic week	Terminate season	Regardless of grade a season is terminated by any abnormality on CT or MRI consistent with brain contusion or other intracranial lesion

(Adapted from Colorado Medical Society: Report of the Sports Medicine Committee: Guidelines for the management of concussion in sports (revised). Denver: Colorado Medical Society, 1991.)

ON-FIELD MANAGEMENT

Preparation and anticipation are the keys to on-field management of head injuries. Every physician and trainer should have a "game plan." This includes making sure that necessary equipment is readily accessible and in good working condition, that a means of transporting the athlete is immediately available, and that the location of the nearest established medical facility is known and a means of communication is established. The most important objective of on-field management is to prevent further injury. Although no single plan or approach is universally accepted, some basic principles apply.

First, every unconscious athlete and any conscious athlete who complains of neck pain, numbness, weakness, or paralysis should be assumed to have a cervical spine injury until proven otherwise. In these instances care must be taken to stabilize the spine until radiographic evaluation can be done (see Chapter 35). Second, the *ABCs* of cardiopulmonary resuscitation must be assessed: airway, breathing, and circulation. Third, once it is established that the athlete is breathing and has a pulse, a baseline neurologic assessment should be performed. The AVPU method (Glasgow coma scale) can be used to assess the level of consciousness: A, *a*lert; V, responds to *v*erbal stimulus; P, responds to *p*ainful stimulus; U, *u*nconscious.

The patient's pupils should be assessed for symmetry and reactivity to light. An asymmetrically dilated pupil in an unconscious athlete suggests that transtentorial herniation has occurred. In this case, the patient should be managed with hyperventilation and immediate transportation to a medical facility.

Fourth, the physician should remember to evaluate the athlete for other injuries and should be aware of the possibility of a skull fracture. A skull fracture should be suspected if there is disruption of the integrity of the scalp. Signs of basilar skull fracture include the presence of postarticular hematoma (Battle's sign), rhinorrhea, otorrhea, periorbital ecchymosis (racoon eyes), and hematotympanum.

If an unconscious athlete is not breathing or does not have a pulse, plans for immediate transportation to a hospital should be made and cardiopulmonary resuscitation initiated. An airway must be established. If the athlete is lying face down, he or she must be brought to a supine position using a log-roll technique (usually performed by a team of five). The leader of the medical support team (usually a physician) should control the head and stabilize the neck while the athlete is rolled onto a spine board.

The face mask (if a helmet is worn) must be removed using bolt cutters or scissors, depending on the type of mask. Rescue breathing can then be given using current recommendations of the American Heart Association. Usually an airway can be established by the jaw-thrust technique. If the jaw-thrust technique is not adequate the head-tilt–jaw-lift technique can be substituted; however, care must be taken not to extend the neck any more than is necessary. If at any time it is felt that the helmet must be removed to establish an airway, the helmet should be removed only with the neck in a neutral position.

If the athlete has remained conscious or rapidly regained consciousness and if a cervical spine injury has been ruled out, the athlete can be taken to the sideline for observation and reevaluation. This secondary evaluation includes determination of orientation to time, person, and place, presence of amnesia and confusion, and observation of gait. At no time should an athlete who has persistent symptoms be permitted to return to play. An asymptomatic athlete is one who has no headache, confusion, dizziness, impaired orientation, impaired concentration, or memory dysfunction *either* at rest or on exertion.

An athlete who develops seizures, focal neurologic signs, or deterioration in mental status while being observed on the sideline should be transported to a medical facility for further evaluation and treatment.

RETURN TO COMPETITION

When an athlete can return safely to competition (particularly contact sports) after an injury is one of the most controversial issues in sports medicine. It is best to be too conservative if there is any doubt that an athlete is ready to return to play. Also, it should be recognized that appearance of some symptoms, such as amnesia, may be delayed by several minutes: thus, a period of observation on the sideline is necessary.[14]

Few sports have set guidelines for return to competition. The New York State Boxing Commission imposes a mandatory 45-day suspension for mild concussions; 60-day suspension for moderate concussions; and 90-day suspension with a requirement for normal results on CT and electroencephalography for severe concussions.[9] In most sports, however, determination of when an athlete can return to play is individualized.

There are several guidelines for return to competition.[8,9] How long the athlete should avoid activity varies among the guidelines, but in all cases higher grades of injury require the athlete to be held out of activity longer. Guidelines from the Colorado Medical Society are included here (see Table 21–1).

The Grade I (mild) concussion is the most common form of concussion—and the most difficult to recognize. It is characterized by confusion without loss of consciousness or amnesia. Frequently, a player who has suffered a Grade I concussion (the "ding" or having one's "bell rung") is brought to the attention of the physician or coach by a teammate. After a first Grade I concussion, return to the game is permissible only if the athlete is asymptomatic. The athlete should be observed both at rest and during exertion (e.g., running in place) over a period of at least 20 minutes. An athlete who suffers a second Grade I concussion in the same contest should be restricted from play that day. Three Grade I concussions in the same season are grounds for terminating play that season. An athlete who experiences headache or other symptoms (dizziness, impaired orientation, impaired concentration, or memory dysfunction) for more than 1 week should be evaluated by CT or MRI.

In a Grade II concussion an athlete experiences confusion and amnesia but no loss of consciousness. The athlete is removed from the contest and is not permitted to return that day. The athlete should be re-evaluated in 24 hours. After a first Grade II concussion, return to competition can be considered after the athlete has been asymptomatic for at least 1 week. After a second Grade II concussion, return to contact play should be deferred at least 1 month and consideration is given to terminating the season. A third Grade II concussion terminates an athlete's season.

A Grade III concussion renders an athlete unconscious. Cervical spine immobilization is indicated, and the athlete should be transported to the nearest hospital for neurologic evaluation and observation. CT or MRI should be performed, when appropriate, to evaluate for brain injury. Neurologic evaluation should be performed daily until all symptoms resolve. After a Grade III concussion, an athlete is usually held out of contact sports at least 1 month. Return to play is permissible after 1 month only if the athlete has been asymptomatic at rest and exertion for at least 2 weeks. CT or MRI is indicated whenever symptoms persist longer than a week. A second Grade III concussion terminates an athlete's season, and future participation in contact sports should be discouraged.

Regardless of grade, a season is terminated by any abnormality on CT or MRI that is consistent with a brain contusion or other intracranial abnormality. Also, return to contact sports is generally contraindicated for any athlete who has suffered a head injury that required intracranial surgery.

Postconcussion Syndrome

Some athletes who have suffered a concussion have persistent symptoms for a period of days to months. Symptoms include headache, dizziness, irritability, fatigue, impaired memory and concentration, and slow decision making. Exercise appears to aggravate some of these symptoms. There is no specific treatment other than rest; however, CT or MRI should be performed to exclude intracranial lesions if symptoms persist. Neuropsychiatric tests are helpful and can be used to monitor recovery. Since the effects of repeated concussions appear to be cumulative, an athlete with a postconcussion syndrome should not return to competition until all symptoms have resolved, both at rest and during exertion.[11]

SECOND-IMPACT SYNDROME

Second-impact syndrome refers to the rapid brain swelling (many times fatal) that occurs when an athlete suffers a second mild head injury while still symptomatic from a first head injury.[15] As an isolated event the second injury would not be sufficient to produce severe pathologic changes. The rapid swelling is the result of autoregulatory dysfunction leading to vascular engorgement of the brain. This phenomenon is a variant of the malignant brain edema syndrome that sometimes occurs in the pediatric age group after severe traumatic brain injury.

PREVENTION

Head injuries are better prevented than treated. There are several ways to prevent head injuries. To some degree, safety can be legislated by requiring athletes in certain sports to wear some type of headgear. Some contact sports, such as football, boxing, lacrosse, and ice hockey, require helmets; other sports, such as soccer and rugby, do not.

The type and condition of the helmet are also important. Helmets with pneumatic pockets are superior to the strap-type suspension. Helmets are most effective when intact and when properly fitted. Defective helmets that have lost their integrity should be replaced. In addition to reducing dental injuries, a well-fitted mouth guard can also reduce concussions.

Changes in the rules of the game can help decrease the incidence of head and neck injuries. Some sports have made important rule changes. For instance, since "spearing" with the head was made illegal in football in 1976, the incidence of serious head and neck injuries has declined approximately 50%.[16] Improved conditioning, primarily strengthening the neck muscles, may also help to reduce the number and severity of head injuries.

Secondary prevention through early diagnosis and management improves survival and quality of life following a serious head injury. Also, understanding when it is safe for an athlete to return to competition can reduce the risk of a subsequent, and sometimes catastrophic, head injury.

REFERENCES

1. Ommaya, A. K., and Gennarelli, T. A.: Cerebral concussion and traumatic unconsciousness: correlation of experimental and clinical observations of blunt head injuries. Brain, *97*:633, 1974.
2. Dempsey, R. J., and Schneider, R. C.: The management of head injuries in sports. In Sports Injuries: Mechanisms, Prevention, and Treatment. Edited by R. C. Schneider, et al. Baltimore, Williams & Wilkins, 1985.
3. Rosenhorn, J., and Gjerris, T.: Long-term follow-up review of patients with acute and subacute subdural hematomas. J. Neurosurg. *48*:345, 1978.
4. Cantu, R. C.: When to return to contact sports after a cerebral concussion. Sports Med. Digest, *10*:1, 1988.
5. Torg, J. S., et al.: The National Football Head and Neck Injury Registry: 14-year report on cervical quadriplegia, 1971 through 1984. J.A.M.A. *254*:3439, 1985.
6. Gerberich, S. G., et al.: Concussion incidences and severity in secondary school varsity football players. Am. J. Public Health, *73*:1370, 1983.

7. Kelly, J. P., et al: Concussion in sports: Guidelines for the prevention of catastrophic outcome. J.A.M.A. *266*:2867, 1991.
8. Cantu, R. C.: Guidelines for return to contact sports after a cerebral concussion. Physician Sportsmed. *14*(10):75, 1986.
9. Wilberger, J. E., Jr., and Maroon, J. C.: Head injuries in athletes. Clin. Sports Med. *8*:1, 1989.
10. Colorado Medical Society: Report of the Sports Medicine Committee: Guidelines for the Management of Concussion in Sports (Revised). Denver: Colorado Medical Society, 1991.
11. Gronwall, D., and Wrightson, P.: Cumulative effects of concussion. Lancet *2*:995, 1975.
12. Levin, H. S., et al.: Magnetic resonance imaging and computerized tomography in relation to the neurobehavioral sequelae of mild and moderate head injuries. J. Neurosurg. *66*:706, 1987.
13. Shell, D., Carico, G. A., and Patton, R. M.: Can subdural hematoma result from repeated minor head injury? Physician Sportsmed. *21*(4):74, 1993.
14. Yarnell, P. R., and Lynch, S.: Retrograde memory immediately after concussion. Lancet *25*:863, 1970.
15. Saunders, R. L., and Harbaugh, R. E.: The second impact in catastrophic contact—sports head trauma. J.A.M.A. *252*:538, 1984.
16. Cantu, R. C., and Mueller, F.: Catastrophic spine injury in football 1977–1989. J. Spinal Dis. *3*:227, 1990.

22 *Angelo Galante*

Facial Trauma

Facial trauma accounts for 1 to 11% of all sports injuries.[1] Injuries to the face are especially common in sports in which balls, racquets, and bats are used, as well as in high-velocity, direct-contact sports (e.g., boxing, karate). Management requires knowledge of anatomy and the ability to make a rapid assessment of the severity of the injury and of the potential for it to progress to serious sequelae. Though there are many types of injuries, the most common ones involve the eyes, nose, and ears.

EYE INJURIES

Sports injuries to the eye are frequently preventable. An excellent example is the rule changes instituted in ice hockey in 1978 and 1980. The new rules require full face protectors that have no opening more than 2 inches in diameter and can withstand the force of a puck traveling 40 to 45 miles per hour. This resulted in the virtual elimination of eye injuries from the sport. The decrease in injuries is estimated to have saved more than $10 million in medical costs each year. Nonetheless, other sports have not adopted this approach, and injuries continue to mount. Some studies have reported sports-related eye injuries as responsible for almost 25% of all ocular trauma.[2]

Sports can be classified according to their risk for eye injuries: sports that do not involve a thrown or hit ball, a stick, or close, aggressive play have low risk; sports involving a high-speed ball or puck have high risk; and combative sports have extremely high risk.

All eye injuries should be treated as serious ones; however, certain findings require immediate attention and further evaluation, possibly by an ophthalmologist. These are blurred vision, loss of visual field, sharp stabbing pain, double vision, abnormal extraocular movement, abnormal pupil, a cut or penetrating wound of the eyelid or eyeball, and abnormal visual acuity.

Many common eye injuries can be managed by a team physician. Corneal abrasions may be caused by a scratch or some foreign material in the eye. Abrasions are characterized by tearing, photophobia, and pain. They are relatively easy to diagnose with the use of fluorescein-impregnated paper strips; defects in the corneal epithelium look bright green under ordinary light and bright yellow under cobalt blue light. Treatment of abrasions involves the use of topical antibiotics, application of a firm sterile pad dressing, adequate analgesia, and re-examination every 24 hours until healing is established. If a foreign body has caused the abrasion, care must be taken to make sure it has been removed. Abrasions caused by a contact lens should not be patched, lest infectious keratitis develop. Topical anesthetics should never be used for corneal abrasions, because the loss of sensation may allow the abrasion to turn into an ulcer.

Burns of the eye are generally confined to sun exposure. This injury occurs most commonly in water and snow sports. Ultraviolet light burns the conjunctiva, resulting in necrosis and loss of individual surface epithelial cells. The most common symptoms are pain and photophobia. The treatment is directed toward pain relief, including systemic analgesics and topical corticosteroids. Once again, topical anesthetics should be avoided. Another less common injury is chemical burns, which are incurred in sports where the lines are drawn with lye rather than paint. As the player hits the line, the lye may enter the eye. The main treatment is copious irrigation with water.

A hyphema, a collection of free blood in the anterior chamber of the eye (Fig. 22–1), is the most common intraocular injury associated with sports. Initially the blood may be dispersed and appear as a haze in the anterior chamber. Examination of the eye reveals an irregular (larger) pupil that is sluggish to react to light. Vision may be blurred. Most of these injuries should resolve within a few days. Patients should be advised to avoid strenuous activity and remain in bed, resting with

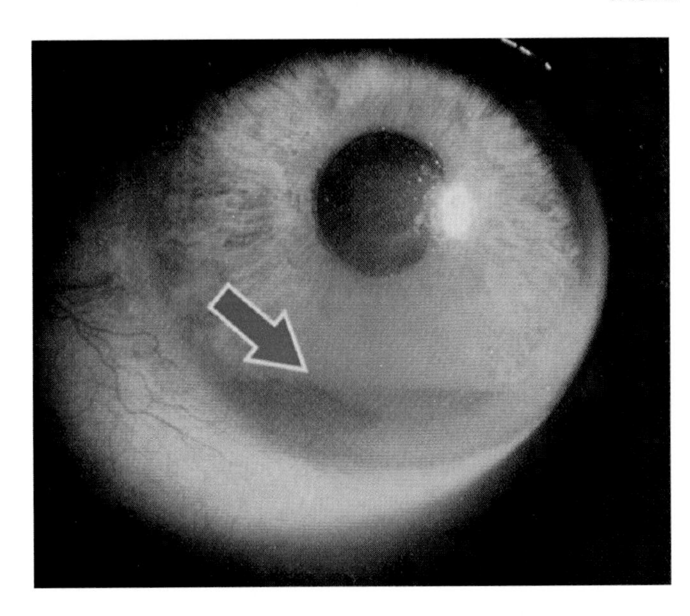

Fig. 22–1. Hyphema is a collection of free blood in the anterior chamber of the eye.

the head of the bed elevated. A topical steroid or cycloplegic may be used to minimize patient discomfort. An antifibrinolytic agent may be used to preserve the clot. Many physicians recommend hospitalization and consultation with an ophthalmologist because rebleeding is common 2 to 5 days after the original bleed, and 25 to 35% of patients also have damage to the other eye. Complications include later development of glaucoma, cataracts, blood staining of the cornea, and rebleeding.

Lacerations of the eye are common sports injuries, and most can be repaired relatively easily; however, three parts of the eye require special care, and consultation may be warranted. The three areas involve important anatomic structures and require exact repair for adequate cosmetic appearance. The areas include those that cross the margin of the lid, those that involve the medial third of the lid (possibly involving the lacrimal area), and corneal lacerations that may result in a ruptured globe.

Subconjunctival hemorrhage results from damage to a conjunctival vessel and results in blood pooling beneath the conjunctiva. These usually resolve within 10 to 14 days without treatment. The patient needs to be reassured of the benign nature of this injury, and an examination should be done to rule out associated injuries such as a ruptured globe.

Posterior segment injuries include retinal detachment, retinal edema, choroid rupture, and hemorrhages. These should be suspected if the patient reports flashes of light or a sensation of a shade or curtain being pulled down over the eye or if examination reveals a decreased pupillary response or a decreased red reflex. These often are the result of severe blunt trauma and may be vision threatening. If a posterior segment injury is suspected, the athlete should be promptly referred to an ophthalmologist.

A one-eyed athlete requires certain special considerations. Such a person is anyone with visual acuity of 20/200 or less in one eye. Most athletes with one eye do not demonstrate disability in their sport; however, the potential exists for injury to the functioning eye. Thus, such athletes should be restricted from extremely high-risk sports. Participation in lower-risk sports requires appropriate eye protection and making sure the athlete understands the potential risks.

EAR INJURIES

The most common external ear injury seen by sports medicine physicians is a hematoma in wrestlers, the so-called *cauliflower ear.* The cauliflower ear results from an auricular hematoma left untreated that becomes organized and evolves to cause a deformity of the ear. The hematoma results from direct trauma to the ear. It is thought that if these injuries are left untreated, blood collects beneath the perichondrium and auricular cartilage; the pressure of the hematoma can cause necrosis and permanent deformation of the ear.

Prompt treatment for auricular hematoma is required to prevent permanent deformity. Initial treatment should include application of ice and aspiration of the hematoma. The athlete should be removed from the area of competition so that strict aseptic technique can be used for aspiration. Infection can lead to necrosis of the cartilage. After aspiration, a pressure dressing must be applied to prevent reaccumulation. This can be accomplished by using a collodion splint or cast formed to the ear or a through-and-through suture using a button for compression. The cast is made from cotton batting and collodion in the form of the ear and ear canal. This is held in place with an external bandage. Plaster of Paris and silicone have also been used to make casts. Infrequently, open drainage is required, and if it is, the patient must take a broad-spectrum antibiotic as prophylaxis against *Staphylococcus aureus* and *Pseudomonas.* The athlete may not participate in sports for 24 hours and should not sleep on the affected ear. Casting is left in place 5 to 7 days. Headgear may help prevent hematomas; however, it does not eliminate the risk of injury. A lubricant such as petroleum jelly should be used at the first sign of redness caused by friction from headgear. It prevents friction burns and decreases progression of existing injuries.

The other commonly encountered ear problem is swimmer's ear (otitis externa). Some athletes involved in water sports are especially prone to this infection, which is caused by bacterial and fungal species and may be painful to the point of disabling. It is believed that the usual protective barrier of the ear is destroyed by excessive swimming. This allows infection to take hold when water, especially chlorinated water, is in the ear for a long time. The ear lining is macerated and the protective keratin layer and normal flora (gram-positive organisms) may be washed away and replaced by gram-negative ones and fungi. The infection then causes a chain reaction of increased wax production, increased canal pH, and multiplication of organisms coupled with canal obstruction to cause inflammation and the classic symptoms of pain, pus, and itching. The patient complains of acute pain, especially after sleeping on that side, decreased hearing acuity, and drainage. On examination, the ear is acutely tender to movement of the pinna or tragus and the canal is narrowed and erythematous.

Otitis externa usually resolves quickly with proper treatment. Corticosteroids or colistin sulfate is usually effective. One must be careful to make sure the tympanic membrane is intact before using any topical treatment. The athlete may need to stop swimming and should be given these instructions on proper ear hygiene:

1. Keep ears dry, avoid water in ears, wear ear plugs, and drain ears of water.
2. Do not use cotton swabs in the ear canal.
3. Never let soap or shampoo in ears.
4. Consider using an aluminum subacetate solution or alcohol drops after swimming, to change pH.
5. Use baby oil as a protective coating.

Occasionally, for severe cases, the use of 3% boric acid or 5% acetic acid with isopropyl alcohol may be necessary. Also, let us not forget that the severity of pain may necessitate strong analgesics.

Other ear injuries include temporal bone fractures and lacerations. If a laceration involves the external ear and cartilage, it should be repaired separately. The athlete should be made aware that perichondritis may result.

NASAL INJURIES

Nasal injuries are frequent in sports. By being located in the midface and extending forward, the nose is significantly at risk for injury. Common injuries include contusions, hematomas, abrasions, lacerations, epistaxis, and fractures, with and without deformities. Because the nose serves in respiration and as a cosmetic element of the face, an injury to the nose must be treated with care.

Epistaxis

The most common problem is the simple nosebleed (epistaxis). But is it really so simple? Epistaxis may occur as a result of local or systemic causes. In athletes, however, most are secondary to trauma. The first order of business is to make the diagnosis and visualize the source of bleeding. The anterior nosebleed, arising from Kiesselbach's plexus (Fig. 22–2) and fed by the anterior and posterior ethmoidal and sphenopalatine arteries, accounts for 90% of epistaxis cases and is relatively easily treated. Once the site is visualized as anterior, ice and compression usually control the bleeding. Otherwise, one could easily cauterize it with silver nitrate sticks or even an electrocautery pen. Occasionally, gauze packing is needed to control the bleeding.

Posterior epistaxis is usually more severe and involves larger nasal branches of the internal maxillary artery or ethmoidal arteries, principally the posterior ethmoidal artery. These bleeds often drain into the throat. Treatment for less severe posterior epistaxis usually requires head elevation and packing with gauze, an inflated Foley catheter, or a specially designed nasal catheter, if available. Once the bleeding is controlled, application of a topical antibiotic is recommended. The patient should be instructed not to blow the nose for

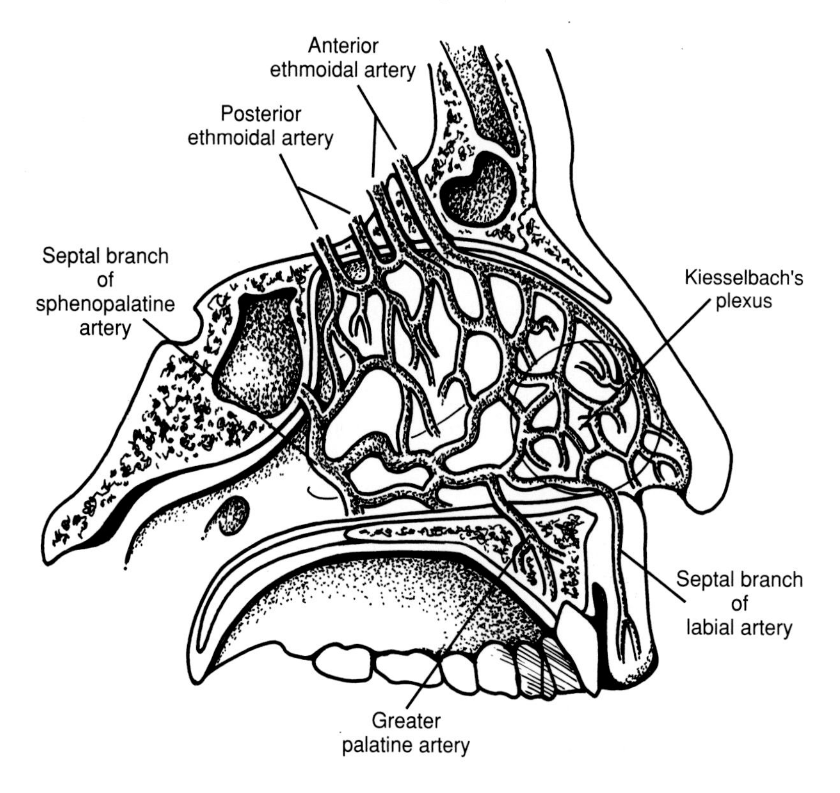

Fig. 22–2. Vascular sources of the nasal cavity.

the first 24 hours. Re-examination should be performed within 2 to 3 days, to check for septal hematoma, a collection of blood between the septal cartilage and the perichondrium. The treatment of major epistaxis is more involved and includes 4 to 10% cocaine for vasoconstriction and lidocaine for anesthesia. These are applied with cotton pledgets left in place 5 to 10 minutes. The nose is then packed with petroleum jelly or iodoform gauze, beginning posteriorly. Packing is left in place 72 hours, and the patient should avoid physical activity and hot beverages and showers until the packing is removed. The nose is examined again after 2 weeks, and the patient is informed of possible complications including sinusitis, otitis media, obstructed eustachian tube, and pressure necrosis to the nasal or nasopharyngeal mucosa. The profuse bleeding that routinely occurs after a fracture is caused by rupture of the anterior ethmoidal artery. For these injuries, reduction and packing are usually required.

Nasal Fractures

The nasal bones are frequently fractured because of their prominent position and thinness. The diagnosis of nasal fractures is primarily clinical. Signs of nasal fracture include epistaxis, swelling of the nasal dorsum, ecchymosis around the eyes, tenderness, fracture visible on radiograph, deformity, and crepitus.

Once the diagnosis is suspected, an examination should be performed to identify the source of epistaxis and to rule out septal hematoma. If left untreated, septal hematoma progresses to necrosis, with resulting airway obstruction, saddle-nose deformity, and, possibly, septal perforation. Treatment of septal hematoma consists of drainage for decompression and nasal packing to prevent recurrence.

Nasal fractures vary, depending on the force and direction of the blow: the nose tolerates frontal blows better than lateral ones. Fractures vary from simple ones, in which only a portion of the nasal bone is fractured, to severe ones, in which the entire nasal-orbital ethmoid complex is fractured and resultant lateral displacement of the medial canthal tendons causes increased distance between the eyes. The cribriform plate may also be fractured, and this can result in leakage of cerebrospinal fluid. Lateral forces usually result in deviated septum and cause inward fracture of the nasal bone on the side of the applied force and outward fracture of the nasal bones of the opposite side.

Once a nasal fracture is diagnosed, it should be adequately reduced as soon as possible. However, a waiting period may be necessary if ecchymosis and swelling delay fracture identification. The maximum time for nasal reduction is usually 4 days for children and 10 to 12 days for adults.

Reduction of nasal fractures can be performed under local or general anesthesia. Closed reduction is used to treat children and unilateral fractures of the nasal bones without major deviation. The nasal bone is elevated with a blunt instrument positioned within the nose. The nasal passage is then packed or the nose splinted to maintain reduction. Intranasal splints are kept in place about 7 to 10 days. Open reduction is indicated in the presence of significant septal displacement or difficulty in maintaining nasal bone reduction. The key to achieving symmetric reduction is to position the nasal septum straight in the midline.

TEETH

Tooth avulsions may occur in contact sports. Prompt treatment may save teeth from being lost. If reimplanted expeditiously a totally avulsed tooth may survive. The tooth must be kept moist and wrapped in a gauze pad and transported with the athlete to a dentist for reimplantation. The likelihood of salvage depends on the length of time the tooth has been out of the socket and the degree to which the periodontal ligament has dried out. The tooth may be rinsed in running tap water to remove loose debris, but the root surface should not be brushed or handled. During transport the tooth must be kept moist. An avulsed tooth should be preserved in a plastic container with whole milk, saliva, or sterile saline solution. After reimplantation, an avulsed tooth needs to be stabilized by splinting to the adjacent teeth for 1 to 2 weeks. Analgesia, a tetanus shot, and antibiotics are indicated.

REFERENCES

1. Sane, J.: Comparison of maxillofacial and dental injuries in four contact team sports: American football, bandy, basketball, and handball. Am. J. Sports Med. *16:*647, 1988.
2. Erie, J. C.: Eye injuries. Prevention, evaluation, and treatment. Physician Sportsmed. *19*(11):108, 1991.

SUGGESTED READINGS

Bakland, L. K., and Boyne, P. J.: Trauma to the oral cavity. Clin. Sports Med. *8:*25, 1989.

Christiansen, T., and Wilson, K.: Facial injuries in sports. Minn. Med. *66:*29, 1983.

Dimeff, R. J., and Hough, D. O.: Preventing cauliflower ear with a modified tie-through technique. Phys. Sportsmed. *17*(3):167, 1989.

Martinez, S. A.: Nasal fractures: Where to go for a successful outcome. Postgrad. Med. *82*(2):71, 1987.

O'Donoghue, G. M., Vaughan, E. D. V., and Condon, K. C.: An analysis of the pattern of facial injuries in a general accident department. Injury *11:*52, 1979.

Peretta, L. J., et al.: Emergency evaluation and management of epistaxis. Emerg. Med. Clin. North Am. *5:*265, 1987.

Schendel, S. A.: Sports-related nasal injuries. Physician Sportsmed. *18*(10):59, 1990.

Schultz, R. C., and de Camara, D. L.: Athletic facial injuries. J.A.M.A. *252:*3395, 1984.

Stevens, H.: Epistaxis in the athlete. Phys. Sportsmed. *16*(12):31, 1988.

Vinger, P. F.: How I manage corneal abrasions and lacerations. Physician Sportsmed. *14*(5):170, 1986.

23 *Mark J. Leski*

Blunt Trauma to the Chest and Abdomen

Few sports injuries are considered life threatening, and this is usually the case for blunt trauma to the chest and abdomen; however, certain injuries can result in shock, and even death. Because the appearance of the athlete after trauma to the chest or abdomen may be misleading, serial examinations, over minutes to hours, may be necessary to adequately evaluate an athlete who has sustained a significant blow to the chest or abdomen. Of utmost importance in evaluating and treating such injuries are the principles of basic acute trauma life support and transfer to an appropriate medical facility, when indicated.[1] To prevent a catastrophe, the physician must maintain a high index of suspicion of serious injury, to recognize and treat the problem in a timely fashion.

MECHANISMS OF INJURY

There are three mechanisms of injury involved in blunt trauma to the chest or abdomen: the direct blow, sudden deceleration, and compressive forces. Direct blows are often responsible for contusions, fractures, and dislocations.[1–4] Sudden deceleration results in severe shear stresses on internal organs and may result in tearing of vascular structures or organs from their attachments.[1,5] Compressive forces increase intrathoracic or intra-abdominal pressure and may result in rupture of hollow or air-filled organs.[1,3,6,7] These forces may also compress solid organs, causing them to fracture.

Contact sports responsible for most chest and abdominal injuries are football, rugby, soccer, and wrestling. Noncontact sports involved in these injuries include downhill snow skiing, water skiing, horseback riding, and others that produce high-speed deceleration injuries. Sports responsible for injury patterns similar to those of general motor vehicle accidents are cycling, three-wheeling, snowmobiling, and dune buggy racing.[6] Cycling is the most common cause of intra-abdominal injury in sports.[6,8]

BLUNT CHEST TRAUMA

Soft Tissue Injuries

Soft tissue injuries about the chest include muscle contusions or disruptions and breast contusions. Muscle contusions are caused by a direct blow to the involved area. The pain is well localized and palpation over the area of trauma detects tenderness. The pain is exacerbated by motion in the involved area. Treatment is application of ice, and possibly compression, for the first 24 to 48 hours after injury. Heat may be applied later, to help resolve hematoma.

Disruption of the pectoralis major muscle can result from a direct blow to the chest (Fig. 23–1).[1,9] Usually, severe pain radiates to the shoulder and upper arm. Passive abduction or active adduction of the arm is very painful, and adduction strength is markedly decreased. Usually a defect is palpable in the pectoralis major, and radiographs may demonstrate absence of the pectoralis major muscle shadow.[1,3] Proximal muscle disruption can often be treated conservatively; however, distal disruptions near the musculotendinous junction usually require surgical repair to restore normal strength and function.[1,9]

In female athletes direct blows to the chest may cause breast contusions. Findings may consist of ecchymosis, pain, and unilateral breast enlargement from hematoma.[2,3] Later, one may see post-traumatic fat necrosis and mammographic changes indistinguishable from those of malignancy.[3] Treatment is application of ice in the first 24 to 48 hours combined with support from a binder or brassiere.[1,4] The athlete should be withdrawn from competition until swelling and inflamma-

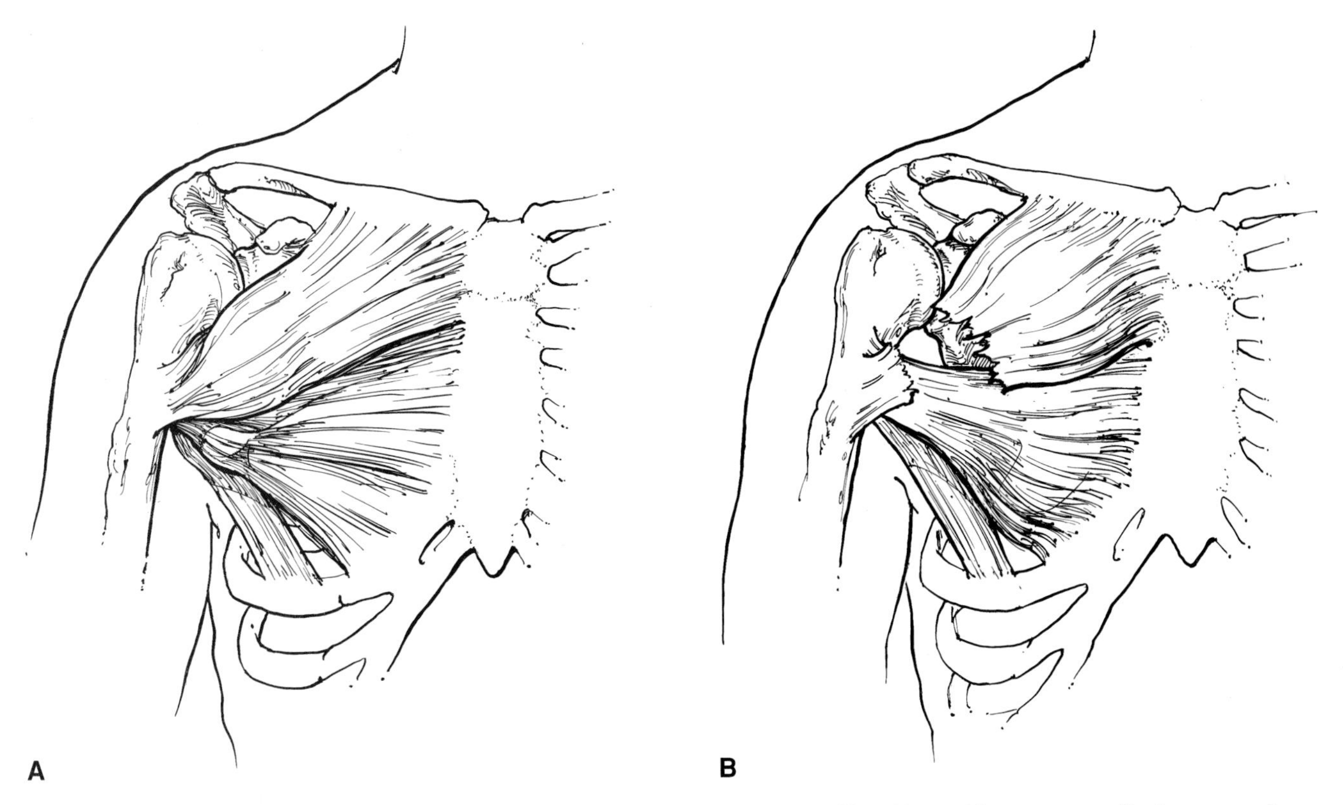

Fig. 23–1. Rupture of the pectoralis major muscle. (*A*) Partial rupture and resultant distal bunching and hematoma; (*B*) distal rupture and resultant proximal mass.

tion subside. When evaluating these patients, the physician should ask about previous breast augmentation and look for bilateral scars that suggest augmentation. Augmented breasts may sustain capsular or implant rupture. With capsular rupture, the breast is softer with a concave profile. Patients with implant rupture may present with gradual or immediate breast decompression and masses adjacent to the breast. Surgical repair is necessary.[2]

Fractures

Rib fractures are not uncommon in collision and contact sports. Rib fractures usually occur in the fifth to ninth ribs at the point of impact or at the posterior angle of the rib (the weakest point) (Fig. 23–2). They are associated with significant pain, often pleuritic in nature and aggravated by movement. Palpation at the site of fracture also elicits pain. The athlete may experience shortness of breath, either from pain or from flail chest secondary to numerous rib fractures. Complications of rib fracture include pneumothorax, hemothorax,[4] lung contusion, liver and spleen laceration, and kidney injury.[3] Fracture of the first three ribs is associated with extreme trauma that may result in great vessel or airway injury. Diagnosis of rib fracture may be made from an anteroposterior chest radiograph or an anterior oblique rib view. One must realize, however, that 50% of rib fractures are not visible on radiographs taken immediately after injury but may become visible 10 to 14 days later. If a rib fracture is found on early radiographs, inspiratory and expiratory films should be obtained to help rule out pneumothorax and hemothorax.[3] Unless the previously mentioned complications are present, treatment of rib fractures is primarily supportive—rest and analgesics. Occasionally, intercostal blocks are used for short-term pain relief.[1]

Clavicular and sternal fractures both result from a direct blow to the affected area and are associated with anterior chest pain. Clavicular fractures are detected clinically by a disruption of the normal contour of the clavicle and by radiographic evaluation (Fig. 23–3).[3] Treatment is usually with a figure-of-eight splint. Sternal fractures are rare and are related to violent traumatic forces.[4] They are often associated with cardiac contusions,[10] so the physician must have a high index of suspicion of this problem if a sternal fracture is found on radiographs.

Separations and Dislocations

Separations and dislocations of the joints about the thoracic cage, common injuries in contact and collision sports, usually result from twisting injuries or an anterolateral blow to the chest.[1,11] Costochondral separation, commonly termed "slipping rib syndrome," is characterized by increased mobility of one or more lower costal cartilages after an episode of trauma. This mobility

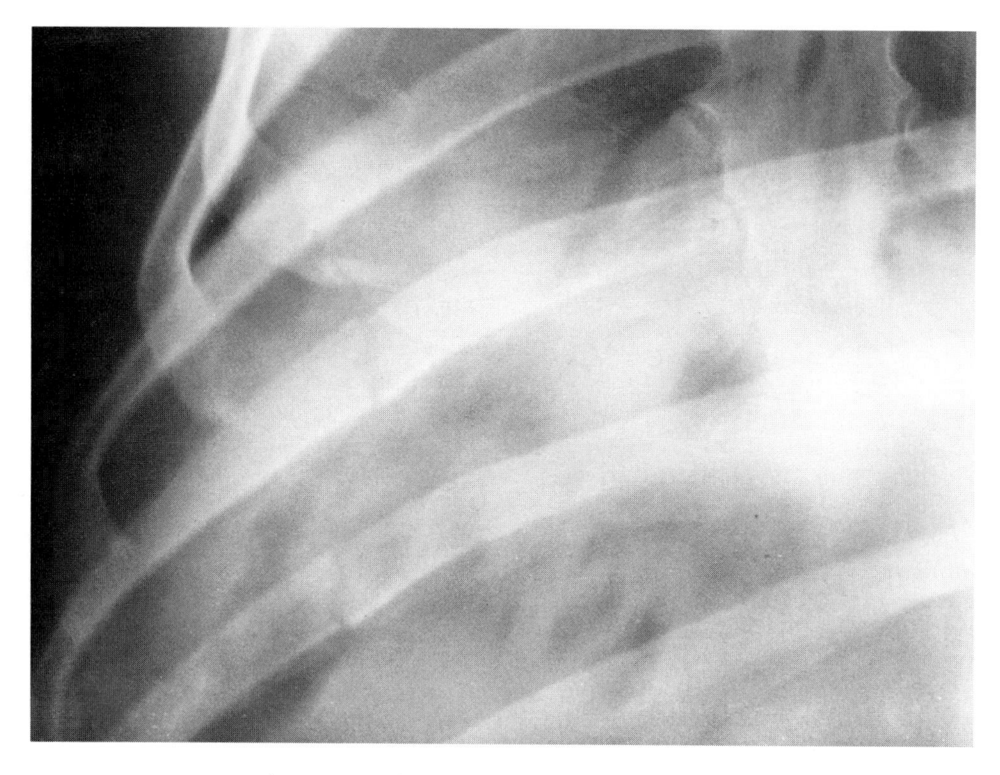

Fig. 23–2. Radiographic appearance of rib fractures.

allows the anterior costal margins to "slip" over one another. The diagnosis is made by physical examination, and findings include pain at the costal margin precipitated by physical exertion and change in position. A deformity may be palpable. Treatment consists of rest, ice, and analgesics.[1]

Sternoclavicular joint dislocations usually result from a fall onto the acromioclavicular joint that transmits the force down the clavicle to the sternoclavicular joint.[1] These injuries may be difficult to detect clinically. The patient may report severe anterior thoracic pain that mimics angina or pleuritic pain.[3] Anterior dislocations

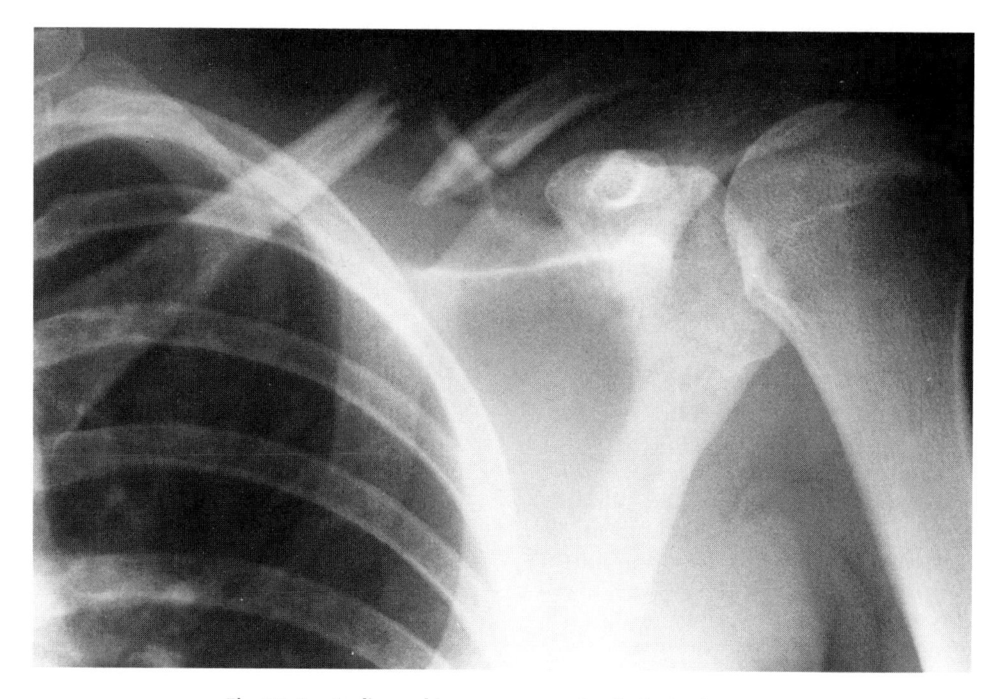

Fig. 23–3. Radiographic appearance of a clavicular fracture.

are the most common, and treatment depends on the severity of injury. Posterior dislocations may be associated with great vessel or airway impingement or disruption and should therefore be considered medical emergencies. The athlete should be transported with the arms against the chest, and vital signs should be monitored en route to an appropriate medical facility.[1] Computed tomography is the best study for imaging the sternal articulations.[3]

Pleural Space Injuries

Pleural space injuries—pneumothorax, hemothorax, chylothorax—are most often associated with pleuritic chest pain and dyspnea.[3] Traumatic pneumothorax may be secondary to a rib fracture[1,3,12] or may result from chest compression against a closed glottis.[3] Physical findings of simple pneumothorax include decreased breath sounds, hyperresonance to percussion, and possibly subcutaneous emphysema, all on the side of the pneumothorax.[1] The best study is the expiratory upright chest radiograph; however, if the patient cannot assume an upright position, a lateral decubitus chest radiograph with the suspected side superior is helpful.[3] Treatment varies, depending on the size of the pneumothorax and the degree of symptoms. A small, asymptomatic pneumothorax may be treated with observation and serial chest radiography, whereas a larger symptomatic pneumothorax requires a chest tube for re-expansion of the lung.[1] Air in the pleural space resorbs at the rate of about 1% per day.

Tension pneumothorax is a life-threatening condition of both respiratory and circulatory compromise. Physical findings in addition to those of simple pneumothorax include distended neck veins, tachycardia, respiratory distress, and possibly hypotension. Upright expiratory chest radiographs demonstrate a collapsed lung with tracheal and mediastinal shift away from the side of the pneumothorax. Immediate treatment is decompression of the tension pneumothorax with a 14-gauge needle inserted in the second or third intercostal space in the midclavicular line. A chest tube is inserted subsequently.[1]

Hemothorax results from laceration or tearing of intercostal or pulmonary vessels; chylothorax results from disruption of the thoracic duct from shear forces.[5] Both result in accumulation of fluid in the pleural space that may compromise respiration if a significant amount of fluid accumulates. In addition to respiratory compromise, circulatory compromise may occur if there is significant hemorrhage into the pleural space. This fluid is seen as a pleural effusion on upright chest radiographs. If the patient cannot sit upright, a lateral decubitus chest film with the suspected side in the dependent position is helpful for identifying the fluid.[3] Acute treatment for a patient who has respiratory compromise is insertion of a chest tube for drainage of the fluid. Intercostal artery laceration and thoracic duct disruption often require ligation or repair when the patient's condition is stable.

Parenchymal Injuries

Parenchymal injuries consist of pulmonary contusion, pulmonary hematoma, and pulmonary embolus. Pulmonary contusions are nonsegmental areas of interstitial and alveolar hemorrhage that produce edema without parenchymal laceration. They are frequently benign, but large contusions can cause ventilation-perfusion mismatch and respiratory failure. Symptoms include rales and cough that may produce blood-tinged sputum. Seventy percent of pulmonary contusions are visible on chest radiographs within 1 hour of injury and are seen as patchy, ill-defined consolidations.[3] Treatment is usually conservative: bronchodilators, nebulizer treatments, and nasotracheal suctioning.

Pulmonary hematomas are macroscopic accumulations of blood in the lung secondary to pulmonary lacerations. This condition frequently causes respiratory compromise and in severe cases may require intubation. The lesions are usually apparent on chest radiographs immediately after trauma and are seen as large consolidations of fluid in the lung parenchyma.[3]

Pulmonary embolus is an infrequent consequence of blunt trauma to the chest. The mechanism for embolus is trauma to the thorax that injures the central vasculature or the heart. This injury precipitates thrombus formation that subsequently may result in pulmonary or systemic embolization. Symptoms include tachypnea, tachycardia, and possibly cyanosis and respiratory failure. Chest pain other than that from the initial trauma is uncommon but may be present. An arterial blood gas test usually shows decreased Pa_{O_2} and oxygen saturation with a relatively normal Pa_{CO_2}. Definitive diagnosis is by ventilation-perfusion scan that demonstrates ventilation-perfusion mismatch.[3] If pulmonary embolus is suspected, intravenous heparin should be given immediately. Other treatments include oxygen therapy, and possibly intubation in cases of respiratory failure.

Mucosal Tears

Mucosal tears are usually associated with deceleration injuries and are found in the trachea, bronchi, and esophagus. Findings are precordial or substernal chest pain, possibly radiating to the shoulders, neck, or back.[3] Findings on chest radiographs include pneumomediastinum with tracheal and bronchial rupture and left-sided pleural effusion with esophageal rupture. Diagnosis of tracheal or bronchial rupture is usually made by bronchoscopy, whereas esophagography with water-soluble contrast medium is the test of choice for esophageal ruptures.

Aortic Rupture

Aortic rupture results from high-speed deceleration injuries. The most common site of rupture is just distal to the left subclavian artery.[1] The patient may describe severe and tearing substernal or back pain.

Some 80 to 90% of these patients do not survive the trip to the hospital. Findings on chest radiographs are a widened mediastinum (mediastinal–transverse chest diameter ratio greater than 0.2:1 at the level of aortic arch), abnormal contour of aortic knob or descending aorta, and depression of left mainstem bronchus greater than 40° below the horizontal plane.[1,3] Treatment is infusion of copious amounts of intravenous fluids, including blood, and immediate surgical repair of the rupture.

Heart Injuries

Injuries to the heart and its vessels are associated with as many as 76% of blunt chest injuries. They result from compression of the heart between the anterior chest wall and the vertebral column.[5,13] Cardiac contusion, the most common heart injury, occurs in as many as 60% of blunt chest trauma cases.[1] The major symptom is chest pain. Cardiac contusion may be the leading unsuspected visceral traumatic injury resulting in death.[3] A high index of suspicion is necessary to make the diagnosis, because the chest pain is often attributed to accompanying musculoskeletal trauma and the electrocardiographic changes and creatine phosphokinase elevation are often nonspecific.[3,14,15] The injury results in transmural myocardial necrosis. Thirty percent of patients with these injuries develop life-threatening complications such as dysrhythmias; congestive heart failure; pericardial effusion with tamponade; pulmonary thromboembolism; and myocardial, papillary muscle, or valve rupture.[3,5] Echocardiography and radionuclide angiography give the most diagnostic information. These studies may demonstrate regional or global depression of ventricular wall motion, decreased ventricular ejection fraction, cardiac chamber enlargement, and pericardial effusion.[3] Cardiac dysrhythmias are the most frequent complication;[5] therefore, patients should have continuous electrocardiographic monitoring.

Coronary artery dissection is a rare complication of blunt chest trauma.[13,16] It may be asymptomatic or result in angina or death.[13] Because the middle one third of the anterior descending coronary artery is located immediately behind the sternum, there is a risk of its being injured by direct trauma to the sternum.[17,18] It is believed that the atherosclerotic arterial wall is ruptured through compressive forces, and this rupture results in hemorrhage into the atheromatous plaque. Coronary artery obstruction then ensues secondary to platelet aggregation, vasospasm, and thrombosis and results in myocardial infarction.[13,16,18] Typical ischemic changes are demonstrated on the electrocardiogram. Treatment is usually conservative medical management if the patient is stable; however, angioplasty or bypass grafting may be indicated if there is ongoing ischemia.[13]

Intraventricular septal defects may occur immediately after or several days after a direct blow to the chest. Acute defects result from compression of the heart between the sternum and spine while the heart is in later diastole or early systole. They are detected by onset of a systolic ejection murmur directly after the traumatic event. Defects that occur later result from necrosis of the septum after cardiac contusion or myocardial infarction and are suggested by delayed appearance of the murmur. The muscular septum near the apex is the most common site of rupture. The triad of chest trauma, systolic murmur, and infarct pattern on electrocardiogram suggests the diagnosis. Complications and prognosis are related to conduction pathway involvement, size of the defect, and other cardiac and noncardiac injuries. Spontaneous healing with medical management and frequent follow up has been noted. Indications for surgery are persistent or progressive heart failure and pulmonary hypertension.[19]

ABDOMINAL INJURIES

Presentation

The pain associated with abdominal injuries may be present immediately, insidiously, or even hours after a blow to the abdomen. Any athlete who complains of persistent abdominal pain should undergo serial physical examinations.[6,20] Once again, a high index of suspicion for serious injury is necessary because an athlete with a serious injury can go into shock quickly.[21] If hemorrhage is slow, the athlete may collapse much later.

Patients with contusions present with pain and tenderness only over the area of impact. The pain is aggravated by tensing underlying muscles, and there is no referred pain. This injury may be difficult to distinguish from, or may coexist with, intra-abdominal injury.[6,20] Patients with intra-abdominal bleeding report intra-abdominal irritation. The pain is often mild, and there may be little tenderness to palpation.[6]

On the other hand, hollow viscus and gland injuries cause chemical and bacterial peritonitis.[20] The pain is severe and initially localized near the injury, but eventually it spreads to the entire abdomen because of diffuse peritonitis. Signs of intraperitoneal injury include abdominal rigidity, involuntary abdominal wall spasm, guarding, referred pain, and loss of bowel sounds. In addition, the pain is aggravated with body movement such as walking, jumping, laughing, and coughing.[6]

With serious abdominal injury and hemorrhage, the patient may be in shock when first seen by the physician. Signs of shock include cool clammy skin, pallor or cyanosis, increased heart rate, decreased blood pressure, thirst, and mental status changes. Immediate treatment consists of placing the patient in Trendelenburg's position, administering intravenous fluids, placing an antishock garment, and transporting to a trauma center. The patient should not be given fluids by mouth.

Evaluation of Injuries

Evaluation of injury starts with a complete history, which usually indicates a blow to the abdomen followed by complaints of abdominal pain. During the physical examination, the physician evaluates the patient for signs of peritonitis and shock, as previously discussed. If examination findings are equivocal or suggestive of peritonitis, diagnostic peritoneal lavage is indicated. This test is 98.5% sensitive for intraperitoneal lesions but less valuable for detecting retroperitoneal injuries. Abdominal computed tomography with intravenous contrast medium is the best imaging study for identifying retroperitoneal injury (kidney, duodenum, pancreas).[6]

Abdominal Wall Injuries

Abdominal wall injuries consist of muscle contusions and rectus sheath hematomas. Contusions to the abdominal muscles may cause long periods of discomfort, debilitation, and inability to compete. Treatment includes rest, ice, and appropriate analgesics.[1]

Rectus sheath hematomas result from rupture of the deep epigastric vessels after significant abdominal wall trauma. Rapid swelling of the abdominal wall may mislead the physician to suspect intra-abdominal injury,[1] but a cross-lateral radiograph of the abdomen may help identify the hematoma. Large hematomas may require evacuation; otherwise, treatment is application of ice, compression, and appropriate analgesics.

Spleen Injuries

The spleen, the most commonly injured abdominal organ,[6,7,22] is more susceptible to injury after a recent (within 6 weeks) viral infection such as mononucleosis, which can enlarge the spleen.[6] Typically, the athlete sustains a blow to the left upper quadrant, left lower ribs, or left back. Pain initially involves the left upper quadrant, and pain may be referred to the left shoulder.[6,22] The pain may progress to diffuse abdominal involvement. Physical examination usually elicits tenderness over the 10th, 11th, and 12th ribs. The patient's pulse is often rapid, and other signs of shock may follow.[6] Diagnosis is suggested by peritoneal lavage, but many centers use computed tomography because it demonstrates superior anatomic detail. If there are no signs of continued bleeding or shock, treatment is bed rest and observation in a facility capable of operating in case the patient takes a downhill turn.[6,22] Most splenic injuries from sports can be sutured if an operation is necessary. Splenectomy is a last resort because it leaves the patient more susceptible to bacterial infections.[6] Any patient suspected of having a spleen injury should receive Pneumovax in case splenectomy becomes necessary.

Liver Injuries

The liver is the second most commonly injured intra-abdominal organ. The mechanism of injury usually involves a blow to the upper midabdomen and right lower chest. The patient may have fractured ribs (10th, 11th, and 12th) on the right. The pain occurs in the right upper quadrant and later may be referred to the right shoulder or diffuse over the entire abdomen. Most blunt injuries to the liver are contusions that result in subscapular hematomas. Findings of the diagnostic peritoneal lavage frequently are negative. If there is no sign of continued hemorrhage or shock, treatment involves bed rest and observation in a facility capable of performing definitive surgery. Most injuries are treated nonoperatively unless the capsule ruptures or continued enlargement of the hematoma is seen on computed tomography.[6]

Pancreas Injuries

The pancreas is not frequently injured in sports. However, when it is, the injury may be life-threatening. Common mechanisms of injury include a blow from a football helmet, bicycle handlebar, motorcycle handlebar, steering wheel, or a karate kick.[6,10] The usual presentation is severe local abdominal or back pain that progresses to diffuse abdominal pain with development of peritoneal signs. Reflex ileus is often present. Diagnostic peritoneal lavage may demonstrate an increased amylase value. Abdominal computed tomography may show a divided pancreas or a mass effect in the area of the pancreas. There are increases in serum amylase and lipase 12 to 24 hours after injury.[23] Treatment is often surgery, especially if there is a severe contusion or division of the pancreas.[6,22]

Hollow Viscus Injuries

Injuries to the intraperitoneal duodenum, small intestine, and colon are uncommon in sports. Athletes with these injuries often have diffuse abdominal pain and tenderness with peritoneal signs. The diagnostic peritoneal lavage may be positive for amylase, food, bilirubin, or organisms (bacteria) found on Gram stain. Abdominal radiography and computed tomography scans may show free air. Treatment is primary repair of the injured structure, with the exception of colon injuries. They may require diverting colostomy.[6]

Retroperitoneal Injuries

Retroperitoneal hematomas are manifested by abdominal pain, with or without radiation. The patient may experience nausea and vomiting several hours to several days after the initial trauma. The upper abdomen is tender to palpation with occasional rebound tenderness. Diagnostic laboratory studies reveal slightly increased white blood cell count, decreased hematocrit if there is a large retroperitoneal bleed, and increased serum amylase and lipase values if the pancreas is injured.[7,24] Abdominal ultrasonography or computed tomography can help make the diagnosis. Management is conservative unless the hematoma is expanding or pulsatile, the gross bladder or kidney injury is seen on intravenous pyelography, the retroperitoneal duodenum is involved, or pancreatic injury is possible.[7]

The retroperitoneal duodenum is susceptible to blunt trauma because it is fixed against the spine. Duodenal obstruction may be secondary to retroperitoneal or intramural hematoma; it is more frequent in children. This injury has a history of blunt trauma to the upper midabdomen, followed by persistent vomiting 1 to 10 days after the injury. An upper gastrointestinal series confirms the diagnosis. The injury usually runs a benign course, and conservative treatment includes nasogastric suctioning and intravenous fluids.[7]

Renal injuries frequently involve a blow to the flank or the lower back. While significant pain may or may not be associated with renal injury, hematuria is almost always present.[22] Diagnosis may be made by ultrasonography, computed tomography, or intravenous pyelography. Arteriography is reserved for suspected vascular pedicle injuries. If there is no evidence of shock, expanding retroperitoneal hematoma, or extravasation of urine on intravenous pyelography, treatment is conservative: observation and appropriate analgesics. Hematuria is monitored for resolution.[22]

Bladder Rupture

Bladder rupture is rare with blunt abdominal trauma. It is frequently associated with pelvic fracture and is more common in vehicular sports. Diagnosis is made by cystography. Intraperitoneal lesions are treated by surgical repair. Small retroperitoneal lesions are treated with Foley catheter or suprapubic cystostomy.[22]

Summary

Serious chest and abdominal injuries from blunt trauma are infrequent in sports. When they do occur, however, they can be life threatening. The team physician needs to have a high index of suspicion for serious chest or abdominal injuries when any athlete is doubled over by a blow, has persistent chest or abdominal pain, or has pain of insidious or late onset. Serial examinations are recommended until pain resolves or a diagnosis is made. Initial management of injuries must revolve around the principles of basic and acute trauma life support. Early recognition of serious injury is mandatory to prevent life-threatening sequelae.

REFERENCES

1. Mellion, M. B., Walsh, W. M., and Shelton, G. L.: The Team Physician's Handbook. Philadelphia, Hanley & Belfus, 1990.
2. Dellon, A. L., Cowley, R. A., and Hoopes, J. E.: Blunt chest trauma: evaluation of the augmented breast. J. Trauma *20*:982, 1980.
3. Groskin, S.: The radiologic evaluation of chest pain in the athlete. Clin. Sports Med. *6*:845, 1987.
4. Sterchi, J. M.: Chest and abdominal trauma. North Carolina Med. J. *41*:518, 1980.
5. Petty, C. S.: Soft tissue injuries: an overview. J. Trauma. *10*:201, 1970.
6. Diamond, D. L.: Sports-related abdominal trauma. Clin. Sports Med. *8*:91, 1989.
7. Gue, S.: Obstruction of second part of duodenum by retroperitoneal haematoma due to blunt abdominal trauma: a report of two cases. Injury *4*:65, 1972.
8. Bergqvist, D., Hedelin, H., Lindblad, B., and Mätzsch, T.: Abdominal injuries in children: an analysis of 348 cases. Injury *16*:217, 1985.
9. McEntire, J. E., Hess, W. E., and Coleman, S. S.: Rupture of the pectoralis major muscle. J. Bone Joint Surg. *54A*:1040, 1972.
10. Schmidt, R. J.: Fatal anterior chest trauma in karate trainers. Med. Sci. Sports Exerc. *7*:59, 1975.
11. Lehman, R. C.: Thoracoabdominal musculoskeletal injuries in racquet sports. Clin. Sports Med. *7*:267, 1988.
12. Belham, G. J., and Adler, M.: Case report. Pneumothorax in a boxer. Brit. J. Sports Med. *19*:45, 1985.
13. Marik, P. E.: Coronary artery dissection after a rugby injury: a case report. South African Med. J. *77*:586, 1990.
14. Kettunen, P., Kala, R., and Rehunen, S.: CK and CK-MB in skeletal muscle of athletes and in serum after thoracic contusion in sport. J. Sports Med. Physical Fitness *24*:21, 1984.
15. Rose, K. D., Stone, F., Fuenning, S. J., and Williams, J.: Cardiac contusion resulting from "spearing" in football. Arch. Intern. Med. *118*:129, 1966.
16. O'Neill, S., Walker, F., and O'Dwyer, W. F.: Blunt chest trauma causing myocardial infarction: An unusual football injury. Irish Med. J. *74*:138, 1981.
17. Espinosa, R., Badui, E., Castaño, R., and Madrid, R.: Acute posteroinferior wall myocardial infarction secondary to football chest trauma. Chest *88*:928, 1985.
18. Gallego, F. G., Marti, J. S., and Blasco, P. P.: Myocardial infarction and subtotal obstruction of the anterior descending coronary artery caused by trauma in a football player. Int. J. Cardiol. *12*:109, 1986.
19. Rosenthal, A., Parisi, L. F., and Nadas, A. S.: Isolated interventricular septal defect due to nonpenetrating trauma. N. Engl. J. Med. *253*:338, 1970.
20. Nolen, W. A.: Athletic injuries: the immediate management of abdominal injuries in athletics. Minn. Med. *48*:1505, 1965.
21. Scharplatz, D., Thurleman, K., and Enderlin, F.: Thoracoabdominal trauma in ski accidents. Injury *10*:86, 1978.
22. Kenney, P.: Abdominal pain in athletes. Clin. Sports Med. *6*:885, 1986.
23. Strauch, G. O.: Clinical findings in abdominal trauma. Radiol. Clin. North Am. *11*:555, 1973.
24. Foley, L. C., and Teele, R. L.: Ultrasound of epigastric injuries after blunt trauma. A.J.R. *132*:593, 1979.

24 R. Todd Dombroski

Genitourinary Problems of Athletes

RENAL INJURIES

The kidneys would appear to be well protected from direct injury. They lie in the retroperitoneum, surrounded by fat. Lateral protection for the upper section of the kidney comes from the rib cage. Anterior protection is provided by the abdominal viscera and the abdominal muscles, posterior protection by the psoas, latissimus, and paraspinal muscles. Despite this protection, the kidney is the most commonly injured urinary tract organ.

Renal injury from blunt trauma can occur in many sports. Physicians covering football, lacrosse, basketball, boxing, wrestling, and hockey should maintain a high index of suspicion for renal injury. Younger athletes are more prone to renal injury because of the relatively large size of their kidneys and the decreased ossification and strength of the rib cage. Approximately 30% of pediatric renal injuries are incurred in sports activity.[1]

Physical findings suggestive of renal damage include tenderness of the flank or upper abdominal region.[2] The pain can be severe, but it generally passes after an hour or two. An example of this is the kidney punch in boxing. The amount of pain depends on the extent of the injury and the condition of the renal capsule. If the capsule is torn, a retroperitoneal hematoma forms. If the capsule is intact, hematuria and localized tenderness may be the only signs. The athlete may experience colic-type pain as the kidney passes clots down the ureter. Flank contusion or ecchymosis may indicate a retroperitoneal collection of blood. A retroperitoneal mass that enlarges is obviously an ominous sign. If urine is extravasated into the perirenal space, this may lead to cellulitis, whose symptoms are malaise, irregular fever, local tenderness, and muscular resistance. Rarely, a renal abscess may result. Secondary adynamic ileus is common after renal injury.

Radiographic findings that are suspicious for renal injury include rib fracture, lumbar transverse fracture, loss of psoas shadow, or a "ground glass" appearance over the site of renal injury.

In laboratory analysis, hematuria is considered the definitive sign of renal trauma, but the degree of hematuria may not indicate the extent of renal injury. To detect microscopic hematuria, a dipstick evaluation is not inferior to a microscopic evaluation, given its 97.5% sensitivity and specificity.[3] Uremia and electrolyte imbalances are later findings of more severe damage.

Renal injury may be graded as renal contusion (Grade I), cortical lacerations (Grade II), deep cortical and calyceal lacerations (Grade III), or vascular pedicle injury (Grade IV) (Fig. 24–1).[4] The diagnosis is often made after intravenous pyelography. Any patient with a history of blunt trauma to the kidneys associated with gross hematuria should undergo intravenous pyelography. If a renal contusion is present, intravenous pyelography may show pelvic-calyceal displacement, a cortical mass effect, or an area of diminished visualization. In the case of renal lacerations, intravenous pyelography will show various degrees of intrarenal dye extravasation. The rare vascular pedicle injury does not allow the dye to "visualize" the kidney. Other conditions in which the kidney cannot be visualized by intravenous pyelography include arterial thrombosis, vascular spasm, and absence of the kidney.

In the majority of cases management of renal injury is conservative. For contusions and minor lacerations, the treatment is strict bed rest, hydration, and analgesics for a few days. It is very important that the athlete refrain from strenuous activities for 2 to 3 weeks. Often, rebleeding from the injury occurs 2 to 3 weeks after the injury as clots resolve. Resuming strenuous activity early increases the risk of rebleeding—and loss of even more training time. Proper rest usually leads to complete recovery. There is some controversy over the conservative management of major lacerations because these can be associated with delayed bleeding (15%) and postinjury hypertension (up to 33%).[5] Surgical intervention

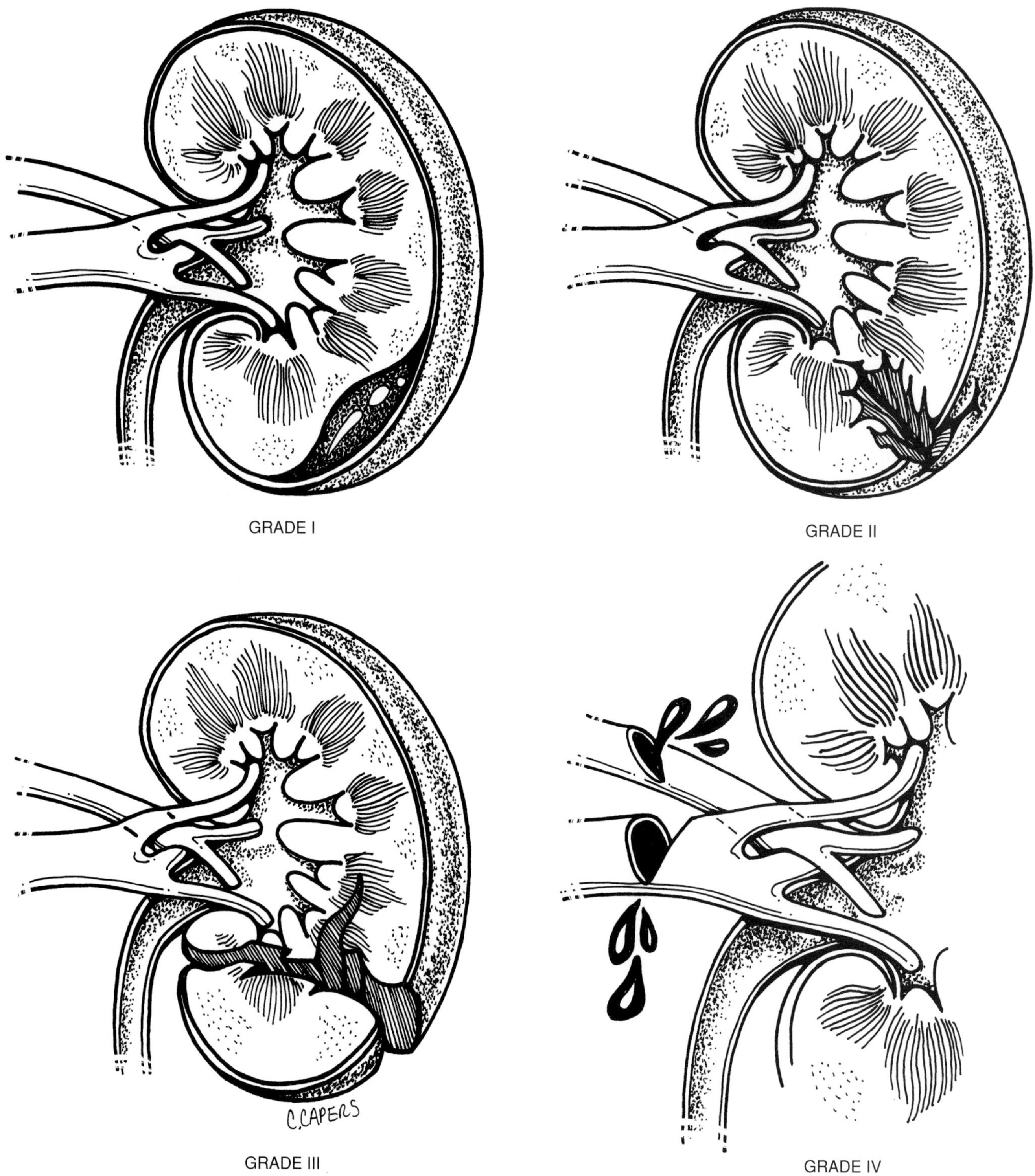

Fig. 24–1. Renal injury may be graded as renal contusion (Grade I), cortical lacerations (Grade II), deep cortical and calyceal lacerations (Grade III), or vascular pedicle injury (Grade IV).

for pedicle injuries and shattered kidneys is well accepted. Careful followup of serial blood pressure measurements and intravenous pyelography at 3 to 6 months after a Grade II or greater renal injury should detect late complications of renal vascular hypertension and hydronephrosis. Intravenous pyelography carries some risk of morbidity, so the risk-benefit ratio should be considered for athletes with microscopic hematuria after renal trauma and for asymptomatic followup.

When the injury is not proportional to the force of the trauma, an underlying renal abnormality should be suspected. Such abnormalities may include horseshoe kidney, megaureter, renal malignancy, and ureteropelvic junction obstruction. Ureteropelvic junction obstruction is usually caused by intrinsic narrowing at the junction of the renal pelvis and the ureter, which impairs drainage of urine from the kidney. A young athlete with a history of intermittent flank pain that is sometimes associated with drinking too much liquid should be restricted from strenuous physical activity until intravenous pyelography can be performed to rule out ureteropelvic junction obstruction.

EXTRARENAL TRAUMA

The ureter is the portion of the urinary tract injured least often. Injuries to the ureter are usually associated with severe abdominal trauma.

Injury to the bladder is also uncommon. It is associated with a pelvic fracture or a direct blow to a full bladder. Bladder injury is manifested as pain, tenderness, muscle guarding, inability to void, pubic ecchymosis, and gross hematuria. To rule out a bladder rupture from a contusion, cystography is the imaging study of choice. Obviously a ruptured bladder requires surgical intervention. A bladder contusion can be treated conservatively with followup urinalysis for hematuria.

Microtrauma of the bladder is well-documented. *Runner's bladder* is gross hematuria after strenuous activity, particularly long-distance running.[6] Routine urinalysis show hematuria in 20% of marathon runners. Cystoscopy reveals a rim of contused bladder tissue. It is postulated that in men, the posterior bladder wall "kisses" the base of the prostate to induce the lesions. Such lesions are self-limited and resolve in about a week. Athletes who are prone to this abnormality are cautioned not to run with a totally empty bladder because this can exacerbate runner's bladder.

Injury to the male urethra can be anterior or posterior lesions. A history of straddle injury, perineal pain, and a bloody meatus indicate anterior urethral trauma, which usually requires surgical repair and realignment. Posterior urethral injury is associated with more severe trauma (usually a pelvic fracture), inability to void, and a "floating" prostate. This can be imaged on a retrograde urethrogram. Immediate surgical intervention is required.

Fortunately, urethral injuries in women are rare and are limited mainly to lacerations; however, female water skiers who fall may experience "forced-water douche," which can injure the urethra and cause delayed salpingitis.

Penile injuries are uncommon and consist mainly of lacerations and contusions from direct forceful contact. Direct blows from other athletes or equipment may cause a contusion that is limited to Buck's fascia and produces a classic butterfly-type pattern of ecchymosis. In many cases, a retrograde urethrogram is required to rule out a urethral tear.

The erect penis is more susceptible to acute trauma. The tunica albuginea, which covers the engorged corpus cavernosum, can fracture (Fig. 24–2). The area of fracture is acutely swollen and ecchymotic, and the penis is usually bent toward the injured side. This is a true urologic emergency that necessitates evacuation of the clot and repair of the tunica tear. It is very difficult to elicit a history of sexual activity just before the injury; the athlete may wish to relate this to a "sporting injury."

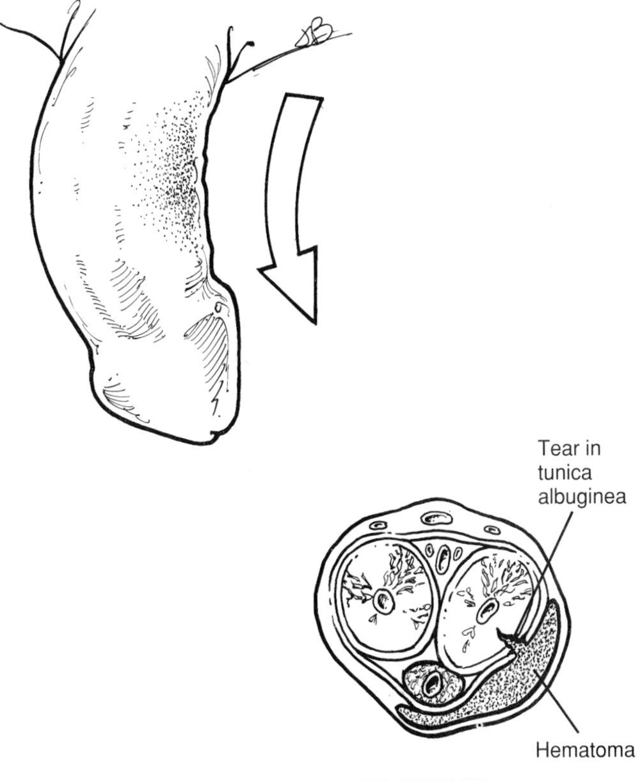

Fig. 24–2. Fracture of the tunica albuginea. On presentation, the penis typically bends toward the side of the injury.

Pressure, irritation, or trauma to the pudendal nerve can result in numbness, tingling, and erectile dysfunction. This has been documented in long-distance cyclists whose racing seats irritate the pudendal nerve. These symptoms resolve spontaneously and can be treated by changing the angle or width of the seat.

The clinical assessment of an athlete with scrotal trauma is often limited because of marked tenderness and swelling. The degree of pain is not a reliable indicator of what structures are involved or how severe the injury is. A contusion of the scrotum from direct blunt trauma causes localized pain, ecchymosis, and scrotal swelling without significant swelling of the testicle. This is treated simply with scrotal support, ice pack, and analgesics. If there appears to be an expanding mass in the scrotum that cannot be transilluminated, if the epididymis cannot be palpated as a distinct structure posterior to the testicle, or if the pain seems out of proportion to the injury, a fracture of the testicle or epididymis must be considered. Ultrasonography of the scrotal contents is the imaging technique of choice. It may show disruption of the tunica albuginea or epididymis. Unfortunately, sonography can produce a false-negative result with these lesions, and a radionuclide testicular scan is not relevant in the acute setting.[7] Therefore, if either clinical examination or ultrasonography prompts surgical exploration, it must not be delayed. If surgery is performed within 72 hours, 90% of all ruptured testes can be saved—as opposed to 55% if surgery is delayed.[7]

A severe blow to the scrotum may result in a dislocation of the testicle to the inguinal, perineal, or crural region. The athlete presents with a swollen hemiscrotum and an absent testicle, findings that warrant prompt referral to a urologist. Sometimes, trauma to the scrotum causes forceful cremasteric contraction that draws the testicle into the inguinal canal. The difference is that the testicle can still be palpated in the inguinal canal. This requires close followup, but it usually resolves spontaneously.

Trauma to the scrotum may also induce a hydrocele or a hematocele (Fig. 24–3). The hydrocele is caused by decreased absorption of the normal tunica vaginalis secretions secondary to trauma, infection, or a tumor. This lesion can be transilluminated through the scrotum. The treatment is scrotal support and analgesics, and a followup ultrasound examination to rule out occult malignancy. A collection of blood between the layers of the tunica vaginalis is a hematocele. Since blood does not transilluminate, ultrasonography is necessary. The usual treatment is surgical exploration, because differentiating an uncomplicated hematocele from a ruptured testicle is very difficult.

Untreated testicular injuries may result in a variety of complications, such as atrophy, necrosis, chronic pain, infection, and sterility. Imaging studies should never delay surgical exploration. A high index of suspicion is vital in minimizing complications.

ATRAUMATIC TESTICULAR PAIN

Testicular pain may be atraumatic. The two causes with the highest associated morbidity are testicular torsion and epididymitis. The classic presentation of testicular torsion is acute testicular pain in an adolescent, sometimes associated with nausea and vomiting. The examination reveals a high-riding testicle, indistinct or abnormally positioned epididymis, and induration of the overlying scrotal skin. Elevation of the testicle does not relieve pain, and the cremasteric reflex is absent. This condition is a true emergency. In almost all cases, prompt urologic evaluation and surgical correction within the first 4 to 6 hours preserve the viability of the testicle. Radionuclide scanning is helpful in distinguishing torsion from epididymitis.[7] Strong clinical suspicion should hold sway over a "negative" scan, and surgical correction should never be delayed to obtain a scan.

Epididymitis also causes pain and induration. The epididymis may be indistinguishable from the testicle; thus it can be difficult, clinically, to rule out testicular torsion. The patient with epididymitis commonly presents with a fever and an elevated leukocyte count. Urinalysis is usually positive for leukocyte esterase, and numerous white blood cells or frank pyuria may be seen. The treatment for acute epididymitis is bed rest, with sitz baths of the scrotum and antibiotics. In men younger than 35 years, the pathogen etiologic is usually *Chlamydia trachomatis* and in older men, *Escherichia coli*. Culture material should also be taken for *Gonococcus* organisms. The treatment for a chlamydia infection is doxycycline, 100 mg twice a day, or tetracycline, 500 mg four times a day.[8]

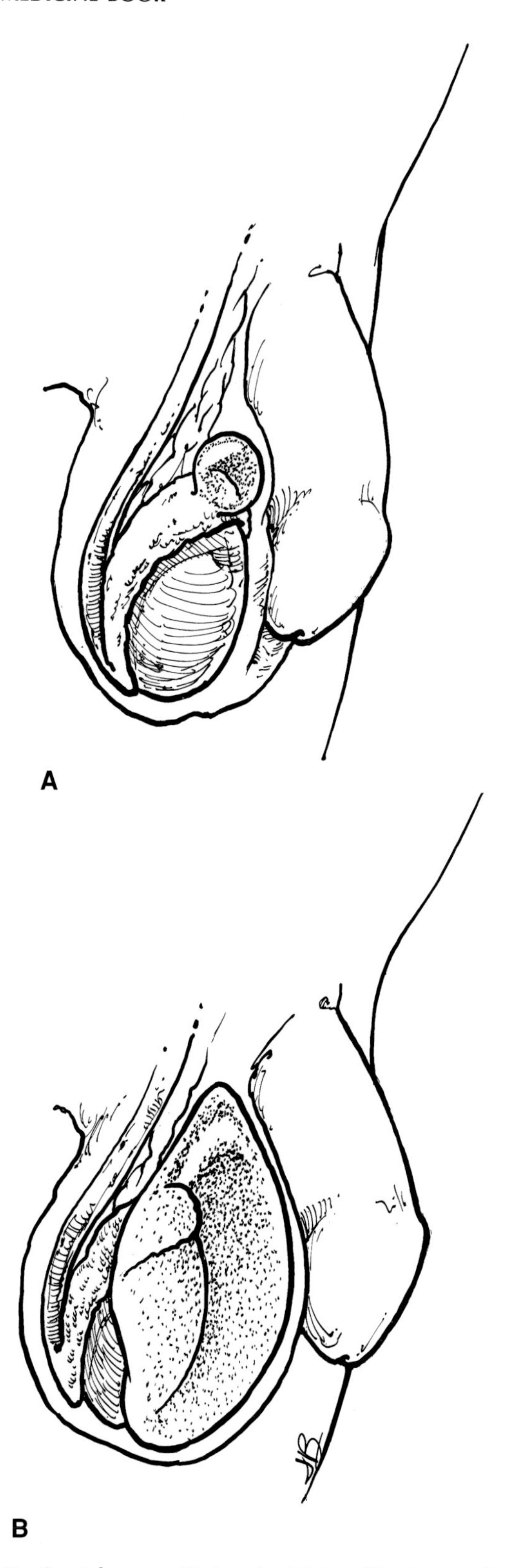

Fig. 24–3. Scrotal masses. Hydroceles (*A*) transilluminate and hematoceles (*B*) do not.

Sexually transmitted diseases may be the most common urologic problem of athletes. The most common sexually transmitted disease is nongonococcal urethritis, usually caused by chlamydia. The treatment is the same as that for epididymitis. Other sexually transmitted diseases include gonorrhea, syphilis, herpes progenitalis, and condylomata acuminata (genital warts).

ATRAUMATIC SCROTAL MASSES

Prompt evaluation of all scrotal masses is essential: the most common malignancy in males 15 to 35 years old is testicular cancer.[9] The major predisposing factor for development of testicular cancer is cryptorchidism. Discovery of an undescended testicle should prompt a urologic referral. Therefore, examination of the scrotal contents during the preseason physical can be life saving. A painless mass that appears to disrupt the integrity of the testicle and is separate from the epididymis and cord is very suggestive of testicular cancer. Ultrasonography of the scrotal contents should accompany early referral to a urologist. A mass that transilluminates is usually a benign lesion; however, even a benign lesion like a hydrocele (which classically transilluminates) can be secondary to an occult testicular cancer. This would also require ultrasonography, and possibly surgical exploration. Given the proximity of the scrotal structures, the rare atypical presentation, and the patient's anxiety, early ultrasonography of the scrotal contents should be emphasized.

A hydrocele (Fig. 24–3) is a cystic mass enveloping the testicle and epididymis that is caused by decreased absorption of the normal secretions of the tunica vaginalis. As stated earlier, when there is no history of trauma or infection, malignancy must be ruled out. The treatment for hydroceles is conservative, and they rarely become large or painful enough to warrant aspiration or surgical correction. A cystic mass in the epididymis is usually a spermatocele, which can be transilluminated. A solid mass within the epididymis is usually a sperm granuloma. Both lesions are benign and require no treatment. Varicoceles, varicosities of the internal spermatic veins, are often described as resembling a "bag of worms" adjacent to the testicle and cord. Varicoceles do not require treatment unless there is a problem with fertility, pain, or decreased testicular size on the ipsilateral side.

HEMATURIA

Much controversy still surrounds the management of hematuria in athletes. First, there is no consensus on the upper limit of normal for red blood cells in the urine. The most commonly accepted upper limit is 3 red blood cells per high-power field, or 1000 per milliliter of urine.[10] Microscopic hematuria is common in the athlete population. It has been reported in virtually all sports and is more prevalent in the running events (marathon running has been reported to cause microhematuria in as many as 50% of runners).[11] The distinguishing feature of exercise-induced microhematuria is that it normally clears in 48 hours. Exercise-induced proteinuria is another common finding on routine screening, which also clears in 48 hours. If the proteinuria does not clear, a 24-hour urine collection for creatinine, calcium, and total protein should be ordered, along with urine microscopy for nephritic sediment and studies of serum blood urea nitrogen and creatinine. Abnormal findings usually warrant referral.

Gardner called this transient and benign hematuria and proteinuria "athletic pseudonephritis."[12] These findings have been attributed to continuous minor renal trauma, increased renal venous pressure, transient renal ischemia, and dehydration. If the urinalysis results return to normal after 48 hours' rest, no further evaluation is required. Proper hydration is the key to preventing these worrisome (yet benign) causes of exercise-induced microhematuria.

Not all dipstick-positive results represent hematuria. The dipstick analysis uses peroxidase, which reacts to any heme group—from intact red blood cells to free hemoglobin or free myoglobin. Overexertion can release free myoglobin into the urine and elevate the serum creatine phosphokinase value. Foot strike hemolysis from strenuous running can cause free hemoglobin secondary to red blood cell trauma. Microscopic urinalysis should reveal disruption of the red blood cells secondary to hemolysis. Red urine is not always hematuria: drugs like phenazopyridine hydrochloride (Pyridium), rifampin, nitrofurantoin, quinine, and phenytoin can discolor the urine, as can some food dyes, beet juice, and vegetable juices.

For gross hematuria, the history of the urine stream can be important.[13] Gross hematuria at the onset of urination suggests a urethral source. Hematuria in the last few drops suggests a prostate or bladder neck source. Hematuria seen throughout urination suggests the bladder, ureters, or kidneys. Passing blood clots indicates nonglomerular bleeding. Large, thick clots are more often associated with bladder injury, whereas small specks or stringy clots indicate that the upper tract is the source of the problem. Cystoscopy in the presence of active bleeding is the best initial study.[13]

Several possible diagnoses are associated with hematuria (Table 24–1). If the cause of the hematuria has not been determined by the history, physical, and associated laboratory testing, the next step is to evaluate the anatomy. Classically, intravenous pyelography would be ordered; however, this study carries a risk of osmotic injury to the kidney. It has been proposed that renal ultrasonography be used because of its lower risk and minimal decrease in diagnostic value.[9] Further evaluation, including the need for cystoscopy, should be referred to a urologist. Followup of these athletes is paramount.

ATHLETES WITH A SINGLE KIDNEY OR TESTICLE

For athletes whose solitary kidney is pelvic, iliac, multicystic, or has an unrepaired anatomic abnormality (such

Table 24–1. History of Hematuria

With	*Consider*
Colicky flank pain	Nephrolithiasis: order an IVP
Male with terminal hematuria and dysuria	Prostatitis: order cultures
Female with dysuria, frequency, urgency	Cystitis: order cultures
Easy bruisability	Blood dyscrasia: order PT/PTT, C3 and C4, and a bleeding time
Recent sore throat, impetigo, cellulitis	PSGN: order an ASO titer
Black or Mediterranean ancestry	Sickle cell anemia: order sickle cell prep or urine electrophoresis
Family history of renal anomalies, e.g. PCKD	Order a renal ultrasound or IVP early
Hypertension and/or edema	Nephritis or vasculitis: order ESR, CBC, ANA, BUN/creatinine, urine sediment for RBC/WBC casts
Any medication, especially anticoagulants	Hematuria secondary to medication*
Over 40 years of age or no other etiology	Carcinoma and referral

(Key: CBC = complete blood count; PT = prothrombin time; PTT = partial thromboplastin time; ASO = antistreptolysin O test; ANA = antinuclear antibody test; ESR = erythrocyte sedimentation rate; IVP = intravenous pyelogram; C3 and C4 are tests for complement; PSGN = post-streptococcal glomerular nephritis; PCKD = polycystic kidney disease)

*may still have an underlying uropathy

as ureteropelvic junction pathology or hydronephrosis), the risk is too great to allow participation in contact sports.[14] Athletes with a normal solitary kidney run a much lower risk of losing the remaining kidney from injury through contact sports. They should, however, be advised against playing contact sports.[15] Athletes who have a solitary testicle should also be advised not to play contact sports. Fortunately, protection for a solitary testicle is available in the form of a scrotal cup, which lessens the chance of significant injury. Just how much a scrotal cup or kidney pad protects an athlete is not well-documented. The rights and responsibilities of coaches, parents, and athletes are still controversial. The physician's concern for an athlete's safety may conflict with the athlete's right to pursue contact sports.

REFERENCES

1. Mandour, W. A., Lai, M. K., Linke, C. A., et al.: Blunt renal trauma in the pediatric patient. J. Pediatr. Surg. *16*:669, 1989.
2. Silen, W.: Cope's Early Diagnosis of the Acute Abdomen. 17th Ed. New York, Oxford University Press, 1987.
3. Mee, S. L., and McAninch, J. W.: Indications for radiographic assessment in suspected renal trauma. Urol. Clin. North Am. *16*:187, 1989.
4. Reid, D. C.: Sports Injury Assessment and Rehabilitation. New York, Churchill Livingstone, 1992.
5. Peterson, N. E.: Complications of renal trauma. Urol. Clin. North Am. *16*:221, 1989.
6. Blacklock, N. J.: Bladder trauma in the long-distance runner. Br. J. Urol. *49*:129, 1977.
7. Noujaim, S. E., and Nagle, C. E.: Acute scrotal injuries in athletes: Evaluation by diagnostic imaging. Physician Sports Med. *17*(10):125, 1989.
8. Berger, R. E.: Chlamydia trachomatis as a cause of acute idiopathic epididymitis. N. Engl. J. Med. *298*:301, 1978.
9. Einhorn, L. H., Crawford, E. D., Shipley, W. U., et al.: Cancer of the testes. *In* Cancer: Principles and Practice of Oncology. 3rd Ed. Edited by V. T. DeVita, Jr., S. Hellman, and S. A. Rosenberg. Philadelphia, J. B. Lippincott, 1989.
10. Sutton, J. M.: Evaluation of hematuria in adults. J.A.M.A, *263*:2475, 1990.
11. Boileau, M., et al.: Stress hematuria: Athletic pseudonephritis in marathoners. Urology *15*:471, 1980.
12. Gardner, K. D., Jr.: Athletic pseudonephritis: Alteration of urine sediment by athletic competition. J.A.M.A. *161*:1613, 1956.
13. Finney, J., and Baum, N.: Evaluation of hematuria. Postgrad. Med. *85*:44, 1989.
14. Dorsen, P. J.: Should athletes with one eye, kidney, or testicle play contact sports? Physician Sports Med. *14*(7):130, 1986.
15. Mandell J., et al.: Sports-related genitourinary injuries in children. Clin. Sports Med. *1*:483, 1982.

25 *Arnold R. Penix*

Stress Fractures

Stress fractures have become an increasingly frequent problem in recreational and competitive athletes, owing largely to the increasing popularity of sports and to individual dedication to maintaining higher levels of personal fitness, for health and social reasons. Unfortunately, our modern conveniences make life very easy, and most people come to sport activities from a very sedentary existence. Our minimally stressed bodies have a high percentage of body fat and low muscle mass, strength, endurance, and bone mass.

We enter a training program in poor physical condition and our muscles respond relatively rapidly to the demands of conditioning. Our bones respond to the increased mechanical demands and begin to remodel their structure, and ultimately increase bone mass to meet the new physical activity levels. But the remodeling process for bone proceeds at a slower pace than conditioning of muscles, and remodeling requires both osteoclastic and osteoblastic activity. The aggregate of events is such that, in some people, the increased mechanical stress on bone outstrips the rate at which bone accommodates biologically. This leads to increased strain in the bone and an accumulation of microfractures. If the process continues, a fracture line may be propagated, and angulation and displacement can occasionally occur. Some authors feel that muscle fatigue contributes to this process.

Stress fractures were first reported in Prussian military recruits in 1855. The fractures were first described as occurring in the metatarsals, and they came to be known as "march fractures." These fractures have remained a problem for the military: until the recent surge of interest in recreational and competitive sports, our greatest experience with the problem was in military recruits. Military studies indicated that the fractures most commonly develop 2 to 3 weeks into basic training, but they can occur much later. These observations led to modification in training schedules for recruits, which have reduced but not eliminated some fractures. Stress fractures still occur frequently, but the specific location of the fractures has changed; today, calcaneal, tibial, and femoral stress fractures are major problems in military recruits.

Over the past 15 years, stress fractures have been diagnosed increasingly in athletes, and currently they may constitute as many as 10% of sports-related injuries. These fractures occur in a wide range of persons, at all ages and all competition levels. Fractures most often occur in weight-bearing bones, but they are not limited to them. Specific fractures may be associated with, but are not exclusive to, particular sports activities. There is an association between gymnastics and pars interarticularis stress fractures. Runners tend to have metatarsal, tibial, and fibular stress fractures. Basketball players may suffer from fracture of the tarsal navicular, and throwing or racquet sports may result in humerus or rib stress fractures. By far, the sport with the highest incidence of stress fractures is running.

PREDISPOSING FACTORS

Individuals with any pre-existing medical condition that reduces bone mass, bone mineralization, or bone quality are at increased risk for stress fracture. Such conditions include nutritional disorders such as rickets, osteomalacia and scurvy; idiopathic osteoporosis; systemic disorders such as rheumatoid arthritis, diabetes mellitus, hyperparathyroidism, and renal osteodystrophy; and congenital defects such as osteopetrosis and osteogenesis imperfecta. When fractures do occur through pre-existing abnormal bone they are most appropriately referred to as insufficiency fractures.

One special concern about stress fractures is their occurrence in female athletes. Until recently, women were relatively excluded from military service and athletic competition. This injustice has been rectified much in recent years, and women are now participating widely in sports and fitness activities and the military. Women have developed stress fractures similar to those of male athletes; however, women appear to be at greater risk for stress fractures. This increased risk of fracture is most commonly associated with amenorrhea and oligomenorrhea seen in highly trained individuals. The precise mechanism of these fractures remains unknown, but they seem to be associated with alteration of endocrine function that is reflected in the menstrual abnormalities, changes in estrogen levels, and decreased bone mineral content. Another reported contributing factor is an association between eating disorders, stress fractures, and amenorrhea. When a female athlete has a stress fracture, endocrine and nutritional factors must be considered. Appropriate nutrition must be ensured, training schedules may need to be reduced to re-establish menstruation, and estrogen replacement may be considered for some.

A pre-existing angular deformity may produce abnormal stress distribution in a bone and predispose a person to stress fracture. Examples of this are varus alignment of the tibia, which has been reported to be associated with stress fracture of the medial malleolus.

PEDIATRIC STRESS FRACTURES

Pediatric stress fractures have been reported to occur at all ages from toddlers to nearly mature adolescents. The incidence is highest among 10- to 15-year-olds, and the site is usually the proximal tibial metaphysis, though stress fractures have been reported in the iliac crest apophysis, patella, and fibula.

Diagnosis of stress fractures is more difficult in children because of the vague history of injury and the advanced radiographic changes associated with reactive bone formation that are usually evident in pediatric stress fractures but absent in adults. Bone scan findings are positive but are of little use in diagnosis because the objective is to distinguish between infection, neoplasia, osteoid osteoma, and fracture. Tomography may be useful as may re-evaluation over a 4- to 6-week period. Biopsy should be performed only after very careful evaluation.

EXAMINATION

Patients with stress fractures complain of pain at the fracture site. The pain is aggravated by sports or activity and usually is relieved by rest. The patient may recently have begun a new training program or changed an older program, leading to development of a stress fracture. Physical examination is usually unrevealing, in that swelling and tenderness are uncommon.

After examination, plain radiography is always indicated. In the early stages of stress fracture, radiographs are normal, and only half of all stress fractures eventually demonstrate radiographic changes. Characteristic changes include cortical lucency or trabecular bone

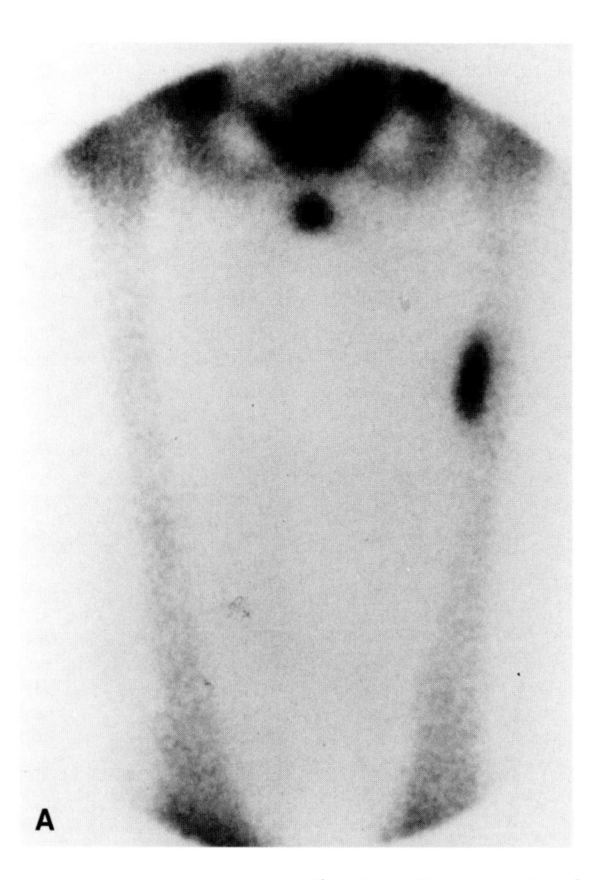

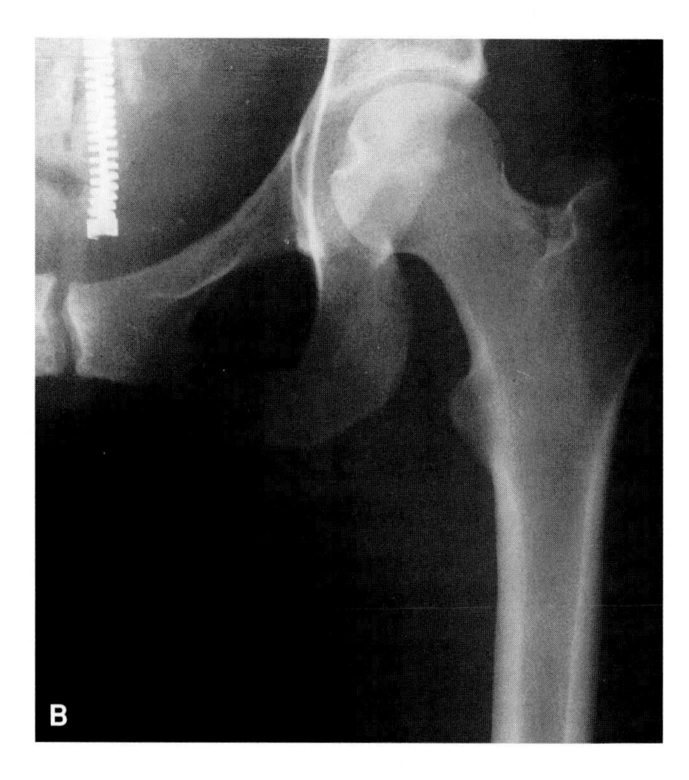

Fig. 25–1. Bone scan (*A*) and radiograph (*B*) of a stress fracture in the midfemur.

compaction with later development of endosteal and periosteal callus. The radiographic changes are usually limited to a single cortex.

If plain radiographs are not sufficient to make the diagnosis, the second step is a bone scan. Bone scans are much more sensitive to active remodeling at the site of the developing fracture and findings are positive much sooner than on radiographs (Fig. 25–1). The scan shows diffuse uptake early on, and a more sharply localized area of uptake in later stages. When a triple-phase bone scan is performed, all three phases of the scan are positive if a stress fracture is present. This is particularly helpful in distinguishing tibial stress fracture from shin splints, which are associated with normal angiogram and blood pool phases of the scan.

An additional study that may be useful is magnetic resonance imaging (MRI), which is extremely sensitive in detecting bone marrow changes. Its use in diagnosing stress fractures has been reported, but its precise role in the diagnosis has not been defined. Early reports indicate that MRI shows anatomic detail better than scans, and it may be even more sensitive. The major objection to MRI is cost and our limited experience with it for imaging fractures.

TREATMENT

The central theme in treating stress fractures is to decrease the offending activity. Most athletes with stress fractures do not have to stop training completely, and alternate conditioning can be continued to avoid deconditioning. Certain fractures may require cast immobilization if displacement is possible or to maintain mobility and control discomfort. Open reduction and internal fixation may be required for certain fractures that are prone to displacement, delayed union, or nonunion.

26

Major Kenneth B. Batts

Dermatologic Problems

Athletic fitness and competitive sports predispose athletes to diverse dermatologic conditions that may limit performance and restrict participation. Many factors, such as heredity, age, sex, skin type, environment, and sporting activity, play a role in common dermatologic conditions of athletes.[1] For a swimmer or wrestler a dermatologic infection or infestation may be as disabling as a meniscal tear of the knee to a football or basketball player.

The skin, our largest organ system, serves as a protective shield, the first line of defense from the external environment. Much like a two-way mirror, the skin also provides the physician with clues to organic disease in the body while regulating body temperature, metabolism, and sensory input. Physicians who care for athletes must recognize the early clinical appearance of skin conditions if they are to provide appropriate treatment, thus limiting disability and recovery time, and ultimately improving performance.

INFECTIONS

Bacterial

Impetigo (Fig. 26–1) is a highly contagious disorder spread by skin-to-skin contact or by fomites from mats, equipment, or towels. Group A β-*hemolytic Streptococcus* organisms produce the characteristic crusted, yellowish, weeping lesions around the mouth and nose, whereas *Staphylococcus aureus* organisms produce blisters (bullous impetigo).[2] Treatment consists of local débridement of the lesions, a 10-day course of topical mupirocin ointment, t.i.d., or oral antibiotics—erythromycin, penicillinase-resistant penicillins, or cephalosporins. Impetigo is common in wrestlers, swimmers, and gymnasts, and participation should be avoided until all lesions have resolved.

Folliculitis (Fig. 26–2), an *S. aureus* infection of the hair follicles, presents as mildly inflamed red papules or, in more severe cases, pustules. Sycosis barbae (pseudofolliculitis) is common in bearded black male athletes: the coarse hairs curl back into the skin. Treatment consists of topical depilatories, acne preparations, and either topical or oral erythromycin or penicillin derivatives. Another type of folliculitis, "hot tub folliculitis," is produced by *Pseudomonas aeruginosa.* The rash is commonly distributed over the skin in areas that contact the occlusive bathing suit. Causative factors include improperly chlorinated water, chemical irritants, and prolonged exposure to high temperatures. Treatment consists of either an anti-*Pseudomonas* penicillin, third-generation anti-*Pseudomonas* cephalosporin, or oral ciprofloxacin. The athlete should not engage in close contact sports until the rash has completely resolved.

Furunculosis (commonly called a *boil*) is a localized staphylococcal abscess of the epidermis found in areas

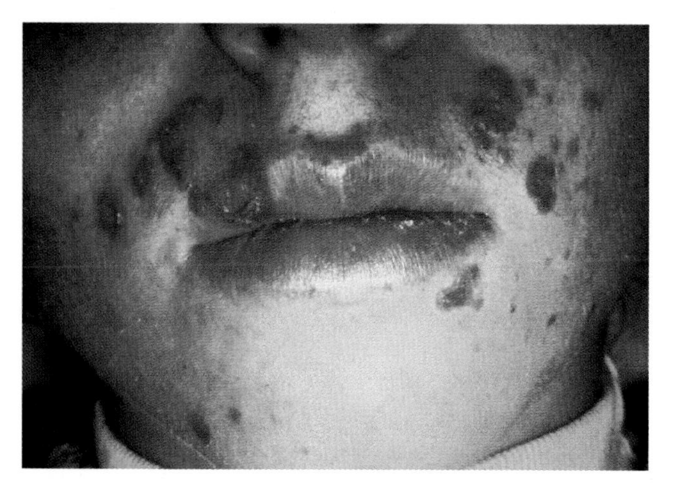

Fig. 26–1. The lesions of vesicular impetigo. (Courtesy of Wade Lillegard, M.D.)

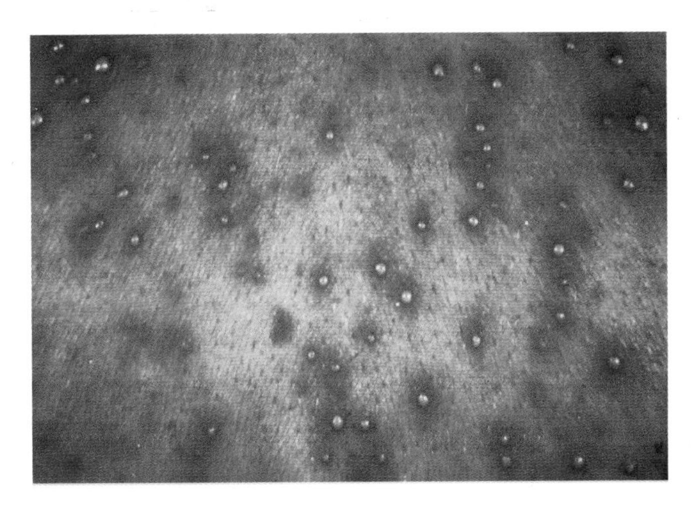

Fig. 26–2. Folliculitis. (Courtesy of Wade Lillegard, M.D.)

of friction such as the axillae, groins, and buttocks. Furuncles usually resolve in a couple of days when treated only with warm compresses. Occasionally, oral erythromycin or penicillin derivatives may be required for 10 days to clear the infection. Since epidemics have been reported among high school football players,[3] participation in close contact sports should be interdicted until the lesions are dry and resolving.

Carbuncles invade deeper into the dermis and occasionally require intravenous antibiotics plus incision and drainage of the area. Bacterial culture of the drainage material is vitally important for appropriate treatment. Recurrent episodes of furuncles and carbuncles may be an early sign of diabetes mellitus.

Erythrasma is a cutaneous bacterial infection of the intertriginous areas caused by *Corynebacterium minutissimum*. In appearance—a well-demarcated, reddish-brown patch—it often resembles tinea cruris. Erythrasma fluoresces coral red under Wood's light, in contrast to tinea, which does not fluoresce.[4] Treatment includes either topical or oral erythromycin for 10 to 14 days and wearing of loose garments for proper aeration of the skin.

Pitted keratolysis is a superficial infection of the weight-bearing surfaces of the feet that mimics tinea pedis. *Corynebacterium* and *Streptomyces* species produce circular pits and longitudinal furrows on the skin surface. The lesions are common in long-distance runners and basketball and tennis players who have hyperhidrosis and wear occlusive footwear. Treatment includes frequent changes of footwear and socks and twice daily application of drying agents such as 20% aluminum chloride (Drysol) and 5% benzoyl peroxide gel in 3% topical erythromycin (Benzamycin).

Viral

Herpes simplex virus is highly contagious and is spread by direct contact from an infected person. Herpes simplex virus type 1 (oral) and type 2 (genital) are large DNA viruses that produce painful vesicles on an erythematous base. "Herpes rugbeiorum" (scrum pox), a common affliction of rugby forwards, is contracted from face-to-face contact in the scrum. "Herpes gladiatorum" (of wrestlers) usually develops on the right side of the face and head, owing to the common lock-up position, in which each opponent's right cheek is pressed against the other's. Serious complications include herpes keratitis and meningitis.

Diagnosis by Tzanck smear or viral culture should not prevent early treatment of herpes-related conditions with drying agents (5 to 10% benzoyl peroxide gel, Campho-Phenique, 4% zinc solutions) and the antiviral drug acyclovir. Topical acyclovir is applied every 3 hours, 6 times a day, for 7 days with a finger cot or rubber glove.[5] Initial episodes of herpetic lesions can be treated with either 200 mg acyclovir, PO, five times a day, or 400 mg, t.i.d., for 7 to 10 days.[6] Athletes who experience more than six recurrences a year can take oral doses of 400 mg b.i.d. routinely while training and competing.[6] An athlete who experiences an outbreak should not be allowed to participate. The NCAA allows athletes to participate if they are free of new or wet lesions for three days before the event.

Molluscum contagiosum is spread by direct inoculation from single or multiple pearly, umbilicated, dome-shaped papules containing poxvirus. Wrestlers are the athletes most often affected by this virus.[2] Therapeutic options include curettage (the quickest, most reliable treatment), cryosurgery with liquid nitrogen, tretinoin, salicylic acid, and laser surgery. Athletes can resume activity 2 to 3 days after curettage.

Verrucae vulgaris (common warts) are epidermal tumors of the papillomavirus that are transmitted from pool decks and shower rooms to the plantar surface of feet and from weight apparatus to the hands. Paring of the wart with a scalpel exposes pinpoint black dots (thrombosed capillaries). This condition must be differentiated from corns and black heel, which are discussed with traumatic skin conditions. Treatment during the season consists of daily application of nonscarring keratolytic agents such as 16% salicylic acid with 16% lactic acid (Duofilm), 40% salicylic acid plaster (Mediplast), or 17% salicylic acid over-the-counter (Compound W). Cryosurgery with liquid nitrogen may produce painful blisters and, so, should be used only after the season.

Fungal

Fungal infections are the most common dermatologic infection of athletes.[4] The dermatophytes, or ringworm fungi, are classified by body region and genera: *Microsporum, Trichophyton,* and *Epidermophyton.* Tinea pedis, or "athlete's foot" (Fig. 26–3), tinea cruris, or "jock itch," tinea corporis (body ringworm), tinea capitis (scalp ringworm), and onychomycosis (nail ringworm) are diagnosed from scrapings of the scaling, hyphae lesions treated with potassium hydroxide (KOH). These infections are spread by direct contact from individual to individual, as well as through moist environments such as locker room floors, showers, and shoes.

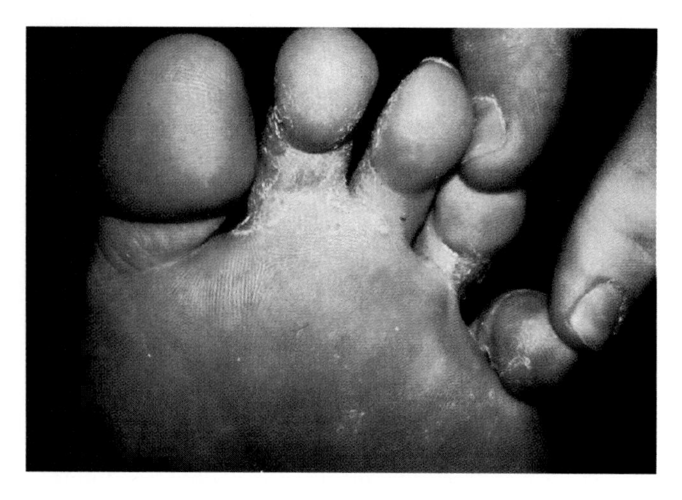

Fig. 26–3. Tinea pedis. (Courtesy of Wade Lillegard, M.D.)

Treatment consists of drying agents (Burow's solution), over-the-counter topical antifungal powders and creams such as miconazole (Micatin), undecylenic acid (Desenex), clotrimazole (Lotrimin, Mycelex), and prescription agents such as econazole (Spectazole) and ketoconazole (Nizoral).[7] For extensive, resistant inflammatory lesions, oral griseofulvin, 250 to 1000 mg daily, is prescribed for several months. Infrequently, for resistant cases of onychomycosis, the athlete may choose to have the toenail removed.

Tinea versicolor is caused by a dimorphic yeast, *Pityrosporum orbiculare.* The infection presents classically as light-colored, scaly patches on the trunk that contrast with unaffected skin, which tans from exposure to the sun. A KOH preparation reveals a "spaghetti and meatballs" smear of the rodlike hyphae and spore clusters. Selenium sulfide shampoo (Selsun) can be applied for 15 minutes daily for 7 consecutive days or for 24 hours once a week for several weeks until all lesions have resolved. Because of the ubiquitous nature of the fungus, the infection is not contagious.

Candidiasis is less common in athletes than tinea infections. *Candida* organisms are found in the intertriginous areas and described as an itchy, erythematous plaque with satellite lesions. It is transmitted from wet shower floors, towels, and equipment. After appropriate diagnosis with KOH smear, treatment consists of topical antifungal imidazole agents (Mycelex, Micatin, Lotrimin). Oral griseofulvin is ineffective for treating Candida infections.

INFESTATIONS

The two common infestations are pediculosis and scabies. Pediculosis is commonly called "crabs" or "lice." Lice are blood-sucking, obligate human parasitic insects.[8] They are spread in sporting events by direct contact and in dressing rooms through towels, clothing, and brushes. Pruritus without a rash and visualization of the nits (eggs) on hair follicles confirm the diagnosis. Treatment options are several shampoos or lotions: lindane (Kwell), permethrin (Nix), pyrethrins (RID), and alathion (Ovide).

Scabies is a highly contagious infestation of *Sarcoptes scabiei* mites. Transmission is by direct contact, and the mites produce erythematous burrows with tiny papules and vesicles in the finger web spaces and axillae and about the waist, ankles, soles of the feet, and genitals. Diagnosis is confirmed by microscopic identification of the mite. Topical shampoos and lotions containing lindane are applied once a week for two consecutive weeks to eradicate the mite. Clothing should be washed in hot, soapy water and stored for 7 to 10 days. Athletes may participate the day after treatment.

ENVIRONMENTAL INJURIES

Exposure to the sun and cold produces painful and disfiguring skin conditions that may limit athletic performance and participation.

Sunburn usually develops 2 to 6 hours after skin exposure to ultraviolet B light and produces a mild erythema with secondary formation of vesicles. Prevention includes proper choice of sunscreen with a solar protection factor (SPF) based on skin type, avoiding peak exposure hours between 11 a.m. and 3 p.m., and covering skin with light, loose cotton garments. Treatment is based on the degree of sunburn and includes the use of cool compresses, topical steroids, oral nonsteroidal anti-inflammatory agents, and oral corticosteroids for severe cases.

The most common superficial cold injury from prolonged exposure to subfreezing temperatures and wind chill is frostnip.[9] Erythema and pain are followed by anesthesia and blistering over exposed areas. These changes are frequently seen on the face and ears of joggers and skiers. Treatment consists of returning to a warm environment and rapidly rewarming the affected area.

Frostbite is a deeper extension of frostnip into dermal and subcutaneous tissues that produces denaturation of cell proteins and formation of extracellular ice crystals. Frostbite develops sequentially by stages: (1) erythema and edema; (2) vesicles and bullae; (3) full-thickness freezing with cold, white, firm skin; and (4) gangrene. The affected skin appears waxy and usually blisters in 24 to 36 hours. Treatment involves active rewarming in baths from 38° to 43°C, analgesics during rewarming, and transfer to a tertiary medical facility experienced in frostbite management.

TRAUMATIC SKIN INJURIES

Blisters (Fig. 26–4) are the most common noninfectious skin problem of athletes.[10] Frictional forces produce an intraepidermal split of the skin, allowing accumulation of serum between layers. Contributing factors include improperly fitted shoes, underlying osseous abnormalities, lack of training for adequate epidermal hyperplasia in areas of maximal pressure, and hyperhidrosis.

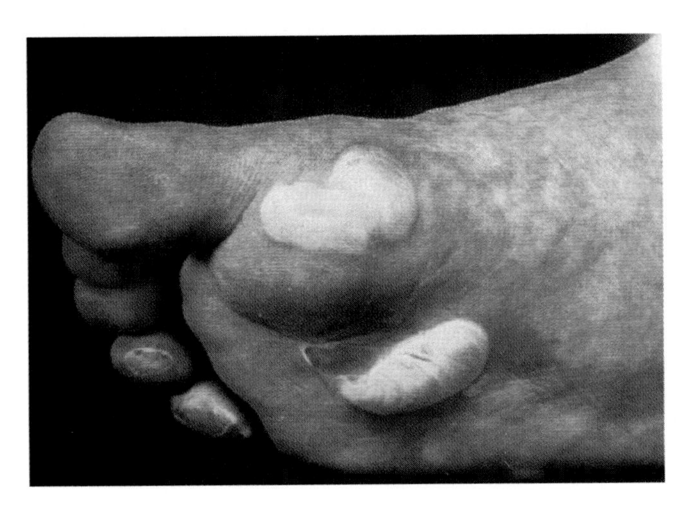

Fig. 26–4. Blisters. (Courtesy of Wade Lillegard, M.D.)

To prevent blister formation, athletes are encouraged to wear properly fitted shoes, talcum powdered socks, and nylon hose. Additional measures include applying benzoin to harden the epidermis over areas of maximum pressure and decreasing friction by lubricating with emollients containing urea, lactic acid, mineral oil, glycerin, or petrolatum. Treatment consists of draining large, tense blisters with a small needle and leaving the roof as a protective layer. Topical antibiotics and an occlusive dressing can be applied to promote epithelialization.

Calluses are a protective response to repeated pressure and friction over bony prominences. Hyperkeratosis commonly develops over the metatarsal and metacarpal heads in association with activities such as gymnastics, dancing, running, and racquet sports. Rowers develop calluses on the skin over the ischial tuberosity of the buttock, a lesion referred to as "rower's rump."

Although calluses are a natural response of the body, they can become tender and painful. Paring with a scalpel blade and sanding with pumice stone after hydration, along with nightly application of topical salicylic acid or lactic acid, are effective therapeutic measures.

Corns are small, painful keratinized lesions, either a soft lesion between the toes or one that has a hard, central translucent core overlying a bony prominence. Corns can be differentiated from plantar warts by the absence of black dots in the central core of corns. Treatment consists of restoring normal function to the foot with properly fitted and padded shoes, paring after hydration, and applying salicylic acid plaster.

Black heel is an asymptomatic formation of black dots or streaks on the posterior or lateral aspect of the heel.[9] The black dots represent rupture of papillary dermal capillaries and extravasation of heme into the epidermis. Paring the skin over the black dots does not produce bleeding and reveals normal skin lines not found in a plantar wart. Also called "calcaneal petechiae," *"talon noir,"* and "basketball heel," the condition is commonly found in basketball, tennis, and racquetball players who routinely make sudden, forceful movements of the feet. Black heel may be prevented by using fitted heel cups, applying moleskin, or adding padding. The lesions resolve spontaneously over time.

Black toe or tennis toe is most common under the first or second toenail.[10] A subungual hematoma forms as a result of sudden or repeated trauma to the nail. Properly fitted shoes, metatarsal pads to achieve plantar flexion of the toes, and relacing shoes during the event may prevent this disorder. To relieve the pain, the nail plate must be punctured with a large-bore needle or wire cautery.

Jogger's nipple is an abrasion of the nipple and areola from friction of coarse, cotton fabric.[11] It occurs more commonly in men than in women because women wear padded support bras. The condition can be alleviated by wearing semisynthetic fabric or silk and applying petrolatum ointment or tape over the nipples.

Athlete's nodules, or "surfer's nodules," are dermal proliferations of collagen from repeated surfboard trauma to the feet and knees. They also occur on the knuckles of boxers and are considered by both athletes to be symbols of achievement and expertise. Available treatment includes use of protective padding, intralesional injection of corticosteroids, and surgical excision.

ACNE

Acne vulgaris is a common, noncontagious skin disorder of adolescents that may persist into adulthood and produce disfiguration of the skin leading to psychological stress. A disorder of the pilosebaceous glands, acne has a multitude of predisposing factors including heredity, increased sebum production, anxiety, hormonal dysfunction, use of topical cosmetics, and abuse of anabolic steroids.[4] Profuse perspiration, coupled with overlying protective equipment (headgear), are factors that exacerbate acne in athletes, especially football and hockey players, and wrestlers.

Noninflammatory lesions, comedones and blackheads, can be followed by inflammatory pustules and cystic acne. Tretinoin (Retin-A) is primarily used once a day for noninflammatory acne. Additional use of topical antibiotics (tetracycline, erythromycin, clindamycin b.i.d.) and benzoyl peroxide gels (2.5 to 10%) have been found effective. Tetracycline, 250 or 500 mg b.i.d., is the most commonly prescribed oral medication for moderate to severe acne.[5] Isotretinoin (Accutane) is reserved for control of severe cystic acne under proper consultation with a dermatologist. Athletes with nodulocystic acne can be treated with intralesional corticosteroids. Triamcinolone acetonide (Kenalog) is injected into the roof of the cyst with a 27- to 30-gauge needle.[5] Acne should not limit participation in sports.

CONCLUSION

Athletes are susceptible to numerous dermatologic conditions that may hinder performance and ultimately restrict participation. As team physicians, trainers, and coaches, we are all responsible for instructing athletes in the importance of proper hygiene. Through early recognition, appropriate intervention, and successful management of dermatologic conditions, the health care team minimizes the amount of time athletes spend away from training and helps them return early to athletic competition.

REFERENCES

1. Bergfeld, W. F.: Dermatologic problems in athletes. Clin. Sports Med. *1*:419, 1982.
2. Schneider, R. C., Kennedy, J. C., and Plant, M. L.: Sports Injuries: Mechanisms, Prevention, and Treatment. Baltimore, Williams & Wilkins, 1985.
3. Sosin, D. M., Gunn, R. A., Ford, W. L., and Skaggs, J. W.: An outbreak of furunculosis among high school athletes. Am. J. Sports Med. *17*:828, 1989.
4. Kantor, G. R., and Bergfeld, W. F.: Common and uncommon dermatologic diseases related to sports activities. Dermatol. Dis. Sport *1*:225, 1990.
5. Habif, T. P.: Clinical Dermatology: A Color Guide to Diagnosis and Therapy. 2nd Ed. St. Louis, C. V. Mosby, 1990.
6. Treatment of sexually transmitted diseases. Med. Lett. *32*:5, 1990.
7. Ramsey, M. L.: Athlete's foot: Clinical update. Physician Sportmed. *17*(10):78, 1989.
8. Rock, B.: Superficial skin infections. Athletic Training *24*:12, 1989.
9. Atton, A. V., and Tunnessen, W. W., Jr.: The athlete and his skin: Sports related cutaneous disorders. Clin. Rev. Allergy *6*:403, 1988.
10. Basler, R. S.: Skin lesions related to sports activity. Prim. Care Clin. Office Pract. *10*:479, 1983.
11. Conklin, R. J.: Common cutaneous disorders in athletes. Sports Med. *9*:100, 1990.

27 *Brian Halpern and Gary Keogh*

Infectious Diseases

It is thought that more than half of the population of the United States exercise regularly. In the past, musculoskeletal injuries were the principal hazard for these athletes. More recently, the interaction between exercise and infectious diseases has been highlighted by increasing publicity about athletes infected with human immunodeficiency virus (HIV). Physicians now are frequently being asked for advice on infection—from professional athletes, high school students, collegians, and the large number of people who participate in recreational sports.

SPECIFIC INFECTIONS

The Common Cold

Colds are often caused by members of two groups of viruses, rhinoviruses and coronaviruses, and less often by other viruses such as parainfluenza virus. Although effective prophylactic therapies have been attempted, there is as yet no treatment for a cold that has already begun. It is a self-limiting disease and infrequently leads to serious complications.[1]

Medications used by many cold sufferers who elect not to go to a physician can contain eight or more ingredients, including antihistamines, decongestants, antitussives, expectorants, analgesics, anticholinergics, bronchodilators, caffeine, and vitamin C. The decongestants are banned by some sports organizations.[2]

Upper respiratory tract infections rarely necessitate interruption of exercise schedules. Incubation for most of the common cold viruses takes 1 to 6 days. The acute symptoms last 2 to 7 days and resolution is complete by 7 to 14 days. Milder colds are characterized by sneezing, watery nasal discharge, nasal congestion, sore or scratchy throat, and a nonproductive cough with little or no systemic involvement.

Upper Respiratory Tract Infections

Epidemiologic findings suggest an increased incidence of upper respiratory tract infections in the week following a marathon race.[3] Other studies have reported mild upper respiratory tract symptoms within 2 weeks of the event. Neiman[3] reported that subjects who ran more than 97 k per week in preparation for a marathon race were twice as likely to suffer respiratory tract infection than those who ran less than 32 k per week. Two reports show that the incidence of these symptoms was more than 50% higher in runners than in age-matched nonrunning controls.[4,5] Less competitive events do not seem to increase respiratory infections, and, indeed, moderate training seems to enhance resistance to infection in both humans and animals.[6]

Fever is often associated with these infections. Exercising with a fever increases cardiac output far more than exercising with a normal basal body temperature. Oxygen consumption and lactate production also increase. These effects of fever lead to decreased strength, aerobic power, endurance, coordination, and concentration and place the athlete at risk for more serious sequelae, i.e., viral myocarditis.[7]

Influenza

Influenza causes more significant morbidity and mortality to high-risk persons. Aspirin should not be given for this infection because it increases viral shedding and also has been associated with Reye's syndrome. Acetaminophen is effective for discomfort and fever. For influenza A, amantadine, 200 mg loading dose followed by 100 mg twice a day for 5 days, is useful in reducing the fever and shortening the duration of the illness by 1 or 2 days. It must be given within the first 24 to 48 hours after symptoms appear. Infection is limited by frequent hand washing, using disposable tissues, and decreased human contact.

Pharyngitis

The agents responsible for the common cold are also the most common causes of pharyngitis: adenovirus, influenza virus, and coxsackievirus. Although they account for only a minority of all sore throats seen clinically, group A β-hemolytic streptococci cause most concern because of the potential for serious sequelae. Group A β-hemolytic streptococci occur mainly in young persons and are very uncommon after age 30 years. The incidence of group A β-hemolytic streptococcal pharyngitis has not changed in recent years, but acute rheumatic fever has recently shown a resurgence.[8]

Although the clinical presentation varies much, the classic presentation of group A β-hemolytic streptococcal infection is severe dysphagia, high fever, exudative tonsillitis, and pharyngitis. A tender larynx or anterior cervical lymph nodes and headache, lethargy, anorexia, abdominal pain, palatal petechiae, and scarlatiniform rash may also be present. Throat cultures have become the standard for diagnosing streptococcal pharyngitis, although only 50% of culture-positive patients are actually "serologically" infected. The rest are presumed to be carriers. There is a 10% false-negative rate for throat cultures.[9] Rapid antigen tests on the market have a specificity of more than 90%, but their sensitivity ranges from 60 to 90%; so when streptococcal pharyngitis is suspected clinically but the rapid test is negative, a throat culture should be obtained.

Treatment of choice for group A β-hemolytic streptococci is oral penicillin V, 250 mg four times daily for 10 days for adults or for children who weigh more than 10 kg. It is effective in preventing rheumatic fever *if* treatment is started within 9 days after the onset of clinical symptoms. If compliance is a problem, injectable benzathine penicillin G is equally effective, 600,000 units for children less than 60 pounds, 900,000 units for children weighing 60 to 90 pounds, and 1.2 million units for children and adults weighing more than 90 pounds. Current recommendations for the management of people who come in contact with group A β-hemolytic streptococci are to take culture material only from those who develop symptoms; if two or more family members have group A β-hemolytic streptococcal disease, consideration may be given to treating the entire family. Individual assessment about the advisability of exercise should be given; the parameters were discussed previously.

Infectious Mononucleosis

Infectious mononucleosis hosts are recognized by general involvement of the lymph system—lymph nodes, spleen, liver, and bone marrow—with Epstein-Barr virus (EBV). EBV is responsible for more than 90% of mononucleosis-like syndromes. The rest are caused by cytomegalovirus, *Toxoplasma* species, hepatitis viruses A and B, and adenovirus. EBV is a double-stranded DNA virus in the herpes family that infects B lymphocytes. The virus persists lifelong in both B cells and salivary glands. Some 70 to 90% of persons shed the virus until 8 to 24 weeks after resolution of the clinical disease. Transmission is by the oral or fecal route, many times through frequent contact such as kissing or sharing utensils. Among college students, numbers of cases are higher in spring and fall. The disease is milder in children, so the majority of them have subclinical infections, whereas most adolescents have mononucleosis syndrome. The incubation period is 20 to 50 days. Onset is insidious, with malaise, headache, and fatigue. Splenomegaly occurs in 45% of patients and hepatomegaly in 35%. Diagnosis is based on a triad of clinical, hematologic, and serologic findings. The minimum hematologic findings include (1) relative lymphocytosis greater than 50% and relative atypical lymphocytosis more than 10% of all leukocytes *or* (2) at least an absolute total lymphocyte concentration of more than 5000 per microliter with more than 1000 per microliter atypical lymphocytes. Lymphocyte atypia of 40% or greater is so specific for infectious mononucleosis that serologic testing is unnecessary. More than 80% of patients with infectious mononucleosis produce high titers and true-positive mononucleosis spot tests during the second week of clinical illness.

The usual clinical course of infectious mononucleosis lasts 2 to 8 weeks. On rare occasions it can take several months to regain the preinfection level of performance. The prevalence of splenic rupture has been quoted at 0.1 to 0.2%. It occurs only in enlarged spleens, though the enlargement may not be palpable. Rupture of the spleen usually occurs 4 to 21 days after the appearance of symptoms and is often associated with trauma, though it can occur spontaneously. Abdominal ultrasound can be used to monitor spleen size. There is no apparent correlation between the clinical severity of infectious mononucleosis and susceptibility to splenic rupture.

A study by Dalrymple[10] among college students showed that students randomly assigned to higher activity levels recovered more rapidly than students treated with bed rest. Permitting daily activities within limits rather than complete rest, which allows deconditioning, seems appropriate, but one should be aware of the possibility of splenomegaly, and no contact activities should be allowed. Training can usually be resumed at around 3 to 4 weeks at a modest level and upgraded, allowing 2 days' rehabilitation for every day of rest. Superimposed infections such as β-hemolytic streptococcal pharyngitis occur in as many as 33% of these cases and should be treated. Use of steroids should be avoided if possible, but it may be needed if airway obstruction, thrombocytopenia, or neurologic sequelae are life threatening.

Viral Hepatitis

Hepatitis may be caused by viral infections such as hepatitis A, B, C, D, or E. Both hepatitis A and hepatitis

B are common in late adolescent and young adult populations and are readily transmitted to those in close contact. Hepatitis C is an important cause of transfusion-related hepatitis. Hepatitis D occurs only in patients with acute or chronic hepatitis B, and hepatitis E is an epidemic form of hepatitis that has characteristics of hepatitis A such as enteric transmission and no chronic phase. It is uncommon in developed countries.

Hepatitis A is probably the most common acute viral hepatitis in young athletes. Since hepatitis A is transmitted principally by the fecal or oral route, sometimes food- or waterborne outbreaks occur. There is no known carrier state for hepatitis A virus. The virus is excreted in the stool before signs and symptoms develop. Viral excretion usually disappears by the time jaundice appears. In the United States about 10 to 20% of persons have evidence of prior infection by age 20 years and about 50% by age 50. Fever, nausea, vomiting, abdominal pain, and anorexia are common prodromal symptoms. Efforts to control exposure to others are important. Immune globulin should be given as soon as possible after exposure, preferably within 2 weeks. For persons traveling to an area where the incidence of hepatitis A is high, pre-exposure prophylaxis is indicated; that is, immune globulin in a single dose for persons who expect to be in the area 3 months or less. Persons with acute hepatitis should be advised to rest until the acute symptoms—fever, nausea, vomiting—have subsided. Work done by Chamers and coworkers indicated that soldiers allowed liberal activity as opposed to bed rest recovered just as quickly.[11] More recent European trials confirmed those findings. Again, individual assessment is important for competitive athletes. A healthy diet and abstinence from alcohol should be advised. There is no necessity for vitamin K unless the prothrombin time becomes significantly prolonged, 1.5 times the upper limit of normal.

Hepatitis B transmission occurs by intravenous drug use, prenatal spread, sexual activity, and exposure to infected blood. With the institution of blood donor screening the other routes of exposure have gained more importance. Only 1% of hepatitis B viral infections are related to transfusions, 35 to 40% of those infected have no identifiable risk factors. The simultaneous presence of hepatitis B surface antigen and hepatitis B core antibody is a sign of ongoing hepatitis B infection. Immunity is indicated by the presence of the antibody to hepatitis B surface antigen, which usually appears 1 to 3 months after recovery. Hepatitis B e antigen is considered a marker of high infectivity and is present during acute hepatitis B viral infections or the early phase of chronic hepatitis. Some 5 to 10% of adults who have had the infection become carriers. Tests for hepatitis B surface antigen should be done at 3 and 6 months to determine this. Twenty-five percent of the carriers develop chronic active hepatitis, and there is an estimated core of a million chronic carriers in the United States.

Again, resumption of competition training is determined by the athlete's response to the infection, return of enzyme levels to normal, and the response to exercise. Vaccine is available, yet the prevalence of hepatitis is increasing in the United States. Athletes who come into close contact with a person with active acute infection can be advised to receive passive immunization with hepatitis B immunoglobulin, followed by hepatitis B vaccine. General sexual precautions for infected persons include use of condoms and avoidance of intercourse during menstruation or intramenstrual bleeding. Casual, nonblood contact does not require active or passive immunoprophylaxis. It is important to bar persons with active infections from certain sports such as wrestling, because transmission has been shown to occur through percutaneous or mucosal contact with infectious body fluids.[12]

Human Immunodeficiency Virus Infection

In the United States, it is estimated that more than one million people are infected with HIV. Boundaries between high-risk groups are becoming less distinct as more women and members of minority groups become infected each year. More than 75% of HIV infections worldwide are acquired through sexual intercourse. Of these, 80% are acquired through heterosexual activity. Acquired immunodeficiency syndrome (AIDS) is a poorly contagious but highly lethal disease associated with the retroviruses HIV 1 and HIV 2. It is not transmitted by casual contact. It is transmitted mainly through blood or sexual contact and perinatally. Transmission via sports contact still represents only a theoretical risk. In sports such as wrestling and football, where bleeding and skin abrasions are common, no transmission has been reported to date. One report about a soccer player in Italy remains unverified.[13]

Occupational HIV exposure represents a small but significant risk to health care workers in sports medicine. The level of risk is unknown, but it is less than the risk of HIV infection by needlesticks from infected patients (approximately 1 in 250).[14] Considering the recognized modes of transmission, emphasis should be placed on the same lines of prevention that are being used in other health care situations, and the risk of transmission via sports should be de-emphasized.

The team physician should concentrate on adequate history and physical examination plus pre- and post-test counseling in risk reduction and guidance. Certain organizations have produced a consensus statement on AIDS in sports.[15] The Centers for Disease Control and Prevention (CDC) Occupational Safety and Health Administration regulations help physicians decide what to do—and what they can and should do in the office. At least half of the one million Americans infected with HIV do not know they are infected according to the CDC. Since there has been no documented case of athlete-to-athlete HIV transmission, the risk remains theoretical.

Against this background, there is no justification for HIV testing before participation in sports if universal precautions recommended by the CDC are followed by health care workers. Some sports carry a higher theoretical risk because of increased prevalence of bleeding—boxing, wrestling, and tae kwon do. A U.S. Olympic Committee report advises testing of athletes in high-risk and moderate-risk sports.[16] Use of gloves is advised when contact with body fluids is possible, as is use of bleach on all surfaces and equipment that may be contaminated by blood. Some changes in rules have resulted; for example, in U.S. wrestling, time outs for bleeding are no longer charged against the athlete.

The decision to continue playing is a difficult one that must be addressed on an individual basis. It should be based on discussion and communication between athlete, trainer, doctor, coach, and family. With the enforcement of the Americans with Disabilities Act, court decisions against discrimination in the workplace among HIV-infected persons have been upheld.

Based on the previously outlined information on the effect of exercise on viral infections and the immune system and the work of Dr. Laperiere in Miami,[17,18] it would seem prudent to recommend that HIV-positive athletes avoid very strenuous exercise, but that moderate exercise be allowed. Besides the effects on the immune system, exercise has been shown to reduce stress, a factor that may affect the progression of HIV infection to AIDS. In 1988, data published by Dr. Laperiere at the Society of Behavioral Medicine showed that a moderate program of exercise influenced CD4 cells to a degree comparable to that of zidovudine (AZT). This area of psychoneuroimmunology is expanding, and questions about how much exercise should be prescribed—and how frequently—for HIV-infected athletes at different stages of progression of HIV infection still need answers. The application of academic research findings to clinical practice must be emphasized, and health care workers at all levels must be educated in the beneficial effects associated with moderate aerobic exercise.[17,18]

Any physician working with an HIV-infected athlete needs to know the basic information for counseling about the disease—its course, prognosis, mode of transmission, and methods of minimizing exposure to teammates. Confidentiality must be assured. Education of coaches, trainers, and other health care members is the responsibility of the physician. The relevant education should emphasize spread by drug use and unsafe sexual practices. Specific drug use, such as sharing needles or injecting anabolic steroids, should be addressed.

Lyme Disease

Lyme disease is a multisystem inflammatory disease caused by the spirochete *Borrelia burgdorferi* and spread by *Ixodes* ticks. The organism has also been demonstrated in other species of ticks and in mosquitoes and deer flies.

The clinical picture, similar worldwide, can be divided into three stages. In Stage I, a localized infection characterized by erythema migrans is usually associated with minor constitutional symptoms and regional lymphadenopathy. About 20% of patients have no characteristic skin lesions. Stage II, disseminated infection, occurs within days or weeks and can involve acute cardiac, neurologic, or musculoskeletal signs and symptoms. The patient can appear quite ill and have debilitating fatigue. Neurologic involvement can include Bell's palsy, radicular neuritis, or lymphocytic meningitis. Cardiac involvement is usually associated with palpitations or fainting due to an arteriovenous nodal block. At this stage cerebrospinal fluid shows pleocytosis of about 100 cells per microliter, predominantly lymphocytes. Cerebrospinal fluid protein is often elevated, and the glucose level is usually normal. Late-stage joint involvement with brief intermittent episodes of arthritis can occur in the second stage. Stage III, chronic infection, follows a latent period of about a year. The nervous system and joints can be involved with polyneuropathy and chronic arthritis. Only 10% of patients with Lyme arthritis go on to develop chronic arthritis, and fewer than 5% of those develop erosive arthritis.[19]

Serologic tests for diagnosis have a high degree of sensitivity and specificity, but because assays are not standardized and differences exist in the interpretation and performance of the tests, many false-negative and false-positive results have been encountered. This has led to overdiagnosis of Lyme disease.[20] Steere's results at the Lyme Disease Center showed that only 20% of patients referred there over the last 5 years had active Lyme disease. Another 20% had in the past had Lyme disease, and the remaining 60% did not have it. Most patients from the 1970s and 1980s are still seropositive today, which suggests that they acquired immunity. The usual test is an enzyme-linked immunosorbent assay (ELISA) test, which detects patients who have Lyme disease or had it in the past. Borderline results should be followed by a Western blot analysis. Antibiotic treatment early in the course of infection can delay or eliminate a diagnostic antibody response. Presently, Lyme borreliosis remains the clinical diagnosis, and testing should be used to confirm the clinical impression. A common dilemma is distinguishing Lyme disease from chronic fatigue syndrome or fibromyalgia. The following points are important to remember:

1. Approximately 80% of patients with Lyme disease have the initial characteristic skin lesion erythema migrans.
2. On neurologic examination, memory loss is usually seen with Lyme disease, whereas concentration problems are associated with chronic fatigue syndrome.
3. Lyme disease patients usually have a problem with somnolence, whereas fibromyalgia or chronic fatigue syndrome patients usually complain of a sleep disorder.
4. Lyme disease patients do not usually have tender points, and the cerebrospinal fluid and electromyography findings are normal with chronic fatigue syndrome or fibromyalgia.

Antibiotic treatment is 90 to 100% effective for erythema migrans and 90 to 95% effective for other acute manifestations. Initial presentation of Bell's palsy, erythema migrans, or arteriovenous first-degree heart block should be treated (in adults who are not pregnant) with doxycycline, 100 mg orally, twice daily for 3 to 4 weeks, or a combination of amoxicillin and probenecid, 500 mg orally three times daily for 3 to 4 weeks. In children 9 years of age or younger the combination of amoxicillin and probenecid is used initially. For patients with central nervous system disease and cerebrospinal fluid abnormalities, second- or third-degree heart block, or with signs of arthritis, ceftriaxone, 2 g intravenously daily for 2 to 4 weeks, is recommended. For children, the dose is 50 to 75 mg/kg body weight daily for 2 to 4 weeks.[21]

Lyme disease seems to be one of the precipitating infections associated with development of chronic fatigue syndrome. Some patients continue after treatment to complain of headaches, musculoskeletal pain, and fatigue. Usually these resolve within 6 to 12 months. Should this longterm problem arise, appropriate therapy is small doses of tricyclic antidepressants, analgesics, and a moderate aerobic exercise program plus supportive care.

A study conducted in Connecticut indicated that the risk of Lyme disease after a deer tick bite was so low that prophylactic antimicrobial therapy was not routinely recommended.[22] Specific endemic areas may be cause for reconsideration of prophylaxis for the deer tick bite. It is important that serologic tests become standardized and that newer tests, for example DNA probes and detection of antigen in urine, should be added to the diagnostic regimen. To remove a tick, it should be grasped firmly with a pair of tweezers close to the site of attachment and firm traction should be applied. Broken-off mouth parts are not cause for undue concern.

The most effective method of prevention is to avoid natural habitats endemic for *B. burgdorferi*–infected *Ixodes* ticks during the feeding season (May through September in the northeast United States). Tick repellents are effective and should be sprayed on shoes and clothes before entering a potentially infested area. Long pants should be worn and all clothes should be removed and washed as soon as possible after leaving the area. Close inspection of the skin is indicated. Removing ticks within 18 hours of attachment usually prevents infection. Tucking long pants into socks, and wearing long sleeves and light-colored clothing are also advisable. It must be stressed that, when treated early, the overwhelming number of Lyme disease patients respond favorably. Exercise prescription must be individualized according to the staging of the disease, completion of therapy, and presence of persistent arthritis, fatigue, or other symptoms.

TRAVEL AND INFECTIOUS DISEASE

As many as 60% of athletes who travel internationally develop diarrhea. Usually it begins in the first week and recovery follows within 2 days. Toxicogenic *Escherichia coli* organisms account for approximately 50% of cases, and these cases respond to standard treatment. Suspicion of other agents, including *Salmonella, Shigella,* and *Campylobacter* species, depends on the clinical course. Advice on the use of local water and consumption of raw vegetables and salads should be given before arrival. Prophylactic therapy using antibacterial agents is recommended less often because of allergic reactions and side effects such as photosensitivity. Prophylactic use of bismuth silicate, two tablets four times daily, does help reduce traveler's diarrhea. Bottled water and boiled water are usually safe. Hand washing with soap and water before eating and peeling fruit are also recommended.

Checks on up-to-date immunizations are mandatory for all traveling athletes. A tetanus booster every 10 years maintains immunity following a primary series. Use of tetanus immune globulin should be restricted to wounds that are "dirty" and for which the circumstances of injury and past treatment are incomplete or unknown. The measles vaccination should be reviewed as there have been sporadic outbreaks of measles at different events. Influenza vaccine is not recommended for healthy athletes. Vaccination may be considered for athletes involved in close contact sports played in fall or winter, to avoid disruption of the season by infection. Vaccination should be considered only if the supply is sufficient to first meet the needs of elderly and chronically ill persons.

REFERENCES

1. Stickler, G. B., Smith, P. F., and Broughton, D. D.: The common cold. Eur. J. Pediatr. *144*:4, 1985.
2. International Olympic Committee List of Doping Classes and Methods. Lausanne, Chateau d'Vidy 1007, 1990.
3. Nieman, D. C., Johansen, L. M., and Lee, J. W.: Infectious episodes in runners before and after Los Angeles marathon. Med. Sci. Sports Exerc. *20*:S42, 1988.
4. Peters, E. M., and Bateman, E. D.: Ultra marathon running and upper respiratory tract infections. S. Afr. Med. J. *64*:582, 1983.
5. Peters, E. M.: Altitude fails to increase susceptibility of ultramarathon runners to post-race upper respiratory infections. S. Afr. J. Sports Med. *5*:4, 1990.
6. Shepherd, R. J., et al.: Physical activity and the immune system. Can. J. Sports Sci. *16*:163, 1991.
7. Sitorius, M.: General medical problems in athletes. *In* The Team Physician's Handbook. Edited by M. Mellion. W. M. Walsh, and G. L. Shelton. Philadelphia, Hanley & Belfus, 1990.
8. Kaplan, E. L., and Hill, H. R.: Return of rheumatic fever consequences, implications, and needs. J. Pediatr. *111*:244, 1987.
9. Sande, M. A., et al. (eds.): Respiratory Infections. New York, Churchill Livingston, 1986.
10. Dalrymple, W.: Infectious mononucleosis. Postgrad. Med. *5*:345, 1964.
11. Chamers, T. C., et al.: Treatment of infectious hepatitis, controlled studies of the effects of diet, rest, and physical reconditioning in the acute phase of the disease and the incidence of relapses and residual abnormalities. J. Clin. Invest. *34*:1163, 1955.
12. Culpepper, L.: Preventing hepatitis B: Focus on women and their families. J. Am. Board Fam. Pract. *6*:483, 1993.
13. Torre, D., et al.: Transmission of HIV-1 infection via sports injury. Lancet *335*:1105, 1990.
14. Henderson, D. K., et al.: Risk of nosocomial infection with human T-cell lymphotrophic virus type III/lymphadenopathy associated virus in a large cohort of intensively exposed health care workers. Ann. Intern. Med. *104*:644, 1986.
15. Goldsmith, M. F.: When sports and HIV share the bill, smart money goes on common sense. J.A.M.A. *267*:1311, 1992.

16. Garal, T., Hrisonalost, and Rink, L.: Transmission of infectious agents during athletic competition, a report to all national government bodies by the U.S. Olympic Committee Sports Medicine and Science Committee. Colorado Springs, U.S. Olympic Committee, 1991.
17. Laperiere A., et al.: Aerobic exercise training and psychoneuroimmunology in AIDS research. *In* Psychological Perspectives on AIDS. Edited by A. Enbalm, and L. Temochok. Hillsdale, NJ, Earlbaum Assoc., 1990.
18. Laperiere, A., Antoni, M. H., and Fletcher, M. A.: Exercise and health maintenance in AIDS. *In* Clinical Assessment and Treatment in HIV. Rehabilitation of a Chronic Illness. Edited by M. L. Galantino. Thorofare, NJ, Charles B. Slack, 1992.
19. Steere, A. C., Schoen, R. T., and Taylor, E.: The clinical evolution of Lyme arthritis. Ann. Intern. Med. *107*:725, 1987.
20. Steere, A. C.: Current understanding of Lyme disease. Hosp. Pract. *28*(4):37, 1993.
21. Burdge, D., and O'Hanlon, D.: Lyme disease. Can. Fam. Physician *38*:1426, 1992.
22. Shapiro, E. D., et al.: A controlled trial of antimicrobial prophylaxis for Lyme disease after deer-tick bites. N. Engl. J. Med. *327*:1769, 1992.

28

John M. Henderson

Amenorrhea, Delayed Menarche, and Osteoporosis

The development of amenorrhea has been linked to intense physical training.[1] Two types of amenorrhea should be understood if physicians are to optimize the care of female athletes. Primary amenorrhea—delayed menarche—is commonly defined as absence of menses by age 16 years. Secondary amenorrhea is defined as missing 3 to 12 consecutive periods. Amenorrhea can cause immediate effects and problems in the distant future. Until recently, amenorrheic athletes did not receive much attention because of the general lack of understanding of the physiology of the condition itself and of its far-reaching complications.

BACKGROUND

The mean age of menarche for girls in the United States is 12 years and 9 months. The initial menses are termed *anovulatory menses,* because no ovum is extruded from a graafian follicle. Menstrual dysfunction in athletes is thought to be caused by inhibition of hypothalamic Gon RH, a gonadotropic-releasing hormone, causing a decrease in luteinizing hormone (LH) and follicle-stimulating hormone (FSH).[2] The hypothalamus is sensitive to the activation of the adrenal axis secondary to strenuous exercise, and this effect is intensified by the calorie drain of vigorous training.[3] These changes manifest as a spectrum of menstrual dysfunctions. *Luteal phase dysfunction* refers to a shortened luteal phase, in which progesterone production is insufficient. In *anovulation* estrogen is unopposed and very long cycles or oligomenorrhea (diminished flow) can result. *Hypoestrogenemic amenorrhea,* a form of hypothalamic amenorrhea, is the most frequently observed problem.

As a general rule of thumb, for each year of training before menarche, menarche is delayed by 5 months.[4–6]

EPIDEMIOLOGY

Both primary and secondary amenorrhea are more common in active women than in the general population. The relationship between activity and amenorrhea is debatable. It is uncertain whether activity (exercise, sports) delays sexual maturation. It is equally uncertain whether women who are successful in sports are those whose sexual maturation was delayed. Additionally perplexing is whether absence or even lightening, of menstrual bleeding is caused by exercise or by a combination of factors.[2]

The prevalence of secondary amenorrhea in athletes is thought to range between 3.4 and 66%, as opposed to 2 to 5% in the general population.[7] Athletes at risk include those involved in strenuous activity such as distance runners, ballet dancers, gymnasts, ice skaters (ice dancers), and cyclists. No data are available on the prevalence of primary amenorrhea, in athletes or in the general population. Again, it is thought to be more common in "high-intensity" athletes, such as volleyball players, figure skaters, gymnasts, and ballet dancers.[6]

COMPLICATIONS

The complications of amenorrhea can reach into a woman's eighth decade. The economic, let alone the medical, burden of these problems can be enormous. Regarding delayed menarche, most studies have addressed university athletes, ballet dancers, or gymnasts. Lowered bone density has been implicated as an effect of primary amenorrhea. Scoliosis and increased incidence of stress fractures have been attributed to this bone weakening.[8] General growth and development are negatively affected by delayed menarche, especially when vaginal atrophy results from hypoestrogenemia.

Secondary amenorrhea can cause infertility and premature osteoporosis, which in turn leads to stress fractures. Theoretical complications related to the hypoestrogenemic state of women with amenorrhea include increased risk of cardiovascular disease. Theoretically, the risks of endometrial hyperplasia and adenocarcinoma can be increased if the amenorrhea is associated with chronic anovulation caused by unopposed estrogen. The female athlete triad of amenorrhea, eating disorders, and osteoporosis is being recognized more often in highly trained female athletes. Any athlete who is found to have one component of the triad should be evaluated for the other two. Low bone mineral density is not limited to the appendicular skeleton of amenorrheic athletes; it is also present in other areas.[9]

EVALUATION

Evaluation for primary amenorrhea should be considered when any athlete reaches her 16th birthday and has had no menstrual bleeding. Evaluation for secondary amenorrhea should be considered after the woman misses three to six periods. After a thorough evaluation, if no other cause of amenorrhea is found, the diagnosis of "athletic amenorrhea" is appropriate. The most common pitfall for physicians who care for women athletes is inappropriately diagnosing menstrual dysfunction without performing a complete evaluation.[10] Other conditions to be considered in the evaluation process are listed in Table 28–1.

For adolescent female athletes, the evaluation may or may not include a pelvic examination, depending on the desires of the athlete and her parents. At times, abdominal palpation and ultrasound evaluation of the pelvis are the most that the athlete or her parents will allow. Often, patient and parental education is the remedy for their hesitance about speculum and bimanual examination.

Table 28–1. Factors often Responsible for Amenorrhea

Familial history of late menarche
Overtraining and/or excessive weight loss
Overwhelming stress (as perceived by the athlete)
Pregnancy—intrauterine or ectopic
Use of androgenic-anabolic steroids
Hypothyroidism or hyperthyroidism
Indeterminate sex syndrome (hermaphroditism)
Chronic illness (Crohn's disease, collagen disorders, renal failure)
Prolactin-secreting tumor (pituitary microadenoma)
Premature ovarian failure
Trisomy (hypergonadotropic hypogonadism)
Delayed growth and development (look at the child's growth charts, bone age, height age)

For many women, the physician's greatest hurdle is to convince the athlete that her amenorrhea is a genuine problem worth concern and the physician's efforts to investigate. The athlete may initially consider her amenorrhea a blessing. The physician's approach should emphasize that a thorough history may uncover the diagnosis without expensive or invasive testing.

History

A thorough history should help separate women who develop amenorrhea because of athletics from those who have another precipitating condition. The gynecologic history should include a complete menstrual history, including age at menarche; frequency, duration, and heaviness of flow; and pelvic pain. The patient should be questioned about the development of secondary sexual characteristics such as breasts, pubic hair, and clitoris. Current and past menstrual patterns associated with exercise or activity should be recorded. Finally, the history should include current method of birth control, history of pregnancy or abortion, and history of infections, especially sexually transmitted diseases.

The physician should also take a thorough activity history, indicating what activities are performed (and their intensity, frequency, duration, and mode). Nutritional factors, including eating disorders; wide swings in weight; and recent changes in weight, height, or body fat content should be investigated.

Other historical factors that could influence the menstrual cycle include perceived stress (work, sport, family, psychiatric history) and other medical problems such as thyroid dysfunction, galactorrhea, hirsutism, acne, colitis, recent trauma, and weight changes.

Physical Evaluation

The physical evaluation should include measuring the patient's height, weight, body mass index (weight/height^2) and percentage of body fat. Blood pressure, temperature, and resting pulse should also be recorded. Resting tachycardia could be a sign of hyperthyroidism, heart disease, or anemia. A good general physical examination should uncover any signs of dysmorphism, chronic illness, anemia, endocrinopathy, heart disease, or masculinization. A pelvic examination can identify questionable sex syndrome, trisomy, pregnancy, and polycystic ovary syndrome.

Common preliminary laboratory tests should be cost effective and should lead to more specific evaluations (Table 28–2). A pregnancy test is in order, as pregnancy is the most common cause of secondary amenorrhea. The thyroid-stimulating hormone assay by radioimmunoassay (RIA) is the single best test for thyroid function. Elevated prolactin is associated with pituitary microadenoma, which could cause pituitary-ovary axis dysfunction. Elevation of FSH could be due to primary ovarian failure. If the athlete is younger than 30 years,

Table 28–2. Laboratory Tests Used to Evaluate Amenorrhea*

Preliminary laboratory tests
- Urine human chorionic gonadotropin, to rule out pregnancy
- TSH by radioimmunoassay, to rule out hypo- and hyperthyroidism
- Prolactin, to rule out pituitary dysfunction
- FSH, to rule out ovarian failure
- Complete blood count, to rule out anemia
- Biochemical profile to evaluate for nutritional status, azotemia, etc.

Secondary laboratory tests
- Bone age determination, to evaluate for developmental delay
- Karyotyping, to evaluate for chromosome abnormality
- Urine hormonal assays, to evaluate for androgens
- Magnetic resonance imaging of brain to evaluate for pituitary adenoma
- Ultrasonography of pelvis, to evaluate for ovarian polycystic disease, presence of uterus, etc.
- Endometrial biopsy, for endometrial timing in evaluation of luteal phase defect
- Bone mass density, to evaluate end-organ comorbidity

* Before initiating any of these tests, a thorough history and examination are mandatory to help choose which test would be most useful and cost effective.

karyotyping is indicated to rule out mosaicism and gonadal malignancy. The incidence of gonadal malignancy is 25% in mosaicism, therefore laparotomy and oophorectomy are indicated.

TREATMENT

Treatment of amenorrhea is based on the perceived necessity for resolution of the problem. Some athletes do not perceive it as a problem, especially if any part of the treatment plan could result in a decrease in athletic performance.

All amenorrheic athletes should at least receive education about their bodies, nutrition, stress reduction, and the potential complications of osteoporosis and infertility. Most should consider reducing their training intensity, which in most women restores normal menstruation.

Athletes with delayed menarche should be considered for management with estrogen supplements. Because they cannot be presumed infertile, contraception should be discussed. It is also worthwhile to screen them for eating disorders (anorexia nervosa and bulimia) and to monitor them for osteoporosis in the future.

Athletes with secondary amenorrhea can be categorized into three treatment groups.[2] Athletes who have a luteal phase defect do not need treatment unless they desire to maintain their fertility. Athletes who exhibit euestrogenic anovulation need a progestational agent, either oral birth control pills or progesterone (Provera) during the last 5 days of their follicular phase (days 10 to 14). Athletes who have hypoestrogenemic amenorrhea can be managed with oral birth control pills, or a combination of estrogen and progesterone, or receive topical estrogen replacement therapy (Table 28–3). The standard contraindications for estrogen replacement should be kept in mind. Athletes who sustain more than one stress fracture or have more than 6 months' amenorrhea should have their bone density tested.

Table 28–3. Medications Useful in the Treatment of Athletic Amenorrhea*

Problem	*Medication and Treatment*
Euestrogenic anovulation	Medroxyprogesterone (Provera), 10 mg per day for days 10 through 14 of the menstrual cycle
Hypoestrogenemic amenorrhea	Sequential estrogen and progesterone: estrogen (Premarin), 0.625–1.25 mg/day for days 1 through 25 *and* medroxyprogesterone (Provera), 10 mg/day for days 19 through 25. *or* transdermal estradiol (Estraderm), 0.05–0.15 mg applied twice a week *and* medroxyprogesterone, 2.5–5 mg per day for days 19 through 25
Progesterone challenge test	Medroxyprogesterone (Provera), 10 mg per day for 5 days
Atrophic vaginitis and dyspareunia associated with hypoestrogenemia	Estradiol vaginal cream (Estrace, 0.01% [each gram contains 0.1 mg of estradiol]) applied every 2–3 days *or* conjugated estrogen cream (Premarin [each gram contains 0.625 mg of conjugated estrogen]) applied every 2–3 days
Birth control pills for contraception	Low-dose sequential dosage forms levonorgestrel and ethinyl estradiol triphasic regimen (Tri-Levlen or Triphasil), *or* norethindrone and ethinyl estradiol (Ovcon), *or* estradiol (Estrace), 1–2 mg/day for days 1 through 25, *and* medroxyprogesterone (Provera), 2.5–5 mg for days 19 through 25

*Information is not meant to be inclusive of all available products.
Manufacturers of prescription drugs in table:
Estrace, Mead-Johnson Laboratories, Evansville, IN
Estraderm, CIBA Consumer Pharmaceuticals, Edison, NJ
Ovcon, Mead-Johnson Laboratories, Evansville, IN
Premarin, Wyeth-Ayerst Laboratories, Philadelphia, PA
Provera, The Upjohn Company, Kalamazoo, MI
Tri-Levlen, Berlex Laboratories, Wayne, NJ
Triphasil, Wyeth-Ayerst Laboratories, Philadelphia, PA

Exercise does promote bone acquisition, so it seems natural to include exercise as part of the prevention and treatment of amenorrhea-induced osteoporosis[11,12]; however, mounting evidence shows that amenorrheic athletes have lower bone mass density in the axial skeleton compared with eumenorrheic athletes.[3,12,13]

Preliminary information indicates that calcium supplements given to amenorrheic adolescents enhance bone mineral acquisition, which may protect against future osteoporotic fracture.[14]

REFERENCES

1. Agostini, R.: Women in sports. *In* The Team Physician's Handbook. Edited by M. Mellion, W. M. Walsh, and G. L. Shelton. Philadelphia, Hanley & Belfus, 1990.

2. Gidwani, G.: The athlete and menstruation. Adolescent Med. *2*:27, 1991.
3. Drinkwater, B., et al.: Bone mineral content of amenorrheic and eumenorrheic athletes. N. Engl. J. Med. *311:*277, 1984.
4. Prior, J. C., Cameron, K., Yuen, B. H., and Thomas, J.: Menstrual cycle changes with marathon training: Anovulation and short luteal phase. Can. J. Appl. Sport Sci. *7*:173, 1982.
5. Frisch, R. E., et al.: Delayed menarche and amenorrhea in ballet dancers. N. Engl. J. Med. *303:*17, 1980.
6. Ayers, J. W.: Hypothalamic osteopenia—body weight and skeletal mass in the premenopausal woman. Clin. Obstet. Gynecol. *28:*670, 1985.
7. Myburgh, K. H., et al.: Low bone mineral density at axial and appendicular sites in amenorrheic athletes. Med. Sci. Sports. Exerc. *25:*1197, 1993.
8. Jones, K. P., Ravnikar, V. A., Tulchinsky, D., and Schiff, I.: Comparison of bone density in amenorrheic women due to athletics, weight loss, and premature menopause. Obstet. Gynecol. *66:*5, 1985.
9. Loucks, A. B., and Horvath, S. M.: Athletic amenorrhea: A review. Med. Sci. Sports. Exerc. *17:*56, 1985.
10. Lehmann, M., Foster, C., and Keul, J.: Overtraining in endurance athletes: A brief review. Med. Sci. Sports Exerc. *25*:854, 1993.
11. Huddleston, A. L., Rockwell, D., Kulund, D. N., and Harrison, R. B.: Bone mass in lifetime tennis athletes. J.A.M.A. *244:*1107, 1980.
12. Nilsson, B. E., and Westlin, N. E.: Bone density in athletes. Clin. Orthop. *77:*179, 1971.
13. Lindberg, J. et al.: Exercise-induced amenorrhea and bone density. Ann. Intern. Med. *101:*647, 1984.
14. Marcus, R., et al.: Menstrual function and bone mass in elite women distance runners. Ann. Intern. Med. *102:*158, 1985.

SUGGESTED READING

FOR FEMALE ATHLETES

Shangold, M.: The Complete Sports Medicine Book for Women. New York, Simon and Schuster, 1992.

FOR PHYSICIANS

American Academy of Pediatrics Committee on Sports Medicine: Amenorrhea in adolescent athletes. Pediatrics *84*:394, 1989.

Gidwani, G.: The athlete and menstruation. Adolescent Med. *2*:27, 1991.

Yeager, K. K., Agostini, R., Nattiv, A., and Drinkwater, B.: The female athlete triad: disordered eating, amenorrhea, osteoporosis. Med. Sci. Sports Exerc. *25*:775, 1993.

29 *Douglas G. Browning*

Diabetes in Athletes

"Sure, it's a disease, but it's a disease that you can handle yourself. My life is no different than anybody else's. The shot to me is nothing. It's my normal routine—like waking up and putting on my pants. You have to be careful with diabetes. It's not a disease that you can take lightly, and if you don't accept it, you are going to have problems. But if you know what it's all about, you can live a full life."

Ron Santo, former Chicago White Sox infielder

Diabetes mellitus, it is estimated, affects as many as 11 million Americans. Type I diabetes affects younger people and requires insulin therapy; Type II diabetes usually appears during middle age or later, is often associated with obesity, and often can be managed with diet and exercise—alone or in combination with oral hypoglycemic medication. The frequency of diabetes guarantees that every provider of health care will have some experience with it, and many of the patients (especially younger Type I diabetics) will be active in sports and athletics. For diabetes patients who are not physically active, exercise may benefit their health, either as a preventive measure or by improving control of the disease. Men who exercise more than five times per week have a 42% lower risk of developing adult-onset diabetes mellitus than men who exercise less than once a week.[1] Until recently, exercise was not emphasized in the management of diabetes, although it has been a component of overall treatment since the 1920s.

More recently, athletes with diabetes mellitus have been able to excel. Ron Santo, diagnosed with Type I diabetes at age 19, was a successful infielder for the Chicago White Sox. Jim "Catfish" Hunter (diagnosed at age 32) pitched for the New York Yankees. Other diabetic professional baseball players include Bill Gulickson (Montreal Expos pitcher), Ty Cobb, and Jackie Robinson. In ice hockey, Bobby Clarke (diagnosed at age 14) played for the Philadelphia Flyers. In football, Wade Wilson (diagnosed at age 26) was a quarterback with the Minnesota Vikings, Calvin Muhammad was a receiver with the Washington Redskins, and Coley O'Brien was diagnosed while he was a quarterback with Notre Dame. Athletes with diabetes have been prominent in almost every other sport as well, including golf, triathlon, marathon, and tennis.

Diabetics, once they achieve good metabolic control, can train essentially as "nondiabetics" do. Blood glucose monitoring may be required to ensure that control is maintained. Urine monitoring for ketones may also be necessary at times, to check for ketonuria. The athlete needs to be aware of the warning signs of high and low blood sugar and ketoacidosis.

More than 50 summer camps now operating in the continental United States have been set up specifically for diabetic children, to allow them to learn to participate in physical activity without worry.[2] The International Diabetic Athletes Association now has chapters in at least 15 cities in the United States as well as in Canada, England, France, Germany, and Japan and other foreign countries.[3]

DIAGNOSIS

Signs of diabetes include polyuria and polydipsia. Rapid weight loss and ketonemia or ketonuria are usually present at the time of diagnosis of Type I diabetes. The diagnosis is confirmed by repetitive measurements of fasting blood sugars higher than 140 mg/dl. The diagnosis of Type II diabetes can be confirmed by an abnormal result on a glucose tolerance test. Health care providers should always keep in mind that diabetes, especially Type II, is associated with increased risk of hypertension, hyperlipidemia, and atherosclerosis.

MANAGEMENT

Consistent good control of blood glucose appears to minimize typical sequelae of diabetes, including retinopathy, microangiopathy, and neuropathy.[4,5] These complications can be reversed, to some degree with prolonged tight blood glucose control. Such control is usually achieved by a combination of appropriate diet, regular exercise, and medical management. Medical management of Type I diabetes usually requires a combination of short-acting (regular) insulin and intermediate- to long-acting (NPH) insulin; whereas Type II diabetes may often be controlled with exercise and diet alone or with the addition of an oral hypoglycemic agent. Monitoring glycosylated hemoglobin allows for monitoring of long-term diabetes control.[6] Increasing exercise and fitness has been associated with decreased levels of glycosylated hemoglobin.[7]

The diabetic's diet should be designed to provide a steady blood glucose level. Well-balanced meals with a preponderance of carbohydrate, some protein, and a small amount of fat (protein and fat buffer entry of glucose into the bloodstream) are recommended. Glycogen (carbohydrate) storage is an insulin-dependent process that requires good diabetes control. A carbohydrate-rich diet promotes glycogen storage.[8] Afternoon and evening snacks may help avoid hypoglycemia, but binge eating should be avoided.

Both types of diabetes predispose to hypoglycemia. Type I patients tend to exhibit ketoacidosis, which is rare in Type II diabetics. Hypoglycemia and ketoacidosis can be minimized with appropriate monitoring of blood glucose and ketones. Type II diabetics can improve their metabolic control by weight loss achieved by dietary control. Exercise is an ancillary measure in weight loss and glucose regulation, but the effect of exercise alone is limited.[9]

BENEFITS OF EXERCISE

The motivation to improve as an athlete may enhance a diabetic's self-management, including the willingness to assess blood glucose more frequently and to pay closer attention to diet. The discipline learned in self-management of diabetes may improve an athlete's ability to perform.

Exercise increases muscle sensitivity to insulin and may decrease insulin production.[10,11] It also increases uptake and utilization of glucose, thus decreasing the blood glucose level. This effect is most pronounced in insulin-treated diabetics and occurs only if therapy is satisfactory; for those with poorly regulated ketotic diabetes, exercise actually accentuates hyperglycemia and may increase ketonuria, particularly if exercise is prolonged.[10,12]

Acute effects of exercise, in both types of diabetics, are well understood, but chronic effects are not, particularly for Type I patients. Anecdotal and biochemical evidence clearly suggests numerous longterm benefits, including weight loss, reduced risk of cardiovascular disease, increased insulin sensitivity, and improved regulation of blood glucose. Recent data show that Type I diabetics who were high school athletes have a significantly lower incidence of cardiovascular disease as adults than those who were not athletes.[13] Participation in team sports in high school or college is not associated with a decrease in the prevalence of microvascular disease (severe retinopathy or blindness) later in life, though in men (but not in women) it is associated with a decreased prevalence of macrovascular disease (i.e., cardiovascular disease and overall mortality).[13] Regular exercise has been proven to reduce blood glucose levels; however, occasional intermittent exercise (e.g., such as the "weekend warrior" achieves) is associated with hypoglycemia during activity, and not with any proven long-term benefit.[14]

Physical trainability and performance are probably optimized when the blood glucose value is consistently "good." Such stability produces more normal substrate utilization, reduced protein degradation (with greater muscle hypertrophy and possibly increased mitochondrial enzymes), greater amounts of glycogen in muscle and liver, and increased volume of body water (increased heat tolerance).

Endurance training increases fat utilization secondary to increases in mitochondrial density and associated enzymes.[12] Training also increases muscle and liver glycogen stores, which allows athletes to be active much longer before they need supplemental carbohydrate. Finally, it reduces blood glucose uptake, which diminishes the likelihood of hypoglycemia. Good control of blood glucose facilitates development of muscle mass. Adequate insulin enhances normal uptake and use of amino acids, whereas inadequate insulin promotes protein degradation and water loss.[12]

The psychological effects of exercise include improved self-esteem and self-confidence. Limitation of activity because of diabetes is a negative reinforcer. Diabetes should not be used—by athletes, parents, or coaches—as an excuse to avoid participation in athletics.

Other benefits of exercise include reduced risk of cardiovascular disease,[6,7,10] reduced levels of total cholesterol and of very–low-density lipoprotein cholesterol, and a small decline in low-density lipoprotein cholesterol. Exercise also increases high-density lipoprotein cholesterol and reduces triglycerides and lowers blood pressure. Exercise also helps manage stress. It increases insulin sensitivity, so the requirement for insulin or oral hypoglycemic medication may decrease. For those who have Type II diabetes, occasionally, glucose control may improve to the point where medication may be discontinued.

CONTRAINDICATIONS FOR EXERCISE

Exercise electrocardiography is warranted (1) if the patient is older than 30 or 40 years, (2) if the duration of diabetes exceeds 10 to 25 years, or (3) if symptomatic atherosclerotic cardiovascular disease is present.[12] It should also be considered if the patient has other primary risk factors for cardiovascular disease.

If the patient exhibits peripheral neuropathy or microangiopathy, exercise that traumatizes the feet should be avoided. Swimming and cycling are good alternatives to walking and jogging. Diabetes patients should examine their feet daily and keep nails carefully trimmed. Blisters, corns, and calluses should be minimized by wearing properly fitting shoes and socks and by periodically filing calluses with a pumice stone. Foot injuries should be treated immediately, to prevent complications.

Proliferative retinopathy precludes strenuous or jarring activity, including weight lifting and contact sports, gymnastics, running, and any activity that raises the heart rate dramatically and raises systolic blood pressure beyond 180 mm Hg. Scuba diving is contraindicated for these persons, because the increased water pressure is a hazard. Exercise while inverted, including some yoga positions, headstands, and hanging upside down, are also potentially dangerous.

EXERCISE GUIDELINES

Good blood glucose control should be established before a diabetes patient starts an exercise program because serum blood glucose levels change dramatically after activity begins (Fig. 29–1). Blood glucose should be measured before, possibly during, and after exercise (Fig. 29–2). This allows the patient and the physician to study the blood glucose response to various exercise conditions with consecutive days of hard training, tournaments, and reduced training days before competition. The higher the blood glucose level at the onset of activity the more it drops during exercise.[15] If the blood glucose value exceeds 250 to 300 mg/dl at the start of exercise, it tends to rise, rather than fall, *during* exercise. If ketosis is present before exercise, ketone production rises.[10,12] These effects are due to the influence of counter-regulatory hormones, such as low insulin, catecholamines, and cortisol.

Pregame anxiety mimics hypoglycemia, leading many diabetic athletes to overeat before competition, to treat

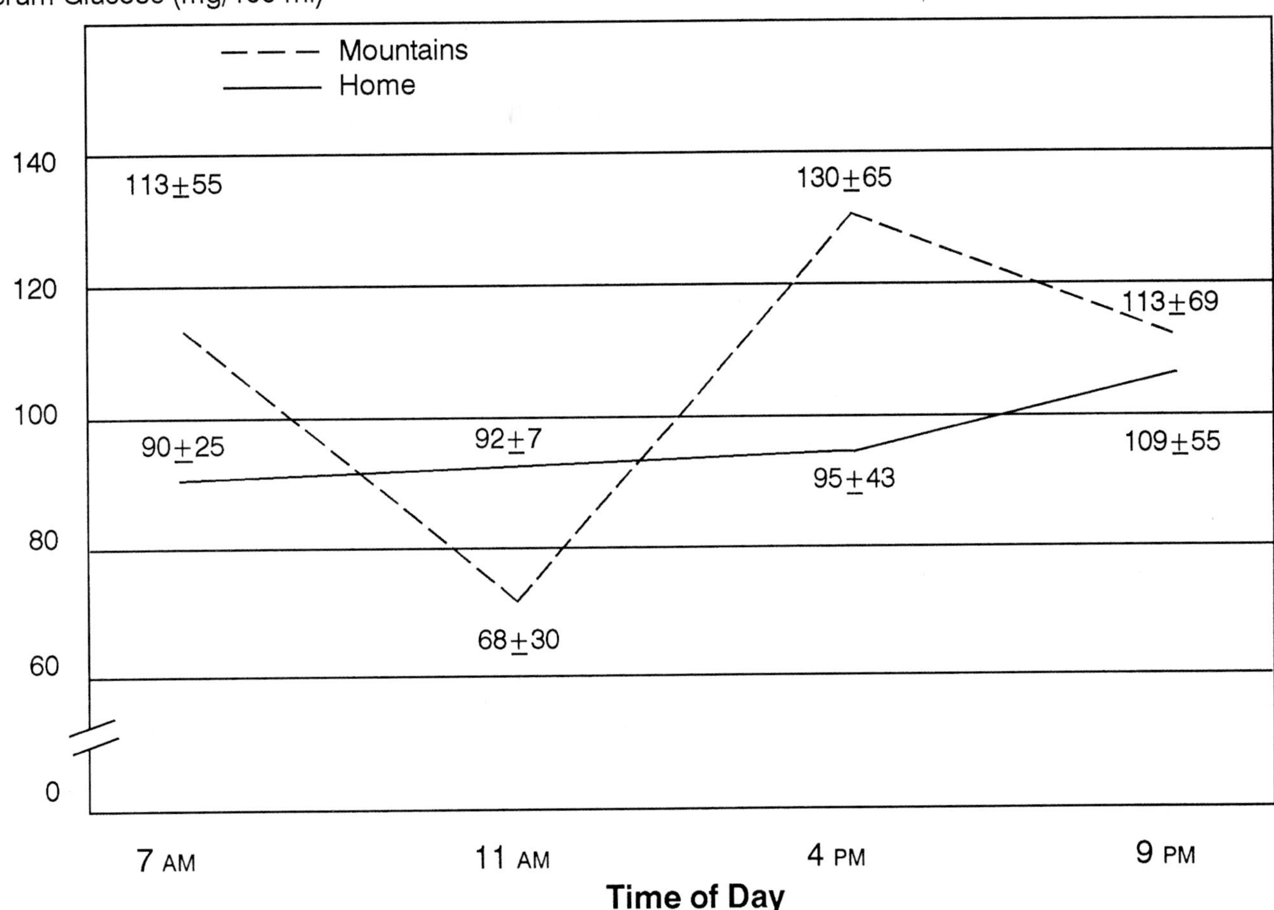

Fig. 29–1. The average serum glucose levels for a 38-year-old, insulin-dependent diabetic man during a 6-day period at home, when he exercised for short periods of time, running 5 miles a day, compared to the averages for a 6-day hiking and backpacking trip that required prolonged daily activity. (Berg, K.: Blood glucose regulation in an insulin-dependent backpacker. Physician Sportsmed. *11*(12):103, 1983.)

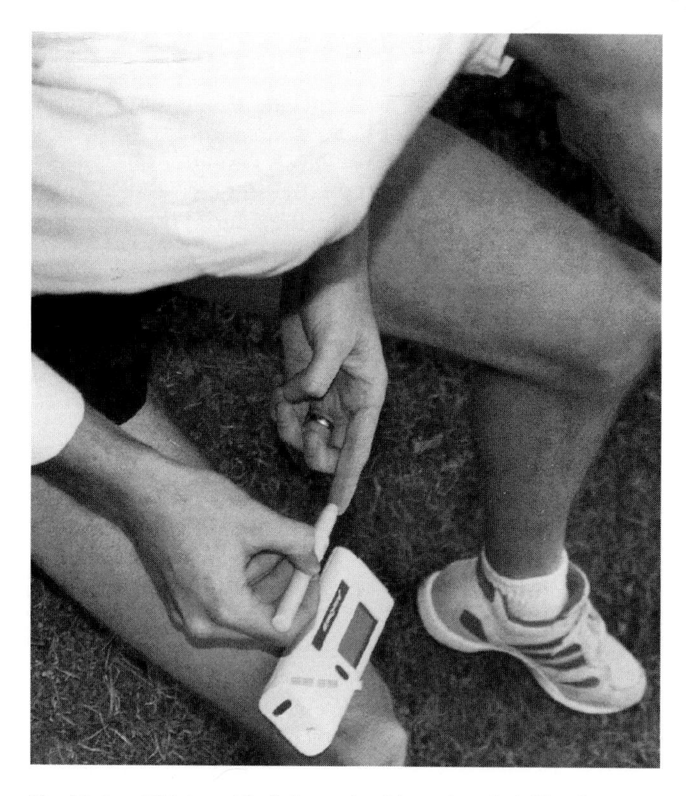

Fig. 29–2. Athletes with diabetes should monitor their blood sugar level before, during, and after exercising.

what they perceive as an insulin reaction. They may exaggerate the needed reduction in the dosage of insulin or oral hypoglycemic medication, again leading to hyperglycemia. These inappropriate steps may lead to accentuated ketoacidosis or poor performance, owing to limited use of muscle glycogen and glucose and reduced blood pH. Before an athlete with diabetes competes in an evening event, he or she should experiment with altering insulin and food intake and then exercising under conditions similar to the competition (e.g., same time and similar energy expenditure). Because insulin sensitivity is affected for at least 4 hours—and as long as 24 hours—after exercise, hypoglycemia may occur during sleep. At times blood glucose may have to be assessed in the middle of the night, to prevent this.

Exercise performed within 1 hour of injection of regular insulin speeds its absorption and reduces the time to peak effect. The same is true for about 2½ hours after injection of intermediate insulin. Type I diabetics typically inject insulin into the thigh, gluteal area, abdomen, triceps, or shoulder. The injection site can be altered, depending on the activity, to prevent this effect.[16,17] If exercise is commonly done soon after injection of regular insulin, no alteration may be needed, because the athlete has probably learned to deal with the effect. Elevation of body temperature also increases the rate of insulin absorption. The duration of warm-up and amount of clothing worn during warm-up should be reasonably consistent if exercise occurs within the first hour after injecting regular insulin.

Consistent daily energy expenditure facilitates blood glucose control. Extra medication or reduction of food intake may be necessary on days of reduced activity, whereas less medication or greater food intake may be appropriate on days of increased training duration or intensity. When exercise lasts several hours (e.g., triathlon, mountaineering, cycling, tournament play), for Type I diabetics the basal dose of insulin should be reduced by as much as 50%. Supplemental food (about one carbohydrate exchange or 60 kcal) can be consumed every 30 to 45 minutes, and blood glucose monitoring during the event may be helpful for diabetics in such sports.

Medication requirements are reduced in the early months of training (a 10 to 40% reduction is typical) and remain lower as long as training continues.[10,18] Mature exercising diabetic athletes usually take less than 0.5 to 0.6 units of insulin per kilogram body weight, whereas the typical dose is 0.5 to 1.0 units per kilogram.[14] Some Type II patients may, eventually, need no oral hypoglycemic medication, owing to the combined effects on insulin sensitivity of fat loss and exercise.

Good blood glucose control facilitates glycogen storage in skeletal muscle. This reduces the likelihood of glycogen depletion after consecutive days of vigorous training or during a prolonged endurance event. Recent evidence suggests that the amount of water stored with skeletal muscle glycogen has a powerful effect on exercise capacity in a hot environment. Many marginally controlled diabetics, particularly, have difficulty exercising in warm environments, partly because of reduced muscle stores of glycogen and water.

AVOIDING HYPOGLYCEMIA ASSOCIATED WITH EXERCISE

It is imperative that the athlete recognize early symptoms of "insulin reaction" or hypoglycemia, including fatigue, weakness, tremor, headache, hunger, or numbness or tingling of the lips or extremities. Someone else who is trained to recognize the signs of hypoglycemia (e.g., a coach or another athlete) should always be around a diabetic athlete. Such signs include staggering gait, slurred speech, clumsy movements (e.g., dropping or spilling things), decreasing performance, confusion, and irritability.

Many diabetics fear that exercise will produce hypoglycemia. The risk of hypoglycemia may be reduced by measuring the blood glucose value before exercise and by following certain precautions. Food should be readily available for supplemental feeding (with the athletic trainer or coach, in the diabetic's locker, on the bus, or on their person, in a pocket of running shorts or in a pack on a bicycle). Additional snacks (fruit, juices, crackers) may be required between a pregame meal and the game, or at halftime or breaks, or after the game. If the preactivity blood glucose value is lower than 100 mg/dl, a pre-exercise snack might be taken. If the glucose level is higher than 100 mg/dl, a small snack may be needed after the activity. If the blood glucose value is higher than 250 mg/dl, exercise should be interdicted until the urine ketone value is negative,[8] because the action of counter-regulatory hormones may cause both the blood glucose and the ketone level to rise during exercise.[12] Active participation in physical activity requires an extra 600 to 800 kcal/hr.[12]

Hypoglycemia is more likely to occur during exercise in the evening and is least likely to occur in the morning, because of a circadian variation in growth hormone level. A diabetic who exercises in the evening should reduce the amount of insulin taken that peaks after eating and during the rest of the evening (by about 20%) *or* more food should be consumed before, and possibly after, exercise. Athletes should consume a light carbohydrate meal 2 hours before the event. To exhibit nearly normal metabolism with activity, diabetics must have available some active insulin to facilitate glucose uptake in the muscle. Those who run early in the morning should take part of their daily insulin as long-lasting insulin the evening before the run; otherwise taking a fraction (25 to 50%) of the usual dose 2½ to 3 hours before exercise is acceptable.[19] The diabetic athlete should avoid exercising in the evening or, if exercise cannot be avoided at this time of day, should develop a plan to meet the reduced insulin need. If an unusually large amount of energy is expended, or if exercise is done in the evening, the athlete should expect possible hypoglycemia at night and the next day. Extra blood glucose monitoring is advisable. A carbohydrate-rich diet restores glycogen to pre-exercise levels within 24 hours.[8]

During and after exercise, hypoglycemia is more common—and more severe—in (1) tightly controlled patients and (2) those who have had Type I diabetes longer than 10 years. In the latter group it occurs even in those who exhibit no clinical signs of autonomic neuropathy.

Insulin that peaks during exercise should be reduced when hypoglycemia occurs with such activity. Short-acting insulin, normally taken before a meal, might not be needed on days of activity, whereas more insulin might be required on nontraining days. The muscles in the region where short-acting insulin is injected should not be exercised for an hour.

Alcohol intake should be avoided during training, because it inhibits enzymes responsible for glycogenolysis and gluconeogenesis, readily causing hypoglycemia.[6] Other drugs and medications should also be reviewed for possible effects on blood glucose.

For the athlete who has become hypoglycemic, a subcutaneous or intramuscular injection of 1 mg of glucagon raises the blood glucose level within minutes. It is advisable to prescribe that a glucagon emergency kit be on hand during physical activity when any diabetic may be at risk for hypoglycemia, particularly when a newly diagnosed diabetic resumes physical activity for the first time. Someone on site, other than the diabetic, should be instructed in administration of the medicine.

CLEARANCE FOR SPORTS

Stable diabetes control—glucose levels between 60 and 300 mg/dl is essential—with no evidence of ketosis, prior to participation in sports. An athlete who is cleared for unlimited participation should exhibit *no* diabetic complications. The athlete should have a thorough understanding of the prevention and treatment of hypoglycemia and should consider wearing a medical alert tag that specifies diabetes. A cautious trial of training and competition should be attempted first, before full clearance for participation is given. Communication with coaches and athletic trainers about management of diabetic athletes is extremely important.[12]

It is easier to control blood glucose in athletes who participate in continuous, progressive, steady, aerobic sports (e.g., cycling, walking, cross-country skiing) than in those whose sport requires short, explosive bursts of energy (e.g., football). Wrestlers may be at greater risk because athletes want to be in the lowest possible weight class. Scuba diving may be ill-advised, owing to the potential for disaster. Skydiving, mountaineering, auto or motorcycle racing, hang-gliding, and windsurfing all may pose hazards particular to diabetes patients. This does not mean that participation in such sports is absolutely contraindicated, only that the athlete and the family should be informed of the risks before participation and should be willing to assume those risks. Diabetics should be advised not to practice alone. Those who participate in marathons and other endurance events, especially, need to have carbohydrates available for consumption during the competition, to avoid hypoglycemia.

Complications of long-term diabetes (15 to 25 years) may delay healing of injuries. Because of this, it may be ill-advised to recommend that a 60-year-old, long-standing diabetic participate in high-risk sports (e.g., downhill skiing).

For endurance events in extremely cold weather (e.g., dog sled race, mountain climbing, cross-country skiing), insulin may be strapped to the body or placed in a prewarmed thermos to prevent freezing. Clinitest tablets are most appropriate for glucose testing in these situations, as they generate their own heat in the test tube.

CONCLUSION

A list of practical recommendations for physical activity for young diabetics regarding insulin, diet, and exercise follows:

1. A good level of metabolic control should be achieved before any physical activity is undertaken. Neither hyperglycemia (>300 mg/dl) nor ketonuria is favorable to exercise.
2. Measurement of blood glucose concentration before, during, and after the activity may be necessary to facilitate good metabolic control without hypoglycemia.

3. A diabetic athlete should always have available some sugar or a glucagon injection kit, and, preferably, both.
4. The intensity and duration of an activity should be increased in a slow, progressive fashion.
5. In the few hours preceding exercise, ingesting slowly absorbed carbohydrates, to replete glycogen reserves in liver and muscle, facilitates maintenance of adequate blood glucose levels.
6. In case of unforeseen physical activity, increasing glucose consumption immediately before, during, and after exercise decreases the risk of hypoglycemia.
7. With planned activities, the insulin dose for the period during and after intense muscle exertion should be reduced. The reduction can vary from 10 to 50%, depending on the intensity of the exercise.
8. Insulin should not be injected at a site that will be intensively involved in muscle activity.
9. Physical exercise should not be performed when the effect of insulin is at its peak.
10. If the activity involves prolonged endurance, ingesting carbohydrates just before, (every 35 to 40 minutes) during, and after the exercise should maintain adequate blood glucose levels.
11. The blood glucose value should be measured before retiring on the evening after major physical activity, to avoid hypoglycemia during the night.
12. Every modification of insulin dose and every change in nutritional status requires evaluation of that change's effect on exercise and performance.
13. Persons who accompany a diabetic athlete should be aware of the procedures for and treatment of severe hypoglycemia (glucagon injection).

FUTURE

New studies indicate the benefit of tight blood glucose control in preventing long-term complications.[4,5] Future management of diabetes may involve more frequent insulin dosing or use of implanted insulin pumps. Finding a cure for diabetes is unlikely in the near future, but further testing and research may lead to better methods of preventing the development of the disease.

REFERENCES

1. Manson, J. E., Nathan, D. M., Krolewski, A. S., et al.: A prospective study on exercise and incidence of diabetes among U.S. male physicians. J.A.M.A. *268*:63, 1992.
2. Murphy, P.: Children with medical conditions *can* go to summer camp. Physician Sportsmed. *15*(7):177, 1987.
3. Thurm, U., and Harper, P. N.: I'm running on insulin: Summary of the history of the International Diabetic Athletes Association. Diabetes Care *15*(Suppl. 4):1811, 1992.
4. The Diabetes Control and Complications Trial Research Group: The effect of intensive treatment of diabetes on the development and progression of long-term complications in insulin-dependent diabetes mellitus. N. Engl. J. Med. *329*:977, 1993.
5. Reichard, P., Nilsson, B. Y., and Rosenqvist, U.: The effect of long-term intensified insulin treatment on the development of microvascular complications of diabetes mellitus. N. Engl. J. Med. *329*:304, 1993.
6. Blackett, P. R.: Child and adolescent athletes with diabetes. Physician Sportsmed. *16*(3):133, 1988.
7. Campaigne, B. N., et al.: The effects of physical training on blood lipid profiles in adolescents with insulin-dependent diabetes mellitus. Physician Sportsmed. *13*(12):83, 1985.
8. Franz, M. J.: Nutrition: Can it give athletes with diabetes a boost? Diabetes Educator *17*:163, 1991.
9. National Institutes of Health Consensus Development Conference on Diet and Exercise in Non-Insulin Dependent Diabetes Mellitus, draft statement. Bethesda, MD, National Institute of Diabetes and Digestive and Kidney Diseases and the National Institutes of Health Office of Medical Application of Research, 1986.
10. Dorchy, H., and Poortmans, J.: Sport and the diabetic child. Sports Med. *7*:248, 1989.
11. LeBlanc, J., et al.: Effects of physical training and adiposity on glucose metabolism and 125I-insulin binding. J. Appl. Physiol. *46*:235, 1979.
12. Hanson, P., and Kochan, R.: Exercise and diabetes. Prim. Care *10*:653, 1983.
13. LaPorte, R. E., Dorman, J. S., Tajima, N., et al.: Pittsburgh Insulin-Dependent Diabetes Mellitus Morbidity and Mortality Study: Physical activity and diabetic complications. Pediatrics *78*:1027, 1986.
14. Robbins, D. C., and Carleton, S.: Managing the diabetic athlete. Physician Sportsmed. *17*(12):45, 1989.
15. Stratton, R., Wilson, D. P., and Endres, R. K.: Acute glycemic effects of exercise in adolescents with insulin-dependent diabetes mellitus. Physician Sportsmed. *16*(3):150, 1988.
16. Etzwiler, D. D.: When the diabetic wants to be an athlete. Physician Sportsmed. *2*(2):45, 1974.
17. Koivisto, V. A., and Felig, P.: Effects of leg exercise on insulin absorption in diabetic patients. N. Engl. J. Med. *298*:79, 1978.
18. Costill, D. L., Cleary, P., Fink, W. J., et al.: Training adaptations in skeletal muscle of juvenile diabetics. Diabetes *28*:818, 1979.
19. Costill, D. L., Miller, J. M., and Fink, W. J.: Energy metabolism in diabetic distance runners. Physician Sportsmed. *8*(10):64, 1980.

30 *Robert O'Neil Snoddy, Jr.*

Exercise-Induced Asthma

Exercise-induced asthma is a common problem: it was described in the second century by Areatus the Cappadocian. Even today, however, often it goes unrecognized. This is unfortunate, because exercise-induced asthma is a condition that, if untreated, may adversely affect an athlete's performance. If the condition is recognized and treated appropriately, however, the results can be excellent. For example, U.S. athletes with a history of exercise-induced asthma won 41 medals in the 1984 Olympics. In the 1988 Summer Olympics, 52 of 667 U.S. athletes had confirmed exercise-induced asthma. The athletes with exercise-induced asthma won medals with the same frequency as those who were unaffected.[1]

For research purposes, exercise-induced asthma is defined as a 10% decrease in forced expiratory volume or peak expiratory flow rate on postexercise pulmonary function tests, as compared with pre-exercise values.[2] Using this definition, exercise-induced asthma is present in 12 to 15% of the general population: 40% of people with "allergies" and 80 to 90% of those who have clinical asthma.[1] Approximately 9% of patients with exercise-induced asthma have no history of allergy or asthma. Exercise-induced asthma is more common in children, but it affects patients of all ages. Some 5000 deaths per year in the United States are attributed to asthma, but exercise-induced asthma is very rarely life threatening.[3]

The pathophysiology of exercise-induced asthma is ill-understood. Several mechanisms have been proposed: (1) the presence of thermally sensitive neuroreceptors in the bronchial epithelium that trigger bronchospasm; (2) a hyperosmolar state caused by water loss in this epithelium that leads to bronchospasm; (3) the release of mediators by epithelial mast cells in response to irritation; (4) vascular hyper-reactivity of the bronchial mucosa; and (5) bronchospasm caused by loss of carbon dioxide owing to hyperventilation. While all of these mechanisms may contribute, it is generally agreed that, overall, respiratory water loss and airway cooling during exercise trigger exercise-induced asthma.[4]

In a patient with exercise-induced asthma, bronchospasm usually begins 10 to 15 minutes after exercise and subsides spontaneously in 30 to 60 minutes.[5] This phenomenon is referred to as the "early response." Some athletes have a second bronchospastic event 4 to 12 hours later, which is called the "late response."

To trigger an episode of exercise-induced asthma, typically, the athlete must exercise enough to raise the heart rate to 170 bpm and must maintain this level 5 to 8 minutes. The severity of exercise-induced asthma varies with the duration and intensity of exercise. Increasing the stimulus results in a progressive decrease in peak expiratory flow rate, but this reduction "plateaus" at about 35%. Prolonged exercise may actually result in less bronchospasm than moderate workouts, however, and the athlete may report an ability to "run through" his symptoms. The severity of an episode of exercise-induced asthma may also be affected by environmental conditions and the state of any underlying lung disease.

The diagnosis of exercise-induced asthma should be considered in patients who present with postexertional cough, chest tightness, shortness of breath, or fatigue. Some athletes may complain of postexertional nasal congestion. The diagnosis should also be considered in athletes who are described by their coaches as responding poorly to conditioning programs. Such athletes are often wrongly accused of being out of shape or "dogging it." Children with exercise-induced asthma may present with postexertional stomachache. Parents of very young children with exercise-induced asthma may report that they cough after a play session or seem to avoid vigorous play.

The initial evaluation of a person suspected of having exercise-induced asthma begins with the history, which should include a description of the symptoms and the circumstances under which they occur. The patient should be asked about allergies and nonexertional asthma or other lung disease. It is important to remember, however, that 9% of patients with exercise-induced asthma have no history of these concurrent conditions.

The physical examination at rest is usually normal, but wheezing and other findings of increased airway resistance may be present after exercise. Baseline pulmonary function tests are usually normal as well, but they may indicate underlying asthma.

A diagnosis of exercise-induced asthma is confirmed in one of several ways. Pulmonary function testing may be performed before and after exercise. The exercise challenge can be accomplished in many ways, but it should be stringent enough so that the athlete reaches 80 to 90% of maximum heart rate and sustains this level for 5 to 8 minutes. A drop in forced expiratory volume of 10 to 15% in the postexercise studies is considered a positive finding. A 25% drop in forced expiratory fraction may indicate small-airway involvement. The pulmonary function tests may need to be performed at intervals for up to 30 minutes after exercise to detect these changes. A negative result on the exercise challenge test does not completely rule out the diagnosis. In some cases, a methacholine challenge test is useful to establish bronchial hypersensitivity. Finally, in a patient with a history typical for the disease, a successful therapeutic trial with an inhaled β-agonist is usually considered sufficient to make the diagnosis informally.

When the diagnosis is exercise-induced asthma, further studies may be indicated, to search for exacerbating factors such as allergies or infection. Before medical therapy is instituted, patients with exercise-induced asthma should be instructed in nonpharmacologic management of the disease. For some patients, such measures may obviate medication.[6] If the patient is a young child, the parents should be included in the education process.

Paradoxically, the initial management of patients with exercise-induced asthma includes judicious use of exercise. Short bursts of exercise lead to reflex bronchodilatation,[7] and trained athletes exhibit a greater degree of exercise-induced bronchodilatation than do sedentary persons. The training effect also increases the athlete's VO_2max, increases work capacity at a given heart rate, and decreases heart rate at a given workload. The patient's maximum voluntary ventilation is also increased, possibly owing to improved efficiency of the respiratory muscles. All of these adaptations contribute to reducing the symptoms of exercise-induced asthma.

Patients with exercise-induced asthma may benefit from choosing an appropriate sport. Sports that involve short bursts of activity followed by periods of rest (e.g., golf, discus throwing, baseball, tennis, circuit weight training) or sports performed in warm, humid environments (e.g., swimming, water polo) may be less "asthmagenic" than other sports. The choice of position within a given sport (e.g., goalie in soccer) may also help. Finally, the choice of geographic location for participation (e.g., Alabama instead of Minnesota) may be important.

During workouts, athletes should be encouraged to breathe slowly through the nose and avoid hyperventilation. They should avoid known allergens and environmental irritants, before and during exercise. In cold, dry environments, wearing a mask or scarf over the mouth and nose may reduce symptoms.

After a bronchospasm episode, most athletes experience a refractory period during which further exercise does not lead to recurrent bronchospasm. This period usually lasts 30 to 90 minutes after the episode of exercise-induced asthma. Athletes with exercise-induced asthma should warm up 45 to 60 minutes before their events to take advantage of this phenomenon. One author suggests that 10 to 12 10-second sprints may induce the refractory state without triggering an episode of exercise-induced asthma.[8]

Finally, patients with clinically significant baseline asthma should have their disease controlled as much as possible before athletic participation. For patients who are not taking maintenance medications and who do not achieve acceptable control with nonpharmacologic therapy, several medical treatment options are available.

The drug of first choice for the treatment of exercise-induced asthma is an inhaled β-agonist.[9] Athletes should use it 10 to 15 minutes before exercising. The drug can also be used to reduce symptoms that occur after exercise. As many as 95% of exercise-induced asthma patients have good results with this treatment. Oral β-agonists are less useful because of longer-delayed action and increased side effects.

Inhaled cromolyn sodium is also effective as a prophylaxis. It should be used 10 to 20 minutes before exercise. It is rated up to 87% effective, but in controlled trials it was less effective than β-agonists. Cromolyn sodium is not useful for reducing symptoms once they have occurred, though its use after an episode of exercise-induced asthma may prevent the "late response." This drug is useful for patients who do not respond to β-agonists and for those who cannot tolerate their side effects. In some patients, cromolyn and β-agonists may be combined. Nedocromil, a drug with properties similar to those of cromolyn, was recently approved by the U.S. Food and Drug Administration.

Theophylline is partially effective for the control of exercise-induced asthma, but side effects usually limit its use. Antihistamines are generally ineffective, though some patients benefit from their use. Anticholinergic drugs, such as inhaled ipratropium, may help limit symptoms once an episode of exercise-induced asthma has been triggered, but these medications are not useful for prophylaxis. Patients with exercise-induced nasal congestion may benefit from a trial of a topical decongestant. Steroids, given either by inhaler or systemically, are of little use in the therapy of exercise-induced asthma.

Calcium channel blockers have been shown to be of some benefit to patients with exercise-induced asthma, but their long-term use has not been thoroughly studied. The clinician may consider giving them to patients with exercise-induced asthma who have another indication for calcium channel–blocker therapy, such as hypertension. Another author has suggested that β-blockers may be useful, but further documentation is not available.

Physicians who care for athletes participating in organized competitions must be aware of the rules and regulations of the governing body regarding participants' use of medications. For example, the International Olympic Committee allows the use of theophylline, cromolyn, and selected β-agonists. Most athletic organizations require advanced written notification if an athlete is using a β-agonist to control exercise-induced asthma.

REFERENCES

1. McCarthy, P.: Wheezing or breezing through exercise-induced asthma. Physician Sportsmed. *17*(7):125, 1989.
2. Anderson, S.: Issues in exercise-induced asthma. J. Allergy Clin. Immunol. *76*:736, 1985.
3. McFadden, E.: Fatal and near-fatal asthma. N. Engl. J. Med. *324*:409, 1991.
4. Afrasiabi, R., and Spector, S. L.: Exercise-induced asthma. Physician Sportsmed. *19*(5):49, 1991.
5. Exercise and asthma, a roundtable. Physician Sportsmed. *12*(1):59, 1984.
6. Katz, R. M.: Prevention with and without the use of medications for exercise-induced asthma. Med. Sci. Sports Exerc. *18*:331, 1986.
7. Haas, F., et al.: Effect of aerobic training on forced expiratory airflow in exercising asthmatic humans. J. Appl. Physiol. *63*:1230, 1987.
8. AAP issues statement on exercise induced asthma in children. Am. Fam. Physician. *40*:314, 1989.
9. Drugs for ambulatory asthma. Med. Lett. *35*:11, 1993.

31

Lawrence D. Rink

Cardiac Problems and Sudden Death in Athletes

In recent years there has been a marked increase in interest in sudden death in athletes. Though this is an unusually rare phenomenon, when a young athlete dies suddenly and unexpectedly, sensational stories make headlines not only in the local newspapers but in the national and international press. The recent deaths of Hank Gathers and Reggie Lewis bring this rare, but tragic, problem to the forefront.[1] Some 25 to 50% of athletes who suffer sudden death have had suspicious symptoms or a history that suggests they could be at risk. Available screening methods should limit the incidence of sudden death in athletes.

DEFINITION OF SUDDEN DEATH

The definitions of sudden death are many. In this chapter, we define *sudden death* as death that occurs within 6 hours of onset of symptoms. Most physicians regard as sudden death one that occurs within 1 hour of event, and the World Health Organization's definition is death within 24 hours of onset of symptoms.

PREVALENCE IN ATHLETES

Sudden death in athletes is always a rare occurrence, but the risk varies according to the athlete's age. Estimates of sudden death in the 1- to 22-year-old age group range between 1.3 and 13.8 in 100,000, and there is marked variability year to year.[2–5] This would amount to about 600 deaths per year in the United States. Sudden death is much more frequent in boys than in girls. The incidence related to sports participation is even lower: sudden death involving athletes in specific sports occur at the rate of one per 50,000 player hours of rugby,[6] one per 13,000 to 26,000 person hours of cross-country skiing,[7] and one jogging death per 7620 joggers (30 to 64 years old) per year, or one per 396,000 person hours of jogging.[8]

DOES EXERCISE INCREASE THE RISK OF SUDDEN DEATH?

Although it is difficult to get exact statistics, it does appear that persons are at higher risk for sudden death during or immediately after exercise than while they are sedentary. Although studies suggest exercise may increase the risk of sudden death, controlled exercise is safe for patients with known coronary artery disease.

CAUSES OF SUDDEN DEATH IN ATHLETES

Accurate information on sudden death in athletes or during exercise is difficult to obtain. In 1931, the American Football Coaches Association initiated the first annual survey of football fatalities. In 1977, the National Collegiate Athletic Association initiated a national survey of catastrophic football injuries. In 1992, this research was expanded to all sports for both men and women at the high school and college levels, and a National Center for Catastrophic Sports Injury Research was established at Chapel Hill, North Carolina.[9] Investigators divide catastrophic injuries into three categories: (1) death; (2) nonfatal injury (i.e., permanent severe functional neurologic disability); and (3) serious injury (i.e., neurologic impairment with complete recovery) (Table 31–1). Catastrophic injuries are classified as direct (injury resulting from participation in the skills of the sport) or indirect (illness or injury caused by systemic failure as a result of exertion while participating).

Table 31–1 Catastrophic Events 1982–1992

	High School	*College*
Direct catastrophes*		
Deaths	67	7
Nonfatal	148	24
Serious	147	57
Total	362	88
Indirect Deaths†		
Heart	114	25
Other	20	12
Total	134	37

*Direct: Injury directly from participation in sport (trauma).
†Indirect: Systemic failure due to exertion or complication of an injury.

Table 31–2 Causes of 200 Cases of Sudden Death in Young Athletes

Diagnosis	*Number*	*(%)*
Hypertrophic cardiomyopathy	44	(22.1)
Coronary artery anomaly	30	(15.1)
Myocarditis	21	(10.5)
Arteriosclerotic coronary artery disease	22	(11.1)
Left ventricular hypertrophy	12	(6.0)
Right ventricular dysplasia	7	(3.5)
Conduction pathology	5	(2.5)
Mitral valve prolapse	9	(4.5)
Ruptured aorta	4	(2.0)
No cause determined	23	(11.6)
Other	22	(11.1)

In high school, indirect deaths now outnumber direct deaths by a ratio of 2:1 over the last 10 years. Most of these deaths in young competitive athletes are due to cardiovascular abnormalities.

The causes of sudden death are relatively consistent in several studies of athletes younger than 35 years (Table 31–2). Atherosclerotic coronary artery disease accounts for almost all sudden deaths in athletes older than 35 years.

Hypertrophic Cardiomyopathy

Hypertrophic cardiomyopathy (HCM) is the most common cause of sudden death in athletes. There are three types of cardiomyopathy (congestive, hypertrophic, and restrictive). Congestive cardiomyopathy is the most common form in adults but is a rare cause of sudden death in athletes. Restrictive cardiomyopathy is a rarely diagnosed form of cardiomyopathy that in retrospective studies has not been listed as a cause of sudden death. Hypertrophic cardiomyopathy is a disease of cardiac muscle that is associated with a hypertrophic left ventricle with areas of myocardial fiber disarray. This diagnosis is made in the absence of other cardiac or systemic disease that could produce this type of left ventricular hypertrophy. The ratio of septal thickness to posterior free wall is usually greater than 1:3 (asymmetric septal hypertrophy). Often the intramural coronary arteries and anterior mitral valve leaflets are abnormally thickened. The left atrium is dilated, the left ventricular cavity small, and there is increased muscle mass. Physiologically, the left ventricular outflow tract is often obstructed, compliance of the left ventricle is decreased leading to abnormal filling of the left ventricle, and mitral regurgitation is observed.[10] Often, there is systolic anterior motion of the mitral valve and early partial closure and reopening of the aortic valve. Occasionally, a plaque is noted on the interventricular septum in the area of the left ventricular outflow tract.

SYMPTOMS OF HYPERTROPHIC CARDIOMYOPATHY

The majority of patients with hypertrophic cardiomyopathy have no symptoms or only mild ones.[11] Death is often sudden and unexpected. If the hypertrophic cardiomyopathy is symptomatic, dyspnea is the most common symptom, followed by angina pectoris, fatigue, presyncope, and syncope. Palpitations and dizziness may also occur. Exertion may exacerbate these symptoms.[12] Sudden death is uncommon in asymptomatic or mildly symptomatic adult patients with hypertrophic cardiomyopathy and relatively mild left ventricular hypertrophy. Sudden death associated with mild localized hypertrophy is more likely to occur in preadolescent children than in adults.

Syncope is thought to be an ominous sign in patients with hypertrophic cardiomyopathy. *Any athlete with hypertrophic cardiomyopathy and syncope should be disqualified from participation in strenuous sports.*

PHYSICAL EXAMINATION FOR HYPERTROPHIC CARDIOMYOPATHY

Examination findings may be normal in asymptomatic patients. Most patients, however, will have a left ventricular lift, a prominent fourth heart sound, and a systolic murmur that is harsh and crescendo-decrescendo in configuration. In some patients, a thrill is noted. A more blowing holosystolic murmur may be heard at the apex that radiates toward the axilla, signifying mitral regurgitation. Several maneuvers that *decrease* preload (Valsalva's maneuver, standing posture, amyl nitrite) *increase* the gradient and the murmur. Maneuvers that *increase* preload, such as squatting, *decrease* the gradient and the murmur. These maneuvers have an opposite effect on persons with valvular aortic stenosis.

Left Ventricular Hypertrophy—Athlete's Heart Syndrome

Left ventricular hypertrophy (LVH) has, on occasion, been the only finding at autopsy in an athlete who succumbed to sudden death (see Table 31–2). Abnormal diastolic function (i.e., decreased compliance of the left ventricle) is usually present in hypertrophic cardiomyopathy and in LVH secondary to hypertension or aortic stenosis. If an athlete has only mild LVH, normal diastolic function, and no symptoms, it is assumed that the risk for sudden death is very low. Unfortunately, if major concerns persist about the diagnosis of athlete's heart syndrome (increased left ventricular wall thickness and size in athletes who perform primarily isotonic or dynamic exercise) versus hypertrophic cardiomyopathy, it may be reasonable to recommend a period of deconditioning. Left ventricular muscle mass and wall thickness should decrease significantly if the athlete does not have hypertrophic cardiomyopathy. This recommendation, however, has not been tested in any prospective studies.

Coronary Arterial Abnormalities

ANOMALOUS ORIGIN OF A MAJOR CORONARY ARTERY

Cheitlin and colleagues first brought attention to this as a possible cause of sudden death in 1974.[13] The investigators evaluated 51 patients with anomalous coronary origins, and 7 of them died suddenly while exercising (in all, the left main coronary artery originated from the right coronary sinus). The origin of the right coronary artery from the left coronary sinus has also been associated with sudden death.[14] The cause of death in these patients is not clear, but is assumed to be the acute take-off angle of the anomalous artery, which is either stretched, compressed between the great vessels, or in some other manner traumatized.

TUNNELED EPICARDIAL CORONARY ARTERIES

At least three different reports have concluded that tunneled epicardial coronary arteries are a cause of sudden death during strenuous exercise;[15,16] however, since such arteries can be a relatively common finding, their significance is still open to question in regard to causing sudden death.

CORONARY ATHEROSCLEROSIS

In athletes over age 30, coronary atherosclerosis causes 90% of sudden deaths. Unfortunately, sudden cardiac death is the first clinical manifestation of coronary artery disease in 25% or more of all coronary heart disease patients.[17] Athletes who die of sudden death with coronary artery disease often at autopsy have evidence of previous myocardial infarction that went undetected. The majority have more than 75% stenosis in at least one vessel, and many have multivessel disease. In a study of nonathletes, Davies reviewed autopsies of 168 consecutive cases of sudden coronary death in London.[18] These patients could be divided into two groups. One group, who had atherosclerosis, developed a new vascular event involving coronary thrombosis, which initiated acute myocardial ischemia (73.3%). The other group had chronic high-grade stenoses due to atherosclerosis plus a previously healed infarction but no recent vascular change (26.7%). It is assumed that most athletes who suffer sudden death from coronary atherosclerosis had no previous symptoms. The athlete's history, electrocardiogram, and echocardiogram may give clues or make the diagnosis if he or she has a history of myocardial infarction. A treadmill test may be abnormal (see Treadmill Testing).

Myocarditis

Several studies have reported myocarditis as a cause of sudden death. Myocarditis may be acute or chronic. Viral infections are the most common cause in North America and Chagas' disease in South America.[17] Many substances may also damage the myocardium (e.g., drugs, lead, catecholamines, allergens). Coxsackie B virus is the most common viral cause.[19] Myocardial damage may be invasive, immune mediated, or toxic.[20] Myocardial involvement may be focal or diffuse, but the lesions are randomly distributed in the heart and clinical effects depend on the location, size, and number of lesions.[19] Cocaine was recently described as a cause of focal myocarditis. Most types of myocarditis have been associated with sudden cardiac death, with or without concomitant cardiac failure.[17] Observers speculated that focal myocarditis was the cause of the sudden death in Reggie Lewis, the Boston Celtics star.[1] Phillips reviewed 19 sudden cardiac deaths that occurred among 1,606,167 U.S. Air Force recruits.[21] Eight recruits had myocarditis (nonrheumatic 4, vaccinia-related 1, rheumatic 3). Viral carditis may damage the conducting system or may be focal, in the myocardium, and result in a propensity to arrhythmias. The risk of potentially lethal arrhythmias is not limited to the acute phase of the disease.[22] The clinical manifestations of myocarditis range from an asymptomatic state to one of fulminant congestive heart failure. In most, the event is self-limited and unrecognized.[23] The physical examination is normal unless there is significant left ventricular dysfunction. The electrocardiogram often is abnormal, with nonspecific ST-T wave changes, atrial and ventricular premature beats, and atrioventricular conduction disturbances.[24]

Diagnosis of myocarditis should be suspected when focal or generalized left ventricular or right ventricular dysfunction is identified by echocardiography. This diagnosis may be suspected if an athlete develops dysrhythmias and has no other evidence of underlying heart disease. Findings on thallium myocardial scintigraphy and magnetic resonance imaging are likely to be abnormal. Right ventricular biopsy may make the diagnosis of myocarditis. The physician should have a high index of suspicion for this disease and suspect it when the athlete has a prolonged respiratory tract infection or develops rhythm or conduction disturbances or a marked unexplained decrease in exercise tolerance.

Mitral Valve Prolapse

Mitral valve prolapse (MVP) is listed in many studies as an uncommon cause of sudden cardiac death (see Table 31–2). This is disturbing to the sports medicine physician, since MVP may affect 15 million Americans.[16] Mitral valve prolapse is, therefore, a common finding among athletes. It was present in 11 of 220 Indiana University athletes that we screened by echocardiography and in 8 of 160 members of the 1992 United States Olympic track and field team, who were studied by echocardiography.[25] Maron found MVP in 14 of 90 athletes who were given special screening because of findings by family history, physical examination, or 12-lead electrocardiography (501 athletes screened).[26]

MVP is manifested by an increased mitral valve leaflet area. The mitral valve is thickened, and myxomatous transformation is often present.[27]

Most patients with MVP are asymptomatic; however multiple symptoms have been attributed to mitral valve prolapse. Atypical chest pain, which is usually sharp, left precordial, and either fleeting or lasting several hours, may be present, although this is much more common in women. It is usually unrelated to physical activity. Dyspnea, fatigue, dizziness, and palpitations have also been attributed to MVP.

On auscultation, a nonejection systolic click remains the hallmark of MVP. The click moves earlier in systole when the patient sits as compared with when he stands. Since few cardiac and extracardiac abnormalities are associated with this type of click, its mere presence is considered diagnostic of MVP.[27] A late systolic murmur is another diagnostic hallmark of MVP. A late systolic murmur, however, can be heard in many other conditions, such as mitral regurgitation secondary to papillary muscle dysfunction or calcification of the mitral valve annulus. If a murmur is heard without a click, echocardiographic confirmation is usually considered necessary.

Although an auscultatory diagnosis should be accepted in most situations, echocardiography has become accepted as a major diagnostic tool for MVP. Many patients, however, have been overdiagnosed with echocardiography. The work of Robert Levine has helped clarify the saddle shape of the mitral valve annulus and has helped us realize that minimal bowing of the anterior leaflet in the apical four-chamber view is a nonspecific finding.[28] Complications from MVP are infective endocarditis, superventricular and ventricular dysrhythmias, transient ischemic attacks, and partial strokes. Sudden death is extremely rare. Approximately 120 cases have been recorded in the literature; most victims are older than 20 years.

If an athlete presents with a typical click, with or without a systolic murmur, but is totally asymptomatic and has no family history of premature death, participation should be allowed if there is no evidence of Marfan's syndrome or significant mitral regurgitation.

The Bethesda Conference recognized the lack of definitive data on athletes with MVP and their fitness for participation in athletics. The Bethesda Conference[29] recommended disqualifying athletes with MVP from strenuous athletic competition if any of the following findings are obtained:

A history of syncope
A family history of sudden death due to MVP
Disabling chest pain or chest pain worsened by exercise
Complex ventricular arrhythmias
Significant mitral regurgitation with moderate or marked cardiomegaly
Marfan's syndrome associated with the MVP

Using these criteria, sports medicine physicians will commonly make the diagnosis of MVP but will rarely have to disqualify an athlete from participation.

Cocaine

Although cocaine was not implicated as a cause of death in the studies presented in Table 31–2, it was implicated in the deaths of basketball star Len Bias and pro football player Don Rogers. It is estimated that as many as 25 million Americans have used cocaine and that one in five of those used it regularly. As many as a million Americans may be addicted to the drug based on reports in 1985,[30] and the number is thought to be higher today. Cocaine has been implicated by clinically- or necropsy-proven cases in causing myocardial ischemia, myocarditis, aortic rupture, systemic hypertension, coronary artery spasm, coronary thrombosis, cardiomyopathy, and ventricular arrhythmias with or without sudden death.[31]

If a team physician suspects an athlete of using cocaine, counseling should be instituted and appropriate drug tests should be obtained. Close attention should be paid to the cardiovascular system before letting this athlete return to play.

EXAMINATION FOR PREVENTION OF SUDDEN DEATH

Evaluation of a symptomatic athlete requires a plan that will arrive at a definitive diagnosis and allow appropriate risk of exercise to be determined. If one were to design a preparticipation examination to exclude an athlete's risk for sudden death, all of the following studies would be performed: history, physical examination, echocardiography, electrocardiography, and exercise treadmill test. If abnormalities were determined, additional studies, such as Holter monitoring, an event recorder, left and right heart catheterization, an electrophysiologic study, magnetic resonance imaging of the heart, chemistry and hematologic profiles, and tilt table testing may have to be included. The expense could be overwhelming. Even performing all these tests would not guarantee a successful outcome for a patient with structural heart disease. The expense of this type of extensive testing cannot be justified for routine screening, or even for the preparticipation screening examination.

History

To rule out causes of sudden death and to detect other cardiovascular abnormalities, the following questions should be asked:

Have you ever felt faint, experienced significant dizziness, lightheadedness, passed out, or lost consciousness during or shortly after exercise?
Have you had chest pain, palpitations, or irregular heartbeats during physical activity?
Do you have palpitations or feel your heart beat irregularly?
Does your heart beat unusually fast for no obvious reason?
Have you ever been told you had a heart murmur, rheumatic fever, high blood pressure, or any other heart problem?
Has anyone in your family died suddenly or had a heart attack at a young age (before age 55 years for males, before age 65 years for females)?
Have you ever taken any illicit drugs?
Are you taking any medications?

A positive response to any of these questions would require further evaluation. For younger athletes, it is important to have the history questionnaire brought home and completed by the athlete and his or her parents or guardians. A study by Resser and coworkers showed that only 39% of the athletes' responses to questions about their history agreed with their parents' version of the child's history.[32]

Physical Examination

Auscultation of the athlete is likely to provide a clue to the diagnosis of hypertrophic cardiomyopathy, valvular heart disease, Marfan's syndrome, or arrhythmias. Auscultation may provide a clue in patients with myocarditis. The success depends on the skills of the examining physician and the amount of time spent in the examination. A quiet examining room improves the accuracy. Clues for hypertrophic cardiomyopathy include a quick carotid upstroke, a bisferious pulse, a systolic murmur that becomes fainter or disappears on squatting and becomes louder on standing, a precordial "ripple," and S_4 gallop.

The typical features of Marfan's syndrome are tall, thin body habitus, subluxation of the lens of the eye, long, supple fingers and joints, high arched palate, an arm span–height ratio greater than 1 and a head to pubis–pubis to foot ratio less than 1. Normal values for these ratios may not be correct for athletes taller than 6 feet 3 inches. Associated auscultatory findings may be aortic diastolic murmur, systolic ejection sound, systolic murmur, either at the left sternal border or the mitral area, and a loud second heart sound. Mitral valve prolapse is suggested by a systolic click (clicks) and varying degrees of mitral regurgitation (systolic murmur). Particular attention must be paid to the second heart sound because the timing of the closure of the aortic and pulmonic valves gives clues to the causes of systolic ejection murmurs. The most common murmur is a soft midsystolic murmur not associated with any cardiac abnormality. This is the innocent murmur or functional murmur seen in 30% of young athletes. Provocation maneuvers (Valsalva's, standing, squatting, amyl nitrite inhalation) can help distinguish causes of systolic murmur. If a diagnosis other than functional murmur is suspected, electrocardiography and echocardiography should be performed to make a definitive diagnosis.

Echocardiography

Echocardiography is the most reliable test to rule out structural cardiac causes of sudden death. The echocardiogram can detect hypertrophic cardiomyopathy, cardiovascular manifestations of Marfan's syndrome, myocarditis (focal or diffuse), MVP, previous myocardial infarctions, congenital heart anomalies, other forms of valve abnormalities, and even some of the coronary artery anomalies. Difficulties with performing routine echocardiography are many: cost, time for test, and deciding which asymptomatic athletes who have an abnormality should be disqualified. The cost of the echocardiogram can be decreased significantly if a "quick look" is obtained by using parasternal, long-axis, and short-axis views with color flow Doppler screening.

Electrocardiography in Athletes

Athletes' electrocardiograms are usually within normal limits but may show rhythm or pattern abnormalities. Sinus bradycardia is a common finding in athletes and is considered normal. The recognized normal sinus rhythm rate of 60 to 100 does not apply to trained athletes. Average daytime heart rates are usually in the 50s (range, 40 to 80) during normal daytime activities and often fall below 40 during sleep.[33–35] The degree of bradycardia is most profound in athletes who participate in aerobic or endurance type sports. Many other "abnormal" electrocardiographic findings may be considered normal variants for an athlete (Table 31–3). It should be noted that the arrhythmias common to athletes (i.e., sinus arrhythmia, bradycardia, junctional rhythm, atrial premature contractions) disappear with exertion and should be considered benign and require no special follow-up.

Electrocardiographic changes suggestive of left ventricular hypertrophy are found more often in athletes. Voltage criteria for left ventricular hypertrophy are frequently observed in distance runners.[36] Other criteria for left ventricular hypertrophy (ST-T wave changes, delayed intrinsacoid deflection, leftward axis, and left atrial abnormalities) are found less frequently.

Electrocardiography is not a good screening study to rule out causes of sudden death in athletes because there are too many false-positive results.

Table 31–3. Electrocardiographic Abnormalities That May Be Normal Variants in Athletes

Sinus bradycardia
Intermittent junctional rhythm
First-degree heart block
Mobitz-I second-degree heart block (Wenckebach's phenomenon)
Incomplete right bundle branch block
Nonspecific T-wave changes
Minor ST segment depression or elevation
Occasional atrial premature and ventricular premature contractions on 24-hour Holter monitoring

Treadmill Testing in Athletes

The predictive power of treadmill testing in young athletes is weak. Exercise testing as a screening procedure in athletes is limited by a lack of adequate personnel to monitor the test, lack of appropriate facilities, cost of the procedure, and lack of knowledge concerning the need and benefits.[37] Routine use of electrocardiographically monitored maximal exercise testing as a screening tool in athletes before participation in sports cannot be recommended. Exercise treadmill testing should be performed in athletes who meet the following criteria:

1. Age older than 35 years and at high risk for cardiac events
2. At any age, symptoms of chest discomfort with exertion, unusual dyspnea, dizziness, lightheadedness, syncope, or palpitations
3. Known cardiovascular disease
4. Abnormal cardiac findings that may indicate a risk for participation in athletics or exercise.

The main indication for exercise testing of an athlete would be to rule out coronary artery disease, whether secondary to atherosclerosis or to congenital anomalies. Unfortunately, in asymptomatic athletes false-positive results are more common than true-positive ones. A positive exercise test in a college athlete is relatively specific (i.e., a normal test is likely to mean a normal examination) but sensitivity and predictive value (percentage of persons with an abnormal test who actually have disease) are low. An athlete who has a positive treadmill test for ischemia by the usual criteria should be evaluated like any other patient and be withheld from competitive athletics until disease is ruled out. Isoelectric or downward sloping ST segment depression greater than 1 mm is rare in athletes and must be evaluated. Disqualification of an asymptomatic athlete based on a single positive treadmill study is not recommended without further studies.

If an athlete is to be given a maximal test, the commonly used protocols by Bruce, Balke, Ellestad, and Naughton may not be appropriate. Athletes often have trouble running on a treadmill at the steep grades (greater than 14°) required during the higher levels of Ellestad and Bruce protocols.

At Indiana University, the author has performed exercise treadmill studies on collegiate basketball players since 1976 (Table 31–4).[38] The protocol described here has been valuable in maximally trained athletes. The athletes do not hold on to hand rails while running, and only grab the hand rails to straddle the treadmill belt to signify their maximal level of exercise tolerance.

Holter Monitors and Event Recorders

Holter monitoring captures 24 hours' continuous electrocardiographic recording. It is indicated for athletes with history of syncope, palpitations, and dizziness, with or without exertion. It rarely identifies a syncopal episode, since these are rare, unpredictable, and may happen weeks or months apart. A 24-hour Holter study documents background rhythm disturbances that have some intermediate diagnostic value.[39] The monitor may be worn on an athlete's back with a figure-of-eight strap during practice in most sports. It is preferable to monitor athletes while they are practicing their specific sport.

The loop electrocardiographic recorder (event recorder) can be used for longer-term monitoring. It stores information from the previous 4 minutes and the subsequent 60 seconds when the button is pressed.[40] In a study of nonathletes with syncope, the loop electrocardiographic recorder was more likely to identify the cause than 24-hour Holter monitoring (~25% vs. 10%).[41]

Tilt Table Testing

Tilt table testing should be performed when an athlete has unexplained syncope and no structural heart disease. Neurocardiogenic syncope (mediated by the vagus nerve) is the most common cause of syncope in patients without structural heart disease.[42] The upright tilt table test is currently the diagnostic standard for this

Table 31–4. Protocol for Exercise Treadmill Testing of 34 Male College Basketball Players

Stage	*I*	*II*	*III*	*IV*	*V*	*VI*	*VII*	*VIII*
Time (sec)	60	120	120	120	60	60	60	60
Speed (mph)	2.5	4.0	6.0	8.0	9.0	10.0	10.0	10.0
Grade (%)	0	0	0	0	2	4	6	8
Mean V_{O_2}(ml/min/kg)	11.0	16.9	32.5	41.3	49.2	54.8	59.3	66.1
Predicted V_{O_2}(ml/min/kg)	10.2*	16.5*	35.4†	46.2†	55.7†	66.5†	71.1†	76.0†

*Walking V_{O_2} = [mph × 26.8 × 0.1] + [% grade (mph × 26.8) 1.8] + 3.5
†Running V_{O_2} = [mph × 26.8 × 0.1] + [% grade (mph × 26.8) 1.8 × 0.5] + 3.5

disorder. The patient is placed at an angle of 80° for 20 minutes and if blood pressure does not drop and no symptoms occur, this may be repeated with low and then high dose isoproterenol infusion. Sensitivity of 75% with unexplained syncope has been reported.[43] Isoproterenol infusion is controversial because it reduces the specificity of the test.[44] With isoproterenol neurocardiac syncope may be incorrectly diagnosed on the basis of a false-positive result while a more serious cause of syncope is overlooked.

Recently, power spectroanalysis of heart ratio variability during tilt table testing was evaluated by Morillo.[45] Although this appears to improve the sensitivity and specificity of the test, further investigation is under way.

DISQUALIFICATION OF THE ATHLETE

The sixteenth Bethesda Conference provided formal guidelines for eligibility for participation of athletes with underlying primary cardiovascular abnormalities. Sports were classified by intensity and types of exercise performed. Recommendations were based on the best scientific information available with a significant dependence on common sense and the *art* of medicine. These are the best set of recommendations available, and this group will meet periodically to re-evaluate them.

There is no official standard or centralized mechanism in the United States for making recommendations on eligibility of athletes with cardiovascular abnormalities to participate. If intensive screening procedures are performed in the preparticipation examination, a few causes of sudden death would likely be identified but many athletes would be unjustly disqualified. A recommendation to disqualify an athlete based on a cardiac abnormality usually requires consultation with a cardiologist. Unfortunately, many cardiologists do not have expertise in sports medicine and require significant guidance from the team physician.

PHYSICIAN'S RESPONSIBILITY

The physician's first responsibility is always to athletes and their families, and the athletic organization that the athlete represents must be secondary. When any medical problem arises with an athlete, the physician discusses it first with the athlete. Only then, with the full knowledge of the athlete, is the situation discussed with the athletic organization. The team physician has final authority about whether an athlete is qualified to participate in an event. The team physician also has a responsibility for obtaining appropriate consultations and following the recommendations of those consultations or obtaining additional expert opinions. The difficulty arises as in the case of Reggie Lewis, when conflicting opinions are obtained. The National Collegiate Athletic Association Sports Medicine Handbook states, "The team physician has the final responsibility to determine when a student athlete is removed or withheld from participation due to injury or illness. In addition, clearance for that individual to return to that activity is solely the responsibility of the team physician or that physician's designated representative."[46] There are additional physician responsibilities to the athlete that could be relieved if the athlete or the minor athlete's parents choose a different primary physician. These points are particularly important when an athlete has a potentially disqualifying or serious cardiac diagnosis.

SUMMARY

Sudden death in athletes remains, fortunately, a rare event. The causes have been well identified and are usually congenital cardiac abnormalities in those younger than 35 years of age and atherosclerotic coronary artery disease in older ones. Education of athletes, coaches, physicians, and trainers is the best way to reduce the incidence of sudden death. Appropriately designed preparticipation examinations will likely decrease the incidence of sudden death in athletes. Routine use of exercise stress test, electrocardiography, and Holter monitoring cannot be recommended. A "quick look" miniechocardiogram may in the future be used to screen large groups of young athletes. New recommendations on eligibility for participation by the American College of Cardiology will be forthcoming. I encourage all team physicians and cardiologists who deal with athletes to have this information available for reference. Some well-known athletes might be alive today if these guidelines had been followed.

REFERENCES

1. "Reggie Lewis." Boston Globe: September 12, 1993: p. 69.
2. Driscoll, D. J., and Edwards, W. D.: Sudden unexpected death in children and adolescents. J. Am. Coll. Cardiol. 5 (Suppl):118B, 1985.
3. Silka, M. J., et al.: Assessment and follow-up of pediatric survivors of sudden cardiac death. Circulation *82:*341, 1990.
4. Klitzner, T. S.: Sudden cardiac death in children. Circulation *82:*629, 1990.
5. Neuspiel, D. R., and Kuller, L. H.: Sudden and unexpected natural death in childhood and adolescence. J.A.M.A. *254:*1321, 1985.
6. Opie, L. H.: Sudden death and sport. Lancet 22(1):678, 1975.
7. Buori, I., Makarainem, M., and Jaaskelainem, A.: Sudden death and physical activity, Cardiology *63:*287, 1987.
8. Thompson, P. D., Funk, E. J., Carleton, R. A., and Sturner, W. Q.: Incidence of death during jogging in Rhode Island from 1975 through 1980. J.A.M.A. *247:*2535, 1982.
9. Cantu, R. C.: Congenital cardiovascular disease—the major cause for athletic death in high school and college. Med. Sci. Sports Exerc. *24:*279, 1992.
10. Wynne, J., and Braunwald, E.: The cardiomyopathy and myocarditis toxic, chemical, physical damage to the heart. *In* Braunwald's Heart Disease. 4th Ed. Edited by E. Braunwald. Philadelphia, W.B. Saunders, 1992.
11. Spirito, P., et al.: Clinical course and prognosis of hypertrophic cardiomyopathy in an outpatient population. N. Engl. J. Med. *320:*749, 1989.
12. Frenneaux, M. P., et al.: Determinants of exercise capacity in hypertrophic cardiomyopathy. J. Am. Coll. Cardiol. *13:*1521, 1989.
13. Cheitlin, M. D., DeCastro, C. M., and McAllister, H. A.: Sudden death as a complication of anomalous left coronary origin from the anterior sinus of Valsalva. A not-so-minor congenital anomaly. Circulation *50:*780, 1974.

14. Roberts, W. C., Siegel, R. J., and Zipes, D. P.: Origin of the right coronary artery from the left sinus of Valsalva and its functional consequences: Analysis of ten necropsy patients. Am. J. Cardiol. *49:*863, 1982.
15. Moral, A. R., Romanelli, R., and Boucek, R. J.: The mural left anterior descending coronary artery, strenuous exercise and sudden death. Circulation *62:*230, 1980.
16. Waller, B. F.: Exercises related sudden death in athletes: The most common causes. *In* Cardiovascular Evaluation of Athletes. Edited by B. F. Waller and W. P. Harvey. Newton, NJ, Laennec Publishing, 1992.
17. Myerburg, R. J., and Castellanos, A.: Cardiac arrest and sudden cardiac death. *In* Braunwald's Heart Disease. 4th Ed. Edited by E. Braunwald. Philadelphia, W.B. Saunders, 1992.
18. Davies, M. J.: Anatomic features in victims of sudden coronary death. Circulation *85*(Suppl. I):I–19, 1992.
19. Weinstein, C., and Fenoglio, J. J.: Myocarditis. Hum. Pathol. *18:*613, 1987.
20. Reyes, M. P., and Lerner, A. M.: Coxsackievirus myocarditis—with special reference to acute and chronic effects. Prog. Cardiovasc. Dis. *27:*373, 1985.
21. Phillips, M., et al.: Sudden cardiac death in air force recruits. J.A.M.A. *256:*2696, 1986.
22. Warren, J. V.: Unusual cardiac death. Cardiol. Ser. *8:*5, 1984.
23. Marboe, C. C., and Fenoglio, J. J.: Pathology and natural history of human myocarditis. Pathol. Immunopathol. Res. *7:*226, 1988.
24. O'Connell, J. B., and Robinson, J. A.: Coxsackie viral myocarditis. Postgrad. Med. J. *61:*1127, 1985.
25. Rink, L. D.: Unpublished data.
26. Maron, B. J., et al.: Results of screening a large group of intercollegiate competitive athletes for cardiovascular disease. J. Am. Coll. Cardiol. *10:*1214, 1987.
27. Jeresaty, R. M.: Mitral valve prolapse: Implications for the athlete. *In* Cardiovascular Evaluation of Athletes. Edited by B. F. Waller and W. P. Harvey. Newton, NJ, Laennec, 1992.
28. Levine, R. A., Triulzi, M. O., Harrigan, P., Weyman, A. E.: The relationship of mitral annular shape to the diagnosis of mitral valve prolapse. Circulation *75:*756, 1987.
29. Mitchell, J. H., Maron, B. J., and Epstein, S. E.: Sixteenth Bethesda Conference: Cardiovascular abnormalities in the athlete: Recommendations regarding eligibility for competition. J. Am. Coll. Cardiol. *6:*1186, 1985.
30. National Institute on Drug Abuse Monograph Series; No. 85–1414, 1985.
31. Waller, B. F.: Cocaine in the cardiovascular system: Relevance to the athlete. *In* Cardiovascular Evaluation of Athletes. Edited by B. F. Waller and W. P. Harvey. Newton, NJ, Laennec, 1992.
32. Resser, W. L., Hoffman, H. M., and Bellah, G. G.: Athletes' examinations. Texas Med. *81:*35, 1985.
33. Ector, H., et al.: Bradycardia, ventricular pauses, syncope, and sports. Laennec, 591–594, 1984.
34. Talan, D. A., et al.: Twenty-four hour continuous ECG recordings in long-distance runners. Chest *82:*19, 1982.
35. Knowlan, D. M.: The electrocardiogram in the athlete. *In* Cardiovascular Evaluation of Athletes. Edited by B. F. Waller and W. P. Harvey. Newton, NJ, Laennec, 1992.
36. Smith, W. G., Collen, K. J., and Thornberg, I. O.: Electrocardiograms of marathon runners in 1962 Commonwealth Games. Br. Heart J. *26:*469, 1964.
37. Rink, L. D., and Knowlan, D. M.: Exercise treadmill testing in athletes. *In* Cardiovascular Evaluation of Athletes. Edited by B. F. Waller and W. P. Harvey. Newton, NJ, Laennec, 1992.
38. Rink, L. D., Dayton, S., Garl, T., and Bomba, B.: Comparison of cardiopulmonary parameters between white and black elite college basketball players (Abstr.). Med. Sci. Sports Exerc. *18:*525, 1986.
39. Gibson, T., and Heitzman, M. R.: Diagnostic efficacy of 24-hour electrocardiographic monitoring for syncope. Am. J. Cardiol. *53:*1013, 1984.
40. Lenzer, M., and Comegno, A.: Long term ambulator ECG monitoring in syncope: The state of the art. Cardiovasc. Rev. and Rep. *5:*11, 1993.
41. Lenzer, M., Pritchett, P. L. C., Pontinen, M., et al: Incremental diagnostic yield of loop electrocardiographic recorders in unexplained syncope. Am. J. Cardiol. *66:*214,1990.
42. Kosinski, D., Wolfe, D. A., and Grub, B. P.: Neurocardiogenic syncope: A review of pathophysiology, diagnosis and treatment. Cardiovasc. Rev. Rep. *5:*22, 1993.
43. Fitzpatrick, A. P., et al.: Methodology of head up tilt testing in patients with unexplained syncope. J. Am. Coll. Cardiol. *17:*125, 1991.
44. Kapoor, W. N., and Brandt, N.: Evaluation of syncope by upright tilt testing with isoproterenol. Ann Intern. Med. *116:*358, 1992.
45. Morillo, C., et al.: Power spectral analysis of heart rate variability during passive tilt identifies patient with neurally mediated syncope. Circulation *86*(Suppl. 1):528, 1992.
46. NCAA Committee on Competitive Safeguards and Medical Aspects of Sports: NCAA Sports Medicine Handbook. 3rd Edition. Mission, KS, National Collegiate Athletic Association, 1987.

III

MUSCULOSKELETAL ASPECTS OF SPORTS

32 *Lee A. Kelley*

Functional Anatomy of the Spine

An understanding of the detailed anatomy of the spine is a prerequisite for treating its disorders. Obviously, a physician who undertakes surgical treatment of the spine must master all aspects of its anatomy, but all evaluation of spinal disorders relies on a determination of aberrations from normal form and function. One's knowledge of the basic elements of functional anatomy of the spine renders more meaningful the findings of clinical evaluation.

THE CERVICAL SPINE

Osteoligamentous Anatomy

The first seven vertebrae (C1–7) of the spinal column comprise the cervical spine (Fig. 32–1). C3 through C7 are very similar in both anatomy and function, but the first two cervical vertebrae are distinctly different from the rest. C1, also known as the *atlas,* is essentially a ring of bone without a true vertebral body (Fig. 32–2). It articulates with the base of the skull by means of two synovial joints formed by the occipital condyles at the base of the skull and the upper portions of the lateral masses of C1. The second cervical segment, the *axis,* includes a true vertebral body and a cephalad projection from its anterior aspect, known as the *dens,* or the *odontoid process* (Fig. 32–3).

C1 and C2 articulate by means of synovial joints formed by the caudad aspects of the lateral masses of C1 and the cephalad aspects of the lateral masses of C2. The joint capsules are quite loose; this allows significant rotation at this level. The odontoid process articulates with the inner aspect of the anterior arch of C1 by means of a true synovial articulation. This joint is stabilized by a transverse ligament that courses posterior to the odontoid process at the level of the anterior arch of C1 and articulates with the posterior aspect of the odon-

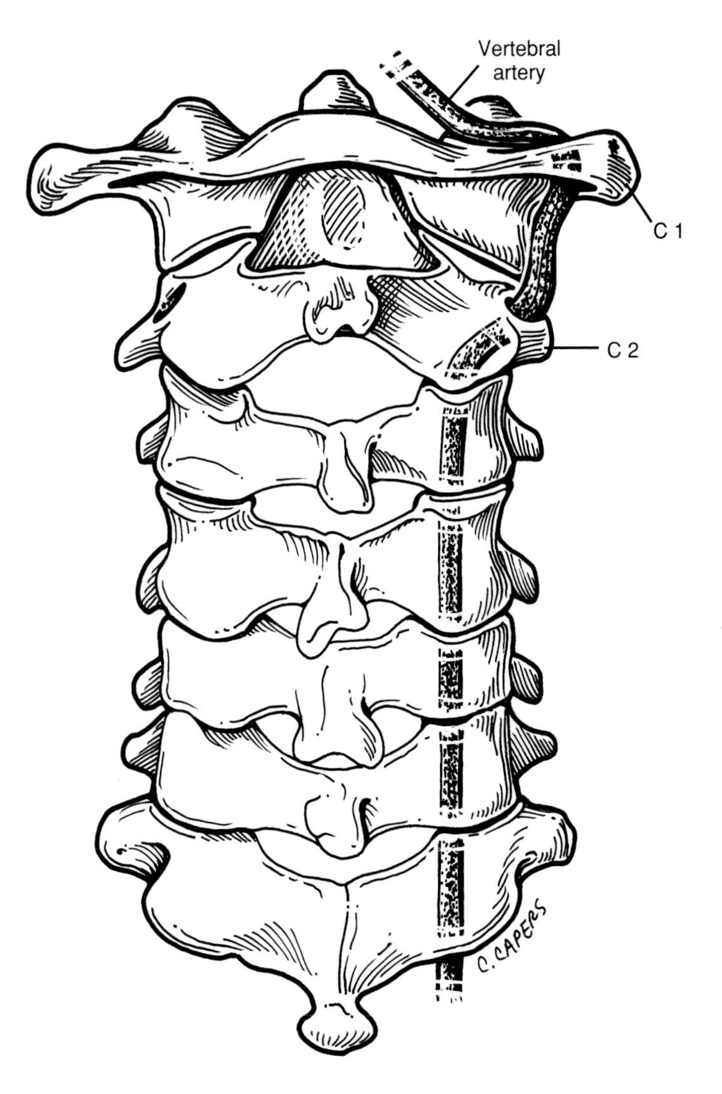

Fig. 32–1. Vertebrae of the cervical spine. Note the morphology and articulation of C1 and C2. The other five vertebrae are very similar to one another.

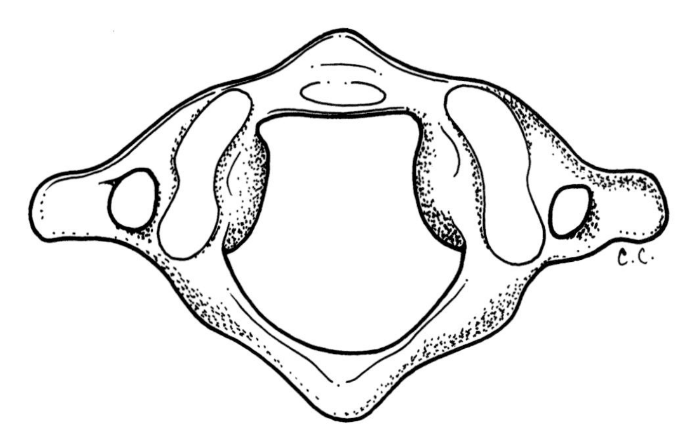

Fig. 32–2. The atlas (C1), is not a true vertebral body.

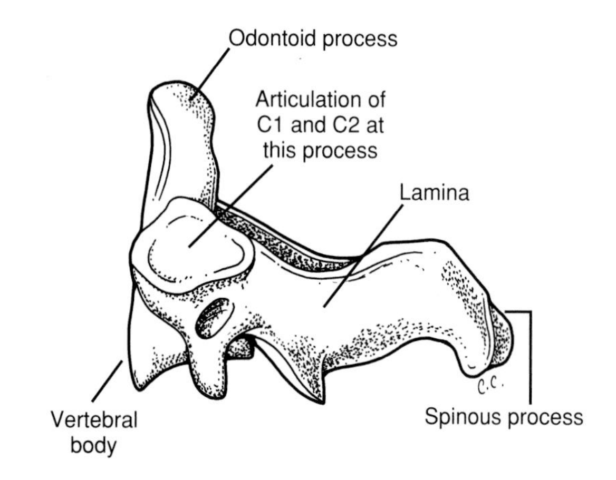

Fig. 32–3. The axis (C2).

toid process by means of a true synovial articulation. Another ligament, the apical ligament, extends from the tip of the odontoid to the base of the skull. The paired alar ligaments extend from the odontoid process to the base of the skull (Fig. 32–4). Approximately 50% of cervical spine rotation occurs at the C1-2 articulation. The remaining 50% of rotation is divided over the remaining five segments of the cervical spine. There is virtually no anteroposterior translation of the C1-2 articulation in the normal spine.

C3 through C7, all very similar, are composed of an anterior vertebral body, which is small and concave along its superior surface. It is somewhat convex along its inferior surface. A transverse process emanates at the level of the pedicle that ultimately forms a portion of a vascular foramen known as the *foramen transversarium,* which transmits the vertebral artery at levels C3 through C6. At C7 this foramen contains only the accessory vertebral vein. The spinal cord is protected within the spinal canal and paired laminae form the roof of the spinal canal. There are two facet articulations at each level that are oriented obliquely and confer stability in the anteroposterior direction by virtue of both orientation and joint capsules. The vertebral bodies of C2 through C7 also articulate with each other by false joints formed by an upward projection from the cephalad end of one vertebral body called an *uncinate process* (Fig. 32–5) that fits into a shallow groove in the vertebral body above, known as the *echancrure.* These are referred to as the *joints of Luschka* or the *neurocentral joints.* These joints form the anteromedial boundary of the neuroforamen; its posterolateral boundary is formed by the facet joint.

An intervertebral disc lies between each pair of vertebral bodies between C2 and C7. Each is bounded circumferentially by an annulus fibrosus and contained within is the nucleus pulposus. A thick anterior longitudinal ligament lies along the anterior vertebral bodies and anterior annulus fibrosus throughout the cervical spine. A thick and strong posterior longitudinal ligament lies along the posterior vertebral bodies and posterior margins of the annulus fibrosus throughout the cervical spine as well (Fig. 32–6). The posterior longitudinal ligament spans almost the entire distance from one neuroforamen to the opposite one at the same level. This is an important influence on the direction of cervical disc herniation.

Some of the ligaments in the cervical spine have already been discussed. The stabilizing ligaments of the atlantoaxial joint and those between the upper cervical spine and the base of the skull were noted previously (see Fig. 32–4). Similarly, the anterior and posterior longitudinal ligaments are significant stabilizing structures in the cervical spine. There is an interspinous ligament between the respective spinous processes of C2 through C7, but there may be no true supraspinous ligament. Rather, there is a blending of fibers in the interspinous ligament with those of a thick midline structure known as the *ligamentum nuchae* that extends from the deep posterior cervical fascia down to the spinous processes of the cervical spine and then blends with the upper thoracic fascia. It should be noted that the ligamentum nuchae extends to the base of the skull posteriorly (Fig. 32–6). A ligamentum flavum extends between the laminae posteriorly at each level in the cervical spine; between the occiput and C1 this is known as the *posterior atlanto-occipital membrane.* At the same level, the posterior longitudinal ligament blends with the cranial dura to form the tectorial membrane. The anterior longitudinal ligament, cephalad to C1, joins the base of the skull as a structure known as the anterior atlanto-occipital membrane. There is no single structure in the lower cervical spine (C3 through C7) that is essential for stability at a given level; however at C1-2, the transverse ligament is largely responsible for anteroposterior stability at that level. Disruption of the transverse ligament by trauma or erosion, as in rheumatoid arthritis, leads to a significant degree of atlantoaxial translational instability.

Musculature

For the sake of simplicity, the cervical spine muscles may be grouped broadly into those of the posterior cervical spine, whose principal function is cervical extension; those of the lateral cervical spine, whose principal

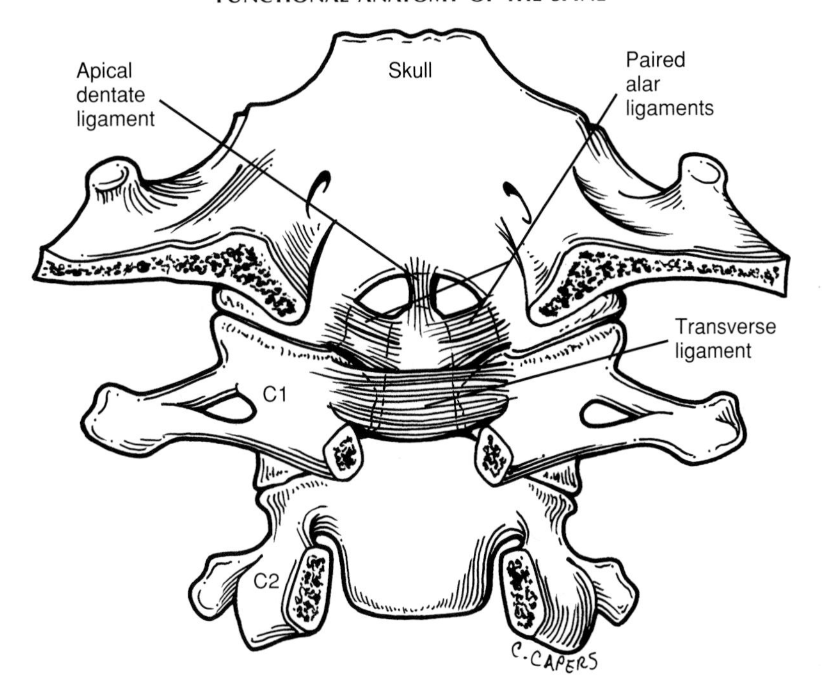

Fig. 32–4. Ligaments of the occiput–C1-C2 complex. The transverse ligament is strongest.

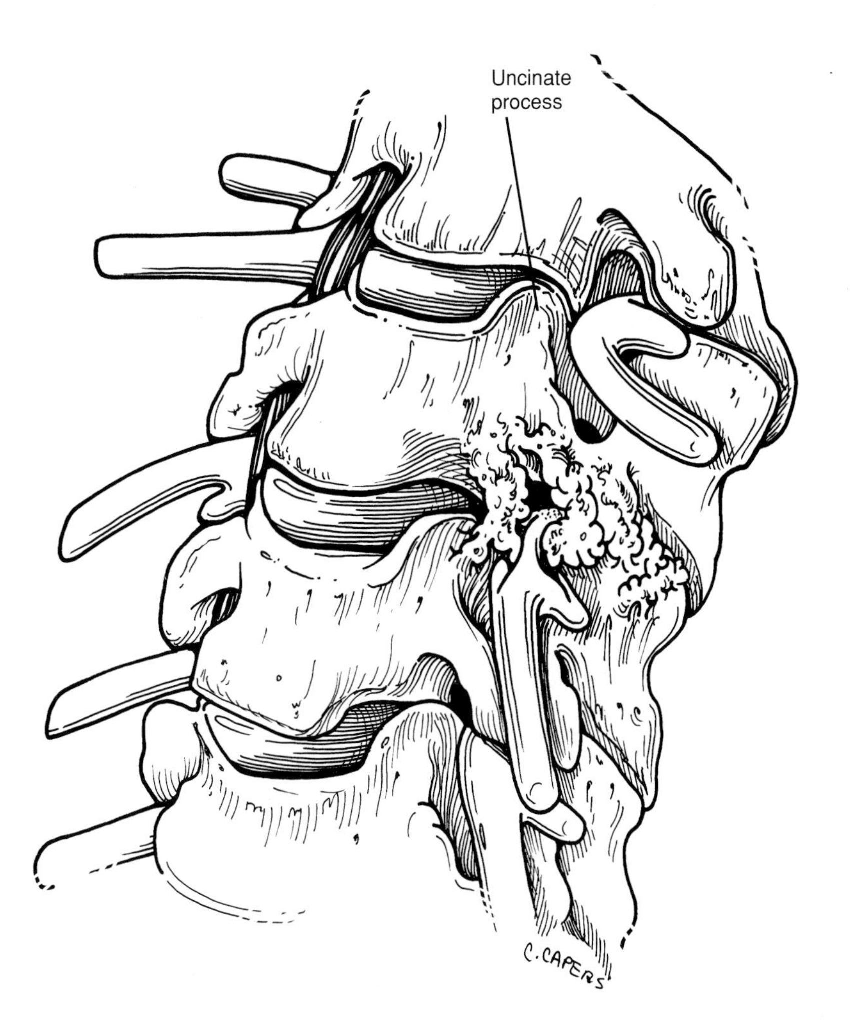

Fig. 32–5. The uncinate process, also known as the neurocentral process, forms the joint of Luschka with the vertebral body above.

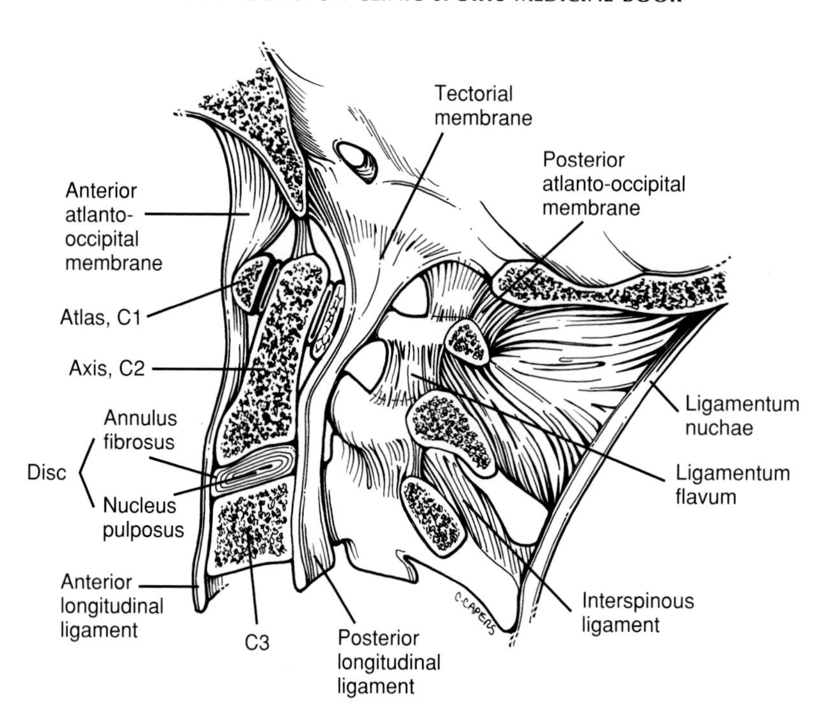

Fig. 32–6. The posterior ligaments of the upper cervical spine.

function is rotation and lateral flexion; and those of the anterior cervical spine, whose main function is flexion. Obviously, there is considerable overlap in these broad groups (Fig. 32–7). The posterior musculature is known as the cervical paraspinal muscles. Listed from superficial to deep ones, these are the trapezius muscles, the splenius capitis, the semispinalis cervicis and capitis, the rectus capitis posterior major, the longus capitis, the iliocostalis cervicis, the multifidi, the intertransversarii, the obliquus capitis inferior and superior, and the inferior oblique muscles. The lateral muscles include the sternomastoid, the levator scapulae, and the splenius cervicis, and the scalenus muscles. The anterior musculature includes the sternocleidomastoid muscles, the longus colli, the longus capitis, and the rectus capitis anterior, as well as some of the strap muscles. In the course of clinical practice, these various muscles generally are not considered as individual muscles but as functional groups. Consideration of these muscles as extensors, flexors, or rotators affords a better understanding of these functional groupings.

Neural and Vascular Structures

It has already been mentioned that the spinal canal is formed by the vertebral bodies anteriorly and the laminae or the neural arches posteriorly. In broad terms, these are the boundaries of the spinal canal. The pedicles support the laminae as walls hold up the roof of a house; thus, they are considered boundaries of the spinal canal as well. There has been considerable discussion about the normal dimensions of the spinal canal, and this has particularly been applied to athletes involved in contact sports. The strict definition of spinal canal stenosis is a spinal canal with a transverse diameter of less than 13 mm. The term *relative stenosis* indicates a spinal canal diameter of 10 to 13 mm. The term *absolute stenosis* describes a spinal canal less than 10 mm in transverse diameter. It has been shown that contact athletes with a narrowed spinal canal are at increased risk for spinal cord injury. Spinal canal dimension can be measured accurately with computed tomography (CT) and somewhat less accurately with magnetic resonance imaging (MRI). These methods should be employed whenever a contact athlete is being evaluated for a significant neck injury. Similarly, osteoligamentous injuries should be sought in contact athletes with neck injury by use of flexion and extension lateral radiographs, and tomography and CT when necessary. Some recent data indicate that pre-existing low-grade instability and ligamentous injury may predispose contact athletes to neurologic injury.

The vertebral artery traverses the foramen transversarium of C3 through C6 (see Fig. 32–1). It is transmitted through a similar type of structure at C2 but lies in a shallow groove along the posterior surface of C1 before entering the foramen magnum, where it contributes to the posterior circulation at the base of the brain in the vertebrobasilar system. Vertebral artery injuries are rare in athletes, as in the general population; vertebral artery involvement in a degenerative process is also rare. The vertebral artery does contribute to the blood supply through vessels to the spinal cord.

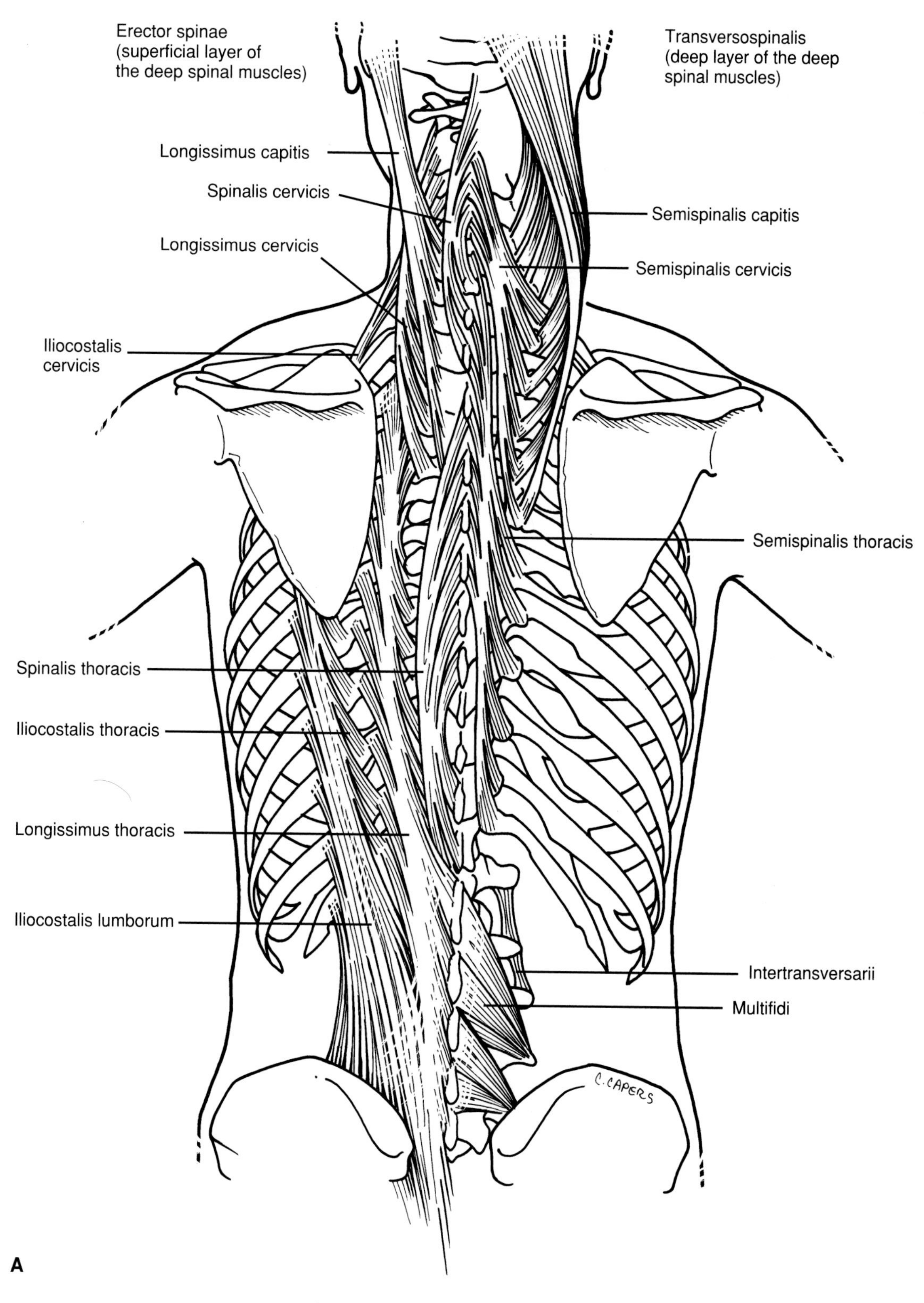

Fig. 32–7. *(A)* **Deeper muscles of the spine.**

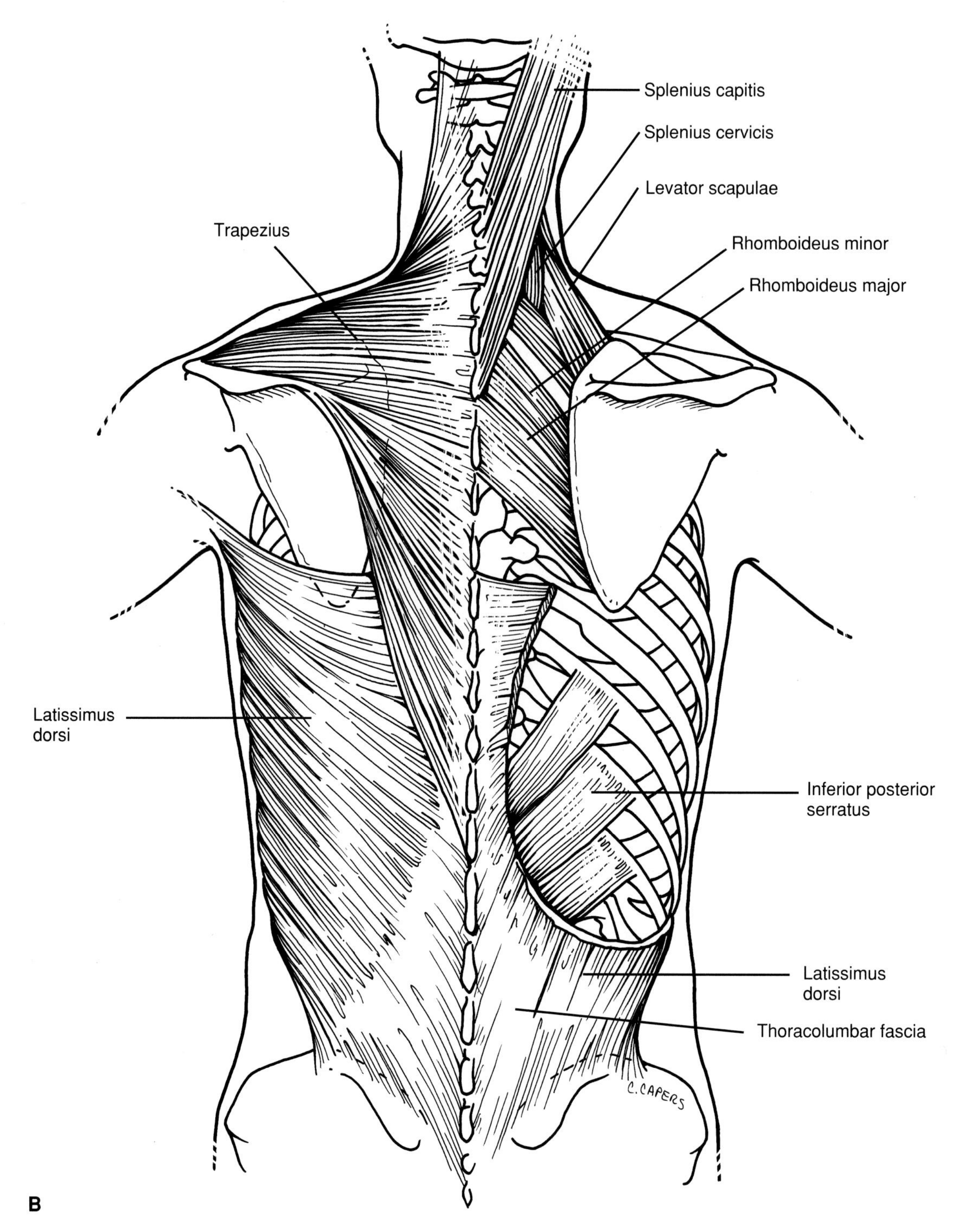

Fig. 32–7. (Continued). ***(B)*** **Superficial muscles of the spine. Note that the trapezius muscle extends to the T12 spinous process.**

THE THORACIC SPINE

Osteoligamentous Structures

The thoracic spine consists of 12 vertebral bodies, each of which articulates with a rib. At the cephalad end of the thoracic spine, the first four thoracic segments bear some resemblance to those in the lower cervical spine (Fig. 32–8). The middle four thoracic vertebral bodies are more typically "thoracic," and the lower four vertebral bodies begin assuming "lumbar" characteristics, in both vertebral body design and facet joint articulations. Each thoracic vertebral segment is composed of a vertebral body; these become successively larger from T1 to T12. There is an intervertebral disc at each level bounded by an annulus fibrosus and an anterior and a posterior longitudinal ligament, as previously described for the cervical spine.

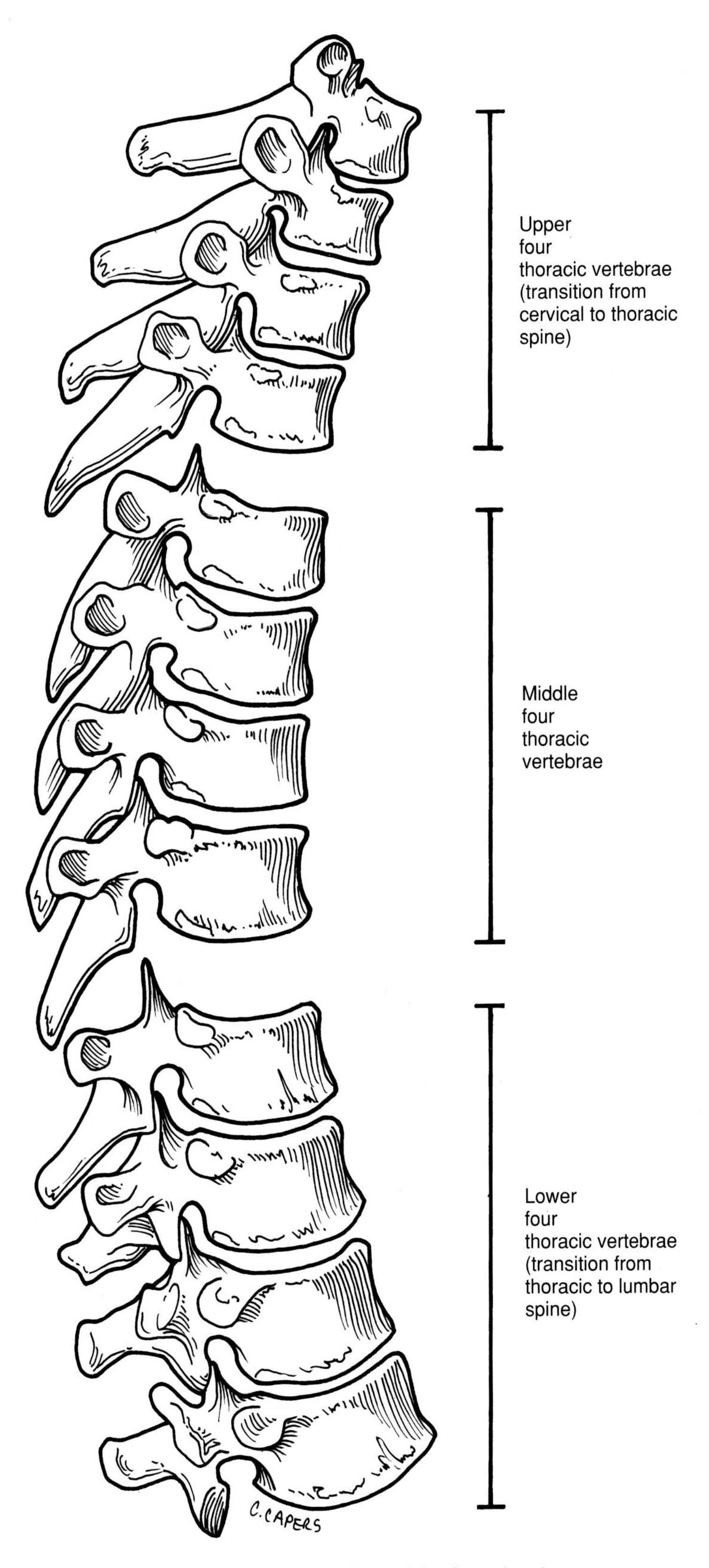

Fig. 32–8. The morphology of the thoracic spine.

Each rib articulates in three places with vertebral components. The rib head articulates with the lower posterior portion of the vertebral body above and the upper posterior portion of the vertebral body below and then with the anterolateral aspect of the transverse process of the vertebral body in the lower segment. The first rib may articulate only with the T1 vertebral body and its transverse process. Similarly, the eleventh and twelfth ribs may only articulate with the respective vertebral body and its transverse process; however, in sum, these rib articulations confer a great deal of stability to the thoracic spine.

The overall shape of the thoracic spine is generally convex posteriorly, a configuration known as *kyphosis.* The cervical spine and lumbar spine are convex anteriorly; that is, the configuration is *lordotic.* The cervicothoracic juncture between C7 and T1 represents the joining of the highly mobile cervical spine with the minimally mobile thoracic spine. Though traumatic injury or degenerative changes may be seen in this area, most such problems are more characteristic of the C5-6 and C6-7 levels. This is not the case at the thoracolumbar junction, where the minimally mobile thoracic spine meets the very mobile lumbar spine. Both compression and burst fractures occur at the lower thoracic spine, and this is where the majority of thoracic disc herniations occur as well. Because the midthoracic spine is situated at the apex of a kyphotic segment, there is some predisposition to fracture in this area. This should be considered when evaluating a painful thoracic spine injury.

Musculature

The trapezius muscle extends from the base of the occiput to T12 in the thoracic spine and is in the most superficial group of muscles (see Fig. 32–7). The levator scapulae and rhomboideus minor and major are situated between the spinous processes of the upper thoracic spine and the medial border of the scapula. These are often strained and represent sources of pain in the upper thoracic spine midline known as the *interscapular region.* The latissimus dorsi is a large superficial muscle found in the middle to lower thoracic spine that extends down into the lumbar spine. Once again, it is commonly injured and when strained often leads to chronic muscle pain. The serratus muscles are found in the intermediate layer of the thoracic spine, and the deeper layers of thoracic spine musculature comprise the iliocostalis, the semispinalis thoracis, the spinalis, the longissimus, and the multifidi. Collectively, the spinalis, longissimus, and iliocostalis muscles are known as the erector spinae or the sacrospinalis. The deep fascia of the thoracic and lumbar spine is common and is referred to as the *thoracolumbar lumbodorsal fascia.*

Neural Elements

The spinal canal of the thoracic spine is continuous with the spinal canal of the cervical spine. It transmits the spinal cord, which tapers to a termination point, generally at the level of L1-2, known as the *conus medullaris.* Stenotic lesions are not usually seen in the thoracic spine, and its general lack of motion makes spinal cord injury at this level less common unless the spine is fractured or violently disrupted. Most painful lesions in the thoracic spine of athletes are myofascial pain syndromes, and they tend to be located either in the interscapular area or at the thoracolumbar junction. Thoracic disc protrusions rarely cause localized thoracic pain. This is discussed further in Chapter 37.

THE LUMBOSACRAL SPINE

Osteoligamentous Structures

The lumbar spine consists of five vertebral bodies that are greater in transverse diameter than in anteroposterior diameter. The vertebral bodies do tend to become progressively larger from L1 to L5. At the thoracolumbar juncture, the facet articulations assume "lumbar" characteristics (Fig. 32–9). Whereas the thoracic articulations are generally located in the coronal plane, the lumbar articulations are located more in the sagittal plane to facilitate flexion and extension motion. The orientation of lumbar facet joints tends to lie oblique to the sagittal plane, which confers anteroposterior stability to the lumbar spine along with its other supporting structures, namely the intervertebral discs and the interspinous and supraspinous ligaments, which connect the spinous processes of L1 through L5.

A thick, strong anterior longitudinal ligament traverses the anterior vertebral bodies from L1 through L5. The posterior longitudinal ligament is incomplete at the posterior margin of the annulus, and this structure tends to become progressively thinner toward the caudal portion of the lumbar spine. This may be a factor in the direction and location of some lower lumbar disc herniations. The remaining posterior ligamentous structures of the lumbar spine include the ligamenta flava, which connect the laminae, and the interspinous ligaments and the supraspinous ligaments, which connect the spinous processes. The facet joint capsules are strong and confer some degree of stability on the facet articulation. The lumbar pedicles are strong and support strong lumbar laminae.

The lumbar spine lordosis varies from person to person, but in general there is a neutral zone of curvature at the thoracolumbar juncture and then the lumbar spine curves into lordosis. The L5-S1 disc lies obliquely in the upright position, and there is a variable amount of shear across this joint. This may be related to the mechanical process of degeneration of this disc. The lumbosacral articulation at L5-S1 is no different from other lumbar articulations. There are variations of normal, however, in which L5 articulates partially or totally with S1. There may be transverse processes of L5 that closely resemble the sacral alae, and there may be a *rudimentary disc* at L5-S1. This is a term applied when the L5-S1 articulation does not move and a disc is present between L5 and S1.

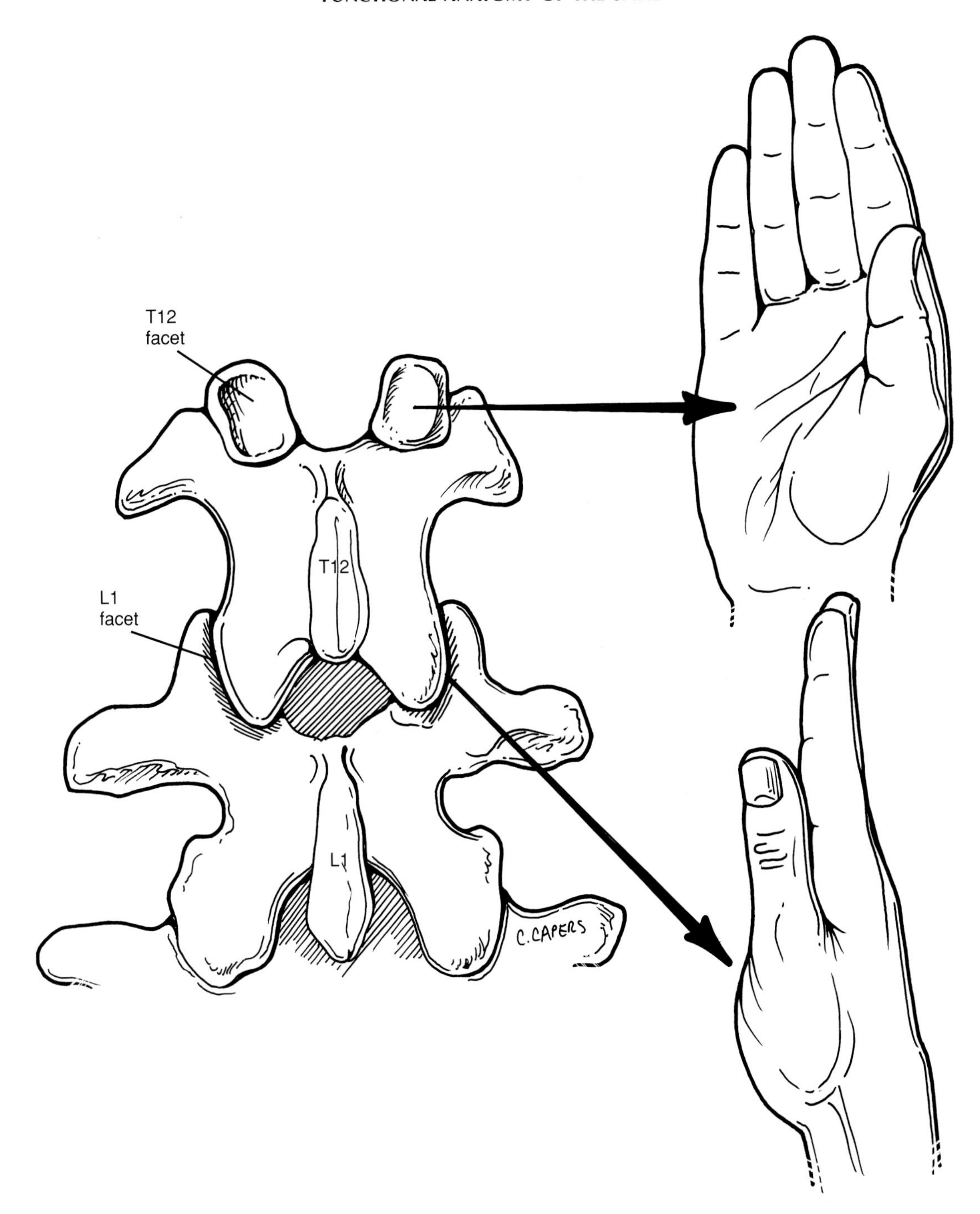

Fig. 32–9. In the transition from thoracic to lumbar vertebra, note the change in orientation of the facet joints.

The disc structures in the lumbar spine are generally no different than those in the remaining portions of the spine. The tough outer annulus fibrosus contains an inner nucleus pulposus. The lumbar discs are larger than the discs in the remaining portions of the spine and must bear more weight. Lumbar disc pressure is greatest with spine flexion, particularly when a person is seated. This is an important fact to remember when evaluating lumbar spine pain, because sitting almost always aggravates low back or leg pain of disc origin.

One aspect of the bony anatomy of the lumbar spine must be understood completely by all who treat spine problems. Paired structures known as the *pars interarticularis* connect the lumbar lamina with the lumbar pedicle (Fig. 32–10). A defect *(spondylolysis)* may develop in this structure in early childhood. On radiographs, it tends to appear as an unhealed fracture, and there is considerable controversy about its exact origin. Over time, osteocartilaginous material fills the defect in the pars interarticularis. This is most common at L5 but can occur at any level in the lumbar spine. The defect may lead to forward slippage of the vertebral body known as *spondylolisthesis.* It may also cause nerve root irritation by compressing the nerve immediately beneath this defect with

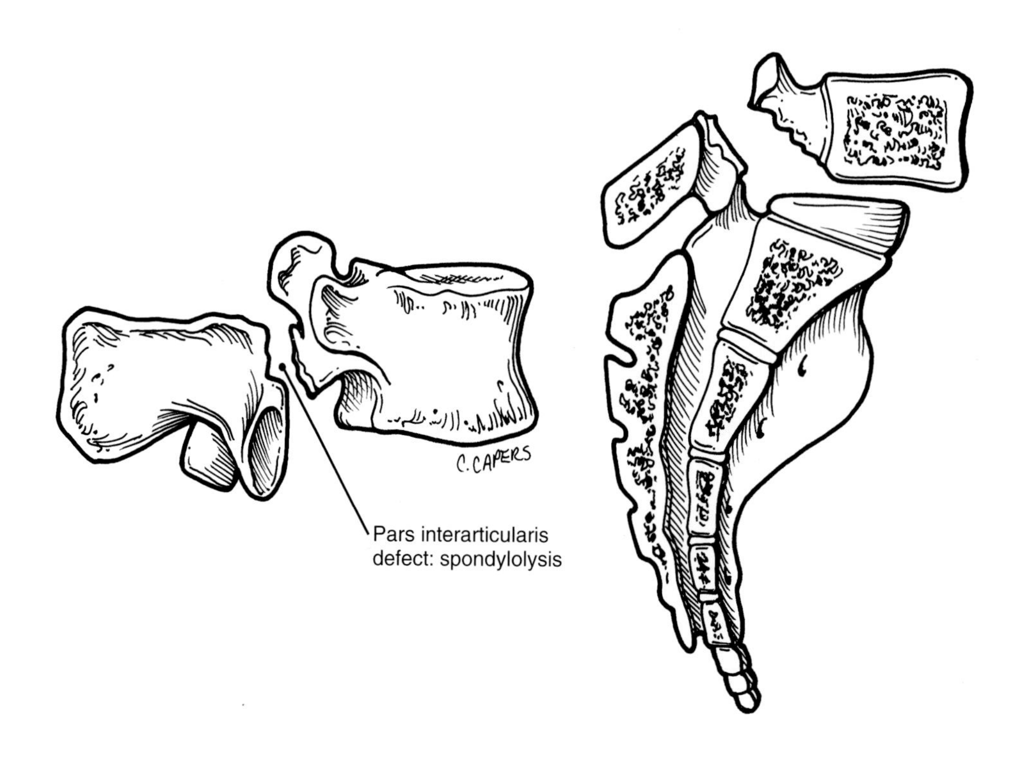

Fig. 32–10. The pars interarticularis connects the pedicle to the lamina. Acquired or developmental defects in the pars interarticularis are the principal lesion that leads to spondylolisthesis in the isthmus.

the hypertrophic osteocartilaginous material. Traumatic injuries to the pars interarticularis may occur in athletes, and generally they tend to occur when the spine is extended. This is well known in football linemen, weight lifters, and gymnasts. If an acute pars interarticularis fracture is suspected, a bone scan frequently confirms it. A longstanding pars defect is demonstrated best on an oblique plain radiograph or an oblique tomogram.

Musculature

The lumbar musculature may be broadly divided into extensors of the lumbar spine or paraspinal muscles and flexors of the lumbar spine, which include the anterior abdominal wall muscles and the flexors of the hips and pelvis. Posteriorly, there is a thick fascial structure that is continuous with the thoracic fascia known as the thoracolumbar fascia (see Fig. 32–7A). Deep to this lie the lumbar paraspinal muscles, which include the interspinalis (immediately adjacent to the spinous process), the multifidi (immediately lateral to the interspinalis), the longissimus (a lateral paraspinal muscle), and the iliocostalis muscles (lateral and confluent with the thoracic spine). The quadratus lumborum lies immediately beneath the iliocostalis muscle, and the intertransversarii laterales and mediales are just deep to the longissimus muscle. The primary anterior musculature is made up of the abdominal wall muscles: the rectus abdominis, internal and external oblique muscles of the abdomen, and the transversus abdominus. The iliopsoas lies deep along the anterolateral vertebral body and acts primarily as a hip flexor, but it may also act to flex the lumbar spine when the hip is locked in full extension.

Lumbar muscle injuries are extremely common and may involve any group of muscles in the lumbar spine. There has been considerable discussion about lumbar facet injuries as the cause of low back pain, and these do exist, but they are difficult to diagnose as a specific entity. Lumbar disc injuries are complex entities that are discussed in Chapter 37.

Neural Elements

Within the spinal canal of the lumbar spine is the conus medullaris, or the caudal tip of the spinal cord at the level of L1-2. The remaining portion of the lumbar spinal canal is occupied by the cauda equina, a collection of lumbar nerves that exit at each level to form lumbar nerve roots. The lumbar nerve roots exit the spinal canal in a very typical fashion. They tend to arise just above the level of a disc and then traverse the disc posteriorly and course caudad in the lateral portion of the spinal canal just beneath the facet articulation. The area beneath the facet articulation is known as the *lat-*

eral recess, or the *subarticular zone.* The nerves then lie in close relation to the pedicle of the exiting vertebral body along its medial aspect and in close relation to the inferior margin of the same pedicle as it exits through the neuroforamen. Therefore, the L5 nerve root arises just above the L4-5 disc. It traverses the posterior aspect of the L4-5 disc. It lies immediately beneath the L4-5 articulation and then lies in contact with the medial and the caudal aspect of the L5 pedicle before exiting the L5-S1 neuroforamen. All of these considerations are extremely important in understanding lumbar nerve root compression, a common problem in patients of all ages.

FURTHER READING

Anderson, J. E. (ed.): Grant's Atlas of Anatomy. 7th Ed. Baltimore, Williams & Wilkins, 1978.

The Cervical Spine Research Society Editorial Committee: The Cervical Spine. 2nd Ed. Philadelphia, J.B. Lippincott, 1989.

Frymoyer, J. W.: The Adult Spine: Principles and Practice. New York, Raven Press, 1991.

Grodinsky, M., and Holyoke, E. A.: Fascial and fascial spaces of the head, neck, and adjacent regions. Am. J. Anat. *63*:367, 1938.

Rothman, R. H., and Simeone, F. A. (eds.): The Spine. 3rd Ed. Philadelphia, W.B. Saunders, 1992.

Watkins, R. G. (ed.): Lumbar Discectomy and Laminectomy. Rockville, MD, Aspen, 1987.

Whitecloud, T. S., and Dunsker, S. B. (eds.): Anterior Cervical Spine Surgery. New York, Raven Press, 1993.

Weinstein, J. N., and Wiesel, S. W. (eds.): The Lumbar Spine. Philadelphia, W.B. Saunders, 1990.

33

Thomas N. Bernard, Jr.

Examining and Imaging the Athlete's Spine

The physical examination, imaging studies, and clinical history are the foundations of accurate diagnosis of an athlete's spine problems. The patient's clinical history should direct the clinician's choice of the type and extent of the physical examination and of imaging studies. The examination begins with the patient's history. The patient's overall behavior and appearance may shed light on the patient's perception of the problem and can alert the examiner to potential behavioral or personality disorders that might ultimately influence the diagnosis and treatment. Patients should be comfortably dressed in an examining gown that allows adequate visualization of the spine and extremities.

CERVICAL SPINE

The examination of the cervical spine begins with inspection of the neck, shoulders, upper back, and extremities for asymmetry of muscle mass, muscle atrophy, and scars. The cervical and upper thoracic paraspinal muscles are palpated for tenderness or spasm. Particular attention should be directed to the levator scapulae, rhomboids, and trapezius muscles, which are common areas of referred pain from cervical syndromes. Palpation of the brachial plexus, cubital tunnel, carpal tunnel, and thoracic outlet completes the initial examination.

The cervical spine is moved actively and passively through the range of motion as the examiner notes, in degrees, the amounts of flexion, extension, lateral bending, and rotation (Fig. 33–1). The examiner should note if the patient experiences pain at any point during the motion examination.

Spurling's maneuver is performed by applying axial compression to the neck in both the neutral position and with the neck in extension, followed by neck extension and rotation to the right and left (Fig. 33–2). This test may elicit localized pain from a cervical facet joint or radicular pain from nerve root irritation.The neurologic examination of the cervical spine includes evaluation of upper extremity motor strength and sensation, spinal reflexes, and, when indicated, certain tests for spinal cord dysfunction. By having the patient actively contract a muscle group against the examiner's resistance, the examiner can evaluate motor strength by manual testing. The upper extremity muscles that are examined to evaluate cervical and upper thoracic nerve root function and the associated cervical reflexes are listed in Table 33–1. Sensation to light touch and pinprick is evaluated over the cervical and upper thoracic dermatomes (Fig. 33–3).

When the clinical history or physical examination suggests an upper motor neuron lesion or spinal cord compression, the patient should be examined for rigidity, spasticity, clonus, and hyper-reflexia in the upper and lower extremities. Other tests for upper motor neuron abnormalities include Lhermitte's sign, Hoffmann's sign, (Fig. 33–4) and the plantar extensor response

Table 33–1. The Predominant Spinal Nerve Root Level and Associated Cervical Reflexes of Upper Extremity Muscles

Muscle	*Spinal Root Level*	*Reflex*
Deltoid	C5	——
Biceps	C5, C6	Biceps
Wrist extensors	C7	Brachioradialis
Wrist flexors	C7, C8	——
Triceps	C7	Triceps
Finger extensors	C7	——
Finger flexors	C8	——
Interossei	T1	——

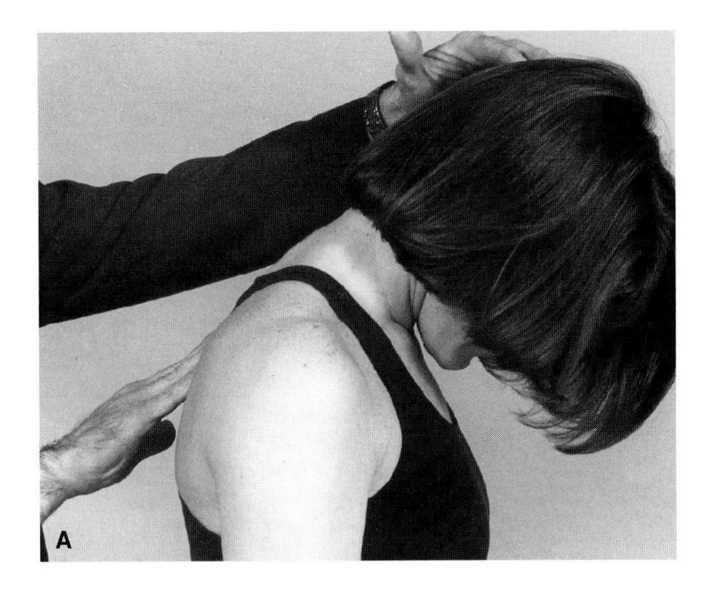

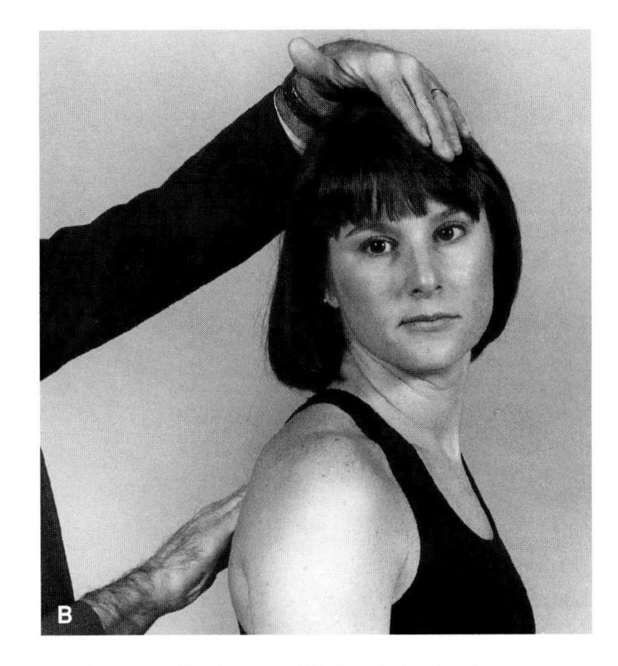

Fig. 33–1. Active and passive range of motion of the cervical spine are determined in degrees of flexion *(A)*, extension, lateral bending, and rotation *(B)*. The examiner should note any restricted range of motion and at what points the patient experiences any symptoms of pain or neurologic changes in upper or lower extremities.

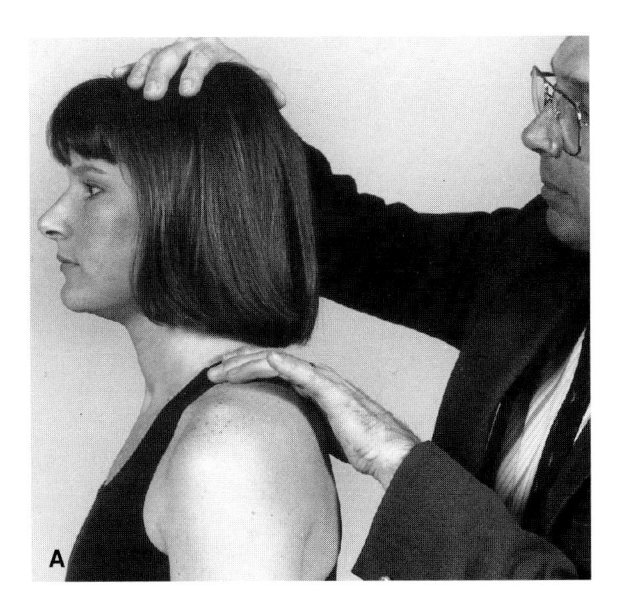

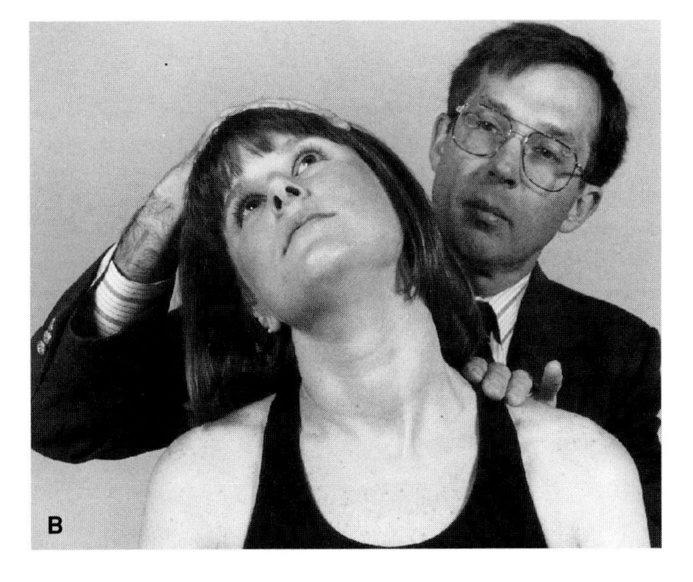

Fig. 33–2. Spurling's maneuver is performed by applying axial compression to the cervical spine in the neutral position *(A)* followed by neck extension and with rotation to both right *(B)* and left. Localized or referred pain may occur if pain is emanating from a cervical facet joint. Radicular symptoms may be elicited with this maneuver in the presence of nerve root irritation.

(Babinski's sign). The shoulder joint should be examined as a part of the cervical spine examination since many cervical spine and shoulder syndromes share common pain pathways.

Cervical Spine Imaging

The clinical history and physical examination dictate the sequence and type of imaging needed. In situations of acute trauma to the cervical spine, a cross-table lateral plain radiograph of the immobilized cervical spine should be the initial film. The C7 vertebra should be clearly seen on this view. Next is the "trauma series," which includes anteroposterior, open-mouthed odontoid, oblique, and physician-controlled flexion and extension lateral views. Patients with documented head injury should have cervical spine radiographs in addition to skull radiographs. In cases other than trauma, anteroposterior and flexion, neutral, and extension lateral radi-

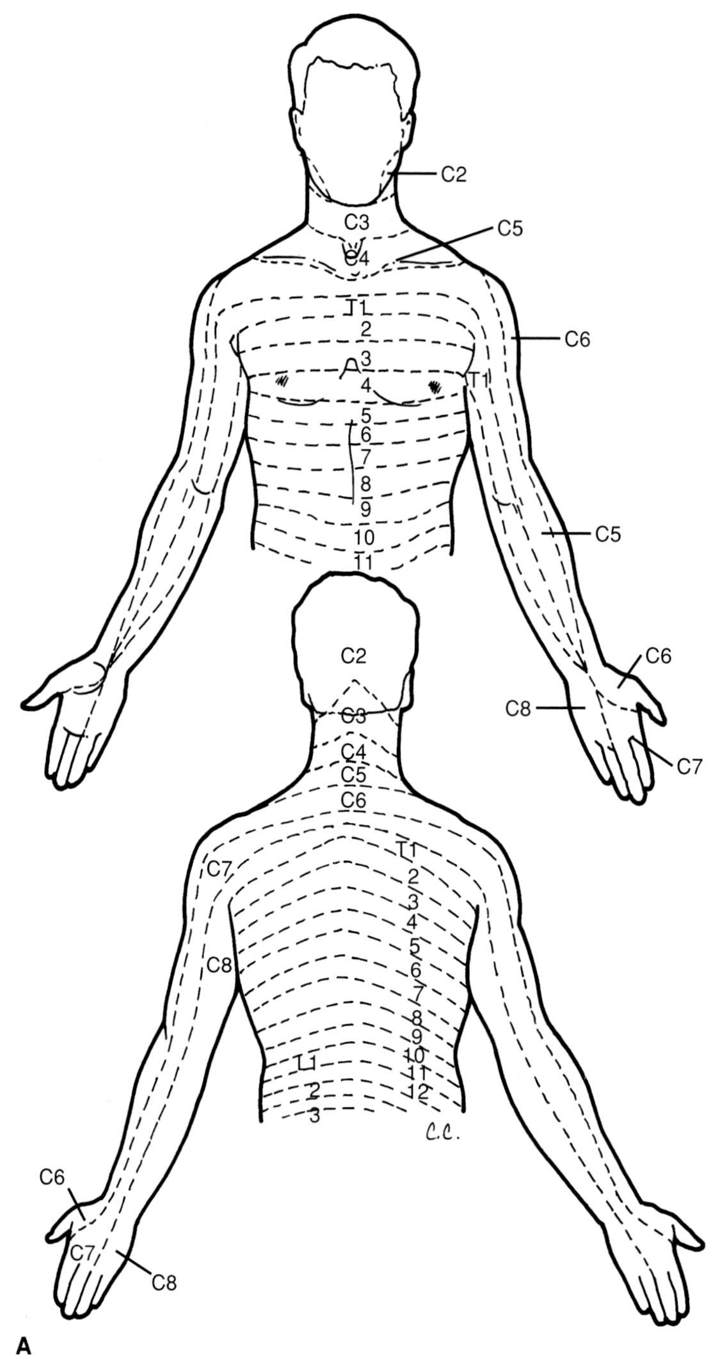

Fig. 33–3. (*A*) **Map of cervical and thoracic dermatomes.**

ographs are adequate for assessing stability of the cervical spine and demonstrating congenital anomalies.

Abnormal plain radiographic findings include loss of cervical lordosis in the neutral position and an atlantodens interval greater than 4 mm in an adult. In adults, prevertebral soft tissue swelling greater than 7 mm at C2 or greater than 22 mm at C6 can indicate significant cervical spine trauma.(1) In children, however, prevertebral swelling may not be a reliable sign.(2) Indicators of cervical spine instability include greater than 3.5 mm forward displacement on a lateral cervical spine radiograph or greater than 11° angulation between adjacent cervical vertebrae (Fig. 33–5).(3,4)

Lateral radiographs of the cervical spine allow measurement of the sagittal diameter of the spinal canal, which may be useful in evaluating cervical spine stenosis. Pavlov's ratio is measured from the middle of the posterior surface of the vertebral body to the nearest point of the corresponding spinal laminar line (Fig. 33–6). A ratio of less than 0.82:1 is thought to indicate cervical spine stenosis.(5–7) Using axial computed tomography (CT) measurements, a midbody measurement of

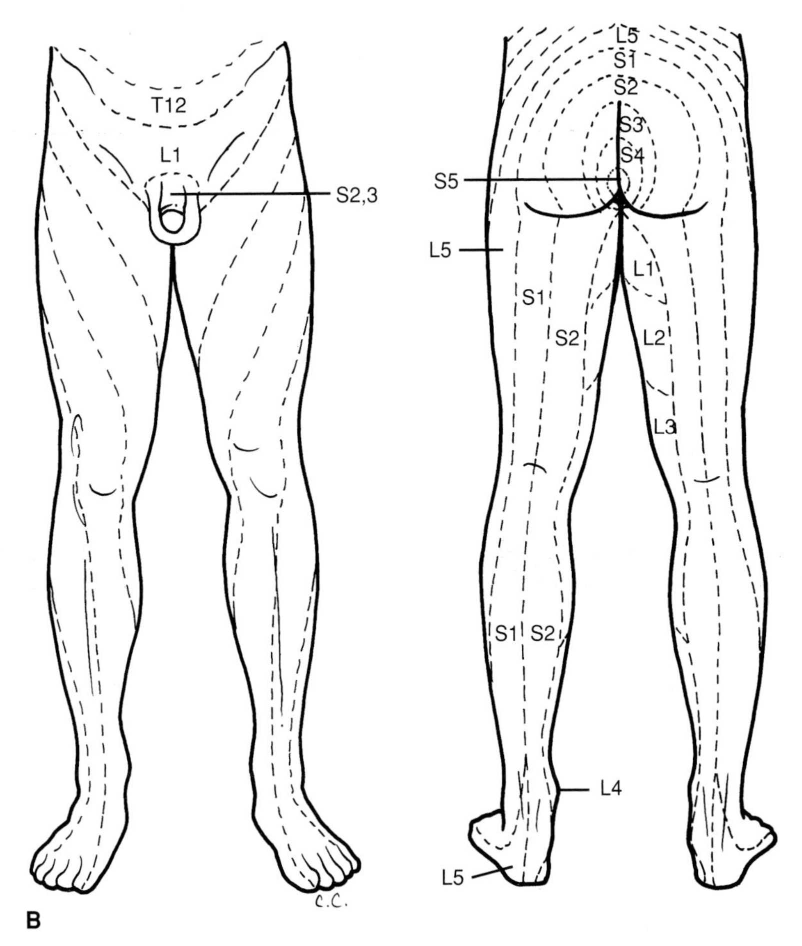

Fig. 33–3. (continued). (*B*) Map of lumbar and sacral dermatomes.

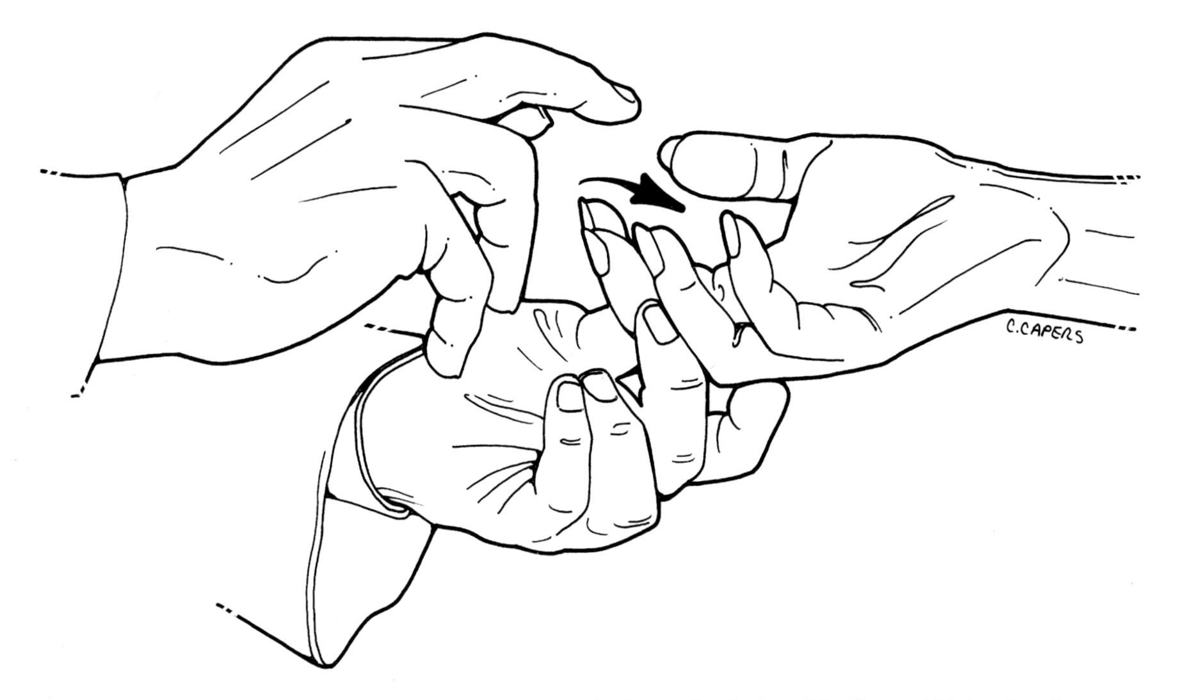

Fig. 33–4. Hoffmann's sign: rapid extension of the fingers leads to reflex flexion of the fingers. This is a sign of upper motor neuron dysfunction.

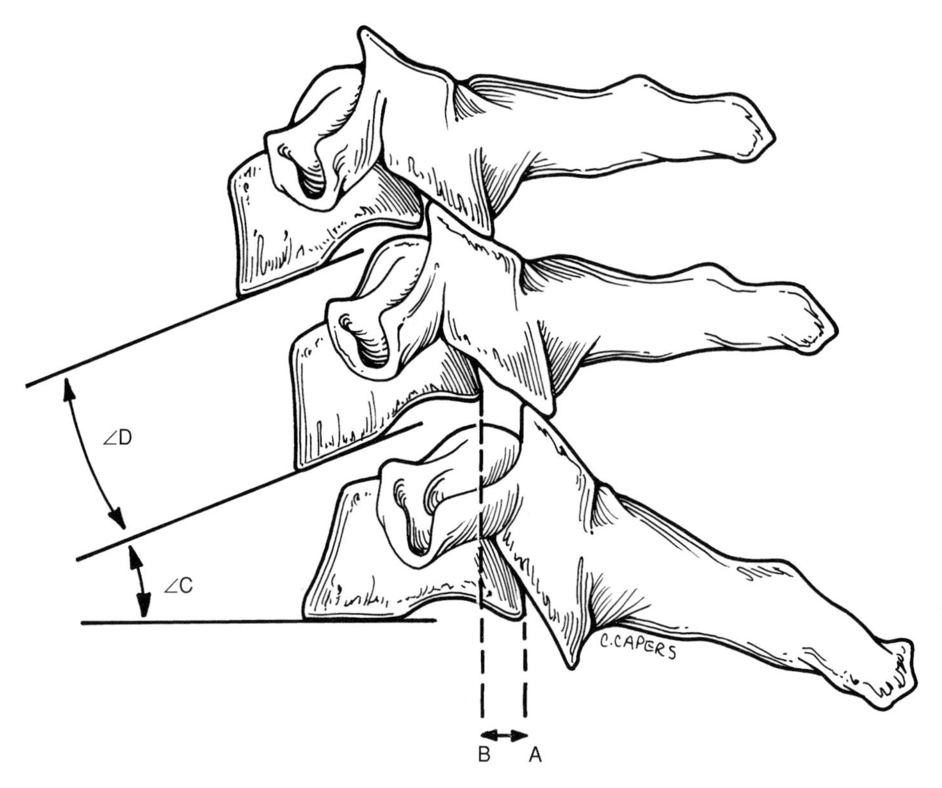

Fig. 33–5. Forward displacement of one cervical vertebra greater than 3.5 mm (the distance between A and B) or angulation between adjacent cervical vertebrae (angle C minus D) more than 11° are findings consistent with cervical instability.

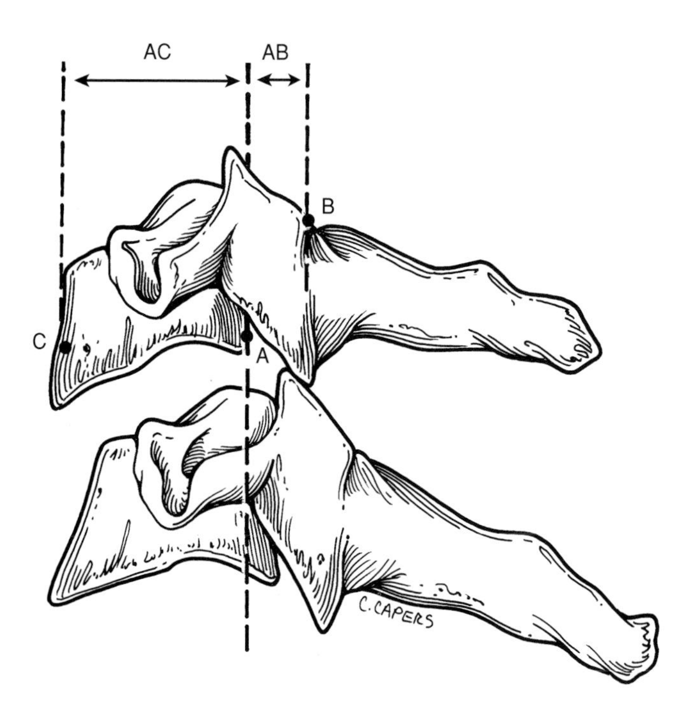

Fig. 33–6. Pavlov's ratio is determined by measuring the distance from the midportion of the posterior cervical body to the spinal laminar line (AB) and dividing this value by the width of the vertebral body (AC).

less than 12.5 mm indicates a marginal-sized spinal canal; however, this method has been criticized because of the observation that increasing cervical lordosis leads to an abnormally high rate of false-positive measurements using this technique. The significance of Pavlov's ratio remains controversial. The overall shape of the cervical spinal canal may be more of a predisposing factor to symptomatic cervical stenosis than the cross-sectional diameter. When quotient produced by dividing the diameter of the sagittal spinal canal by the transverse diameter is less than 0.6, the athlete may be predisposed to spinal cord injury if sufficient trauma occurs (Fig. 33–7).[8]

A history of numbness or weakness in both upper extremities or a combination of numbness or weakness in both upper and lower extremities should raise suspicion of a significant neurologic event. A clear distinction must be made between spinal cord contusion and brachial plexus contusion (or "stingers"). When the clinical history and physical findings suggest that the injury was the result of spinal cord contusion, the radiographic findings inform the decision to allow the athlete to continue in contact sports or to forbid such activity. These findings include loss of cervical lordosis on a neutral lateral radiograph, a Pavlov's ratio less than 0.82:1 at any motion segment between C3 and C7, an absolute vertebral sagittal diameter less than 12.5 mm

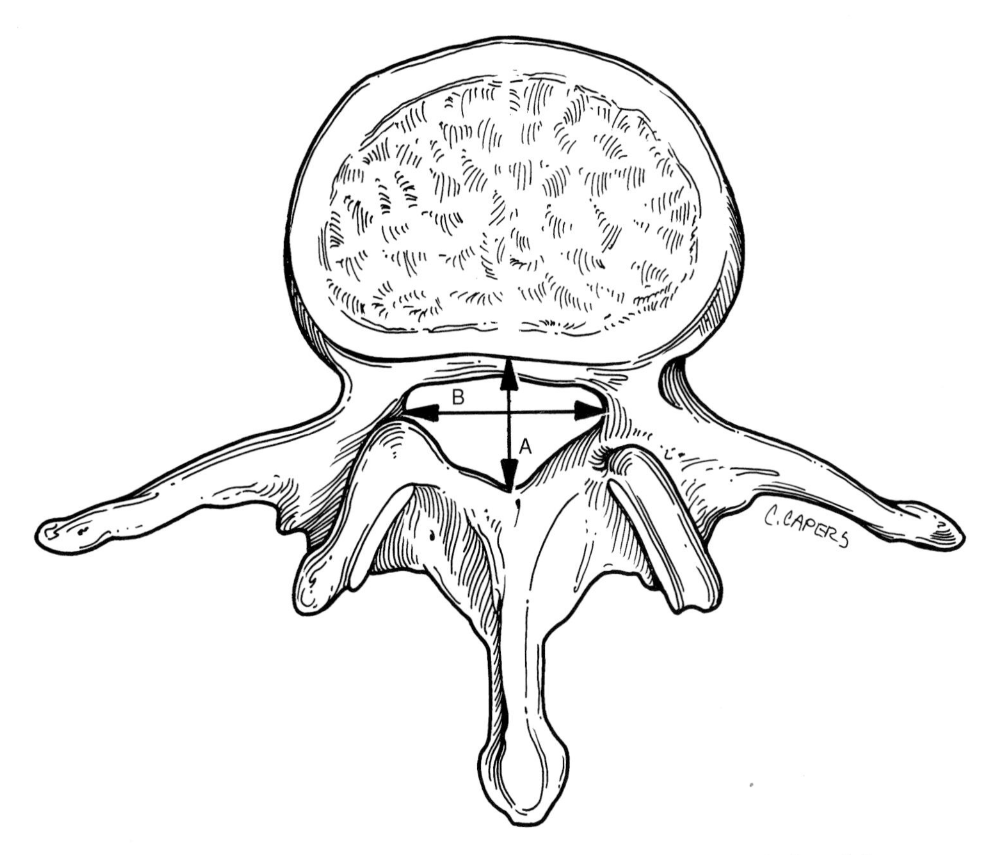

Fig. 33–7. The ratio of the sagittal spinal canal diameter (*A*) divided by the transverse spinal canal diameter (*B*) may be a more sensitive indicator of a spinal canal configuration that predisposes to spinal cord injury. A ratio of less than 0.6 is abnormal.

on CT with cervical lordosis eliminated, and a transverse diameter ratio of less than 0.6:1 between any motion segment from C3 to C7.

A nonenhanced CT image should be obtained to evaluate any acute fracture or to resolve any questionable anomaly seen on plain radiographs. CT with bone-window settings using both sagittal and coronal reformations provides the best means for assessing bony abnormalities in the cervical spine.

Magnetic resonance imaging allows visualization of the spinal cord, cervical disc, and the occipitocervical junction. Cervical magnetic resonance imaging (MRI) should be the primary test when evaluating for cervical radicular syndromes. Intrathecally enhanced CT would be a secondary imaging study to evaluate equivocal findings on cervical MRI.

THORACIC SPINE

The thoracic spine should be inspected with the patient standing in the neutral position. The examiner notes any asymmetry or cutaneous abnormalities such as hairy patches or midline dimples that might suggest an underlying spinal dysraphism. Spinal balance is determined by noting the position of the C7 spinous process relative to the first sacral spinous process. The patient is examined in forward flexion, extension, and lateral bending. When evaluating patients with increased thoracic kyphosis, the distinction between a postural round back deformity and Scheuermann's deformity may be made by noting whether there is a sharp break in the kyphotic angle when the patient is in the forward flexed position. The paraspinal muscles overlying the thoracic posterior facet joints should be palpated for areas of tenderness.

The neurologic evaluation of the thoracic spine is limited to evaluating the thoracic dermatomes by light touch and pinprick. The superficial abdominal reflex is performed with the patient supine on the examining table. Each quadrant of the abdomen is stroked with the end of a neurologic hammer or pin wheel noting whether the umbilicus deviates toward the point being stroked. Absence of the abdominal reflex in the upper quadrants indicates an upper motor lesion from T7 to T10, whereas absence of the reflex in the lower quadrants indicates a lesion between T10 and L1.[9]

Thoracic Spine Imaging

Standing anteroposterior and lateral plain radiographs are used to evaluate sagittal and coronal plane deformity. The normal range of thoracic kyphosis is 20° to 40°.[10] Any wedging of three adjacent vertebrae greater than 5° with the presence of Schmorl's nodes or end-plate irregularity may suggest Scheuermann's kyphosis. Radionuclide imaging and MRI of the thoracic spine should be considered to evaluate any unexplained thoracic pain or upper motor neuron abnormalities affecting the lower extremities.

LUMBAR SPINE

The examination of the lumbar spine begins with observing the patient's posture and gait and inspecting the lumbar region for deformity or asymmetry. The peripheral pulses should also be examined. The paraspinal muscles are palpated for tenderness or spasm. Other areas that should be palpated during the lumbar evaluation include the sacral sulci, coccyx, and greater trochanters. The lumbar paraspinal region is palpated for trigger points, subcutaneous fat nodules, and any step-off between lumbar spinous processes that might suggest spondylolisthesis. The lumbar spinous processes are then gently rocked from side to side to evaluate the lumbar facet joints. The muscles of the buttocks and lower extremities are palpated for motor point tenderness. Thigh and calf circumference, leg length, and hamstring tightness are measured. The patient's range of motion in flexion, extension, and lateral bending are noted in degrees (Fig. 33–8).

The neurologic examination of the lumbar spine includes evaluation of lower extremity motor strength, sensation to light touch and pinprick, spinal reflexes, and signs of nerve root tension. The lower extremity muscles, along with the predominant spinal nerve root and associated reflex, are listed in Table 33–2. The lumbar and sacral dermatomes are examined by light touch and pinprick, according to the scheme shown in Figure 33–3.

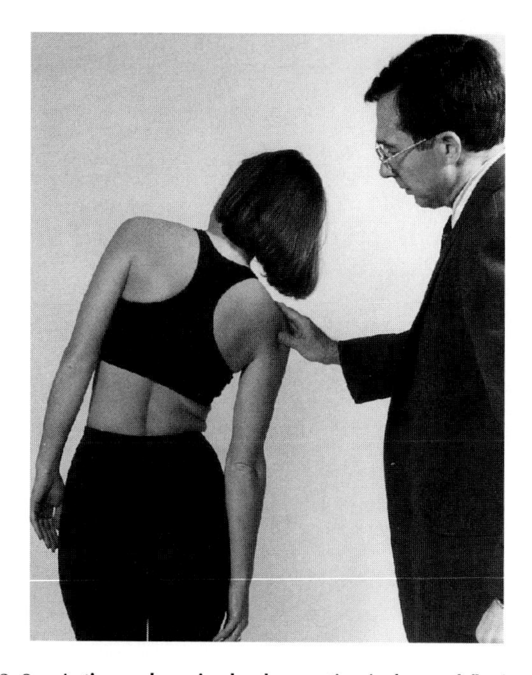

Fig. 33–8. Active and passive lumbar motion in forward flexion, extension, and lateral bending are noted in degrees.

Table 33–2. The Predominant Spinal Nerve Root and Associated Reflexes of Lower Extremity Muscles

Muscle	*Spinal Root Level*	*Reflex*
Iliopsoas	T12, L1, L2, L3	——
Quadriceps femoris	L2, L3, L4	Patella
Hip adductor	L2, L3, L4	——
Tibialis anterior	L4	——
Extensor hallucis longus	L5	——
Peroneus longus, brevis	S1	Achilles
Gastrocnemius, soleus	S1, S2	——
Gluteus maximus	S1	——

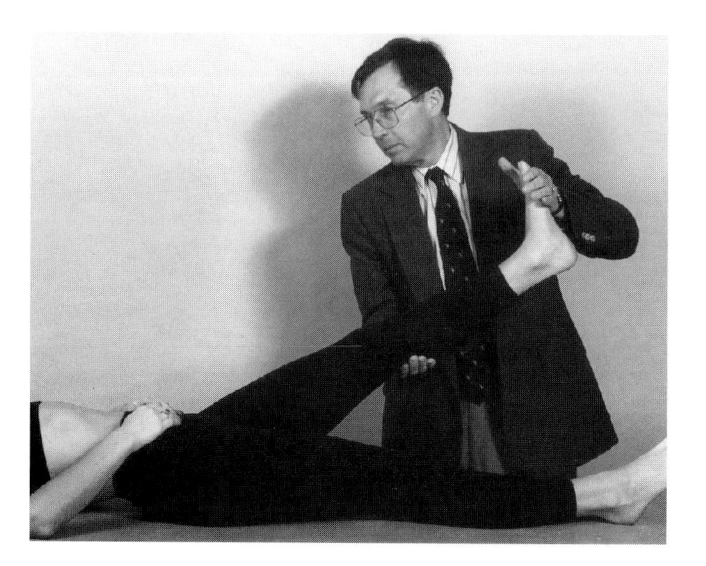

Fig. 33–9. Fajersztajn's maneuver.

Among the various sciatic nerve stretching maneuvers, the straight leg–raising maneuver is probably best known. This is performed with the patient in the supine position and is considered positive when there is reproduction of radicular pain and not purely lower back pain. Foot dorsiflexion (Fajersztajn's maneuver) may exacerbate a positive response during the straight leg–raising maneuver (Fig. 33–9).[11] Hamstring tightness may be an obstacle to performing the maneuver. In this case, the popliteal compression test or Cram's maneuver can be performed to isolate the sciatic nerve, and it may be more specific for nerve root irritation (Fig. 33–10).[12] The accuracy of the sciatic nerve root tension signs is not affected by the angle at which the test is positive but by whether familiar leg pain is reproduced.

The femoral nerve tension test may be performed with the patient prone or on one side. The patient extends the hip and then flexes the knee. The less familiar sitting straight leg–raising test (Deyerle's and May's test) may be used to confirm a supine straight leg–raising test. Contralateral nerve root tension signs are very suggestive of nerve root entrapment or disc herniation.

The prone knee flexion test of Herron and Pheasant is performed with the patient prone and the knee flexed.[13] With maximal knee flexion, the lordosis of the lumbar spine is accentuated, and this may enhance

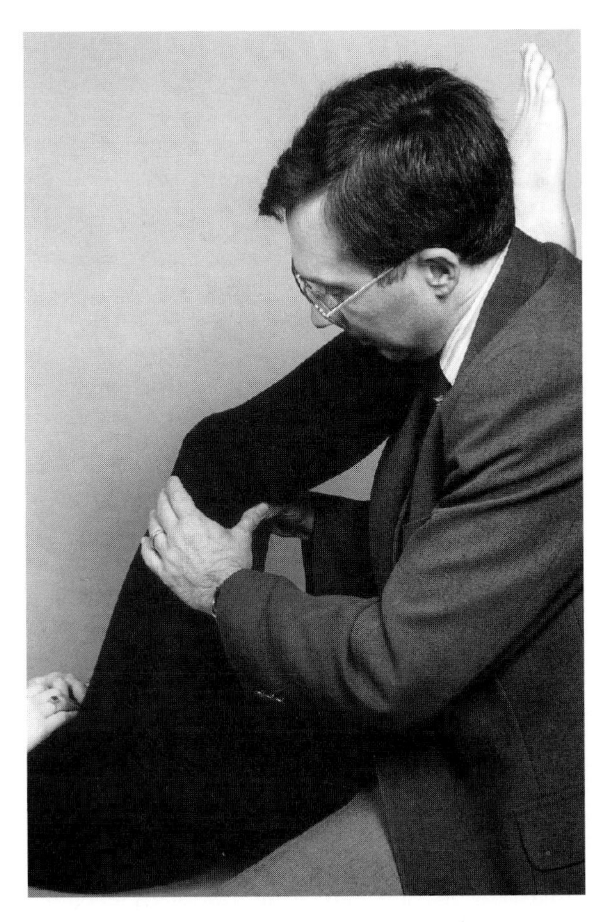

Fig. 33–10. Cram's maneuver, or popliteal compression test, is performed with the hamstrings relaxed.

reflex suppression or motor weakness secondary to spinal stenosis or lumbar disc herniation.

Signs of nonorganic pain include a positive pain response to axial loading of the spine in the standing position, rotating the upper torso without moving the lumbar spine, a reverse straight leg–raising sign, and a negative sitting straight leg–raising sign in the presence of a markedly positive supine straight leg–raising sign.

Lumbar Spine Imaging

Plain radiographic evaluation of the lumbar spine should include anteroposterior, lateral, oblique, and Ferguson's (30° cephalad tilt) views of the lumbosacral junction. These views will identify any transitional motion segments and reveal abnormalities in the pars interarticularis. Radionuclide scanning should be obtained to confirm any occult fractures and to identify whether a pars interarticularis defect is acute. To evaluate the lumbar compartment for disc herniation, spinal stenosis, or intrathecal lesions, MRI is the primary test. Nonenhanced CT is superior to MRI for evaluating bony anomalies in the lumbar spine. Intrathecally enhanced CT may be indicated to evaluate equivocal findings on MRI or nonenhanced CT. Lumbar discography may be of value to confirm whether disc abnormalities are clinically significant.

REFERENCES

1. Charlton, O. P., Gehweiler, J. A., and Martinez, S.: Roentgenographic evaluation of cervical spine trauma. J.A.M.A. *242*:1073, 1979.
2. Boger, D. C.: Cervical prevertebral soft tissues in children: An unreliable soft tissue indicator of cervical spine trauma. Contemp. Orthop. *5*(4):31, 1982.
3. White, A. A., Johnson, R. M., Panjabi, M. M., and Southwick, W. O.: Biomechanical analysis of clinical stability in the cervical spine. Clin. Orthop. *109*:85, 1975.
4. White, A. A., Southwick, W. O., and Panjabi, M. M.: Clinical instability in the lower cervical spine: A review of past and current concepts. Spine *1*:15, 1976.
5. Pavlov, H., Torg, J. S., Robie, B, and Jahre, C.: Cervical spinal stenosis: Determination with vertebral body ratio method. Radiology *164*:771, 1987.
6. Torg, J. S.: Pavlov's ratio: Determining cervical spinal stenosis on routine lateral roentgenograms. Contemp. Orthop. *18*(2):153, 1989.
7. Torg, J. S., Vegso, J. J., O'Neill, M. J., and Sennett, B.: The epidemiologic, pathologic, biomechanical, and cinematographic analysis of football-induced cervical spine trauma. Am. J. Sports Med. *18*:50, 1990.
8. Matsuura, P., et al.: Comparison of computerized tomography parameters of the cervical spine in normal control subjects and spinal cord–injured patients. J. Bone Joint Surg. *71A*:183, 1989.
9. Hoppenfeld, S.: Physical Examination of the Spine and Extremities. New York, Appleton-Century-Crofts, 1976.
10. Lowe, T. G.: Current concepts review Scheuermann disease. J. Bone Joint Surg. *72A*:940, 1990.
11. Scham, S. M., and Taylor, T. K. F.: Tension signs in lumbar disc prolapse. Clin. Orthop. *75*:195, 1971.
12. Cram, R. H.: A sign of sciatic nerve root pressure. J. Bone Joint Surg. *35B*:192, 1953.
13. Herron, L. D., and Pheasant, H. C.: Prone knee-flexion provocative testing for lumbar disc protrusion. Spine *5*:65, 1980.

34 Barry L. White

Stingers and Burners

Ask any football coach about a "stinger" or "burner" and he or she will most likely be familiar with them because of the frequency with which athletes experience them in practices and in games.[1–10] A defensive end coach sees these "hotshots" much more often than a quarterback coach.[2,4–7] A wrestling coach or weight lifting coach also likely knows about these "zingers" but sees them far less frequently. Gymnasts, boxers, backpackers, dirt bikers, and other athletes and outdoorsmen also occasionally have these "nerve concussions."[6,7,9] What are stingers or burners (also known by the other terms in quotes above)?

Stinger or *burner, hotshot, zinger,* and *nerve concussion* are terms for an intensely painful sensory paresthesia that lasts a few seconds to a few minutes and is accompanied by weakness in one upper extremity.[2] The weakness is of variable severity and can persist 15 minutes or longer.[5] Even though all stingers start out with almost exactly the same symptoms in most cases, the underlying injury can be quite different in severity and can affect either the brachial plexus or the nerve root.[4,11]

These symptoms are most often experienced unilaterally and indicate an injury no more proximal than the nerve root. If the symptoms appear simultaneously in both upper extremities, they are most often caused by a spinal cord injury and must be treated extremely cautiously as a medical emergency.[12]

The typical unilateral syndrome of the stinger or burner has a wide spectrum of resulting injury: a single transient nerve irritation with no residual deficits; those that recur as many as 50 times during a season with no residual deficits; complete avulsion of the nerve roots at the level of the spinal cord that results in catastrophic permanent anatomic and functional deficits to the upper extremity.[13,14] The result of the collision that causes the stinger syndrome depends on the scientific formula of mass times acceleration (size multiplied by speed) and the position of the structures (head, neck, and shoulder) involved at the instant of impact (Fig. 34–1).[10]

It is imperative for clinicians, trainers, coaches, and athletes to understand that all stingers are not the same. They are symptoms of a neurologic insult to either the nerve root or the brachial plexus that must be evaluated systematically to determine the extent of each injury and the appropriate treatment. Also, these professionals must try to prevent any recurrent injury, since recurrent stingers may result in more severe residual injury.[8] The purposes of this chapter are these:

1. To make it clear that resulting weakness after a stinger or burner is most likely nerve injury
2. To describe the underlying pathophysiology
3. To describe a method of classifying the injury and its severity
4. To suggest methods of treatment
5. To present criteria for return of athletes to competition
6. To suggest methods that will make recurrent injury less likely.

The primary goal for all concerned is to understand that stingers and burners are syndromes of nerve injury, so any residual weakness should be viewed as the result of nerve damage until it is proven otherwise. The athlete must be held from further contact sports until that weakness (nerve damage) is diagnosed, treated, and resolved.[1,2,4–6,8,10] The following sections of this chapter clarify this position.

CASE PRESENTATION

The following case presentation is included to emphasize the importance of the team approach to the health care of the athlete and the need for coaches and team health care professionals to communicate effectively. It

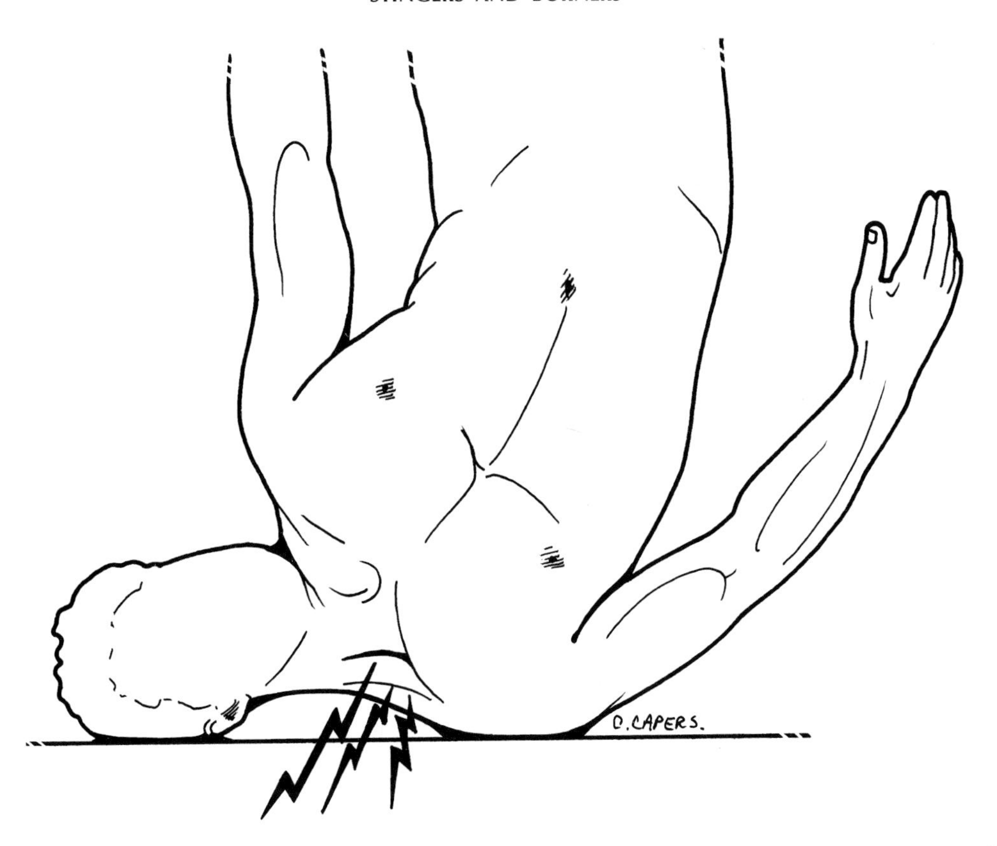

Fig. 34–1. The neck-shoulder angle is forced beyond normal range of motion by shoulder depression with cervical hyperextension with lateral bending toward the contralateral shoulder.

is most important for all coaches to understand that, in the absence of a trained sports medicine clinician, weakness following a stinger or burner must be considered the result of a nerve injury and players must avoid further contact until they are evaluated and released by the team physician. Any athlete who reports a stinger or burner should be evaluated immediately by the appropriate team sports medicine staff, and the results of that evaluation must be effectively reported to the player, trainer, and coach.

In the 1988 college football season, just at game time of the season opener, the head trainer pointed out to the team sports medicine clinician a senior football player who had experienced a right upper extremity stinger during a full-contact practice a few days earlier. The player, who was an extremely aggressive linebacker, came over for evaluation and demonstrated the following signs:

Range of motion: Full cervical range of motion without pain, less than 90° shoulder abduction and flexion against gravity without pain on the involved side
Strength (Manual muscle test): 5/5 (normal) on the uninvolved side, 3−/5 (could not hold against any resistance) on the involved side's deltoids and shoulder external rotators, 3+/5 biceps (able to move elbow through range and hold against minimal resistance) with no other significant weakness
Sensation: Normal, bilaterally, to light touch
Reflexes: 2+ for all upper extremity reflexes except for the involved side biceps, which was 1+.

The defensive coach was told by the clinician that the player had a weak shoulder and should not play until evaluated further after the game. The clinician left the player's shoulder pads off, so the injured player missed the first game of his senior year.

The injured linebacker came in for clinical evaluation the following week as requested. His right deltoid, external rotators, and biceps were still significantly weak. His strength in those muscles was less than good (4−/5). The player did have electrophysiologic studies that demonstrated a mild to moderate acute upper trunk brachial plexus injury with some nerve damage to the muscles that were weak on clinical evaluation. The site of the injury appeared to be the upper trunk of the brachial plexus distal to the dorsal root ganglion. There were no findings of cervical spine or nerve root injury.

The player was given a routine of light weight exercises and running. He was followed at weekly intervals until the fourth week of the season, at which time his strength was normal (equal to the left side). Electromyography showed no injury potentials (fibrillations and positive sharp waves at rest), and his recruitment pattern was near normal. In the fourth game of the season the linebacker was allowed to play with extra padding under his shoulder pads and a neck roll. He went on to have a great season, and subsequently played semi-professional football with no recurrent stingers or residual weakness. He did miss the first three games of the season because the team physician diagnosed the problem and effectively communicated to the coaches and player its seriousness. The player and coaches were able to accept the no-play status because the team physician made it clear that weakness following a stinger means nerve injury. The player was fortunate in this case because everyone worked together and his injury was easily resolved with rest.

MECHANISM AND FREQUENCY OF INJURY IN DIFFERENT CONTACT SPORTS AND AT DIFFERENT LEVELS OF COMPETITION

The stinger and burner syndrome is a very common complaint in American-style tackle football, but it is also reported in wrestlers, weight lifters, boxers, mountain climbers, backpackers, snow skiers and sledders, dirt bikers, and equestrian athletes.[5,6,8,9,13,15] Since most of the available literature on this syndrome deals with football injuries, that is the main focus here. The mechanism of burners usually involves the athlete's shoulder colliding with another athlete, the ground, or another fixed object and depressing the shoulder at the same time the cervical spine is hyperextended, hyperflexed, or laterally flexed to the opposite side. This results in a shoulder-neck angle beyond the normal range, which stretches the brachial plexus on the side of the contact.[2,4–7,10,16] The upper trunk of the brachial plexus or the C5-C6 nerve roots are injured. Nearly 50% of some collegiate football varsity teams' players may suffer this injury during a 4-year period. Five to ten percent of these may be serious enough to cause neurologic deficits that last several hours or longer.[1,5]

Vereschagin and coworkers[2] studied 446 football players at high school, junior college, and university levels of competition during 1989 and found the following incidences of exposure at practice and during games: university, 0.41%; junior college, 0.04%; high school, 0.02%. Articles by Hunter and Vereschagin present numbers of burners by position, and it is clear that defensive ends, linebackers, and defensive backs are more likely to receive stingers than other players.[2,7] Our 1993 fall sports physical examination of approximately 1000 freshmen-through-senior high school football players reported that 24 of them had previously had stingers and that no residual weakness was demonstrated on muscle testing of the shoulder abductors.

PATHOPHYSIOLOGIC BASIS OF STINGERS AND BURNERS

The symptoms of severe burning, stinging paresthesia, and anesthesia in one upper extremity radiate from the shoulder distally through the arm as far as the fingers. The burning and the accompanying weakness, most often of the shoulder abductors, external rotators, and elbow flexors (all upper trunk brachial plexus, C5-6–innervated muscles) are from a neural injury (Fig. 34–2). Symptoms can last a few seconds or years.[1,13,14]

The extent of the damage to the neural elements determines the severity and duration of the symptoms. The classification that we will use is an electrophysiologic method that correlates to Sunderland's classification system:

1. *Transient neurapraxia* (no structural damage and paresthesia and weakness that resolve in minutes) is a transient block of the neural conduction owing to temporary loss of the myelin (Schwann cell) function (a transient mechanical deformity or ischemia) around the axon. Most often it takes just minutes for this process to be resolved, so it is most likely a mechanical and vascular response of the neural elements with no structural damage. After myelin function is restored, the player is symptom free; although there is often soreness and bruising about the shoulder and soreness at the supraclavicular triangle (Erb's point) for days, during which Tinel's sign can be elicited.[7] This correlates to the "nerve pinch" and "nerve concussion" coined by Clancy and Hunter, respectively.[5,7]

2. *Neurapraxia* (numbness resolves in minutes but there is a degree of muscle weakness for up to 6 weeks) is an injury to the myelin sufficient to cause the body to actually absorb the injured cells and synthesize new Schwann cells, which then go through a maturation process to replace the damaged ones. This reparative phase takes varying periods, depending on the number of Schwann cells damaged and their location. Most often the neural function is back to a normal state within 2 to 6 weeks. During the period of dysfunction, the severity and the distribution of the neurapraxia can be estimated by the difference in muscle strength between the noninjured and the injured extremity. This can be documented electrophysiologically by nerve conduction studies, which should correlate with the motor weakness estimated by manual muscle testing.[4,6,11]

3. *Axonotmesis* (clinically evident when the athlete still has weakness after 6 weeks' compliance with a rehabilitation program) occurs when the injury is sufficient to cause damage to the axon and the myelin, which results in actual degeneration of the motor unit organization (nerve and its muscle fibers), which causes the clinically detected weakness. The extent of this injury can be documented by nerve conduction studies during the first 2 to 3 weeks. During this degenerative phase, the findings in the electrophysiology laboratory should correlate to the weakness found clinically. An electromyographic needle examination after about 2 to 3 weeks demonstrates fibrillations or positive sharp waves in the weak muscles that were formerly innervated by the damaged axons. This type of nerve injury usually regenerates to proximal muscles within 5 or 6 months.[17]

4. *Neurotmesis* (extensive injury in which an athlete who complies with the rehabilitation program continues to have residual weakness after 6 months) is damage of the axon, surrounding myelin, and adjacent connective tissue, sometimes including the epineurium (outer connective tissue covering of nerve) that is so extensive that regeneration is very poor and loss of function is permanent. This classification can be made only when it is evident that there is no return of function within a reasonable period (6 months to 1 year).[13] Nerve conduction studies are helpful in demonstrating the relatively low evoked amplitudes when compared with the normal side.[11] Electromyography demonstrates fibrillations and fewer motor units firing once the degenerative process is complete (in about 2 to 3 weeks).[3,11] During the regeneration phase, the structures of the involved axons are too severely damaged to allow regeneration, and the proximal nerve stumps may form neuromas as the regenerating nerve fibers are unable to grow

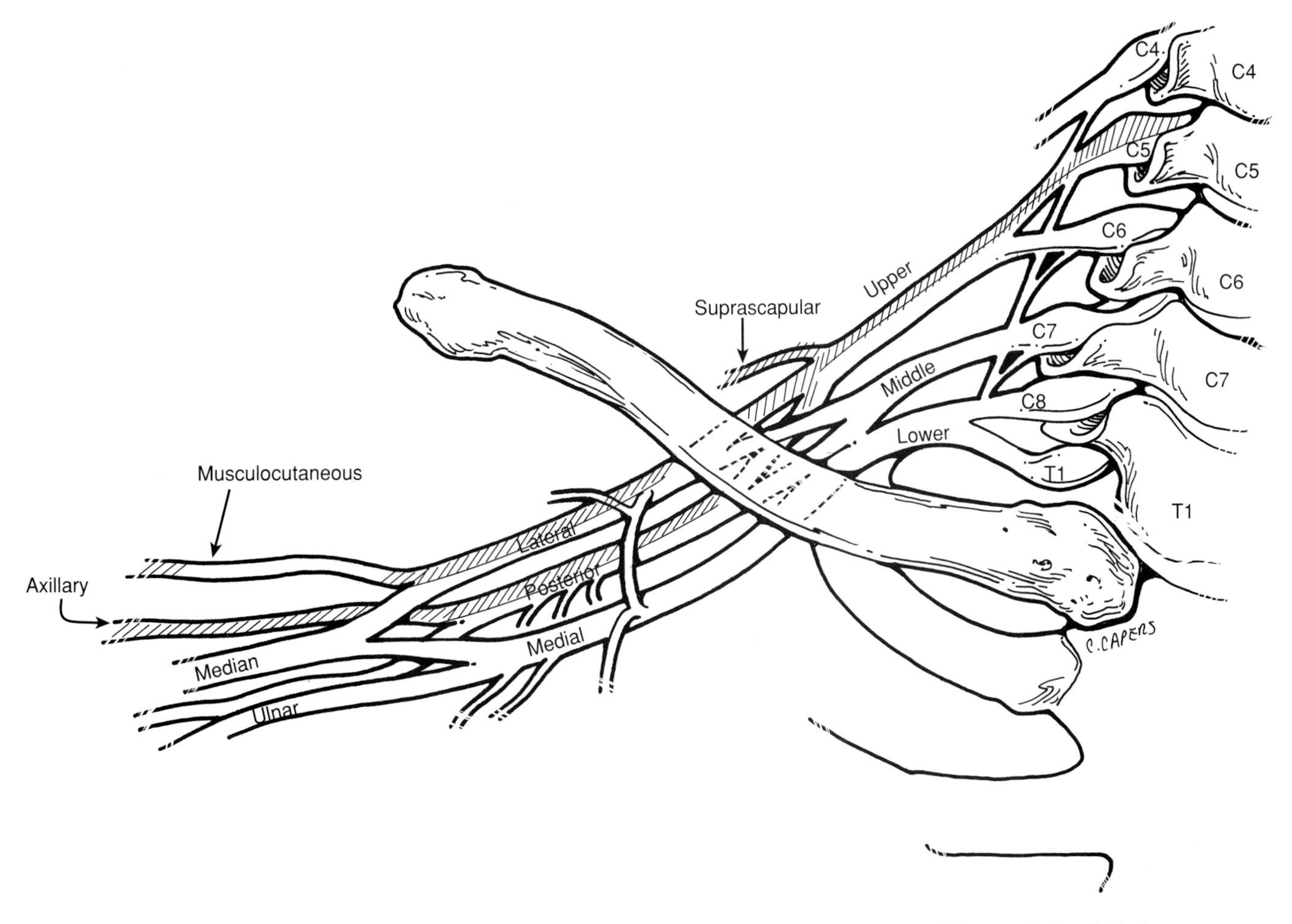

Fig. 34–2. Nerves involved in the most common patterns of delayed weakness after traction injury to the brachial plexus. The weak muscles allow the clinician to track the site of injury: C5, rhomboid minor and major; C5-6, supraspinatus and infraspinatus (suprascapular nerve), coracobrachialis, biceps, and brachialis (musculocutaneous nerve), deltoid and teres minor (axillary nerve), and serratus anterior (long thoracic nerve). Very often, the serratus anterior is spared, which indicates that the injury is distal to this point.

through the scarring at the site of injury.[13] The only increase of strength comes from collateral sprouting of spared axons into the denervated muscle fibers to create larger than normal numbers of muscle fibers per motor axon. This process is represented by giant potentials on electromyography. Some increased strength may be appreciated because of hypertrophy of other uninjured motor units and substitution of uninjured muscles.[11]

METHODS OF EVALUATION AND TREATMENT

At the Time of Symptoms

For a coach, trainer, or team physician, it is not difficult to spot a stinger because the athlete often runs off the playing field holding a limp arm to his side.[10] The person responsible for the athlete's care should immediately ask where it hurts and how the injury was sustained. The player removes as much of the uniform and protective gear as possible to allow inspection of the cervical spine, shoulders, and arms.[10] The following examinations should be performed and appropriately documented:

Active range of motion of the cervical spine and upper extremities
Manual muscle testing of both upper extremities
Gross sensation to light touch in dermatomes C5-T1
Reflexes of the biceps, triceps, and brachioradialis.

If all these findings are normal and the pain has resolved, the player can be put back in the game once the protective gear is checked and modified with additional shoulder padding and a neck roll.[1,7,10] While on the sidelines, the player should have any area of tenderness, such as that over the supraclavicular triangle, iced. He should be checked repeatedly throughout the rest of the game for sequelae or recurrence of stinger symptoms.[10]

Immediately After the Competition

After the competition, the player should be re-evaluated in the locker room with the same tests done on the field but in greater detail.[1,10] Any loss of motion in the cervical spine with pain and radicular symptoms of sensory disturbance or weakness should prompt referral for imaging studies to rule out vertebral injury and disc injury. If soreness on palpation in the supraclavicular triangle is the only symptom, the athlete should ice that area for up to 72 hours. Further participation in contact sports is interdicted until the player is re-examined by an appropriate health professional to ensure that no weakness has developed.[10]

Before Exposure to Further Contact

The athlete should receive another evaluation of range of motion, strength, sensation, and reflexes before being exposed to further contact. In the event of any detectable weakness, the athlete should be restricted from any exposure to further injury until that weakness has resolved (since the weakness represents a nerve injury). Once there is evidence of increasing strength, the player should begin a conservative weight training program until his strength is equal bilaterally. The shoulder pads should be adapted to decrease shoulder depression and cervical deviation. The goal is to prevent recurrent injury, since subsequent injuries tend to be more severe. In cases of unresolved weakness, sensory changes or recurrent stingers, further evaluation is appropriate, and forbidding further contact is in the best interest of the player's health.

PREVENTION

Rules were changed in 1979 to prevent use of the head for spearing or butting in football because of the large number of cervical injuries, but stingers and burners still occur.[7] A high-quality shoulder pad is helpful in absorbing the compression forces received in aggressive shoulder tackling. Once a football player receives a stinger or burner, additional padding to the shoulder pads and a neck roll are helpful.[1,7,10]

REHABILITATION

Because muscles and bones protect the brachial plexus and nerve roots from injury, soreness from strain and contusion of the scalene, trapezius, and levator scapulae muscles is often associated with a stinger or burner. Immediate ice to those structures minimizes bruising. After the first 72 hours, heat should be applied—by moist heat packs or other heat modalities. Range of motion and light stretching exercises help the athlete regain full pain-free range of motion. Once pain-free range of motion of the cervical spine and involved shoulder are normal, a slowly progressive strengthening exercise program should be started to build up the muscles that stabilize the neck and scapula, the posterior, lateral, and anterior neck muscles and the trapezius and deltoids.

These strengthening exercises should be continued during the season and in the off season because it has been documented that stingers and burners often recur, and the recurrences are sometimes followed by increased neurologic deficits.[13] Adapting the player's equipment has also been suggested.

REFERENCES

1. Speer, K. P., Bassett, F. H.: The prolonged burner syndrome. Am. J. Sports Med. *18:*591, 1990.
2. Vereschagin, K. S., Wiens, J. J., Fanton, G. S., and Dillingham, M. F.: Burners, don't overlook or underestimate them. Physician Sportsmed *19*(9):96, 1991.
3. Robertson, W. C., Eichman, P. L., and Clancy, W. G.: Upper trunk brachial plexopathy in football players. J.A.M.A. *241:*1480, 1979.
4. Poindexter, D. P., and Johnson, E. W.: Football shoulder and neck injury: A study of the "stinger." Arch. Phys. Med. Rehabil. *65:*601, 1984.
5. Clancy, W. G., Brand, R. L., and Bergfield, J. A.: Upper trunk brachial plexus injuries in contact sports. Am. J. Sports Med. *5:*209, 1977.
6. DiBenedetto, M., and Markey, K.: Electrodiagnostic localization of traumatic upper trunk brachial plexopathy. Arch. Phys. Med. Rehabil. *65:*15, 1984.
7. Hunter, H. C.: Injuries to the brachial plexus: Experience of a private sports medicine clinic. J. Am. Osteopath. Assoc. *81:*757, 1982.
8. Hu, R., et al.: Burners in contact sports. Clin. J. Sports Med. *1:*236, 1991.
9. Collins, K., Storey, M., Peterson, K., and Nutter, P.: Nerve injuries in athletes. Physician Sportsmed. *16*(1):92, 1988.
10. Hershman, E. B.: Brachial plexus injuries. Clin. Sports Med. *9:*311, 1990.
11. Wilbourn, A. J.: Electrodiagnostic testing of neurologic injuries in athletes. Clin. Sports Med. *9:*229, 1990.
12. Maroon, J. C.: "Burning hands" in football spinal cord injuries. J.A.M.A. *238:*2049, 1977.
13. Kline, D. G., and Lusk, M. D.: Management of athletic brachial plexus injuries. *In* Sports Injuries: Mechanisms, Prevention, and Treatment. Edited by R. C. Schneider, J. C. Kennedy, and M. L. Plant. Baltimore, Williams & Wilkins, 1985.
14. Bonney, G.: Prognosis in traction lesions of the brachial plexus. J. Bone Joint Surg. *41B:*4, 1959.
15. Bateman, J. E.: Nerve injuries about the shoulder in sports. J. Bone Joint Surg. *49A:*785, 1967.
16. Barnes, R.: Traction injuries of the brachial plexus in adults. J. Bone Joint Surg. *31B:*10, 1949.
17. Rorabeck, C. H., and Harris, W. R.: Factors affecting the prognosis of brachial plexus injuries. J. Bone Joint Surg. *63B:*404, 1981.

35 *Reynold L. Rimoldi*

Cervical Injuries

Although motor vehicle accidents are the chief agent of catastrophic cervical spinal cord injuries, athletic activity has accounted for as many as 14% of such injuries: football,[1-6] rugby,[7] ice hockey,[8,9] gymnastics,[10-14] and water sports.[15,16] Injuries to the cervical spine and brachial plexus include strains, sprains, neurapraxia, and fracture-dislocations, with and without neurologic sequelae. The frequency of various types of injury is inversely related to their severity. In other words, most injuries are myoligamentous sprains or strain syndromes. It is estimated that 50% of all collegiate football players have at least one significant injury during their playing career.[17] These include brachial plexus neurapraxia and cervical radiculopathy. Nonfatal, permanent cervical spinal cord injuries occur at a frequency of 1 in 7000 in football and gymnastics and 1 in at least 92,000 participants in men's basketball.

The mechanism that produces cervical injuries with associated neurologic trauma is hyperflexion plus axial loading. Epidemiologic and cinematographic analyses have demonstrated that direct axial loading secondary to making initial contact with the crown of the helmet has led to the majority of cervical spinal cord injuries associated with football. Most players who have sustained cervical spinal cord injuries as a result of football played the position of defensive back, and the incident occurred while making a tackle. Furthermore, all of the tackles were made in similar fashion: using the helmet as a battering ram.

In 1975, the National Football League (NFL) established the Head and Neck Injury Registry.[3,4] Studies of NFL injuries before 1975 show a decreasing trend in closed head injuries but an increasing trend in cervical spine injuries. Refinements in helmet design led to the decrease in head injuries, but at the same time this more durable, lighterweight helmet began to be used as a tackling or striking weapon, which accounts for the increased incidence of cervical spine injuries. Torg and coworkers estimate that 52% of the severe cervical spine injuries occurring in professional football between 1971 and 1975 were secondary to a "spearing" type tackle.[3] According to statistics from the University of Alabama National Spinal Cord Injury Statistics Center, football ranked 13th as a cause of spinal cord injury in 1992. Football accounted for 0.7% of all catastrophic spinal cord injuries.

Among college and high school players, 78% of injuries resulting in quadriplegia occurred while the player was making a tackle. Between 50 and 75% of players who sustained severe spinal cord injuries were defensive backs, if all levels (high school, college, professional) were considered.[3]

The National Collegiate Athletic Association has rules opposing head-on tackling, or "spearing." Since the advent of these rule changes, the rate of catastrophic cervical spine injuries has decreased.

The mechanism of injury for most cervical spine injuries is compressive flexion, as described by Allen and Ferguson.[18] This type of injury involves compressive failure of the anterior vertebral column, which is demonstrated by a decrease in anterior column height (Fig. 35–1). As the force vector and momentum increase, failure progresses through the middle column in the form of tension failure. Further progression of the force vector results in retropulsion of the middle column at the involved motion segment. This retrolisthesis accounts for the associated spinal cord injury. The lateral radiograph provides the most information about this injury; although anteroposterior radiographs can show a vertical fracture line, yielding the so-called crush cleavage injury. This injury is

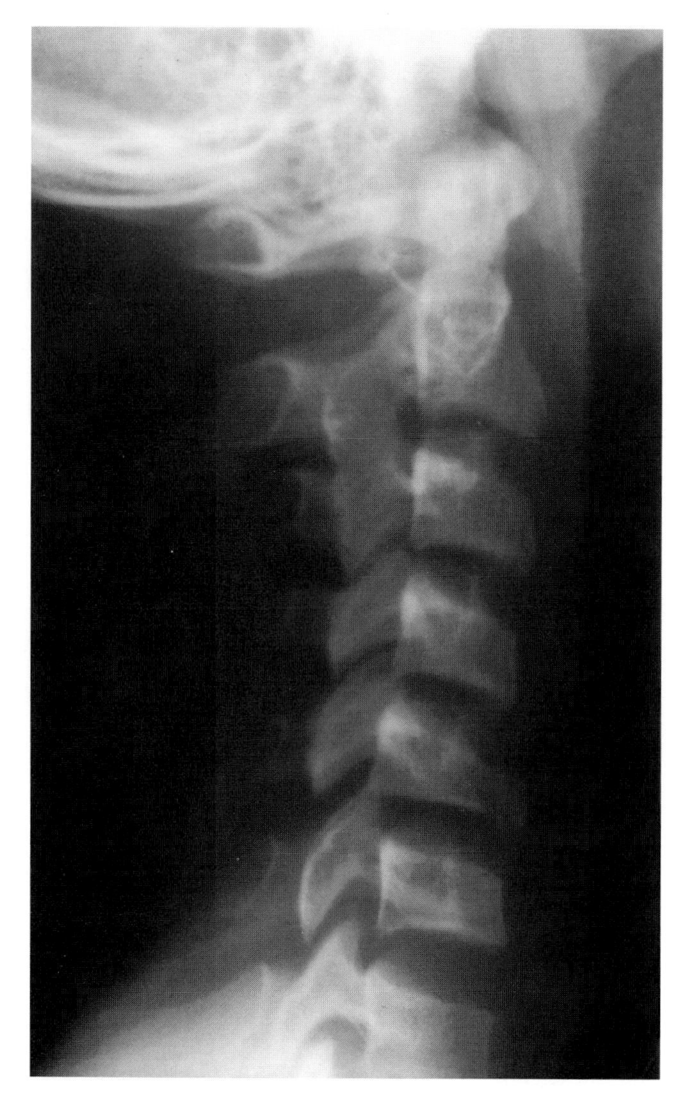

Fig. 35–1. Lateral radiograph shows a compressive flexion injury of C5.

readily apparent after reviewing the computed tomographic (CT) image of the lesion (Fig. 35–2). As the energy absorbed increases, more retropulsion is observed, which increases the incidence—and severity—of spinal cord injury.

The other common mechanism of injury, vertical compression, leads to symmetric failure of both the anterior and the middle column that results in symmetric decrease of the cervical vertebral body height. Lateral radiographs reveal a concavity at the superior or inferior end-plate of the involved vertebra, and as the force vector increases, retropulsion of bone into the canal occurs. Higher stages of compression flexion injuries may produce chronic instability from ligamentous disruption posteriorly (Fig. 35–3), but the majority of the axial-loading vertical compressive injuries do not.

Trampolines and springboards have caused most cervical spine injuries in the gymnast population.[10–12,14,19] Most of these lesions occur at the middle to lower cervical spine and are axial loading injuries. Torg has strongly recommended complete abandonment of trampolines and springboards.

Diving injuries are more often associated with recreational activity. At Rancho Los Amigos Medical Center, 8% of all patients admitted with cervical spine injuries and quadriplegia were injured diving into shallow water (5 feet deep or less). The injuries consist of compressive flexion, vertical compression, and compressive extension mechanisms. To prevent these injuries, people are advised not to dive in unfamiliar water until the water is surveyed. Water that is cleared for diving purpose should be at least twice the diver's height. Also, one should not dive into the ocean, surf, or body surf in water that does not have a base depth of at least 12 feet, regardless of whether the bottom is sand or reef.[15]

Cervical spine injuries are being incurred more frequently during ice hockey, and the compressive flexion mechanism is noted most often. The most common mechanism is riding an opponent into the boards while cross-checking. The frequency of injuries has increased since helmets became mandatory for all players. This is similar to the history noted in football players in the 1960s and early 1970s: with helmet improvements and availability of face masks, the number of cervical injuries increased. Although penalties are assessed for cross-checking in the National Hockey League, they are not severe enough to discourage the practice. Before a serious attempt can be made to eliminate cervical injuries, rigid restructuring of rules on fighting and clashes that can result in catastrophic injury must be undertaken.

SCREENING HISTORY AND PHYSICAL EXAMINATION

One of the most important questions is whether any candidate may safely take part in contact athletics. This question is best addressed by considering probable risk to the player.

A lateral cervical spine view should be obtained. The probability of a player developing future problems should be considered when any radiographic evidence of instability exists or when the participant's spinal canal measures less than 10 mm from the posterior vertebral body of C5 to the spinolaminar line on the radiograph. An athlete with a mobile os odontoideum should not participate in contact sports. Patients with a history of fractures involving two columns, cervical fusion, or decompression are not permitted to play, not because of the previous injury but because of the excessive stress placed on the adjacent intervertebral motion segment. Avulsion fractures of the cervical spinous processes or compression injuries involving less than 20% of the anterior vertebral body height must be thoroughly assessed for instability on lateral cervical spine radiographs in flexion and extension. If the spine is stable,

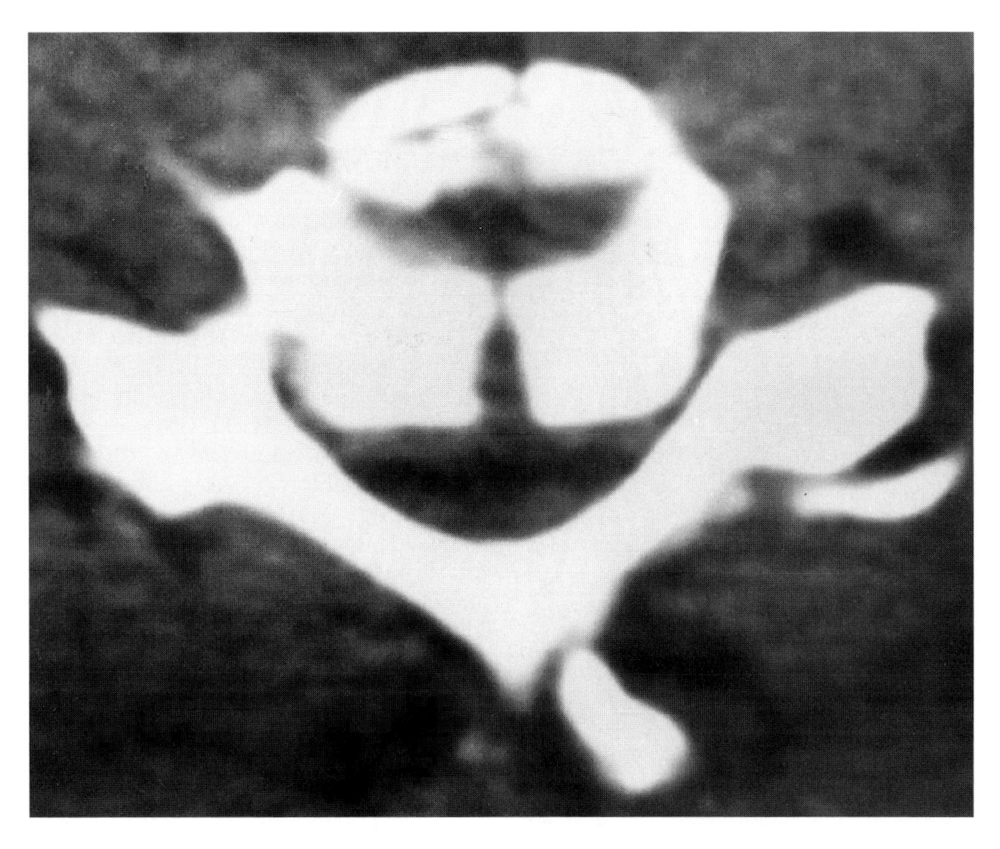

Fig. 35–2. CT shows a crush cleavage injury.

the athlete can be allowed to play with minimal risk to the cervical region.

CERVICAL STRAINS AND SPRAINS

Traumatic cervical strains are the most frequent cervical injury of competitive athletes. Studies of these types of injuries show that they are more frequent in muscles that span more than one joint. In the cervical area, these muscles include the semispinalis cervicis, which arises on the transverse processes of the thoracic and lower cervical vertebrae and inserts on the spinous processes of the upper cervical vertebrae. This is the deep muscle group. Also involved is the erector spinae group, which consists of the iliocostal, the spinalis, and the longissimus cervicis, which are more superficial. These muscles have greater numbers of Type II fibers, also called *oxidative fibers.* They contain larger amounts of oxidative enzymes and are capable of faster contractions. They have poor endurance qualities and are more susceptible to injury. Once strain injuries occur, they are likely to recur, owing to poor rehabilitation practices. Stronger muscle groups are at less risk for injury. It has been suggested that joint inflexibility predisposes to muscle injury, but this has not been demonstrated conclusively.

High-intensity forceful contraction in an eccentric manner occurs when the muscle is loaded but the fibers are undergoing lengthening. A player using his helmet as a tackling device may sustain a flexion moment about the cervical region, thus undergoing eccentric contraction. High-intensity forceful contraction in an eccentric mode has been shown to increase muscle soreness. This mechanism has been associated with strain injuries.

Recent studies have shown that transient weakness of as much as 50% occurs after prolonged eccentric contraction. These injuries occur at the musculotendinous junction in response to powerful eccentric contractions. Studies in rabbits showed that muscles stretched into the plastic region of the load deformation curve showed disruption at the musculotendinous junction; histologically, an inflammatory reaction was noted, with fibrotic scar formation. Other studies have suggested that initial activation allows a muscle to absorb more energy; thus, a relaxed muscle is injured before an activated muscle. This suggests that weakness and fatigue predispose a muscle to injury-producing loads. It seems reasonable that the warm-up process is an important measure for reducing muscle injuries.

Immobilization, often required for short periods after a strain-type injury, may also influence the reinjury rate of muscle. Immobilization has been shown to affect the number of muscle fiber sarcomeres. Muscle fibers add more sarcomeres at the musculotendinous junction if immobilization occurs in a position that lengthens the muscle. It has been suggested that there is less susceptibility to reinjury if the injured muscle is immobilized in its lengthened position.

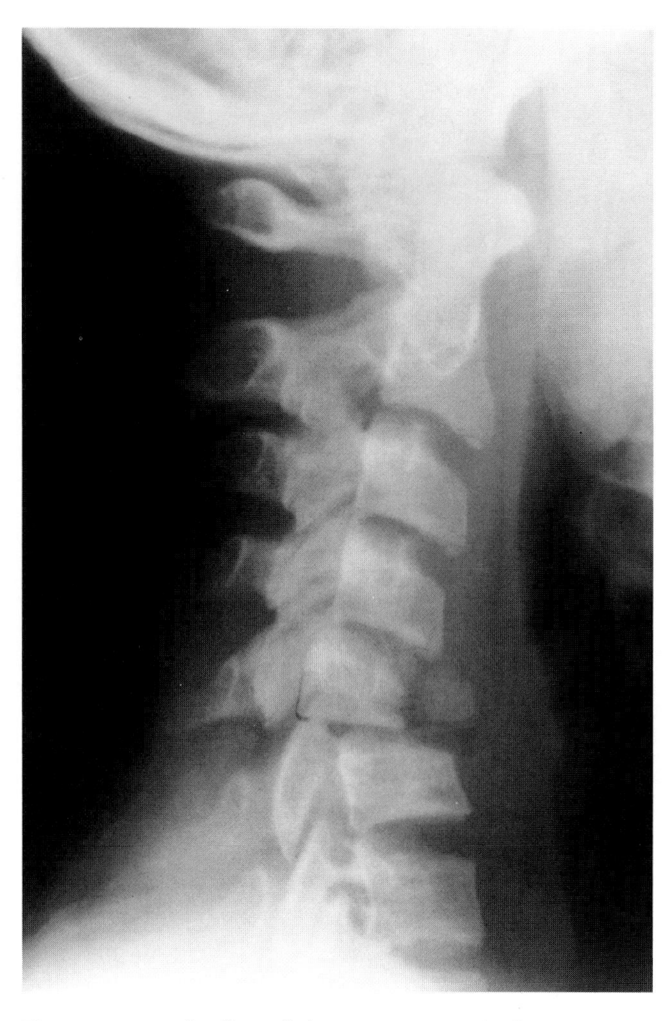

Fig. 35–3. Lateral radiograph demonstrates posterior ligament disruption.

Cervical sprains suggest injury to the ligamentous structures of the cervical spine. These may present in the same fashion as a strain, but more severe (Grade III) injuries can present as cervical subluxation or frank dislocation, with catastrophic neurologic sequelae. The more common injuries consist of partial tears (Grade I and Grade II injuries). Players present with limitation of cervical motion. There are no neurologic sequelae with Grade I and II sprains.

Lateral cervical radiographs that include flexion and extension views are needed to evaluate patients with persistent symptoms. Most patients are adequately treated with immobilization, rest, nonsteroidal anti-inflammatory medications, range of motion exercises, and cervical strengthening.

Cervical strains or injuries to the cervical paraspinous muscles are the most common types sustained by athletes. These injuries are usually produced when the cervical paraspinal muscles are overloaded eccentrically. Often, the precipitating event is not apparent to the injured player. Symptoms may "peak" 24 hours after the game. Treatment consists of ice, nonsteroidal anti-inflammatory medication, and cervical flexibility and strengthening exercises.

TREATMENT ON THE FIELD AND FOLLOWUP

The classification by Allen is an excellent one to use, not only to understand the mechanism of injury but to formulate a treatment plan.[18] Care of the injured athlete begins the moment the player is injured. The patient is evaluated on the field by the orthopedist or athletic director. If the athlete runs off the field, questioning and examination are completed on the sidelines. If the athlete remains down on the field, the team physician or athletic trainer must rule out an unstable cervical spine injury before the player can be moved. The patient's condition is thoroughly assessed. Questions about pain, tingling, numbness, blackouts or dizziness, and memory assessment to check for a closed head injury are mandatory. Any patient with neck and arm pain or findings suggesting a closed head injury must be assumed to have an unstable cervical spine injury until it is proven otherwise.

A player who can walk alone or with assistance off the playing field is immediately assessed for residual sensory or motor deficits. This is done cursorily on the sidelines; then, a thorough examination is done in the locker room. Radiographic examination is mandatory before contact activities are resumed. If the patient remains down, an adequate airway must be established or maintained. The patient is log rolled if prone, the mouth is cleared, and a neurologic examination is performed. If there is evidence of cervical tenderness or abnormal neurologic findings, the patient should be properly transported. The physician must maintain head control during the procedure. If a backboard is available, the patient is log rolled onto it and five people (two on each side and one to stabilize the head) transport the athlete off the field. Lacking a backboard, two people are positioned on either side at the shoulders, two at the waist, and one at the feet. The carriers lock arms under the supine patient and begin removing the patient from the field. The physician or trainer controlling the head must place his or her arms so that the hands are grasping the trapezius muscle and the forearms are supporting the posterior head and neck (Fig. 35–4). The helmet is not removed on the field.

Once the patient is on the sidelines or in the locker room, the physical examination is carried out in a more detailed fashion. Numbness, tingling, weakness, and pain in the arms are contraindications to returning to the field. Decreased cervical range of motion with pain, also an indication for removal from play, often indicates an occult, potentially catastrophic injury. An athlete whose symptoms resolve and who demonstrates full range of motion can return to play. A player should not return to the playing field if painful limited range of motion or a neurologic deficit persists. If lower extrem-

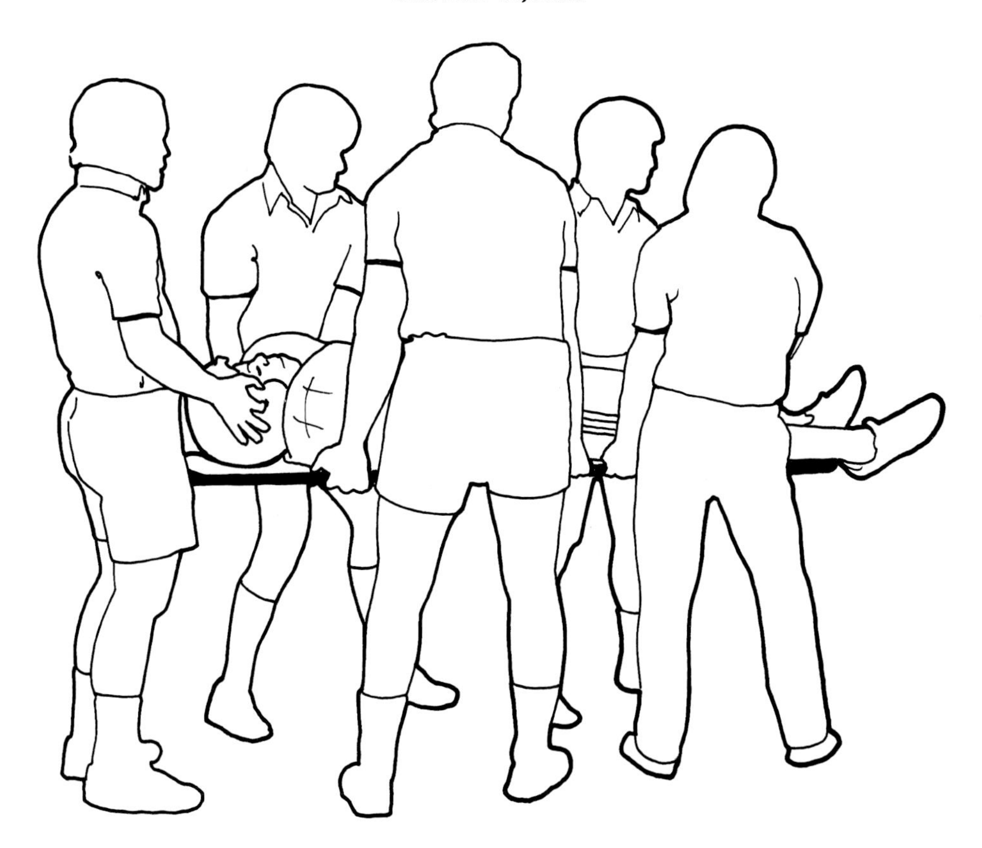

Fig. 35–4. Technique for transport off the field.

ity findings are noted, the patient should be kept out until a full radiographic evaluation is completed, even if the symptoms later resolve.

A lateral cervical spine radiograph is taken with the helmet in place if there are abnormal findings on physical examination (Fig. 35–5). It is imperative that all seven cervical vertebrae be visualized. Although the swimmer's view may assist visually, more often than not Boger straps are necessary, especially in patients with muscle spasms that often accompany acute cervical injury. The lateral cervical spine film is meticulously inspected. All vertebrae from C1 to C7 are viewed. In addition to the obvious signs of disabilities that are readily observed, subtle signs of injury should also be sought. The prevertebral or retropharyngeal soft tissue shadow can be the only clue to a cervical spine injury. This shadow should be no more than 4 mm directly anterior to the C3 vertebral body. The posterior aspect of the vertebral bodies and the spinolaminar line should be continuous. If the radiograph is clear and normal, the helmet can be removed in the locker room. The decision to remove the helmet can be made only after a lateral radiograph shows normal findings.

If radiographs are not available on site, the patient must be transported with the helmet in place. The athlete is placed on a backboard while the physician or trainer stabilizes the head and neck at all times. Tape reinforcement of the helmet to the backboard with adjacent sandbags helps maintain stabilization during transport to the medical facility. The helmet is removed with a cast saw or with two assistants placing lateral traction via the ear holes and the physician supporting the head and neck in the previously described cradle position. The two assistants can now safely withdraw the helmet by maintaining the traction and providing a superior force to remove the helmet. Bolster supports are placed to prevent hyperextension. A full examination is then done. The examiner should inspect for ecchymosis and swelling. After the examination is completed, the remaining trauma series radiographs of the cervical spine are obtained. These include the anteroposterior, openmouthed, and oblique radiographs. Once they have been evaluated, flexion and extension lateral views should be obtained. A predens interval (the space between the posterior aspect of the atlas, or first cervical vertebral body, and the anterior aspect of the odontoid process of the axis, or second vertebral body) greater than 3 mm in the flexion view and available space for the spinal cord less than 13 mm suggest, respectively, C1-2 instability and a dens fracture. Any difference in angulation greater than 11° or translation greater than 3.5 mm in these views suggests instability. If no abnormality is noted and the patient has neurologic or radicular findings, magnetic resonance imaging is mandatory. Some physicians prefer to wait to perform this test, to see if symptoms resolve.

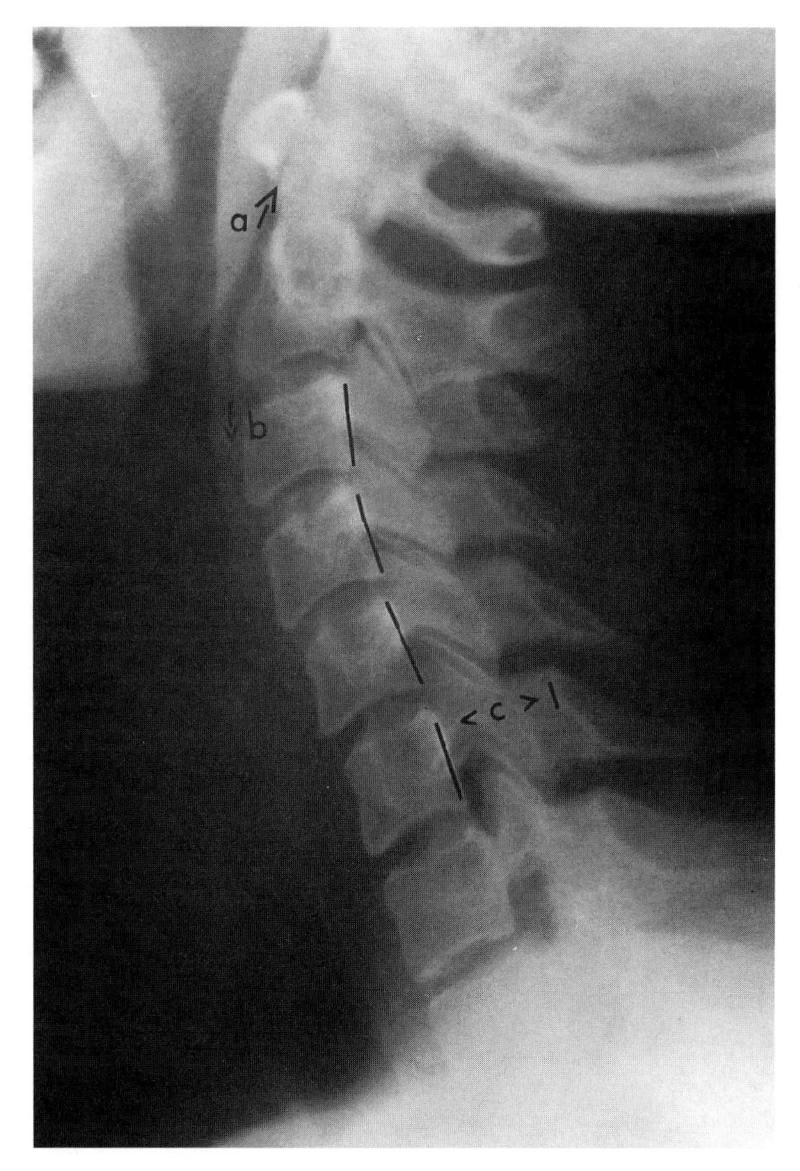

Fig. 35–5. **Normal lateral cervical spine radiograph shows landmarks: *(a),* predens interval; *(b),* convex curve; *(c),* sagittal diameter of the spinal canal.**

SUMMARY

Neck-strengthening exercises, conditioning, and education in proper blocking and tackling techniques are important in the prevention of cervical spinal cord injuries. Using the helmet as a battering ram in a spearing maneuver places the player at an increased risk for cervical injury. The incidence of cervical injuries has increased as the quality of helmets has improved. Epidemiologic studies and direct observation have demonstrated that incidents resulting in severe cervical neurotrauma are a direct result of leading the "hit" with the helmet. Therefore, the importance of instruction in proper technique becomes apparent, especially at the high school level.

REFERENCES

1. Schneider, R. D.: Serious and fatal neurosurgical football injuries. Clin. Neurosurg. *12:*226, 1966.
2. Torg, J. S., et al.: Spinal injury at the level of the third and fourth cervical vertebrae from football. J. Bone Joint Surg. *59A:*1015, 1977.
3. Torg, J. S., et al.: National football head and neck injury registry: Report on cervical quadriplegia, 1971 to 1975. Am. J. Sports Med. *7:*127, 1979.
4. Torg, J. S., et al.: The National Football Head and Neck Injury Registry. Report and conclusion 1978. J.A.M.A. *241:*1477, 1979.
5. Torg, J. S.: Epidemiology, pathomechanics, and prevention of athletic injuries to the cervical spine. Med. Sci. Sports Exerc. *17:*295, 1985.
6. Torg, J. S., et al.: Severe and catastrophic neck injuries resulting from tackle football. J. Am. Coll. Health Assoc. *25:*224, 1977.

7. Burry, H. C., and Gowland, H.: Cervical injury in rugby football: A New Zealand survey. Br. J. Sports Med. *15:*56, 1981.
8. Feriencik K.: Trends in ice hockey injuries: 1965 to 1977. Physician Sportsmed. *7*(2):81, 1979.
9. Tator, C. H., et al. : Spinal injuries due to hockey. Can. J. Neurol. Sci. *11:*34, 1984.
10. Ellis, W. G., et al.: The trampoline and serious neurological injuries. J.A.M.A. *174:*1673, 1960.
11. Evans, R. F.: Tetraplegia caused by gymnastics. Br. Med. J. *2:*732, 1979.
12. Rapp, G. F.: Problems with the trampoline. Pediatr. Ann. *7:*730, 1978.
13. Torg, J. S., and Das, M.: Trampoline-related quadriplegia: Review of the literature and reflections on the American Academy of Pediatrics position statement. Pediatrics *74:*804, 1984.
14. Zimmerman, H. M.: Accident experience with trampolines. Res. Q. *27:*452, 1956.
15. Albrand, O. W., and Walter, J.: Underwater deceleration curves in relation to injuries from diving. Surg. Neurol. *4:*461, 1975.
16. Kewalramani, L. S., and Taylor, R. G.: Injuries to the cervical spine from diving accidents. J. Trauma *15:*130, 1975.
17. Clancy, W. G., Brand, R. L., and Bergfield, J. A.: Upper trunk brachial plexus injuries in contact sports. Am. J. Sports Med. *5:*209, 1977.
18. Allen, B. L. Jr., Ferguson, R. L., Lehmann, T. R., and O'Brian, R. P.: A mechanistic classification of closed, indirect fractures and dislocations of the lower cervical spine. Spine *7:*1, 1982.
19. Rapp, G. F., and Nicely, P. G.: Trampoline injuries. Am. J. Sports Med. *6:*269, 1978.

36

J. Kenneth Burkus

Thoracic and Lumbar Spine

Back pain and injuries are common complaints in athletes that must be evaluated with great care. The young athlete with back pain may have a stress fracture or an occult spinal deformity. Often, the origin of the complaint is initially unclear. Subsequent physical examination and diagnostic tests are frequently necessary to establish the cause of persistent spine symptoms.

SCOLIOSIS

Scoliosis, a spine deformity common in adolescents,[1] is a curvature of the spine in the frontal plane (Fig. 36–1). Typically adolescent idiopathic scoliosis involves a right thoracic and left lumbar curve pattern.[2] It is thought that scoliosis is hereditary. Close to 80% of adolescents with scoliosis have a relative who also had scoliosis. Adolescent idiopathic scoliosis is found in both boys and girls; its prevalence in high school–aged adolescents ranges from 2 to 3%. Smaller curves, those measuring less than 10°, occur as often in boys as in girls, but larger curves are more common in girls. Women also require treatment for scoliosis curves seven times more frequently than men.

Adolescent idiopathic scoliosis is not painful. If an adolescent presents with a painful spinal curvature, its cause should be investigated. Painful disc herniations, muscle contusions or spasms, or fractures often cause the patient to "list" and cause the spine to curve. Spinal cord tumors and primary bone tumors of the spinal column (osteoid osteomas or osteoblastomas) may also be the cause of painful scoliosis.

Participation in athletics has not been shown to increase the risk of progression of a spine deformity. Rather, the increase in curvature occurs at the time of the most rapid adolescent skeletal growth. Younger athletes with scoliosis are more likely to show progression

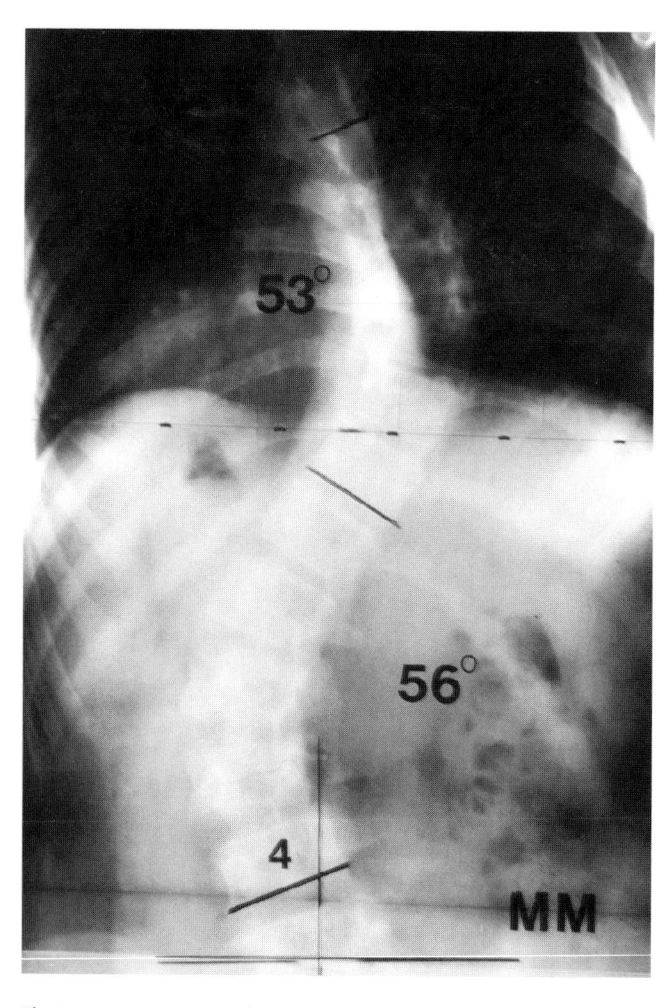

Fig. 36–1. Anteroposterior radiograph of the thoracic and lumbar spine shows a pattern typical of adolescent idiopathic scoliosis. There is a 53° right thoracic curve and a 56° left lumbar curve, but no evidence of vertebral malformations.

than older ones; the incidence of progression decreases as athletes age. The athlete's stage of physical maturation, the initial size of the scoliotic curve, and the curve pattern are also important factors in predicting if the spinal curvature will increase.

Athletes with adolescent idiopathic scoliosis can safely participate in contact and noncontact sports. The curve pattern should be followed closely with serial physical examinations and radiographs. All adolescents diagnosed with scoliosis should have an anteroposterior and a lateral spine radiograph. The radiographs should be of diagnostic quality, to rule out congenital abnormalities of the spine. Vertebral malformations in the thoracic and lumbar spine are frequently associated with abnormalities in the cervical spine and the neural axis. Physicians should be aware of this and look for cervical abnormalities. Such congenital abnormalities may place the athlete at risk for a devastating neurologic injury. Athletes with certain patterns of congenital vertebral malformations may need to be restricted from participation in specific sports activities.

Adolescent idiopathic scoliosis is treated by observation with serial examinations and radiographs if the magnitude of the curves is less than 25°. It is treated by bracing if the curves are between 20° and 40°. Surgery is recommended for curvature greater than 50°. Adolescents who have undergone spinal fusion for scoliosis may return to competitive noncontact sports. The level of participation in sports depends on the extent and type of spinal fusion.

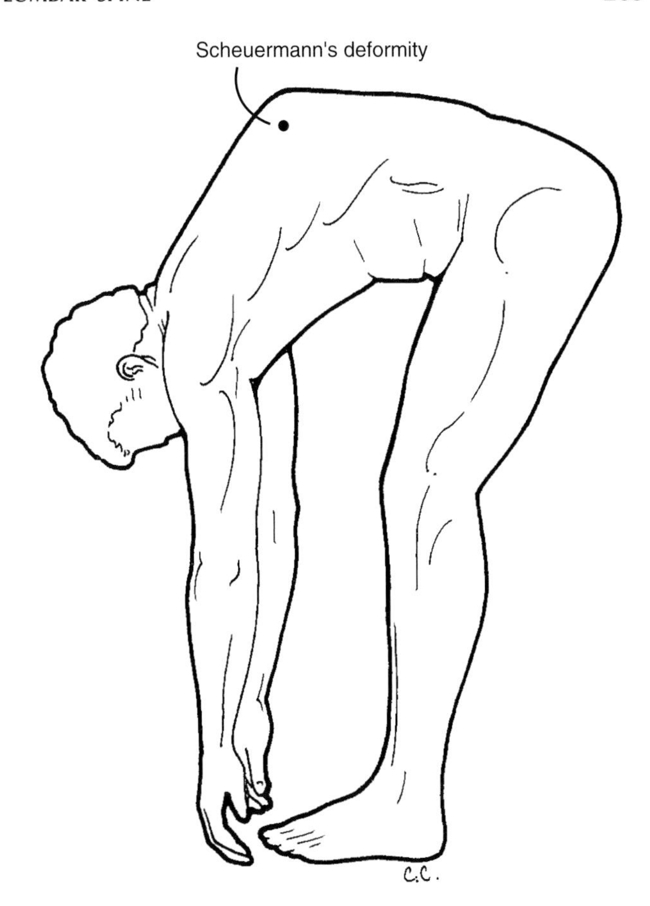

Fig. 36–2. Scheuermann's disease results in an increase in local kyphosis, which can be seen when the patient bends forward.

KYPHOSIS

The thoracic spine normally has a kyphotic sagittal contour. Growing adolescents normally have a range of 20° to 45° of kyphosis in the thoracic region. The thoracolumbar junction should be neutrally aligned, and any degree of kyphosis at the thoracolumbar junction or in the lumbar spine is abnormal.

Scheuermann's disease affects adolescents nearing the growth spurt.[3] The spine's sagittal balance is offset by a progressive increase in kyphosis at the midthoracic spine or at the thoracolumbar junction. The increase in kyphosis results from wedging of the vertebral bodies. Asymmetric growth and development of the anterior and posterior portions of the vertebral body leads to a trapezoidal configuration of the vertebral body and an associated increase in the local kyphosis (Fig. 36–2). Wedging of the vertebral bodies is also associated with irregularities of the vertebral end-plates, Schmorl's node formation, and disc space narrowing. Lateral radiographs demonstrate the bone changes, which are easily confused with fractures. Magnetic resonance imaging (MRI) of the spine can distinguish between acute injuries and the chronic changes in vertebral bodies associated with Scheuermann's disease.

The clinical presentation of kyphosis is different in the thoracic and in the thoracolumbar region. In the thoracic spine, the deformity develops spontaneously and is not associated with any specific injury or activity; at least three adjacent vertebral bodies are usually affected. The deformity commonly has its apex in the midthoracic region (T7–T9), and it is not associated with pain. This spine deformity occurs at or before puberty in approximately 5% of adolescents. It is more common in girls than in boys.

Scheuermann's disease in the thoracolumbar and lumbar spine commonly presents with involvement of only one or two vertebral bodies. In these caudal regions of the spine, the increase in local kyphosis is often painful and is associated with trauma and with certain sports activities.[4] In the thoracolumbar and lumbar spine, kyphosis is twice as common in boys as in girls and is more frequent in young athletes who participate in rowing, weight lifting, and gymnastics.[5]

Treatment of the deformity depends on its magnitude, its flexibility, and the adolescent's state of physical maturation. Patients with thoracic Scheuermann's disease and with at least 9 months' growth remaining can be treated with hyperextension exercises and a brace. Exercise routines should include pelvic tilts to reduce lumbar lordosis, hyperextension stretching to overcome contractures, and thoracic extension exercises to develop the thoracic extensor muscle groups. Restriction of athletic activities, including contact sports, is not recommended.

Patients with thoracolumbar and lumbar kyphosis should be treated with a molded hyperextension thoracolumbar standing orthosis brace and should avoid activities and exercises until they are pain free. The period of reduced activity may take up to 3 months. Once the patient is relieved of back pain, he or she can begin hyperextension stretching and exercise routines. Athletes with thoracolumbar and lumbar kyphosis should avoid activities that involve repetitive flexion and extension of the spine. Surgery may be indicated for patients who show progression of the deformity or persistent pain after nonoperative treatment.

THORACIC DISC HERNIATION

Disc herniations are rare in the thoracic spine. They occur in fewer than 0.3% of the population, and they are involved in fewer than 1% of all surgical disc procedures.[6–8] Thoracic disc herniations occur with equal frequency in men and women and are most common during the fourth through the sixth decades of life. Thoracic disc herniations occur most frequently in the lower thoracic spine between T9 and T12 but may occur at any level.

The diagnosis of thoracic disc herniation is difficult to make because of the variable clinical presentation. Symptoms may occur insidiously over the course of weeks to months; additionally, most patients do not have a history of a specific traumatic or exertional event related to the onset of their symptoms.

Patients with thoracic disc herniations usually complain of poorly localized thoracic backache, lancinating anterior chest pain, and nonspecific lower extremity pain. Painful symptoms vary from cramping to burning or dull aching. Sensory complaints, including numbness, coldness, and paresthesia, may involve the lower extremities. Lower extremity weakness is also a common complaint. Bladder and bowel dysfunction occurs in approximately a third of patients. Neurologic findings vary and depend on the level of the disc herniation in the spinal column and the size, position, and composition of the herniated disc fragment. Spasticity and gait abnormalities, including a wide-based, ataxic stance, can be seen. The treatment of thoracic disc herniations depends on the duration of the patient's symptoms, the physical findings, and the neuroradiographic findings.[9,10] Patients with thoracic backache alone and no objective neurologic deficits can be successfully treated with a brace, nonsteroidal anti-inflammatory agents, and observation for at least 6 weeks. The majority of these patients do not require surgery; however, if symptoms recur after this conservative treatment regimen, disc excision and local fusion may be required.[11,12]

Surgery is indicated for patients with a neuroradiologically discrete thoracic lesion and an objective neurologic deficit or incapacitating pain and discomfort. Patients with radiating pain but no muscle wasting or gait abnormalities can also initially be treated with nonoperative measures. Patients with evidence of muscle weakness or wasting, gait abnormalities, or bladder and bowel dysfunction require surgical intervention without trial of conservative treatment. Delay in treating significant neurologic deficits is not warranted.

FRACTURES

Fractures of the thoracic and lumbar spine may result from a direct blow to the axial skeleton. Fractures of the transverse processes or the posterior spinous processes are stable injuries. They are painful because of the soft tissue attachments and the associated soft tissue injury. These fractures need not be treated with a cast or a brace; rather they can be treated by a reduction in activities. Isolated posterior spinous process fractures may result from a flexion injury. Similarly, transverse process fractures may be secondary to torsional injuries. These fractures resulting from hyperflexion or torsional injury may be associated with significant ligamentous injury and instability.[13–15] Such injuries may require longterm immobilization or surgery.

Compression fractures result from axial loading of the spine.[13,16] The anterior portion of the vertebral body is disrupted, and there is a variable injury to the posterior ligamentous complex. Stability and treatment options are established by findings on plain radiographs and physical examination. On physical examination, the posterior spinous processes should be carefully palpated in addition to the interspinous ligament. If there is a significant step-off or a significantly painful interspinous interval, a posterior ligamentous injury is present. In these cases, the patient should be treated with a molded hyperextension brace or cast. If there is no posterior ligamentous injury, the patient can be treated with a thoracolumbar corset or a hyperextension brace.[17]

Compression fractures associated with loss of height of the anterior vertebral cortex greater than 50% on plain radiographs are unstable.[13,16] These fractures often require surgical stabilization in addition to a brace or cast.

Burst fractures[13,14] and fracture-dislocations[15,16] involve an injury pattern to anterior and posterior portions of the vertebral body and the posterior ligamentous complex (Fig. 36–3). These are severe and unstable injuries that commonly require surgical treatment.

SPONDYLOLYSIS AND SPONDYLOLISTHESIS

Spondylolysis and spondylolisthesis are common causes of back pain in children and adolescents, and they occur most frequently in the lower lumbar spine. Spondylolysis is a defect in the posterior arch of a vertebra (Fig. 36–4). This loss of bone integrity occurs at the pars interarticularis, the area of the posterior arch linking the lamina to the superior articular facet. With loss of the posterior stabilization of the spine, the vertebral body can subluxate forward, causing spondylolisthesis (Fig. 36–5). Spondylolysis is most frequent in children

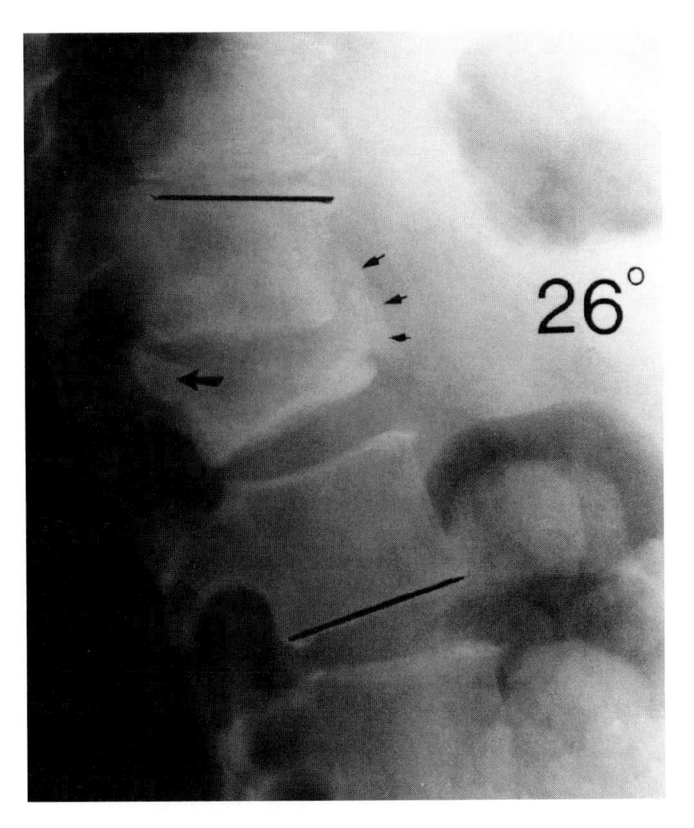

Fig. 36–3. Lateral radiograph of the thoracolumbar junction shows a burst fracture of L1. There is severe collapse of the anterior portion of the vertebral body *(small arrows)* and retropulsion of bone from the vertebral body into the spinal canal *(large arrow)*. The local kyphosis is 26°.

between age 6 and 10 years. The defect is often asymptomatic. Forward slippage of the vertebral body and progression of the spondylolisthesis most often occurs between age 10 and 15 years.(18–21)

Spondylolysis and spondylolisthesis occur in approximately 5% of the population. They are associated with certain sports activities and occupations. Pars lesions occur in more than 20% of female gymnasts and their prevalence is greater among adolescents who participate in diving, power weight lifting, football, wrestling, high jumping, and rowing than in the general population.(22,23) Repetitive flexion and extension activities involving the lumbar spine have been considered the reason for the pars interarticularis injury. It has been proposed that repetitive extension of the spine results in microtrauma to the pars interarticularis. The repetitive trauma causes stress fractures within the pars.

Low back pain is the most common presenting clinical complaint of athletes with spondylolysis and spondylolisthesis.(24,25) The pain is usually localized to the low back area but may be referred into the buttock and posterior thighs. Rarely does the pain radiate below the knee and into the calf and foot. The pain is exacerbated with activities and partially relieved with rest. Hamstring tightness manifested by the athlete's limited flexibility and inability to bend and touch his or her toes is common. These symptoms may result from a specific traumatic event or they may develop insidiously.

Physical examination of an athlete with spondylolisthesis shows paravertebral muscle spasm, hamstring tightness, and a palpable step-off in the posterior spinous processes. These patients usually have no neurologic

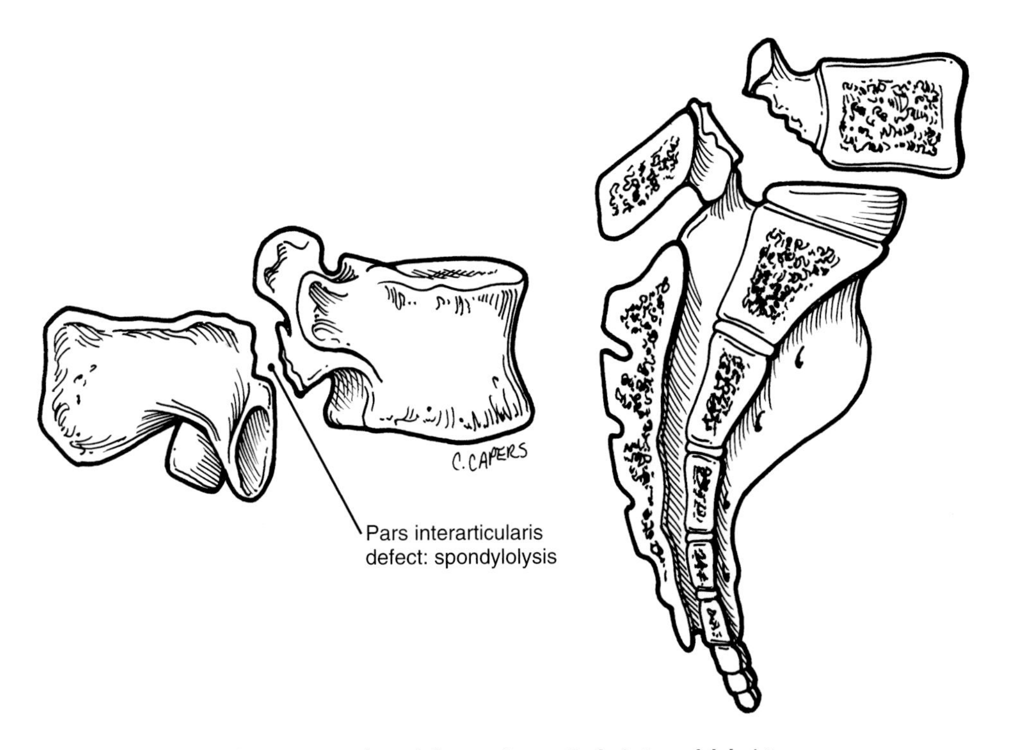

Fig. 36–4. Defect of the pars interarticularis (spondylolysis).

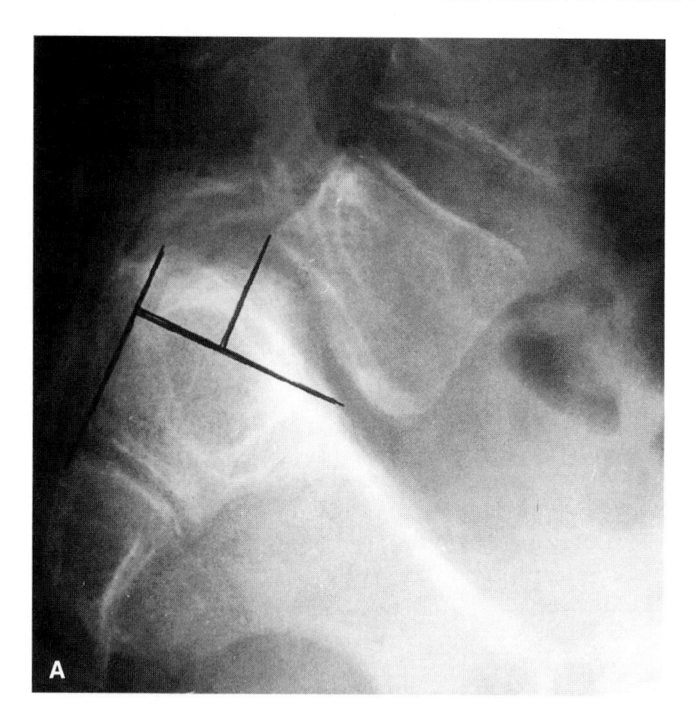

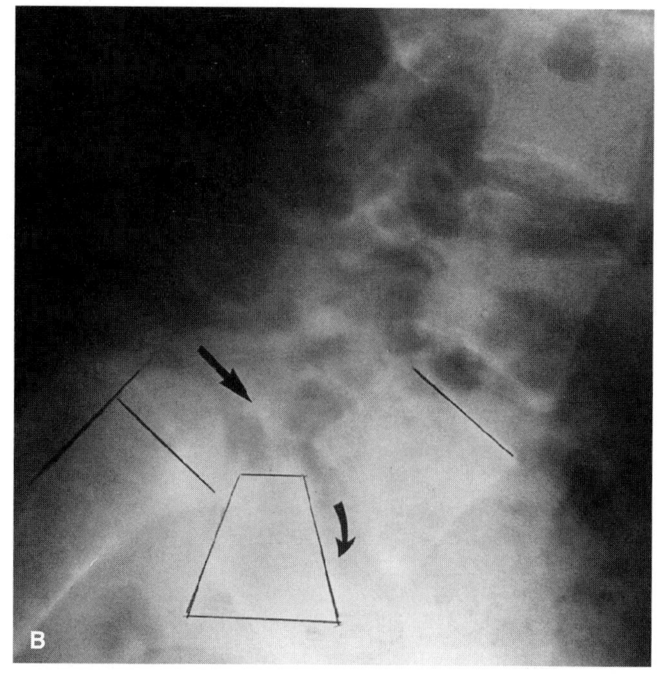

Fig. 36–5. *(A)* **Lateral radiograph of the lumbosacral spine demonstrates a spondylolisthesis deformity of L5 on the sacrum. There are several radiographic risk factors for progression of the deformity: anterior subluxation greater than 40% and significant rounding (doming) of the sacrum.** *(B)* **Lateral radiograph of the lumbosacral spine shows significant progression of the untreated spondylolisthesis deformity** *(arrows)***. There has been progression in the anterior subluxation of L5 on the sacrum and an increase in the kyphotic angulation between the olisthetic vertebral body and the sacrum.**

symptoms. They may stand with a list to one side or have some evidence of scoliosis. A painful list should not be confused with primary scoliosis. This scoliosis pattern is not structural but is secondary to the muscle spasm associated with the spondylolisthesis.

The diagnosis of spondylolysis and spondylolisthesis can be made with plain radiographs.[26] A lateral view of the lumbosacral spine demonstrates any forward subluxation of the vertebral body. Oblique radiographs profile the pars interarticularis and show any defects; however, plain radiographs cannot rule out the possibility of a developing stress fracture. A technetium bone scan can show an early stress injury to the pars interarticularis and computed axial tomography may show a fracture defect before plain radiographs do.

The treatment of an athlete with spondylolysis and spondylolisthesis depends on their age, symptoms, and the magnitude of the deformity. Symptomatic spondylolysis is rare; 5% of the general population has a pars defect. Adolescents who become symptomatic and who continue to have pain with activity can be successfully treated with bed rest, reduction of physical activities, and use of a molded body brace. Complete resolution of symptoms usually takes approximately 8 to 12 weeks. Once symptoms resolve and the athlete has been adequately reconditioned, he or she may return to all activities, including contact sports. If the athlete remains symptomatic following an adequate period of conservative therapy, spinal fusion may be necessary. The patient may be a candidate for direct repair of the pars interarticularis defect.

The treatment of an athlete with spondylolisthesis is more complex.[20,27] Spondylolisthesis often progresses during the adolescent growth spurt. Skeletally mature persons rarely show a significant increase in the deformity. There are several other risk factors for progression, in addition to age. Female patients are at greater risk for progression, as are those with recurrent episodes of back pain. Radiographic findings associated with progression include anterior subluxation of 50% or more of the vertebral body, a domed or rounded sacrum, and an increase in the slip angle or lumbosacral kyphosis (see Fig. 36–5).

The treatment of athletes with spondylolisthesis depends on the severity of symptoms and the degree of slippage. Adolescent athletes with subluxation greater than one third of the vertebral body may require surgical treatment even if they are not symptomatic. Symptomatic athletes with subluxation of 33% or less can be successfully treated with restriction of activities and a molded lumbosacral brace. Once the symptoms have resolved, the athlete may start a reconditioning program and return to all activities, including contact sports. These athletes should be followed with serial lumbosacral radiographs every 6 months, or sooner if the low back symptoms return.

Athletes who have persistent symptoms or recurrence of symptoms after conservative treatment may require surgery. Those with subluxation greater than one third or those that show progression of vertebral body slippage may require surgical stabilization, even if they are asymptomatic.

REFERENCES

1. Lonstein, J. E., and Carlson, J. M.: The prediction of curve progression in untreated idiopathic scoliosis during growth. J. Bone Joint Surg. *66A:*1061, 1984.
2. Weinstein, S. L., Zavala, D. C., and Ponseti, I. V.: Idiopathic scoliosis: long-term follow up and prognosis in untreated patients. J. Bone Joint Surg. *63A:*702, 1981.
3. Lowe, T. G.: Scheuermann disease. J. Bone Joint Surg. *72A:*940, 1990.
4. Blumenthal, S. L., Roach, J., and Herring, J. A.: Lumbar Scheuermann's: A clinical series and classification. Spine *12:*929, 1987.
5. Micheli, L. J.: Low back pain in the adolescent: differential diagnosis. Am. J. Sports Med. *7:*362, 1979.
6. Albrand, O. W., and Corkill, G.: Thoracic disc herniation. Treatment and prognosis. Spine *4:*41, 1979.
7. Bohlman, H. H., and Zdeblick, T. A.: Anterior excision of herniated thoracic discs. J. Bone Joint Surg. *70A:*1038, 1988.
8. Maiman, D. J., Larson, S. J., Luck, E., and El-Ghatit, A.: Lateral extracavitary approach to the spine for thoracic disc herniation: Report of 23 cases. Neurosurgery *14:*178, 1984.
9. McAllister, V. L., and Sage, M. R.: The radiology of thoracic disc protrusion. Clin. Radiol. *27:*291, 1976.
10. Ross, J. S., et al.: Thoracic disc herniation: MR imaging. Radiology *165:*511, 1987.
11. Middleton, G. S., and Teacher, J. H.: Injury of the spinal cord due to rupture of an intervertebral disc during muscular effort. Glasgow Med. J. *76:*1, 1911.
12. Sekhar, L. N., and Jannetta, P. J.: Thoracic disc herniation: Operative approaches and results. Neurosurgery, *12:*303, 1983.
13. Denis, F.: The three column spine and its significance in the classification of acute thoracolumbar spine injuries. Spine *8:*817, 1983.
14. Denis, F.: Spinal instability as defined by the three-column spine concept in acute spinal trauma. Clin. Orthop. *189:*65, 1984.
15. Nicoll, E. A.: Fractures of the dorso-lumbar spine. J. Bone Joint Surg. *31B:*376, 1949.
16. Holdsworth, F. W.: Fractures, dislocations, and fracture-dislocations of the spine. J. Bone Joint Surg. *45B:*6, 1963.
17. Young, M. H.: Long-term consequences of stable fractures of the thoracic and lumbar vertebral bodies. J. Bone Joint Surg. *55B:*295, 1973.
18. Boxall, D., Bradford, D. S., Winter, R. B., and Moe, J. H.: Management of severe spondylolisthesis in children and adolescents. J. Bone Joint Surg. *61A:*479, 1979.
19. Burkus, J. K., and Denis, F.: Thoracic disc disease. *In* Chapman, M.W. (ed.): Operative Orthopaedics, 2nd Ed. Philadelphia, J.B. Lippincott, 1993.
20. Burkus, J. K., Lonstein, J. E., Winter, R. B., and Denis, F.: Long-term evaluation of adolescents treated operatively for spondylolisthesis. J. Bone Joint Surg. *74A:*693, 1992.
21. Hensinger, R. N., Lang, J. R., and MacEwen, G. D.: Surgical management of spondylolisthesis in children and adolescents. Spine *1:*207, 1976.
22. Jackson, D. W., Wiltse, L. L., and Cirincione, R. J.: Spondylolysis in the female gymnast. Clin. Orthop. *117:*68, 1976.
23. Wiltse, L. L., and Jackson, D. W.: Treatment of spondylolisthesis and spondylolysis in children. Clin. Orthop. *117:*92, 1976.
24. Newman, P. H.: A clinical syndrome associated with severe lumbosacral subluxation. J. Bone Joint Surg. *47B:*472, 1965.
25. Seitsalo, S., Österman, K., Hyvärinen, H., and Poussa, M.: Severe spondylolisthesis in children and adolescents. J. Bone Joint Surg. *72B:*259, 1990.
26. Wiltse, L. L., and Winter, R. B.: Terminology and measurement of spondylolisthesis. J. Bone Joint Surg. *65A:*768, 1983.
27. Pizzutillo, P. D., Mirenda, W., and MacEwen, G. D.: Posterolateral fusion for spondylolisthesis in adolescence. J. Pediatr. Orthop. *6:*311, 1986.

37 *Lee A. Kelley*

Disc Disorders of the Spine

Intervertebral disc disorders in the cervical and the lumbar spine are extremely common. Everyone develops some degree of degenerative change in at least some of the discs in these areas. Degenerated discs occasionally become symptomatic. It is not as common to see obvious degenerative changes in the thoracic discs, and they rarely become symptomatic. It is important to understand the process of disc degeneration and what symptoms may result. Since all orthopedic surgeons must be able to recognize the various causes of neck and lower back pain, it is important to develop a systematic approach to the evaluation of these problems.

The manifestations of disc disorders in the three areas of the spine—cervical, thoracic, and lumbar—are not significantly different. In each area, pain can be caused by the degenerative process of the disc itself, compression of nerve roots by disc material or osteophytes that result from the degeneration of the disc, or central compression of the spinal cord or cauda equina.

CERVICAL DISC DISORDERS

Six intervertebral discs extend from C2-3 through C7-T1. The structure of the intervertebral disc involves a layered outer fibrous covering called the *annulus fibrosus.* This connects circumferentially to the vertebral body just above and the one just below the vertebral end-plate (Fig. 37–1). Within the annulus fibrosus is a semisolid material known as the *nucleus pulposus.* In very young persons, this material is nearly liquid, but with aging it begins to dehydrate and becomes more solid.

Over time, the annulus fibrosus may develop small tears within the concentric layers of its outer covering. The combination of changes within the annulus fibrosus and the nucleus pulposus ultimately lead to a loss of disc height. Settling of the disc space causes a loss of congruence of the articulation of the facet joint (Fig. 37–2). This ultimately leads to the development of some degree of abnormal motion, antero-posterior translation, and sagittal angulation, between the two vertebral bodies that border the disc above and below. This segmental instability is evidenced on plain films by traction osteophytes, horizontally projecting bones spurs located within 2 mm of the vertebral end-plate (Fig. 37–3).

In the cervical spine, as the intervertebral disc settles further, congruence is also lost in the false articulations known as the neurocentral joints or the joints of Luschka. Osteophytes frequently begin to form in the area of the neurocentral joints and within the facet joints because of this loss of articulation. Since osteophytes form anteriorly and posteriorly within the neuroforamen, the exiting nerve root can potentially be compressed from either direction (Fig. 37–4). In the cervical spine, this process of generalized degenerative changes is known as *cervical spondylosis.* It is the most common cause of neck pain and radicular arm pain in middle-aged or older patients.

In younger patients, true disc herniation may be either an isolated entity or one associated with some of the more advanced spondylotic changes. These are termed *soft disc herniation* when the nerve root compression is caused by disc material extending into the spinal canal or neuroforamen. *Hard disc* is a term used to describe nerve root or spinal cord compression caused by osteophytic projections in the cervical spine.

Clinical Diagnosis

The single most important item in assessing a patient with neck or arm pain is obtaining the appropriate information on a history. Patients tend to be vague about the site of pain in the neck or the arm; it is important to have them localize exactly the pain in the neck and have them trace with the opposite upper extremity

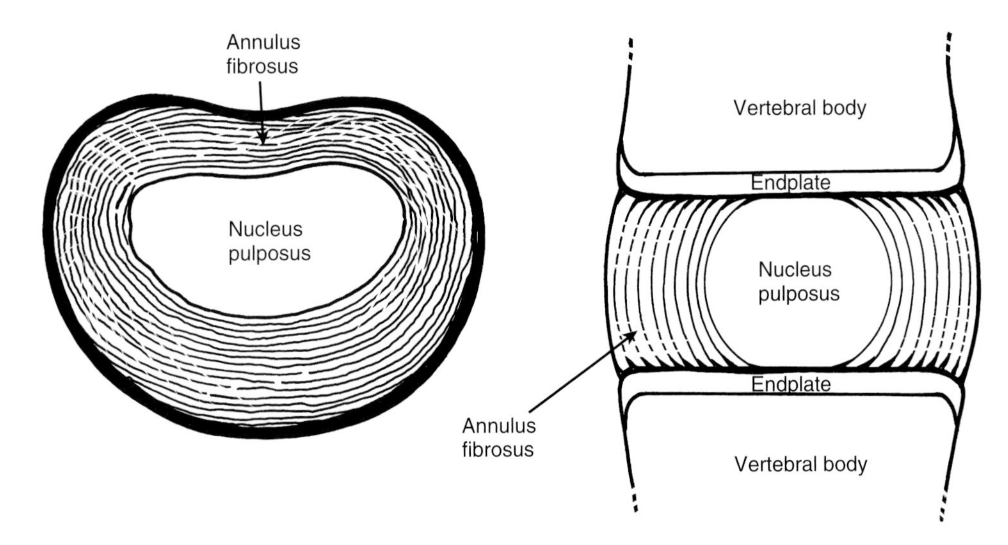

Fig. 37–1. Cross section *(left)* and sagittal section *(right)* through an intervertebral disc.

the precise location of the pain down the arm. Arm pain related to nerve compression in the neck frequently follows a dermatomal pattern, though it is well known that the dermatomes in the upper extremity overlap considerably. The history should note what type of injury led to the onset of the pain. When evaluating an athlete, it is important to try and elicit as much detail as possible on this part of the history. For instance, a head-down open field tackle by a defensive back is known to impart a great deal of force to the cervical spine. This is the most common mechanism of serious cervical spine injuries. In other cases, the history may show that the patient was struck directly on the neck by an object, a mechanism that is much less likely to lead to a true neurologic problem.

The examiner should also catalog what activities aggravate pain. Nerve root pain in the arm is frequently exacerbated by cervical extension, and in particular by simultaneous rotation and extension of the neck. Cervical flexion may also increase nerve root pain, but much less often than cervical extension does. Almost every form of neck pain seems to be aggravated by holding the head in the flexed position for long periods or holding the head in a fixed position for a long time, as when driving or looking at a computer screen.

It is important to note in the history the presence or absence of complaints associated with spinal cord problems. These include a change in bowel or bladder habits and change in gait. The typical gait associated with myelopathy is a wide-based, uneven gait. Lower extremity pain generally is not associated with cervical spine problems.

Once all items of the history have been documented, a detailed physical examination is very important. One should note tenderness to palpation about the posterior cervical paraspinous muscles and in the trapezius muscles and interscapular areas. Regions of muscle spasm, either localized or generalized, should be noted. The cervical range of motion should be carefully measured in flexion-extension and in right and left rotation. It

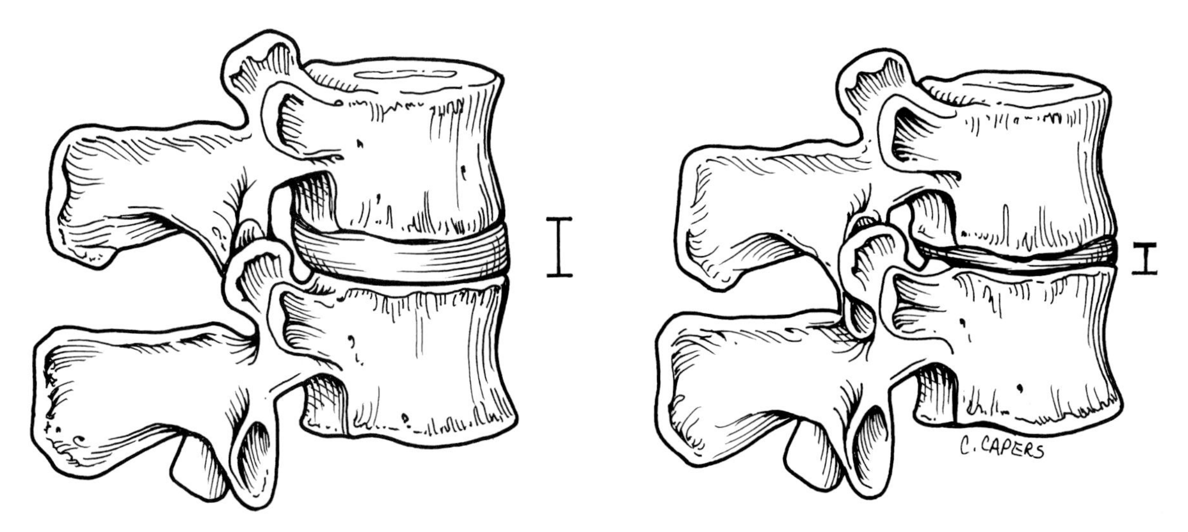

Fig. 37–2. Facet articulations are "designed" to conform with normal disc height *(left)*. With disc degeneration *(right)*, facet congruence is lost.

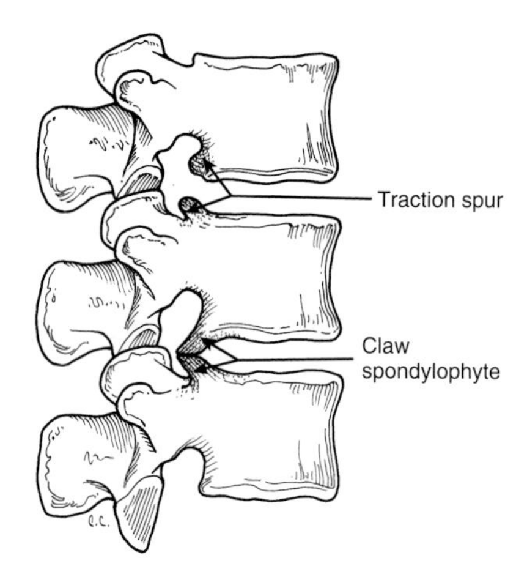

Fig. 37–3. Traction spurs occur 2 to 3 mm from the vertebral end-plate, at the attachment point of the annulus fibrosus. The claw spondylophyte is actually within the anterior longitudinal ligament.

should also be noted which of these motions elicit pain. A provocative test known as Spurling's maneuver should be performed. Next, motor examination of the upper extremities is carried out. Generally, shoulder abduction is a C5 function, elbow flexion a C6 function, elbow extension C7, wrist extension C6, wrist flexion C7, finger flexion C8, and motions of the hand intrinsic muscles a T1 function. The deep tendon reflexes of the upper extremity are then measured. Testing for ankle clonus is necessary because this is also a long tract finding that indicates spinal cord compression. Babinski's signs are measured in each lower extremity.

Other physical findings go along with cervical myelopathy or cervical radiculopathy. With a positive arm abduction test result, pain radiating into the arm is relieved by placing the arm on top of the patient's head with the shoulder in maximal abduction. This finding indicates nerve root compression. Another commonly discussed sign is Lhermitte's sign, a shocklike sensation in the trunk or limb following a quick extension or flexion of the neck. This is said to be present in approximately 25% of patients with myelopathy secondary to cervical spondylosis.

Imaging Studies

Some of the plain film findings have already been discussed—narrowing of the disc space, formation of traction osteophytes, loss of congruence of the facet articulations, and uncovertebral osteophytes. The facet changes may be better appreciated on oblique views, and the uncovertebral joint changes are best appreciated on the anteroposterior view. It is important to note

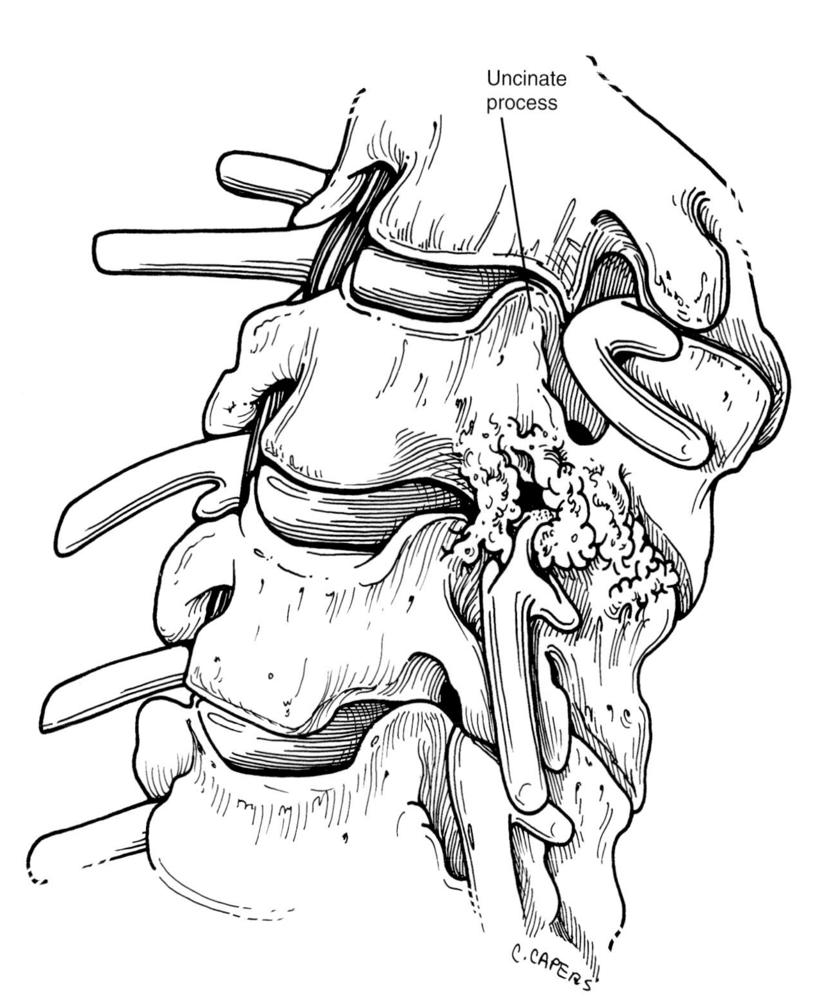

Fig. 37–4. Compression of cervical nerve root in the neuroforamen. Note anteromedial osteophytes from the uncovertebral joint and posterolateral osteophyte from the facet joint.

on the lateral radiographs whether cervical lordosis has been lost, which may occur in an acute muscle strain from spasm or may represent the sum of multiple spondylotic changes.

There is an important finding on the lateral radiographs that can indicate a significant degree of congenital narrowing of the spinal canal. Generally, the cervical lamina is seen between the spinous process and the cervical facet joint on the lateral view. Specifically, it is the area of bone between (1) the spinolaminar line formed by the junction of the spinous process and the upper lamina and (2) the posterior aspect of the facet joint. In patients with significant congenital narrowing of the spinal canal, the spinous process appears to emanate from the upper end of the facet without any intervening lamina (Fig. 37–5). When this is noted on a plain film study in a patient with neck or arm pain, (Fig. 37–6) evaluation of the spinal canal with computed tomography (CT) or magnetic resonance imaging (MRI) should follow.

Significant instabilities between vertebral bodies should be visible on plain films. It is not uncommon to see low-grade translations of 1 to 2 mm as a result of disc and facet degeneration. These generally do not increase significantly on flexion radiographs and may reduce on extension views. If there is any suspicion of ligament injury in association with an acute spine injury, flexion and extension views should be obtained to evaluate for subtle instability. Routine use of flexion and extension lateral radiographs of the cervical spine is not necessary.

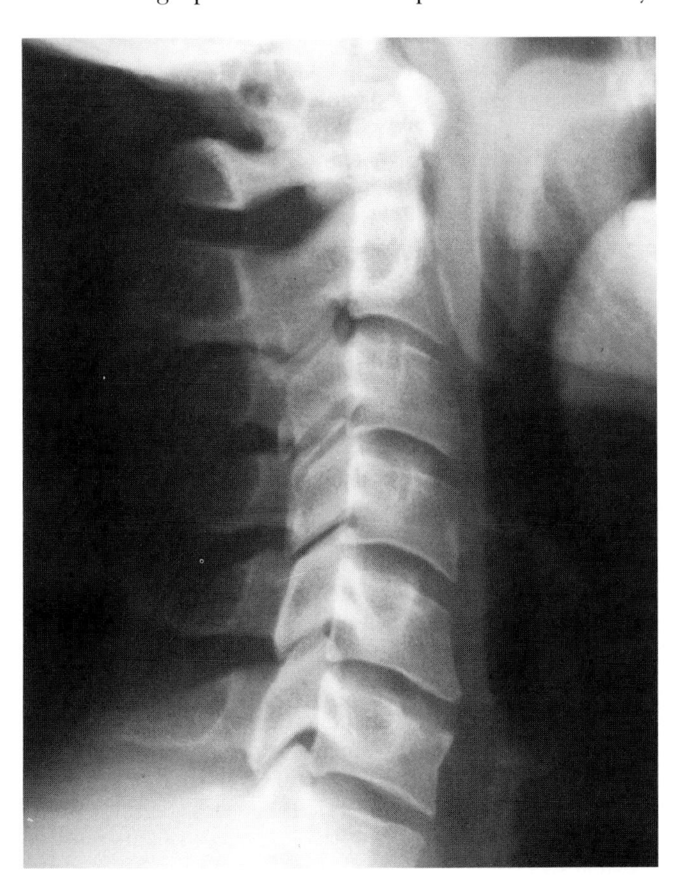

Fig. 37–5. Note the decreased distance from the spinolaminar line to the posterior vertebral body.

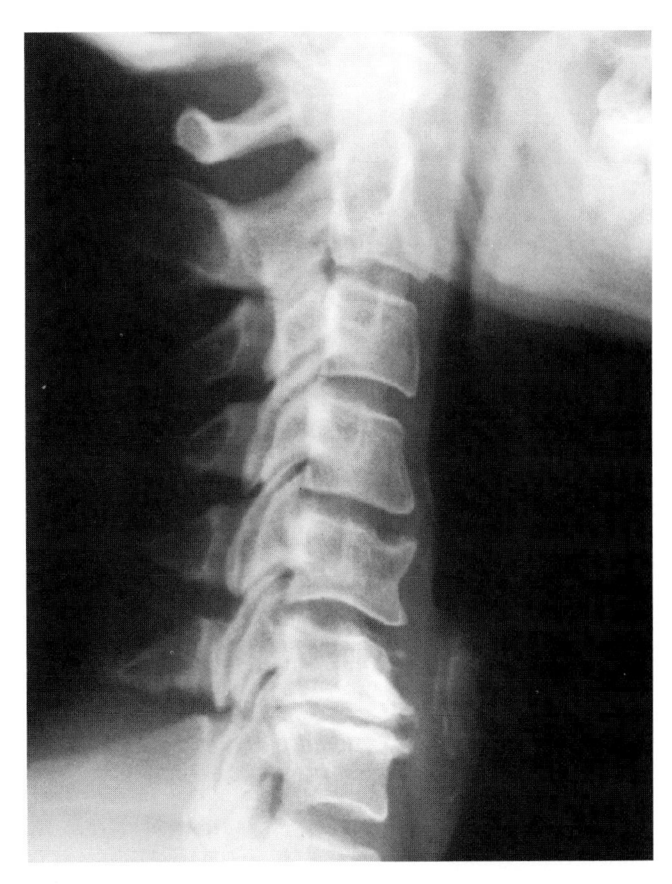

Fig. 37–6. Typical changes of spondylosis are seen at C6-7. Note the narrowed disc space and anterior and posterior osteophytes.

For persistent neck or arm pain or any indication of spinal cord involvement, advanced diagnostic studies should be undertaken: cervical myelography with post-myelography CT or MRI of the cervical spine. In my opinion, both the MRI and the postmyelography CT are excellent tools for evaluating central spinal canal stenosis. It should be noted that measurements of spinal canal diameter on MRI may not be as accurate as those obtained from CT. MRI has the added advantage of evaluating the bone marrow elements in patients who may have neck pain of causes other than degenerative disease.

Electromyography (EMG) and nerve conduction studies of the upper extremities may be employed to distinguish cervical radicular pain from peripheral nerve pain. Since many cases of cervical radicular pain involve the sensory elements of the nerve only, EMG changes are not always evident, even in the presence of significant cervical radiculopathy. Nerve conduction velocities, however, are generally abnormal in the presence of peripheral neuropathy.

Treatment

The initial treatment of cervical radicular pain is the same, whether it is believed to be the result of soft disc herniation or cervical spondylosis. Restriction of activity should be recommended. This includes any activity that consistently causes radiating pain into the upper extremities. In general, high-impact exercise is restricted and patients should be advised against running and playing such sports as basketball and tennis. Certain types of weight lifting consistently aggravate cervical radicular pain; in general, overhead lifting activities such as military press repetitions and overhead pull-down weight-lifting exercises are restricted. Patients should also be advised against performing squatting exercises with weights across the shoulders. In many cases, sitting pectoral exercises using significant quantities of weight aggravate neck and upper extremity pain. Patients may be allowed to perform supine bench press exercises and semireclined, curl-type exercises with the elbow stabilized against a pad. Competitive athletes such as football players and baseball players should be restricted from play until symptoms have subsided in the upper extremity. It may not be necessary for all of the axial neck pain to have resolved before the athlete is allowed to resume participation in noncontact sports.

Along with activity modification, anti-inflammatory medications are usually the first line of treatment. The preferred initial medication is a nonsteroidal anti-inflammatory medication such as naproxen or ibuprofen. This should be given on a regular daily basis, not only when pain is perceived to be a problem.

The initial treatment of upper extremity radicular pain should include cervical traction. This is generally used both in physical therapy and at home with a home cervical traction unit. It is common to begin using 8 to 10 pounds of weights and progress up as high as 12 pounds if necessary. It is very important to instruct the patient in proper orientation of the neck while traction is being applied. Traction with the neck in neutral position or slight flexion frequently brings relief of upper extremity radicular pain; if, however, the neck is in extension, it may actually exacerbate the pain.

It has become customary to use epidural steroid injections in the form of injected Depo-Medrol. This may be used in place of oral corticosteroid medication or it may be used as a further conservative measure, even after suboptimal response to oral corticosteroids. Cervical epidural steroid injections are administered by pain treatment specialists, generally anesthesiologists. These are given one at a time at intervals of 3 to 4 weeks, and the response to each is measured before follow-up injection is considered. Some articles in the anesthesiology literature indicate that epidural steroid injections should be given to all patients in a series of three. There is no clinical support for this contention at this time. I feel it is best to administer one injection, and if improvement appears to continue over time, it is best to have the patient take anti-inflammatory medication every day and to continue activity modifications and daily traction until all symptoms have subsided.

Physical therapy plays a vital role in treatment of most neck and upper extremity pain syndromes. It is important to instruct patients in proper daily exercises for strengthening the cervical muscles, generally isometric exercises. Stretching exercises should also be included. Newer techniques focus on postural modifications to affect pain control. Chin tucks have been popular for this reason and have been effective in many patients. Physical therapy may be most valuable when the upper extremity radicular pain begins to resolve and the pain becomes more axial in the trapezius and posterior cervical paraspinal muscles. At this point, aggressive attention to exercise, stretching, and postural modifications frequently affords significant benefits.

Surgical treatment is reserved for patients whose radicular symptoms have remained intractable and disabling. A minimum period of 6 weeks of nonoperative treatment should be afforded to all patients before consideration is given to surgical treatment. There are exceptions to this rule, of course. Sometimes pain is so severe that it is not possible to prolong conservative treatment 6 full weeks. Though traditional teaching has indicated that a progressive neurologic deficit is a reason for urgent surgery, there is no good evidence that soft disc herniations of the neck that involve a single nerve root lead to permanent upper extremity muscle weakness. It is not unusual to see a significant loss of muscle tone in the triceps or biceps muscle from posterolateral disc protrusion. In time, these muscles recover strength, with or without surgery. The primary indication for surgical treatment remains intractable upper extremity pain. The preferred surgical treatment is anterior cervical disc excision and interbody fusion using autogenous iliac crest bone. There is significant evidence in the literature that anterior cervical disc excision without fusion produces longterm results equal to those of anterior cervical disc excision and fusion when treating soft disc herniations. However, cervical spondylosis responds much better to anterior cervical disc excision and fusion than anterior cervical excision without fusion. For cervical radicular pain secondary to soft disc herniation or spondylosis, surgical treatment through a posterior approach by laminoforaminotomy generally produces results equal to those of anterior procedures. Fusion is not necessary for treating radicular pain syndromes from the posterior approach. It is a matter of personal preference and training which of these approaches is undertaken when surgical treatment is necessary for radicular pain.

When athletes present with radicular pain syndromes in the upper extremities, it is sometimes difficult to distinguish a cervical nerve root lesion from a peripheral nerve lesion or brachial plexus injury, particularly in football players. Initial evaluation should, of course, consist of a detailed history and a physical examination. Brachial plexus stretch injuries may occur when the head and shoulder on the ipsilateral side to the injury are pulled in opposite directions during the course of a tackle or a fall. Cervical nerve root injuries may occur when the head and shoulder are compressed toward each other in a tackle or fall. In either case, physical findings help to determine the presence of an ongoing cervical nerve root lesion. The first priority in a contact athlete is to determine the presence or absence of any obvious abnormalities on plain film studies of the cervical spine. MRI of the cervical spine detects the presence or absence of intracanal lesions. If this proves to be negative, ongoing conservative treatment is certainly the choice, and the abovementioned plan can be used for a long time.

THORACIC DISC DISEASE

Thoracic disc herniation is much less common than cervical or lumbar disc herniation. It is believed that thoracic disc herniations are more commonly caused by degenerative changes than by trauma. This fact distinguishes this entity from lumbar disc herniation. This is not a common entity in athletes, but it should be considered when thoracic or lumbar pain is severe and does not respond to conservative measures. It should also be considered when neurologic changes in the lower extremities suggest spinal cord compression.

Pathophysiology

Degenerative changes almost always precede thoracic disc herniation. It is unusual for thoracic disc herniation to occur in the absence of some associated posterior osteophytes of the disc space. Thoracic disc herniation is commonly associated with plain film radiographic evidence of calcification in the disc space or of Scheuermann's disease. The fact that these rare disc herniations are almost never seen in young patients lends further support to the idea that degenerative changes are the cause.

Clinical Presentation

Although localized pain to the midthoracolumbar lumbar area may be present, it is well known that with thoracic disc herniation, the symptoms may not indicate the source of the problem. Low back pain is not an uncommon finding, and pain may be referred along thoracic dermatomes. The groin area is in the T12-L1 dermatome and may be involved. When a patient complains of paresthesia-type symptoms along the rib cage, thoracic disc herniation should certainly be considered. Classic findings involve back pain, lower extremity paresthesia, and long tract signs in the lower extremities. Gait alteration (a more wide-stance gait) or physical findings associated with spinal cord compression, including hyper-reflexia, ankle clonus, and positive Babinski's sign in the lower extremity may be observed. It should be part of a routine examination of the lower back to assess the lower extremities for these findings. No symptoms are truly typical of this entity. In Bohlman's series, the typical symptoms in 19 patients were listed in decreasing order of frequency: (1) nonspecific pain in the back, chest, or lower limb, (2) increasing weakness in the lower limb, (3) numbness in either the chest or lower extremities, (4) ataxia, (5) bowel and bladder problems, and (6) paresthesia.

It should be noted that the differential diagnosis of thoracic disc herniations includes tumors of the spinal cord as well as demyelinating disease, vascular lesions of the spinal cord, intercostal neuritis, costochondritis, and rib lesions.

Diagnostic Findings

It has already been mentioned that plain film findings of thoracic disc herniation may demonstrate calcification of a disc space or associated findings of Scheuermann's disease. Localized kyphosis and posterior osteophytes may also be observed at the thoracic disc levels. Confirmatory radiographic testing may include thoracic myelography and postmyelography CT; however, thoracic MRI is extremely reliable and should be the definitive investigative study whenever thoracic disc herniation is suspected (Fig. 37–7). It should be noted that thoracic discs may herniate in three directions: centrad, centrolaterad, or posterolaterad. Obviously, central herniation may be the most dangerous type if it is large enough to cause cord compression. Centrolateral disc herniation may cause a combination of findings associated with spinal cord compression and thoracic root compression, including a sensory change in a thoracic dermatome. Posterolateral herniations typically compress the thoracic roots and cause paresthesias in the distribution of the given thoracic root. The majority of thoracic disc herniations occur at the thoracolumbar junction. In two recent large series of thoracic disc herniations, more than half occurred between T10 and L1. In a good lumbar MRI study, the sagittal views visualize the spine to the level of T10 or T11, and this area should be inspected closely during the course of routine evaluation of a lumbar MR image. It is extremely rare to see multiple thoracic disc herniations in one patient.

Treatment

Initial treatment of thoracic disc herniation depends largely on its size, location, and associated symptoms. A large central thoracic disc herniation with physical findings confirming spinal cord compression should be treated surgically. The preferred method, anterior transthoracic disc excision and interbody fusion, is described in detail by Bohlman. It is also acceptable to excise the disc through a posterior transpedicular approach. When a thoracic disc herniation is centrolateral, it may be treated conservatively, as long as there are no positive findings of spinal cord compression. Conservative measures include activity modifications and anti-inflammatory medications. Lateral thoracic disc herniations ordinarily are not associated with any signs of spinal cord compression. These may be associated with symptoms that closely correlate with the compressed thoracic root. They may also be asymptomatic.

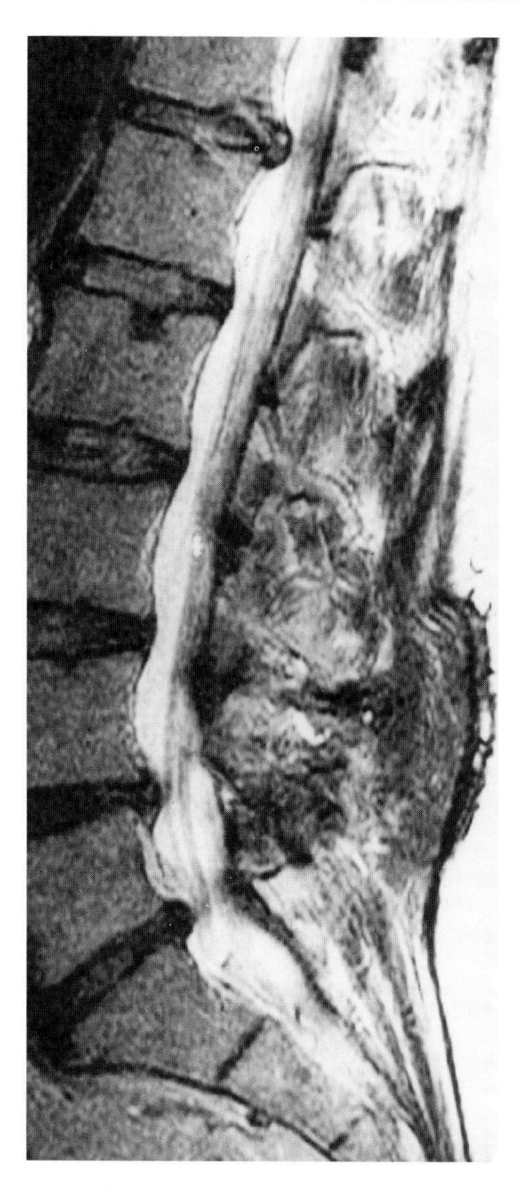

Fig. 37–7. MRI shows thoracic disc herniations at T11-12 and T12-L1. There is, at least, bulging of the L4-5 and L5-S1 discs.

Surgical treatment generally is not indicated for such herniations unless the symptoms are severe and persistent. Conservative treatment—time, anti-inflammatory medications, pain medication, and activity modifications—usually lead to resolution of the initial symptoms of posterolateral thoracic disc herniation. If the patient is an athlete with a posterolateral disc herniation, activities may be resumed as soon as these symptoms have largely subsided.

LUMBAR DISC HERNIATION

Lumbar disc problems are so common that every physician or trainer involved in the care of athletes encounters some such problems on a regular basis. Fortunately, most problems are transient and respond to conservative measures over a relatively short time. It is important to make a thorough initial evaluation in the performance athlete so that appropriate treatment may be instituted promptly without a prolonged period of empiric methods. It is very important to realize that the average person may be treated with a much more conservative approach when symptoms indicate lumbar disc herniation because recovery time frequently is not a factor. For elite athletes, and in particular professional athletes, often the luxury of prolonged conservative treatment is not an option.

Pathophysiology

The lumbar discs are very similar to cervical discs in overall structure. The outer annulus fibrosus contains the semisolid nucleus pulposus. The intervertebral articulations in the lumbar spine are similar to those in the cervical spine, except that uncovertebral joints are absent in the lumbar spine. Macnab termed the linkages in the lumbar spine "three-joint articulations." Two of the three joints are the facet joints posteriorly, the third is the disc. Each three-joint articulation constitutes a motion segment, and numerous biomechanical studies detail the forces and force transitions involved in each motion segment of the lumbar spine during the course of normal movement, with and without loading.

The lumbar spine is subject to much greater forces than the cervical spine, in all directions. In addition, the orientation of the L5-S1 disc and, in some persons the L4-5 disc, imposes additional shear stress across these structures, which contributes to the degenerative changes observed in these discs. In general, lumbar disc degeneration begins in the fourth or fifth decade of life, but in many persons changes are noted even earlier. The advent of MRI has shown that many asymptomatic teenagers and persons in their early twenties show changes in disc interspaces suggestive of early degenerative change.

Lumbar disc herniation, which is also a sequela of disc degeneration, describes extrusion of the inner nucleus pulposus into the spinal canal. Lumbar disc herniations are most commonly posterolateral and involve a single lumbar nerve root (Fig. 37–8). The levels commonly involved are L5-S1 and L4-5. Because the posterior longitudinal ligament is relatively strong in the midline of the lumbar spine but does not always extend across the entire width of the lumbar disc space, lumbar disc herniations tend to follow a more posterolateral course. There are many instances of central disc herniation in the lumbar spine, however, and the symptoms may be severe low back pain or unilateral or bilateral leg pain or both back and leg pain. Large central disc herniations in the lumbar spine may cause significant compression of the cauda equina, and only this type of disc herniation is "dangerous" from a neurologic standpoint. Posterolateral disc herniation most commonly causes leg pain in a dermatomal distribution; and though the pain can be a significant problem as far as it limits activity, it is

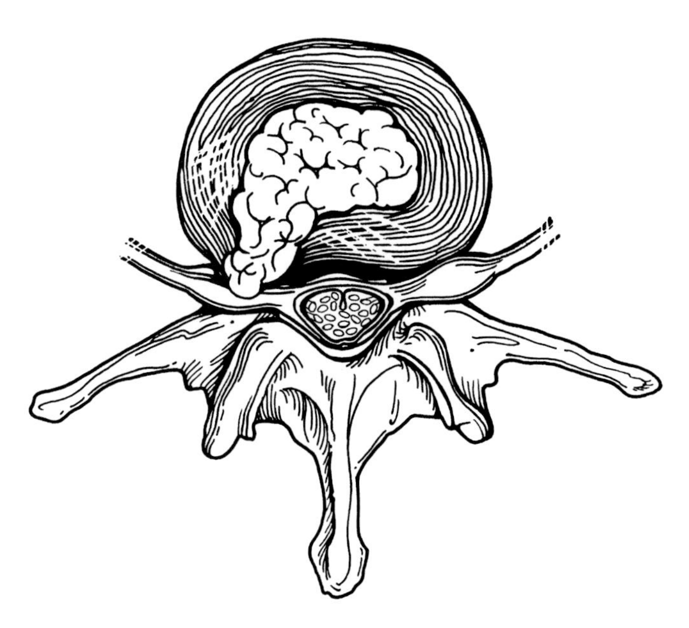

Fig. 37–8. Posterolateral lumbar disc herniation with compression of lumbar nerve root.

extremely unusual for permanent motor deficits to result from posterolateral disc herniation. It is uncommon to see lumbar disc herniations at L1-2 or L2-3. Trauma may ultimately lead to herniation of a degenerated disc in the lumbar spine, but it is not always associated with a specific incident of injury—e.g., with lifting.

Clinical Findings

It is essential, in taking a history, to distinguish between axial back pain, which is generally in the midline lumbar and lumbosacral spine, and pain that radiates into the buttock or lower extremities. Although axial back pain may be the initial presenting symptom of lumbar disc herniation, with nerve root compression some pain almost always radiates into the buttock and the lower extremity. The exception is central disc herniation in the lower lumbar spine, and it is for this reason that even axial back pain, if persistent, must be considered as a possible sequela of lumbar disc protrusion. It is much more common to see axial back pain in relation to strain injuries of the lower back and pain of degenerative disc origin, the so-called discogenic-type pain.

When a patient complains of pain radiating into the buttock and lower extremity, the examiner should have the patient indicate the exact location of the pain throughout the entire course of the extremity. This is the only way a dermatomal association may be made to establish the level of nerve root involvement. One should elicit in the history whether back or leg pain has a mechanical basis. In the broadest terms, this means that the pain is aggravated by activity and relieved by rest or certain posture modification.

It is important to document what level of activity the patient can tolerate, given the current complaints of pain. A runner who has radiating leg pain only after reaching the 5- to 7-mile mark is in a different category than a patient who cannot walk 50 feet because of leg pain. It is important to document which activities predictably exacerbate the pain. In almost all forms of compressive nerve root disorders, any strenuous physical activity intensifies pain.

It is also important to document in the history any antecedent low back or lower extremity radicular pain. The patient should be questioned about a subjective feeling of weakness and about any recent change in bowel or bladder habits.

The physical examination should proceed in an orderly manner. The lumbosacral posture should be recorded and any areas of tenderness on palpation should be noted. The site of localized muscle spasm that is palpable should be recorded. The patient should be asked to bend forward while standing and extend the lumbosacral spine as far as is tolerable and to bend to the right and left. If the patient leans or lists to one side, this should be noted, because its association with nerve root irritation is well-known.

Motor functions should be tested in the lower extremities by asking the patient to stand on one foot at a time and lift the heel off of the ground. This tests the strength of the gastrocsoleus complex and is a well-accepted test for the integrity of the S1 nerve root. The patient should then be asked to walk on the heels with the toes off the floor, which tests the strength of ankle dorsiflexion and is generally considered a test of L5 nerve root integrity, though the L4 nerve root also plays a part in ankle dorsiflexion. Great toe extension is generally considered an L5 motor test. Resisting knee extension is an L3 and partial L4 motor test. Hip abduction should be measured against resistance. This is also an L5 motor function test. Hip flexion in the sitting position is generally considered a test of the L1 motor function. The deep tendon reflexes of the patellar tendons measure the L4 reflex and the Achilles tendon reflexes measure the S1 reflex arc. Sensation should be tested along the lower extremity dermatomes. The straight leg raise test should be performed in both lower extremities with the patient supine. The degree of elevation at which pain radiates into the lower extremity is recorded. Low back pain with straight leg raise is not considered a positive straight leg raise finding.

The positive findings strongly associated with lumbar disc herniation are (1) radiating lower extremity pain that follows a dermatomal distribution, (2) any evidence of motor weakness involving a muscle innervated by a nerve root correlating to the dermatomal distribution in which the pain is located, (3) a reflex change similarly associated with the nerve root involved according to the dermatomal distribution of the pain, (4) a positive straight leg raise test that occurs between 30° and 50° elevation, (5) decreased sensation in a dermatomal distribution correlating to the site of the pain. It is very rare to see all five of these associated findings in a single patient with leg pain; however, the presence of a dermatomal pain distribution along with a positive straight leg raise is generally considered a reliable indication of a herniated lumbar disc unless this can be otherwise disproved. Obviously, if a patient gives any history of bowel or bladder disturbance associated with severe back or lower extremity pain, one should proceed immediately to evaluate the lumbar spine with imaging studies under close neurologic observation. The loss of perineal sensation in the same scenario is an ominous sign that generally indicates cauda equina syndrome. These are surgical emergencies for which no conservative treatment is indicated.

Imaging Studies

The initial imaging studies should always be anteroposterior and lateral plain radiographs of the lumbar spine. Oblique radiographs are taken to evaluate the pars interarticularis and facet articulations in the lumbar spine. If there is any suspicion of spondylolysis in the lower lumbar spine, oblique views should be obtained. I do not feel that these are necessary in the initial evaluation of each patient with low back pain or lower extremity radicular pain. Plain film findings include disc space narrowing, an indication of degenerative change in the disc. Anterior and posterior osteophytes are also associated with disc degeneration. The facet joints should be inspected for the presence of degenerative changes and in "contact athletes" with severe back pain. The possibility of facet fracture or an acute pars interarticularis fracture should be considered. These latter entities, however, may require bone scintigraphy and CT for definitive evaluation.

Subsequent imaging studies of the lumbar spine may involve lumbar myelography plus postmyelographic CT to assess for lumbar disc herniation. MRI has become the definitive study for evaluating the lumbar spine for disc disorders, and any patient who has persistent severe back pain or persistent lower extremity radiating pain after conservative measures have been used for an appropriate time should be evaluated with CT or MRI to assess for possible lumbar disc protrusion (Fig. 37–9). The role of lumbar myelography in younger patients with possible disc disease is reserved for patients who present with radicular symptoms for which MRI fails to demonstrate compression. Lumbar myelography with postmyelographic CT is an excellent way to determine if, in fact, disc disease or another lesion is compressing nerve roots in the lumbar spine.

In some persons the diameter of the spinal canal in segments of the lumbar spine is small. Areas of small canal diameter may involve only a single level of the lumbar spine or several levels (Fig. 37–10) . Small canal diameter may affect the degree of symptoms that arise from a disc herniation. In the face of decreased spinal canal diameter, a relatively small disc herniation may be more symptomatic than a similar herniation in a spinal canal of normal diameter (Fig. 37–11). Throughout the spine the average canal diameter is 17 mm, and spinal canal stenosis is defined as a diameter smaller than 13 mm.

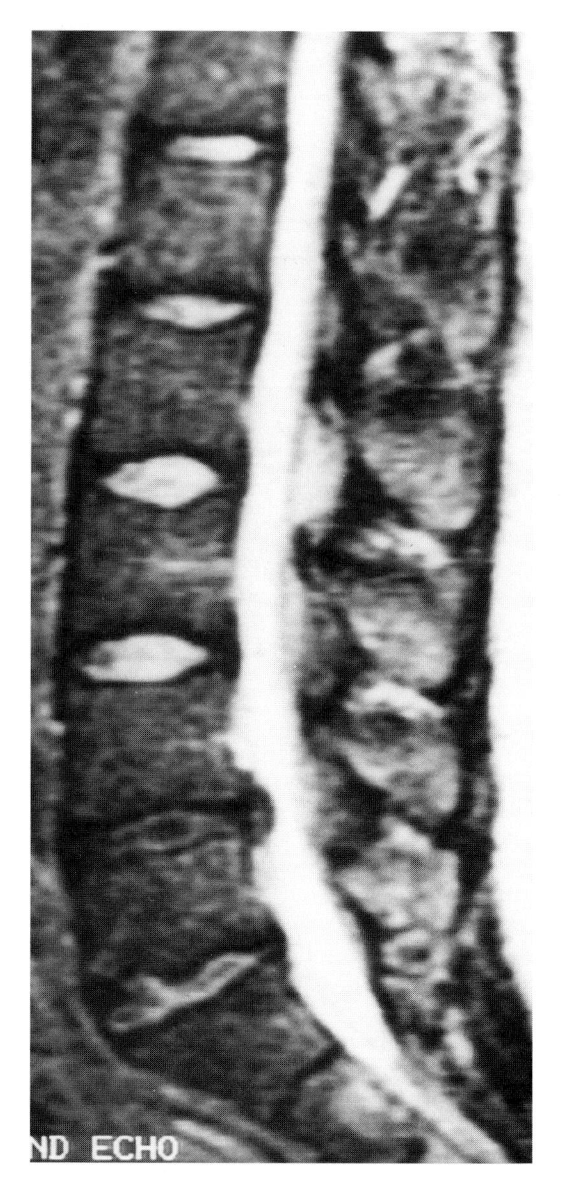

Fig. 37–9. **Lumbar MRI showing L4-5 disc herniation in sagittal section.**

Treatment

A patient who presents with low back and lower extremity radicular pain or with radicular pain alone should be treated with the same conservative measures outlined in the section on cervical disc disease. Initially, activity modifications are recommended and athletic involvement is limited or avoided entirely. It is essential to have the patient rest until the radicular leg pain has almost completely resolved; then, aggressive measures may be pursued to help resolve the axial low back pain, which frequently follows resolution of lower extremity radicular pain. Oral nonsteroidal anti-inflammatory medications are the first step in treatment. For severe radiating leg pain, a 6-day course of oral cortisone may be used as well. It is common practice to confirm the presence of a disc herniation with an imaging study such as CT or MRI before giving a lumbar epidural

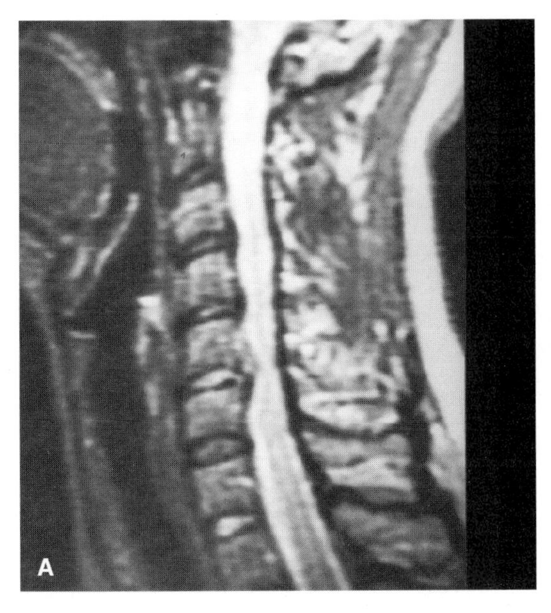

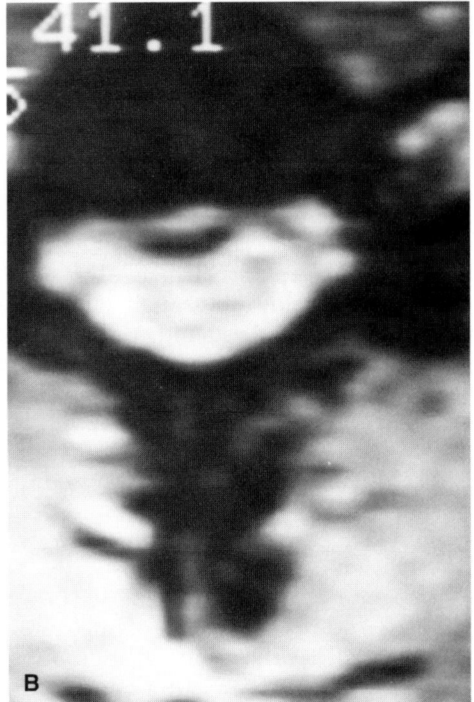

Fig. 37–10. *(A)* **Sagittal MRI shows decreased spinal canal diameter at the lower end.** *(B)* **Axial (transverse) MRI section also shows decreased canal diameter.**

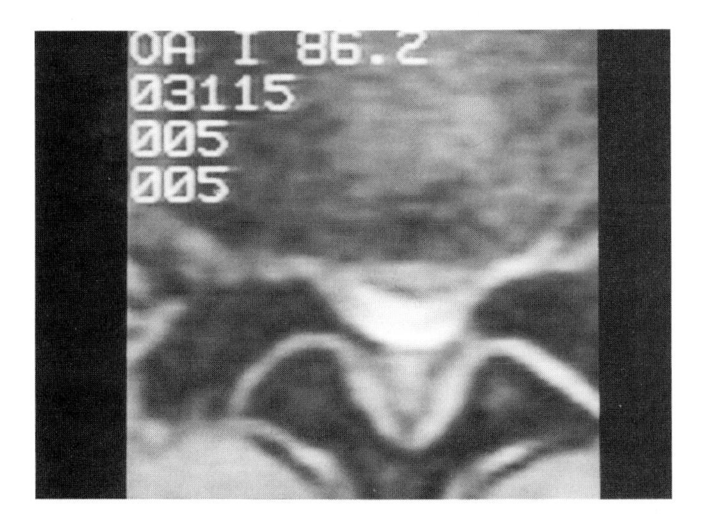

Fig. 37–11. Lumbar MRI showing L4-5 disc herniation centrally and to the left. Note the decreased spinal canal diameter.

steroid injection, but in a young person with clear evidence of lumbar disc herniation and radicular leg pain, it is reasonable practice to give an epidural steroid injection even without an advanced imaging study. Every attempt should be made to supervise the patient through a conservative treatment program for at least 6 weeks. Once the radiating leg pain has become "centralized" a physical therapy regimen should commence that involves conditioning exercises of the flexor muscles of the spine as well as the spinal extensor muscles. Lower extremity stretching and strengthening exercises are usually included in the low back exercise program.

Obviously, certain cases of lumbar disc herniation warrant a much abbreviated course of conservative care. Large disc herniations in high-demand athletes may be treated surgically from the outset because symptoms are likely to continue and the athletic patient may lose an inordinate amount of time in the course of attempting to prolong conservative care.

Surgical Treatment

Surgical treatment for lumbar disc herniations involves unilateral exposure of the spine at the level of disc herniation and a small laminotomy with disc excision. It is often necessary to perform a minimal medial facetectomy to decompress the nerve root completely. There has been considerable discussion about the relative merits of microdiscectomy and of standard laminotomy and disc excision. It is important to understand that the initial description of microdiscectomy involved removal of the ligamentum flavum unilaterally without significant laminotomy or medial facetectomy. This minimally invasive surgical procedure was supposed to have the advantage of a shorter recovery period and less epidural scarring, though these results were never demonstrated in a prospective clinical study. It was later shown that the original microdiscectomy technique often failed because of persistent lateral recessed stenosis in which the nerve root remained entrapped beneath the articular facet. This led to a change in the technique of microdiscectomy. The current technique involves a smaller incision than is usually used in standard laminotomy and disc excision. Laminotomy and medial facetectomy are performed with microscopic magnification, and the disc is then removed. In essence, this is no different from a standard laminotomy. Though the incision may be smaller, no difference has been demonstrated in outcome or recovery time. It is still the standard of care, even in athletes, to perform limited unilateral exposure and laminotomy with disc excision for the surgical treatment of lumbar disc herniation.

Other methods of treating disc herniation have been popular in the past but have very limited indications. These include chymopapain injection into the disc, percutaneous nucleotomy, and, more recently, laser discectomy. All three of these methods tend to accomplish the same objective, removal of a portion of the inner nucleus pulposus with subsequent shrinkage or subsidence of the disc protrusion into the spinal canal. The indications for use of any of these indirect methods involve a contained disc herniation (meaning that the disc is still within the outer annulus fibrosus and has not herniated into a subligamentous or intracanal position) and pain almost entirely in the leg, without a strong component of back pain. Finally, physical findings should demonstrate "classic" disc herniation of dermatomal radicular pain in a patient with a positive straight leg raise. Obviously, if one follows strictly the recommendations for these indirect procedures, only a small number of patients are candidates for such treatment. It is important to realize that a significant number of patients' pain probably will resolve with conservative measures if a disc herniation is contained and not extremely large.

Rehabilitation after surgical treatment of lumbar disc herniation should proceed incrementally, beginning in the immediate postoperative period. For the first 2 weeks postoperatively, the patient is not allowed any strenuous activity. For the second 2 weeks, the patient is allowed to walk for exercise and to engage in most activities of daily living. Beginning 4 weeks after operation, an athletic patient may begin training on a stationary bicycle and perhaps begin to work out on a stair stepper. Most athletic patients are capable of swimming for exercise 4 weeks after surgery. Beginning 6 weeks after surgery, low back–strengthening exercises are begun and the other exercises previously mentioned are increased to involve a more strenuous workout. Running usually is not allowed until the 2- to 3-month point. Contact athletes may return to contact sports at 6 months after operation, although some have returned after only 3 months. It is absolutely essential that an aggressive rehabilitation program, as outlined above, be undertaken by athlete patients, to ensure satisfactory postoperative recovery.

FURTHER READING

Abitbal, J., and Gerfin, S.: Surgical management of cervical disc disease; anterior cervical fusion. Semin. Spine Surg. *1:*233, 1989.

Bell, G.: Diagnosis of lumbar disc disease. Semin. Spine Surg. *1:*8, 1989.

Benjamin, V.: Diagnosis and management of thoracic disc disease. Clin. Neurosurg. *30:*577, 1983.

Bohlman, H. H., and Zdeblick, T. A.: Anterior excision of herniated thoracic discs. J. Bone Joint Surg. *70A:*1038, 1988.

Brinckmann, P.: Injury of the annulus fibrosus and disc protrusions. Spine *11:*149, 1986.

The Cervical Spine Research Society Editorial Committee: The Cervical Spine. 2nd Ed. Philadelphia, J. B. Lippincott, 1989.

Dillin, W. H.: Conservative management of acute back pain and sciatica. Semin. Spine Surg. *1:*18, 1989.

Frymoyer, J. W. (ed.): The Adult Spine: Principles and Practice. New York, Raven Press, 1991.

Macnab, I., and McCulloch, J.: Backache. 2nd Ed. Baltimore, Williams & Wilkins, 1990.

Mochida, J., et al.: Percutaneous nucleotomy in lumbar disc herniation: Patient selection and role in various treatments. Spine *18:*2212, 1993.

Rothman, R. H., and Simeone, F. A. (eds.): The Spine. 3rd Ed. Philadelphia, W. B. Saunders, 1992.

Sakou, T., et al.: Percutaneous discectomy in athletes. Spine *18:*2218, 1993.

Watkins, R. G. (ed.): Lumbar Discectomy and Laminectomy. Rockville, MD, Aspen, 1987.

Weber, H: Lumbar disc herniation: A controlled prospective study with ten years of observation. Spine *8:*131, 1983.

Weinstein, J. N., and Wiesel, S. W. (eds.): The Lumbar Spine. Philadelphia, W. B. Saunders, 1990.

White, A., Rothman, R., and Ray, C.: Lumbar Spine Surgery. St. Louis, C. V. Mosby, 1987.

Whitecloud, T. S., and Dunsker, S. B. (eds.): Anterior Cervical Spine Surgery. New York, Raven Press, 1993.

38 *Thomas A. Boers*

Mechanical Low Back Pain

Back pain is a common malady of athletes in all sports. For many top athletes—Jack Nicklaus, Lee Trevino, Joe Montana, Daryl Strawberry, and Larry Bird to name just a few—back pain has influenced their careers. A wide variety of health care professionals concern themselves with the treatment of lower back pain. The philosophy set forth here is a purely mechanical approach for a purely mechanical problem.

Although back problems are no different in athletes than in the rest of the population, their care can be quite different. The demands to continue sports participation or finish the season and the pressure of "no play, no pay" can put heavy burdens on the athlete and the therapist.

ETIOLOGY

Mechanical low back pain is directly related to the function of the spine and is caused by overload. Causes are divided into several categories based on the structures involved: soft tissue injuries; soft tissue injuries plus joint dysfunction; or soft tissue injuries, joint dysfunction, and positive neurologic findings.

Every joint has limits to the amount of stress load it can handle—at one time and over time. The difference between acute and chronic low back pain is that, in the first, the patient associates the onset of pain with a particular incident. Often, minor trauma or day-to-day activities can instigate acute low back failure. The cause here is the accumulation of events that finally lead to the acute episode. Rarely is one trauma alone responsible for the back failure. The phenomenon is very similar to the way chronic tendinitis can lead to tendon rupture.

The body has the capability to store fatigue stress, especially when there is insufficient time to recuperate. Poor endurance can finally lead to the stress exceeding the tolerance level, resulting in mechanical failure.

The reactions range from muscle and ligament strain or joint dysfunction to a herniated nucleus pulposus. Strained muscles and ligaments can be restored in time with rest and proper exercise. When joint dysfunction occurs, the body protects the motion segment with muscle guarding. This constant protection of the motion segment creates an inflammatory reaction that maintains the arthrokinematic reflex. This reflex is controlled by the nerve supply of the involved facet joints. The reflex can result in massive spasms in the acutely injured low back or in a minimal reaction of the muscles, as in chronic injuries.

Exercises that force motion in the dysfunctional segment can actually aggravate the situation. By restoring the function first and then exercising to maintain it, the dysfunction can be resolved. As long as the arthrokinematic reflex is present, motion is limited, which can limit the athlete's performance.

SACROILIAC JOINT

Biomechanics

Much has been written about the biomechanics of this complicated joint. Biomechanists still have not reached a consensus on where the axis of rotation is located.

The rather immobile sacroiliac joint is located between a fairly mobile lumbar spine and a very mobile hip joint. The function of the sacroiliac joint is related to both areas. The joint acts like a buffer zone that enables forces to be transmitted from the femur to the ilium to the lower back as well as from the lower back to the ilium to the femur. The absorption of forces in the sacroiliac joint reduces the stress on the pelvis. It makes a relatively rigid system more pliable, preventing injuries to the pelvis, but the total amount of motion in the sacroiliac joint is rather limited and practically immeasurable.

The often overlooked symphysis pubis plays a role very similar to that of the sacroiliac joint by enhancing overall pelvic mobility. The sacroiliac joint consists of two poles running in different planes (Fig. 38–1). The purpose of the different planes is to increase the stability of the joint and minimize the function (the small amount of motion in the joint). The function in one pole automatically limits function in the other.

The superior pole stands more vertical and is often shorter than the inferior pole. It runs posterosuperior to anteroinferior. The inferior pole runs from posteroinferior to anterosuperior. The inferior pole is slightly curved, with the concavity facing inferiorly.

There is a distinct relationship between the inferior pole and the hip joint. The outline of the inferior pole echoes the shape of the acetabulum, which lies just inferior and anterior to it.

When the pelvis (i.e., ilium) moves anterior or posterior over the femoral head, the inferior pole, which runs in the same direction, can absorb and reduce forces on the pelvis. The instantaneous axis of rotation of the frontal axis of the sacroiliac joint is in the same plane as the axis of the hip joint.

The superior pole plays a similar corresponding role with the L5–S1 junction. Maximum extension in the lumbar spine opens up the anterior disc space between L5 and S1. The sacrum tilts forward and inferiorly, precisely in the direction of the superior pole (Fig. 38–2). The instantaneous axis of rotation for flexion and extension has to be inferior to the sacroiliac joint. In this manner, maximum flexion and extension of the hip and the lumbar spine are accommodated in the sacroiliac joint while a high degree of stability is maintained.

The minor motion in the sacroiliac joint is critical to adequate functioning of the kinematic chain consisting of the lumbar spine, sacroiliac joint, and hip joint. Dysfunction, meaning limited joint function, of the sacroiliac joint automatically involves the hip and lumbar spine. This can explain the diversity of symptoms seen with sacroiliac joint dysfunction. Isolated joint dysfunc-

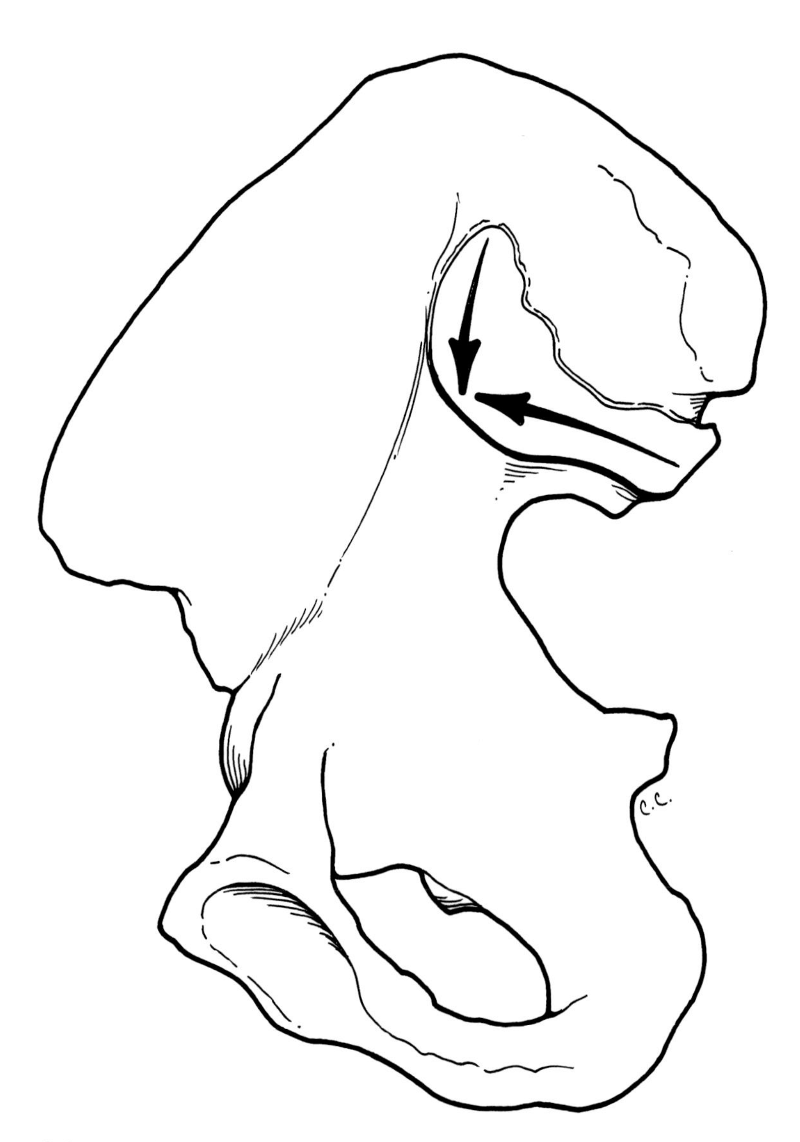

Fig. 38–1. **Medial view of the right ilium shows the superior and inferior poles of the sacroiliac joint** ***(arrows).***

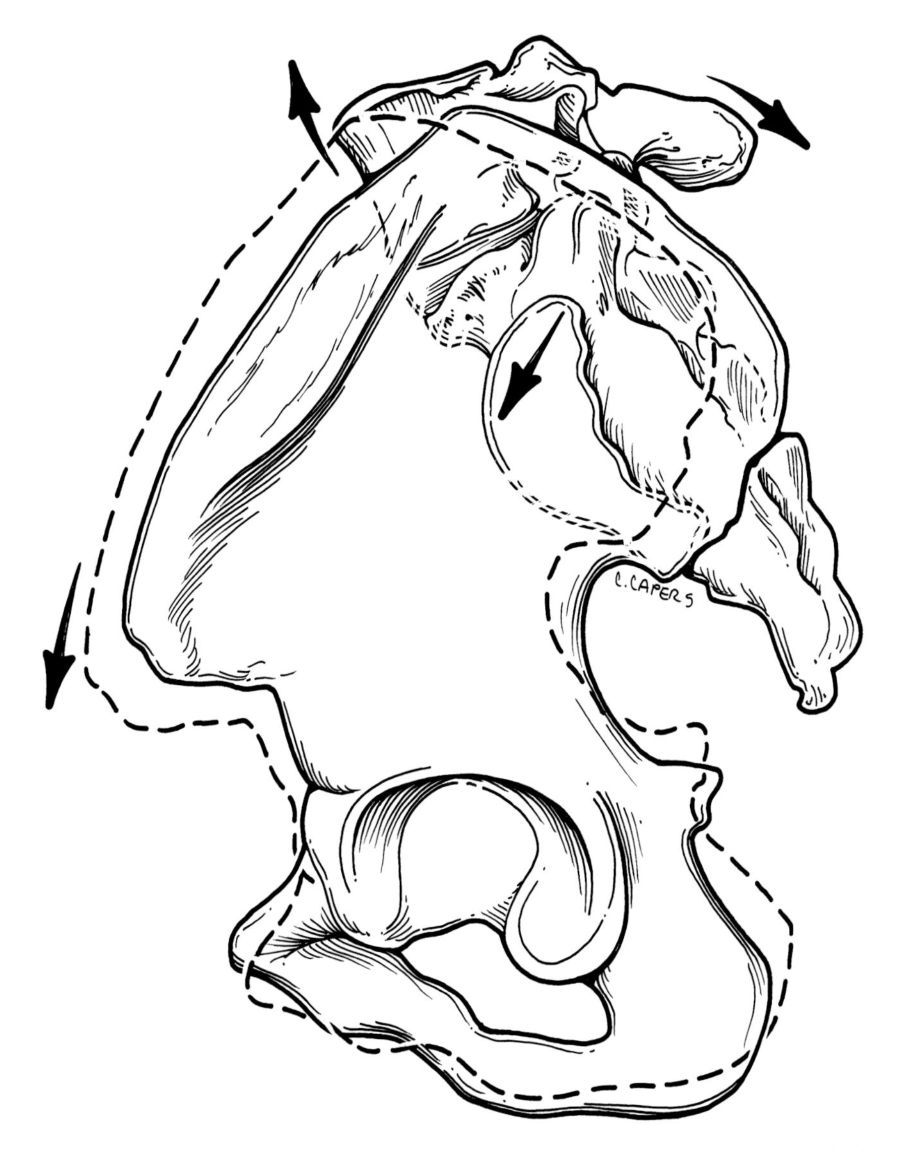

Fig. 38–2. Lateral view of the left ilium shows the movement of the sacrum during extension of the lumbar spine. The sacrum tilts forward and inferior in the same plane as the superior pole.

tion in the sacroiliac joint is therefore unlikely. The joint is not capable of functioning on its own because of lack of direct muscle activity on the sacroiliac joint.

The arthrokinematic reflex is the key means of recognizing sacroiliac joint dysfunction. Measuring joint function clinically is impossible, because the motions are so small. A normal amount of asymmetry is also present in the pelvis, which makes matters even more complicated. The position of the pelvis certainly does not indicate by itself whether sacroiliac joint dysfunction is present. Function and position, by definition, are not related.

Clinical Evaluation

The sacroiliac joint is evaluated with the patient in three positions: standing, sitting, and supine. The evaluation should indicate which sacroiliac joint is dysfunctional and in which direction.

STANDING EVALUATION: THE LATERAL SIDE BENDING TEST (FIG. 38–3).

This test gives a global look at the function between lumbar spine, sacroiliac joint, and hip joint in a fully loaded position. The test is performed with the patient standing with the feet side by side. The patient is asked to bend to each side. During lateral bending to the right side, the right posterior iliac spine should move to the left and up. This prevents the center of gravity from falling outside the patient's support base. With dysfunction in the lumbar spine or sacroiliac joint this shift does not occur.

SUPINE EVALUATION: THE ROTATION TEST AND THE ROTATION STRESS TEST

The rotation test indicates if sacroiliac joint dysfunction is present and which side is involved. The hip joint is used to elicit motion in the sacroiliac joint. If sacroil-

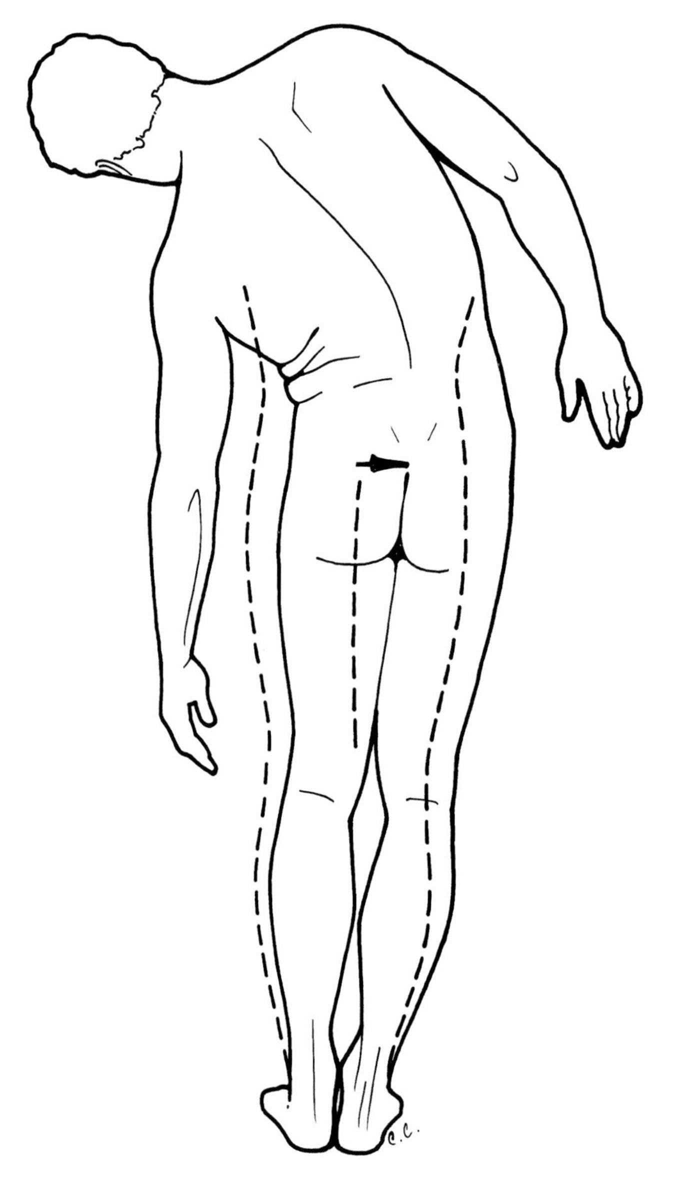

Fig. 38–3. Lateral side bending test. The arrow shows the lateral and upward movement of the iliac spine as the patient bends to the side.

iac dysfunction is present, a positive arthrokinematic reflex should be noted on the side of the dysfunction. There should be increased resistance against maximum rotation of the hip. Note that asymmetric antetorsion of the hip needs to be excluded because this can give a false impression of increased resistance against external rotation of the hip.

In the rotation stress test (Fig. 38–4), the examiner lifts the patient's leg by the ankle and externally rotates the femur until a closed packed position (natural limit of rotation) has been reached. The examiner then forces the femur past the closed packed position and external rotation is continued so that the ilium also externally rotates. During the external rotation of the ilium, it also tilts caudally. The ilium actually moves laterally during this maneuver and causes the leg to appear longer when returned to the neutral position. This apparent lengthening is not seen when the sacroiliac joint is dysfunctional because motion is prevented by the arthrokinematic reflex. The rotation stress test does not measure movement in the sacroiliac joint itself but tests the ability of the pelvis to move, indicating normal function of the sacroiliac joint.

The rotation stress test is also performed with internal rotation. In this test, shortening of the leg is noted in a normally functioning sacroiliac joint and is absent with dysfunction on that side.

SITTING EVALUATION

Knowing the side of the dysfunction does not indicate its direction. The main directions to test are flexion and extension. In a normally functioning pelvis, both ilia move anteriorly and craniad with extension of the lumbar spine and pelvis. They tilt posteriorly and caudad with flexion. The direction of the dysfunction reveals itself by an increased asymmetric position of the pelvis in the closed packed position as compared with the middle position (Fig. 38–5).

The correction of the dysfunction depends on the following factors: side of dysfunction (determined by rotation stress test), direction of dysfunction (determined by sitting maximum extension/flexion test), asymmetric position of the pelvis, and type of dysfunction:

I. Right sacroiliac dysfunction as indicated by failure of the right ilium to extend. Findings of rotation stress test are positive. Extension dysfunction is shown by increased asymmetry in extension in the sitting position. The left ilium appears more anterior and craniad as compared with the right ilium.

II. Right sacroiliac dysfunction as indicated by the sacrum not extending on the right side. Results of the rotation stress test are positive. Extension dysfunction is seen with increased asymmetry in extension in the sitting position. The left ilium appears posterior and caudad as compared with the right one.

III. Flexion of the right sacrum is limited. Right sacroiliac joint dysfunction is shown by a positive rotation stress test. Flexion dysfunction is seen with increased asymmetric position in flexion in the sitting position. The left ilium appears anterior and craniad as compared with the right one.

IV. Flexion of the right ilium is limited. Right sacroiliac joint dysfunction is shown by a positive rotation stress test. Flexion dysfunction is seen with increased asymmetric position in flexion in the sitting position. The left ilium is posterior and caudad as compared with the right one.

Specific Manipulation

The treatment of the dysfunction is a logical consequence of the limitation. The ilium or sacrum is moved

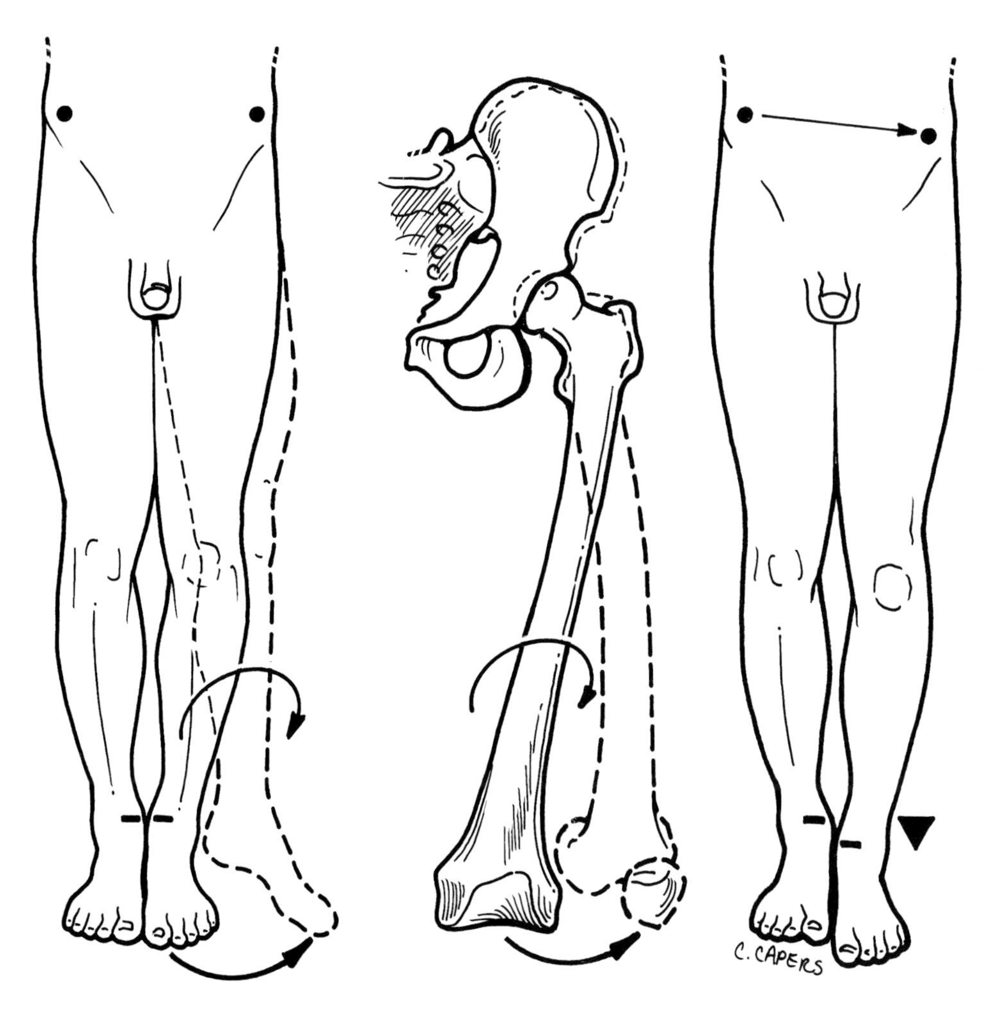

Fig. 38–4. The rotation stress test demonstrates the movement of the ilium during external rotation in the closed packed position (center). Movement in the sacroiliac joint causes the leg to appear longer.

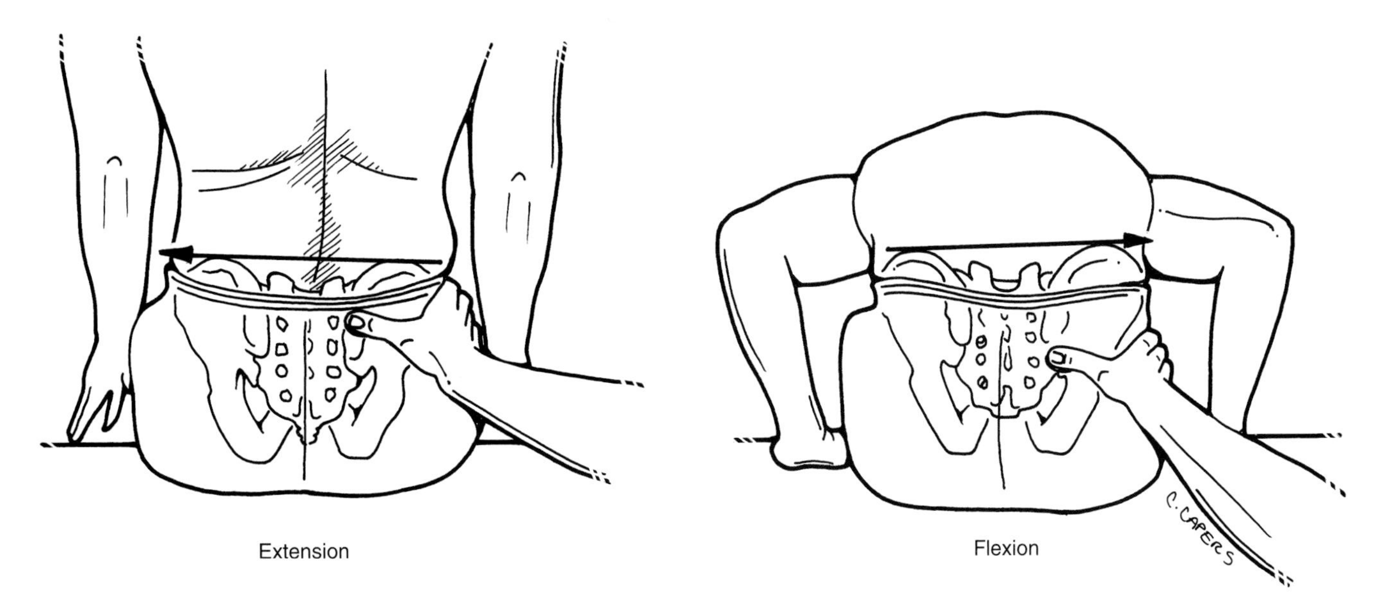

Fig. 38–5. The examiner feels the position of the ilium in the neutral and flexed position. Asymmetry in the closed packed position (flexion) reveals the direction of the dysfunction.

in the direction in which the arthrokinematic reflex is protecting the joint(s). Results should be immediate after the specific manipulation. There should be normal lengthening and shortening with the rotation stress test.

SPECIFIC POINTS ON MANIPULATION

1. Physiologic function always occurs with both participating parts of the joint. Imitating the normal physiologic motion causes the least unnecessary stress to the joint, facilitating the specific manipulation.
2. To overcome the arthrokinematic reflex, a gentle specifically directed force in a maximum relaxed position is used. A high-velocity manipulation has the tendency to make the patient protect the dysfunctional joint even more, resulting in soft tissue overstretching. When the joint can move into the fully closed packed position, the arthrokinematic reflex disappears.
3. Physiologic function always occurs under compression of the muscles that cross the joint. The therapist applies compression to the joint to increase synovial fluid output, thus lubricating the joint.
4. Traction has the opposite effect of compression. It also puts more unnecessary tension on the soft tissues involved in joint dysfunction.

Postmanipulation Protocol

Restoring joint function itself is only a small part of total recovery. After restoration of joint function is indicated by absence of the arthrokinematic reflex, the patient must maintain the restored function. Specific exercises are prescribed for this. It should be noted that the inflammatory reaction that accompanies the dysfunction does not change immediately after the specific manipulation. It may take several days for joints to adjust. It is important, particularly during the early phase, that the function is maintained without overloading the joint. The patient needs to avoid prolonged static positioning.

The postmanipulation protocol may last approximately a week, after which cardiovascular exercises are added to the program. A full reconditioning program is instituted after the joint or joints have remained loose 2 weeks. The reconditioning program includes continued flexibility, strengthening, and cardiovascular exercises. The main emphasis is on regaining maximum cardiovascular output.

THE LUMBAR SPINE

Evaluation

Normal function of the lumbar spine is characterized by maximum motion within the facet joints, appropriate muscle flexibility and strength, and sufficient cardiovascular strength to maintain the function over the necessary period of time.

Kinesiology

The lumbar facet joints work within a kinematic chain; movement in one facet automatically triggers motion in the others in the kinematic chain. The facet joints do not act independently but are part of a sequence; thus, dysfunction in one part disturbs the whole sequence. It is the overall movement that is limited, not just a particular facet joint. In this manner, peripheral joint dysfunction can differ from true spinal dysfunction. The segmental facet motion depends on several factors. The position of the articular process determines in which plane the motion takes place. The amount of segmental motion depends on the combination of left and right facet joints.

L5-S1 Articulation

The position of the facet joint differs from level to level and from person to person. In general, the articular process of the L5-S1 junction stands in a more frontal plane than the levels above. This allows for more rotation, but at the cost of decreased lateral flexion. The flexion-extension ratio between L5-S1 and L4-5 is similar.

L4-5 Articulation

The L4-5 junction has an articular process just like the levels above but in a more sagittal orientation. This results in less rotation but a somewhat better ratio for lateral flexion. The stability of the lumbosacral articulation is enhanced because L5-S1 is capable of more rotation and L4-5 of more lateral flexion. This intrinsic stability means that there is less need for muscular stabilization than if each segment had motion potential in all three planes.

The stability of the bottom two levels is also controlled by the orientation of the iliolumbar ligaments. The two lower vertebrae are directly connected to the sacrum by the iliolumbar ligaments. The upper part passes from the transverse process of L4 caudolateral and dorsal to the sacral crest. The lower part originates from the lower part of the transverse process of L5 and passes caudal and lateral to the iliac crest anterior and medial to the upper part.

The middle and upper lumbar facet joints are positioned in a predominantly sagittal plane. This alone allows for small articular movements, mainly in flexion and extension, and to a lesser degree in lateral bending and rotation.

The muscles of the lumbar spine act in groups, rather than in an isolated fashion. The muscles act on several segments at a time. The innervation is also regulated on

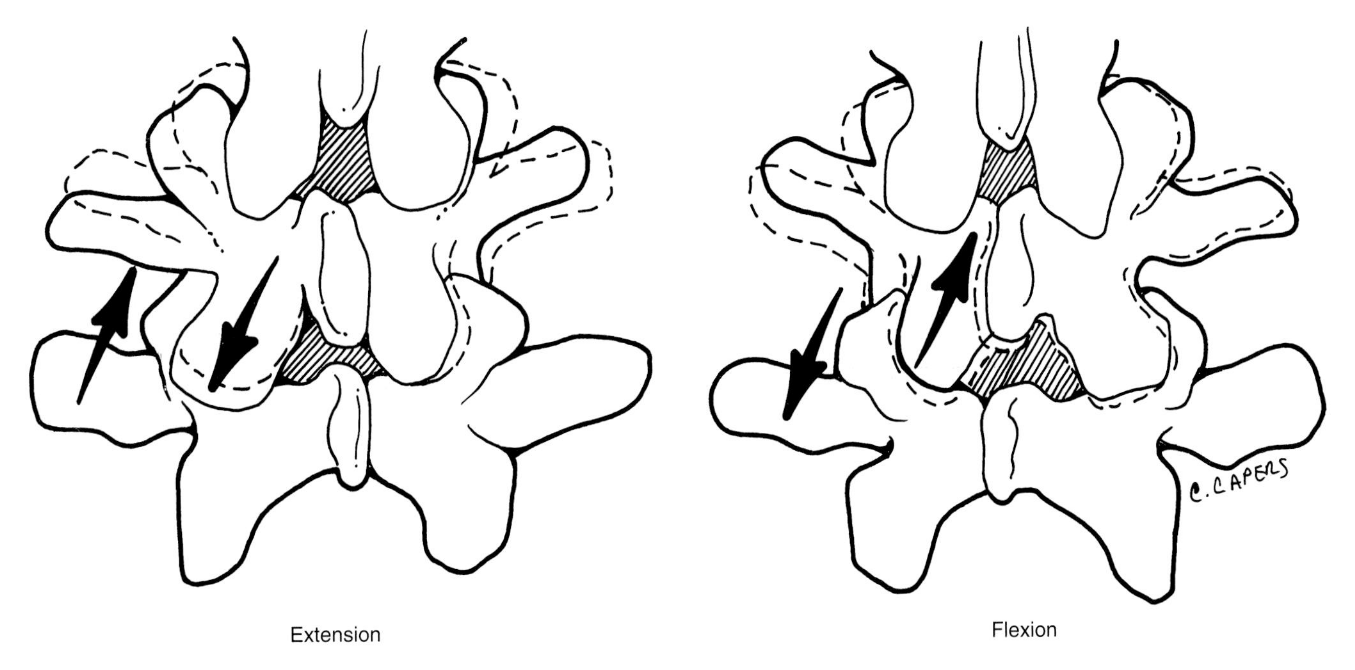

Fig. 38–6. Each segment in the lumbar spine is tested in full extension and flexion.

a segmental basis. The muscles are innervated by the same nerves that innervate the facet joint they act upon.

Examination

Joint dysfunction in the lumbar spine occurs by overloading of the facet joints. The lumbar spine is examined on a segmental basis. This can cause many difficulties because of (1) the lack of consistency between segments and (2) individual variability. Averages of degree per segment are known but are little help on an individual level. Therefore, each segment is brought into its closed packed position in flexion and in extension. The examiner palpates for the arthrokinematic reflex by overpressing (gently pushing the joint in a closed packed position) each segmental level. The examination is performed with the patient seated because loading the lumbar spine facilitates the arthrokinematic reflex. Each segment is palpated over the facet area. In extension, the superior articular process is pushed anterior in relation to the inferior articular process of the vertebra above. By overpressing in the anterior direction, a closed packed position is either reached or is prevented by a muscle response. In flexion, the superior articular process is brought posterior and the inferior articular process of the vertebra above is brought anterior (Fig. 38–6). It is important to avoid maximal lengthening of the muscles during this facet testing.

The examiner checks joint dysfunction in flexion and in extension on the right and on the left facet joint. Dysfunction can occur at any location or a combination of sites.

Treatment

A specific manipulation is used to restore the maximum function of the facet joint. After the manipulation, the function of the segment is restored, and it should be possible to load it in the closed packed position. During the manipulation, the articular processes involved are brought into the restricted direction until the closed packed position has been reached. The patient is treated lying on the side. The force used is gentle and it is applied only on the involved vertebrae; no lever arms are used. The gentle manipulating force also prevents additional tightening of the muscles. The specific manipulation is three dimensional, following the articular surfaces of the joint. During the manipulation, compression is applied to stimulate synovial output because the distraction forces "dry out" the articular surface. It also unnecessarily tightens the joint capsule and ligaments. All segments involved are treated.

The postmanipulation protocol involves the same components as for sacroiliac joint manipulation. The patient begins with exercises to maintain function and gradually adds general flexibility and strengthening exercises. Finally, the reconditioning phase starts.

39 *George M. McCluskey III*

Functional Anatomy of the Shoulder

The anatomy and biomechanics of the shoulder girdle are complex and ill-defined. Functionally, the shoulder is composed of four joints: acromioclavicular, sternoclavicular, glenohumeral, and scapulothoracic. Each has individual functions, but they work together to provide the strength and stability required of the shoulder.

BONES

Scapula

The scapula is a thin, triangular bone that has several prominent bony processes and thickened areas that serve as muscle attachment sites and provide an opposing articular surface for the humeral head. The glenoid, acromion, coracoid, spine of the scapula, and lateral border of the scapula compose the bulk of the weight of the scapula.

The scapula is oriented 30° anteriorly on the posterior chest wall. The anterior surface of the scapula, the shallow, concave subscapular fossa, serves as the origin for the subscapularis muscle (Fig. 39–1). The posterior, or dorsal, scapula is divided into two areas by the scapular spine, a horizontal projection of bone that extends from the medial scapular border to the glenoid neck. The posterior and superior continuation of the lateral scapular spine is called the *acromion.*

Above the prominent scapular spine is the supraspinatus fossa, which houses the supraspinatus muscle. The suprascapular notch, located just medial to the base of the coracoid on the superior aspect of the scapula, is an indentation of the bone. The transverse scapular ligament forms the roof of this notch, above which lies the suprascapular artery and below which runs the suprascapular nerve.

Below the spine of the scapula, the infraspinatus fossa houses the infraspinatus muscle. The thickened lateral scapular border serves as the attachment site for the teres minor and the long head of the triceps brachii.

The acromion is a continuation of the scapular spine that has no direct attachment to the body of the scapula. It serves as the roof of the coracoacromial arch and as an attachment site for the coracoacromial ligament anteriorly and for the deltoid and trapezius muscles posteriorly and laterally. Developmentally, the acromion has two centers of ossification that generally unite by age 21 years. Persistence of the epiphyseal line occurs in 3% of persons and has been implicated in the impingement syndrome.

The coracoid process is a thick projection of bone forward and laterad from the scapular neck. It serves as an attachment for the coracoclavicular, coracohumeral, and coracoacromial ligaments. The coracobrachialis and short head of the biceps brachii originate from the anterior coracoid tip, and the pectoralis minor inserts along the medial coracoid process.

The glenoid neck and cavity comprise the lateral angle of the scapula. The articular surface of the glenoid is oriented in 5° to 8° retroversion with respect to the scapula. The shallow glenoid is slightly concave and is deepened minimally by the surrounding glenoid labrum. It articulates with the humeral head, forming the glenohumeral joint.

Clavicle

The clavicle is located between the sternum and the acromion. Functionally, it suspends or connects the upper extremity to the axial skeleton and serves as an important attachment site for the deltoid, trapezius, pectoralis major, and sternocleidomastoid muscles. The clavicle is S shaped, like a crankshaft. The medial two thirds is triangular with anterior convexity, and the posterior third is flat and convex in the posterior direction.

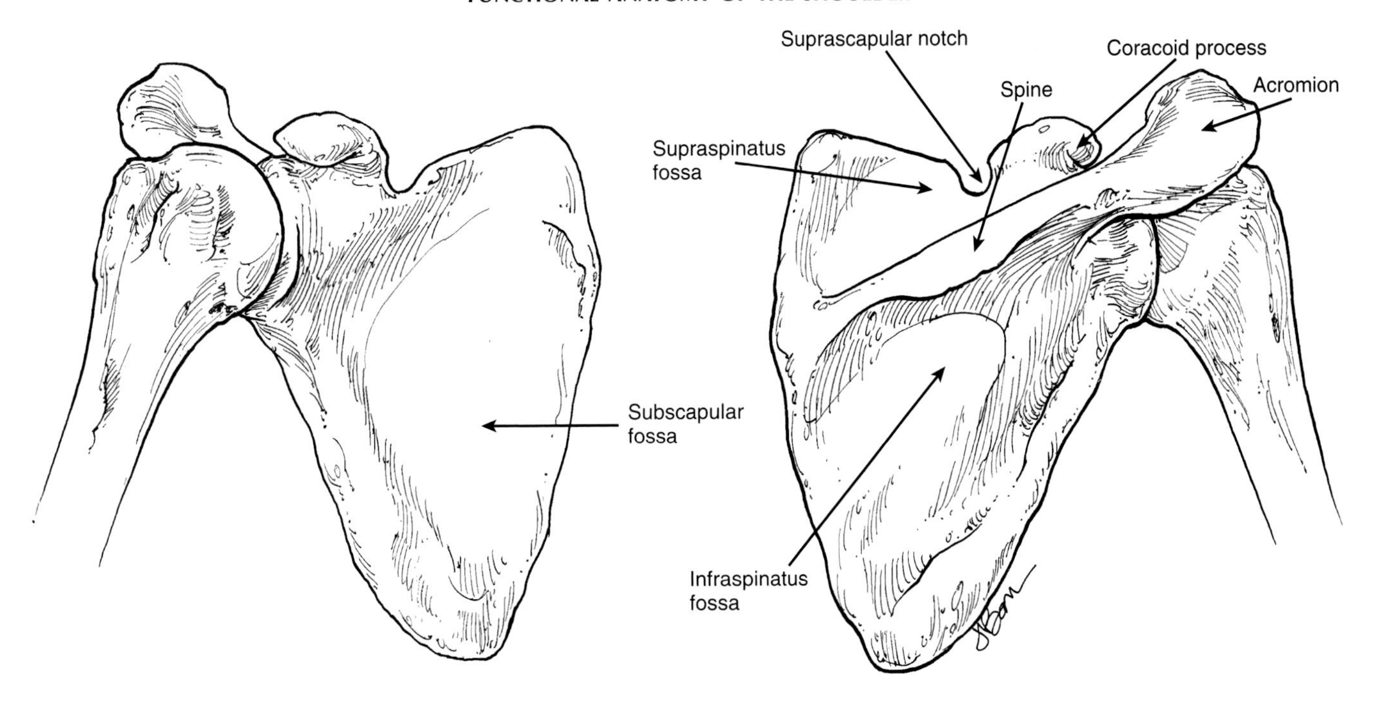

Fig. 39–1. ***(A)*** **Anterior and** ***(B)*** **posterior views of the scapula and the proximal humerus.**

The medial end of the clavicle is a portion of the sternoclavicular joint. It has close anatomic relationships with the first cervical rib, the subclavian artery, and the subclavian vein. The middle third of the clavicle, related anatomically to the axillary artery and the brachial plexus, is the most common site of clavicle fractures. The lateral third of the clavicle, articulating with the acromion, makes the acromioclavicular joint. The clavicle is the first bone in the body to ossify. Its medial end is usually the last epiphysis to close, at or about age 25 years.

Proximal Humerus

The proximal third of the humerus comprises the humeral head, the greater and lesser tuberosities, and the bicipital groove. The humeral head articulates with the glenoid cavity of the scapula and is retroverted 30° to 35° in relation to the humeral shaft. The anatomic neck of the humerus, which lies just below the inferior articular surface of the humeral head, serves as the attachment site for the glenohumeral joint capsule. The greater tuberosity projects laterally with the supraspinatus, infraspinatus, and teres minor muscles inserting into well-defined facets on the greater tuberosity. The lesser tuberosity lies below the anterior aspect of the anatomic neck and receives insertions from the subscapularis muscle and the anterior capsular ligamentous complex.

The bicipital or intertubercular groove is an anterior sulcus in the proximal humerus just lateral to the midline in which the long head of the biceps tendon rests. It separates the greater and lesser tuberosities and serves as an attachment site for the latissimus dorsi, pectoralis major, and teres major. Proximally, the transverse humeral ligament forms the roof of the bicipital groove at the tuberosity level and demarcates the intra-articular and extra-articular portions of the biceps tendon. The surgical neck of the humerus, the area of the proximal humerus just below the greater and lesser tuberosities, is often a site of fracture.

MUSCLES

Deltoid Muscle

The deltoid muscle is a triangular muscle that gives the tip of the shoulder its rounded appearance. It is divided into anterior, middle, and posterior thirds; the function of each portion depends on its anatomic location (Fig. 39–2). The anterior third of the deltoid originates from the lateral third of the clavicle and assists in flexing the arm in the plane of the scapula and in internal rotation. The middle portion of the deltoid originates from the lateral acromion and is involved in elevation of the arm in any plane. The posterior third arises from the scapular spine and is involved in posterior elevation and external rotation of the arm. The deltoid muscle is the primary abductor of the arm, particularly above 90° elevation.

The deltoid muscle is innervated by the axillary nerve and receives its blood supply principally from the posterior humeral circumflex artery. The axillary nerve and posterior humeral circumflex artery both exit the quadrangular space posteriorly, in the interval between teres

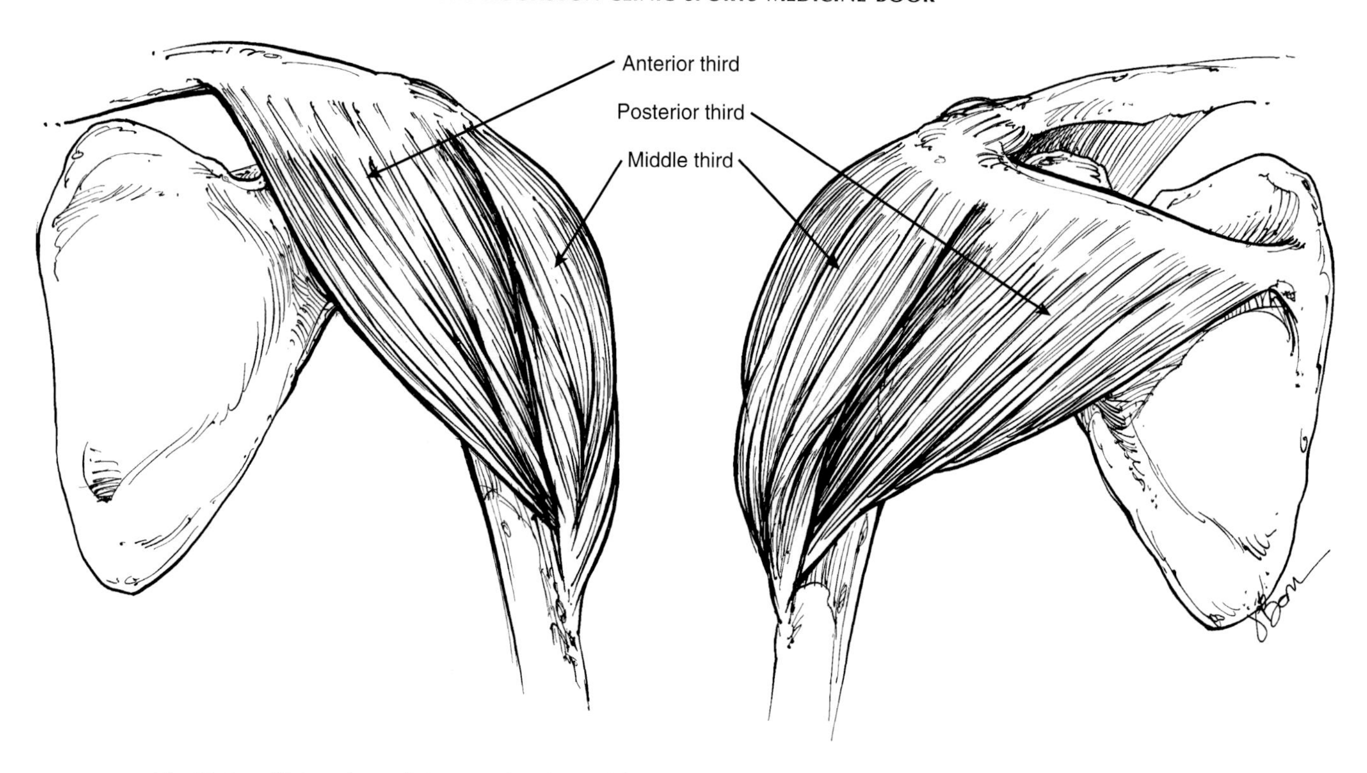

Fig. 39–2. *(A)* Anterior and *(B)* posterior views of the shoulder demonstrate the middle and posterior portions of the deltoid muscle.

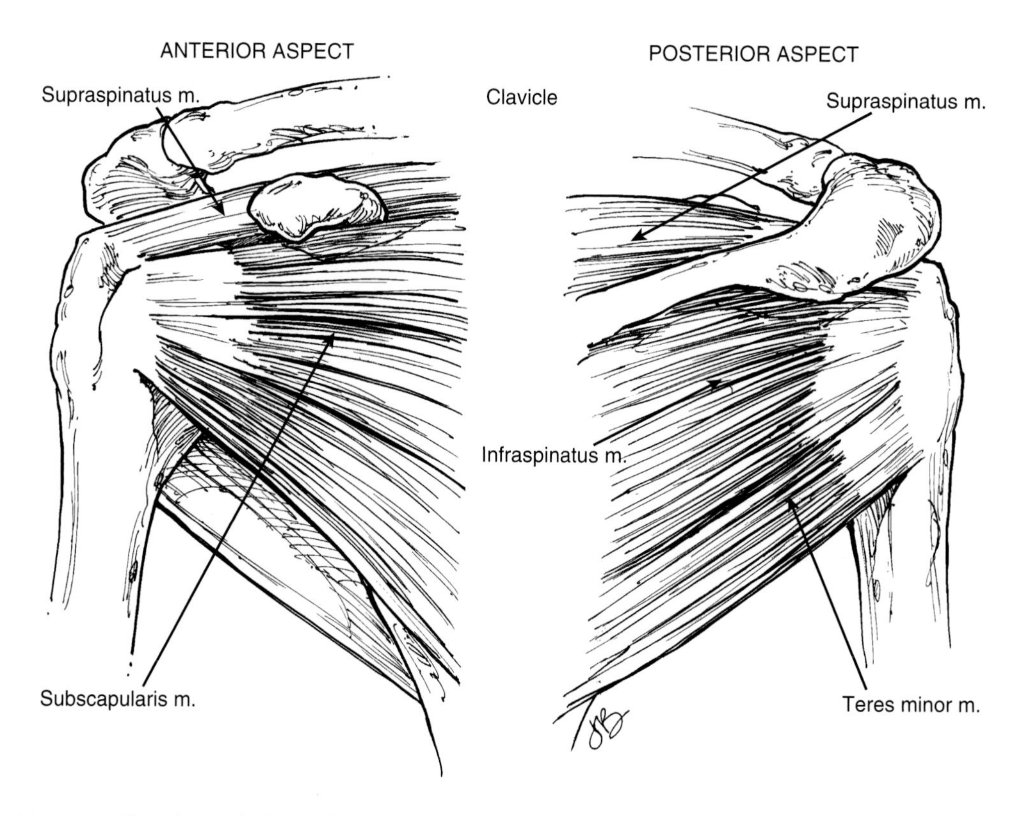

Fig. 39–3. *(A)* The subscapularis muscle originates from the subscapularis fossa on the scapula and inserts into the lesser tuberosity. The supraspinatus lies above the humeral head, inserting into the greater tuberosity. The rotator interval is between the anterior portion of the supraspinatus and the superior portion of the subscapularis. *(B)* The external rotators: The infraspinatus arises below the scapular spine in the infraspinatus fossa and inserts into the posterior facet of the greater tuberosity. The teres minor inserts below the infraspinatus on the greater tuberosity.

minor, teres major, long head of the triceps, and humeral shaft.

Rotator Cuff

The rotator cuff includes the supraspinatus, infraspinatus, teres minor, and subscapularis muscles. These muscles have individual and collective functions (Fig. 39–3). The rotator cuff acts in synchrony to provide optimal function and movement of the shoulder joint. The supraspinatus originates from the supraspinatus fossa on the scapula and inserts on the superior facet of the greater tuberosity. The infraspinatus muscle arises from the infraspinatus fossa on the scapula and inserts on the middle facet of the greater tuberosity posteriorly. The supraspinatus and infraspinatus are innervated by the suprascapular nerve. The teres minor arises from the lateral border of the scapula and inserts posteriorly into the inferior facet of the greater tuberosity. The teres minor is an important landmark for approaches to the posterior shoulder girdle because of its anatomic relationship to the quadrangular space, through which the axillary nerve and posterior circumflex artery run. The teres minor is supplied by the posterior branch of the axillary nerve. The subscapularis arises from the anterior or deep surface of the scapula in the subscapularis fossa and inserts into the lesser tuberosity of the humerus. Some fibers of the subscapularis blend with the anterior capsule as it inserts into the tuberosity. The subscapularis muscle is supplied by the upper and lower subscapular nerves.

The rotator cuff provides dynamic stability to the glenohumeral joint against subluxation or dislocation tendencies of the humeral head on the glenoid. The supraspinatus acts in concert with the long head of the biceps tendon to provide an important humeral head–depressing action that helps to prevent superior migration of the humeral head during abduction (Fig. 39–4). The supraspinatus helps to steer the humeral head into the glenoid, providing a fulcrum by which the deltoid can elevate the arm. The subscapularis, an important anterior stabilizer of the shoulder, acts in concert with other important anterior shoulder girdle muscles. The infraspinatus and teres minor provide most of the posterior stability to the shoulder. The supraspinatus and middle deltoid provide stability against inferior subluxation of the humeral head along with the triceps, biceps, and coracobrachialis.

The rotator cuff is essential in providing active movement and strength to the glenohumeral joint. The infraspinatus and teres minor provide external rotation and extension for the shoulder. The infraspinatus provides 90% of external rotation strength. The subscapularis rotates internally and adducts the humerus. The supraspinatus assists the deltoid in abduction of the arm.

The *rotator interval* is the area between the anterior border of the supraspinatus and the superior border of the subscapularis, which is covered by a thin, fibrous tissue.[1] The long head of the biceps tendon and the cora-

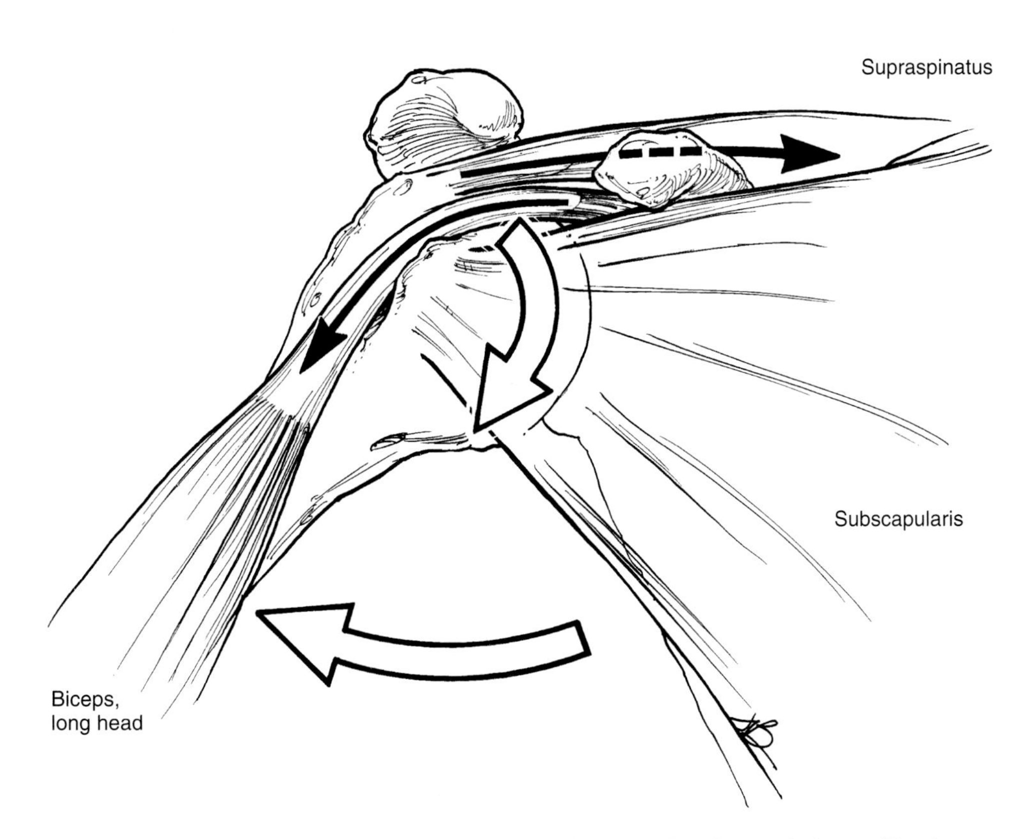

Fig. 39–4. The supraspinatus and long head of the biceps work to depress the humeral head.

cohumeral ligament lie under this thin tissue, in the rotator interval. This interval is an important entry point into the glenohumeral joint for some intra-articular procedures. Release of the rotator interval is important in rotator cuff surgery, as the retracted supraspinatus tendon is often scarred. Release of the rotator interval, including the coracohumeral ligament, is also important for mobilization of the retracted supraspinatus muscle and tendon.

Pectoralis Major

The pectoralis major, a large muscle that covers most of the anterior thorax, has several points of origin. The clavicular portion arises from the medial clavicle. The sternocostal portion of the pectoralis major originates from the costal border of the sternum and its associated ribs. These two principal portions insert along the lateral border of the bicipital groove as a broad tendon.

The principal functions of the pectoralis major are adduction and internal rotation of the proximal humerus. It also participates in flexion (upper fibers) and extension of the arm (inferior fibers). The pectoralis major is innervated by the lateral and medial pectoral nerves. The main blood supply to the pectoralis major comes from a branch of the thoracoacromial artery.

Biceps Brachii

The biceps brachii, an important muscle that acts on the shoulder and elbow, has a long head and a short head. The long head of the biceps tendon arises intra-articularly from the supraglenoid tubercle at the superior aspect of the glenoid. This "long-head biceps tendon" then exits the glenohumeral joint and runs down the proximal humerus in the bicipital groove.

The short head of the biceps tendon arises from the tip of the coracoid process. The common distal biceps tendon inserts into the bicipital tubercle on the radius and into the lacertus fibrosus on the anteromedial aspect of the elbow. The chief functions of the biceps are flexion and supination, principally at the elbow. The long head of the biceps tendon functions as a humeral head depressor, along with the rotator cuff. The innervation to the biceps brachii is the musculocutaneous nerve.

Trapezius Muscle

The trapezius muscle is a superficial, large, fan-shaped muscle in the posterior shoulder girdle and neck region. The trapezius has a long origin, from the superior nuchal line of the occipital portion of the skull down to the inferior thoracic vertebral spinous processes. The upper third of the trapezius inserts on the distal third of the clavicle; the middle third, into the acromion and the scapular spine; and, the lower third, into the medial aspect of the scapular spine. Collectively, these muscles function to suspend and retract the scapula. Other important functions of the trapezius include elevation of the lateral angle of the scapula, which is particularly important during abduction of the arm.

The trapezius is innervated by the eleventh cranial nerve (the accessory nerve) and by branches of the ventral rami of the third and fourth cervical nerves. The principal arterial blood supply to the trapezius includes the transverse cervical artery and the dorsal scapular artery.

Serratus Anterior

The serratus anterior is a scapular stabilizing muscle that originates from the anterolateral aspect of the upper eight ribs. Its muscle fibers run posteriorly, to insert along the costal surface of the scapula at its medial vertebral border and at the inferior angle of the scapula. The principal function of the serratus anterior is to protract the scapula, particularly at the inferior angle. This allows the scapula to rotate upward during abduction.

The serratus anterior is supplied by the long thoracic nerve, a structure that is particularly vulnerable (1) during surgical procedures about the thorax such as radical mastectomy, (2) to infections, and (3) to some injuries to the upper extremity.

Rhomboids

The rhomboid minor and -major are scapula-stabilizing muscles. The rhomboid minor originates from the spinous processes of the seventh cervical and first thoracic vertebrae. It inserts along the medial border of the scapula at the base of the scapular spine. The rhomboid major arises from the spinous processes of vertebrae T2 through T5. It inserts along the medial border of the scapula from the base of the spine to the inferior angle. The interval between these two muscles is often difficult to delineate. The principal function of the rhomboid muscles is to retract and elevate the scapula. The primary innervation to the rhomboids is the dorsal scapular nerve.

Levator Scapulae

The levator scapulae muscle is a scapular stabilizer that originates from the transverse processes of the first through the fourth cervical vertebrae and inserts along the superior medial angle of the scapula. The principal function of this muscle is to elevate the superior angle of the scapula, allowing upward rotation of the bone. The levator scapulae is innervated by the dorsal scapular nerve and by branches from the cervical plexus.

Latissimus Dorsi

The latissimus dorsi covers a large portion of the back. It arises from the spinous processes of the sixth through the twelfth thoracic vertebrae and from the spinous processes of the lumbar vertebrae and from the inferior three ribs. The latissimus dorsi spirals around the teres major muscle and inserts along the medial wall and floor of the bicipital groove of the humerus, along with the teres major tendon.

The principal functions of the latissimus dorsi are adduction and internal rotation of the arm. It also assists in extension of the arm. Its innervation comes via the thoracodorsal nerve.

CORACOACROMIAL ARCH

The coracoacromial arch is the area above the supraspinatus and infraspinatus tendons. Its boundaries include the acromion, the coracoacromial ligament, the acromioclavicular joint, and the coracoid process. The floor of this arch contains the subacromial bursa, which lies just above the supraspinatus tendon. Certain anatomic and mechanical variations in the coracoacromial arch have been implicated in outlet impingement, as described by Neer. Any structure that compromises the space in this coracoacromial arch may lead to degeneration of the supraspinatus tendon and the creation of a rotator cuff tear.

STERNOCLAVICULAR JOINT

The sternoclavicular joint is a diarthrodial synovial joint that connects the medial end of the clavicle to the manubrium and to the cartilage of the first rib. The joint is divided into two compartments by an intra-articular disc and is surrounded by a strong, fibrous joint capsule that is reinforced by a series of strong ligaments (Fig. 39–5). The anterior and posterior sternoclavicular ligaments provide the most stability to this joint, particularly in the posterior direction. The interclavicular ligament provides superior stability, running from one sternoclavicular joint to the other across the top of the sternum, to which it also attaches. The costoclavicular ligaments connect the cartilage of the first rib to the undersurface of the medial clavicle and resist lateral and medial displacement and forward rotation of the clavicle on the thorax.

Important structures situated posterior to the sternoclavicular joint include the trachea, the esophagus, and major vessels at the base of the neck. These structures make posterior dislocation of this joint and surgical procedures here dangerous. The sternoclavicular joint is the only joint that connects the arm to the body.

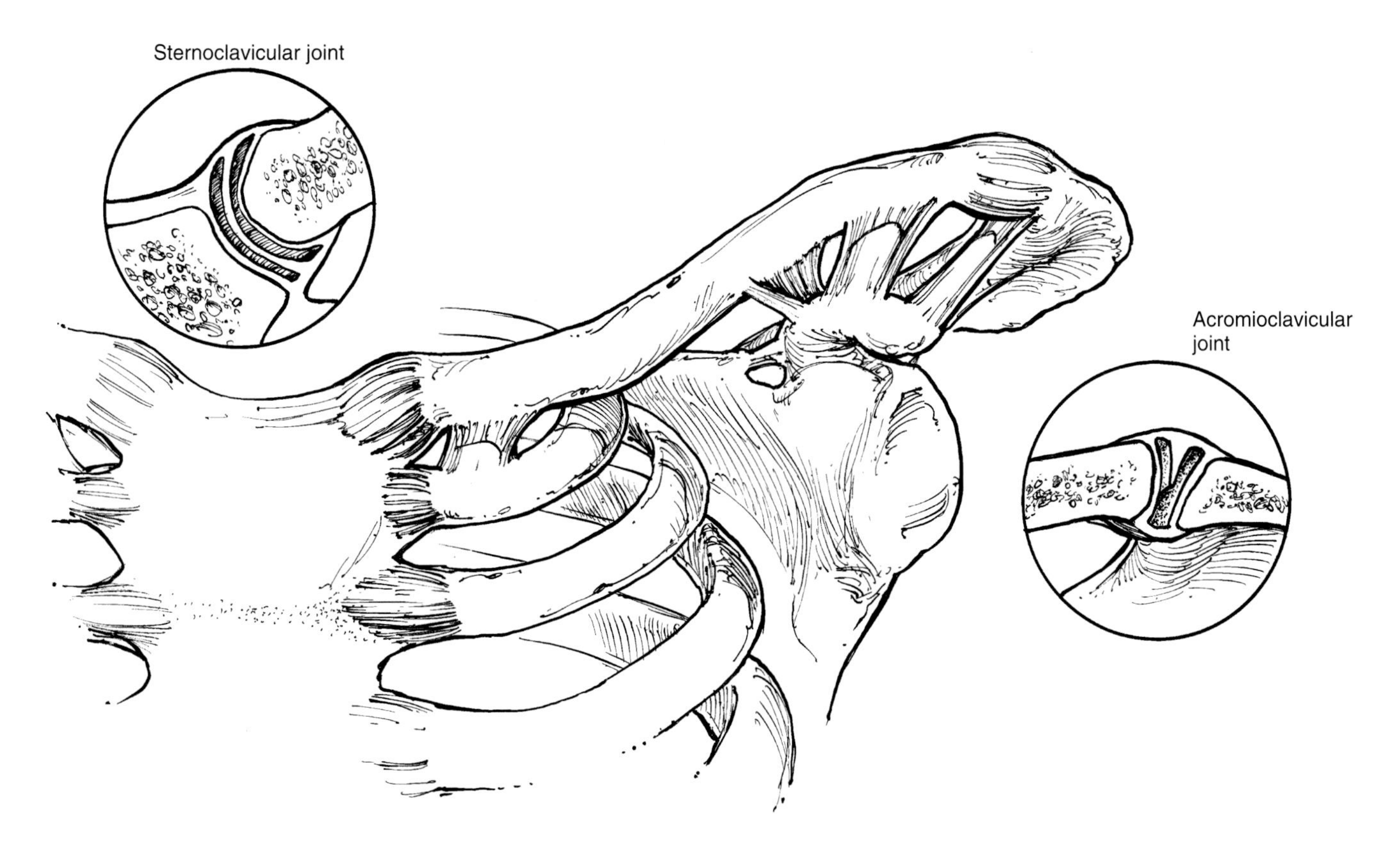

Fig. 39–5. The sternoclavicular joint is divided into two compartments by an intra-articular disc and is surrounded by a strong, fibrous capsule with supporting ligaments. The acromioclavicular joint is stabilized by coracoclavicular ligaments and by a strong fibrous capsule and supporting acromioclavicular ligaments. An intra-articular disc is sometimes present.

Significant rotation occurs at the sternoclavicular joint: the clavicle rotates upward approximately 40° during the first 90° of shoulder flexion.

ACROMIOCLAVICULAR JOINT

The acromioclavicular joint is a diarthrodial joint involving the distal end of the clavicle and the medial acromion (see Fig. 39–5). The inclination of the distal clavicle varies considerably. The stability of this joint is provided by the acromioclavicular ligaments, the coracoclavicular ligaments, and muscle fascia of the deltoid and trapezius muscles. The acromioclavicular ligaments primarily prevent anterior translation of the clavicle. The coracoclavicular ligaments (conoid and trapezoid) provide most of the inherent stability to the acromioclavicular joint, particularly preventing inferior and posterior translation of the scapula on the clavicle. In a complete dislocation, disruption of both the acromioclavicular and coracoclavicular ligaments renders the joint unstable.

GLENOHUMERAL JOINT

The glenohumeral joint is designed for function, not for stability. This joint enjoys more global motion than any other in the body. Its bony architecture provides no inherent stability because the spherical humeral head is three times the size of the shallow glenoid. The glenohumeral capsule is redundant and voluminous, to allow global shoulder motion. Openings in the capsule are found superiorly, to allow the biceps tendon to pass intra-articularly, and anteriorly, for communication with the subscapularis bursa. The anterior capsule is much thicker than the posterior capsule, and the three glenohumeral ligaments provide static stabilizing forces to prevent abnormal glenohumeral translation (Fig. 39–6). The glenohumeral ligaments are condensations or thickenings of the anterior capsule and demonstrate considerable variability. The posterior capsule has no named glenohumeral ligaments.

The superior glenohumeral ligament originates at the superior glenoid tubercle, just posterior to the long head of the biceps tendon, and inserts on the humeral head at the superior aspect of the lesser tuberosity. This ligament primarily resists inferior subluxation when the arm is carried at the side.

The middle glenohumeral ligament originates on the superior aspect of the glenoid and glenoid labrum and blends in with the subscapularis tendon 2 cm medial to its insertion on the lesser tuberosity. It has much variability in size, and in some shoulders is absent. At 45° abduction, this ligament limits anterior translation and external rotation of the humeral head.

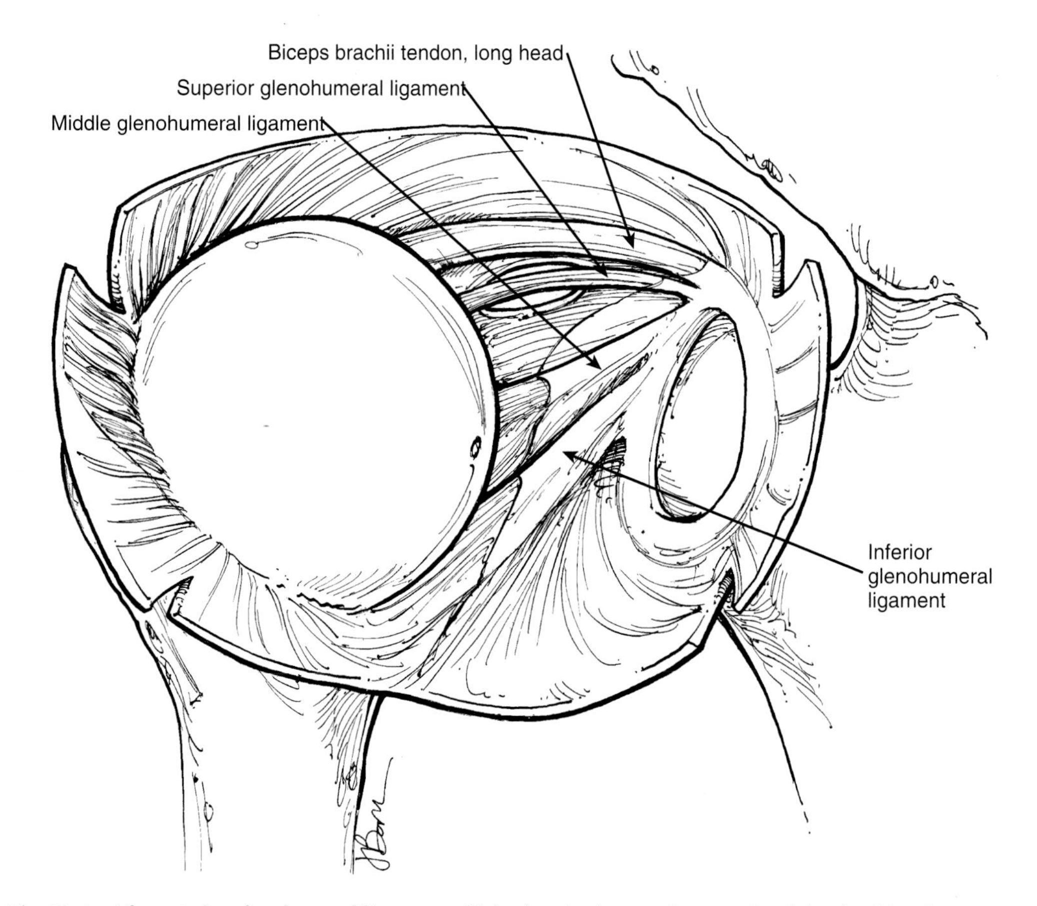

Fig. 39–6. The anterior glenohumeral ligaments, thickenings in the anterior capsule of the shoulder, demonstrate considerable variability. The inferior glenohumeral ligament is the principal static stabilizer of the shoulder.

The inferior glenohumeral ligament is the primary static stabilizer of the shoulder between 45° and 90° abduction. It originates along the anterior glenoid rim and the glenoid labrum and inserts along the inferior margin of the humeral articular surface and the anatomic neck of the humerus. It has been described by Schwartz and Warren as having a thickened anterior band, an inferior axillary pouch, and a thinner posterior band.[2] Turkel divides the inferior glenohumeral ligament into three components: the superior band and the anterior and posterior axillary pouches.[3]

Pollock and coworkers have demonstrated in laboratory studies that capsule injury occurs initially when stresses that are sufficient to cause subluxation and dislocation of the humeral head are applied to the anterior stabilizing structures of the shoulder.[4] In some cases, tearing of the glenoid labrum also occurs as an end response, and the capsular mechanism fails first. This may to some extent explain the frequent failure of surgical repairs of glenoid labrum tears in patients who demonstrate anterior instability of the shoulder.

NERVES

Brachial Plexus

The brachial plexus is the constellation of the anterior primary rami of the fifth through the eighth cervical nerves plus the first thoracic nerve, with some contribution of fibers from the fourth cervical nerve. The brachial plexus extends from the scalenus anterior to the axilla (see Chapter 34). Each of the nerve roots from C5 to T1 is divided into an upper, a middle, and a lower trunk. Each trunk gives off an anterior and a posterior division. The six divisions then form a posterior, a lateral, and a medial cord. All cords are formed superior to the clavicle, above the first rib. As they descend below the clavicle, each cord gives off multiple branches. The lateral one forms the musculocutaneous nerve and the lateral root of the median nerve. The medial cord forms the ulnar nerve and the medial root of the median nerve. The posterior cord forms the axillary and radial nerves. Several terminal branches of the brachial plexus arise from the roots and the cords of the plexus and are divided into supraclavicular and infraclavicular branches.

Axillary Nerve

The axillary nerve arises from the posterior cord of the brachial plexus from the C5 and C6 nerve roots. The axillary nerve courses below the subscapularis muscle and the anteroinferior capsule of the glenohumeral joint and runs with the posterior circumflex humeral vessel to the quadrilateral space posteriorly. Before the quadrilateral space, an anterior articular branch exits to supply the glenohumeral joint. At the quadrilateral space, the axillary nerve divides into an anterior and a posterior branch. The posterior branch innervates the teres minor and the posterior third of the deltoid and then terminates as the lateral brachial cutaneous nerve, supplying skin over the lateral aspect of the deltoid muscle. The anterior branch runs along the deep surface of the deltoid approximately 2 inches below the acromial edge, to innervate the anterior two thirds of the muscle. This branch must be protected when a deltoid-splitting incision is made.

Suprascapular Nerve

The suprascapular nerve arises from the superior aspect of the upper trunk. The nerve courses along with the inferior belly of the omohyoid muscle to the suprascapular notch and then passes below the transverse scapular ligament, entering the supraspinatus fossa. The supraspinatus muscle is innervated with two branches, and the nerve then winds around the lateral aspect of the scapular spine to innervate the infraspinatus muscle in the infraspinatus fossa. Articular branches are given off to the acromioclavicular and glenohumeral joints.

Musculocutaneous Nerve

The musculocutaneous nerve originates from the lateral cord of the brachial plexus and penetrates the deep surface of the coracobrachialis muscle, on average, 5 cm from the tip of the coracoid process. This nerve has been found to enter the muscle as close as 1.5 cm to the coracoid tip. The musculocutaneous nerve innervates the coracobrachialis, the long head of the biceps brachii, and the brachialis muscle. It then terminates as the lateral antebrachial cutaneous nerve in the forearm.

Arteries

The principal arterial supply to the shoulder girdle comes from the axillary artery, which is a continuation of the subclavian artery (see Chapter 46). The proximal border of the artery is located at the outer border of the first rib, and its distal extent is the lower border of the teres major muscle, beyond which it becomes the brachial artery. The axillary artery is divided by the pectoralis minor tendon into three portions. The portion of the artery proximal to the pectoralis minor tendon has one branch, the superior thoracic artery. The second portion of the axillary artery, which lies directly behind the pectoralis minor tendon, has two branches, the thoracoacromial and the lateral thoracic artery. The third position of the axillary artery lies distal to the pectoralis major tendon and contains three branches: the subscapular artery, the anterior circumflex humeral artery, and the posterior circumflex humeral artery. The axillary vein runs along with the axillary artery and is located anterior and inferior to it. Clinically significant branches of the above-named arteries include the four branches of the thoracoacromial artery. The acromial branch runs with the coracoacromial ligament to the acromion and sends branches to the deltoid muscle. It must be coagulated when excising the coracoacromial ligament. The deltoid branch runs in the deltopectoral interval, along with the cephalic vein. The pectoral branch lies between the pectoralis major and -minor muscles. The clavicular branch supplies the sternoclavicular joint. The circumflex scapular artery, a branch of the subscapular artery, passes through the triangular space and supplies the dorsal musculature on the scapula.

REFERENCES

1. Neer, C. S. II: Shoulder Reconstruction. Philadelphia, W. B. Saunders, 1990.
2. Schwartz, R. E., O'Brien, S. J., Warren, R. F., and Torzilli, P. A.: Capsular restraints to anterior-posterior motion of the shoulder. Orthop. Trans. *12*:727, 1988.
3. Turkel, S. J., Panio, M. W., Marshall, J. L., and Girgis, F. G.: Stabilizing mechanisms preventing anterior dislocation of the glenohumeral joint. J. Bone Joint Surg. *63A*:1208, 1981.
4. Pollock, R. G., et al.: The mechanical properties of the inferior glenohumeral ligament. Presented at American Shoulder and Elbow Society Annual Meeting, New Orleans, Louisiana, 1990.

40 *Joseph A. Martino*

Physical Examination of the Shoulder

The cornerstone of proper treatment of all shoulder problems is an accurate diagnosis. Most shoulder injuries can be identified by a thorough history and physical examination, without relying on costly, and often unnecessary, sophisticated tests. Occasionally, additional investigative methods, such as arthrography, computed tomography, magnetic resonance imaging, and electromyography are required to clarify a complicated diagnosis. The appropriate use of these methods should be reserved for complex situations and only when indicated.

HISTORY

The history-taking portion of interviewing a patient is analogous to the questions asked by a detective attempting to solve a crime. Each answer provides a clue that prompts yet another question. Questions are asked until the interviewer has a precise understanding of the events related to the shoulder problem. During this phase of the evaluation, the examiner must avoid the pitfalls of jumping to conclusions and focusing too quickly on the shoulder. Patients with disabling shoulder pain occasionally have cervical spine disorders, so these are initially included in the differential diagnosis of a shoulder problem.

At the onset of every patient interview at the Hughston Clinic, four basic questions are asked: What? How? Where? When? These simple questions provide a basis for determining the cause of the problem. The *what* is the predominant symptom. The direction of all further questions is based on this first answer. The answer is usually summarized as pain, instability, weakness, or deformity—affecting the right or the left shoulder. *How* is how the patient's problem developed. Was the onset insidious or related to a specific injury, traumatic event, or repetitive motion? *Where* establishes the location of the patient at the time of onset of the problem—on the football field, at work, or in a motor vehicle accident. *When* the problem began identifies it as acute (occurring within the past 6 weeks) or chronic (of more than 6 weeks' standing).

For example, a 24-year-old professional baseball pitcher presents with the sensation of a "dead arm," his dominant arm. Symptoms were first noted 3 weeks earlier while he was practicing during the off season. The patient does not recall any specific injury to the affected shoulder.

What: Dominant arm, "dead" sensation.
How: Pitching.
Where: Practice.
When: Three weeks ago.

He relates that the sensation occurs during the overhead phase of throwing and has begun to slow his fastball. The symptoms suggest a diagnosis of anterior instability, which is confirmed by physical examination.

In addition to the basic four questions, the examiner must establish the patient's age, medical and surgical history, occupation, and type and level of athletic participation. Questions about hand dominance, previous injuries, and the degree to which the underlying problem affects the individual's performance are also relevant. The presence of pain, instability, weakness, swelling, loss of motion, popping, and catching, and the relationship of symptoms to activity provide essential information as well.

Stiffness

Stiffness is defined as reduced motion. Shoulder stiffness is often accompanied by pain in the shoulder girdle. A common cause of shoulder stiffness is adhesive capsulitis, an idiopathic fibrosis and contracture of the glenohumeral joint capsule. This insidious problem is associated with a family history of diabetes, connective tissue disorders, and vascular disturbances and is usually observed in patients older than 30 years. The initial presentation may involve shoulder pain that gradually progresses to stiffness without pain.

PHYSICAL EXAMINATION

After obtaining the history, a systematic physical examination is performed. A detailed knowledge of the anatomy of the shoulder girdle is required to properly complete this phase of investigation. In addition, the cervical spine and the elbow should be examined when investigating a complaint about the shoulder. Performing a thorough physical examination requires diligence and practice, which eventually helps to establish experience. The three basic goals of a physical examination are observation, palpation, and rotation. Although the examiner may be biased by the information obtained from the medical history, a standardized format for performing the physical examination should be used to ensure completeness and to develop one's skills. This format should include initial impression, inspection, palpation, range of motion, neurovascular examination, and special tests.

Initial Impression

Ideally, observation of the patient should begin at the time of injury. On occasion, this opportunity presents itself to the alert sideline team physician. Being on the sidelines at a sporting event affords the clinician a rare chance to observe the actual force and mechanics involved in producing an injury, thus assisting in the assessment of the patient.

Inspection

An accurate physical examination requires that the patient be comfortable and that the upper torso and both shoulders be exposed to allow an adequate examination. Under field conditions, this may require that the patient be transported to a locker room to allow equipment removal and facilitate positioning on an examining table. In the clinical setting, body habitus should be observed as the patient enters the examining room. This includes shoulder symmetry during arm motion while walking; jerky or distorted movements are noted.

Adequate exposure of the shoulders under well-lit conditions is vital. The personal dignity of female patients can be preserved by using a gown fitted around the torso that covers the breasts but leaves the shoulders and back exposed, thus allowing complete visualization of the shoulders. The patient's upper body and shoulder girdles should be observed from the back, sides, and front. Ecchymosis, abrasions, swelling, scars, atrophy, and asymmetry should be noted. The simplest way to detect the presence of abnormalities is bilateral comparison, which should be used throughout the examination.

Specific attention should be directed toward determining atrophy of the muscle groups. Abnormal contour of the shoulder should also be noted; this can be caused by a fracture or dislocation of the humerus. A high-riding distal clavicle may represent an acromioclavicular joint separation, or possibly a clavicle fracture. The outline of the scapula as viewed posteriorly should be noted. Asymmetry of this outline may indicate winging of the scapula because of weakness of the serratus anterior muscle, which is innervated by the long thoracic nerve, or the trapezius muscle, which is innervated by the spinal accessory nerve. Prominence of the spine of the scapula occurs in association with supraspinatus and infraspinatus atrophy, which may be observed in patients with chronic rotator cuff tears. In addition, suprascapular nerve entrapment can also cause atrophy of the supraspinatus and infraspinatus, especially in association with repetitive overhead activities such as volleyball.

Bone Palpation

It is helpful to begin with palpation of the uninjured shoulder first. During the process of palpating the shoulder, the clinician should observe the shoulder for tenderness, swelling, deformities, and temperature differences. The examiner stands behind the patient, who is preferably sitting comfortably, and gently places the index and long fingers on the anterolateral aspect of the patient's acromion, a useful landmark and reference point. Palpating the adjacent acromioclavicular joint the examiner notes any swelling, deformity, tenderness, or crepitus. The acromioclavicular articulation is easily palpated in a lateral to medial direction while the patient flexes and extends the shoulder. Next, the index and long finger are placed adjacent to the suprasternal notch, which is medial and superior to the deltoid and clavicle. The sternoclavicular joint lies immediately lateral to the suprasternal notch, and both sides are palpated simultaneously.

The examiner's attention turns to the anterolateral portion of the acromion while he palpates laterally to the greater tuberosity, located inferiorly with the patient's arm in neutral rotation. The examiner should discern a slight step-off between the anterolateral acromial border and the greater tuberosity. Once this landmark has been palpated, the examiner asks the patient to externally rotate the arm 15°. The examiner should advance the index finger anterior and medial, to locate the intertubercular groove, which is where the biceps tendon normally passes, and then continues to palpate medially until a second projection is felt, the lesser tuberosity. Careful palpation in smooth succession should allow the examiner to distinguish the greater and lesser tuberosities as well as the biceps tendon within the intertubercular groove (Fig. 40–1).

The last bony region that requires palpation is the

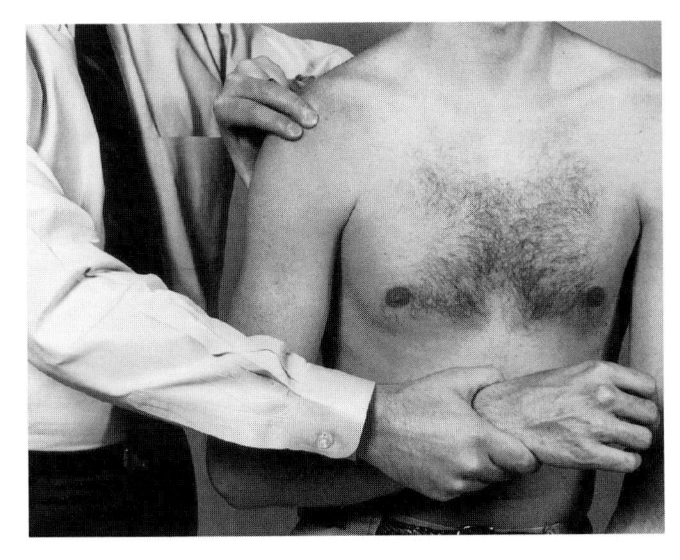

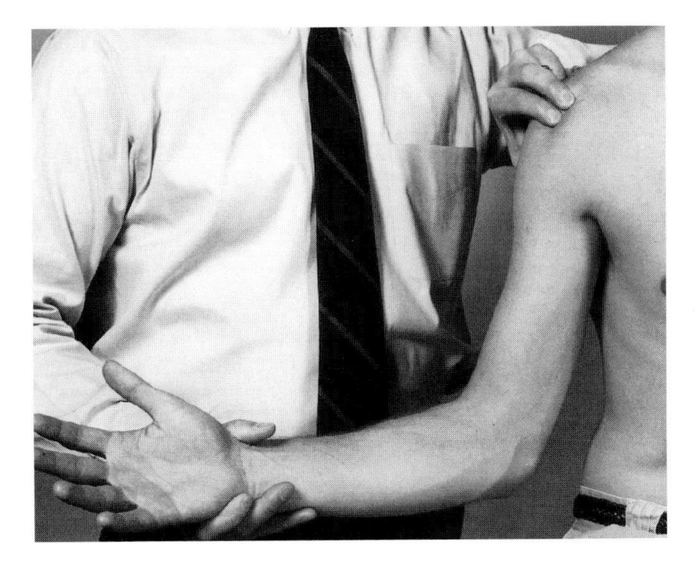

Fig. 40–1. Palpation of the greater and lesser tuberosities and biceps tendon in internal *(A)* and external *(B)* rotation.

scapula. The examiner begins by running the thumb over the posterolateral portion of the acromion and continues over the scapular spine in a medial direction, noting that these two anatomic landmarks form a continuous arch. The spine of the scapula terminates just below the superior medial angle of the scapula, which should be covered by the levator scapulae muscle. Last, the medial border of the scapula is traced downward to the inferior angle, which curves sharply upward and lateral at the level of the seventh rib. At this point, the examiner should observe the latissimus dorsi, teres major, and teres minor muscles.

Soft Tissue Palpation

A methodic examination of the relevant soft tissue structures attached to the shoulder girdle is based on four clinical zones: the rotator cuff, the subacromial bursa, the axilla, and the major muscles of the shoulder girdle. Each zone should be examined for muscle tone, tenderness, swelling, and atrophy or hypertrophy relative to the opposite side. The precise location of any tenderness should be noted during the examination.

ROTATOR CUFF

The four muscles that constitute the rotator cuff are the supraspinatus, infraspinatus, teres minor, and subscapularis. The clinical importance of the rotator cuff relates to its ability to initiate motion and control position of the humerus within the glenoid, thus facilitating fluid shoulder motion.

To palpate the rotator cuff muscles the patient should be seated with the arm at the side. The examiner palpates the lateral acromion and the greater tuberosity. Once these landmarks have been located, the examiner passively extends the shoulder by holding the patient's flexed elbow and moving it posteriorly. This maneuver rotates the rotator cuff from its position beneath the acromion. With the index finger of the opposite hand, the examiner then palpates the rounded contour between the anterolateral acromion and the greater tuberosity, revealing the exposed insertions of the supraspinatus, infraspinatus, and teres minor muscles. By positioning the patient's arm in external rotation, the examiner may then direct his or her index finger medially to the insertion of the subscapularis muscle on the lesser tuberosity. Tenderness during palpation may indicate inflammation of the rotator cuff, possibly related to a complete or partial tear. Occasionally, the examiner discerns a palpable defect caused by a complete tear of the rotator cuff. The most common site of a rotator cuff tear is the insertion of the supraspinatus muscle.

SUBACROMIAL BURSA

Irritation of the subacromial bursa frequently accompanies several clinical problems associated with the shoulder. After palpation of the rotator cuff portion of the subacromial bursa, the adjacent subdeltoid bursa should be palpated while the patient's arm is still extended and externally rotated. The bursa extends from the anterior edge of the acromion laterally to the intertubercular groove. The subdeltoid portion of the bursa extends laterally, separating the anterior deltoid from the rotator cuff. Gentle range of motion during palpation may reveal crepitation and allows the examiner to feel a thickening of the bursal tissues. Any swelling or tenderness should be appreciated as well.

AXILLA

While the patient sits with his or her arm passively abducted, the examiner faces the patient and gently palpates the thoracic region. The pectoralis and latissimus muscles cross the thorax in the area adjacent to the axilla before inserting onto the proximal humerus. Tenderness or palpable defects may represent rupture of these powerful muscles. Abduction of the arm accentuates the profile of both muscles. The latissimus dorsi can be palpated with the thumb and index finger in the posterior wall of the axilla. The pectoralis muscle can be palpated at its insertion on the humerus. The examiner should note the muscle tone and the presence of pain or a defect. Although uncommon, rupture of the pectoralis has been reported to occur at the musculotendinous junction adjacent to this insertion.

After evaluating these muscle groups, the examiner palpates the axilla, allowing deep probing of the axillary lymph nodes and the serratus anterior muscles. While palpating the axillary zone the examiner should also feel for the brachial artery pulse, which lies within the lateral quadrant of the axilla.

MAJOR MUSCLES OF THE SHOULDER GIRDLE

The first area to be approached is the neck, beginning with the sternocleidomastoid muscles. The sternocleidomastoid muscles are palpated bilaterally from the base of each muscle located on the medial third of the clavicle and the manubrium to its insertion on the mastoid process of the skull. The muscle can be palpated more easily by having the patient rotate the head from side to side.

While still positioned behind the patient, the examiner palpates the trapezius muscles bilaterally. He begins by grasping the superior portion of the trapezius at its origin on the base of the occiput then gently sweeps across this broad muscle toward its insertion sites on the clavicle, acromion, and scapular spine. The trapezius extends inferiorly to its distalmost insertion on the spinous process of T12, overlying the rhomboid muscles.

The rhomboid major and minor muscles are palpated simultaneously from their origin on the spinous processes of C7 to T5, obliquely downward to the medial border of the scapula. This muscle group can be distinguished from the overlying trapezius muscle by placing the patient's arm behind the back with the elbow flexed and the shoulder internally rotated (Fig. 40–2). In this position, the patient pushes the affected arm posteriorly, thus contracting the rhomboid major and minor muscles.

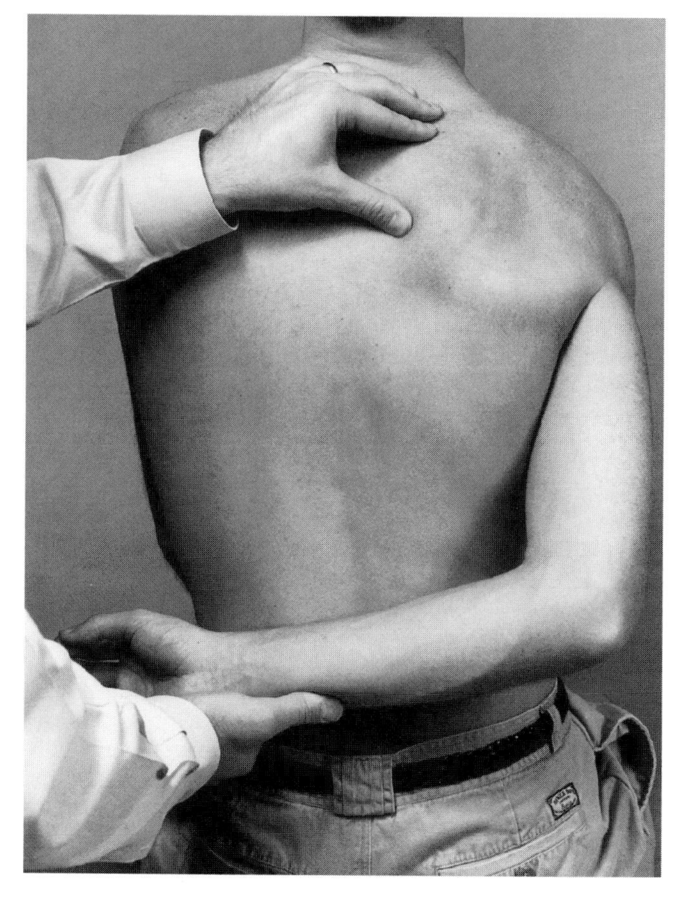

Fig. 40–2. Palpation of the rhomboid major and minor muscles.

Still behind the patient, the examiner addresses the serratus anterior muscles, which run along the medial border of the axilla from ribs one through eight. This muscle group allows scapular protraction, which is required for reaching. Tenderness in the distribution of this muscle is common in those who play sports that require repeated overhead reaching, such as tennis.

Next, the examiner moves to the side of the patient and palpates the acromion. The lateral portion of the acromion is a useful landmark for systematic palpation of the anterior, middle, and posterior head of the deltoid muscle. The anterior head originates from the lateral concavity of the clavicle, adjacent to where the pectoralis major ends, and it is responsible for the normal contour of the shoulder. Progressing laterally across the acromion, the middle head, and subsequently the posterior head, may be palpated sequentially. Specific attention is given to atrophy, diminished tone, and tenderness.

Still positioned at the patient's side, the clinician palpates the belly of the biceps muscle with the patient's arm flexed 90°. Proximal rupture of the biceps tendon presents as a palpable defect in the muscle belly because of the balling up of the long head of the biceps. The long head of the biceps tendon normally passes through the intertubercular groove, between the greater and the lesser tuberosity. It is easier to palpate by positioning the patient's arm in 15° of external rotation. Tenderness in this area may be due to bicipital tendinitis, irritation of the subacromial and subdeltoid bursa, or rotator cuff tendinitis. Specific localization of the tenderness helps identify the cause. It is important to mention that it is not uncommon for inflammation and irritation to occur simultaneously in these three structures.

The final soft tissue structure to be palpated is the pectoralis major muscle, which originates on the clavicle and sternum. Still at the patient's side, the examiner places a thumb in the patient's axilla and sweeps the forefingers across the two heads of the pectoralis major in a broad arc from the medial two thirds of the clavicle and the sternum. Next the muscle is palpated as it inserts onto the lateral lip of the intertubercular groove on the humerus. Traction injuries may produce tearing, or even rupture, of this powerful muscle, usually at the musculotendinous junction.

Range of Motion

Range of motion is an important parameter to quantify because it provides an objective measure for comparison later. No other joint in the body allows the freedom of motion observed in the shoulder. Comparison with the contralateral shoulder is essential. In active range of motion testing the patient uses the muscles to perform the motion; in passive range of motion testing the examiner moves the joint. Passive testing is usually reserved for situations in which the patient has difficulty performing active range of motion. The six motions involving the shoulder girdle are abduction, adduction, forward elevation, extension, external rotation, and internal rotation.

Recording shoulder motion in an organized manner requires a methodic approach to ensure consistency. To begin, the patient sits with arms at the sides in neutral abduction and rotates the arm in external and internal rotation. This position allows maximum internal and external rotation because the passive restraint provided by the glenohumeral ligaments is relaxed with the arm in neutral abduction. If the examiner is treating an injured athlete under field conditions, the patient may be examined in a supine position. Limitation of external rotation may indicate posterior shoulder dislocation. Maximum internal rotation is measured by recording the highest spinous process level that the patient's thumb can actively reach (Fig. 40–3). This is also a measure of shoulder extension. This maneuver may be difficult for the patient to perform if an associated elbow injury is present and should be substituted with measurement of internal rotation in the forward plane.

The next motion to be tested involves forward flexion in the plane of the scapula, also referred to as elevation in the plane of the scapula. This motion is the most important for providing a functional arc because it represents maximum elevation. With the patient in an upright or supine position, upward excursion of the arm is measured approximately 30° lateral to the patient's midline, halfway between the sagittal and the coronal plane. It is important to note that both glenohumeral and scapulothoracic motion are being observed during this sequence in a ratio of 2:1. Stabilizing the patient's scapula with one hand while the patient is upright allows selective measurement of glenohumeral elevation. This technique can help identify a frozen shoulder. It is also important to note that the natural rhythm of motion associated with forward elevation requires scapular rotation as well as glenohumeral motion because humeral elevation is blocked by the acromion.

Abduction and adduction can be measured next with the patient positioned upright. Abduction is measured in the coronal plane by raising the patient's arm with the elbow flexed 90°. When the arm reaches 90° of abduction, the patient's arm must be externally rotated to allow clearance of the tuberosities beneath the acromion, termed "Codman's pivotal paradox" (Fig. 40–4). Adduction is best measured by crossing the patient's arm in front of the thorax. Pain within the

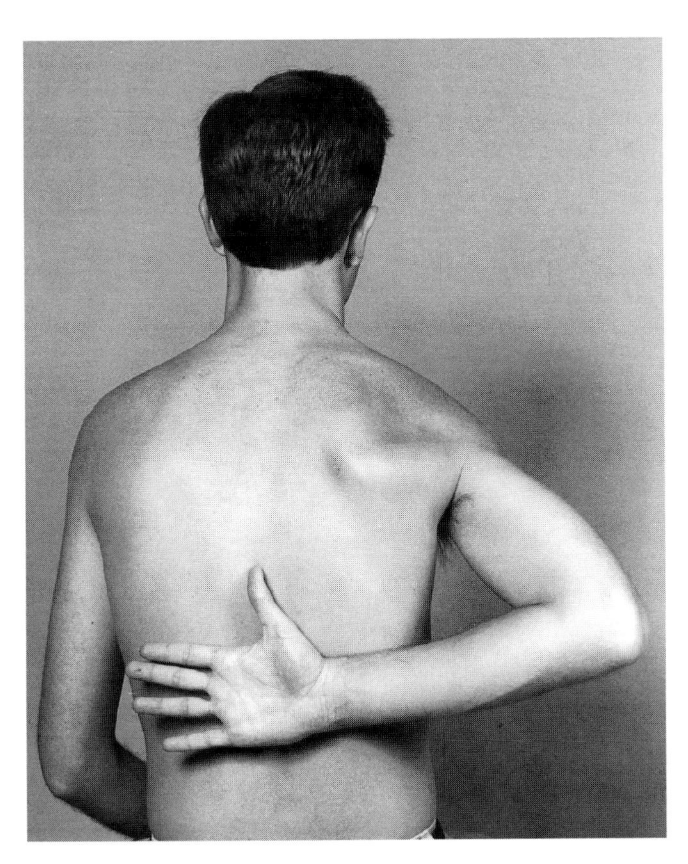

Fig. 40–3. Measurement of maximum internal rotation.

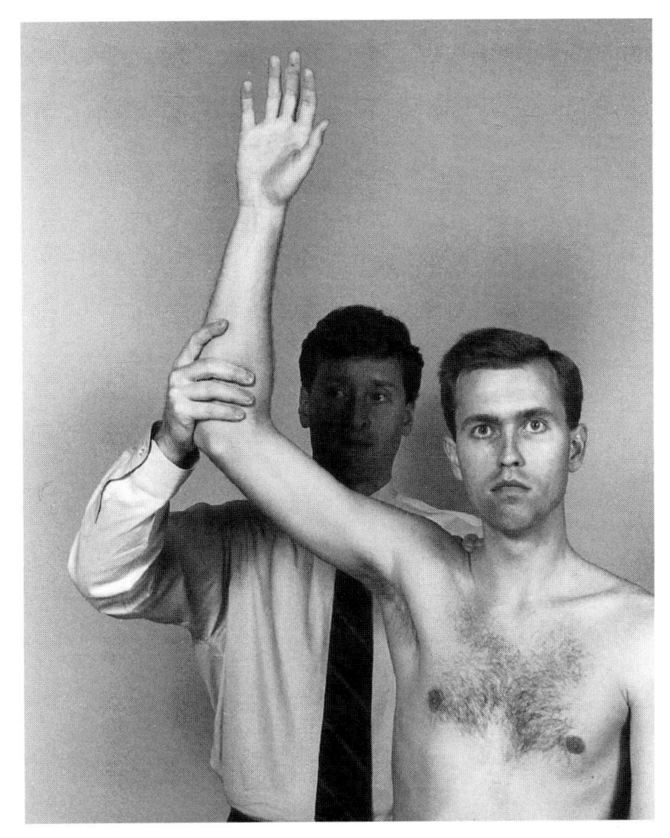

Fig. 40–4. Codman's pivotal paradox.

region of the acromioclavicular joint may be elicited with this maneuver, which merits further investigation. Most sports or daily activities involving overhead activity require the arm to be raised in the scapular plane, which is halfway between full forward flexion in the sagittal plane and pure abduction in the coronal plane. Therefore, the most functionally important range of motion is elevation in the plane of the scapula and not—the common misconception—abduction.

Neurovascular Examination

Examination of the shoulder is not complete until neurovascular status is determined. When responding to an acute shoulder injury in a sideline situation the neurovascular status of the patient must be established. Once airway, breathing, and circulation have been established, the degree of consciousness and presence of neck pain must be determined. After this, a basic neurologic examination of the patient's upper extremities should be performed bilaterally. The neurologic examination is essentially identical in field conditions and in the office setting. A standard muscle strength grading system is used:

Grade 5: Normal strength with resistance
Grade 4: Good strength with slightly less resistance
Grade 3: Fair strength with motion against gravity only
Grade 2: Poor strength, motion only with gravity eliminated
Grade 1: Trace evidence of active muscle contraction
Grade 0: No evidence of contractility.

Motor Strength

Trapezius motor function is tested by having the patient perform a shoulder shrug, against which the examiner applies downward resistance with the hands placed directly over both trapezius muscles. Next, deltoid function is tested by having the patient abduct the arms against resistance bilaterally. To isolate the patient's supraspinatus muscle, resistance is measured with the patient's arm elevated to 90° in the plane of the scapula with the arm internally rotated so that the patient's thumb points downward (Fig. 40–5). Next, the patient should perform a pushup away from a wall so the rhythm of scapular motion can be observed. Asymmetry may indicate either rhomboid or serratus anterior muscle weakness, which is not uncommon in "overhead" athletes with shoulder problems.

Isolated measurement of the posterior deltoid is accomplished by resisting the patient's efforts to direct the elbow posteriorly with the arm in neutral abduction and 90° elbow flexion. Still positioned behind the patient, the examiner measures resisted external rotation and internal rotation with the arm in neutral abduction. Weakness with resisted external rotation in this position may indicate an injury to the infraspinatus muscle (innervated by the suprascapular nerve) or the teres minor muscle (innervated by the axillary nerve). Weakness with resisted internal rotation may indicate an isolated injury to the subscapularis muscle, innervated by the upper and lower subscapularis nerves.

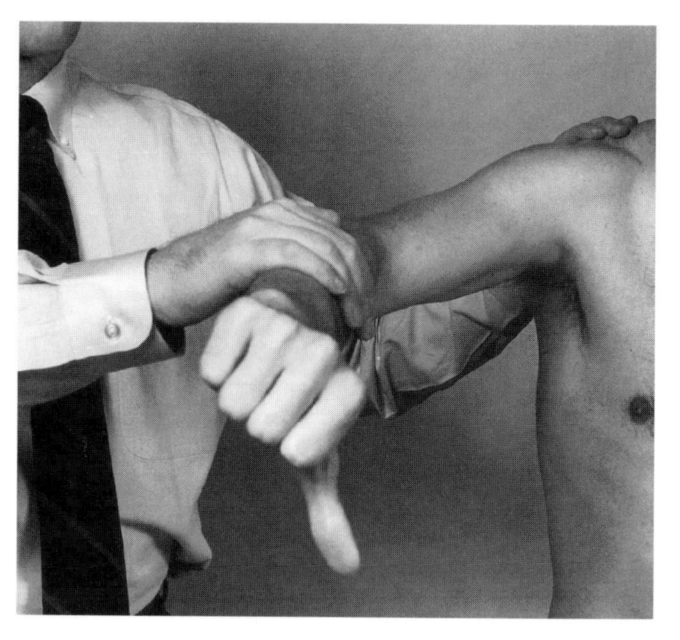

Fig. 40–5. Testing of the supraspinatus muscle.

Next, triceps and biceps function are evaluated from in front of the patient, whose arm is in neutral abduction. Resisted extension and flexion of the patient's elbows, as well as resisted supination of the forearm, provide an indication of triceps and biceps strength. Pain in the region of the intertubercular groove with resisted supination may indicate bicipital tendinitis (Yergason's test), a finding occasionally associated with rotator cuff tendinitis.

Finally, the patient's motor strength is evaluated by resisted wrist flexion and extension and by abduction of the digits and thumb extension. Weakness of any of these functions may indicate a nerve injury in the brachial plexus or cervical spine, which would require further investigation (see Chapter 33).

Sensory Examination

The sensory innervation of the upper extremity and shoulder is organized into dermatomes. The dermatomes should be tested bilaterally using light touch and sensitivity to sharp sensation. Beginning from the top of the patient's shoulder, the dermatome innervated by the C4 nerve root is tested. Next, the lateral arm is tested, which is innervated by C5. Specific attention should be directed to sensation in the region of the lateral deltoid, innervated by the sensory branch of the axillary nerve. Presence of sensation in this site indicates that the axillary nerve is intact. It is important to test the function of the axillary nerve before and after attempts at reducing shoulder dislocations. The medial arm is innervated by the T1 nerve root, and the axillary dermatome by the T2 nerve root. A more detailed description of the remaining dermatomal distribution of the upper extremity is covered in Chapter 33.

Reflexes

Testing the spinal reflexes provides a useful, objective method for determining neurologic injury. Deep tendon reflexes are recorded as being normal, decreased, or increased by using bilateral comparison. The triceps reflex (C7 nerve root) is tested by gently tapping the posterior elbow in the region of the triceps insertion with the arm supported by the examiner's other hand. The biceps reflex (C5 nerve root) is tested by supporting the patient's supinated forearm and tapping with a thumb over the cubital fossa. Last, the brachioradialis reflex (C6 nerve root) is tested by supporting the patient's arm in a similar manner and tapping the brachioradialis tendon near its insertion on the distal radius.

SPECIAL TESTS

Several tests are designed specifically to analyze certain pathologic conditions of the shoulder. Such clinical tests are usually reserved for the office. Significant injuries observed from the sideline should be subject to a basic evaluation and to referral for routine radiographs before performing special testing under more controlled conditions. Specific tests for shoulder impingement and instability are described in later chapters.

SUGGESTED READINGS

Codman, E. A.: Normal motions of the shoulder joint. *In* The Shoulder: Rupture of the Supraspinatus Tendon and Other Lesions in or about the Subacromial Bursa. Boston, Thomas Todd, 1934.

Cofield, R. H., and Irving, J. F.: Evaluation and classification of shoulder instability with special reference to examination under anesthesia. Clin. Orthop. *223*:32, 1987.

Hawkins, R. J., and Hobeika, P.: Physical examination of the shoulder. Orthopedics *6*:1270, 1983.

Hawkins, R. J., and Murnaghan, J. P.: The shoulder. *In* Adult Orthopaedics. Vol. 2. Edited by R. L. Cruess and W. R. J. Rennie. New York, Churchill Livingstone, 1984.

Hoppenfeld, S.: Physical Examination of the Spine and Extremities. Norwalk, CT, Appleton-Century-Crofts, 1976.

Jobe, F. W., and Jobe, C. M.: Painful athletic injuries of the shoulder. Clin. Orthop. *173*:117, 1983.

Neer, C. S. II: Shoulder Reconstruction. Philadelphia, W. B. Saunders, 1990.

Neer, C. S. II, and Welsh, R. P.: The shoulder in sports. Orthop. Clin. North Am. *8*:583, 1977.

Rockwood, C. A. Jr. and Matsen, F. A., III (eds): The Shoulder. Vol 1. Philadelphia, W. B. Saunders, 1990.

41

George M. McCluskey III and Steven D. Levin

Imaging of the Shoulder

Diagnostic imaging of the shoulder has progressed tremendously over the last several years. Many sophisticated modalities are now available for diagnosing shoulder problems, but standard radiography is still the first investigative study to be used. Shoulder radiographs provide essential information to the clinician, such as the presence of bony lesions and evidence of and the direction of dislocation.

PLAIN RADIOGRAPHY

Standard Views

A standard series of three radiographs should routinely be taken when evaluating a patient's shoulder problems. This series includes a true anteroposterior (AP) view, a true scapular lateral view, and an axillary lateral view.[1]

AP radiographs of the shoulder have been described based on the position of the x-ray beam relative to the plane of the body and to that of the scapula. The difference between the two planes reflects the position of the scapula relative to the plane of the body: the scapula is oriented 30° to 45° from the frontal plane of the body.[2] Thus, a scapular AP film provides a true AP view of the glenohumeral joint (Fig. 41–1). Scapular AP views of the shoulder joint provide excellent visualization of the glenohumeral relationship in the frontal plane.

The standard AP view is taken with the x-ray beam perpendicular to the thorax. This does not provide as good a view of the true glenohumeral joint; however, it does visualize the relationship of all the bony elements of the shoulder in a true AP direction.

The true scapular lateral view is also commonly referred to as the scapular Y view or the trans-scapular view. This view demonstrates the relationship of the humeral head to the glenoid. Normally the head is centered on the glenoid at the intersection of the Y formed by the coracoid process, scapular spine, and body of the scapula (Fig. 41–2). In dislocations about the shoulder, the humeral head may be situated anterior, posterior, or inferior to the glenoid fossa.

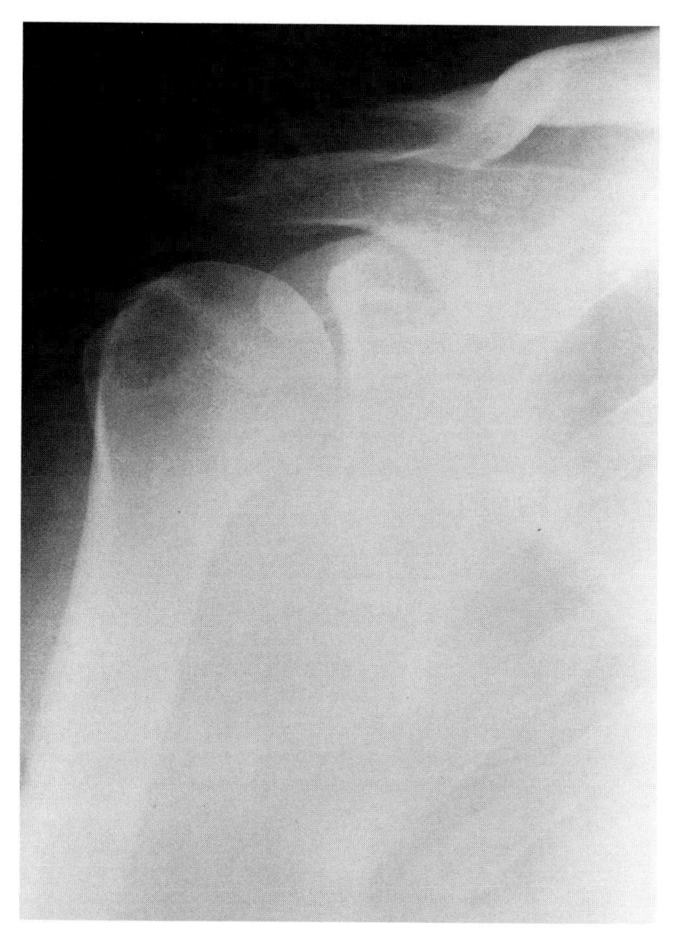

Fig. 41–1. A true AP view.

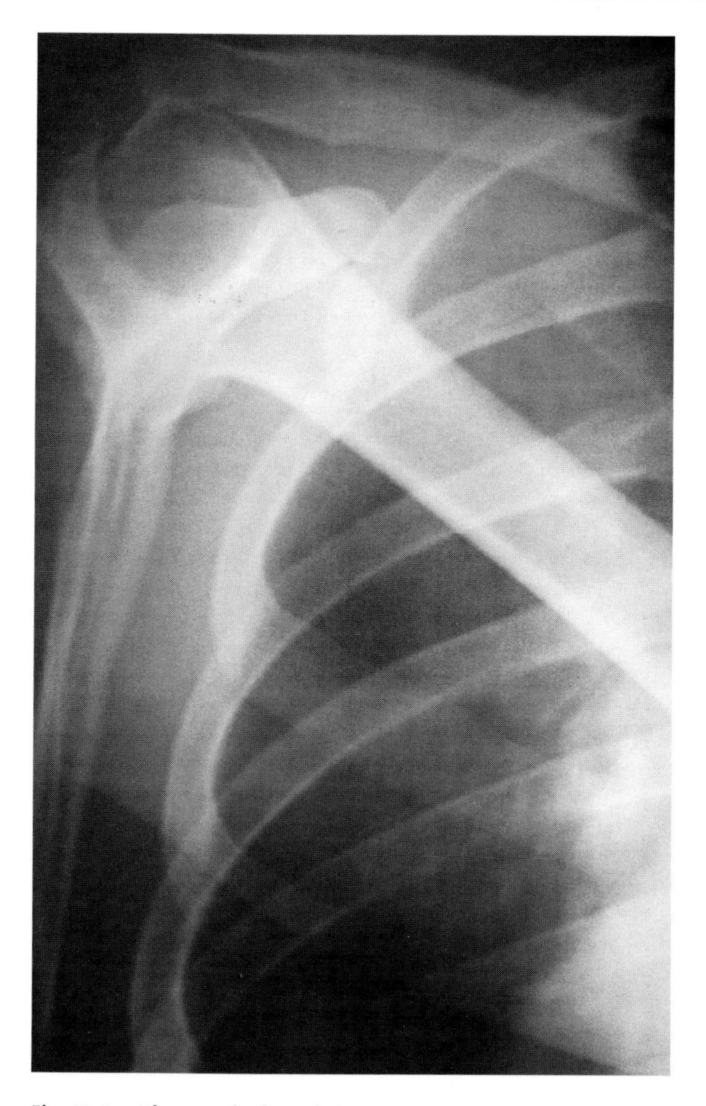

Fig. 41–2. The scapular lateral view.

The supraspinatus outlet view, as described by Neer, is useful for visualizing an impingement lesion, rotator cuff disease, or acromioclavicular joint pathology.[3] This view best defines the acromial morphology. The patient is positioned for a true scapular lateral radiograph with the x-ray beam tilted 10° caudad. Many surgeons obtain this outlet view routinely, rather than the scapular lateral view, as part of their standard series.

The axillary lateral view is useful in evaluating the glenohumeral joint and detecting the presence of an os acromiale or acromial fracture (Fig. 41–3). The cassette is placed superior to the shoulder with the patient erect and the arm abducted 75° to 90°. The x-ray beam is directed into the axilla superiorly.

Special Views

VELPEAU'S AXILLARY LATERAL

When the patient with an acute shoulder injury cannot abduct the arm for a routine axillary lateral radiograph, Velpeau's axillary lateral view is used to view the shoulder in this plane. This view is taken with the arm in a sling or immobilizer, or with the arm held across the chest in internal rotation. The standing patient leans backward against the table about 20°, and the x-ray beam is directed inferiorly from the top of the shoulder toward the cassette placed under the shoulder on the table.

TRAUMA AXILLARY LATERAL

The trauma axillary lateral view can be taken with an acutely injured patient in the supine position. A foam pad is placed under the elbow, which is flexed 20° as the arm is held across the chest. The cassette is placed superior to the shoulder, and the x-ray beam is angled into the axilla, toward the cassette.

WEST POINT LATERAL

The West Point lateral radiograph is used principally to evaluate patients with anterior instability of the shoulder. It affords accurate identification of bony abnormalities of the anterior glenoid rim (Bankart's lesion) in patients with suspected glenohumeral anterior instability. The patient lies prone with the involved shoulder raised on a small pad and the arm hanging over the table. The head is turned toward the contralateral shoulder, and the cassette is placed along the superior aspect of the involved shoulder. The x-ray beam is angled toward the axilla, 25° downward and 25° mediad.

STRYKER NOTCH VIEW

The Stryker notch view is valuable for assessing traumatic anterior instability of the shoulder and a Hill-Sachs lesion in the posterolateral aspect of the humeral head (Fig. 41–4). The supine patient places the hand of the involved side on the top of the head. The cassette is placed under the shoulder with the x-ray beam aimed 10° cephalad and centered over the coracoid process.

ZANCA'S VIEW

Zanca's view is useful for evaluating the acromioclavicular joint and distal clavicle. A standard AP view of the shoulder is taken with the x-ray beam angled 10° cephalad.

REDUCED VOLTAGE VIEW

The acromioclavicular joint can be visualized well with a routine AP view of the shoulder and the intensity of the voltage decreased by 50% compared with that used to visualize the glenohumeral joint.

ANTEROPOSTERIOR STRESS RADIOGRAPHS

Stress radiographs of the shoulder are indicated for suspected Type I or II acromioclavicular joint separations. An AP view of both shoulders should be taken, using a single cassette if possible. The patient stands with 10 to 15 pounds of weight strapped around each wrist (*not* held in the hands). The coracoclavicular dis-

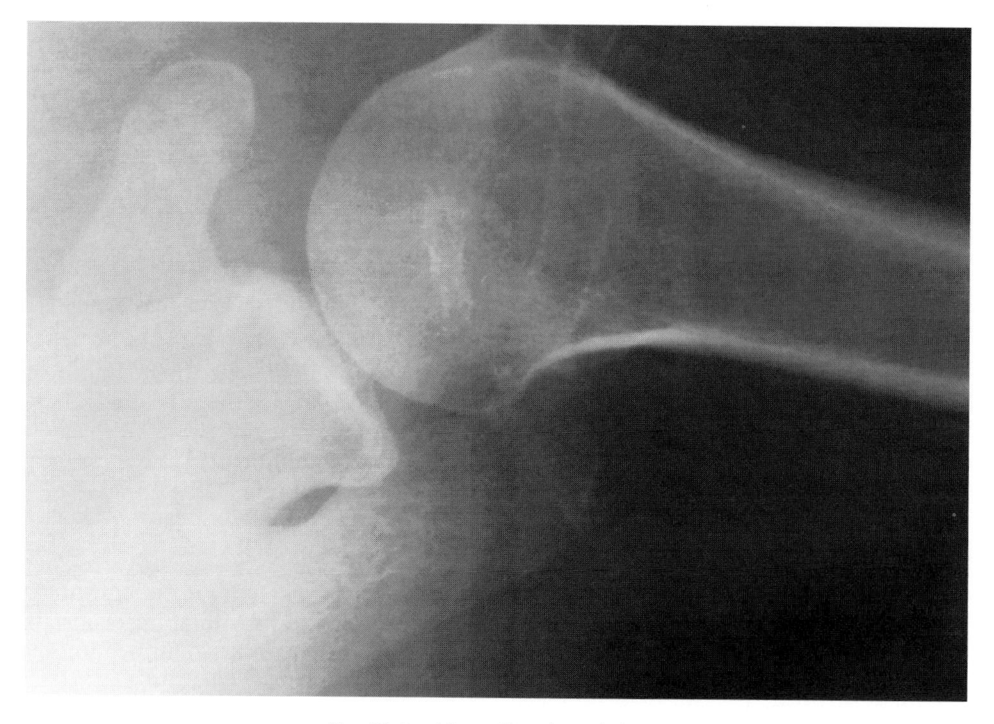

Fig. 41–3. The axillary lateral view.

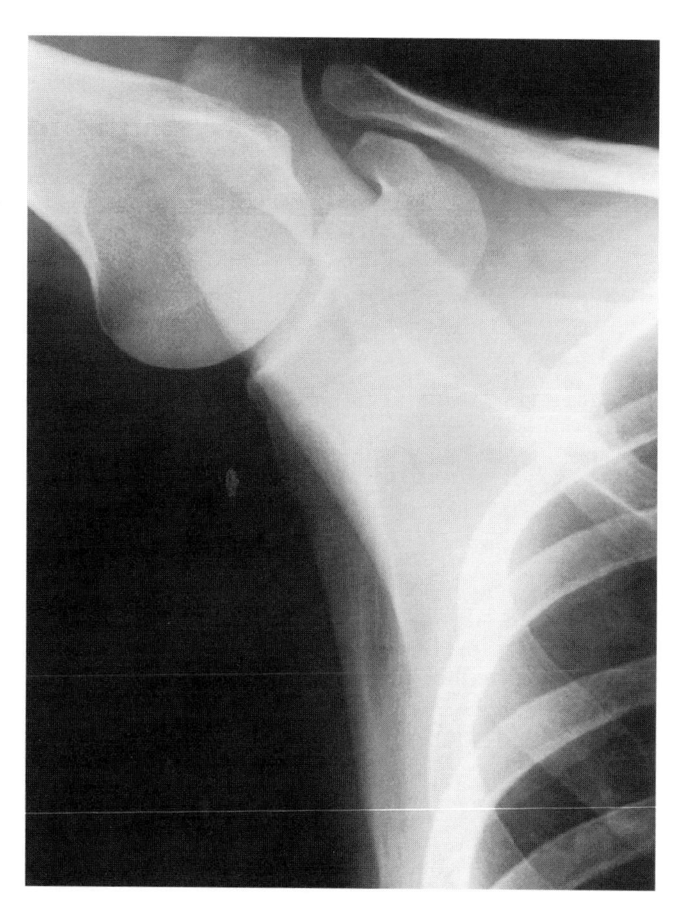

Fig. 41–4. Stryker notch view.

tance is measured on both sides for comparison. With acromioclavicular separation, the distance is greater on the injured side than on the normal one.

SERENDIPITY VIEW

The sternoclavicular joint is best evaluated initially with the serendipity view. An 11- by 14-inch nongrid cassette is placed under the supine patient to include both shoulders, chest, and neck. The x-ray beam is angled 40° cephalad, toward the manubrium and sternum.

ARTHROGRAPHY

The arthrogram has long been considered the best means for evaluating full-thickness tears of the rotator cuff. Its specificity and sensitivity for detecting full-thickness tears exceeds 90%. Articular surface partial rotator cuff tears may also be seen with single-contrast arthrograms, but less reliably than full tears. Adhesive capsulitis may also be diagnosed with this method.[4]

The size of the rotator cuff tear is difficult to assess accurately in most studies. The geyser sign—contrast extending up into the acromioclavicular joint—indicates a large or massive rotator cuff tear (Fig. 41–5). When contrast material is present posteriorly in the internal rotation AP view, extension of the tear into the external rotators is predictable.

Recently, the glenoid labrum has become the focus of much clinical attention. This fibrocartilaginous struc-

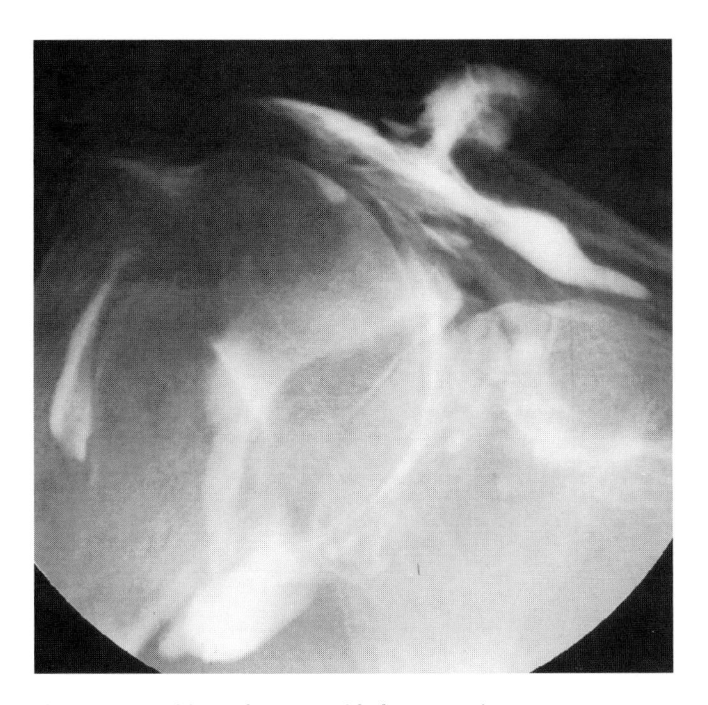

Fig. 41–5. Positive arthrogram with the geyser sign.

ture does not show up on standard radiographs, so double-contrast arthrography has become an important tool in diagnosing lesions. (Single-contrast arthrography has been largely unsuccessful because pooling of examination contrast material results in unclear images.)[4,5] Double-contrast arthrography relies on the use of both air and contrast material to improve visualization of intra-articular structures.

COMPUTED TOMOGRAPHY

Computed tomography (CT) has been a useful adjunctive study in patients with specific skeletal disorders involving the shoulder girdle. CT is especially important when evaluating proximal humeral fractures and fracture-dislocations of the glenohumeral joint and the acromioclavicular joint. In patients with glenohumeral instability, CT can be helpful in determining the size of associated glenoid rim fractures and of humeral head defects in chronic anterior and posterior dislocations of the shoulder. Many studies have alluded to the superior quality of bone resolution with CT as compared with that for standard radiography.[6–8] CT offers other advantages over standard radiography, including lower radiation dose, more comfortable patient positioning, imaging in different planes at one sitting, and the capability for coronal and sagittal reformatting. The notable disadvantages are greater cost to the patient and inability to image soft tissue.

Double-Contrast CT Arthrography

Danzig and colleagues first used CT arthrography in 1982 to help clinicians document intra-articular soft tissue lesions associated with glenohumeral instability.[9] Deutsch and colleagues combined CT arthrography with double-contrast arthrography to further elucidate structural damage to the labrum, articular cartilage, capsular structures, and biceps tendon.[10]

The technique of double-contrast arthrography involves injection of 1 to 4 ml of contrast material and 10 to 15 ml of room air into the shoulder joint. After limited exercise, images are obtained with the patient supine and the shoulder in neutral position or in slight internal rotation to relax the anterior structures. Multiple cuts of the area of concern are taken in 2- to 3-mm increments. Reconstruction in the sagittal or coronal planes can then be obtained.

The labrum is triangular, with a smoothly rounded anterior apex. The posterior labrum has a more blunted contour in CT arthrography. The base of the labrum is continuous with the articular cartilage of the glenoid. Capsular insertions are clearly identifiable and usually are continuous with the bony attachment of the labrum.[6] Unstable shoulders may demonstrate tearing or absence of the labrum, capsular detachment from the glenoid, or capsular redundancy (Fig. 41–6).

CT arthrography offers advantages over standard arthrotomography, such as ease of administration, decreased radiation, and less patient discomfort. Some of the disadvantages include high cost and complications of dye reactions.

Double-Contrast Arthrotomography

Because of the inadequate results of single- and double-contrast arthrography for imaging the glenoid labrum, arthrotomography has been introduced. It offers the advantage of more complete visualization of the entire labrum. The disadvantages of this technique are awkward and uncomfortable positioning of the patient (a prone oblique position with the affected shoulder adjacent to the cassette). The technique often takes longer than an hour. Also, the patient is exposed to a great deal of radiation. Several clinical studies have reported excellent diagnostic accuracy for this technique. These analyses have documented sensitivities and specificities between 85 and 100% for evaluation of labral disorders. Because of the aforementioned disadvantages, however, magnetic resonance imaging (MRI) and CT scan seem to have overtaken its usefulness.

ULTRASONOGRAPHY

In recent years, a number of centers have begun using ultrasound to evaluate the rotator cuff. In these centers, the accuracy of the study approaches that of arthrography for detection of full-thickness rotator cuff tears. It is most accurate for moderate to large-sized tears and less accurate for small or partial tears. Ultrasonography is quick and inexpensive to perform and has no known risks. Its main disadvantages are (1) limited resolution; (2) a significant learning curve for performing the

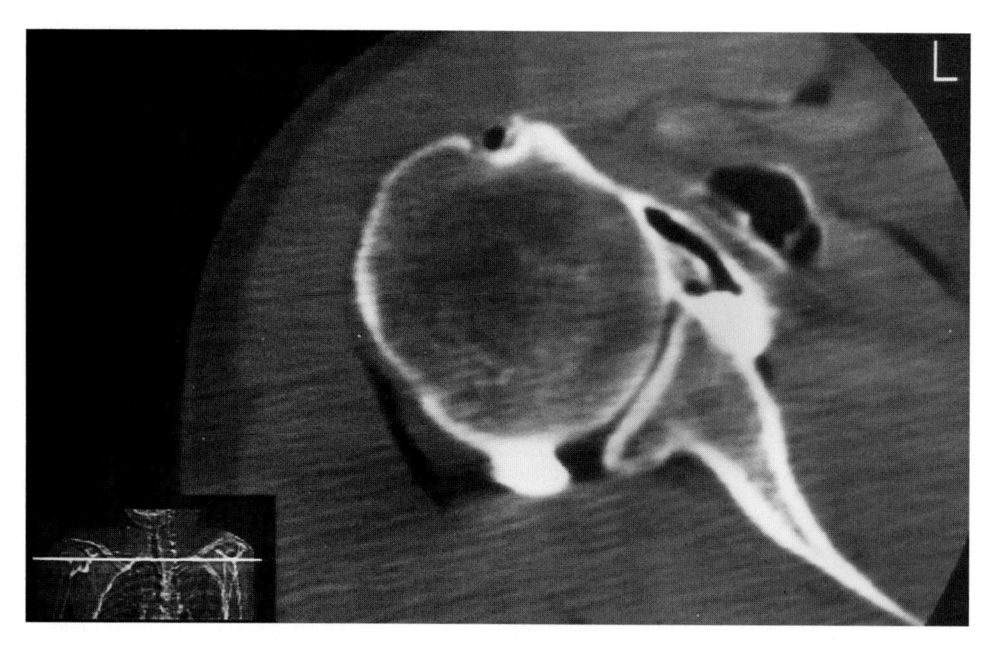

Fig. 41–6. CT arthrogram shows a labral tear.

study and interpreting results; and (3) difficulty in differentiating between small full-thickness tears, incomplete tears, and postoperative scarring in rotator cuff tendons. Ultrasonographic findings are much more operator dependent than those of other imaging techniques.

MAGNETIC RESONANCE IMAGING

The imaging modality that is most extensive and provides the most information about the shoulder is MRI, a noninvasive technology that is excellent for diagnosing many shoulder disorders, including impingement and rotator cuff disease. Images are taken in three planes while the patient lies supine with the upper extremity in the neutral position. Coronal images are best for examining the rotator cuff, as they run in the plane of the tendon. The reported accuracy of MRI for full-thickness tears of the rotator cuff ranges from 95 to 100%.

Two major types of signals are elicited on MRI, T1- and T2-weighted images. T1-weighted images demonstrate bright or white signals in fatty structures such as bone marrow or subcutaneous tissue. Muscle and hyaline cartilage have intermediate signal intensity or gray, signals. T2-weighted images show fat-containing structures with some signal loss, and water-filled structures appear brighter. Bone, labrum, capsule, and ligaments have low signal intensity and therefore appear black on T1- and T2-weighted images.

The diagnosis of a rotator cuff tear is made when loss of continuity of the tendon seen on the T1-weighted image is complemented by a bright fluid signal on the T2-weighted image (Fig. 41–7). Evolution of rotator cuff disease from rotator cuff tendinitis and inflammation to tendon degeneration and partial-thickness tears may be determined by MRI scanning. MRI may also help to predict surgical outcome in patients with large to massive-sized rotator cuff tears when significant fatty infiltration and muscle atrophy of cuff muscles are seen on preoperative studies. The size and shape of the acromion and the acromioclavicular joint may also be readily seen on MRI, and these parameters have diagnostic value for rotator cuff problems.

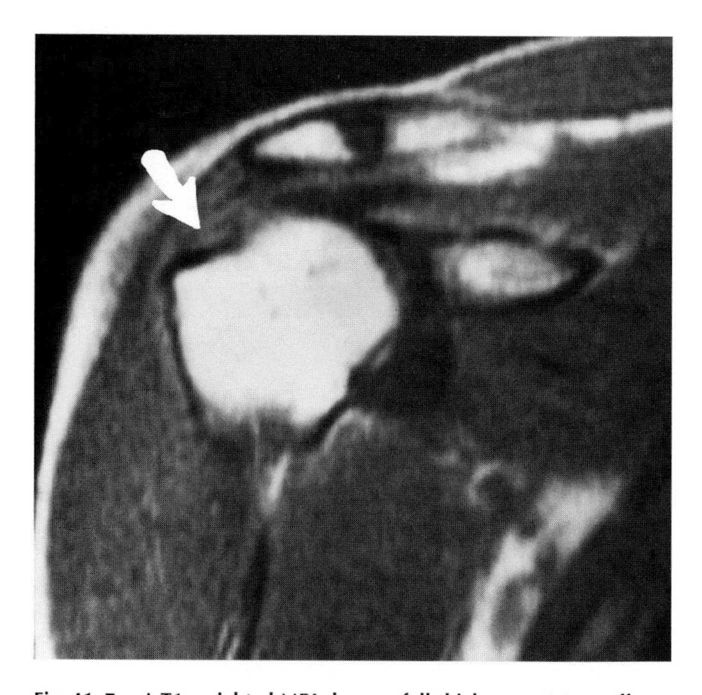

Fig. 41–7. A T1-weighted MRI shows a full-thickness rotator cuff tear as a "divot" in the humeral head *(arrow).*

Although many earlier studies demonstrated poor sensitivity and specificity for evaluating glenoid labrum tears, newer, more sophisticated scanners show greater promise. In evaluating the shoulder capsule complex, the axial imaging plane is the most useful. MRI can demonstrate pathologic lesions associated with anterior instability, including the Hill-Sachs lesion and fractures of the anterior inferior glenoid rim.

MRI can also be useful in evaluating other shoulder disorders, including biceps tendon disorders, post-traumatic degenerative disease, and other arthritic conditions of the glenohumeral joint, osteonecrosis, and tumors about the shoulder.

Disadvantages of MRI include its cost relative to that of ultrasonography or arthrography. Some claustrophobic patients have difficulty tolerating the close quarters MRI requires. Motion artifact can also interfere with image quality.

MRI is currently the diagnostic tool of choice for evaluating most shoulder disorders.[11] Its use will likely increase in the future as it offers clear delineation of soft tissue, noninvasive technique, and lack of radiation.

REFERENCES

1. Altchek, D. W. and Dines, D. M.: The surgical treatment of anterior instability: selective capsular repair. Operative Techniques in Sports Medicine *1*:285, 1993.
2. Matsen, F. A. III, Thomas, S. C., and Rockwood, C. A., Jr.: Glenohumeral instability. *In* The Shoulder. Vol 1. Edited by C. A. Rockwood, Jr. and F. A. Matsen III. Philadelphia, W. B. Saunders, 1990.
3. Neer, C. S. II: Shoulder Reconstruction. Philadelphia, W. B. Saunders, 1990.
4. Goldman, A. B., and Ghelman, B.: The double-contrast shoulder arthrogram. Radiology *127*:655, 1978.
5. Tijmes, J., Loyd, H. M., and Tullos, H. S.: Arthrography in acute shoulder dislocations. South. Med. J. *72*:564, 1979.
6. Deutsch, A. L., Resnick, D., and Mink, J. H.: Computed tomography of the glenohumeral and sternoclavicular joints. Orthop. Clin. North Am. *16*:497, 1985.
7. Randelli, M., and Gambrioli, P. L.: Glenohumeral osteometry by computed tomography in normal and unstable shoulders. Clin. Orthop. *208*:151, 1986.
8. Hill, J. A., Tkach, L., and Hendrix, R. W.: A study of glenohumeral orientation in patients with anterior recurrent shoulder dislocations using computerized axial tomography. Orthop. Rev. *18*:84, 1989.
9. Danzig, L., Resnick, D., and Greenway, G.: Evaluation of unstable shoulders by computed tomography. Am. J. Sports Med. *10*:138, 1982.
10. Deutsch, A. L., et al.: Computed and conventional arthrotomography of the glenohumeral joint: Normal anatomy and clinical experience. Radiology *153*:603, 1984.
11. Tsai, J. C., and Zlatkin, M. B.: Magnetic resonance imaging of the shoulder. Radiol. Clin. North Am. *28*:279, 1990.

42

Mark R. Brinker and Steven H. Weeden

Fractures About the Shoulder

CLAVICLE FRACTURES

Fractures of the clavicle traditionally have been classified by configuration: greenstick, oblique, transverse, and comminuted fractures. Fractures may also be classified by anatomic site. Clavicular shaft fractures of children usually are not formally classified. Because of the thick periosteum, most clavicular shaft fractures in children are nondisplaced or minimally angulated greenstick fractures. Fractures in adults are often displaced and over-riding.

Fractures in children commonly result from a fall on the point of the shoulder or on the outstretched hand. The most common mechanism of clavicle fractures in adults is a fall on an outstretched hand.[1] The incidence of clavicular fractures is high in hockey and lacrosse players, owing to direct blows to the clavicle.[2] In nonathletes, this mechanism of clavicular fracture is rarely observed.

Older children and adults with clavicle fractures often have signs of crepitus, swelling, and tenderness. Athletes usually report a clear history of either direct or indirect injury to the shoulder. The patient usually presents holding the involved extremity elevated to reduce pain. Pulmonary, muscular, vascular, and neural injuries may also be associated. Standard radiographic evaluation of clavicular fractures includes a routine anteroposterior (AP) view of the clavicle and a 45° cephalic tilt view.

Most orthopedic surgeons prefer nonoperative treatment for essentially all clavicular fractures. Immobilization for comfort is all that is required. The nondisplaced fracture may only require treatment with a sling and application of ice. A figure-of-eight harness helps reduce displaced fractures and may be useful in the initial treatment. Operative management may be indicated for (1) débridement of an open fracture, (2) patients with neurovascular compromise that does not resolve with closed reduction, (3) patients with several, irreducible displaced fragments, and (4) mediastinal compression associated with a posteriorly displaced medial clavicular fracture.[3,4] Fractures of the distal third of the clavicle have different healing responses because of the involvement of the coracoclavicular ligaments. Type I fractures are more common; these occur between the acromioclavicular joint and the coracoclavicular ligaments. They are stable and require only a sling. Type II fractures occur medial to or through the coracoclavicular ligaments and are unstable. They often require operative stabilization. Type III fractures, which involve the articular surface of the distal clavicle, are often missed and present with late sequelae. Type IV and V fractures are uncommon (Fig. 42–1).[5,6]

In treating athletes with clavicular fractures it is often wise to discuss treatment with the trainer and coaches. A clear explanation of the possible complications is also necessary. A thorough clinical examination, along with radiographic views of the clavicle demonstrating solid bone union, should be documented over time before an athlete is released to competitive activity.

Athletes are at risk for numerous complications resulting from clavicle fracture. Nonunion is a rare but serious complication.[7] Inadequate immobilization has long been recognized as a cause of nonunion. Radiographic evaluation of a healing fracture may be desired before mobilization is allowed. Malunion may present a cosmetic or functional problem. Many authors have suggested osteotomy, internal fixation, and bone grafting for clavicular malunion.[8] Post-traumatic arthritis may occur at the clavicular articulations. Often, post-traumatic arthritis is the result of an unrecognized Type III distal clavicle fracture. Associated injuries in clavicular fractures include rib fractures, pneumothorax or hemothorax, tears in the trachea or main bronchi, and neurovascular injuries.

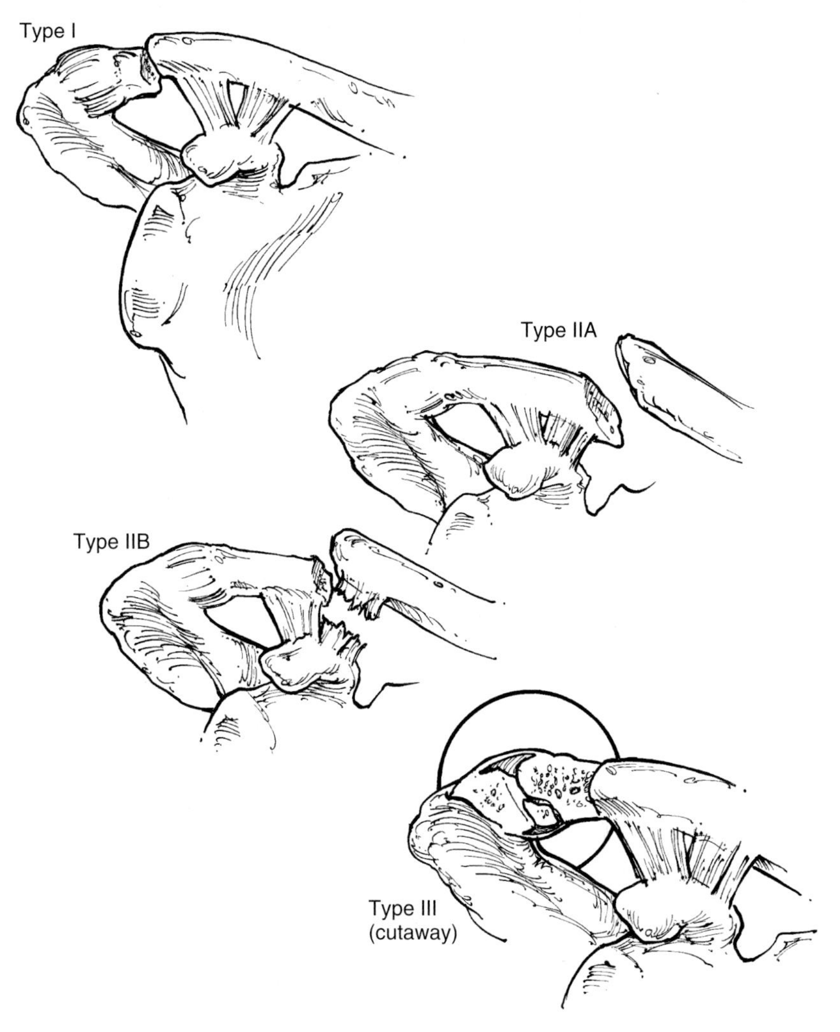

Fig. 42–1. Distal clavicle fractures. Type I occur between the acromioclavicular joint and the coracoacromial ligaments. The intact ligaments hold the fragments in place. Type IIA fractures occur medial to the coracoacromial ligaments. Type IIB fractures involve a tear of the coracoacromial ligaments. Type III involve only the articular surface of the clavicle. (Drawn from Rockwood, C. A. Jr., and Green, D. P. (eds.): Fractures in Adults. 3rd Ed. Vol I. Philadelphia, J. B. Lippincott, 1991 p. 935-937.)

SCAPULAR BODY, ACROMION, AND CORACOID FRACTURES

Fractures of the scapula are usually classified by anatomic site. The neck and body are the areas most often fractured. Three types of scapular fractures have been described:[9] Type I, fractures of the scapular body; Type II, fractures of the apophysis, including the coracoid and acromion; and Type III, fractures of the superior lateral angle, including the neck and glenoid.

A second classification system for scapular fractures, described by Thompson and coworkers,[10] is based on their series of fractures from blunt trauma and also consists of three classes: Class I, coracoid and acromion fractures and small fractures of the scapular body; Class II, glenoid and neck fractures; and Class III, major scapular body fractures. Either system may be used to assess scapular fractures in athletes.

No true classification scheme has been described for scapular fractures in children. Fractures in young athletes are usually classified by anatomic site. An accurate assessment of scapular fractures in children demands a clear understanding of the ossification centers in the scapula, including their locations and at what age fusion occurs. Identification of the various growth centers in the scapula, acromion, and coracoid may be confusing, and they can be mistaken for a fracture.

The mechanisms of injury of scapular, acromial, and coracoid fractures are numerous. Sports-related fractures of the scapular neck are often associated with direct trauma or a fall on the point of the shoulder or an outstretched arm (axial loading). Scapular body fractures during athletic activity usually result from direct trauma, often with high energy. Sudden muscle contraction may contribute to displacement of scapular body fracture fragments. Fractures of the acromion commonly result from a direct superior blow. In most acromial fractures the fracture line is lateral to the acromioclavicular joint and minimal displacement occurs. The acromion may also fracture as a result of axial loading through the humeral head. Coracoid fractures may be isolated, as from a direct blow to the coracoid during a sporting event, or they may be associated with acromioclavicular dislocation while the coracoclavicular ligaments remain intact.[11,12] In adolescents, injury to the acromioclavicular joint is not uncommon during athletic activity, and an associated coracoid fracture must be ruled out.

The athlete with a scapular fracture typically holds the arm adducted and protects it from movement; abduction is usually especially painful. Local tenderness, ecchymosis, and hematoma may be found overlying and adjacent to the fracture site. Deep inspiratory pain is typically associated with a coracoid or scapular body fracture. Patients with a fracture of the acromion may exhibit pain on attempted abduction of the arm, a flattened shoulder, localized pain, swelling, and tenderness. With coracoid fractures, acute injury is associated with local pain, tenderness, and pain on adduction of the shoulder and flexion of the elbow. Severely displaced coracoid fragments may be palpated close to the axillary fold.[13] Subtle or occult neurologic deficits may be overlooked initially during the evaluation of a coracoid fracture. These neurologic deficits may result from direct trauma to the coracoid that causes the fractured part to contuse the cords of the brachial plexus that lie beneath. If the suprascapular nerve is injured in the notch during a fracture, its paralysis may be mistaken for a tear of the rotator cuff; electromyograms may be useful for identifying an athlete with a suprascapular nerve injury.

Initial radiographic evaluation of athletes with suspected scapular, acromial, and coracoid fractures should include an AP view of the shoulder, a tangential oblique view of the scapula, and an axillary view. Tangential and anteroposterior radiographs may be useful in demonstrating fracture of a scapular body or neck. Acromial fractures are confirmed on AP and axillary lateral views of the shoulder. In young athletes one must be careful not to confuse an acromial epiphysis or os acromiale with a fracture.[14] A 30° caudal tilt and a supraspinatus outlet view may be helpful for assessing acromial fractures. In younger patients plain films of the contralateral shoulder joint may inform the evaluation. If a coracoid fracture is suspected, an axillary lateral radiograph is essential to avoid missing the lesion. The Stryker notch view and Goldberg's posterior oblique 20° cephalic tilt view may also aid in the visualization of a coracoid fracture. In selected cases, computed tomography (CT) may be useful for defining the fracture pattern.

Indications for surgical fixation of a scapular fracture in an athlete are rare. In adults, significant trauma is required to fracture the scapula. Athletes who suffer high-energy trauma (e.g., in motorcycle or automobile racing) may be more likely to sustain a scapular fracture than those involved in other sporting events. For most scapular neck fractures, reduction of the fracture and restoration of the glenoid to its anatomic position are not necessary. The shoulder may be placed in a sling to immobilize it for comfort. A scapular body fracture usually does not require operative intervention because the surrounding muscles provide an excellent environment for healing. Pain management is important during the healing process. Ideally, rehabilitation should result in restoration of full range of motion.

Several treatment methods are available for athletes with an acromial or coracoid fracture. A nondisplaced acromial fracture responds well to symptomatic treatment and immobilization in a sling. Some clinicians prefer a tension band wire for fixation of displaced acromial fractures. Rehabilitation is begun immediately after an isolated acromial fracture. Rehabilitation includes passive range of motion exercises, progressing to isometrics and, after fracture healing, active resistance exercises. For athletes with an isolated coracoid fracture, most authors believe that no specific treatment is needed, since anatomic alignment is not essential for adequate healing and future competition. Open reduction of coracoid fractures may be indicated if displacement is significant,[15] or in cases of complete third-degree acromioclavicular separation combined with a significantly displaced coracoid fracture. If suprascapular nerve or brachial plexus entrapment is suspected, early exploration may be necessary to avoid future complications that could affect athletic performance.

Diagnosis of a scapular fracture may be delayed because of associated injuries. Diagnosis may also be delayed while emergent care is provided for life-threatening injuries sustained during severe trauma. Rib fractures, pneumothorax, pulmonary contusion, clavicular fracture, spine damage, and neurovascular damage have all been reported as associated injuries.[10, 16] Rotator cuff disruption is frequently associated with fractures of the acromion and scapula. Complications may include neurovascular injury, loss of function, and loss of anatomic symmetry about the shoulder. Bone irregularities may cause the soft tissues to impinge on the ribs and result in pain, crepitus, and limitation of motion.

GLENOID FRACTURES

Ideberg's classification (Fig. 42–2) of glenoid fractures is frequently used by clinicians:[17,18] Type I, fractures with avulsion of the anterior margin; Type II, transverse fractures through the glenoid fossa with an inferior triangular fragment displaced with the humeral head; Type III, oblique fractures through the glenoid exiting at the midsuperior border of the scapula and often associated with an acromioclavicular fracture or acromioclavicular dislocation; Type IV, horizontal fractures exiting through the medial border of the body; and Type V, combined Type IV fractures plus a fracture separating the inferior half of the glenoid. In child athletes, glenoid fractures can be divided into two types, (1) those associated with dislocation of the glenohumeral joint and (2) those that extend from fractures of the scapular neck, which are often comminuted.[19]

The mechanism of injury and clinical presentation of glenoid fractures are similar to those for scapular, acro-

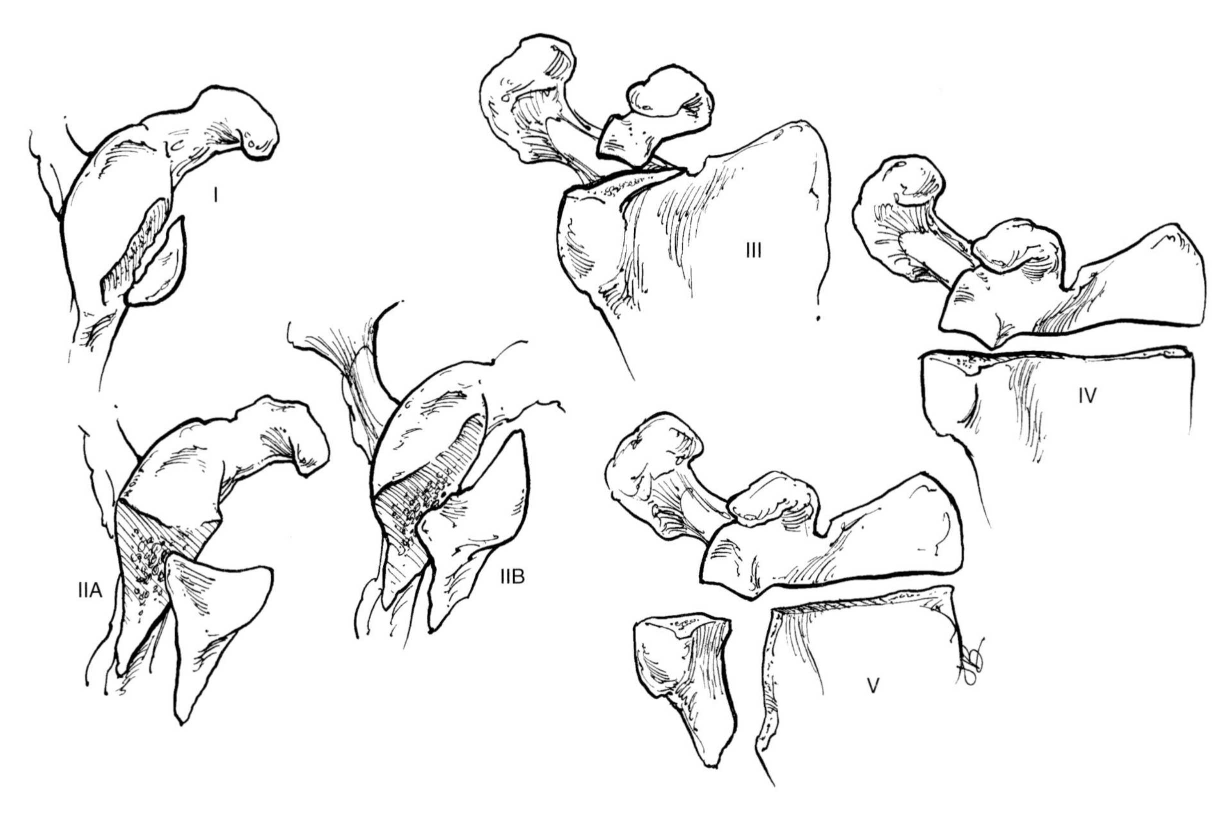

Fig. 42–2. Ideberg's classification of intra-articular fractures of the glenoid. (Drawn from Rockwood, C. A. Jr., and Green, D. P. (eds.): Fractures in Adults. 3rd Ed. Vol I. Philadelphia, J. B. Lippincott, 1991, p. 1003.)

mial, and coracoid fractures. During sporting events, injury by direct force is produced by falling onto the point of the shoulder with the arm at the side in an adducted position (Fig. 42–3). Type I glenoid fractures frequently occur with dislocations and subluxations. A posterior shoulder dislocation may result in a posterior rim glenoid fracture. An anterior shoulder dislocation may cause a glenoid fracture by knocking off a glenoid fragment, with or without an avulsion force from the surrounding capsular structure. Type V glenoid fractures typically result from violent trauma about the shoulder. AP, tangential scapular lateral, and axillary lateral radiographs, and often CT are necessary to confirm a glenoid fracture. Other views may be desired in selected cases or when the aforementioned views are not diagnostic.

Knowledge of both closed and open treatment methods is required to ensure early return to athletic activity after a traumatic glenoid fracture. If a large glenoid fragment is displaced, open reduction with screw fixation may be desired. Aggressive surgical repair of displaced glenoid fragments is indicated to avoid recurrent instability. Open reduction and fixation of Ideberg's Type I glenoid fractures may obviate reconstruction with fragment fixation or bone graft. The indications for operative management of Type II through V glenoid fractures are less clear. When surgery is performed, an anterior approach is best for anterior glenoid rim and coracoid fractures, and a posterior approach for glenoid neck and fossa fractures. For most glenoid fractures in athletes, CT is helpful in determining fragment size and humeral head position. When a large anterior glenoid fracture is treated nonsurgically, followup radiographs with physical examinations must be performed frequently, to assess fracture healing and joint stability. An adolescent athlete with a minimally displaced glenoid fracture can be treated conservatively with a good prognosis for full return of function. Older children with a fragment of 1 cm or larger should be treated like adults, with replacement of the fragment plus anterior shoulder reconstruction.

For glenoid fractures, the complications and associated injuries are similar to those for other shoulder fractures. Pneumothorax, rib fracture, spine damage, shoulder dislocation, and other associated injuries may be seen in athletes with glenoid fractures. Fracture of the clavicle is frequently associated with a glenoid or scapular neck fracture. Brachial plexus injury must always be ruled out when acute shoulder trauma is observed. Attention to life-threatening injuries should be the immediate priority and should guide fracture repair. In children, severe traumatic anterior dislocation of the shoulder with fracture and displacement of the anterior glenoid rim is extremely rare. If this injury occurs in a child, recurrent subluxation and dislocation of the shoulder may occur. In every athlete with a glenoid fracture, assessment of shoulder stability is important, to ensure future competitiveness.

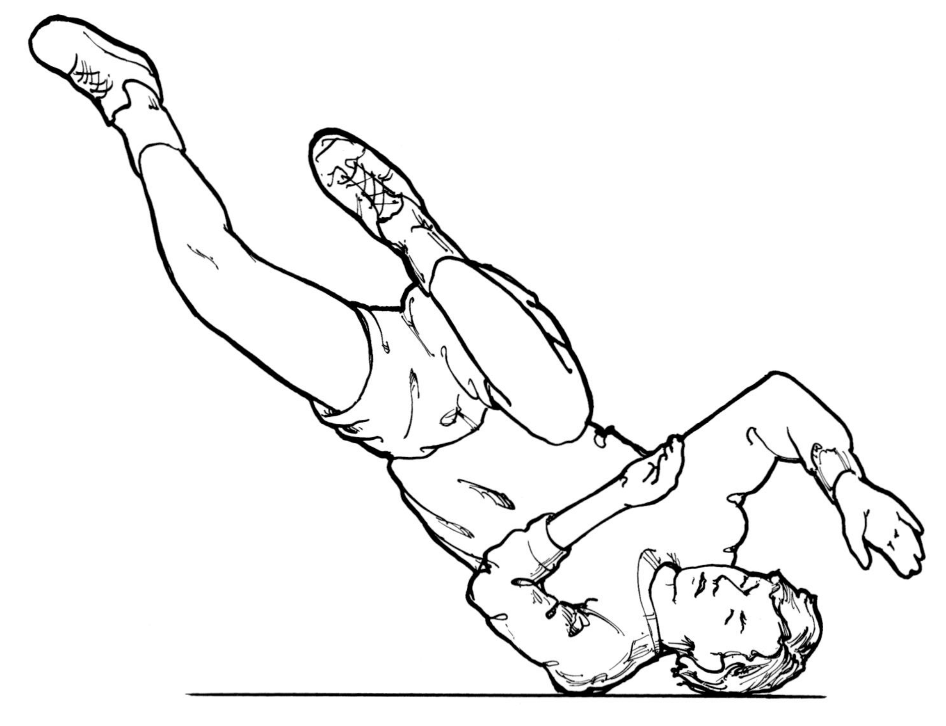

Fig. 42–3. Common mechanism of shoulder fracture in athletes. (Drawn from Rockwood, C. A. Jr., and Green, D. P. (eds.): Fractures in Adults. 2nd Ed. Vol I. Philadelphia, J. B. Lippincott, 1984, p. 867.)

PROXIMAL HUMERAL FRACTURES

A fracture classification system based on anatomy and biomechanical forces is necessary for proper diagnosis and clinical management of proximal humeral fractures. The Neer classification of proximal humerus fractures takes into account both the anatomy and the forces that result in displacement of fracture fragments.[20] A fragment is considered displaced when there is more than 1 cm of separation between fragments or a fragment is angulated more than 45° from other fragments. Radiographic studies of the proximal humerus may show a displaced fracture of two, three, or four parts. Head-splitting fractures of the proximal humerus, usually the tuberosities or surgical neck, are also considered by Neer, as are dislocations of fractured bone.

Any sporting event in which a significant force is transmitted to the proximal humerus can result in a fracture. A fracture usually occurs when an athlete throws the arm into an abducted, extended, and externally rotated position to break a fall. Transmission of force toward the shoulder joint may lead to a fracture. Such fractures typically occur in structurally weak anatomic areas; namely, the metaphysis in a young child and the physis in older children. One example of proximal humeral fractures is "Little League shoulder," believed to result from prolonged pitching, which causes a fracture through the physis of the proximal humerus. Stress fractures through the physis of the proximal humerus in Little League pitchers have also been described.[21] Fractures may also occur with falls directly on the lateral side of the shoulder. During such an event, the major deforming force is imparted directly to the epiphysis and developing growth plate. Older children can sustain a proximal humeral fracture by falling on an outstretched hand.

Pain, swelling, dysfunction and tenderness about the shoulder joint should raise suspicion of a proximal humeral fracture. Proximal humerus fracture-dislocations are often missed on the initial examination. Crepitus and local ecchymosis may be present, the latter occurring 24 to 48 hours after the injury. The diagnosis is best made with proper radiographic studies. A detailed neurovascular examination is indicated whenever the proximal humerus is fractured because of the proximity of the brachial plexus and axillary vessels.

Radiographic evaluation of suspected proximal humeral fractures must be accurate, to ensure correct diagnosis and proper treatment. The trauma series is the best first study for diagnosis of proximal humeral fractures. The three separate perpendicular planes provided by the trauma series allow for accurate fracture classification and assessment of displacement in athletes.

Proximal humeral fractures in athletes deserve individual consideration because they can impair the ability to compete. The majority of proximal humeral fractures are minimally displaced and can be managed with initial immobilization and early motion. In a minimally displaced proximal humeral fracture, range of motion exercises can be started early (i.e., within 10 days, if pain allows). Closed reduction is usually inadequate for two- or three-part fractures. Open reduction with internal fixation via screws, wires, or suture material is the treatment of choice for two- and three-part fractures.[22,23]

During fixation of a three-part fracture, care must be taken to avoid denuding the fracture fragments of their blood supply. Certain three-part proximal humeral fractures require a humeral head prosthesis, and four-part fractures and head-splitting fractures commonly require one. Children with proximal humeral fractures rarely require operative treatment.

Rehabilitation of an athlete with a proximal humeral fracture is essential for a successful outcome. Passive assisted exercises should be started early, when the fracture or fracture repair is stable. With a minimally displaced proximal humeral fracture, exercises may begin as early as the seventh day. To promote relaxation, warm-up should be accomplished with either a hot shower or a heating pad, followed by stretching. Early rehabilitation of a proximal humeral fracture in an athlete consists of physician- or physical therapist–assisted elbow flexion and extension, pendulum exercises, and supine lateral rotation. As the injured arm gains strength, exercises to ensure restoration of full abduction, external rotation, and internal rotation are extremely important. Exercises are routinely performed three or four times per day. Isometrics are generally started at 3 to 4 weeks. During rehabilitation, light weights may be used as early as 3 months. If pain is excessive during exercise or after weight lifting, the load should be decreased or the weight lifting discontinued. The use of a physical therapist for guidance and management of proximal humeral rehabilitation usually enhances the athlete's compliance, motivation, and future ability to compete. Without proper exercise, even perfect closed reduction or surgical repair does not achieve optimum results.

Complications following proximal humeral fractures include avascular necrosis, brachial plexus injury, myositis ossificans, frozen shoulder, infection, pneumothorax and pneumohemothorax, nonunion, malunion, and others. Hardware failure is another potential complication. Growth deformities in children range from a small decrease in degrees of arc of motion to limb length inequalities and angular deformity.[24–26] Careful followup of athletes, plus knowledge of frequent and infrequent complications, allow early detection and prevention of potentially harmful fracture complications.

REFERENCES

1. DePalma, A. F.: Surgery of the Shoulder. 3rd Ed., Philadelphia, J. B. Lippincott, 1983.
2. Silloway, K. A., et al.: Clavicular fractures and acromioclavicular joint injuries in lacrosse: Preventable injuries. J. Emerg. Med. *3*:117, 1985.
3. Curtis, R. J. Jr.: Operative management of children's fractures of the shoulder region. Orthop. Clin. North Am. *21*:315, 1990.
4. Mital, M. A., and AuFranc, O. E.: Venous occlusion following greenstick fracture of clavicle. J.A.M.A. *206*:1301, 1968.
5. Parkes, J. C., and Deland, J. T.: A three-part distal clavicle fracture. J. Trauma *23*:437, 1983.
6. Dameron, T. B. Jr., and Rockwood, C. A. Jr.: Fractures and dislocations of the shoulder. *In* Fractures in Children. Edited by C. A. Rockwood Jr., K. E. Wilkins, and R. E. King. Philadelphia, J. B. Lippincott, 1984.
7. Marsh, H. O., and Hazarian, E.: Pseudarthrosis of the clavicle. J. Bone Joint Surg. *52B*:793, 1970.
8. Bateman, J. E.: The Shoulder and Neck. Philadelphia, W. B. Saunders, 1978.
9. Zdravkovic, D., and Damholt, V. V.: Comminuted and severely displaced fractures of the scapula. Acta Orthop. Scand. *45*:60, 1974.
10. Thompson, D. A., Flynn, T. C., Miller, P. W., and Fischer, R. P.: The significance of scapular fractures. J. Trauma *25*:974, 1985.
11. Bernard, T. N. Jr., Brunet, M. E., and Haddad, R. J. Jr.: Fractured coracoid process in acromioclavicular dislocations. Clin. Orthop. *175*:227, 1983.
12. Zettas, J. P., and Muchnic, P. D.: Fractures of the coracoid process base in acute acromioclavicular separation. Orthop. Rev. *5*:77, 1976.
13. Rowe, C. R.: Fractures of the scapula. Surg. Clin. North Am. *43*:1565, 1963.
14. Liberson, F.: Os acromiale: A contested anomaly. J. Bone Joint Surg. *19*:683, 1937.
15. Rowe, C. R. (ed.): The Shoulder. New York, Churchill Livingstone, 1988.
16. McLennan, J. G., and Ungersma, J.: Pneumothorax complicating fractures of the scapula. J. Bone Joint Surg. *64A*:598, 1982.
17. Ideberg, R.: Unusual glenoid fractures: A report on 92 cases. Acta Orthop. Scand. *58*:191, 1987.
18. Ideberg, R.: Fractures of the scapula involving the glenoid fossa. *In* Surgery of the Shoulder. Edited by J. E. Bateman and R. P. Welsh. Philadelphia, B. C. Decker, 1984.
19. Rockwood, C. A. Jr., Wilkins, K. E, and King, R. E. (eds.): Fractures in Children. 3rd Ed. Philadelphia, J. B. Lippincott, 1991.
20. Neer, C. S. II, and Horowitz, B. S.: Fractures of the proximal humeral epiphysial plate. Clin. Orthop. *41*:24, 1965.
21. Cahill, B. R., Tullos, H. S., and Fain, R. H.: Little league shoulder. J. Sports Med. *2*:150, 1974.
22. Ahovuo, J., Paavolainen, P., and Björkenheim, J. M.: Fractures of the proximal humerus involving the intertubercular groove. Acta Radiol. *30*:373, 1989.
23. Hagg, O., and Lundberg, B.: Aspects of prognostic factors in comminuted and dislocated proximal humeral fractures. *In* Surgery of the Shoulder. Edited by J. E. Bateman, and R. P. Welsh. Philadelphia, B. C. Decker, 1984.
24. Langenskiold, A.: Adolescent humerus varus. Acta Chir. Scand. *105*:353, 1953.
25. Lucas, L. S., and Gill, J. H.: Humerus varus following birth injury to the proximal humeral epiphysis. J. Bone Joint Surg. *29*:367, 1947.
26. Baxter, M. P., and Wiley, J. J.: Fractures of the proximal humeral epiphysis. J. Bone Joint Surg. *68B*:570, 1986.

43 *David B. Keyes*

Soft Tissue Injuries to the Acromioclavicular and Sternoclavicular Joints

ACROMIOCLAVICULAR JOINT

The acromioclavicular joint is a diarthrodial joint (see Fig. 39–5) surrounded by a thin capsule that is circumferentially reinforced by the acromioclavicular ligament. The coracoclavicular ligament, a very strong ligament, runs from the undersurface of the clavicle to the coracoid process. It has two parts, the conoid and the trapezoid ligament.

Mechanism of Injury

The most common mechanism of injury to the acromioclavicular joint is direct trauma. Typically, this occurs when the athlete falls onto the point of the shoulder. The acromion is driven downward, rupturing the ligaments in a predictable pattern, as discussed below.

Classification

Acromioclavicular joint injuries are classified according to the amount of displacement and damage to the ligaments and surrounding muscles. The progression of injury starts with a sprain of the acromioclavicular ligament. As the force continues, the acromioclavicular ligament tears, and then the coracoclavicular ligament, and finally the scapular attachments of the deltoid and trapezius muscles.

The most basic classification divides injuries of the acromioclavicular joint into three grades.[1] A Grade I injury is an incomplete tear of the acromioclavicular ligament. The coracoclavicular ligament and the deltoid and trapezius muscles remain intact. A Grade II injury is associated with complete disruption of the acromioclavicular ligament but not complete separation of the joint surfaces. The coracoclavicular ligament remains essentially intact, as do the deltoid and trapezius muscles. A Grade III injury involves a complete tear of both the acromioclavicular ligament and the coracoclavicular ligament. There is some detachment of the deltoid and trapezius muscles from the scapula. Rockwood has established a classification with six types that is useful clinically (Fig. 43–1).[2] The first three types are the same as the three grades established by Tossy and coworkers described above.[1] The three types Rockwood adds are variations of the Type III (or Grade III) injury. The Type IV injury is a Type III injury in which the clavicle dislocates posteriorly instead of superiorly. Type V injury is a severe form of the Type III injury in which there is extensive disruption of the deltoid and trapezius muscles. Type VI injury involves complete disruption of the acromioclavicular ligament and coracoclavicular ligament with inferior dislocation of the clavicle.

Incidence

Acromioclavicular joint injuries are quite common. They frequently affect athletes, especially male athletes. Incomplete injuries (Types I and II) are much more common than complete ones (Types III, IV, V, and VI). Type VI injuries are exceedingly rare.

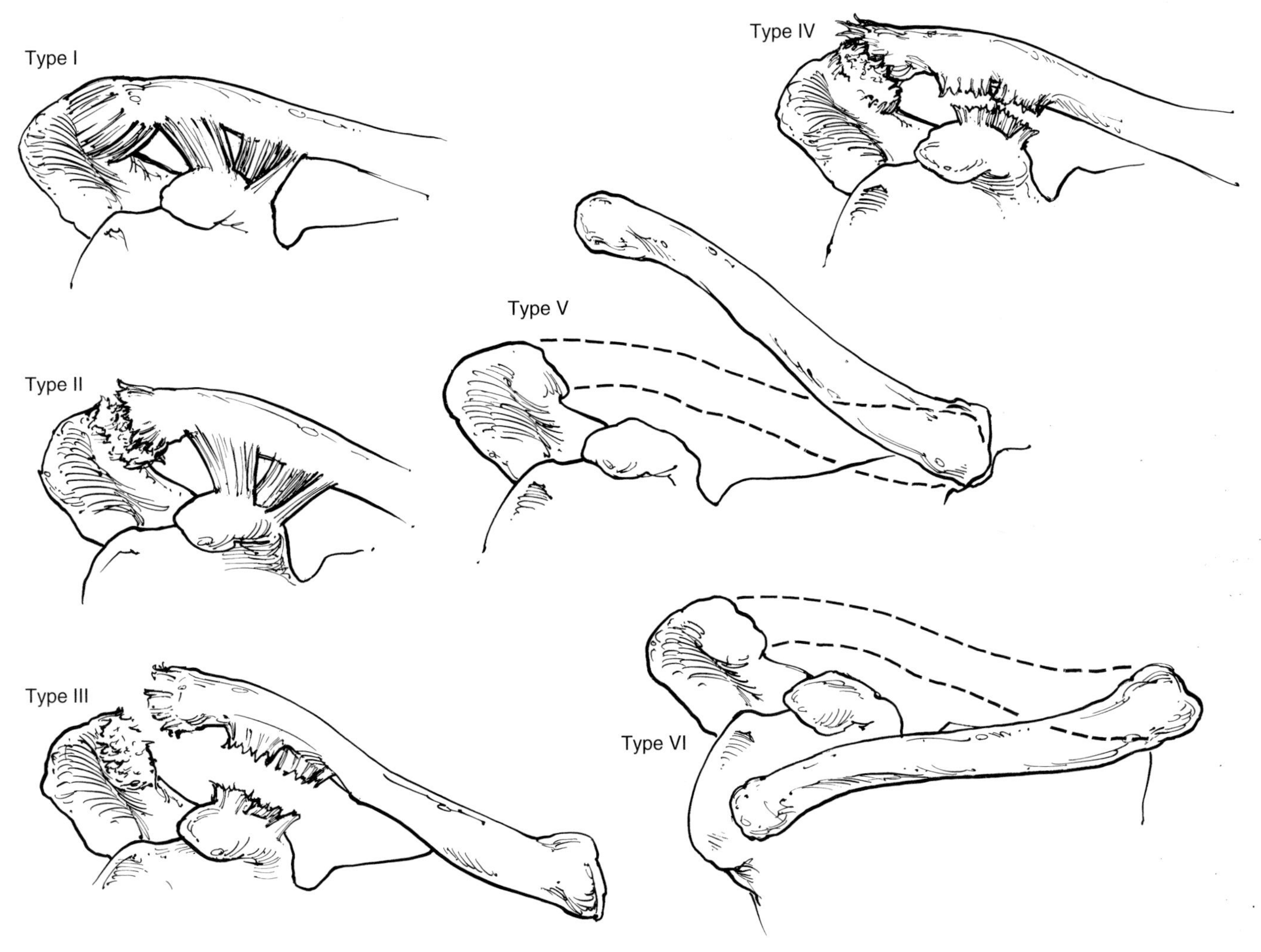

Fig. 43–1. Classification of acromioclavicular injuries. Type I, the acromioclavicular and coracoclavicular ligaments are not disrupted. Type II, acromioclavicular ligament disrupted, but the coracoclavicular ligament is intact. Type III, both acromioclavicular and coracoclavicular ligaments are disrupted. Type IV, both ligaments are disrupted and the distal end of the clavicle is displaced posteriorly. Type V, both ligaments are disrupted and the muscles are detached. Type VI, both ligaments are disrupted, and the end of the clavicle is dislocated inferiorly. (Drawn from Rockwood, C. A., Jr., and Green, D. P.: Fractures in Adults. 2nd Ed. Vol. 2. Philadelphia, J. B. Lippincott, 1984, p. 871.)

Clinical Presentation

With a Type I injury, the only sign may be point tenderness over the acromioclavicular joint. The joint remains stable and the athlete often reports only mild discomfort at the extremes of motion. With a Type II injury, there is more tenderness over the acromioclavicular joint and moderate swelling. Physical examination may reveal some laxity in the joint and a slight step-off may be felt between the acromion and the clavicle. Type III injury is characterized by even more tenderness and swelling. The clavicle is displaced superiorly in relation to the acromion. The athlete complains of pain and limited motion. Type IV injury has the same features as Type III, but the clavicle is displaced posteriorly or posterosuperiorly. Type V injury is a severe form of Type III in which the distal clavicle is displaced superiorly, occasionally with tenting of the skin. With Type VI injury, the acromion is prominent because the clavicle is displaced inferiorly. There may be severe swelling and associated neurologic or vascular injuries.

Radiographic Evaluation

An anteroposterior view of the shoulder should be taken with the beam at a 15° cephalic inclination, so that the acromioclavicular joint is displaced off the spine of the scapula. Although stress views are not routinely used, they can help distinguish Type II injury from Type III. The stress view should be taken with 10 to 15 pounds of weight tied to the wrist, *not* held in the hand. This allows the shoulder muscles to relax and avoids falsely reducing the amount of coracoclavicular separation. To check for posterior displacement, an axillary lateral or Alexander's lateral radiograph must be obtained. Alexander's view is taken with the patient standing. The patient shrugs the shoulder forward while holding the injured arm across the chest. The shoulders should be 30° to 35° off the cassette with the x-ray tube angled 15° caudad and directed at the coracoid.[3]

With Type I injury, radiographs are normal. With Type II injury, slight elevation of the clavicle and slight widening of the acromioclavicular joint may be observed. Stress views do not show a significant change in the elevation of the clavicle. In a Type III injury, the clavicle is displaced superiorly and the coracoclavicular distance is 25 to 100% greater than in the normal shoulder. In a Type IV injury, the clavicle is displaced posteriorly on the axillary or Alexander's lateral view (Fig. 43–2). There may be only slight elevation on the anteroposterior view, and there is usually widening of the acromioclavicular joint. In a Type V injury, the clavicle is displaced superiorly and the coracoclavicular distance is 100 to 300% greater than in the normal shoulder. With a Type VI injury, the clavicle is displaced inferior to the acromion or coracoid process.

Treatment of Acute Injuries

With a Type I injury the injured joint may initially be placed in a sling, to rest it. Ice and analgesics lessen the discomfort. As the symptoms subside, active range of motion is allowed as tolerated, and sports may be resumed as tolerated.

A Type II injury is also treated nonoperatively. The only point of controversy is which of the conservative options is best. Each embodies one of two philosophies. The first advocates accepting any clavicular displacement. A sling followed by early range of motion is used, as for Type I injuries. The second suggests using a device such as the Kenny Howard sling to hold the clavicle in reduced position. This requires a significant amount of continuous force over the distal clavicle for several weeks. It may cause skin ulcers under the shoulder strap, and I no longer recommend this type of treatment. Sports can be resumed when the range of motion is full and painless. A protective pad placed on the top of the shoulder of athletes involved in contact sports may be useful to prevent pain and further injury to the ligaments.

Type III injury is the most controversial, from a treatment standpoint. Many authors recommend conservative treatment for these injuries.[4,5] In a retrospective review of conservatively treated Type III acromioclavicular dislocations, Wojtys and Nelson found that strength and endurance levels of the injured and uninjured shoulder were not significantly different.[6] Tibone and coworkers also found no significant strength deficit in the 6 motions tested.[7] In a comparison of surgical and nonsurgical treatment of complete acromioclavicular dislocations, Galpin's group found nonoperative treatment gave equal or superior results and allowed earlier return to work.[8] Larsen and colleagues, who also compared surgical and nonsurgical treatment, found no difference in the clinical result between the two groups and reported more rapid return to work for those treated nonoperatively.[9] Sports may be resumed using the criteria discussed for Type II injuries.

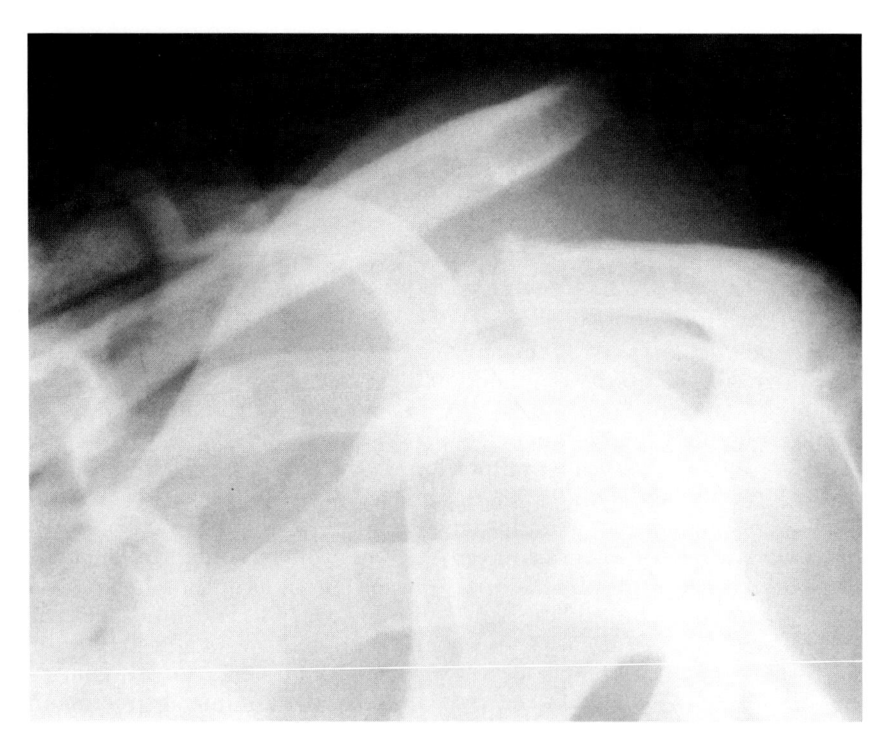

Fig. 43–2. Alexander's view shows posterior displacement of the clavicle.

While the current trend nationally is to treat Type III injuries nonoperatively, at the Hughston Clinic, the Tossy Type III injury, including Rockwood Types IV, V, and VI, is commonly treated with open reduction and internal fixation unless there was some complication or the patient does not desire operative treatment. Rockwood also recommends surgery for active patients and for those who do heavy labor. He believes this produces a stronger shoulder that holds up better under repetitive stress.

If a Type III complete dislocation of the acromioclavicular joint is treated nonoperatively, and, so, not reduced, with repetitive activity the residual joint instability may produce a dull ache in the shoulder and neck. Patients also frequently complain of the deformity. Furthermore, the resultant malfunction rarely allows an athlete to resume using the shoulder in throwing sports.

Myriad techniques are available for operative repair of acromioclavicular dislocations. All include repair of the deltotrapezius fascia, and many include repair of the coracoclavicular ligament. At the Hughston Clinic an 18-gauge wire, nonelastic nylon type suture, or braided triple strand of #0 polydioxanone suture (PDS) is used to form a double loop around the coracoid and the clavicle for fixation of the acromioclavicular reduction.[10,11] This allows some rotation of the clavicle without subluxation of the joint. Also, the torn acromioclavicular ligament and muscle avulsions (deltoid, trapezius) are repaired. Generally, an athlete with this type of repair and fixation is allowed to return to contact sports after 6 weeks. The experience at the clinic has been that these athletes have no rerupture, even when they later fall, or appear to fall, again on the point of the shoulder.

Another fairly popular form of fixation is a screw through the clavicle into the coracoid (commonly termed the *Bosworth technique*).[12] This gives rigid fixation of the clavicle to the scapula. After the ligaments heal, the screw is removed. The resultant hole leaves the clavicle weak for a time, until bony filling occurs.

In the past, transarticular Kirschner wires or screws have been used for fixation of the reduction. This generally resulted in poor stabilization, and it disrupted the joint surfaces. Also, the pins sometime broke at the joint margin and migrated.[2,13–16] This type of fixation is not recommended.

Late Complications

Historically, Type II subluxations give the poorest results, with frequent recurring pain owing to restraint of the unstable joint. Also, this instability of the opposing surfaces produces wear and tear with chronic arthritis. This arthritis may require acromioclavicular joint arthroplasty (excision of the distal end of the clavicle).

If Tossy Type III dislocations are treated nonoperatively, fatigue, aching, and soreness in the shoulder and neck muscles may result with excessive use. The patient usually complains of comparative weakness (owing to the altered biomechanics), an unsightly deformity, and an inability to excel in throwing sports and archery.

In the records of the Hughston Clinic late complications, pain, or arthritis are minimal when Type III dislocations are treated with reduction, repair, and double-loop fixation. Radiographs in the late followup period may show much soft tissue calcification; however, this usually is not disabling and does not constitute an "arthritic joint." The patient should be informed about this, so that if radiographs are taken elsewhere the reader will not be alarmed by the appearance of severe arthritic changes.

STERNOCLAVICULAR JOINT

The sternoclavicular joint is a diarthrodial joint formed by the sternal end of the clavicle, the lateral aspect of the sternum, and the cartilage of the first rib.[17] The joint is incongruous because the articular surface of the medial clavicle is much larger than that of the sternum. Therefore, responsibility for the stability of the joint falls to the soft tissues: the intra-articular disc, the costoclavicular ligament, the interclavicular ligament, and the capsular ligament. The capsular ligament, a thickening of the joint capsule, is much stronger anteriorly than posteriorly.

The medial clavicular epiphysis does not appear before age 18 years and may not unite until age 25 years.[12] This is important because many so-called sternoclavicular dislocations are really Salter-Harris Type I or II fractures.[2]

Mechanism of Injury

The most common mechanism of injury to the sternoclavicular joint is an indirect force. If a posteriorly directed force is applied to the anterolateral aspect of the shoulder, anterior instability of the sternoclavicular joint may result. If an anteriorly directed force hits the posterolateral shoulder, posterior instability may result. The sternoclavicular joint can also be dislocated from a direct force such as a posteriorly directed force to the anteromedial clavicle.[18] While significant trauma is usually required, spontaneous atraumatic anterior subluxation has been described.[19]

Classification

These injuries are best classified according to the position that the displaced clavicle assumes, anterior or posterior. The injury may result in a sprain, subluxation, or dislocation of the sternoclavicular joint.

Incidence

The sternoclavicular joint is injured much less often than the acromioclavicular joint. Anterior dislocations are much more common than posterior dislocations.

Clinical Presentation

The patient usually presents with the arm held adducted and internally rotated. Pain can be mild, moderate, or severe, depending on the degree of displacement. There is a variable amount of swelling, which may obscure any deformity. In anterior dislocations, the medial clavicle can be quite prominent. In posterior dislocations, the normal prominence of the inner clavicle is lost.

Posterior dislocation may result in difficulty swallowing or breathing if there is compression of the esophagus or trachea. The physical examination should also include assessment of venous and arterial circulation because the posteriorly displaced clavicle can compress the major vessels in the mediastinum.

Radiographic Findings

The diagnosis of sternoclavicular dislocation is readily made by physical examination. This is fortunate because routine radiographs of the sternoclavicular joint are difficult to interpret. The 40° cephalic tilt radiograph can be quite helpful in confirming the diagnosis. The x-ray tube is tilted 40° cephalad from the vertical plane. The clavicle appears anteriorly in the case of anterior dislocation and posteriorly in the case of posterior dislocation. Computed tomography (CT) is the best radiographic technique for diagnosing subluxation or dislocation of the sternoclavicular joint. It is also useful for studying the vital soft tissue structures in the mediastinum.

Treatment

A sprain results in pain without joint instability. It is managed with ice for 12 to 24 hours and immobilization in a sling for a few days. Range of motion is allowed as tolerated. When full, painless range of motion is regained, sports may be resumed. This usually takes 1 to 2 weeks.

Subluxation of the sternoclavicular joint is also treated expectantly. A figure-of-eight clavicle strap may be used, in an attempt to reduce the sternoclavicular joint, or a simple sling may be used until the pain subsides. Again, motion is allowed as tolerated. Noncontact sports are allowed when full, painless range of motion is restored. Contact sports are allowed 6 to 8 weeks after the injury.

Acute anterior sternoclavicular dislocations are usually quite easy to reduce. Unfortunately, the reduction is usually unstable and the joint redisplaces. Because of this, some authors accept the deformity and do not even attempt reduction.[20] Most, however, recommend attempting closed reduction because of the ease with which it is accomplished.[2,13,21] The patient is placed supine and given a muscle relaxant and a narcotic intravenously. Folded towels are placed between the shoulder blades. The arm is abducted to 90° and fully extended as gentle traction is placed on the arm. The medial clavicle is then pushed back into place. If the sternoclavicular joint stays reduced, it can be held with a figure-of-eight clavicle strap for 4 to 6 weeks. More commonly, the sternoclavicular joint is again displaced after traction is released. If this occurs, the arm is placed in a sling for 2 weeks, followed by range of motion exercises as tolerated. While a cosmetic deformity may persist, it seldom interferes with function. As noted previously, in patients younger than 25 years, these are usually Salter-Harris Type I or II fractures and not dislocations, so they can heal and remodel.

There is seldom an indication for open reduction and never an indication for closed reduction and percutaneous pin fixation. There are many reports of complications from pin migration, including laceration of the heart and death.[16,22] Sports are resumed according to the same criteria listed for subluxation of the sternoclavicular joint.

In acute posterior dislocation, attention should first be directed to any sign of injury to mediastinal structures. Any sign of neurovascular, tracheal, or esophageal compression requires consultation with the appropriate specialist.

In contrast to anterior sternoclavicular dislocation, the reduced joint is usually stable in posterior dislocation. It is reduced in a manner similar to the technique described for anterior dislocation, but the force is directed anteriorly. If the clavicle cannot be pulled anteriorly with the fingers, a towel clip can be placed around the medial portion. The towel clip can then be used to pull the clavicle anteriorly. This should be done in the operating room using sterile technique. The sooner closed reduction is attempted, the easier it is to perform. After 48 hours, closed reduction is seldom possible.[18] Because of the risk of compression of the mediastinal structures, open reduction is necessary if closed reduction is unsuccessful. After reduction, the shoulders are immobilized in a figure-of-eight clavicle strap or a spica cast. Immobilization should continue for 4 to 6 weeks, and contact sports are interdicted for an additional 6 to 8 weeks. Late complications are rare.

REFERENCES

1. Tossy, J. D., Mead, N. C., and Sigmond, H. M.: Acromioclavicular separations: Useful and practical classification for treatment. Clin Orthop. *28*:111, 1963.
2. Rockwood, C. A. Jr.: Subluxations and dislocations about the shoulder. *In* Fractures in Adults. Vol. 2. 2nd Ed. Edited by C. A. Rockwood, Jr., and D. P. Green. Philadelphia, J. B. Lippincott, 1984.

3. Waldrop, J. I., Norwood, L. A., and Alvarez, R. G.: Lateral roentgenographic projections of the acromioclavicular joint. Am. J. Sports Med. *9*:337, 1981.
4. Glick, J. M., et al.: Dislocated acromioclavicular joint: Follow-up study of 35 unreduced acromioclavicular dislocations. Am. J. Sports Med. *5*:264, 1977.
5. Bjerneld, H., Hovelius, L., and Thorling, J.: Acromioclavicular separations treated conservatively. Acta. Orthop. Scand. *54*:743, 1983.
6. Wojtys, E. M., and Nelson, G.: Conservative treatment of grade III acromioclavicular dislocations. Clin. Orthop. *268*:112, 1991.
7. Tibone, J., Sellers, R., and Tonino, P.: Strength testing after third-degree acromioclavicular dislocations. Am. J. Sports Med. *20*:328, 1992.
8. Galpin, R. O., Hawkins, R. J., and Grainger, R. W.: A comparative analysis of operative versus non-operative treatment of grade III acromioclavicular separations. Clin. Orthop. *193*:150, 1985.
9. Larsen, E., Bjerg-Nielsen, A., and Christensen, P.: Conservative or surgical treatment of acromioclavicular dislocation. J. Bone Joint Surg. *68A*:552, 1986.
10. Warren, R. F., Hawkins, R. J., and Noble, J. S.: Suture repair technique for acute and chronic acromioclavicular joint dislocations. Presented at American Academy of Orthopaedic Surgeons Annual Meeting, Tape VT-23119, San Francisco, 1993.
11. Bearden, J. M., Hughston, J. C., and Whatley, G. S.: Acromioclavicular dislocation: Method of treatment. J. Sports Med. *1*:5, 1973.
12. Bosworth, B. M.: Acromioclavicular separation. Surg. Gynecol. Obstet. *73*:866, 1941.
13. Rockwood, C. A. Jr., and Matsen, F. A. III (eds.): The Shoulder. Philadelphia, W. B. Saunders, 1990.
14. Richards, R. R.: Acromioclavicular joint injuries. AAOS Instr. Course Lect. *42*:259, 1993.
15. Taft, T. N., Wilson, F. C., and Oglesby, J. W.: Dislocation of the acromioclavicular joint. J. Bone Joint Surg. *69A*:1045, 1987.
16. Lyons, F. A., and Rockwood, C. A. Jr.: Migration of pins used in operations on the shoulder. J. Bone Joint Surg. *72A*:1262, 1990.
17. Pick, T. P., and Howden, R. (eds): Gray's Anatomy. 15th Ed. New York, Bounty Books, 1977.
18. Selesnick, F. H., Jablon, M., Frank, C., and Post, M.: Retrosternal dislocation of the clavicle. J. Bone Joint Surg. *66A*:287, 1984.
19. Rockwood, C. A. Jr., and Odor, J. M.: Spontaneous atraumatic anterior subluxation of the sternoclavicular joint. J. Bone Joint Surg. *71A*:1280, 1989.
20. Bigliani, L. U.: Shoulder: Trauma. *In* Orthopaedic Knowledge Update 2. Park Ridge, IL, American Academy of Orthopaedic Surgeons, 1987.
21. Warren, R. F.: The acromioclavicular and sternoclavicular joints. *In* Surgery of the Musculoskeletal System. 2nd Ed. Edited by C. M. Evarts. New York, Churchill Livingstone, 1990.
22. Daus, G. P., Drez, D., Jr., Newton, B. B. Jr., and Kober, R.: Migration of a Kirschner wire from the sternum to the right ventricle. Am. J. Sports Med. *21*:321, 1993.

44 *Bernard G. Kirol, Robert M. Shalvoy, Franklin D. Wilson, and David Harsha*

Shoulder Instability

Acute Glenohumeral Instability

Bernard G. Kirol

The shoulder is the most frequently dislocated large joint in the body. Little inherent bony stability is present at the glenohumeral articulation, which can be described as similar to a golf ball on a tee. Here, soft tissue structures are more important than bony structures in resisting instability. The capsuloligamentous complex has a wide range of motion and is subjected to considerable stress. The inferior glenohumeral ligament provides the most stability when the arm is in the vulnerable position of abduction and external rotation.[1] The fibrocartilaginous glenoid labrum is firmly attached to bone below the level of the glenoid equator and also contributes to stability. Rotator cuff and periscapular musculature dynamically positions and stabilizes the shoulder joint.

CLINICAL HISTORY

The clinical history should focus on the athlete's mechanism of injury to determine the arm position and magnitude of force that was present during the instability episode. Anterior dislocation, by far the most common type,[2] occurs when the arm is in abduction, extension, and external rotation. If the injury occurs while the arm is flexed and adducted, a posterior dislocation may occur. Seizures also commonly result in a posterior dislocation. In an acute shoulder injury, a violent mechanism of injury, such as contact during a football game, is more likely to produce a dislocation, while a noncontact injury sustained throwing a baseball is more likely to produce a subluxation.

PHYSICAL EXAMINATION

Physical examination of the acute anteriorly dislocated shoulder is usually sufficient to make the diagnosis. The shoulder is very painful with spasm of the surrounding musculature. The patient holds his or her arm in an externally rotated, mildly abducted posture. The humeral head can usually be palpated in the anteriorly dislocated position. Neurovascular examination is mandatory, and the examiner should pay special attention to the presence of distal pulses, as well as to the function of the axillary nerve, the nerve most commonly injured during an anterior dislocation.[3]

Recognition of a posterior dislocation requires a higher index of suspicion. The patient holds the arm across the body in an adducted and internally rotated position, similar to the position held as a player comes off the field after many types of shoulder injuries. Closer examination will reveal an inability to externally rotate the arm past 0°, a palpable posterior prominence, and a more noticeable coracoid process on the dislocated side.

RADIOGRAPHIC EVALUATION

Radiographs are an essential part of the clinical evaluation of a shoulder dislocation. They are used to 1) confirm the direction of dislocation; 2) identify any associated fractures; and 3) reveal possible barriers to reduction. Three radiographic views are commonly taken. The first is an anteroposterior view in the plane of the scapula, which will show the humeral head completely out of the socket (Fig. 44–1). With posterior shoulder dislocations, the humeral head may overlap glenoid surfaces, making recognition difficult. Second, a lateral view in the plane of the scapula, or "Y" view, is taken. The humeral head will be located anterior to the glenoid in an anterior dislocation and vice versa in a posterior dislocation. The third view obtained is an axillary view. Although the arm cannot easily be abducted very far, every attempt should be made to obtain this view because it shows any humeral head compression fractures (e.g., Hill-Sachs lesion) or glenoid rim fractures (e.g., Bankart lesion) as well as an anteriorly or posteriorly dislocated humerus. After the dislocation is reduced, a postreduction series of radiographs is always obtained to ensure the adequacy of reduction and to document any fractures that may have occurred during the reduction.

TREATMENT

Acute Traumatic Anterior Dislocations

Acute traumatic anterior dislocations should be reduced as quickly and atraumatically as possible. Early relocation reduces the amount of compression on neurovascular structures. Before any reduction attempt, the patient must be as relaxed as possible. Otherwise, the dislocation may be irreducible unless excessive force is used, resulting in additional trauma to the joint surfaces. Usually, narcotic sedation is used in a monitored environment. However, if a patient is relaxed enough, reduction without sedation may be attempted. Although radiographs are preferable before the relocation, physicians covering sporting events may be able to perform a reduction easily on the scene before excessive spasm compromises their effort.

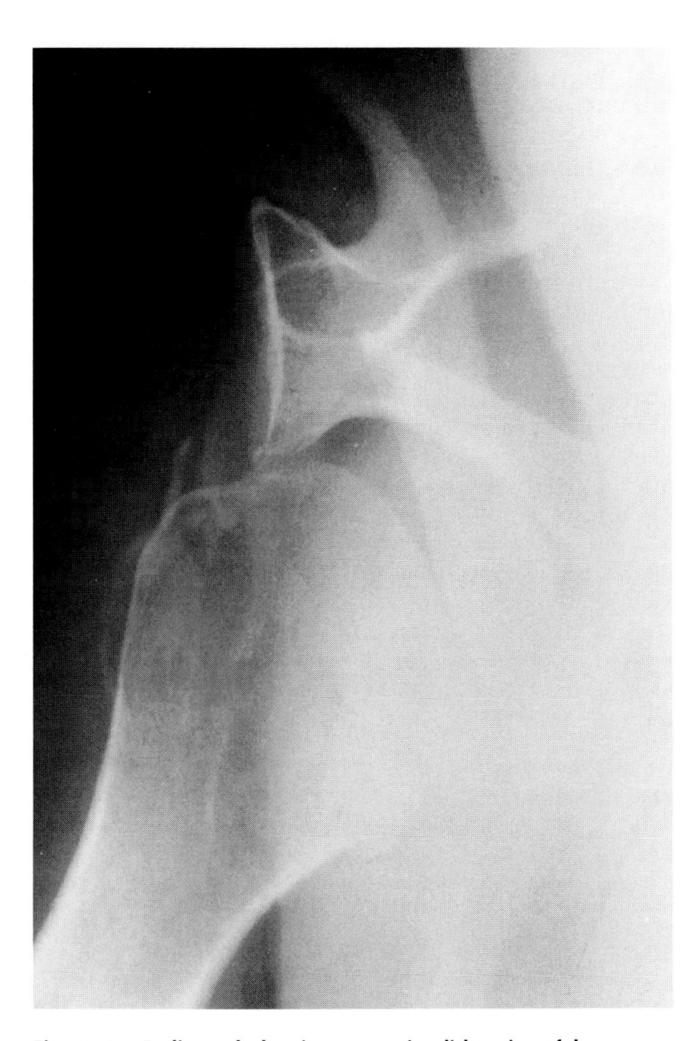

Fig. 44–1. Radiograph showing a posterior dislocation of the humeral head.

The abduction and external rotation technique is one of the more effective methods of reduction to use on the field. This can be done with the patient supine or prone. While abducting and externally rotating the arm, use your thumb to push the humeral head back in place. Another method, traction and countertraction (Fig. 44–2), is useful if an assistant and a table are available. In this method, longitudinal traction is applied to the arm in line with the deformity while the arm is gently externally rotated. Countertraction is applied using a sheet wrapped around the chest. Finally, the Hippocratic method is another useful single-person technique. With the patient supine pull in-line traction on the injured arm using external rotation as needed, while placing your foot along the chest wall just below—never in—the axilla.

Postreduction management includes the use of a sling for comfort. Circumduction exercises are begun once initial spasm subsides during the first few days, and the sling is soon discarded. Range of motion exercises, working toward increasing abduction and external rotation as well as rotator cuff strengthening, are instituted. When the patient has full range of motion and strength, he or she may return to competition. A brace that limits abduction and external rotation may be used for return to some sports (e.g., football lineman or fullback) for added protection. A change in position may also be considered. For example, a two-way starter at fullback and linebacker might be limited to playing the offensive position only. This will help prevent the abduction and external rotation stress imposed during tackling.

Acute Traumatic Posterior Dislocations

The same general principles that apply to posterior dislocation also apply to anterior dislocations: neurovascular injury must be ruled out, the timing of the reduction is important, the patient must be relaxed before reduction is attempted, and the proper radiographs must be obtained. Patients with acute posterior dislocations have considerably more pain and usually require narcotic pain relief before reduction.

Reduction takes place with the patient supine. Traction is applied with the arm adducted in line with the deformity, using internal rotation as necessary while lateral traction is simultaneously applied to the upper humerus by an assistant. Care must be taken to avoid externally rotating the arm so forcefully as to produce a humeral head or glenoid fracture.

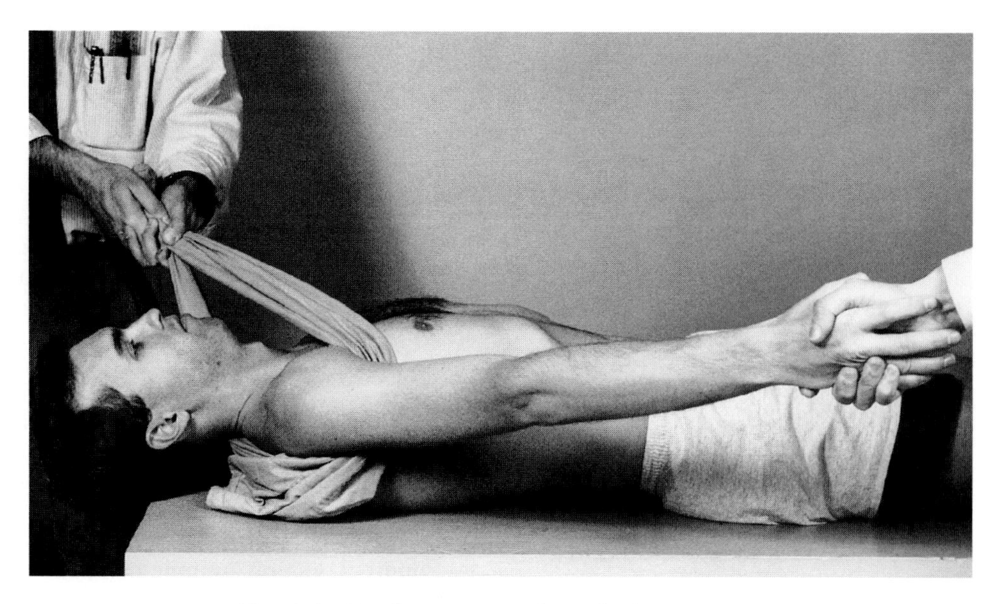

Fig. 44–2. Traction-countertraction reduction maneuver.

If the glenohumeral joint is stable after reduction, a sling and swathe are applied. An abduction/external rotation brace should be used if the shoulder tends to subluxate or redislocate. Wrist and elbow movement should begin immediately. Range of motion and rotator cuff strengthening exercises should be started in the stable shoulder once initial discomfort subsides. The athlete may return to competition when full range of motion and strength return. No effective brace exists for return to sports after a posterior dislocation.

PROGNOSIS

Recurrent dislocation is the most common complication after an acute traumatic anterior shoulder dislocation. The patient's age at the time of dislocation is the major predictor of the incidence of recurrence. In patients under 20 years of age this incidence is usually reported to be between 80 and 100%. In patients over 40 years of age, the incidence of recurrence drops to between 10 and 15%. The athletic population is at greater risk for redislocation than nonathletes.[4]

Several authors have noted that the difference in the redislocation rates is not affected by the type or length of immobilization.[5,6] Neither shoulder dominance nor shoulder strength seems to play a role. However, recurrences are more common in men than women by a factor of four to one. The recurrence rate also increases with the increasing severity of the initial dislocation trauma.[7] In a young athlete, the chance of a dislocation producing an unstable shoulder is extremely high.

Fractures may be associated with dislocations that result from high-energy trauma. Glenoid rim and humeral head compression fractures are associated with both anterior and posterior dislocations. Greater tuberosity fractures are usually associated with anterior dislocations, and lesser tuberosity fractures with posterior dislocations. Greater tuberosity fractures seen with anterior dislocations occur more often in elderly patients. When such a fracture is present in a young athlete, the redislocation rate is much lower than in cases without accompanying fracture. Anatomic considerations offer an explanation for this phenomenon. In an isolated anterior dislocation, the capsuloligamentous structures, and often the labrum, are torn from their bony attachments, rendering the ligaments less competent. If avulsion of the greater tuberosity occurs before extensive soft tissue injury, the fracture may heal with the ligaments intact, helping to prevent future dislocations.

Because recurrence is so common in the athletic population, rehabilitation alone is not always successful in producing a stable shoulder joint. Surgery can even be performed as an initial treatment of choice if soft tissue interposition is blocking the initial reduction, or if a significantly displaced tuberosity or glenoid rim fracture is present. Likewise, surgery may ultimately be necessary in the patient with an acute traumatic dislocation that fails rehabilitation and redislocates. Anterior shoulder reconstruction surgeries are usually directed toward tightening the capsuloligamentous structures and reattaching the torn labrum (if present) at the front of the shoulder joint.

REFERENCES

1. Turkel, S. J., Panio, M. W., Marshall, J. L., and Girgis, F. G.: Stabilizing mechanisms preventing anterior dislocation of the glenohumeral joint. J. Bone Joint Surg. *63A*:1208, 1981.
2. Cave, E. F., Burke, J. F., and Boyd, R. J. (eds.): Trauma Management. Chicago, Year Book Publishers, 1974.
3. Blom, S., and Dahlback, L.: Nerve injuries in dislocations of the shoulder joint and fractures of the neck of the humerus. Acta Chir. Scand. *136*:461, 1970.
4. Simonet, W. T., and Cofield, R. H.: Prognosis in anterior shoulder dislocation. Am. J. Sports Med. *12*:19, 1984.

5. McLaughlin, H. L., and Cavallaro, W. U.: Primary anterior dislocation of the shoulder. Am. J. Surg. *80*:615, 1950.
6. Hovelius, L., et al.: Recurrences after initial dislocation of the shoulder: Results of a prospective study of treatment. J. Bone Joint Surg. *65A*:343, 1983.
7. Rowe, C. R., and Sakellarides, H. T.: Factors related to recurrences of anterior dislocations of the shoulder. Clin. Orthop. *20*:40, 1961.

SUGGESTED READINGS

Matsen, F. A. III (ed.): The Shoulder. A Balance of Mobility and Stability. Rosemont, IL, American Academy of Orthopaedic Surgeons, 1993.
Rockwood, C. A., Jr., and Matsen, F. A. III (eds.): The Shoulder. Philadelphia, W. B. Saunders, 1990.

Recurrent Glenohumeral Instability

Robert M. Shalvoy

Recurrent instability of the glenohumeral joint is a challenging problem with many recent developments that have led to an evolution of treatment. Recurrent instability defines a state in which the humeral head is insufficiently contained by the restraints of the shoulder. The result is a spectrum of disorders ranging from recurrent frank dislocations of the joint, to gross subluxations of the humeral head, to more subtle subluxations that, over time, present as shoulder pain and weakness, impairing function and performance.

Management of the chronically unstable shoulder requires an understanding of the various forms of the problem and how they occur. A thorough assessment of the athlete and proper diagnosis open the gate to the most appropriate treatment and allow for an efficient return to competition.

The problem of recurrent dislocations after trauma is only part of the problem of recurrent shoulder instability. Progressive instability from repetitive microtrauma, such as swimming or pitching, and instability without trauma in the hypermobile individual can lead to a number of disorders all involving the inability to appropriately contain the humeral head within the shoulder complex. Likewise, results are not assessed simply in terms of recurrent dislocations but by function, including a return to athletic performance. Matching treatment to the specific problem is the surest guarantee of a good result.

CLASSIFICATION

Classifying recurrent shoulder instability allows for a better understanding of an individual's prognosis, treatment, and proper follow-up. Subgroups are used to define the direction, cause, and degree of instability, as well as the patient's control or volition. *Direction* refers to the location of the humeral head in reference to the glenoid. It can be anterior (most common), posterior, inferior, or multidirectional. The *cause* of instability can be traumatic, as in a previous primary dislocation, or the cumulative result of repetitive microtraumatic events, such as pitching. It can also be atraumatic, as in hyperplastic, hyperlax individuals with instability. The *degree of instability* describes a state of frank dislocations or varying amounts of joint subluxation. *Patient control* is determined by whether the events are voluntary and controlled, or involuntary in occurrence.

No category or subgroup stands on its own. One must understand the place and relative importance of each category to make a complete assessment of what can be a complex as well as a subtle problem. Matsen has generalized recurrent instability into two groups using the acronyms TUBS and AMBRI.[1] TUBS (Traumatic, Unidirectional, Bankart, Surgery) refers to those patients with a history of *trauma* resulting in a *unidirectional* instability. Because anterior dislocation is most common, these shoulders have *Bankart* lesions or ruptures of glenohumeral ligaments at the glenoid rim that require *surgery*. Conversely, AMBRI (Atraumatic, Multidirectional, Bilateral, Rehabilitation, Inferior capsular shift) describes *atraumatic* instability that is more commonly *multidirectional* as well as *bilateral*. *Rehabilitation* is the treatment of choice for this type of instability, but if surgery is necessary an *inferior capsular shift* should be done.

ANATOMY

Stability of the shoulder depends on several anatomic factors, some of which are static and others dynamic. Static stabilizers include the glenoid, labrum, glenohumeral ligaments, and coracohumeral ligament. The dynamic stabilizers of the shoulder are the rotator cuff, the subscapularis, and the long head of the biceps. Anatomic variations as well as injury to these structures can lead to recurrent instability.

With many variables working in a delicate balance, any one of these stabilizers may be deficient, resulting in instability. When viewed arthroscopically tearing of the labrum is the most visible change. The tear is located inferiorly and is caused by shearing loads of the humeral head as it translocates. Detachment of the thickened anterior inferior quadrant where the inferior glenohumeral ligament attaches constitutes a classic Bankart lesion, which indicates anterior inferior instability. The next most visible lesion is the Hill-Sachs lesion, a compression fracture of the posterior aspect of the humeral head. When the humeral head is translocated anteriorly, the edge of the lesion can be seen to correspond with the anterior inferior edge of the glenoid. Stretching of the middle glenohumeral ligament and stretching or tearing of the inferior glenohumeral ligament are also seen arthroscopically. In cases of posterior instability stretching of the posterior capsule is seen. Other changes associated with instability include superior labral tears at the biceps attachment, rotator cuff tears, and changes in the articular surface.[2]

PRESENTATION

The symptoms of chronic anterior instability include pain and apprehension as well as instability or giving way of the shoulder, especially during abduction and external rotation. This describes the most common form of recurrent subluxation in the throwing arm of baseball pitchers. Repetitive stress from throwing causes attenuation of the anterior capsule and eventual subluxation. During the wind-up phase, pain and clicking may be present anteriorly. Often, however, the pain may be located posteriorly or associated with the follow-through phase of pitching. Pain in the posterior area of the shoulder can be associated with posterior instability as well as anterior instability. Any pain that is associated with a particular phase of throwing is generally due to underlying instability.[3] It is not uncommon for pitchers with instability to develop a secondary impingement syndrome with signs and symptoms of both conditions present, making the diagnosis of instability more difficult or at least more subtle.

Athletes with posterior instability also present with pain that may be located posteriorly or anteriorly. Symptoms can be reproduced through adduction, flexion, and internal rotation of the arm. This may be seen in pitchers as well as in the lead arm of batters. Offensive linemen in football, freestyle swimmers, and tennis players with strong backhand strokes are also susceptible to posterior instability.

Multidirectional instability almost always has some component of inferior instability. For that reason, in addition to symptoms of anterior or posterior instability, patients frequently present with pain and clicking while the arm is in the dependent position, and commonly exhibit a sulcus sign. Generally, these patients are more continuously disabled in terms of their activity than would be the case in a unidirectional instability.

PHYSICAL EXAMINATION

The examination starts with a general observation, looking for asymmetry or atrophy of the shoulder and its musculature. An assessment for generalized ligamentous laxity includes evaluation of the contralateral shoulder, as well as evaluation of the knees, elbows, and metacarpophalangeal joints of the hand for hyperextension as well as the thumbs for hypermobility. The cervical spine should be evaluated to rule out cervical disc disease and cervical radiculopathy.

Examination of the shoulder starts with palpation to elicit areas of tenderness. The rotator cuff and subacromial space may be tender anteriorly, posteriorly, or laterally. The biceps tendon and the glenohumeral interval, both anteriorly and posteriorly, may be tender as well. Range of motion is assessed to evaluate shoulder flexion, abduction, and rotation. Rotation should be checked in both 0° and 90° of shoulder abduction. Patients with anterior instability commonly lack external rotation in abduction secondary to apprehension; however, losses of up to 20° in abduction are common. A complete motor examination should be performed to assess any weakness and rule out a neurogenic cause of shoulder pain or weakness. Particular attention should be paid to the external rotators, i.e., the rotator cuff, to assess integrity and strength. The most important part of the examination is a series of stress tests to evaluate joint stability in various directions. These are best performed in both the sitting and supine positions.

Load-and-Shift Test

The load-and-shift test can be used to test for both anterior and posterior instability. A force is applied in line with the humerus to compress the glenohumeral joint. With the opposite hand, the examiner cradles the glenohumeral joint with the thumb in front and the remaining four fingers behind. The arm is then levered or translated anteriorly and posteriorly, back and forth, assessing for a "clunk" as the humeral head exits the glenoid, or for the reproduction of the patient's symptoms (Fig. 44–3). The zone of instability can be uncovered by varying humeral abduction and adduction.

Apprehension Test

The apprehension test is performed with the patient's arm in abduction and external rotation. The examiner pushes anteriorly on the posterior humeral head (Fig. 44–4A). The patient experiences pain if the joint is unstable and apprehension if it is prone to recurrent dislocations.

Relocation Test

The relocation test is performed in conjunction with the apprehension test. A posteriorly directed force is

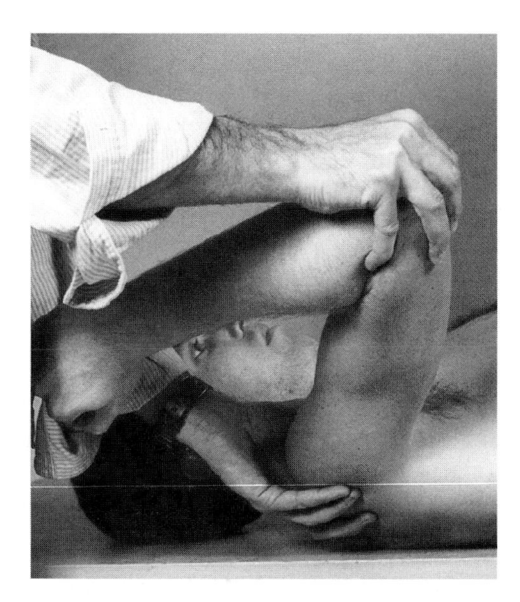

Fig. 44–3. The load-and-shift or "clunk" test.

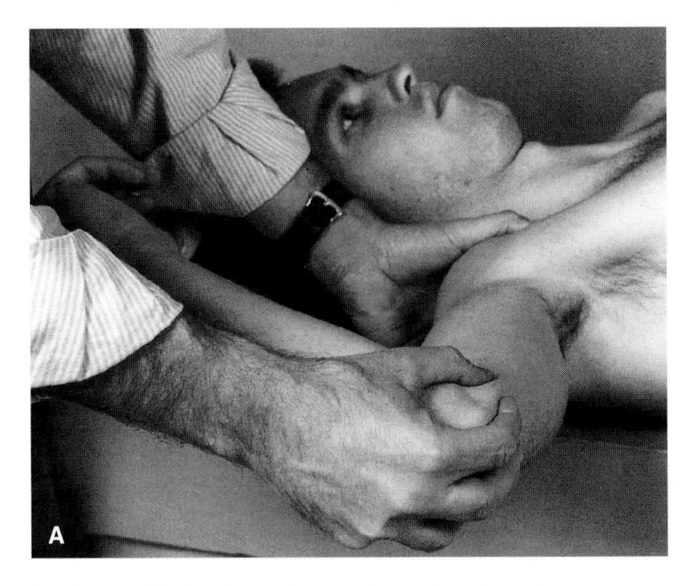

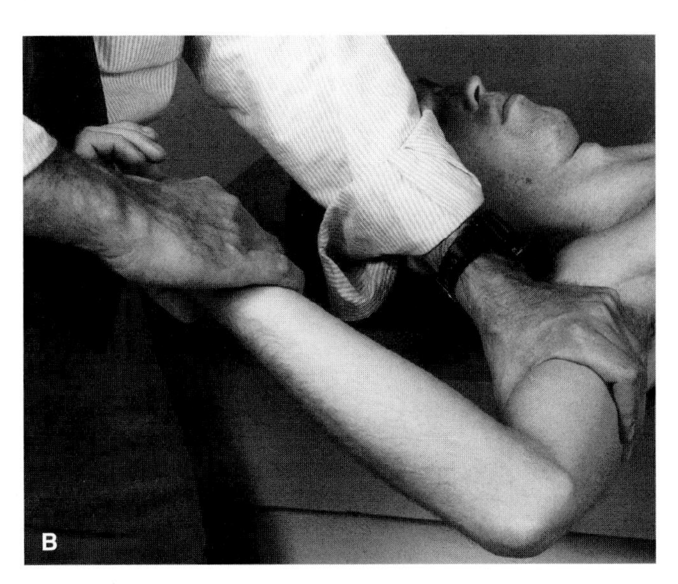

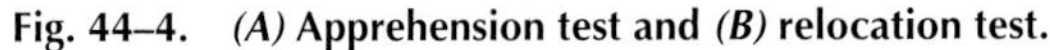
Fig. 44–4. ***(A)*** **Apprehension test and** ***(B)*** **relocation test.**

now placed on the humeral head from the front (Fig. 44–4B). Patients with pain from the apprehension test will see their pain resolved, allowing for greater external rotation with less pain.

Sulcus Sign

The sulcus sign is used to test for inferior instability. A downward force is applied through the humerus while the patient is in a sitting position. The lateral acromion is observed and palpated for an opening, or sulcus, created by inferior translation of the humeral head. This is commonly seen in multidirectional instability.

RADIOLOGIC STUDIES

Routine evaluation includes an anteroposterior, axillary, and subacromial outlet view. When recurrent instability is suspected, special views can be obtained to reveal the underlying pathologic causes. For example, the West Point view provides a tangential view of the anterior inferior rim of the glenoid, where a Bankart lesion would be found.[4] The Stryker notch view is obtained with the patient supine and the film cassette under the shoulder. This view demonstrates defects in the humeral head, such as a Hill-Sachs lesion.[5]

The computed tomography (CT) arthrogram can reveal further detail of glenoid rim defects and other bony abnormalities. It is an excellent test for labral damage and may show changes in the anterior capsule as well. Magnetic resonance imaging (MRI) is a relatively new method for imaging the glenohumeral joint. It can be used to evaluate bony pathologic changes as well as labral tears and capsular injury.

TREATMENT

Any treatment plan for recurrent instability must be thoroughly customized to meet the needs of the patient. The direction, cause, and degree of instability must be taken into account, as well as the sport activity of the patient and the expectations or level of performance anticipated. Timing within the framework of the athletic season must also be considered in forming a treatment plan.

Anterior Instability

All forms of instability initially should be treated to reduce any inflammation present. This is followed by treatment to strengthen the dynamic stabilizers of the shoulder. In the case of anterior instability, emphasis is placed on strengthening the subscapularis and the infraspinatus of the rotator cuff.

Traumatic instability is frequently associated with treatable pathologic changes identifiable on radiographs, CT arthrograms, or MRI, or via arthroscopy. Athletes with recurrent dislocations are best treated surgically at the end of the season. Those with subluxations may respond to a supervised rehabilitation program to strengthen the dynamic stabilizers. Surgical repair is indicated for those who fail to improve.

Surgery should directly address the pathologic structures. The Bankart procedure is used to reattach the glenohumeral ligaments to the anterior inferior glenoid rim. The anterior capsule is commonly reefed, and the results are excellent for eliminating recurrent dislocations, apprehension, and pain.[6]

Athletes involved in collision sports such as football and basketball respond well to a Bankart procedure or similar repairs that reduce capsular volume. Throwing athletes require special consideration because external rotation must be preserved along with muscle function. Arthroscopic reconstruction may be indicated if the injury occurs near the end of the playing season. While arthroscopic surgery minimizes surgical trauma, long-term results have yet to approach the success of open reconstruction.[7] Jobe has described a capsulolabral reconstruction for throwing athletes that, when performed with capsular repair, reinforces the labrum without excessive shortening. The subscapularis is split and not detached, enhancing proprioception and function.[3]

The athlete's demands and expectations vary by season, especially in the scholastic population. This should be taken into account when devising a treatment program. A Bankart procedure necessary for treating a football injury may prevent that athlete from pitching during the following baseball season.

Patients with repetitive microtrauma and atraumatic instability rarely present with dislocation. Subluxation is a more common problem with these patients, and supervised rehabilitation is recommended. Arthroscopy may be indicated to assess and treat secondary damage, such as labral tears and rotator cuff tears. Controlling symptoms in this manner may be necessary for the rehabilitation program to be successful. For those who fail to improve through rehabilitative exercise, surgery is indicated. Surgery is aimed at reducing capsular volume and tightening attenuated tissues, and Neer's capsular shift addresses both with excellent results.[8] In throwing athletes, Jobe's capsulolabral reconstruction is the treatment of choice for achieving stability and preserving function.

Multidirectional Instability

Multidirectional instability usually is atraumatic and associated with hypermobility. It should always be treated with rehabilitative exercise to stabilize the shoulder girdle and strengthen the dynamic stabilizers. Surgery is reserved for those who fail conservative treatment and demonstrate continued impairment.

Repetitive microtrauma may be superimposed on a hypermobile shoulder with multidirectional instability. This may create symptoms of a unidirectional instability (anterior or posterior). A thorough physical examination should differentiate the two.

Global shoulder strengthening is necessary to stabilize the joint. Treating one component or direction of instability results in accentuating the others. Surgery for failed rehabilitation must likewise treat the entire problem. Neer's capsular shift is designed to eliminate capsular redundancy anteriorly, inferiorly, and posteriorly, effectively treating multidirectional instability.[8] A Bankart or anterior repair, however, will accentuate posterior instability. Jobe's capsulolabral reconstruction is indicated in throwing athletes with multidirectional instability, because inferior redundancy is adequately controlled.

Posterior Instability

Posterior instability is relatively rare, and surgical indications are even rarer. Evidence of multidirectional instability should be sought. Athletes with symptoms of posterior instability should be diligently rehabilitated with strengthening of the scapular stabilizers and rotator cuff, especially the infraspinatus and teres minor. Surgical repair is reserved for the most severe cases, as results have been less than encouraging.[9]

RETURN TO PLAY

The criteria for safe and effective return to activity are full range of motion without pain and adequate shoulder strength. Patients with recurrent dislocations may continue to play in season if these criteria are met. A protective harness may be worn to reduce further episodes although some function will be compromised. Athletes undergoing rehabilitation programs may continue to be active as long as symptoms are controlled. Rest may be necessary before strengthening can be successful. Pitchers may need to change positions and swimmers change their events as long as symptoms persist.

Postoperatively, athletes need a mandatory rest period to allow healing, followed by a four- to six-month rehabilitation program before returning to competition. Throwing athletes require a specific return-to-throw program initiated following rehabilitation to gradually develop their throwing ability.[10] Surgery for posterior instability may require six to twelve months before the athlete can return to competition.

REFERENCES

1. Matsen, F. A., III, Thomas, S. C., and Rockwood, C. A., Jr.: Anterior glenohumeral instability. *In* The Shoulder. Edited by C. A. Rockwood, Jr., and F. A. Matsen, III. Philadelphia, W. B. Saunders, 1990.
2. Caspari, R. B., and Geissler, W. B.: Arthroscopic manifestations of shoulder subluxation and dislocation. Clin. Orthop. *291*:54, 1993.
3. Jobe, F. W., and Kvitne, R. S.: Shoulder pain in the overhand or throwing athlete. Orthop. Rev. *18*:963, 1989.
4. Rokous, J. R., Feagin, J. A., and Abbott, H. G.: Modified axillary roentgenogram. Clin. Orthop. *82*:84, 1972.
5. Engebretsen, L., and Craig, E. V.: Radiologic features of shoulder instability. Clin. Orthop. *291*:29, 1993.
6. Rowe, C. R., Patel, D., and Southmayd, W. W.: The Bankart procedure: A long-term end-result study. J. Bone Joint Surg. *60A*:1, 1978.
7. Esch, J. C.: Surgical arthroscopy of the shoulder: Anterior instability. *In* Arthroscopic Surgery. The Shoulder and Elbow. Edited by J. C. Esch and C. L. Baker. Philadelphia, J. B. Lippincott, 1993.
8. Neer, C. S., and Foster, C. R.: Inferior capsular shift for involuntary inferior and multidirectional instability of the shoulder. J. Bone Joint Surg. *62A*:897, 1980.
9. Tibone, J. E., and Bradley, J. P.: The treatment of posterior subluxation in athletes. Clin. Orthop. *291*:124, 1993.
10. Jobe, F. W., Tibone, J. E., Jobe, C. M., and Kvitne, R. S.: The shoulder in sports. *In* The Shoulder. Edited by C. A. Rockwood, Jr., and F. A. Matsen, III. Philadelphia, W. B. Saunders, 1990.

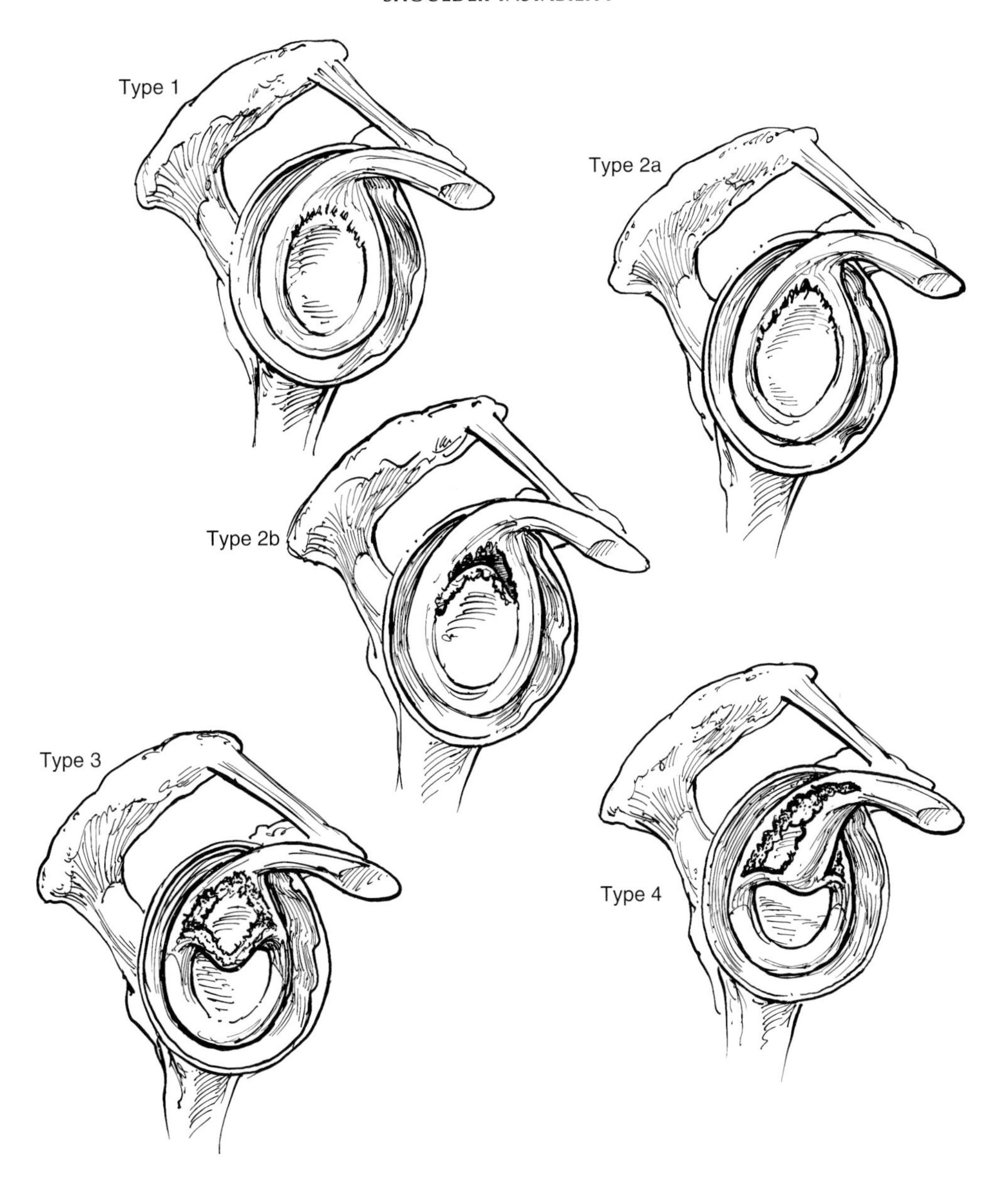

Fig. 44–5. **Type 1 lesion *(upper left)* with fraying of the superior labrum. Type 2a lesion *(upper right)* with fraying, as in Type 1, together with partial separation of the underlying labrum. Type 2b lesion *(center)* with separation of the superior labrum from the underlying glenoid. Type 3 lesion *(lower left)* with a displaced bucket-handle tear that leaves the biceps tendon intact. Type 4 lesion *(lower right)* with a bucket-handle tear that extends into the biceps tendon.**

SLAP Lesions of the Shoulder

Franklin D. Wilson and David Harsha

Superior labrum anterior posterior (SLAP) tears of the glenoid labrum are a unique constellation of shoulder injuries. They represent a set of labral injuries first described by Snyder et al. in 1990.[1] Four types of SLAP tears have been identified (Fig. 44–5). A Type 1 lesion involves fraying of the superior labrum. A Type 2 tear, the most common type, has fraying of the labrum as in a Type 1 injury, as well as separation of the labrum from the underlying glenoid. We have found some variation in Type 2 lesions with a gradation in their severity. What we have called a "Type 2a" lesion involves fraying similar to Type 1 injuries, plus a partial separation of the labrum from its underlying attachment. A "Type 2b" lesion involves total separation or avulsion of a significant portion of the labrum from the glenoid. Type 3 lesions present as bucket-handle tears of the superior labrum with central displacement of the tear into the joint space. Peripheral portions of the labrum remain intact. Finally, a Type 4 lesion involves a bucket-handle tear of the superior labrum that extends into the biceps tendon. The biceps tendon and torn labrum can displace into the joint space.

SLAP lesions may occur as isolated tears or in combination with associated conditions. Conditions often found in conjunction with SLAP tears include acromioclavicular arthritis, rotator cuff tears (partial or complete), and glenohumeral instability.

HISTORY

SLAP lesions are usually caused by an acute traumatic event. Several mechanisms of injury have been described.[1–3] Falling on an abducted, forward flexed arm, violent throwing events, catching heavy objects, and "jerking" traction injuries all have caused SLAP tears. Each of these actions occur in sports and places high demands on the shoulder with the potential for mechanisms of injury as noted above.

Patients frequently complain of pain associated with overhead movements in abduction, external rotation, and extension, such as with a tennis serve or throwing a baseball. In our experience, patients often complain about losing their ability to throw a ball well or hit an effective serve. We have also noted that athletes will voluntarily change positions, e.g., from second base to outfield, to accommodate deficiencies caused by their injury. Night-time pain as well as pain when lifting heavy objects may also be reported. Occasionally, patients may experience numbness and tingling or describe a history of instability.

PHYSICAL EXAMINATION

A thorough physical examination is indicated in all patients with shoulder complaints. It is important to document range of motion, areas of tenderness, and special test findings. Common examination findings in patients with SLAP tears include positive impingement tests, instability on load-and-shift maneuvers, rotator cuff weakness, and positive apprehension testing. A new test called the labral apprehension sign has also been developed.[2] This maneuver is performed by abducting the arm to 130° and externally rotating the shoulder to 90°. The examiner then places one hand posterior to the glenohumeral joint while the other hand grasps the elbow. An apprehension maneuver is then performed by pushing forward on the glenohumeral joint (Fig. 44–6). Apprehension or pain is interpreted as a positive result. A positive response to the traditional load-and-shift test is also sometimes found in the presence of SLAP tears.[4]

It is important to remember that associated conditions may be found in combination with SLAP lesions. Appropriate testing for the conditions noted above should be done as part of the routine shoulder evaluation.

DIAGNOSTIC TESTING

We have found that the use of the impingement test, i.e., subacromial injection of bupivacaine, can be very helpful when the labral apprehension sign and impingement sign are both present. Eradication of the impingement sign in the presence of continued positive labral testing has been helpful in sorting out a confusing picture of shoulder pain from SLAP lesions associated with the impingement syndrome.

Plain films of the shoulder should always be obtained to aid in sorting through the possibilities of associated injury. These should include an anteroposterior film in internal and external rotation, an axillary view, and an Alexander's view. This will allow the identification of such problems as Hill-Sachs lesions, acromioclavicular arthritis, and sclerosis of the greater tuberosity in rotator cuff disease.

Reliable imaging of SLAP lesions has proven difficult. This is due to the varying attachment of the central labrum to the glenoid.[5] Conventional MRI has not thus far been able to reliably distinguish normal variant from pathologic tear. This has lead to the use of CT arthrography. Hunter and colleagues have had favorable results in determining both presence and type of SLAP tear with

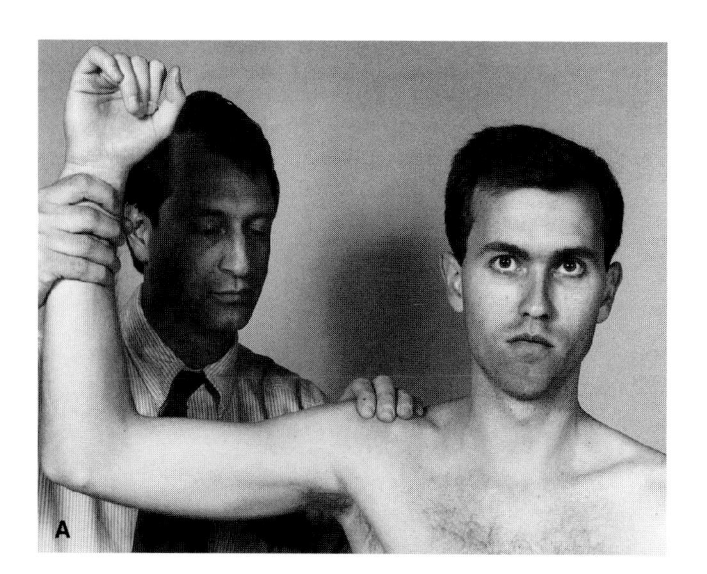

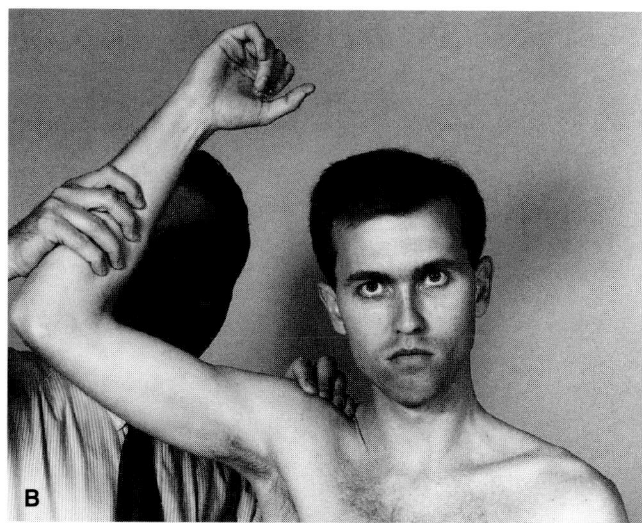

Fig. 44–6. ***(A)*** **Standard apprehension test for anterior instability with the arm in 90° of abduction, 90° of external rotation.** ***(B)*** **Labral apprehension sign with the arm at 130° of abduction, 90° of external rotation. The examiner's hands are placed as shown, pushing forward on the humeral head while stabilizing the elbow with the other hand.**

CT arthrograms.[6] Magnetic resonance arthrography may eventually prove very useful as techniques improve.

Examination under anesthesia at the time of arthroscopy may also prove helpful in identifying underlying instability. At this time, it is unclear what role instability plays regarding SLAP tears. However, Pappas and colleagues have previously noted "functional" instability from labral tears.[7] An isolated flap tear of the labrum can cause functional instability. If mechanical instability is found at examination under anesthesia, associated instability may be the cause of impingement pain. A Bankart lesion, if found at the time of arthroscopy, should be repaired along with appropriate treatment of any SLAP lesion present.

Finally, arthroscopy remains the "gold standard" for identification of SLAP lesions. It is important, however, that arthroscopy be used both as a diagnostic and a treatment tool simultaneously.

TREATMENT

SLAP lesions of all grades require surgical treatment. Therefore, primary care physicians should refer patients to an orthopedic surgeon familiar with treatment of SLAP lesions. The type of treatment required is determined at the time of surgery, and depends on the type of tear and associated injury. Type 1 lesions are treated with debridement of the frayed edges of the labrum. Type 2 lesions are treated with debridement as well as stabilization of the biceps complex. In addition, the superior neck of the glenoid is abraded to a surface of bleeding bone to stimulate healing of the labrum to the glenoid. Stabilization of the complex is currently accomplished with sutures or absorbable tacks (Suretac). In the past, staple fixation was used. However, because of the frequent need for removal of staples due to pain or damage caused by the staple, staples are no longer recommended. In clinical research by Wilson and Harsha, second-look arthroscopies for staple removal showed the SLAP tears to be well healed.[2] Therefore, we feel that suture fixation will provide excellent stabilization of unstable SLAP tears without the need for re-operation, as is necessary with staples. Type 3 and 4 lesions require repair or resection of the torn portions of the biceps and labrum. If the biceps complex is then considered to be unstable, suture or tack fixation is required, as in Type 2 lesions. It is critical that associated lesions be identified and treated at the time of surgery, if full recovery is to be possible.

After surgery, the patient is allowed to do protected Codman exercises for 1 to 3 weeks followed by physical therapy for active range of motion and strengthening.

In our experience, early identification and treatment of SLAP tears results in excellent function and high potential for return to previous level of function.

REFERENCES

1. Snyder, S. J., et al.: SLAP lesions of the shoulder. Arthroscopy *6*:274, 1990.
2. Wilson, F. D., and Harsha, D. M.: Evaluation and treatment of SLAP lesions of the shoulder. Unpublished data.
3. Andrews, J. R., Carson, W. G., Jr., and McLeod, W. D.: Glenoid labrum tears related to the long head of the biceps. Am. J. Sports Med. *13*:337, 1985.
4. Mellion, M., Walsh, W. M., and Shelton, G. L.: The Team Physician's Handbook. Philadelphia, Hanley & Belfus, 1990.
5. Detrisac, D. A., and Johnson, L. L.: Arthroscopic Shoulder Anatomy: Pathologic and Surgical Implications. Thorofare, NJ, SLACK Inc., 1986.
6. Hunter, J. C., Blatz, J. B., and Escobedo, E. M.: SLAP lesions of the glenoid labrum: CT arthrographic and arthroscopic correlation. Radiology *184*:513, 1992.
7. Pappas, A. M., Goss, T. P., and Kleinman, P. K.: Symptomatic shoulder instability due to lesions of the glenoid labrum. Am. J. Sports Med. *11*:279, 1983.

45 George M. McCluskey III and Thomas K. Miller

Shoulder Impingement and Rotator Cuff Lesions

Rotator cuff lesions are a common cause of shoulder pain and dysfunction in athletes. The spectrum of rotator cuff lesions ranges from acute reversible tendinitis, to chronic tendinitis with fibrosis and partial disruption of tendon fibers, to full-thickness retracted tendon tears, to massive tears with associated glenohumeral arthropathy.

The close relation between impingement syndrome and rotator cuff disease is well-established. Impingement syndrome is the condition that results from repeated abrasion or load to the rotator cuff (particularly the supraspinatus tendon) beneath the coracoacromial arch.[1] The concept of impingement requires an understanding of the balance between the coracoacromial arch, rotator cuff, and glenohumeral joint and capsule. Impingement syndrome occurs when the rotator cuff tendons are compromised beneath the coracoacromial arch.

PATHOPHYSIOLOGY

Primary causes of rotator cuff failure include intratendinous and extratendinous factors. *Secondary* factors, including glenohumeral instability, may also be related to rotator cuff injuries. Outlet impingement, as described by Neer,[1,2] occurs when narrowing of the supraspinatus outlet leads to mechanical irritation of the rotator cuff. The supraspinatus outlet includes the area just beneath the anterior one third of the acromion, the acromioclavicular joint, and the coracoacromial ligament. The floor of this space is formed by the supraspinatus tendon and the subacromial bursa. Narrowing of this space occurs with anterior acromial spur formation, various shapes and slopes of the acromion, and acromioclavicular joint arthritis with distal clavicle spurring.

Based on bone anatomy, impingement can be secondary to congenital or developmental abnormalities in the acromion or to a previous greater tuberosity fracture. Bigliani and coworkers have classified the acromion by shape: Type I, flat; Type II, curved; Type III, an anterior beak (Fig. 45–1).[3] A significant leading edge prominence, either because of a Type III acromion or an anterior spur, is associated with increased risk of impingement of the supraspinatus tendon against this bony prominence. Anterior extension of the acromion beyond the anterior border of the clavicle may also result in bony impingement of the rotator cuff.[4]

The os acromiale, an unfused acromial epiphysis, is present in approximately 3% of patients over age 25.[5] If the anterior acromial fragment tilts downward at the level of fibrous union, it can produce outlet impingement. Arthritic changes involving the acromioclavicular joint may narrow the supraspinatus outlet and lead to impingement and rotator cuff lesions. Preoperatively, the acromioclavicular joint must be evaluated so that any bony excrescences can be properly identified and treated.

The critical zone, as described by Codman,[6] lies just medial to the site of insertion of the supraspinatus tendon on the greater tuberosity. This area has been determined by some investigators to be hypovascular, and it is thought that supraspinatus tears usually begin in this avascular area. Codman also described "rim rents" on the articular surface of the rotator cuff at its attachment to the greater tuberosity.[7] These microtears may coalesce and lead eventually to a complete tear of the tendon with superior migration of the humeral head against the undersurface of the acromion.

Overuse injury of the arm can occur in patients, particularly athletes who perform repetitive overhead movements. Repetitive microtrauma to the rotator cuff secondary to repetitive overhead motion can cause cuff

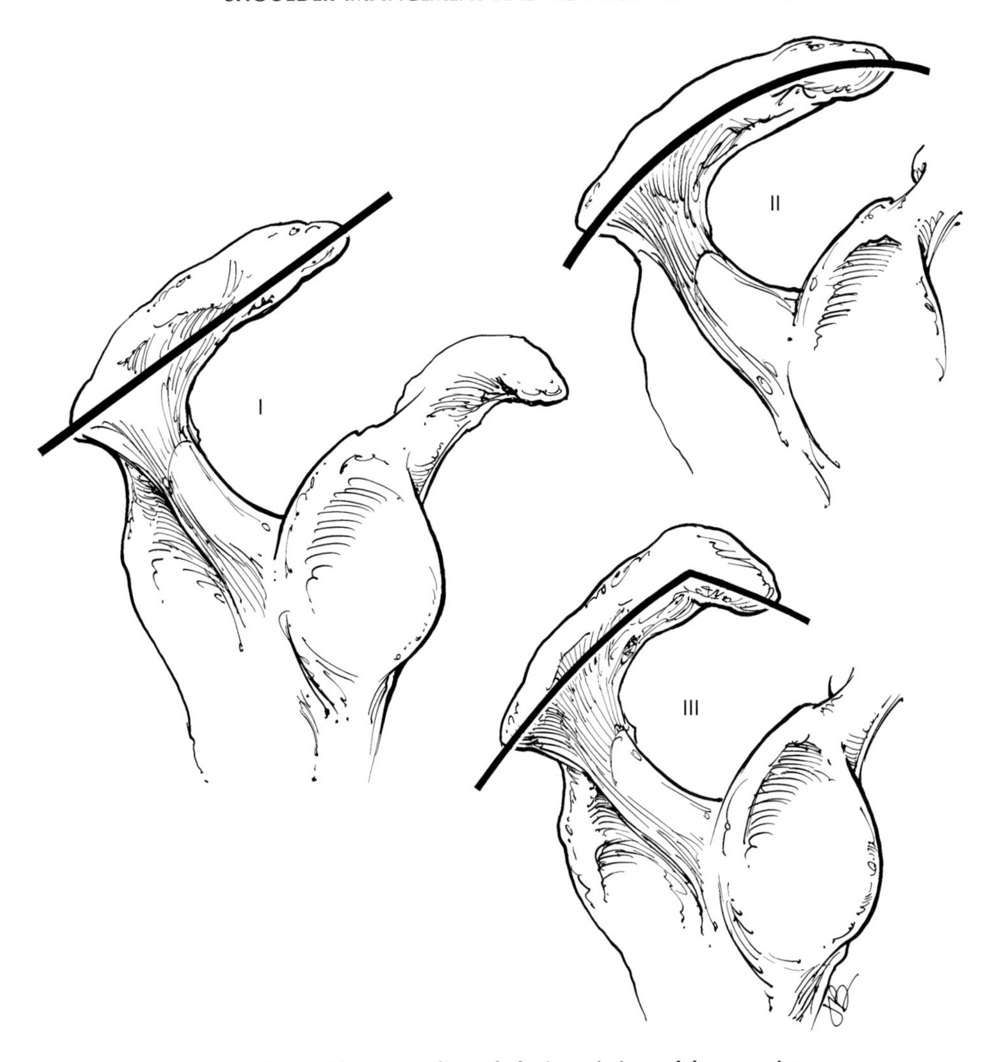

Fig. 45–1. The range of morphologic variations of the acromion.

tendinitis and inflammation that decreases the volume of the subacromial space and potentiates the impingement process.

Altered scapular mechanics can modify the presentation of the leading edge of the coracoacromial arch to the rotator cuff. Winging of the scapula results in lateral displacement and, more important, in anterior tilt of the scapula and "closure" of the coracoacromial arch. Persons with abnormal scapular mechanics may have impingement in the face of normal capsular status and normal rotator cuff strength but a functionally compromised arch.

Major trauma is an infrequent cause of a rotator cuff tear. In most cases, a patient experiences minor trauma to the shoulder, which may produce an acute extension of a pre-existing chronic tear. Symptoms include sudden acute onset of pain with more profound weakness than was previously experienced.

Glenohumeral Instability

Glenohumeral instability is a common cause of impingement syndrome and rotator cuff lesions in younger patients, particularly those involved in throwing or overhead sports. Rotator cuff tears may result when capsular injury leads to overuse of the cuff muscles as they attempt to stabilize the joint in the absence of competent static stabilizers. Fatigue and wear of the cuff muscles lead to loss of the normal head-depressing function of the rotator cuff and impingement of these tendons under the acromion. Patients with multidirectional instability often experience impingement symptoms as the unstable humeral head is displaced superiorly and anteriorly with overhead activity of the arm (Fig. 45–2). Treatment should be directed at the underlying shoulder instability.

CLASSIFICATION

Neer classified impingement in three stages. The first stage, characterized by edema and hemorrhage,[2] is usually seen in younger patients, especially those who excessively use the arm overhead. In Stage II, seen in the 25- to 40-year-old group, fibrosis and tendinitis are common findings, owing to mechanical inflammation. Stage III, usually seen in older patients, involves tears of

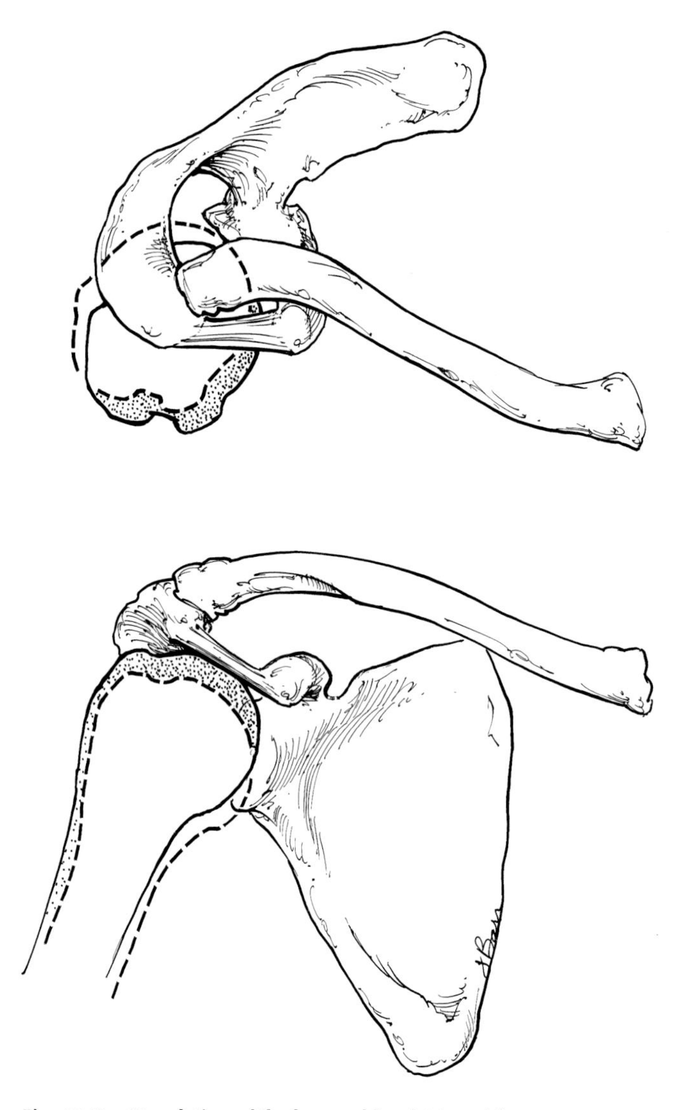

Fig. 45–2. Translation of the humeral head (*dotted line* represents original position) with weakened rotator cuff leads to impingement.

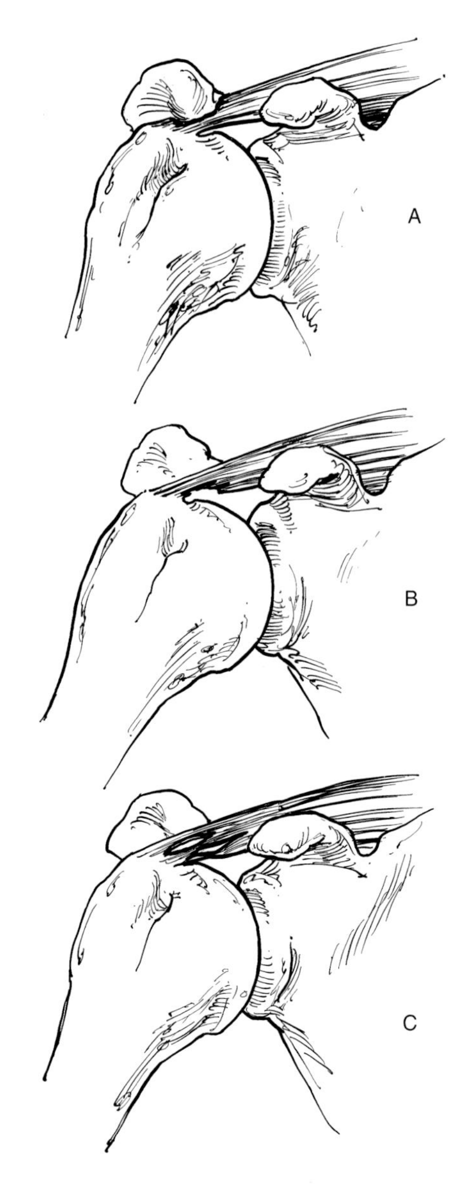

Fig. 45–3. Classification of rotator cuff tear. *(A)* Bursal surface tear, *(B)* articular surface tear, *(C)* intratendinous tear.

the rotator cuff, biceps lesions, or bony alteration at the anterior acromion and greater tuberosity. Since athletes place more stress on their shoulders than nonathletes, these stages of impingement may progress more rapidly in the athlete.

Rotator cuff tears can be divided into partial and complete lesions, depending on the degree of fiber disruption. Partial rotator cuff tears, more frequent than complete tears,[8–10] are divided into bursal surface, articular surface, and intratendinous tears (Fig. 45–3). Authors disagree on the frequency of the types of partial tears. Intratendinous tears cannot be visualized by arthrography or arthroscopy. Bursal surface tears are often disguised by overlying bursal tissue at arthroscopy, whereas articular surface tears are easily visualized. In most reports, articular surface tears far outnumber bursal surface tears.[9–11]

Complete tears of the rotator cuff are marked by total disruption of cuff fibers from the bursal surface to the articular surface. These tears are described and classified according to the size of the tear (the distance of the avulsed tendon edge from its normal humeral attachment), the number of torn tendons, and the quality of the tendons. The size of the tear or the degree to which it is retracted is graded as small (less than 1 cm), moderate (1 to 3 cm), large (3 to 5 cm), or massive (greater than 5 cm). Matsen has classified full-thickness tears into Stage I, involving the supraspinatus tendon only; Stage II, involving the supraspinatus and infraspinatus tendons; Stage III, involving the supraspinatus, infraspinatus, and subscapularis tendons; and, Stage IV, rotator cuff arthropathy.[12]

Classifying full-thickness cuff tears has important implications for treatment options and prognosis for pain relief and restoration of strength and function in the shoulder, following nonsurgical or surgical treatment.

CLINICAL FEATURES

In contrast to the extreme pain of an acute subacromial bursitis or calcific tendinitis or the trauma-related history of an acute rotator cuff tear, impingement problems usually are manifested in intermittent shoulder pain and stiffness of progressively increasing frequency and severity. The symptoms are usually associated with certain athletic activities and, in more chronic situations, with activities of daily living.

Activities that elicit pain typically involve overhead or across-body movement or throwing (impingement with or without deceleration pain). Lifting in a "thumb down" position (supraspinatus load) usually exacerbates symptoms. Night pain and morning stiffness are common, but not diagnostic. Although point tenderness, especially at the leading edge of the acromion, is common, generalized shoulder pain or discomfort extending to the level of the deltoid insertion also may be seen.

Complaints are to some degree sport specific. Swimmers may note discomfort related to either length of workout or intensity, overdistance and repeat intervals being the common causes. In athletes involved in climbing and kayaking, activities that cause direct impingement may produce pain. Affected throwing athletes typically describe the sensation of the arm slipping during cocking or pain during follow-through and deceleration. Their symptoms are velocity- or intensity related.

Patients with rotator cuff tears and those with impingement usually report the same symptom pattern. Pain with activity and weakness in the arm are common symptoms. In addition, rotator cuff disease often is associated with crepitation, grinding, and popping. The degree, or severity, of the pain is not predictive of the size of the tear.

It is important to determine the patient's activity level—at work and in recreation—as well as the duration of symptoms. Less active persons who do not use the arm at shoulder level or higher and those whose symptoms are less than 3 to 6 months old require less aggressive treatment and workup. On the other hand, active persons who play overhead sports routinely and have had symptoms for more than 3 months require early intervention with diagnostic tests and treatment to minimize the period of dysfunction.

It is important to obtain history—surgery, physical therapy, medications, injections. Additionally, any previous diagnostic tests, such as electromyography, cervical radiography, or other ancillary tests (magnetic resonance imaging or arthrography), should be obtained for review and interpretation.

PHYSICAL EXAMINATION

Pertinent findings on the physical examination of the shoulder depend to some extent on the degree of cuff damage. Symptoms range from mild tenderness, weakness, and pain on impingement tests (Fig. 45–4) to profound atrophy and inability to raise the arm actively. Superior subluxation of the humeral head is associated with massive rotator cuff tears.

Tenderness is generally localized to the greater tuberosity and subacromial bursa. The biceps tendon is often inflamed and painful to palpation, and in some cases the long head of the biceps tendon may be ruptured. The upper third of the trapezius and the insertion of the deltoid on the humerus may be tender, owing to referred pain and compensatory overuse of these muscles.

Range of shoulder motion should be measured and recorded systematically. The examiner must be certain that motion is not hindered because of pain. If so, ablation of pain must be obtained by injecting xylocaine into the subacromial bursa. Active range of motion is

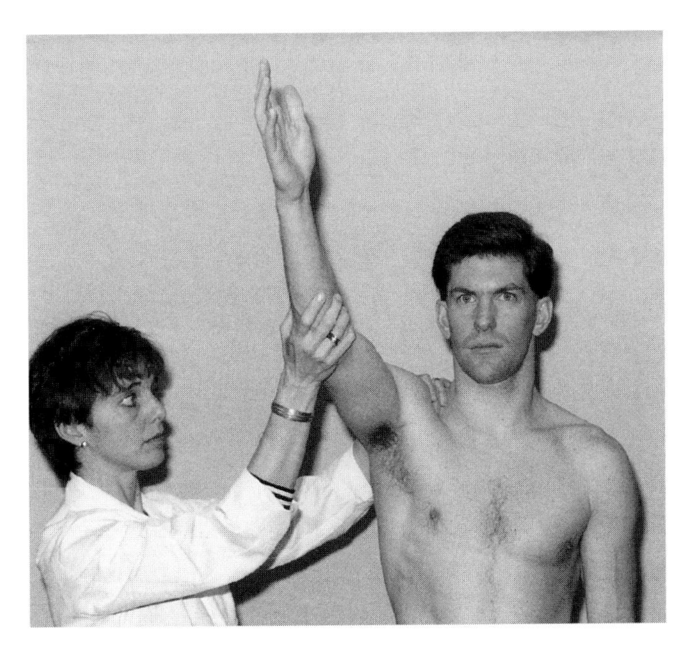
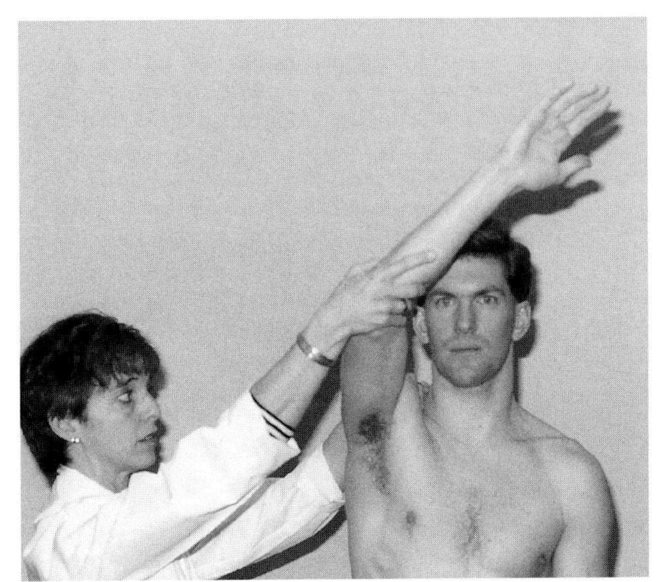

Fig. 45–4. Impingement sign.

often painful throughout its arc whereas passive motion is generally painful only at the extremes of the range. Stiffness of the shoulder often occurs in patients with partial tears or longstanding large complete tears. Shoulder stiffness must be differentiated from adhesive capsulitis.

Strength testing is usually the most revealing indicator of the size of a cuff tear. Supraspinatus weakness in forward flexion and abduction is very sensitive for rotator cuff tear if pain has been ablated with a local anesthetic. The degree of weakness correlates well with the size of the tear. Concomitant weakness in external rotation suggests involvement of the infraspinatus as well. Some patients with massive tears, cannot hold the arm passively in a position of external rotation. The strength of the deltoid, internal rotators, and biceps should also be measured.

Scapular mechanics should also be tested—for passive range of motion of the scapula and for scapular position under load, as with a wall pushup or abduction against resistance, looking for asymmetric motion or tilt.

The acromioclavicular joint should be closely examined for tenderness and for evidence of previous subluxation or spurring. Horizontal and overhead adduction cause pain at this joint. Overlooked pathologic changes of the acromioclavicular joint are a primary cause of failure of surgery for impingement and rotator cuff disease.

RADIOGRAPHIC EVALUATION

Plain Radiography

Plain radiographs of the shoulder afford valuable insights into the diagnosis of rotator cuff disease and must be performed on every patient. Standard views should include a true anteroposterior view of the glenohumeral joint (in the plane of the scapula, not of the chest) in internal and external rotation, a supraspinatus outlet view, and an axillary view.

The true anteroposterior view of the shoulder helps the examiner determine the acromiohumeral distance, which is narrowed in association with some larger tears, acromial spurring and sclerosis, glenohumeral arthritis, and reactive changes at the greater tuberosity (including cyst formation and sclerosis). The supraspinatus outlet view, a true lateral scapular view with the tube tilted 10° caudad, identifies acromial shape and distal clavicular spurring (Fig. 45–5). The axillary view helps to identify os acromiale and narrowing of the glenohumeral joint.

A special view of the acromioclavicular joint is useful in many cases to demonstrate osteolysis of the distal clavicle and degenerative changes in the acromioclavicular joint. This view is taken in the anteroposterior plane with a 20° cephalic tilt.

Arthrography

For many years, arthrography has been used in the diagnosis of rotator cuff lesions. The test is relatively inexpensive and easy to perform and interpret and its accuracy rate is 95%. Unfortunately, a negative arthrogram does not exclude a partial bursal surface or intratendinous tear. Leakage of radiographic dye from the glenohumeral joint into the subacromial space indicates a full-thickness tear (Fig. 45–6). The size of the tear is not always related to the amount of dye leakage. Articular surface partial rotator cuff tears display a thin stream of dye into the tendon defect but no extravasation into the bursal space.

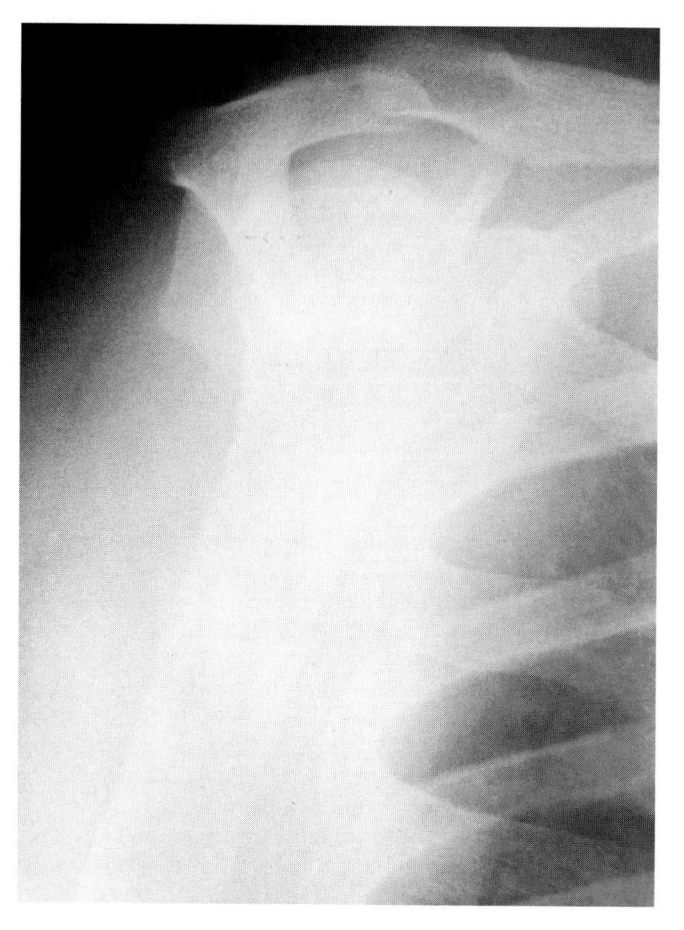

Fig. 45–5. Supraspinatus outlet view.

Magnetic Resonance Imaging

MRI has improved our ability to image the cuff. More definitive information about the rotator cuff is available on MRI, including increased accuracy in diagnosing full-thickness tears (about 98 to 99%), bursal and intratendinous partial tears, rotator cuff tendinitis, impingement lesions with acromial and distal clavicle spurring, and hypertrophy of the acromioclavicular joint capsule. Muscle atrophy and other bone anomalies (os acromiale) are also easily demonstrated. MRI is more expensive than other imaging modalities and is used principally when the diagnosis cannot be made or confirmed by other methods such as physical examination, plain radiography, or arthrography.

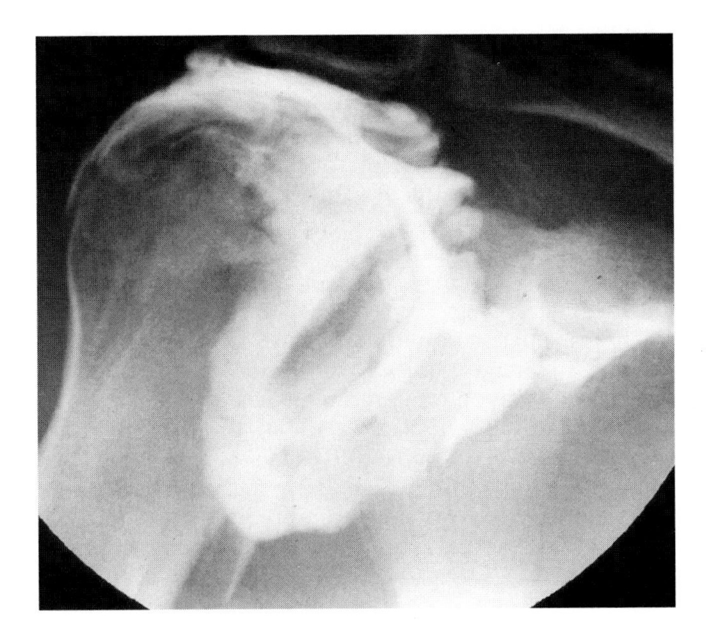

Fig. 45–6. Arthrogram of a full-thickness rotator cuff tear.

TREATMENT

Most patients without rotator cuff tears can be adequately treated with nonsurgical measures. These include patients with Neer Stage I and early Stage II impingement lesions that have not developed actual fiber disruption in the rotator cuff. A smaller percentage of patients with late Stage II and Stage III lesions respond to conservative treatment, and many eventually require surgical intervention. Accurate diagnosis and staging of the rotator cuff lesion is imperative because the treatment and prognosis are different for rotator cuff tendinitis and for partial, complete, or massive rotator cuff tears. Most authors recommend conservative nonsurgical treatment for all patients, initially, except for those with massive cuff avulsions and associated fractures that require early, more aggressive treatment.[1,13,14]

Control of inflammation may require reduction or elimination of the exacerbating athletic activities (decreased yardage or reduction of intervals in swimming, fewer pitches or longer rest intervals in throwing). Modification of technique may also decrease rotator cuff compromise: no "thumb lead" on water entry in swimming, changes in paddling technique or paddle type in kayaking and canoeing, evaluation by coaches (especially if pre- and postinjury videotapes are available) of throwing athletes.

Local steroid injections have been valuable when used judiciously to treat rotator cuff lesions in patients with tendinitis and partial tears.[15–17] Most patients get temporary pain relief from the reduced inflammation, and this is often enough to allow them to participate in and benefit from an exercise program to optimize motion and strength. These injections should not be given to patients with complete rotator cuff tears, especially if surgery is eventually anticipated. For patients who undergo rotator cuff reconstruction, frequent steroid injections (four or more) are reported to weaken cuff tissue and give overall poorer results than when frequent injections are avoided.[18]

Nonsteroidal anti-inflammatory medications are frequently used to treat impingement syndrome and rotator cuff lesions, although good clinical studies justifying this routine use of the medication are not available. Most patients get some analgesic benefit from these medications, but the side effects can be problematic. They must be used cautiously and under the strict supervision of the treating physician.

The goals of any exercise program for patients with rotator cuff disease are to decrease inflammation, restore normal range of motion, and optimize rotator cuff, deltoid, and scapular muscle strength. Every patient must have an individualized program designed to meet specific needs and present physical capabilities. Personal communication and understanding between patient, surgeon, therapist, and trainer is necessary to maximize the benefit of such a program.

Return to activities should be restricted until the range of motion is restored and both rest- and activity-related pain have been eliminated; in addition, provocative tests such as rotator cuff load or impingement testing should not reproduce the pain. Resumption of activities should be gradual (slow increase in distance or velocity of throwing, gradual increase in yardage and addition of interval work for swimmers). Load or volume of work may need to be modified in response to intermittent recurrence of symptoms during this time frame. Careful attention should be paid to mechanics, to remedy "bad habits." As long as impingement or tendinitis symptoms do not recur, work load can be increased until the athlete has returned to full and unrestricted activities. Flexibility and strengthening exercises should, however, be continued after return to full and unrestricted activities to prevent recurrence of symptoms.

Although in the majority of athletes impingement symptoms resolve and they are able to return to competitive activities, some do not benefit from conservative treatment. In most cases, patients with rotator cuff lesions who do not make appropriate progress in a well-supervised therapy program should be considered for further diagnostic workup or even surgical intervention. Those with significant abnormalities in acromial morphology or radiographic changes showing sclerosis of the acromion or hypertrophy of the greater tuberosity might be expected to be less responsive to conservative measures. Patients with a documented intact rotator cuff but persistent symptoms (no signs of rotator cuff tear on arthrography or MRI but abnormal examination) may benefit from therapeutic subacromial injections of corticosteroids. After control of inflammation by injection, treatment then relies on resumption of conservative measures. Failure to respond beyond this level often necessitates surgical intervention.

Surgical options may be arthroscopic, open, or a combination of the two, depending on the bone and soft tissue conditions anticipated or encountered during surgery. Shoulder arthroscopy involves inspection of both the glenohumeral and the subacromial space.[20] This is typically done via a posterior arthroscopic portal and an anterior working portal. Arthroscopic evaluation of the glenohumeral joint may reveal previously undiagnosed glenohumeral damage, including biceps tendon lesions, labral tears, or incomplete lesions of the rotator cuff. In addition, glenohumeral stability (degree of humeral head translation, glenohumeral ligament laxity) may be assessed arthroscopically. After glenohumeral assessment and attention to glenohumeral lesions, the arthroscope is directed into the subacromial space. Bony landmarks are identified (leading edge of the acromion, glenohumeral ligament, acromioclavicular joint) and subacromial decompression and débridement can be performed most reliably for bursal scarring, Type II acromial shape, or "incomplete" rotator cuff lesions. Larger bone lesions are usually addressed by limited open procedures and bony resection of the leading edge of the acromion, as described by Rockwood.[6] The surgical technique is performed via a small anterior incision over the leading edge of the acromion followed by deltoid interval splitting (between the anterior and the middle third of the deltoid) with minimal release of the deltoid origin. This approach allows for resection of large Type III acromions, acromial prominence beyond the anterior edge of the clavicle, and calcification of the coracoacromial ligament. This approach also allows for repair of rotator cuff tears, when necessary. If decision making for surgical intervention is to be informed, it is essential to distinguish between primary and instability-dependent impingement. Patients with apprehension signs or signs of labral pathology or instability can be expected to develop more problems if their complaint is addressed by decompression alone without attention to underlying instability.

Surgical Treatment of Symptomatic Rotator Cuff Lesions

Surgery for a rotator cuff tear relieves pain, but it does not predictably improve function or strength. The overall surgical result depends on many factors, some controlled by the patient, some by the surgeon, and some by the nature of the disease. They include quality of the repair, quality of the tissues, interval from injury to repair, size and extent of the tear, associated neurologic injury and deltoid function, and a disciplined postoperative therapy program.

Surgical results are better when the surgery is done earlier, because muscle atrophy and contracture, development of arthritic changes, and progressive shoulder stiffness make the surgery and rehabilitation more technically difficult and the results less predictable. Accurate preoperative diagnosis and careful consideration of the patient's overall medical condition are paramount before surgery is considered.

PARTIAL ROTATOR CUFF TEARS

The treatment of partial-thickness rotator cuff tears depends on factors such as the size of the tear, acromial shape, and the patient's age and activity level. For partial rotator cuff tears involving less than 50% of the tendon in patients with a Type II or Type III acromion, the arthroscopic or open acromioplasty for decompression and débridement of the rotator cuff tear is appropriate. A young throwing athlete with this problem should be evaluated thoroughly to see whether instability is contributing to the problem.

In an active younger patient with a partial rotator cuff tear involving more than 50% of the tendon's thickness, open acromioplasty with rotator cuff repair is the preferred choice of treatment. Alternatively, arthroscopic acromioplasty and rotator cuff repair or arthroscopic acromioplasty with an open minideltoid split approach to rotator cuff repair has been used by some surgeons. Older, less active patients with large partial-thickness tears may require only arthroscopic acromioplasty and cuff débridement if their symptoms are minimal.

COMPLETE ROTATOR CUFF TEAR

Symptomatic complete tears of the rotator cuff should be repaired or reconstructed. Acromioplasty should accompany the repair if the patient has outlet impingement or a Type II or Type III acromion. Distal clavicle excision is also recommended if preoperatively there is clinical or radiographic evidence of acromioclavicular joint arthritis or to facilitate surgical exposure for mobilization of a retracted supraspinatus tendon.

Complete mobilization of retracted tendons is usually performed with routine extra-articular techniques, including release of the coracohumeral ligament and incision of the rotator interval. Occasionally, intra-articular mobilization is necessary when the retracted tendons are scarred. Transposition of the subscapularis muscle is occasionally used to compensate for a deficient supraspinatus tendon.

A bone trough made in the sulcus between the lateral humeral articular surface and the superior aspect of the greater tuberosity and sutures placed through drill holes in bone that will advance the tendons into the created trough is usually necessary to accomplish rotator cuff repair. Meticulous deltoid repair is mandatory to avoid deltoid pull-off and atrophy.

MASSIVE ROTATOR CUFF TEARS

Some patients with massive rotator cuff tears have achieved satisfactory results with mobilization of the rotator cuff tendons and acromioplasty[19,20]; however, many patients with massive retracted rotator cuff tears involving multiple tendons cannot be satisfactorily repaired. These patients have usually been treated successfully with open or arthroscopic rotator cuff débridement and acromioplasty. Functional improvement is minimal in these patients because of continual rotator cuff deficiency, and a limited-goals type of rehabilitation program is appropriate for them.

REFERENCES

1. Neer, C. S. II: Anterior acromioplasty for the chronic impingement syndrome in the shoulder. A preliminary report. J. Bone Joint Surg. *54A*:41, 1972.
2. Neer, C. S. II: Impingement lesions. Clin. Orthop. *173*:70, 1983.
3. Bigliani, L. U., Morrison, D., and April, E. W.: The morphology of the acromion and its relationship to rotator cuff tears. Orthop. Trans. *10*:228, 1986.
4. Rockwood, C. A., and Lyons, F. R.: Shoulder impingement syndrome. Diagnosis, radiographic evaluation, and treatment with a modified Neer acromioplasty. J. Bone Joint Surg. *75A*:409, 1993.
5. McCluskey, G. M. III; Butler, J. B. V. V: Os Acromiale: Incidence and preliminary results of surgical excision of the meso-acromion. 1992. The Hughston Clinic Research project. Unpublished data.
6. Codman, E. A.: Rupture of the supraspinatus tendon. *In* The Shoulder: Rupture of the Supraspinatus Tendon and Other Lesions in or about the Subacromial Bursa. Malahar, FL: Robert E. Krieger, 1934, (Suppl. ed.).
7. Codman, E. A.: The Shoulder: Rupture of the Supraspinatus Tendon and Other Lesions in or about the Subacromial Bursa. Boston, Thomas Todd, 1934.
8. Yamanaka, K., Fukuda, H., Hamada, K., and Mikasa, M.: Incomplete thickness tears of the rotation cuff. Orthop. Traumatol. Surg. 26:713, 1983.
9. Fukuda, H., et al.: The partial thickness tear of the rotator cuff. Orthop. Trans. 7:137, 1983.
10. DePalma, A. F.: Surgery of the Shoulder. 2nd Ed. Philadelphia, J. B. Lippincott, 1973.
11. Petterrson, G.: Rupture of the tendon aponeurosis of the shoulder joint in anterior inferior dislocation. Acta Chir. Scand. 77(Suppl.):1, 1942.
12. Matsen, F. A. III, and Arntz, C. T.: Rotator cuff tendon failure. *In* The Shoulder. Rockwood, C. A., and Matsen, F. A., III (eds). Philadelphia, W. B. Saunders, 1990.
13. McLaughlin, H. L.: Rupture of the rotator cuff. J. Bone Joint Surg. *44A*:979, 1962.
14. Rowe, C. R.: Ruptures of the rotator cuff: Selection of cases for conservative treatment. Surg. Clin. North Am. *43*:1531, 1963.
15. Coomes, E. N., and Darlington, L. G.: The effects of local steroid injection for supraspinatus tears. Controlled study. Ann. Rheum. Dis. *35*:943, 1976.
16. Lee, P. N., et al.: Periarthritis of the shoulder. Ann. Rheum. Dis. *33*:116, 1974.
17. Hollingworth, G. R., Ellis, R. M., and Hattersley, T. S.: Comparison of injection techniques for shoulder pain: Results of a double blind, randomised study. Br. Med. J. 287:1339, 1983.
18. Watson, M.: Major ruptures of the rotator cuff: The results of surgical repair in 89 patients. J. Bone Joint Surg. 67B:618, 1985.
19. Hawkins, R. J., Misamore, G. W., and Hobeika, P. E.: Surgery for full-thickness rotator-cuff tears. J. Bone Joint Surg. 67A:1349, 1985.
20. Apoil, A. and Augerean, B.: Anterosuperior arthrolysis of the shoulder for rotatory cuff degenerative lesions, In Surgery of the Shoulder. Edited by M. Post, B. F. Morrey, and R. J. Hawkins. St. Louis, Mosby-Year Book, 1990.

46

Stephen H. Liu

Neurovascular Compression Syndromes About the Shoulder

Athletes suffering from compression of the neurovascular structures of the shoulder often develop symptoms during or after sports. Symptoms vary, depending on what anatomic structures (artery, vein, nerve) are compressed and on the location of the compression. Patients with vascular compression complain of upper limb heaviness, fatigue, and claudication.[1] Swelling, discoloration, and ulceration may be present. Arterial insufficiency usually produces symptoms of coldness, numbness, and exertional fatigue, whereas venous obstruction causes upper limb edema, heaviness, and cyanosis.

Compression of the lower trunk of the brachial plexus frequently results in pain and paresthesia from the neck and shoulder down to the medial aspect of the hand associated with weak grasp and difficulty with fine finger movements. In contrast, compression of the upper trunk of the brachial plexus results in more obscure symptoms, with pain proximal in the neck and shoulder region. These symptoms resemble those of cervical disc herniation.

When both neurologic and vascular structures are involved, the pattern of symptoms may be mixed. A detailed physical examination, with emphasis on the cervical spine and the shoulder girdle, and the use of three specific tests (Adson's, costoclavicular, hyperabduction) are essential to localizing the anatomic site of the compression.

CLINICAL TESTS

Adson's test is used to demonstrate compression of the subclavian artery by the scalenus anticus muscle.[2,3] The patient inhales deeply, extends the neck, and turns the chin toward the affected shoulder. Diminution of the radial pulse or change in blood pressure indicates scalenus anticus syndrome. In the costoclavicular maneuver,[3] the patient thrusts the shoulder backward and down, similar to a military brace position. This maneuver decreases the space between the clavicle and the first rib, compressing the neurovascular structure in this area. In the hyperabduction maneuver,[4] the patient takes a deep breath and turns the head to the opposite side as the affected arm is abducted and externally rotated (Fig. 46–1). This test is specific for neurovascular compression in the subcoracoid region, with compression of the second part of the axillary artery under the pectoralis minor muscle.

These tests are not 100% sensitive or specific. Several studies have reported that for more than 50% of normal asymptomatic persons Adson's test is positive.[5,6] Thus, a test should be considered truly positive only when the maneuver reproduces the symptoms.

ANCILLARY STUDIES

Whenever neurovascular compromise is suspected, plain radiographs of the cervical spine should be taken to seek cervical or first thoracic ribs. Although cervical ribs are commonly associated with neurovascular injuries, fewer than 10% of patients with these bone abnormalities have symptoms.[7] The cervical rib originates from the transverse process of C7 and attaches directly to the first rib.[2,6] An anteroposterior (AP) view may also show abnormalities or fractures of the first rib or clavicle that can constrict the neurovascular structures.

Electrodiagnostic studies are useful in ruling out peripheral lesions distally (e.g., carpal tunnel syndrome, ulnar nerve neuropathy) or in the differential diagnosis of cervical radiculopathy. Noninvasive and invasive vas-

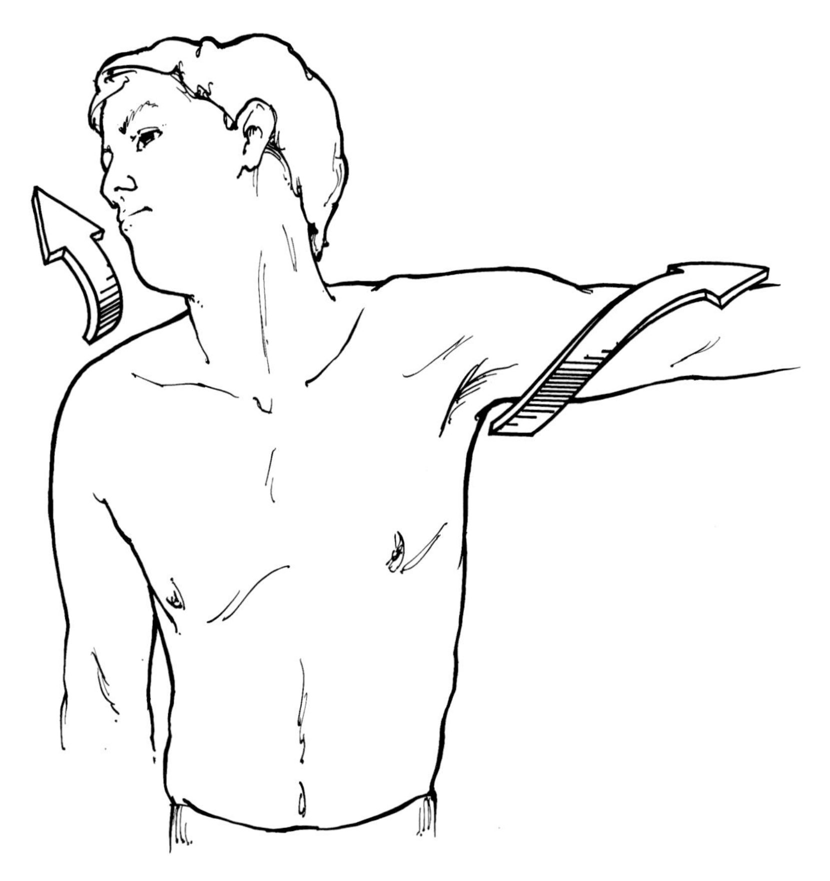

Fig. 46–1. Wright's maneuver.

cular examinations also can be used to diagnose neurovascular compression syndrome.[3,4,8,9] Digital subtraction angiography may be used in place of arteriography in certain patients; however, definitive diagnosis of vascular compromise requires venograms and angiographic studies of the subclavian and axillary arteries. When performing these studies, it is important to do them with the affected arm and the normal arm in the position associated with symptoms.

SPECIFIC SYNDROMES

Thoracic Outlet Syndrome

Thoracic outlet syndrome is an ill-defined term that describes the signs and symptoms attributed to compression of the neurovascular structures from the neck to the axilla. The neurovascular structures in this area lie close to one another, and thus are subject to varying degrees of compression of the brachial plexus and subclavian arteries.

In the past, structural and congenital abnormalities have been blamed for the thoracic outlet syndrome. Although these abnormalities contribute to thoracic outlet syndrome, we now recognize that trauma and dynamic changes in the shoulder secondary to throwing mechanics are common causes of thoracic outlet syndrome.[10,11] Injuries to the shoulder muscles can cause functional impairment in association with secondary neurovascular compression. In addition, exuberant callus formation or malunion after a clavicle fracture may result in reduction of the costoclavicular space and subsequent thoracic outlet syndrome.[12]

CLINICAL PRESENTATION

Symptoms of thoracic outlet syndrome depend on the degree to which particular neurovascular structures are compromised. In throwing athletes, the neurovascular symptoms of thoracic outlet compression are usually associated with specific throwing activities. The symptoms can be elicited by reproducing the activity and are often relieved by rest.

Initial treatment of thoracic outlet syndrome is nonoperative. Most patients can be treated effectively with nonsteroidal anti-inflammatory medications, local trigger point injections, and by abstaining from the precipitating activities. Patients with vascular problems should have the appropriate studies and followup treatment. The rehabilitative program should include correcting any postural abnormalities and strengthening the shoulder girdle and scapular musculature. It is important not to aggravate the symptoms with any of the exercises. Congenital abnormalities such as cervical ribs or fibrous bands at C7 are difficult to treat with exercise. Increasing cervical spine flexibility with various cervical stretches may help decrease compression.

Surgical intervention is reserved for those who continue to experience functional impairment and pain despite a well-directed rehabilitation program. Surgical treatment depends on what particular condition is causing the syndrome; it can take the form of excision of the cervical rib, scalenotomy, or release of fibromuscular bands.[3]

Axillary Artery Occlusion

Axillary artery occlusion occurs secondary to repetitive overhead activities requiring hyperabduction and external rotation of the shoulder joint. Part of the axillary artery is occluded by pressure from the overlying pectoralis minor when the arm is brought overhead.

Symptoms associated with axillary artery occlusion include pain, tenderness over the pectoralis minor area, claudication, fatigue, decreased distal pulses, and cyanosis. These symptoms can be reproduced when the arm is hyperabducted and externally rotated. Definitive diagnosis usually requires angiographic demonstration of thrombosis with complete arterial occlusion or an aneurysmal dilatation of the artery.

Surgical intervention is usually necessary for treating axillary artery occlusion. Common procedures include thrombectomy, sympathectomy, segmental excisions, bypass or vascular graft, and anastomosis or angioplasty.[8,11,13,14]

Effort Thrombosis

Effort thrombosis is named because of its frequent association with repetitive, vigorous activity or blunt trauma that directly injures the subclavian and axillary veins. Compression of the axillary vein can occur at various locations along its anatomic course. The most significant compression occurs in the costoclavicular space (Fig. 46–2), especially after a combined maneuver of hyperextension of the neck and hyperabduction of the arm or assumption of the military brace position. Compression can also occur between the costocoracoid ligament and the first rib, the subclavian muscle, and the first rib—or, more commonly, between the clavicle and the first rib. Symptoms usually occur within the first 24 hours after trauma or activity. Symptoms are limited to the affected upper extremity; most often they consist of a dull, aching pain and swelling. The pain is associated with numbness and heaviness in the upper extremity and activity-related fatigue.

Physical examination reveals edema involving the entire upper extremity. The skin may be mottled and cold, and superficial veins may be prominent, but pulses are usually normal. Occasionally, a tender cordlike structure is palpable in the examination. These physical findings may become prominent during overhead activities. The diagnosis of effort thrombosis is frequently made by a detailed history and physical examination and is confirmed by venography. Typically, a thrombus is

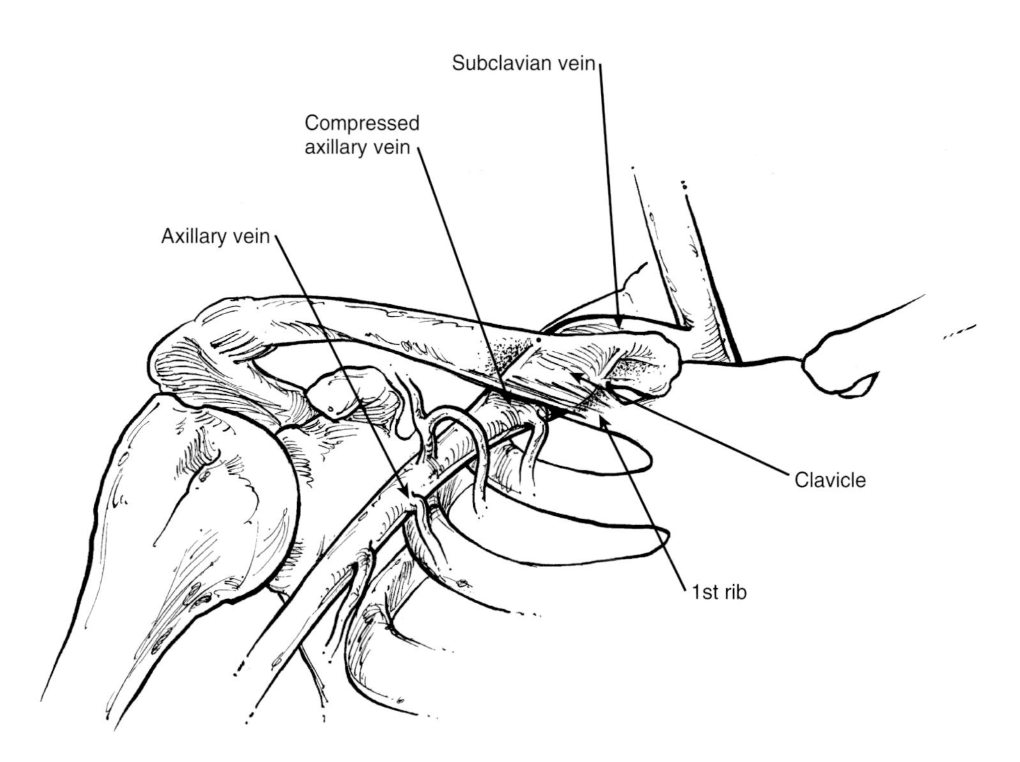

Fig. 46–2. Anatomy of the subclavian and axillary veins, depicting the area of thrombosis and increased venous collateralization.

found that occludes the axillary or subclavian vein. Collateralization and recanalization of the thrombosed vein may be extensive.[14,15]

Treatment of effort thrombosis should be directed toward alleviating the symptoms with the ultimate goal of returning the athlete to his or her previous activities. Although rest and elevation of the arm usually resolve acute pain and swelling within 3 to 4 days, 60 to 85% of patients treated conservatively may experience residual symptoms.[16]

Anticoagulation therapy with heparin, followed by warfarin, are often used in the acute phase to prevent progression of the thrombus, and streptokinase has been indicated for the lysis of intravenous clots.[14,15] This fibrinolytic therapy is effective with acute clots but ineffective with longstanding clots. Surgical intervention with early thrombectomy and simultaneous decompression of the thoracic outlet has been reported to have good longterm results.[17–19]

Although the syndrome is rare, throwing athletes are clearly at risk for effort thrombosis. Physicians should be familiar with the signs and symptoms of this condition, so that vascular occlusion in the proximal upper extremity can be diagnosed promptly and not overlooked.

Quadrilateral Space Syndrome

The quadrilateral space, located over the posterior scapula and subdeltoid region, consists of the teres minor superiorly, the long head of the triceps medially, the teres major inferiorly, and the surgical neck of the humerus laterally (Fig. 46–3). Through this space, the axillary nerve and the posterior humeral circumflex artery exit. Fibrous bands in this space can compress neurovascular structures when the arm is abducted and externally rotated. This syndrome has been reported in throwing athletes.[11,13,17]

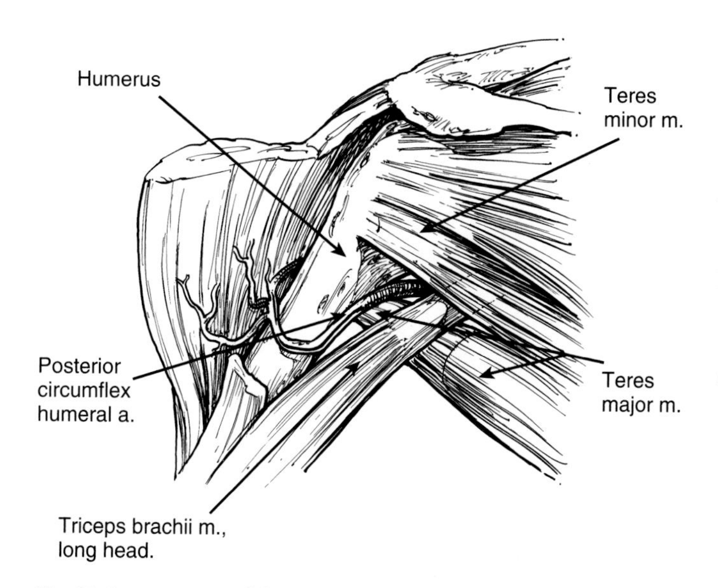

Fig. 46–3. Anatomy of the quadrilateral space.

Symptoms usually include pain and paresthesia in the upper extremity without associated trauma. The pain is poorly localized and activated by abduction and external rotation of the humerus, and it often interferes with throwing.

On physical examination the shoulder of patients with quadrilateral space syndrome is usually normal, although exquisite point tenderness may be noted over the affected quadrilateral space. Findings of neurologic examination, electromyography, and nerve conduction studies are normal.

The diagnosis is based on a subclavian arteriogram performed with both arms held at the patient's side and then in an abducted, externally rotated position. The arteriogram shows the obvious posterior humeral circumflex artery when the humerus is at its side but occlusion of the artery when the humerus is abducted and externally rotated. Treatment of quadrilateral space syndrome includes treatment of the symptoms and reassurance. Gradual strengthening of the rotator cuff and stretching of the shoulder structures may help to alleviate the symptoms; however, for symptomatic patients, Cahill recommended surgical decompression of the quadrilateral space through a posterior approach.[9]

Because neurovascular compression syndromes are rare in throwing athletes, diagnosis of these conditions requires (1) a thorough history and physical examination with emphasis on specific tests (Adson's, costoclavicular, Wright's), and (2) ancillary studies, including cervical radiography, chest radiography, Doppler measurements, venography, and arteriography.

Once the diagnosis is confirmed, the initial treatment usually is conservative, including postural and shoulder girdle strengthening exercises and abstaining from the precipitating activities. Cervical decompression to enlarge the floor of the thoracic outlet is indicated for chronically symptomatic patients. Vascular occlusion can be treated with anticoagulation or thrombolytic therapy. Surgical intervention includes thrombectomy, sympathectomy, segmental excision, or vascular bypass graft.

When throwing athletes present with upper extremity pain, neurovascular compression syndrome of the shoulder should be considered in the differential diagnosis. Awareness of these clinical syndromes facilitates diagnosis and treatment. Subsequently, the athlete will be able to return to his or her previous activities without prolonged delay or unnecessary disability.

REFERENCES

1. Lord, J. W., and Rosati, L. M.: Thoracic-outlet syndromes. Clinical Symposia 23(2):3, 1971.
2. Adson, A. W., and Coffey, J. R.: Cervical rib: Method of anterior approach for relief of symptoms by division of scalenus anticus. Ann. Surg. *85*:A39, 1927.
3. Baker, C. L., and Thornberry, R.: Neurovascular syndromes. *In* Injuries to the Throwing Arm. Edited by B. Zarins, J. R. Andrews, and W. G. Carson, Jr. Philadelphia, W. B. Saunders, 1985.

4. Wright, I. S.: The neurovascular syndromes produced by hyperabduction of the arm. Am. Heart J. *29*:1, 1945.
5. Riddell, D. H., and Smith, B. M.: Thoracic and vascular aspects of the thoracic outlet syndrome, 1986 update. Clin. Orthop. *207*:31, 1986.
6. Sellke, F. W., and Kelley, T. R.: Thoracic outlet syndrome. Am. J. Surg. *156*:54, 1988.
7. Brown, C.: Compressive, invasive referred pain to the shoulder. Clin. Orthop. *173*:55, 1983.
8. Tullos, H. S., et al.: Unusual lesions of the pitching arm. Clin. Orthop. *88*:169, 1972.
9. Cahill, B. R.: Quadrilateral space syndrome. In Management of Peripheral Nerve Problems. Edited by G. E. Omer. Philadelphia, W. B. Saunders, 1980.
10. Karas, S. E.: Thoracic outlet syndrome. Clin. Sports Med. *9*:297, 1990.
11. Nuber, G. W., et al.: Arterial abnormalities of the shoulder in athletes. Am. J. Sports Med. *18*:514, 1990.
12. Bateman, J. E.: Nerve injuries about the shoulder in sports. J. Bone Joint Surg. *49A*:785, 1967.
13. Rohrer, M. J., et al.: Axillary artery compression and thrombosis in throwing athletes. J. Vasc. Surg. *11*:761, 1990.
14. Sotta, R. P.: Vascular problems in the proximal upper extremity. Clin. Sports Med. *9*:379, 1990.
15. Vogel, C. M., and Jensen, J. E.: Effort thrombosis of the subclavian vein in a competitive swimmer. Am. J. Sports Med. *13*:269, 1985.
16. Redler, M. R., Ruland, L. J., and McCue, F. C.: Quadrilateral space syndrome in a throwing athlete. Am. J. Sports Med. *14*:511, 1986.
17. Adams, J. T., and DeWeese, J. A.: Effort thrombosis of the axillary and subclavian veins. J. Trauma *11*:923, 1971.
18. Campbell, C. B., et al.: Axillary, subclavian and brachyiocephalic vein obstruction. Surgery *82*:816, 1977.
19. Aziz, S., Straehley, C. J., and Whelan, T. J., Jr.: Effort-related axillosubclavian vein thrombosis. A new theory of pathogenesis and a plea for direct surgical intervention. Am. J. Surg. *152*:57, 1986.

47 *James R. Andrews and Timothy B. Sutherland*

Arthroscopy in the Management of Athletic Shoulder Disorders

The treatment of athletic shoulder injuries is challenging and fraught with difficulty. The diagnostic and therapeutic options facing the sports medicine physician are many and new ones are devised almost daily. Shoulder arthroscopy, popularized in the last decade, offers significant advances in both the diagnosis and treatment of complex shoulder injuries.

The arthroscope is a secondary tool used for the diagnosis of elusive shoulder disorders and for the treatment of many common athletic shoulder problems that are refractory to conservative treatment. The indications for shoulder arthroscopy continue to evolve as our understanding of the benefits and limitations of surgical shoulder arthroscopy expand. In the past few years we have learned as much about the limitations of arthroscopy as about the benefits. Indications for shoulder arthroscopy in athletes include the evaluation and treatment of labral tears, rotator cuff tendinitis and tearing, impingement, glenohumeral instability, and thrower's exostosis. Arthroscopic surgery is often preferable to open surgery because it not only decreases surgical trauma but also allows more rapid healing, more aggressive rehabilitation, and earlier return to competitive sports. Arthroscopy also allows more complete visualization of intra-articular and bursal lesions, aiding in both diagnosis and treatment of athletic shoulder injuries. Disadvantages of shoulder arthroscopy include technical difficulty, necessity for special equipment, and risk of fluid extravasation. Relative contraindications for arthroscopy include conditions that require open surgery, adhesive capsulitis, significant degenerative joint disease, and lack of expertise.

BASIC SETUP

Two standard approaches to shoulder arthroscopy exist: the lateral position and the beach-chair position. We will first review the setup for our preferred approach: the lateral decubitus position.[1]

After general anesthesia is administered, the patient is positioned in the lateral decubitus position and is supported by a bean bag or kidney rest.[2] The arm is then suspended from the overhead pulley system in about 30° to 70° of abduction and 15° of forward flexion. The suspension rope is secured to a free-hanging 10- to 20-pound weight. After the shoulder is prepared and draped in a sterile fashion, with a sterile surgical marking pen the bony anatomic landmarks are outlined: the anterolateral and posterolateral corners of the acromion, the acromioclavicular joint, and the coracoid process.

The posterior portal is identified by palpating the posterior "soft spot" over the glenohumeral joint. This point is approximately 2 to 3 cm inferior and 1 cm medial to the posterolateral corner of the acromion; it is the interval between the infraspinatus and the teres minor. Gentle internal and external rotation of the arm can help locate this interval. A spinal needle is then inserted into the soft spot and directed anteriorly toward the coracoid process. Forty to fifty milliliters of saline is used to distend the joint, and free backflow from the needle ensures proper placement. The needle is then removed, and a small skin incision is made. The arthroscopic cannula and dull trocar are advanced to the glenohumeral joint. The tip of the trocar is used to palpate the rim of the glenoid, and the cannula is inserted just lateral to the posterior rim. The posterior portal allows good visualization of the biceps tendon, anterior labrum, subscapularis tendon, and glenohumeral articular surfaces.

To clear debris and allow visualization of the posterior joint and use of operating instruments, an anterior portal is established. The anterior portal allows more careful examination of the posterior rotator cuff, posterior labrum, and anterior inferior capsular structures. This portal is established halfway between the coracoid process and the anterolateral corner of the acromion. A spinal needle is passed into the joint and visualized with the arthroscope. The needle should pass just below the biceps tendon, through the rotator cuff interval, when viewed within the joint. Complete diagnostic glenohumeral arthroscopy includes viewing from both the anterior and the posterior portal, to allow visualization of the entire joint.

After glenohumeral arthroscopy is completed, subacromial bursoscopy is performed. The operator advances into the bursa a cannula and trocar, taking care that the cannula is not posterior to the bursal curtain, medial under the acromioclavicular joint, or lateral under the deltoid muscle. Before inserting the arthroscope, the operator checks the general position of the cannula by lining up a second cannula of identical length on the outside of the shoulder.

Subacromial bursoscopy is then accomplished in an organized, systematic fashion. The coracoacromial ligament, acromion, rotator cuff, and acromioclavicular joint are carefully identified and examined for evidence of abnormality. If necessary, a lateral portal is then established, which is used for both instrumentation and visualization of the subacromial bursa. Motorized "débriders" and burs are used through the lateral portal to remove bursal scar and accomplish subacromial decompression. If necessary, the arthroscope may be inserted through the lateral portal, both to increase visualization of the distal clavicle and acromioclavicular joint and to evaluate the adequacy of subacromial decompression. A spinal needle is inserted approximately 1 cm posterior and 3 cm distal to the anterolateral acromion. This is identified with the arthroscope, and access to all involved structures is ensured. A small incision is then made, and the arthroscopic cannula and trocar are inserted into the bursa. A small, full-radius débrider is commonly used to resect the abundant bursal tissue and allow complete examination of the subacromial structures. After appropriate diagnostic and surgical intervention, the arthroscope and cannula are removed.

The upright, or beach-chair, position is also used for shoulder arthroscopy.[2,3] Scalene block anesthesia is often used. The operating table is adjusted so that the patient's torso is 70° to the horizontal. A small pad is placed under the medial border of the scapula, and the patient is placed with the shoulder free over the edge of the table. The arm is allowed to hang free at the side, and an arm board is used at the side of the table. The anatomic landmarks are carefully marked, and the posterior, anterior, and lateral portals are established, as described for the lateral decubitus position. Careful needle localization is encouraged for the development of the anterior and lateral portals because the soft tissues of the shoulder are in a slightly different position in the beach-chair position than in the lateral decubitus position.

SPECIFIC LESIONS

Labral Tears

Preoperative evaluation aims to distinguish between isolated and instability-associated labral tears, since the treatments of the two are radically different. The history is crucial for glenoid labral tears. Typically, patients with isolated tears describe pain, with or without a sense of catching, clicking, or popping about the shoulder. The mechanical symptoms are secondary to the interposed labral flaps or bucket- handle tears that interfere with the glenohumeral articulation. During the physical examination, the examiner should attempt to reproduce mechanical symptoms with the "clunk test".[4,5] History and complete examinations are also done, to rule out any associated instability pattern.

If rehabilitation fails to restore the desired level of function of an athlete with an isolated labral tear, diagnostic and therapeutic arthroscopy is considered. A careful preoperative examination with general anesthesia should be done, to rule out associated instability. Diagnostic arthroscopy also includes specific evaluation for evidence of instability. Labral detachment below the equator of the glenoid, posterior humeral head articular changes (Hill-Sachs lesion), or evidence of significant capsular stretching should be sought. If an isolated labral lesion is found, resection is accomplished through hand and motorized instruments (Fig. 47–1). The goal is to contour the labrum to restore a stable peripheral rim. Caution must be taken to avoid overzealous débridement of the anterior or posterior labrum, which can lead to overt instability. Followup data are limited, but early studies indicate good results if débridement is limited to functional tears. The surgeon must maintain a high index of suspicion for occult instability and perform careful preoperative evaluation; examination under anesthesia and arthroscopic examination are crucial.

Glenohumeral Laxity

After the administration of general anesthesia, a complete and recorded examination is done on both shoulders.

Diagnostic arthroscopy is then undertaken. The glenohumeral joint is carefully assessed for evidence of capsuloligamentous disruption. The glenoid labrum is carefully probed for detachment from the glenoid or from the anterior capsule. The posterior humeral head is carefully assessed for Hill-Sachs lesions (Fig. 47–2). Depending on the degree of anterior instability, the decision is then made to proceed with arthroscopic sta-

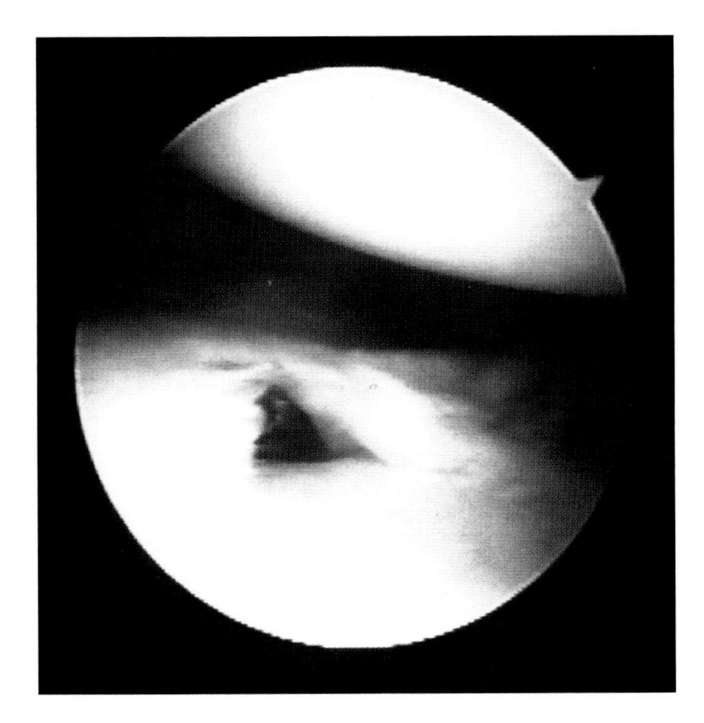

Fig. 47–1. Anterior superior labrum tear.

bilization or with open anterior capsular reconstruction. Our indications for arthroscopic stabilization include anterior labral detachment with the capsule attached to the labrum, a small Hill-Sachs lesion or none, and minimal capsular laxity. Contraindications to arthroscopic stabilization include lesions of athletes involved in collision sports, large Hill-Sachs lesions, arthroscopic evidence of capsular laxity, or evidence of multidirectional instability on physical examination (positive sulcus sign). Many techniques have been described for arthroscopic stabilization.[6–8] These include suture, staple, and absorbable tack fixation. We currently prefer to use the absorbable arthroscopic tack. After an appropriate lesion has been identified, two anterior portals are created for visualization and instrumentation of the anterior glenoid neck. With the arthroscope in the anterosuperior portal, instruments are introduced through the anteroinferior portal, and the anterior glenoid neck is débrided to bleeding bone. A grasping instrument is then inserted through the anterosuperior portal, and a Kirschner wire and cannulated drill are inserted through the anteroinferior portal. The Kirschner wire is then placed through the labrum and into the débrided glenoid neck. The neck is drilled, and the drill bit is removed, leaving the Kirschner wire in place. The bioabsorbable tack is placed over the Kirschner wire, reapproximating the capsulolabral complex to the glenoid neck. The repair is then carefully probed under direct visualization, using both the anterior and posterior portals. If possible, two tacks are used, and the labrum is approximated as close as possible to the glenoid rim.

Postoperative rehabilitation involves approximately 4 weeks' immobilization with gentle range of motion exercises. A graded program is then instituted to restore motion and strength and to prepare the athlete for return to sports. We use the arthroscopic approach only for carefully selected patients. Arthroscopic stabilization techniques have a slightly higher recurrence rate than open techniques, and less secure fixation in the arthroscopic technique necessitates less aggressive postoperative rehabilitation. Competitive athletes can ill afford failure, and recurrence often signals the end of a career. For these reasons, even with today's state-of-the-art arthroscopic technology, most athletes with significant instability are treated with open reconstruction.

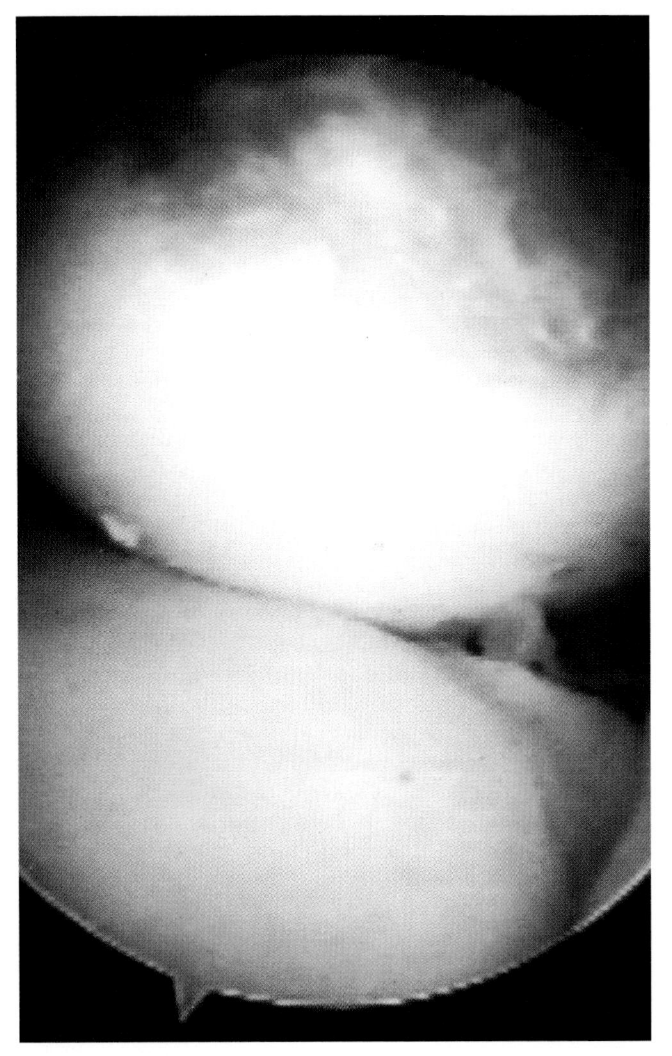

Fig. 47–2. Posterior Hill-Sachs lesion with anterior translation of the head of the humerus.

Arthroscopy and arthroscopic stabilization of acute shoulder dislocations remain controversial. Although arthroscopic stabilization of acute dislocations has been shown to decrease anterior instability significantly,[9] it is difficult to predict which athletes will develop symptomatic anterior instability after a traumatic dislocation. We currently do not recommend routine arthroscopy and surgical stabilization for first-time shoulder dislocations. We would, however, consider this more aggressive course for traumatic dislocation of the dominant arm of a throwing athlete. Diagnostic arthroscopy with arthroscopic stabilization of anterior labral detachments remains an option in this high-demand patient population.

Rotator Cuff Disease

Initial treatment of primary compression should be conservative. Education in avoidance of provocative activities, nonsteroidal anti-inflammatory medications, steroid injections, strengthening exercises, and stretching exercises should be offered. If the patient's symptoms do not respond to conservative treatment, surgical arthroscopy is considered. After complete examination under anesthesia, diagnostic glenohumeral arthroscopy is done to rule out evidence of occult instability, tensile cuff lesions, or degenerative joint disease. Typically impingement patients have a normal glenohumeral joint. The arthroscope is then introduced into the subacromial bursa. Typical findings of impingement include proliferative bursitis and hypertrophy of the coracoacromial ligament (Fig. 47–3). Arthroscopic evidence of abrasion on the undersurface of the acromion and the superficial rotator cuff should be evident. Without evidence of mechanical abrasion the diagnosis of subacromial impingement should be suspect. If evidence of impingement exists, arthroscopic acromioplasty is done. Using a lateral portal, a soft tissue débrider and motorized bur are used to accomplish anteroinferior acromioplasty.[1] Adequacy of acromioplasty is confirmed by the thickness of the anterior periosteal sleeve, identification of the distal clavicle, and increased clearance between the acromion and the rotator cuff. The acromioclavicular joint is then assessed, and any inferior osteophytes are removed using the motorized bur. If evidence of acromioclavicular arthritis was present preoperatively, an arthroscopic distal clavicle excision is done using a portal just anterior to the acromioclavicular joint.

The integrity of the rotator cuff is assessed next. Partial-thickness bursal tears are débrided. Full-thickness cuff tears are carefully evaluated, and the tear type, quality of cuff tissue, and patient characteristics inform the treatment decision (Fig. 47–4).

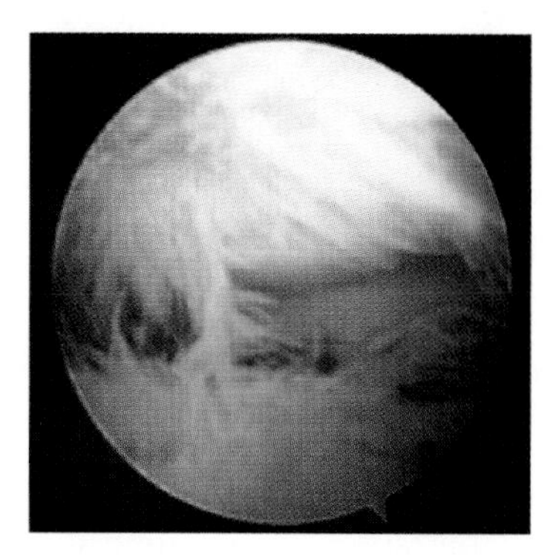

Fig. 47–3. Typical findings of impingement include proliferative bursitis and hypertrophy of the coracoacromial ligament.

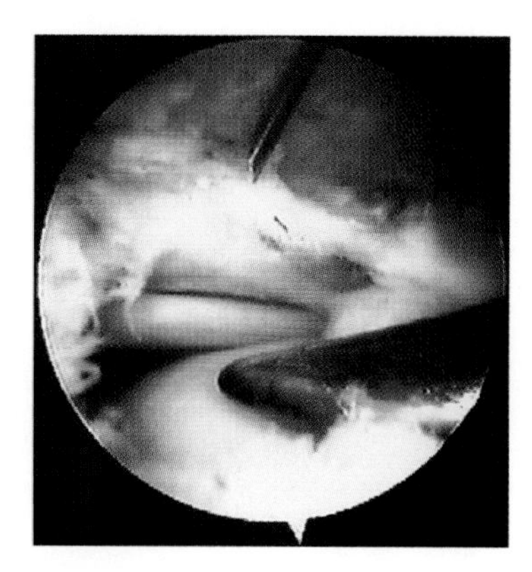

Fig. 47–4. A full-thickness rotator cuff tear.

With young, active patients, we repair full-thickness cuff tears. We use a "mini-open" approach for these patients. We use the arthroscope to evaluate the glenohumeral joint and the bursa and then perform arthroscopic acromioplasty. A small skin incision is used at the lateral edge of the acromion to expose the deltoid muscle and the acromion. The deltoid is split between its anterior and middle thirds, and the rotator cuff is exposed. The cuff is mobilized and repaired to a bony trough adjacent to the articular surface. Postoperatively, patients are treated with early mobilization, dynamic strengthening, and sport-specific exercises.

Arthroscopic decompression and débridement alone are considered for certain full-thickness rotator cuff tears. Older patients with massive irreparable tears or with the primary complaint of pain without objective or subjective weakness are offered débridement. These patients are treated postoperatively with rapid mobilization and an aggressive strengthening program that emphasizes restoration of transverse and coronal force couples.

Secondary Compression Cuff Disease

Initial treatment of patients with rotator cuff lesions caused by shoulder instability includes aggressive rehabilitation emphasizing dynamic stabilization of the glenohumeral joint. If conservative treatment fails, examination under anesthesia and arthroscopic glenohumeral and bursal evaluation help define the underlying problem. If the patient demonstrates evidence of anterior instability, stabilization, either arthroscopic or open, must be carried out. Secondary compressive disease may also be secondary to tensile failure of the rotator cuff. Repetitive tensile loading of the cuff, like that associated with violent deceleration of the throwing arm, can exceed the ability of both the dynamic cuff stabilizers and the static capsuloligamentous stabilizers and can lead to secondary impingement. Again, treatment is initially conservative. If this fails, arthroscopic débridement of the tensile tear is performed, with subacromial decompression or anterior stabilization, as necessary.

Tensile Lesions

Tensile lesions in an athlete's shoulder usually occur as undersurface cuff tears or lesion of the biceps-labrum complex.[3,10] The mechanism of injury in primary tensile failure is deceleration of the rotator cuff as it resists horizontal adduction, internal rotation, anterior translation, and distraction forces that occur during the deceleration phase of throwing.[6,11] Partial tears secondary to repetitive microtrauma are seen in the undersurface of the supraspinatus and posterior cuff tendons. Tensile lesions can also be secondary to anterior laxity when increased forces are placed on the posterior rotator cuff musculature.

On physical examination these patients often have minimal weakness and pain primarily over the supraspinatus and infraspinatus tendons and the posterior capsule. Advanced imaging with computed tomography (CT) arthrography or saline magnetic resonance imaging (MRI) may reveal partial tearing of the undersurface.

Initial treatment involves aggressive rehabilitation with strengthening of the rotator cuff and scapular stabilizers. If the patient does not improve, diagnostic and therapeutic arthroscopy can be considered. Arthroscopy usually reveals partial tearing of the undersurface of the rotator cuff at or near its insertion into the humerus and involves the supraspinatus and the posterior cuff. Arthroscopic débridement is done with a motorized shaver to healthy cuff tissue. Débridement should be done from both the anterior and the posterior portal, to ensure adequate débridement. Subacromial bursoscopy is then performed. The subacromial space is usually normal, but occasionally, in chronic conditions, secondary impingement may be present. In these patients, secondary decompression should be done.

Débridement of partial-thickness tears seems to decrease pain to the point where aggressive rehabilitation can be successfully completed. If instability is present, the primary lesion should be addressed in addition to cuff débridement.

Thrower's Exostosis

Posterior glenoid exostosis was initially described by Bennett in 1941.[12] These patients, most often throwing athletes, present with diffuse posterior shoulder symptoms and point tenderness over the posterior inferior glenoid. The cause of these lesions is thought to be traction or pulling of the posterior inferior capsule on the glenoid during followthrough. The exostosis is located approximately at the 8:00 o'clock position on the right glenoid and is probably a reaction to repeated microtrauma with tearing of the posterior and inferior capsule from its glenoid insertion. The lesion is well-defined using the Stryker notch view with careful examination of the inferior glenoid (Fig. 47–5). The exostosis is best visualized from the anterior portal using the 70° arthroscope. Arthroscopically, the glenoid exostosis is usually found in conjunction with posterior labral and undersurface cuff tearing. Resection can be done in symptomatic patients using motorized instruments to reflect the posterior and inferior capsule and excise the exostosis.[1] Resection is followed by aggressive rehabilitation to restore motion, strength, and dynamic stability. Arthroscopic resection performed on several pitchers alleviated symptoms and allowed them to return to competitive pitching.

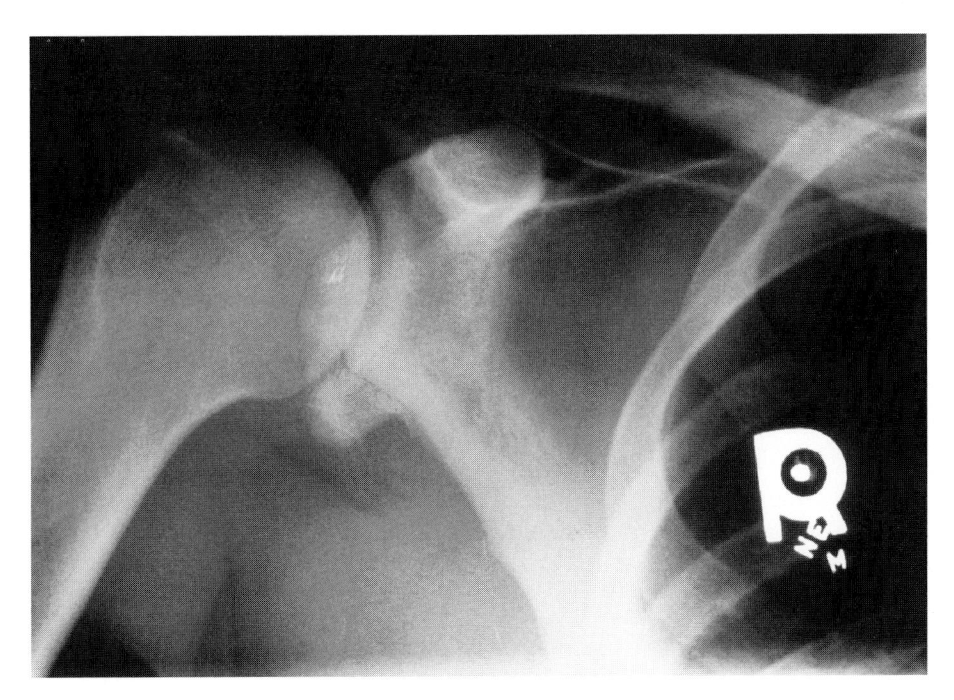

Fig. 47–5. Thrower's exostosis.

REFERENCES

1. Andrews, J. R., Carson, W. G., Jr., and Ortega, K.: Arthroscopy of the shoulder: Technique and normal anatomy. Am. J. Sports Med. *12*:1, 1984.
2. Altchek, D. W., Warren, R. F., and Skyhar, M. J.: Shoulder arthroscopy. *In* The Shoulder. Edited by C. A. Rockwood, Jr. and F. A. Matsen III. Philadelphia, W. B. Saunders, 1990.
3. Andrews, J. R., and Angelo, R. L.: Shoulder arthroscopy for the throwing athlete. *In* Operative Techniques in Shoulder Surgery. Edited by L. E. Paulos and J. E. Tibone. Gaithersburg Maryland, Aspen, 1991.
4. Andrews, J. R., Kupferman, S. P., and Dillman, C. J.: Labral tears in throwing and racquet sports. Clin. Sports Med. *10*:901, 1991.
5. Andrews, J. R., and Gillogly, S.: Physical examination of the shoulder in throwing athletes. *In* Injuries to the Throwing Arm. Edited by B. Zarins, J. R. Andrews, and W. G. Carson, Jr. Philadelphia, W. B. Saunders, 1985.
6. Caspari, R. B.: Arthroscopic reconstruction for anterior shoulder instability. *In* Operative Techniques in Shoulder Surgery. Edited by L. E. Paulos and J. E. Tibone. Gaithersburg, Maryland, Aspen, 1991.
7. Johnson, L. L.: Shoulder arthroscopy. *In* Arthroscopic Surgery, Principles and Practice. Edited by L. L. Johnson. St. Louis, C. V. Mosby, 1986.
8. Morgan, C. D., and Bodenstab, A. B.: Arthroscopic Bankart suture repair: Technique and early results. Arthroscopy *3*:111, 1987.
9. Arciero, R., Whazler, J., Ryan, J., and McBride, J.: Arthroscopic Bankart repair for initial anterior shoulder dislocations. Presented at American Orthopaedic Society for Sports Medicine Specialty Day. San Francisco, 1993.
10. Andrews, J. R., Broussard, T. S., and Carson, W. G., Jr.: Arthroscopy of the shoulder in the management of partial tears of the rotator cuff: A preliminary report. Arthroscopy *1*:117, 1985.
11. Andrews, J. R., Carson, W. G., Jr., and McLeod, W. D.: Glenoid labrum tears related to the long head of the biceps. Am. J. Sports Med. *13*:337, 1985.
12. Bennett, G. E.: Shoulder and elbow lesions of the professional baseball pitcher. J. A. M. A. *117*:510, 1941.

48

Tim L. Uhl

Rehabilitation After Injury or Surgery of the Shoulder

Several key components are involved in starting an athlete on a rehabilitation program for a shoulder injury. The first is knowledge of the anatomy of the human shoulder complex; but knowing the muscles, their actions, and their attachments is not enough to thoroughly rehabilitate an athlete to return to a particular sport. Understanding the biomechanics and stabilizing effects of the bony geometry, ligaments, and musculature of the arm while performing a particular action of a sport is the foundation on which a rehabilitation program is built.

The second component is understanding the normal mechanics of a particular sport. It is important to observe several hundred repetitions of a particular motion, to be able to identify early pathomechanical or subtle adaptive changes that indicate that an injury is present or is developing. This commonly occurs in microtraumatic or overuse injuries, as a response to excessive stress or to tight or weakened tissue. It is most prevalent among athletes in sports that involve repetitive overhead movements, such as baseball, tennis, swimming, and volleyball.

When an acute injury to the shoulder occurs, it is critical to understand the sport, to determine what position the arm was in and to identify what structures were stressed at the time of injury. For example, if a wrestler falls on his arm and reports that it felt as if it popped out while in a half-Nelson, the clinician should suspect anterior shoulder instability, since the arm was positioned in abduction and external rotation for this hold.

The third component is understanding the physical and mental requirements of the sport. Different level athletes require different levels of rehabilitation. A recreational tennis player participating at a 3.0 level and a collegiate tennis player are going to have different muscle capacities. The college athlete is probably going to produce higher-velocity serves and respond to high-speed serves with larger ballistic capabilities of the muscles than the 3.0 player, even though they are playing the same sport. When setting up a rehabilitation program for a particular athlete, the goals of the program must be consistent with the athlete's goals, not with the goals of the coach or parents who are supporting the athlete. Understanding the psychology of the athlete in rehabilitation is critical to a successful rehabilitation program.

The final, and probably most critical, component is communication between the physician and the treating athletic trainer or physical therapist. For example, if an orthopedic surgeon feels that the tissue was attenuated at the time of surgery, a slower rehabilitation protocol might be best, so as not to damage the repaired structures. Therefore, communication between physician, coach, and athlete or parent in rehabilitating the athlete frequently rests on the shoulders of the treating therapist or trainer. With all parties communicating, a sports medicine team approach is promoted that we have found to be the most successful way to rehabilitate any patient.

PHASES OF SHOULDER REHABILITATION

Most shoulder rehabilitation programs can be divided into phases. Ours is divided into three: Phase I, the acute phase or immediate postinjury or postsurgery phase; Phase II, the subacute phase or strengthening and endurance phase; and Phase III, the advanced, sport-specific rehabilitation phase.

With some injuries a patient can go through all three phases in a week or two. Other injuries may require a patient to go through rehabilitation for a full year to a year and a half to advance through all three phases. Generally, rehabilitation protocols are physician- or clinic specific and do not take into consideration extraneous variables such as patient motivation, severity of injury, and quality of tissue, which are all important factors in developing a rehabilitation program.

Set time frames for rehabilitation protocols are difficult to follow for the variety of patients seen. One common denominator of all athletic injuries is the healing phases. The three phases of the rehabilitation program generally follow three healing phases. The first phase, the inflammatory phase, begins immediately after injury and lasts 5 to 6 days. It is characterized by hematoma formation, warmth, redness, and pain. The fibrin clot is formed while removal of damaged tissue is initiated during this phase. The tensile strength of the tissue is very low, since the fibrin clot is the principal source of strength. Therefore, the exercises performed during this phase must be light, to protect the low tensile strength of the injured tissue.

The second phase is called the proliferation phase, it begins on the fourth or fifth day after injury and winds down in approximately 3 weeks. It is characterized by contraction of the wound edges, deposition of extracellular matrix and collagen, and capillary growth. This is the critical phase in which to align new tissue in the correct planes by early motion; however, the tensile strength of the tissue is still weak and cannot withstand large forces. Therefore, exercises to stretch and strengthen the injured tissue must be monitored closely so as not to aggravate the healing tissue.

The third or final phase, the maturation phase, begins at approximately 3 weeks and may last 12 months or more. This is when the definitive scar tissue is formed. Type I collagen is still being laid down; however, tensile strength is increasing faster than the net volume of collagen. Normal stresses of athletic activity are tolerated as the tissue continues to strengthen. The progressive intensity of the exercises allows the healing tissue to accommodate increasing stresses.[1]

Phase I

The primary goals during Phase I are controlling inflammation and pain, protecting damaged or repaired tissue, preventing loss of motion, and minimizing loss of strength of injured and surrounding structures.

Several electromodalities and thermomodalities are available to help control pain and inflammation. These techniques are discussed in detail in a later chapter. The most commonly used modality in our practice is still good old-fashioned ice. Ice is used for two reasons: (1) it is effective in controlling inflammation and pain and (2) it is economical and convenient for athletes to use at home.

An important technique in controlling pain that is frequently overlooked is positioning of the shoulder. Frequently, patients complain of hand swelling, neck pain, and pain at rest in the shoulder after an acute trauma. Kaltenborn recommends the resting position of the shoulder be 55° abduction, 30° horizontal adduction, and 0° rotation.[2] This position minimizes tensile strain in the supraspinatus tendon while preventing the "wringing out" of the tendon's vascular supply.[3] This position also minimizes inferior capsule tightness by keeping a mild stretch on the capsule. Positioning the patient in 30° to 45° recumbency to rest or to sleep has generally been found more comfortable for patients during the acute stage.

The exercises listed in Table 48–1 are commonly used in our athletic shoulder rehabilitation program. Not all exercises are used each time and there are other exercises that can be incorporated as necessary and appropriate.

Generally, all exercises are performed for 10 to 50 repetitions, two or three times a day. These exercises are limited by pain during this phase and are modified if they seem to be aggravating the injury. A general rule of thumb is to expect discomfort for a few hours after exercise; however, if pain and discomfort last 24 to 48 hours after exercise, the exercise should be discontinued or modified.

Phase II

The goals for Phase II rehabilitation are to regain full passive and active range of motion of the shoulder, regain nearly normal strength of the shoulder, and regain normal aerobic conditioning level and the rest of the body's normal strength and endurance levels.

In Phase II we work on fatigue-resistant Type I muscle fibers with high repetitions and low resistance (Table 48–2). Using a heavy weight is a common mistake in rehabilitation. Unfortunately, it causes larger muscle groups around the shoulder to compensate for the weakened rotator cuff and does not strengthen the cuff muscles.

Some excellent articles have been written on the electromyographic activity of the rotator cuff associated with a variety of shoulder exercises.[4–6] The incorporation of this valuable research gives a scientific basis for the core

Table 48–1. Phase I Exercises

Pendulum
Stick or T-bar exercises (passive to active assisted range of motion)
- Flexion
- Abduction in the plane of the scapula (scaption)
- Abduction
- Internal rotation at 0° and 90°
- External rotation at 0° and 90°

Rope and pulley (passive to active assisted range of motion)
- Flexion
- Abduction in the plane of the scapula (scaption)
- Abduction

Active range of motion
- Elbow/wrist/hand

Shoulder isometrics (arm at 0°, elbow at 90°)
- Flexion-extension
- Abduction-adduction
- Internal-external rotation

Scapular retraction and depression

Table 48–2. Phase II Exercises

- Stretching exercises to obtain terminal range of motion
- Stick or T-bar
  - Supine external rotation at 135° to 180° abduction
  - Side-lying internal rotation at 90° abduction
  - Internal rotation pulling the arm up the back
- Progressive resistive exercises
  - "Core exercises"
    - Prone horizontal abduction (supraspinatus)
    - Prone external rotation at 90° abduction (infraspinatus)
    - Prone extension (teres minor)
    - Pushup plus (serratus anterior)
    - Press-up/sitting dips (pectoralis minor)
    - Rowing (rhomboids)
    - Scaption (trapezius)
  - Supplemental shoulder exercises
    - Standing
      - Flexion
      - Abduction
      - Internal/external rotation at 0° to 90° with a pulley or rubber tubing
      - Diagonal patterns with a pulley or rubber tubing: flexion–abduction–external rotation, extension–adduction–internal rotation
    - Side-lying external rotation at 0°
    - Prone flexion
  - Elbow-strengthening exercises
    - Biceps curls
    - Triceps extensions
    - Weight room exercises (modified range of motion not allowing elbows past the plane of the shoulder)

exercises prescribed for strengthening the periscapular and rotator cuff muscles.

Blackburn and coworkers described the core exercises for the rotator cuff in throwing athletes.[4] Prone horizontal abduction (Fig. 48–1) works the supraspinatus muscle; prone external rotation at 90° of abduction (Fig. 48–2) works the infraspinatus muscle; and prone extension (Fig. 48–3) works the teres major muscle.

Townsend and colleagues also did research based on muscle firing patterns in the shoulder and added core exercises for strengthening the scapular muscles.[5] The *pushup plus* consists of a normal pushup adding maximum shoulder and scapular protraction with elbows fully extended to strengthen the serratus anterior. Elevation of the arm in the scapular plane with the arm in neutral rotation works the middle trapezius. The press-up, or sitting dip, is done by having the patient sit with hands on the table surface on either side of the hips. The patient lifts his or her body off the table, thus exercising the pectoralis minor muscle. Rowing is performed by both arms pulling against resistance toward the body, pinching the shoulder blades together to exercise the rhomboid muscles.

Several options are available to the treating physical therapist or athletic trainer for resistive exercises—manual resistance, water, rubber tubing, weights, and isokinetics. Any mode of resistive training can be effective, but the key is the experience of the treating clinician and deciding what works best for the individual athlete and the particular situation.

These exercises are progressive resistive exercises, so people progress at their own rate. Generally, all exer-

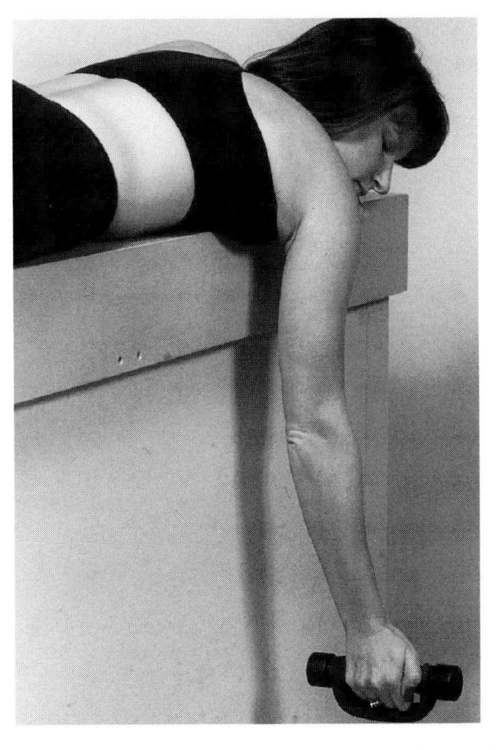

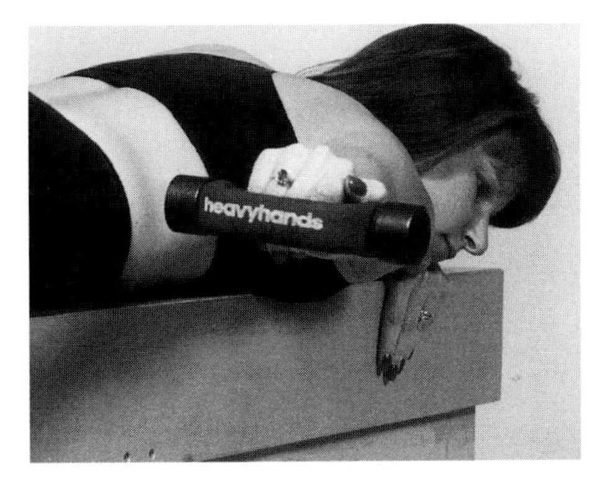

Fig. 48–1. Prone horizontal abduction is done with the arm in external rotation, so that the thumb points away from the body. The arm is lifted into horizontal abduction until it is parallel to the floor and makes a 90° to 100° angle with the body of the axilla. The arm is held in this position for 3 seconds and then returned to the resting position.

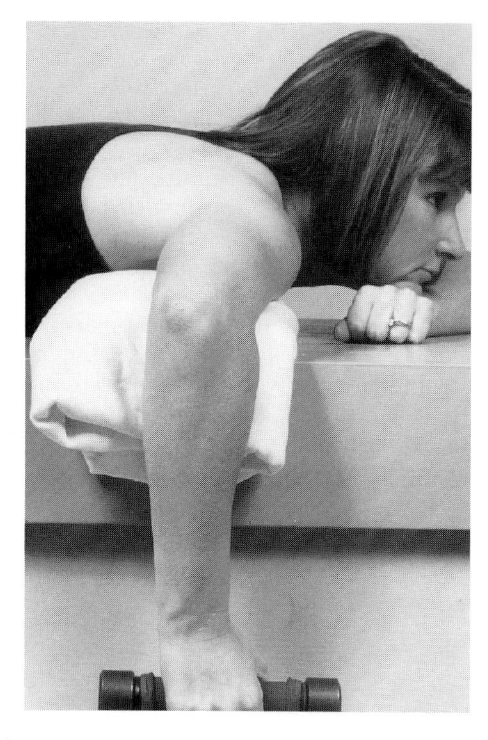

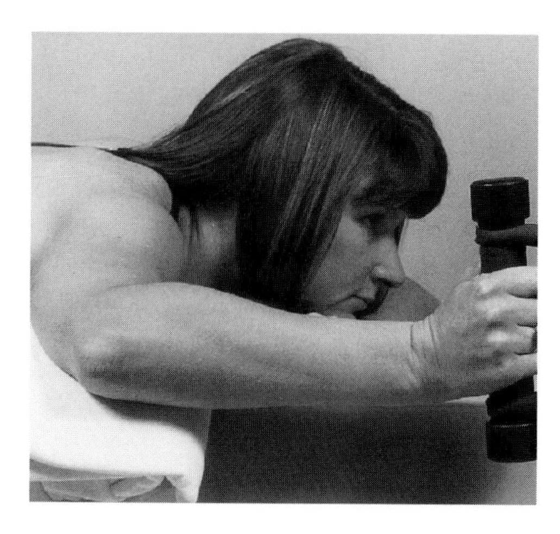

Fig. 48–2. Prone external rotation is done with the upper arm supported on the table and the elbow at the edge of the table. The forearm is externally rotated until it is parallel with the floor. The arm is held in this position for 3 seconds and then returned to the resting position.

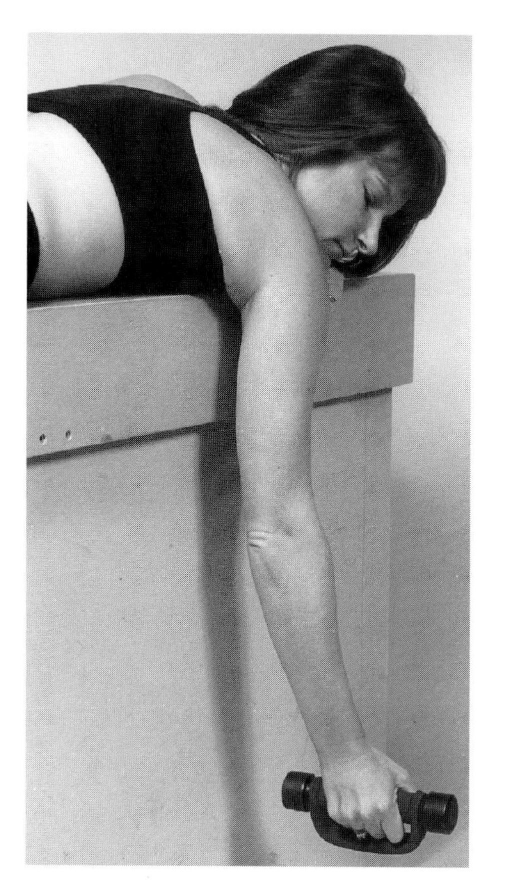

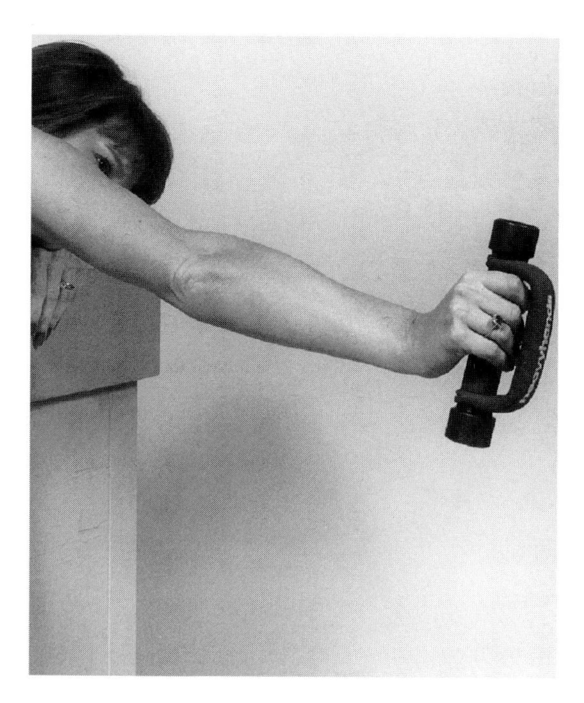

Fig. 48–3. Prone extension is done with the arm externally rotated so that the thumb points away from the body. The arm is extended until parallel with the floor and held in this position for 3 seconds. The arm is then returned to the resting position.

cises are started with no resistance until proper technique is attained. Incremental progression works well with injured tissues. For example, patients may start with a 1-pound weight and gradually increase the number of repetitions as they feel comfortable. Once the designated repetitions can be done, a 2-pound weight can be used, dropping the number of repetitions back to 10. The progressive increase in repetitions begins again.

Phase II exercises are performed one or two times a day, 10 to 50 repetitions, as tolerated. As the resistance increases and as the athlete progresses to Phase III and more sport-specific activities, resistive training is cut back to two to three times per week. For most of the exercises resistance is kept low (1 to 3 pounds) to prevent substitution of larger muscles for the commonly involved rotator cuff muscles. Any exercise that seems to aggravate the shoulder should be modified or discontinued.

Phase III

In this phase, the goals are to prepare the shoulder for high-velocity ballistic concentric and eccentric stress and to return the athlete to full sports participation. The SAID principle (*s*pecific *a*ctivity to *i*mposed *d*emand) is the focus of this phase, no matter what sport or activity the athlete wants to perform. This requires that the treating therapist or trainer have a good understanding of the mechanics of the sport and be creative with the rehabilitation program to help the athlete achieve the ultimate goal.

Many injuries of the shoulder commonly seen in sports are caused by excessive eccentric loads on the musculotendinous junctions and ligamentous tissue about the shoulder. After the tissue is repaired or healed, which usually occurs during Phase I and II, the capacity for these tissues to handle high-velocity loads must be regained during Phase III. The focus of this phase's exercises are to progressively increase the eccentric and concentric load capacity of the shoulder.

There are no set criteria for initiation of Phase III activities; each situation is different. Generally, we like to see full pain-free active range of motion of the shoulder complex and minimal, if any, side-to-side difference in manual muscle tests of rotator cuff and periscapular musculature. Some clinicians like to use an isokinetic strength test to determine progression of exercises.

EXERCISES

Flexerciser Rod and Body Blade are devices that can be used to facilitate dynamic cocontraction of the musculature about the shoulder by using oscillatory motions. The arm can be in any position while the oscillatory motions are performed—in flexion-extension, abduction-adduction, or internal-external rotation. These exercises are generally performed in sets of three to five times for 10 to 30 seconds per position or motion. The arm can be moved while the oscillations are occurring from a position of strength to a position of weakness and then return to initial position.

Inertial exercise is another technique for facilitating concentric and eccentric strengthening of the musculotendinous unit. The Impulse is the device we use, and it can be set up to work any motion of the upper arm specific to the athlete's sport. The principle of inertial exercise is that, as the mass decreases, acceleration forces increase. Therefore, in a rehabilitation program, a weight of 10 to 15 pounds is started with and the patient works toward weights of 1 to 2 pounds, thus attaining greater acceleration and deceleration speeds to duplicate forces that shoulder would have to tolerate to return to sports. This type of exercise is generally performed for 1 to 3 sets of 30 seconds for each prescribed motion.

Plyometric training is another technique used in this phase. Plyometrics have been used for years for lower body power training in track and field events. This has been so effective that upper body plyometrics have received much attention by trainers and therapists over the last 5 years. A weighted medicine ball of 2 to 12 pounds has many applications in rehabilitation of shoulder injuries. A general rule of thumb of plyometric progression is two-handed activities to one-handed activities and simple, pain-free motions to functional, more difficult and stressful motions.

The focus of this rehabilitation technique is quickness of reversing catching to throwing; often a rebounder is used so athletes can work at their own pace. This reversing phase is known as *the amortization phase.* The shorter this phase is, the greater eccentric stress and concentric force production is developed in the shoulder musculature. For the individual sport, this might require a variety of positions to exercise the appropriate musculature. Three to five sets of 10 to 30 repetitions is a standard prescription for each motion.

The most important aspect of the Phase III rehabilitation is the progressive return to sports participation. This critical step from rehabilitation to normal performance should in all sports be closely supervised by a certified athletic trainer or physical therapist. The following passage describes a return-to-throwing program commonly used at our clinic.

INTERVAL THROWING PROGRAM

The interval throwing program is designed to allow the athlete to work two times a day at a submaximal level, trying never to fatigue the arm but to get a light workout. This enables the arm to gradually become stronger and more conditioned to the act of throwing. The program should begin with thorough stretching of the throwing extremity and application of moist heat. It should be followed by ice, as necessary. Even though the athlete *could* throw harder, that is not the idea of this program. It is slow buildup and conditioning of the arm that will allow the athlete to progress and to not reinjure the shoulder.

The athlete throws 2 days in a row and rests a day. One interval equals one set of long tosses and one set of short tosses with two intervals being thrown in a day. Each throwing session begins with several minutes of 10-foot tossing, to get the arm warmed up for the long tosses. The long toss set may start with throws that will just roll to a partner and graduate to one hop and then on the fly. The athlete may gradually work up to the long toss distance. We give the athlete a time limit and a number of tosses to reach. In the guidelines given below, which are based on rehabilitation for a college or professional pitcher, the athlete stops after the time limit or the number of tosses has been reached, whichever comes first.

Phase I: The long toss set is 5 minutes or 25 throws at 90 feet, with intensity to tolerance. The short toss set is 5 minutes or 50 throws at 30 feet working at half speed.
Phase II: The long toss set is 5 minutes or 25 throws at 120 feet, with intensity to tolerance. The short toss set is 5 minutes or 50 throws at 60 feet working at half speed.
Phase III: The long toss set is 5 minutes or 25 throws at 150 feet. The short toss set is 5 minutes or 50 throws at 60 feet at three-quarters work speed.
Phase IV: The long toss set is 5 minutes or 25 throws at 180 feet. The short toss set is 5 minutes or 50 throws at 60 feet with three-quarters work speed and throws off the mound.
Phase V: The long toss set is 5 minutes or 25 throws at 210 feet. The short toss set is 5 minutes or 50 throws at 60 feet with one-half to three-quarters speed and throws off the mound, throwing breaking balls.
Phase VI: The long toss set is 5 minutes or 25 throws at 250 feet. The short toss set is 5 minutes or 50 throws at 60 feet or more at three-quarters to full speed with throws off the mound, throwing breaking balls.

SPECIFIC DIAGNOSES

Rotator Cuff Tendinitis, Bursitis, Impingement Syndrome

Rotator cuff tendinitis, bursitis, and impingement syndrome generally are treated in similar fashion. Initially, for approximately 2 weeks, the acute inflammatory process is controlled with relative rest from activities that exacerbate symptoms. This is followed by Phase I exercises and pain and inflammation control. Once full active range of motion is achieved, Phase II strengthening activities are performed for the next 4 weeks.

Precautions should be taken when performing the exercises in this phase. Any motions that cause impingement or aggravate the shoulder should be stopped or modified. Commonly, the exercise of prone external rotation is modified to side-lying external rotation with the arm abducted no more than 20° until rotator cuff muscles are stronger. Activities with the arm below 90° of elevation are usually tolerated better initially, and the patient gradually works up to overhead reaching activities. Phase III activities can usually be started at 6 weeks, as long as symptoms are resolving. The objectives should be to develop eccentric strength of the posterior cuff and scapular musculature plus posterior cuff flexibility, to complete the rehabilitation program and prevent injury. Having the patient lie on one side with the shoulders turned so that the affected scapula is stabilized against the table surface allows passive stretching in internal rotation (Fig. 48–4).

If patients do not respond to rehabilitation in approximately 3 months, they probably need débridement and decompression, either open or arthroscopic. Since, generally, no tissue repair is performed in this surgical intervention, passive range of motion, active assisted range of motion, and other Phase I exercises can be started on the first day after surgery. Phase I exercises are generally performed for 2 to 3 weeks at whatever level pain tolerance dictates. Phase II is then initiated, focusing on the core rotator cuff and scapular exercises for 4 to 6 weeks. Phase III exercises are combined with those of Phase II as soon as the athlete has full pain-free active range of motion and as long as the activities do not increase symptoms. Commonly, athletes can return to modified or full athletic competition in approximately 2 to 3 months.

Rotator Cuff Tears

Initially, rotator cuff tears are treated conservatively, with the phased rehabilitation program, for 6 weeks to 3 months. If the patient does not regain normal strength and has recurring irritation, surgical intervention is required. For partial rotator cuff tears, open or arthroscopic débridement and decompression is the treatment of choice. The postoperative rehabilitation program is the same one described above, and the athlete is generally ready for competitive sports in 2 to 4 months.

Complete rotator cuff tears require open surgical intervention. A period of 4 to 6 weeks is needed for collagen healing to mature before active range of motion exercises can begin. Therefore, Phase I is extended to 4 to 6 weeks with assisted exercises, such as stick and rope and pulley, performed primarily in a passive manner. Active assisted exercises using these devices are instituted as soon as healing constraints allow, and the focus is on technique of motions performed, so substitution patterns are not developed. Phase II low resistive isometric or isotonic exercises are started at approximately 6 weeks, to restore normal function and strength of the rotator cuff muscles.

Phase III activities are generally started 4 to 6 weeks after the core program is instituted, to allow development of strength. Patients with complete rotator cuff tears may take 4 to 6 months, sometimes longer, to work up to sport-specific activities.

Glenoid Labral Tears

Glenoid labral tears are treated very much like rotator cuff tendinitis. The differences are that stabilization of the glenohumeral joint by the rotator cuff and scapular muscles seems to be the key to successful nonoperative treatment. Labral tears can be associated with ligamentous compromise, so, positions that cause pain or stress to damaged tissue should be avoided or minimized. If enhancing muscle control through rehabilitation cannot obviate the pain or stress associated with certain positions or motions that are required for athletic competition, surgical intervention may be indicated.

Patients who undergo labral débridement with no ligamentous or labral repair generally follow the rehabili-

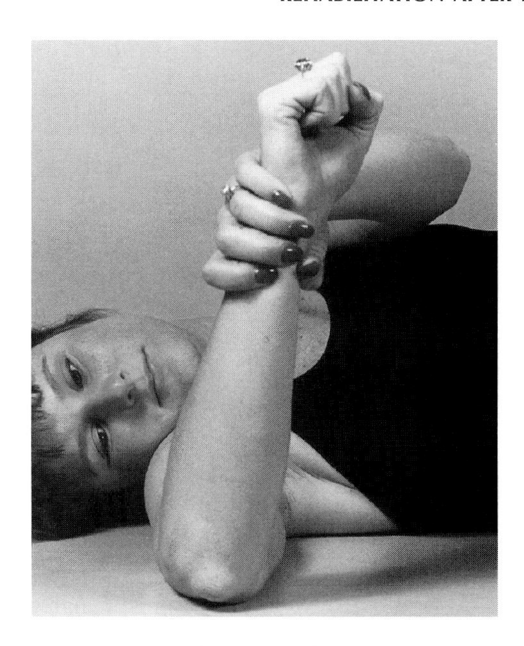

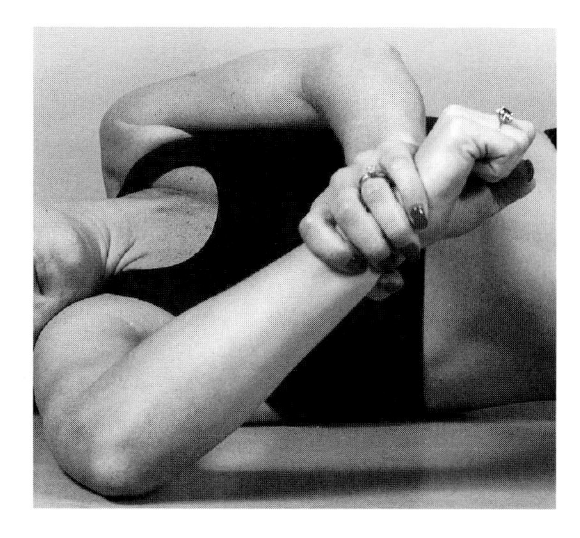

Fig. 48–4. Side-lying internal rotation is done with the arm positioned in 90° abduction. The patient gently internally rotates the arm with the opposite hand to the point of stretch but not of pain. This position is held for 15 to 20 seconds and the arm then is returned to the starting position.

tation program outlined above for patients who undergo rotator cuff débridements. For patients who have labral repairs for Bankart and superior labrum anterior posterior (SLAP) lesions, we usually keep the shoulder immobilized for 4 to 6 weeks for healing. The shoulder is usually held in internal rotation; therefore, external rotation motions are generally the most difficult to regain. SLAP lesion repairs generally involve the long head of the biceps, so active and resistive elbow flexion exercises and passive shoulder extension exercises are guarded for 4 to 6 weeks. Patients treated with these repairs generally progress through Phase I in 2 to 4 weeks after the immobilization period. Phase II and III take approximately 6 to 8 weeks, each, to complete.

Glenohumeral Instability

Determining the cause of the instability assists greatly in establishing realistic expectations for rehabilitation. Burkhead and Rockwood published results where 87% of AMBRI (Atraumatic, Multidirectional, Bilateral, Rehabilitation, Inferior capsular shift) type patients responded positively to nonoperative treatment and only 18% of TUBS (Traumatic, Unidirectional, Bankart, Surgery) type patients got better with nonoperative treatment.(8) Focusing on Phase II and III exercises, and specifically on dynamic stabilization of the glenohumeral joint by the rotator cuff and scapular muscles, seems to be the key to nonoperative treatment.

Many surgical interventions are available to correct shoulder instability. The most common surgical intervention for athletes, especially those who reach overhead, is capsular reconstruction. Postoperatively, the shoulder is relatively immobilized for 3 to 6 weeks and isometric shoulder exercises are instituted at 2 to 3 weeks. Phase I active assisted range of motion exercises are commenced after the immobilization phase. Active assisted range of motion exercises are the focus, so that muscles about the shoulder protect the repaired capsular tissue. Frequently, gradual return of external rotation and elevation range of motion over a 3-month period is prescribed. For example, after inferior capsular shift surgery for a multidirectional instability, external rotation is limited to 30° for 6 weeks and 50° for 9 weeks after the immobilization period, while elevation is limited to 130° for 6 weeks and 150° for 9 weeks after the immobilization period. This protects the repaired tissue from being stretched too soon.

Phase II exercises are commenced within the available range of motion of the shoulder by 2 to 4 weeks after the immobilization period. The patient's pain tolerance, reaction to the exercise, and individual technique for performing the exercises guide the progression. If scapular stabilization exercises and normal scapulohumeral patterns can be incorporated into the program early, the patient has less chance of developing poor biomechanical motions in the shoulder. Phase III exercise usually is added 3 to 4 months postoperatively and is practiced for 3 to 4 months, so the total rehabilitation process averages 6 to 9 months after operation.

The phased rehabilitation program is designed to be modified for the specific needs of the athlete. These exercises have been used with great success over the years to deal with all types of patients. Because new information on the shoulder comes out continuously, the treating clinician must stay in tune with the current literature. When, however, a difficult problem arises, it is always good practice to return to the basics: Listen to the patient. Think about the anatomy and mechanics of the problem area and of the entire body. Then, discuss it as a team, to resolve the problem.

REFERENCES

1. Leadbetter, W. B., Buckwalter, J. A., and Gordon, S. L. (eds.): Sports-Induced Inflammation: Clinical and Basic Science Concepts. Park Ridge, IL, American Academy of Orthopaedic Surgeons, 1990.
2. Kaltenborn, F. M.: Manual Therapy of External Joints. 3rd Ed. Oslo, Olafnorlis Vokhandel, 1983.
3. Rathbun, J. B., and Macnab, I.: The microvascular pattern of the rotator cuff. J. Bone Joint Surg. *52B*:540, 1970.
4. Blackburn, T. A., McLeod, W. D., White B., and Wofford, L.: EMG analysis of posterior rotator cuff exercises. Athletic Training *25*:41, 1990.
5. Townsend, H., Jobe, F. W., Pink, M., and Perry, J.: Electromyographic analysis of the glenohumeral muscles during a baseball rehabilitation program. Am. J. Sports Med. *19*:264, 1991.
6. Moseley, J. B., Jr., et al.: EMG analysis of the scapular muscles during a shoulder rehabilitation program. Am. J. Sports Med. *20* :128, 1992.
7. Wilk, K. E., et al.: The strength characteristics of internal and external rotator muscles in professional baseball pitchers. Am. J. Sports Med. *21*:61, 1993.
8. Burkhead, W. Z. Jr., and Rockwood, C. A., Jr.: Treatment of instability of the shoulder with an exercise program. J. Bone Joint Surg. *74A*:890, 1992.

49 *Kurt E. Jacobson*

Functional Anatomy and Biomechanics of the Elbow

The unique qualities of the elbow joint make it well-suited for its specialized function in the upper extremity. The shoulder determines the spacial position of the limb, and the elbow then regulates the limb length and height to optimize hand position and function. During high-load, complex motions such as overhand throwing, the elbow integrates the function of the shoulder and hand, allowing the athlete to propel the ball at high speeds and deliver it precisely to a target. The elbow functions by taking advantage of the concerted activity of its musculotendinous and bony structures.

ANATOMY

The bony anatomy of the elbow permits flexion and extension as well as pronation and supination. It provides a stable base to accept varus, valgus, and axial forces during functional activities. There are three separate articulations at the elbow joint: the humeroulnar, humeroradial, and radioulnar joints.

Humeroulnar Joint

The distal end of the humerus widens in the mediolateral plane and is made up of the medial and lateral condyles. The capitellum and trochlea are the articulating surfaces of the lateral and medial condyles, respectively. The trochlea is shaped like an asymmetric spool, with a groove bounded by medial and lateral ridges. The proximal end of the ulna articulates with the groove, whereas the medial and lateral ridges of the trochlea give stability.[1] In the anteroposterior plane, the articular surface of the distal humerus lies, on average, in 6° of valgus (Fig. 49–1A).[2] From the lateral perspective there is 30° to 45° of anterior angulation (Fig. 49–1B). Axially, the articulating surface lies in 3° to 8° of internal rotation with respect to the epicondylar axis.[3]

On the proximal ulna, the olecranon and coronoid processes create the sigmoid notch. From the lateral perspective the articular surface of the ulna has 30° to 45° of posterior angulation to match the 30° to 45° of anterior angulation of the distal humerus (Fig. 49–1C). This relationship enhances the bones' stability in the extended position. The articular surface of the proximal ulna also averages several degrees of valgus in relation to the axis of the shaft.

The combined valgus angles of the distal humerus and proximal ulna articular surfaces determine the carrying angle of the extremity (Fig. 49–1D). The carrying angle is the angle formed by the long axes of the humerus and the ulna with the elbow fully extended. This angle averages 10° to 15° and is usually a few degrees larger in women than in men. This angle allows loads to be carried with the elbow in extension without requiring active abduction of the shoulder. The relative degree of valgus of the elbow decreases during pronation, as the radial shaft rotates over the ulna.

Normal anatomic variations in the angulation of the articulating surfaces account for the different degrees of extension or recurvatum of the elbow, as well as relative varus-valgus angulation in extension and flexion. Injury to the condyles, such as supracondylar or condylar fractures, may also change the articular angles or axial alignment.

Humeroradial Joint

The capitellum is almost ball shaped and is separated from the trochlea by a groove (see Fig. 49–1A). The

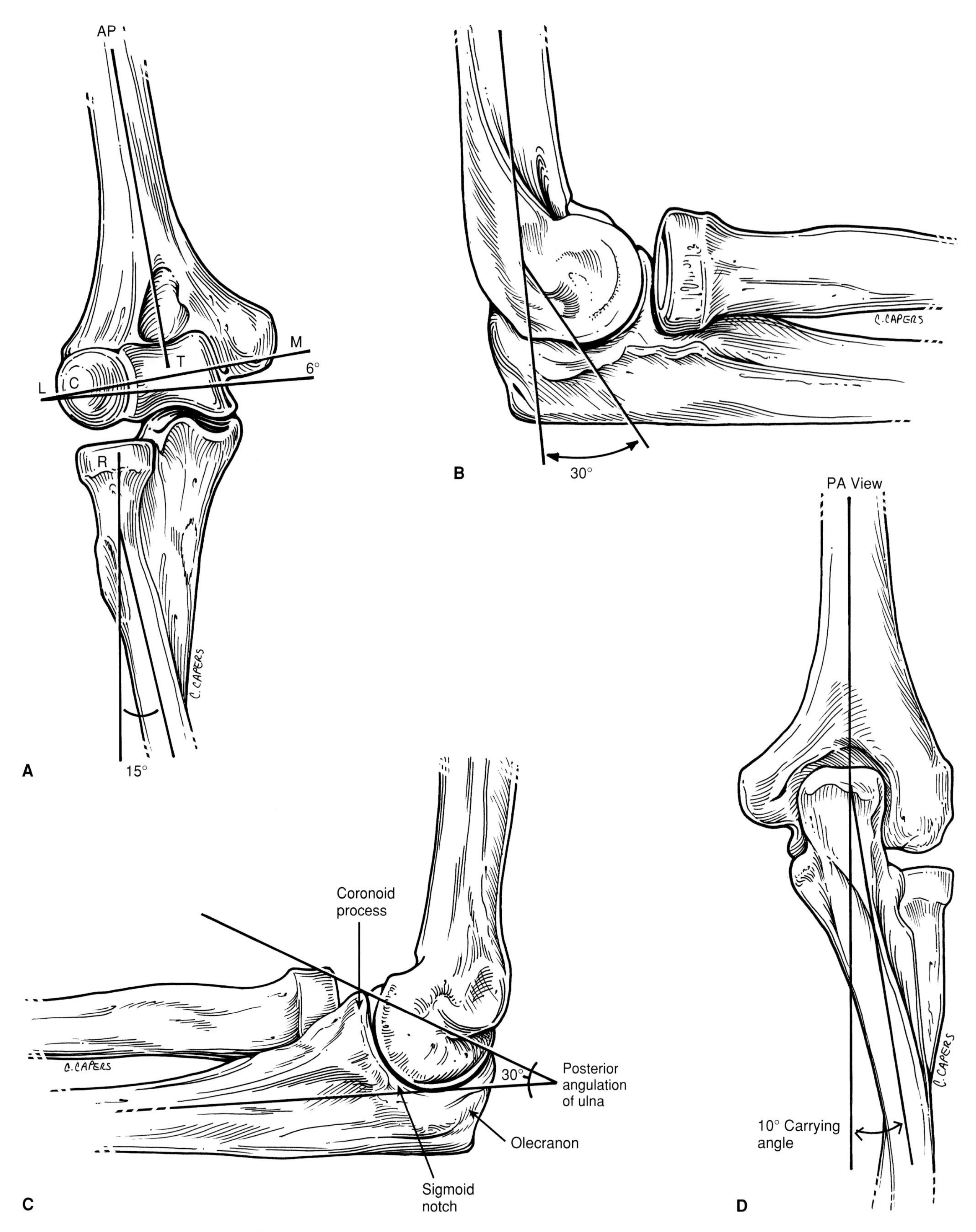

Fig. 49–1. Humeroulnar joint. *(A)* The articular surface of the distal humerus lies, on average in 6° of valgus. (Key: L, Lateral condyle; C, Capitellum; T, trochlea; M, medial condyle; R, radius.) *(B)* The articular surface of the distal humerus has 30° to 45° angulation. *(C)* From the lateral view, the ulna has 30° to 45° of posterior angulation to match the angulation of the distal humerus. *(D)* The carrying angle is formed by the long axes of the humerus and the ulna with the elbow fully extended.

shallow, cup-shaped radial head articulates with the capitellum. The radial neck is angled, on average, 15° in relation to the radial shaft (Fig. 49–2A).[2] The humeroradial (radiocapitellar) joint is subject to both axial and valgus loading. Rotational motion occurs at the radiocapitellar joint during pronation and supination over an arc of 160°.

Proximal Radioulnar Joint

On the lateral aspect of the coronoid process, the radial notch articulates with the margin of the radial head. The annular ligament secures the joint via its attachment to the anterior and posterior notch margins (Fig. 49–2B).

Elbow Motion

Flexion and extension of the elbow occur between the humeroulnar and humeroradial joints, over an arc of 160°. The axis of rotation is central within the trochlea and capitellum, in line with the anterior surface of the distal humeral shaft. The instant center of motion varies only 2 to 3 mm during the helical motion of the flexion arc. Extension is limited by the olecranon process, anterior capsule, and elbow flexor muscles. Flexion is limited by anterior muscle bulk, the posterior capsule, and triceps contraction.

Pronation and supination occur through an axis from the center of the radial head to the distal articular surface of the ulna (Fig. 49–3). The average arc of pronation is 70°; that of supination, 80° to 85°.

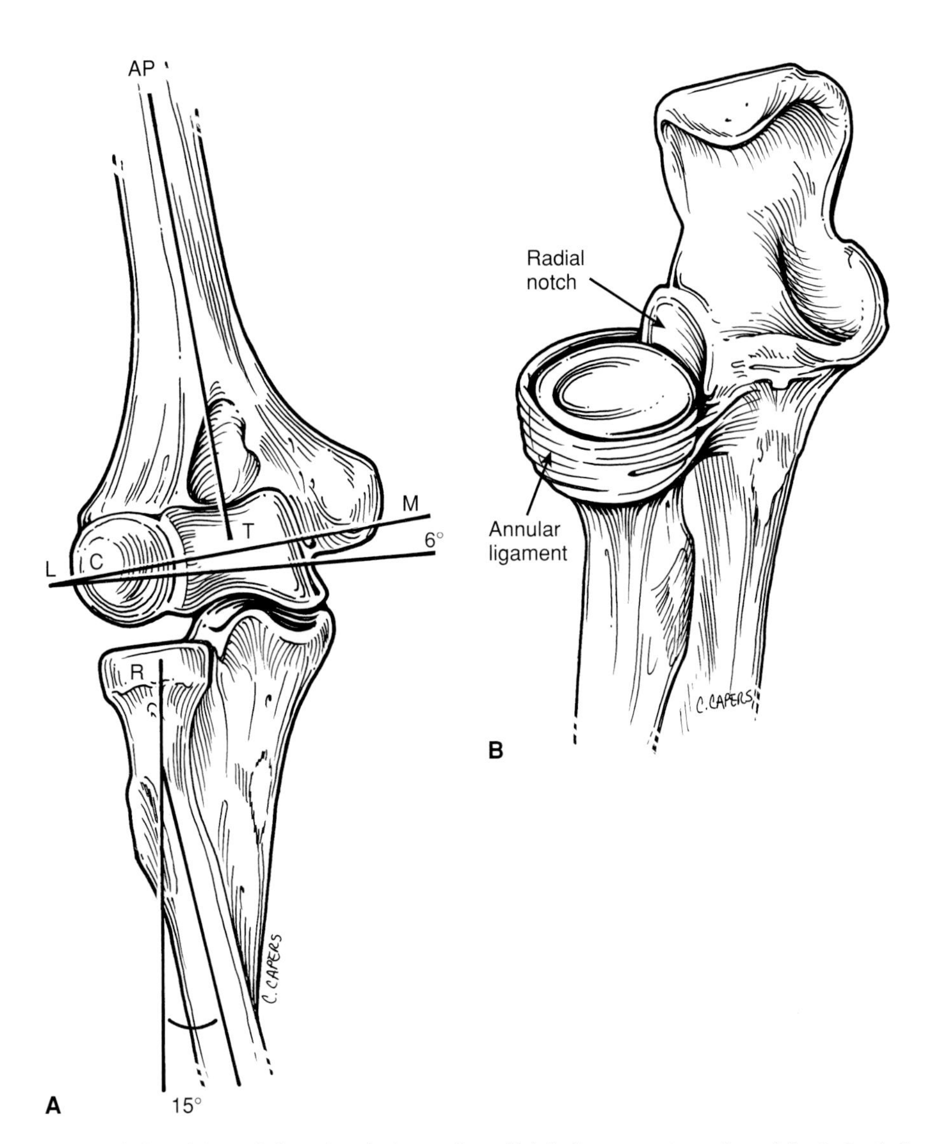

Fig. 49–2. ***(A)*** **The radial neck is angled 15° in relation to the radial shaft. (Key: L, Lateral condyle; C, Capitellum; T, trochlea; M, medial condyle; R, radius.)** ***(B)*** **The radial notch articulates with the margin of the radial head. The annular ligament secures the joint.**

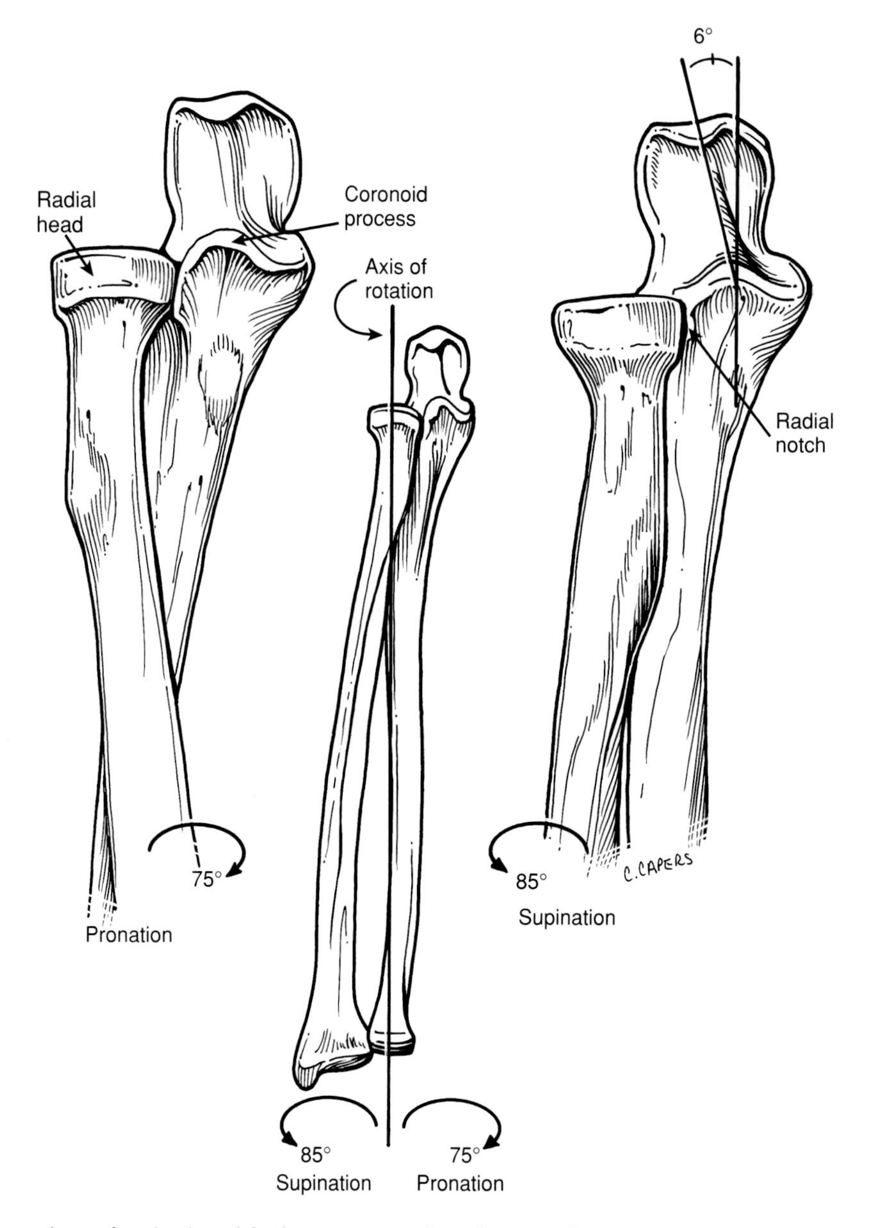

Fig. 49–3. Pronation and supination of the forearm occurs through an axis that extends from the center of the radial head to the distal articular surface of the ulna.

The inherent stability of the elbow is due in large part to its unique interlocking bony anatomy. The bony articulations provide approximately 50% of the elbow's stability under varus-valgus loads; the trochlea and ulnar fossa provide the primary foundation. Posterior displacement of the ulna with reference to the humerus is blocked by the coronoid process. In the flexed position, the capitellum and radius resist valgus stress and posterior dislocation. Over the last 30° of extension the olecranon locks in its fossa, providing valgus stability.

The motion required for activities of daily living is flexion and extension over a range of 100° (30° to 130°) and supination and pronation over a range of 100° (50° to 150°). Limitations of these motions may require compensation by shoulder abduction and rotation as well as trunk and head movement.

Soft Tissue

The soft tissue structures about the elbow provide 50% of the restraining force in extension and 25% in flexion.[2] The medial collateral ligament, an important stabilizer against valgus stress, is composed of two primary bundles as well as an additional transverse component (Fig. 49–4A). The anterior oblique bundle is the primary medial stabilizer and is tight over much of the arc of motion. The posterior oblique bundle is less important and is taut only in flexion. The transverse component appears to serve little function. Morrey has shown that, because the origins of the anterior and posterior bundles do not lie on the axis of rotation, a cam effect is created that allows for varied tension of the ligament fibers over the arc of motion.[2]

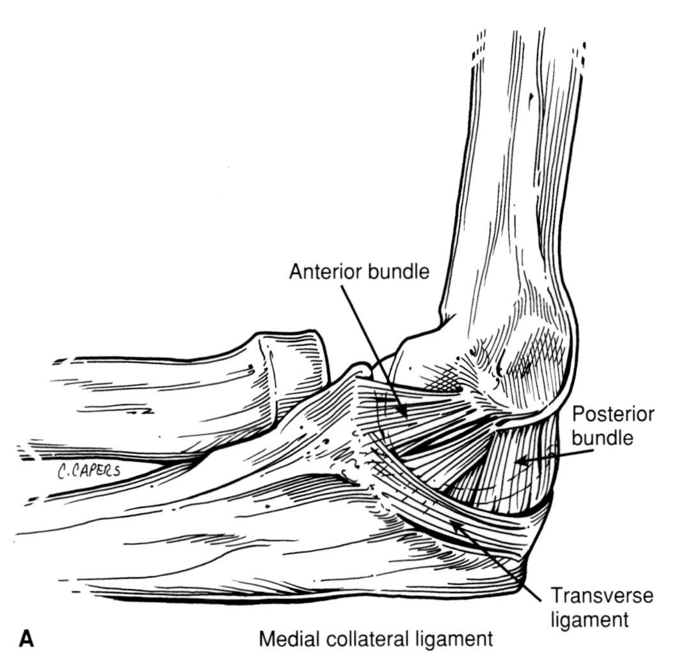

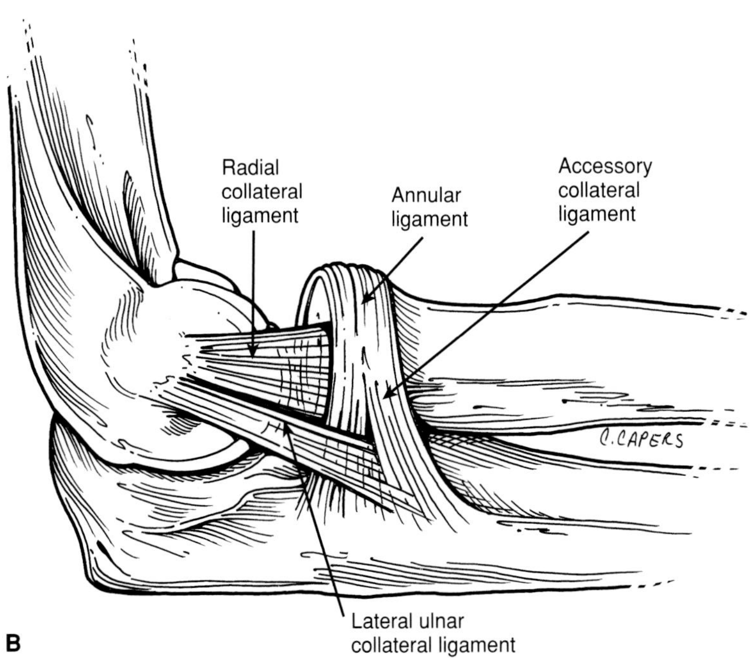

Fig. 49–4. *(A)* **The medial collateral ligament is made up of an anterior oblique bundle and a posterior oblique bundle, along with a transverse component.** *(B)* **The lateral collateral ligament originates on the lateral epicondyle and inserts distally into the annular ligament and the proximal ulna.**

Laterally, the elbow has much less in the way of soft tissue supports. The lateral collateral ligament takes origin from the lateral epicondyle and inserts distally into the annular ligament and proximal ulna (Fig. 49–4B). Additional support comes from the anconeus muscle and the thin radial collateral ligament. Recently, Morrey described the clinical presentation of posterolateral elbow instability that follows significant injury to the lateral collateral ligament.

Other important soft tissue structures include the anterior capsule, which provides stability in extension; the annular ligament, which allows pronation and supination of the radial head without displacement; and the interosseous membrane, which damps the natural diastasis of the radial and ulnar shafts during pronation and supination. Additionally, the interosseous membrane resists longitudinal translation of the radial and ulnar shafts.

Muscles

Flexion of the elbow is accomplished primarily by the brachialis and biceps muscles, which are both innervated by the musculocutaneous nerve. The brachialis usually receives additional innervation from the radial nerve. The biceps can assist when the forearm is in neutral position or is supinated, but it provides little force in pronation. The radially innervated brachioradialis assists elbow flexion when the forearm is in neutral position or pronated. Maximal flexion force is generated at 90° of flexion with the forearm neutral or supine.

Extension of the elbow is accomplished by the triceps, the medial head being the most important element. The anconeus assists in all positions, particularly as the elbow is pronated and supinated.

Pronation is accomplished primarily via the median-innervated pronator quadratus and pronator teres. Supination is initiated by the release of pronation, supplemented by the action of the supinator, brachioradialis, and biceps muscles. Medially, the elbow flexor pronator group helps resist valgus loads and pronates the forearm.

Vascular Supply

The arterial supply of the elbow joint is anastomotic. The proximal descending sources are the radial and medial collateral branches of the deep brachial artery plus the superior and inferior ulnar collateral branches of the brachial artery. Distal ascending sources include the ulnar recurrent branches of the ulnar artery, and the radial recurrent branch of the radial artery, and the interosseous recurrent branch of the posterior interosseous artery. These vessels provide a generous blood supply and, because of the anastomotic pattern, rarely permit joint ischemia (Fig. 49–5).

Nerves

The elbow joint receives innervation via branches from the musculocutaneous, radial, ulnar, and median nerves (Fig. 49–5). Because of their position, the nerves that cross the joint have certain predispositions to injury. Medially, the ulnar nerve may be injured as it courses posterior to the medial epicondyle in the ulnar groove. Laterally, the posterior interosseous branch of the radial nerve may become entrapped as it passes the arcade of Frohse owing to muscle impingement by the extensor carpi radialis brevis or the supinator. The median nerve may be at risk anteriorly with supracondylar fractures or anterior dislocations.

BIOMECHANICS

Elbow Joint Forces

Because of the biomechanics of the elbow joint with the long lever arm of the forearm, small loads applied to the hand produce large joint reaction forces in the elbow. Typical joint reaction forces occur during eating and dressing (300 N), getting out of a chair (1700 N medially, 800 N laterally), and pulling a table (1900 N).

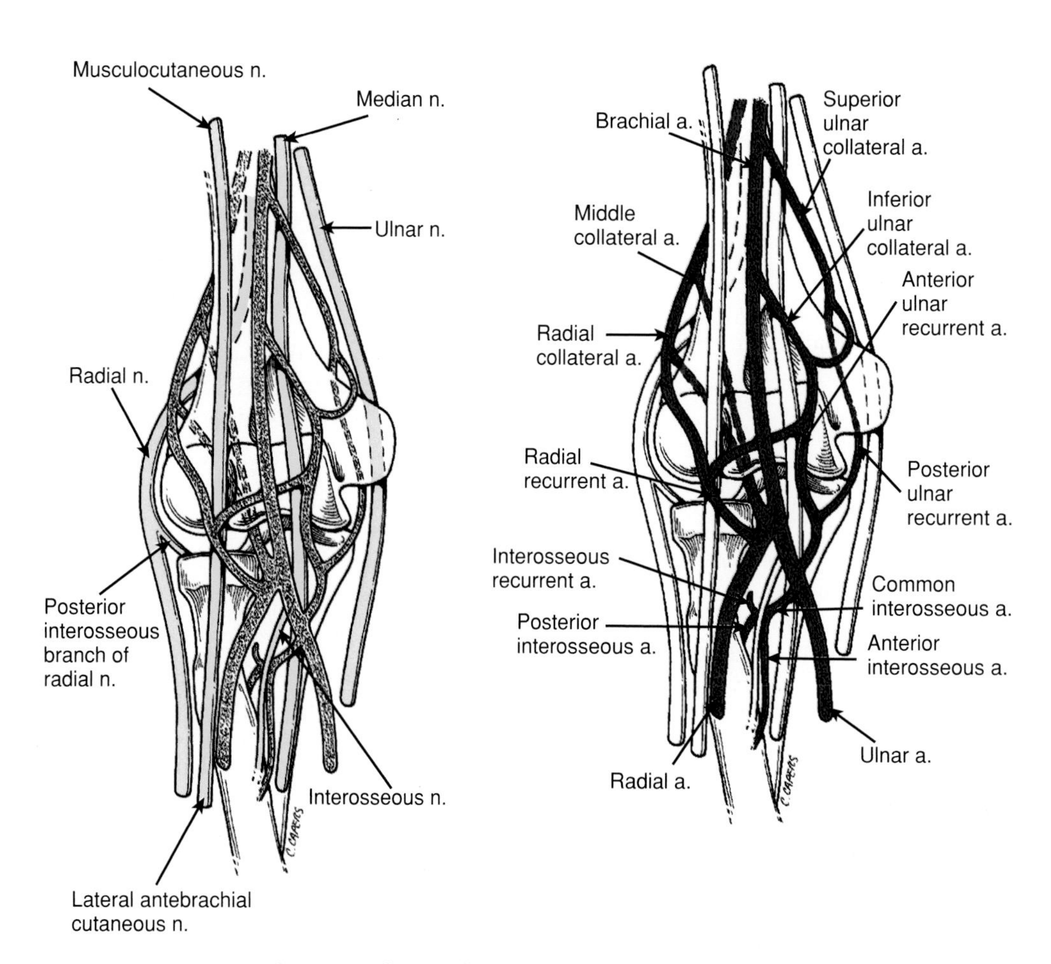

Fig. 49–5. The vascular and nerve supplies to the elbow.

Morrey has shown that, when the elbow is extended and axially loaded, 60% of the load is borne by the humeroradial joint and 40% by the humeroulnar joint. With repeated valgus stress to the elbow, acquired medial collateral ligament laxity allows increased load to the radiocapitellar joint. Common clinical evidence of this is valgus extension overload in pitchers.

The medial collateral ligament accepts tremendous loads during pitching with progressive recruitment of collagen fibers as the load is applied. As additional fibers are recruited, the ligament stiffens to accept the load and shares stresses with the bones and muscles. Deficiencies in any component (ligament, bone, or muscle) therefore increase stress on the other structures.

Throwing

The elbow joint functions as a stable articulation between the upper arm and the forearm in the throwing athlete. During the act of throwing, it is subject to extreme valgus torque and extension forces that can exceed physiologic levels and produce acute or chronic pathologic changes. The act of throwing can be viewed in five phases: (1) wind-up, (2) cocking, (3) acceleration, (4) deceleration, and (5) follow-through.

WIND-UP

During the wind-up phase, no significant forces are applied to the elbow joint. There is posturing of the trunk and shoulders and weight is shifted to the backmost leg. The elbow flexes with the forearm pronated, but no load is applied to the elbow joint.

COCKING

The trunk, shoulder, arm, and forearm are positioned to launch the acceleration forces of the throw. The humerus abducts to 90° and is brought into full external rotation. The elbow stays flexed and is not significantly loaded. Muscle activity principally involves wrist extensors and pronators of the forearm to position the arm for the next phase of throwing.

ACCELERATION

During this phase the ball is accelerated from resting position to speeds approaching 80 to 90 mph in a time frame estimated to be between 50 and 80 milliseconds. The acceleration begins with a forward weight shift and twisting of the trunk. Tremendous momentum generated from the trunk then passes distally through the shoulder, upper arm, elbow, forearm, wrist, and hand, until the ball is launched. The humerus is accelerated anteriorly and rotated internally. Early in acceleration, the forearm, wrist, hand, and ball remain essentially in the same position, which results in the generation of tremendous forces at the elbow, with valgus torque and later extension. The medial ligaments see tensile forces, and laterally the radiocapitellar joint is loaded. After initial acceleration, the humerus is then decelerated by the teres minor and posterior cuff muscles. As the humerus slows, the momentum is transferred across the elbow joint, with increased rates of internal rotation. As the ball accelerates, a tremendous centrifugal force generated across the elbow causes the joint to extend. As the elbow reaches nearly full extension, the elbow flexors fire in an eccentric mode, to slow the rate of extension. The biceps and brachialis prevent forceful hyperextension of the elbow joint. During this phase significant compressive and shear forces are generated at both the radiocapitellar joint and the olecranon fossa. The arm, hand, and ball reach maximum velocity at the end of the acceleration phase and enter the release point. The posture and position of the hand and fingers determine the type of pitch at release by imparting varying degrees of momentum to the ball.

DECELERATION

During the deceleration phase the tremendous amount of force generated in the arm is decelerated by the active contraction of the muscles about the shoulder, arm, and forearm. The powerful external rotators of the shoulder and posterior portion of the deltoid actively contract to decelerate the upper arm. Deceleration occurs with specific motions, such as glenohumeral internal rotation, glenohumeral distraction, and elbow extension.

FOLLOW-THROUGH

The trunk continues its forward rotation while following the decelerating arm in a way that reduces the overall contraction force and prolongs the time available to complete the deceleration, thus limiting soft tissue stresses overall.

The pattern of throwing, as well as sport-specific factors (football, softball, etc.), can significantly affect the manner and magnitude of force application.

SUMMARY

A knowledge of the functional anatomy of the elbow and of the biomechanics of common activities makes it possible to predict, diagnose, and treat common elbow problems.

REFERENCES

1. Milch, H.: Fractures of the external humeral condyle. J.A.M.A. *160*:641, 1956.
2. Morrey, B. F.: The Elbow and Its Disorders. 2nd Ed. Philadelphia, W. B. Saunders Co., 1993.
3. London, J. T.: Kinematics of the elbow. J. Bone Joint Surg. *63A*:529, 1981.

SUGGESTED READINGS

Celli, L. (ed.): The Elbow: Traumatic Lesions. New York, Springer-Verlag, 1991.

Gray, H.: Anatomy of the Human Body. 30th American Edition. Edited by C. D. Clemente. Philadelphia, Lea & Febiger, 1985.

Zarins, B., Andrews, J. R., and Carson, W. G. Jr. (eds.): Injuries to the Throwing Arm. Philadelphia, W. B. Saunders, 1985.

50

William W. Peterson

Physical Examination and Ancillary Tests of the Elbow

Evaluation of an elbow injury depends on correlating the athlete's symptoms and history with a careful physical examination and appropriate radiographic and ancillary tests. The first step in this evaluation is to obtain an accurate history. It is necessary to determine not only if the athlete has pain but also if there are other symptoms such as weakness, swelling, loss of motion, locking, or areas of paresthesia. The location of the problem should be noted and correlated with the underlying anatomic structures. It is important to determine if these problems are aggravated by certain elbow or arm movements and if there is a relation to specific sport activities. Next, it is necessary to determine when and how the problem began. Did it begin suddenly, with a specific activity or injury, or did it begin gradually? The response of the injury to previous treatment, including rest or modification of activities, should be assessed. It is important to determine if the athlete's technique or training predispose him or her to injury or overuse problems. Finally, injured athletes should be questioned about their goals and expectations for returning to active sports participation. After a thorough history is obtained, it should be possible to construct a differential diagnosis.

A systematic physical examination should include general inspection of the elbow, range of motion measurements, palpation for areas of tenderness, evaluation of strength, provocative tests, determination of stability, and neurovascular examination of the extremity. Inspection of the elbow may reveal abnormal axial alignment that is due to either angular or rotational deformities. Angular deformities (cubitus varus or valgus) can be detected by determining the carrying angle of the arm, the angle formed by the forearm and the humerus when the elbow is extended. Although normal variation is considerable, the mean carrying angle for men is 10° and for women 13°.[1] Most abnormalities of axial alignment are related to previous trauma or fractures, but some ligamentous injuries, such as valgus extension overload, can cause abnormalities as well.

Inspection also reveals swelling, whether localized or generalized throughout the soft tissues. Localized swelling may represent fluid in the olecranon bursa or a joint effusion if it is in the area of the "soft spot" between the lateral epicondyle, tip of the olecranon, and radial head. The examiner should also look for muscle atrophy and hypertrophy. Measurements of arm and forearm circumference can be useful to determine muscle size. Any asymmetry between the injured and the uninvolved arm should be evaluated. Finally, scars related to previous injury or surgery should be noted, particularly if additional surgery is anticipated.

The range of elbow motion should be measured. Normal values are approximately 0° of extension to 150° of flexion, and about 70° pronation and 85° supination with the elbow flexed to 90° (hyperextension may be a normal finding if bilateral). Both active and passive range of motion should be assessed; a significant difference between the two sets of values suggests that pain is inhibiting active movement or that there may be a problem with the muscles about the elbow. During evaluation of range of motion, joint crepitus should be sought. Crepitation can result from intra-articular loose bodies, defects in the articular surface, or degenerative changes in the elbow. A mechanical block to elbow movement or rotation can be a sign of an intra-articular loose body.

Next, the elbow should be carefully and systematically palpated to determine areas of tenderness. These findings must be interpreted in terms of the underlying bone landmarks and the musculotendinous structures and ligaments. On the lateral aspect of the elbow, the epicondyle and extensor tendon origin should be examined for areas of tenderness consistent with lateral epicondylitis. This lesion must be distinguished from tenderness over the radial tunnel, which lies just anterior to the lateral epicondyle and continues to the level of the supinator. Abnormalities of the radial tunnel can be associated with compression neuropathy of the radial nerve and its terminal motor branch, the posterior interosseous nerve. Swelling or tenderness in the area of the "soft spot" is associated with conditions that cause hemarthrosis or synovial inflammation. Occasionally, loose bodies are palpable in this area.

The medial side of the elbow also needs to be systematically palpated. Tenderness over the medial epicondyle and flexor origin must be distinguished from tenderness just posterior to the epicondyle in the area of the medial collateral ligament. If the ligament is injured, applying valgus stress with the elbow flexed 20° to 30° causes intense pain in this area (Fig. 50–1). Tenderness, and especially the presence of distal tingling from percussion (Tinel's sign) over the ulnar nerve as it travels through the cubital tunnel behind the medial epicondyle, can be a sign of an ulnar nerve compression syndrome. Also, any tendency toward nerve subluxation in and out of the cubital tunnel with elbow flexion and extension should be assessed. Compression neuropathies of the median nerve at the elbow are less common, but they can be seen in athletes who engage in repetitive forceful movements. The nerve can be compressed as it passes between the two heads of the pronator teres muscle, and this area should be examined for tenderness and tested for Tinel's sign by percussion.

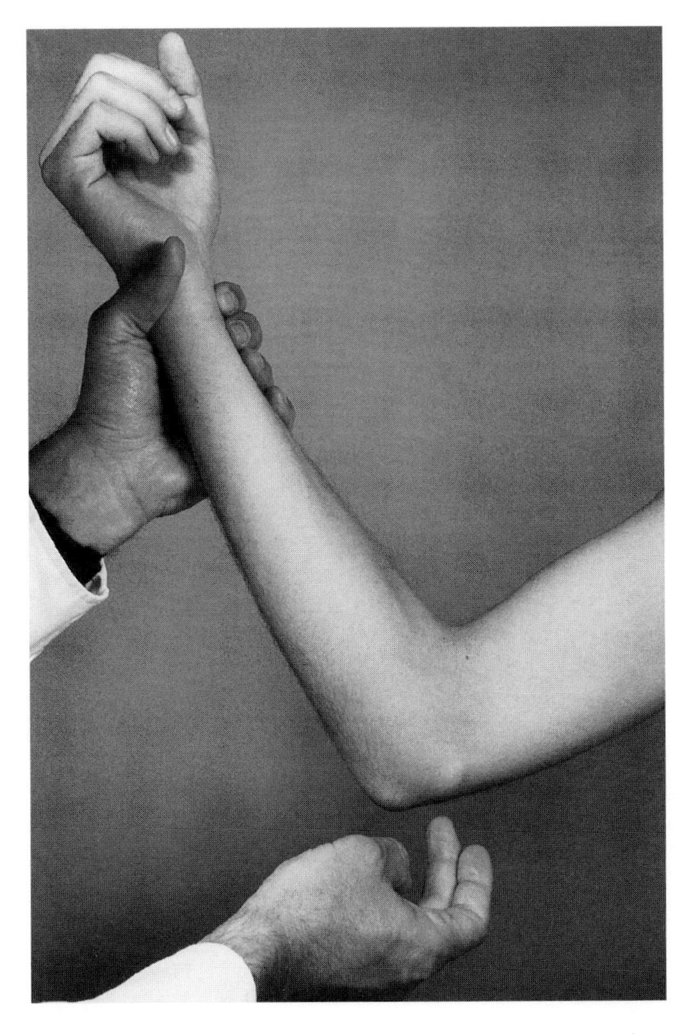

Fig. 50–1. Tinel's sign. Percussion over the ulnar nerve as it travels through the cubital tunnel reproduces symptoms in nerve distribution.

Finally, the posterior and anterior elbow should be examined for tenderness or swelling. Activities that subject the elbow to repetitive valgus stress or forceful extension, such as throwing, may produce problems posteriorly in the area of the olecranon or triceps tendon. Anteriorly, the antecubital fossa should be examined by palpation of the biceps tendon and the area of the anterior capsule. Although the anterior compartment is not a common site of problems, injuries can occur in sports that require hyperextension, such as gymnastics.

Precise measurement of elbow strength is not possible in a clinical setting, but gross estimates should be made. More important are various provocative tests that can help localize the source of an athlete's problem. Resisted wrist extension or radial deviation that stresses the extensor carpi radialis longus and -brevis causes pain over the lateral epicondyle and extensor origin in a patient with lateral epicondylitis. Similarly, pain medially with resisted wrist flexion may suggest medial epicondylitis. Other specific muscles can be tested to determine if the pain is reproduced, suggesting tendinitis or muscle strain.

Provocative tests can be performed for various nerve compression disorders about the elbow. Compression of the median nerve in the proximal forearm (pronator syndrome) may be aggravated by tests such as resisted pronation of the extended forearm (which stresses the pronator teres), resisted elbow flexion and forearm supination (which stresses the lacertus fibrosus), and resisted flexion of the proximal interphalangeal joint of the long finger (which stresses the flexor digitorum sublimus arch). Another proximal median nerve compression disorder is the anterior interosseous syndrome, which may be manifested by an unusual posture of pinch with hyperextension of the distal interphalangeal joint of the index finger and interphalangeal joint of the thumb owing to weakness of the flexor digitorum profundus to the index finger and the flexor pollicis longus. A provocative test for ulnar nerve compression at the elbow is increased numbness in the ulnar nerve digits with maximum elbow flexion and supination. Finally, the flexor-pronator test is a provocative test for radial nerve compression at the radial tunnel. This test is performed by flexing the wrist to tighten the extensor carpi radialis brevis and pronating the forearm to tighten the supinator, which increases compression of the radial nerve.[2]

Accurate evaluation of elbow stability can be difficult. During extension, the elbow is extremely stable because the olecranon is locked into the olecranon fossa of the humerus. Therefore, collateral ligament stability must be assessed with the elbow flexed approximately 20° to 30° to relax the anterior capsule and free the olecranon from its fossa. Varus stress is best applied with the humerus in full internal rotation, whereas valgus stress is best applied with the humerus in external rotation, to help minimize the effect of shoulder rotation. Abnormal joint opening is significant as is pain during the stress tests. Stress radiographs can be obtained to quantitate elbow instability.

Finally, examination of the elbow is not complete without a careful neurovascular evaluation of the arm. Function of the ulnar, median, and radial nerves can be impaired by various elbow disorders. Also, a primary nerve problem, such as one of the various nerve entrapment syndromes, can present as pain or weakness around the elbow. Therefore, careful assessment of strength and sensation in the forearm and hand is necessary. Also, the brachial pulse in the antecubital fossa and the distal radial and ulnar pulses at the wrist must be palpated.

Once a careful history and physical examination have been performed appropriate radiographic and ancillary tests can be obtained. Routine radiographic evaluation of the elbow should include an anteroposterior view in

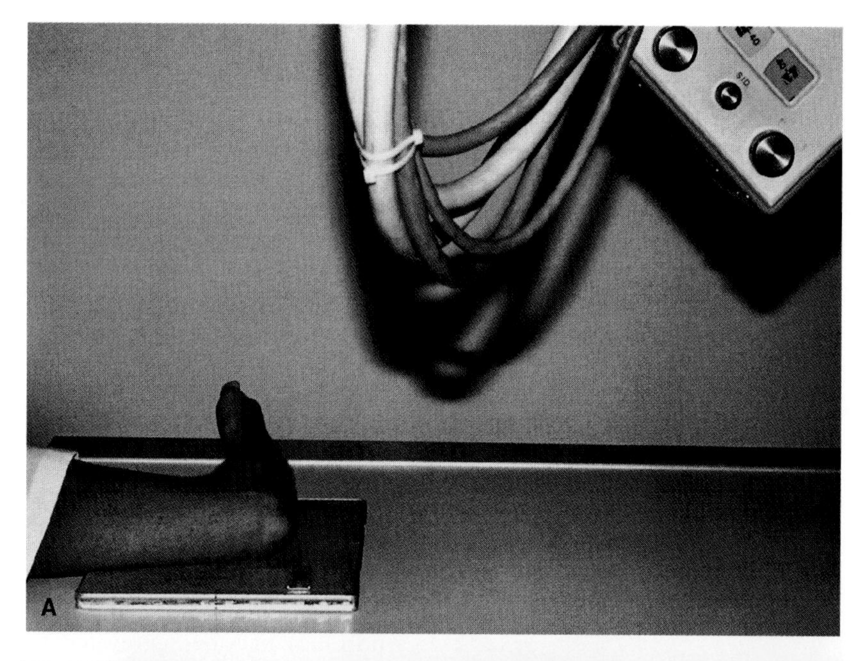

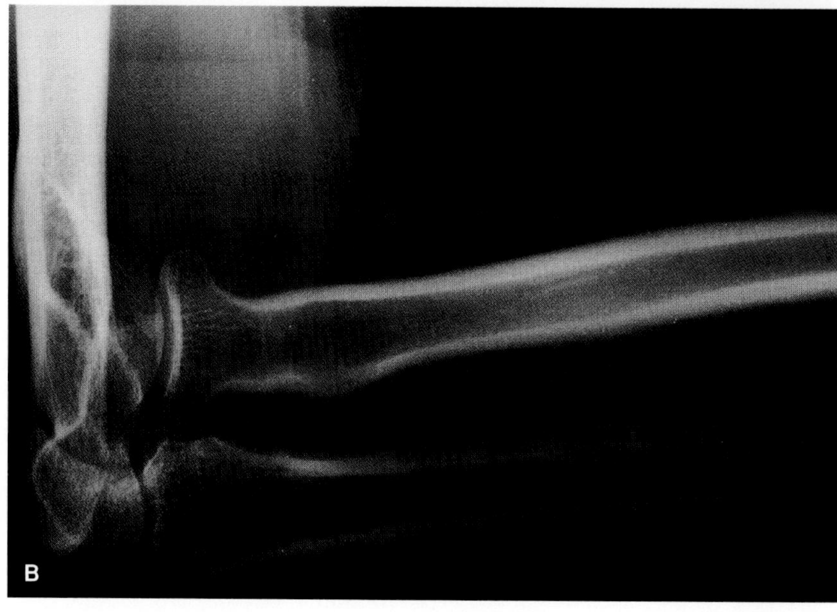

Fig. 50–2. *(A)* For the radial head–capitellum view, the arm is positioned as for a routine lateral projection, but the x-ray tube is angled 45°. *(B)* This view gives a good image of the radial head and capitellum and can demonstrate subtle injuries to these structures.

full extension and a lateral view with the elbow flexed 90°.[3,4] Oblique views are often part of the standard elbow examination. A lateral oblique view (obtained with the elbow extended, the arm externally rotated about 40°, and the forearm supinated) helps visualize the radiocapitellar joint, medial epicondyle, and radioulnar joint.[3,4] A medial oblique view (also obtained with the elbow extended but with the arm internally rotated about 45° and the forearm pronated) improves visualization of the trochlea, olecranon, and coronoid.[3,4]

Additional views are often helpful for visualizing specific areas. The radial head–capitellum view (Fig. 50–2) can help to demonstrate subtle injuries to the radial head and capitellum (such as fractures or osteochondritis dissecans). It is obtained by positioning the arm as for a routine lateral projection but angling the x-ray tube 45° (see Fig. 50–2).[5] Damage to the olecranon or epicondyles can be evaluated with an axial view, obtained by flexing the elbow 45° and directing the x-ray beam perpendicular to the humerus.[3,4] Osteophytes of the olecranon, loose bodies between the olecranon and the capitellum, and soft tissue abnormalities adjacent to the epicondyles can be seen. A similar view, the cubital tunnel view (elbow maximally flexed and externally rotated 15°) profiles the cubital tunnel.[6]

Radiographs must be evaluated systematically. The lateral view should be carefully reviewed for displacement of the anterior or posterior fat pad (Fig. 50–3). The presence of the posterior fat pad, not normally seen because of its position within the olecranon fossa, indicates intra-articular fluid. The anterior fat pad may be seen in normal elbows, but if it is displaced anteriorly that also indicates a joint effusion. A joint effusion may be caused by inflammation of the joint (including infection) or a traumatic hemarthrosis, which would suggest an occult fracture.[7] The radiographs should be evaluated for fractures, osteophytes, loose bodies, osteochondritis dissecans, and soft tissue calcification. Knowledge of the separate epiphyseal centers is essential to proper interpretation of radiographs of a skeletally immature athlete. Abnormalities such as fragmentation of the medial epicondyle or widening of the distance between the medial epicondyle and the humeral metaphysis may be seen in "Little Leaguer's elbow."

Specialized radiographic studies can be obtained, if needed, to make a diagnosis or further evaluate a particular problem. Stress views can be helpful in evaluating for ligamentous laxity. These can be made with fluoroscopic guidance, to achieve proper positioning and to detect subtle degrees of instability. Another technique for assessing elbow stability is to obtain a gravity stress view to evaluate for medial joint opening. To quantitate elbow instability, stress radiographs can be obtained using Telos equipment. Telos instrumentation allows proper positioning of the elbow joint while a measured amount of stress is applied. Radiographs can then be obtained that can be used to measure the degree of joint laxity. Arthrograms, often combined with conventional tomography or computed tomography (CT), can be quite valuable in detecting loose bodies or capsular tears that can occur with ligament injuries.[8,9] CT arthrography is also helpful in assessing the integrity of articular surfaces in patients with osteochondritis dissecans or osteochondral fractures (Fig. 50–4). A technetium-99m bone scan is quite sensitive for detecting abnormal activity associated with occult fracture, stress injuries, or osteochondritis dissecans. Finally, magnetic resonance

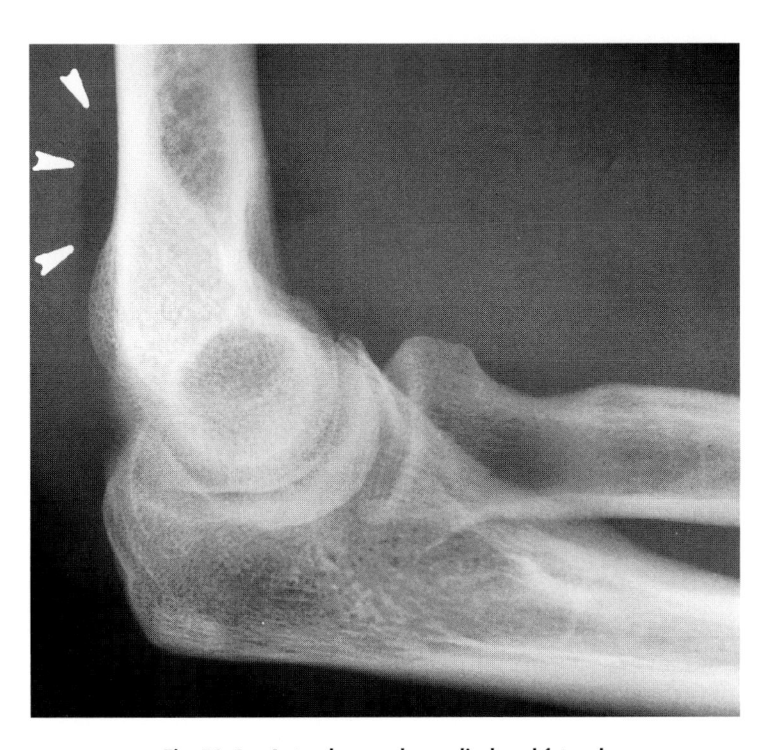

Fig. 50–3. Lateral x-ray shows displaced fat pad.

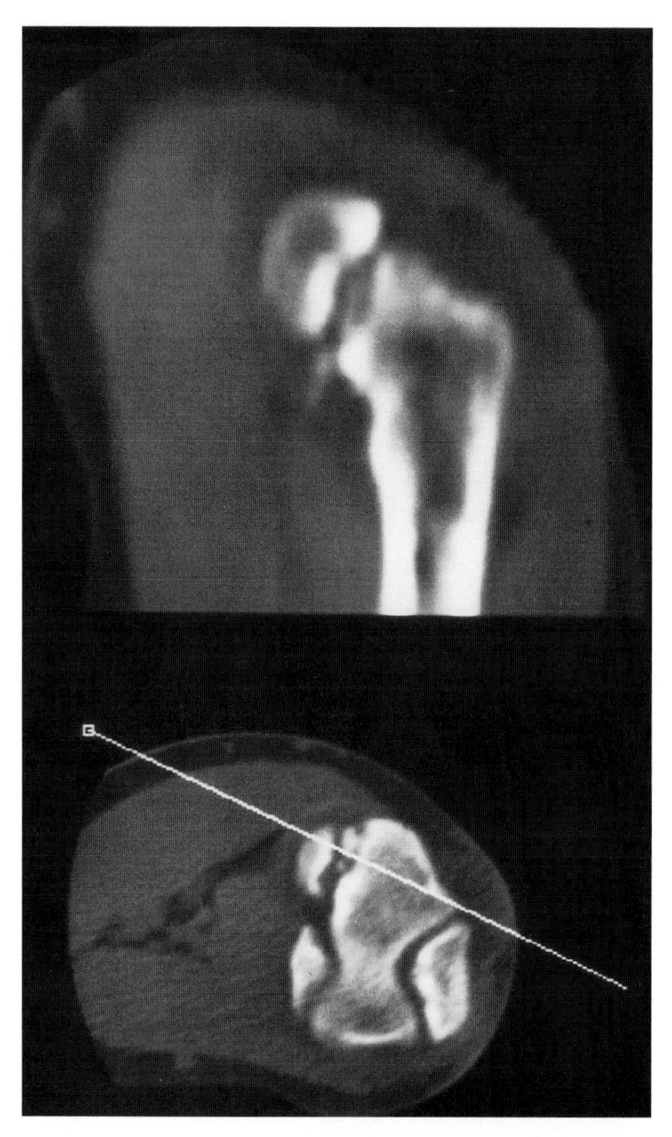

Fig. 50–4. CT arthrogram shows osteochondritis dissecans.

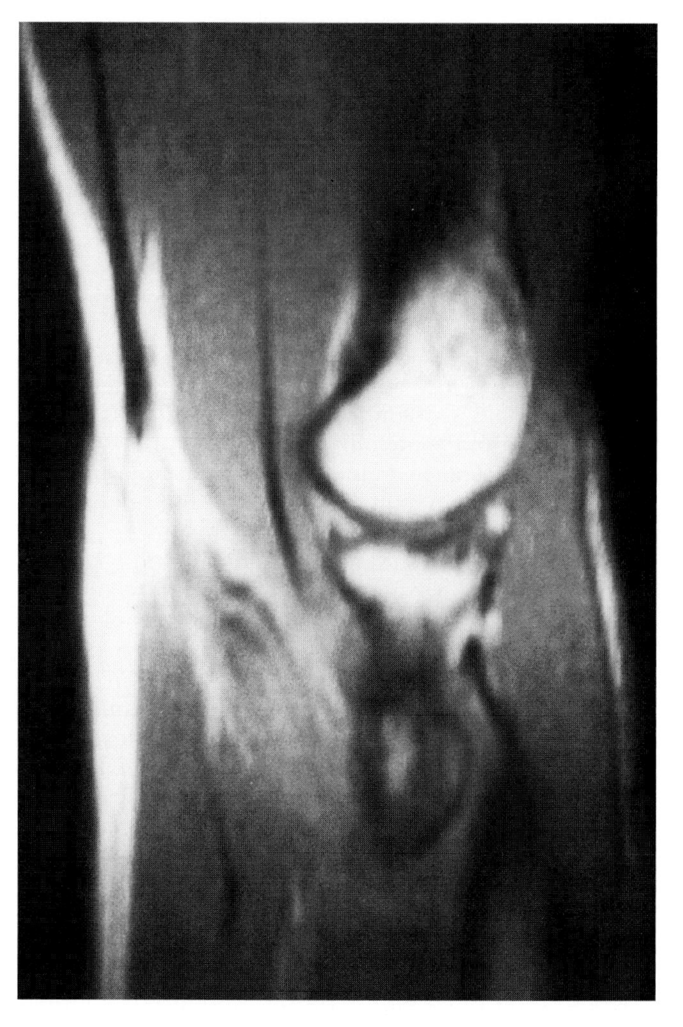

Fig. 50–5. MRI can be helpful in evaluating soft tissue injuries. Here, the image shows hemorrhage about the musculotendinous junction of the biceps tendon.

imaging (MRI) may be helpful in evaluating some conditions, especially soft tissue injuries, that may occur about the elbow. Disorders such as osteochondritis dissecans and Panner's disease may be identified by MRI before any abnormalities can be seen on plain radiographs. MRI can also be helpful in evaluating the soft tissues around the elbow and identifying ligamentous or tendinous strains or ruptures (Fig. 50–5).

Certain elbow conditions may require other ancillary tests to make an accurate diagnosis. Electrodiagnostic testing (electromyography and nerve conduction velocity studies) is necessary to evaluate associated nerve injuries. The nerve most commonly affected is the ulnar nerve as it passes through the cubital tunnel behind the medial epicondyle; however, the median, radial, and musculocutaneous nerves can also be injured as they pass into the forearm. In rare cases, arteriography or venography may be needed to exclude a vascular lesion. Finally, systemic diseases, such as the various rheumatic conditions and gout, can present as problems of the elbow, and appropriate laboratory studies are helpful.

Accurate diagnosis of elbow injuries depends on careful correlation of the athlete's history and symptoms plus a systematic examination of the elbow and appropriate radiographic and ancillary tests. Failure to do this may lead to improper treatment and cause further injury or delay the athlete's recovery and return to sports participation.

REFERENCES

1. Volz, R. G., and Morrey, B. F.: The physical examination of the elbow. *In* The Elbow and Its Disorders. Edited by B. F. Morrey. Philadelphia, W. B. Saunders, 1985.
2. Eversmann, W. W. Jr.: Entrapment and compression neuropathies. *In* Operative Hand Surgery. 3rd Ed. Edited by D. P. Green. New York, Churchill Livingstone, 1993.
3. Ballinger, P. W.: Merrill's Atlas of Radiographic Positions and Procedures. 6th Ed. St. Louis, C. V. Mosby, 1986.

4. Bontrager, K. L., and Anthony, B. T.: Textbook of Radiographic Positioning and Related Anatomy. 2nd Ed. St. Louis, C. V. Mosby, 1987.
5. Greenspan, A., and Norman, A.: The radial head, capitellum view: Useful technique in elbow trauma. AJR *138*:1186, 1982.
6. St. John, J. N., and Palmaz, J. C.: The cubital tunnel in ulnar entrapment neuropathy. Radiology *158*:119, 1986.
7. Murphy, W. A., and Siegel, M. J.: Elbow fat pads with new signs and extended differential diagnosis. Radiology *124*:659, 1977.
8. Eto, R. T., Anderson, P. W., and Harley, J. D.: Elbow arthrography with the application of tomography. Radiology *115*:283, 1975.
9. Singson, R. D., Feldman, F., and Rosenberg, Z. S.: Elbow joint: Assessment with double-contrast CT arthrography. Radiology *160*:167, 1986

51 *David L. Higgins*

Fractures About the Elbow

In athletes, elbow fractures can be secondary to acute trauma or to overuse. The acute traumatic injuries—supracondylar, condylar, epicondylar, olecranon, radial head and neck fractures—are caused by a direct blow or a fall on an outstretched upper extremity. The overuse injuries—capitellum osteochondral fractures, radial head fractures, medial epicondyle fractures, coronoid fractures—can be caused by falls or by chronic stress, especially in throwing athletes. Some of these fractures are more common in certain age groups. Certain fractures that are more common in athletes are discussed in greater detail.

MEDIAL EPICONDYLE FRACTURES

Medial epicondyle fractures in athletes are most often associated with a fall or overuse. In the general population, medial epicondyle fractures are commonly associated with elbow dislocations (i.e., more than 50% of medial epicondyle fractures), so physicians must be aware of the additional injuries that often occur when the mechanism is a fall.[1] Sometimes there is spontaneous reduction before the patient is seen. Regardless of the mechanism of injury, this fracture usually occurs in teenagers because their medial epicondyle has not yet fused with the distal humerus.[2]

The avulsion fracture of the medial epicondyle can be secondary to a fall on the extended upper extremity, but more often it is secondary to chronic valgus overload of the elbow in adolescent throwing athletes. The pull of the forearm flexor group and the normal valgus elbow anatomy produce the fracture through the epicondylar apophysis (Fig. 51–1). In a skeletally mature athlete, a fall that produces these forces would probably cause an injury to the medial collateral ligament rather than avulsion of the bone.

During the cocking phase of throwing, the athlete positions the elbow in valgus and flexion and creates a distraction force medially. This puts stress on the medial epicondyle. During the acceleration phase, an excessive valgus load is placed on the elbow and there is excessive muscle contraction of the flexor muscle mass. This also creates greater stress at the medial epicondyle. Thus excessive throwing by the adolescent can lead to medial epicondyle fatigue fractures.

The diagnosis of medial epicondyle fractures is best made by a thorough history and physical examination. The pain is often localized to the medial aspect of the elbow, but it may be diffuse. In the absence of a traumatic event, it is important to find out the pitching history (e.g., innings per week, types of pitches thrown). For the contact athlete it is important to determine the exact mechanism of injury. The greater the force involved, the better reason to suspect elbow dislocation.

An avulsion fracture causes tenderness over the medial epicondyle and a variable amount of swelling. Because the ulnar nerve lies close to the medial epicondyle, a thorough neurologic examination must be done. Range of motion may be limited because of pain. In contact athletes, this may be due to more extensive injury or because the medial epicondyle fragment is entrapped in the elbow joint.

Anteroposterior, lateral, and oblique radiographs should be obtained for all elbow injuries. Because of the radiolucent physis in a skeletally immature athlete, comparative views of the normal elbow may be needed to distinguish minimally displaced fractures in this group. The fracture usually involves only the epicondyle, but a small portion of the metaphysis may be attached. The epicondyle is displaced distally (Fig. 51–2). The fracture usually occurs through the apophysis, which in the majority of cases is the weakest area, but it may occur through the epiphysis. The fragment may become

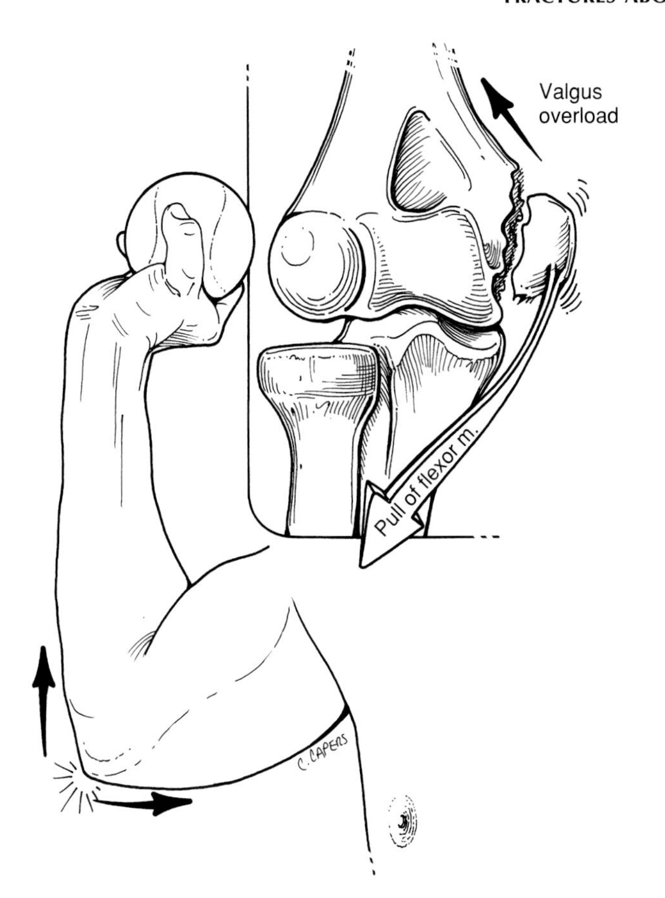

Fig. 51–1. Mechanism of injury of an avulsion fracture of the medial condyle. The pull of the forearm flexor group and the normal valgus elbow anatomy produce the fracture through the epicondylar apophysis.

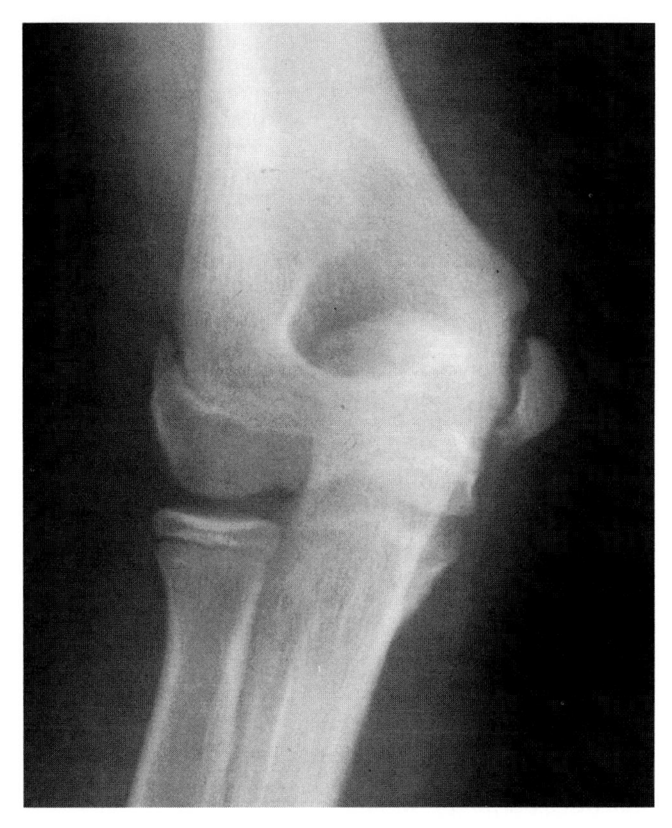

Fig. 51–2. Radiograph shows a medial epicondylar fracture.

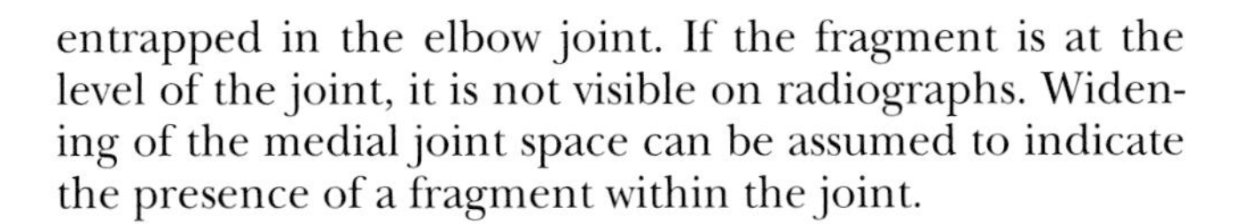

entrapped in the elbow joint. If the fragment is at the level of the joint, it is not visible on radiographs. Widening of the medial joint space can be assumed to indicate the presence of a fragment within the joint.

Treatment

Most medial epicondylar fractures can be managed nonoperatively. The decision for nonoperative versus operative treatment depends on several variables: amount of fracture displacement, valgus instability, whether the fragment is entrapped in the joint, and ulnar nerve injury.

Nondisplaced and minimally displaced (2 to 3 mm) fractures are treated with immobilization with a posterior splint. Active assisted range of motion exercises are started as early as 4 to 5 days after injury. Once swelling and tenderness are minimal, the splint is discarded. Return to sports is allowed when full range of motion and full strength are restored.

Displaced fractures not associated with valgus instability, an entrapped fragment, or ulnar nerve injury are also treated nonoperatively. The posterior splint may be worn longer, but use of the splint should still be kept to a minimum to attain full range of motion. Many reports support nonoperative treatment.[3,4] The results of conservative treatment are (at least) equal to or better than those for open reduction and fixation.

If the fragment is entrapped in the joint, as determined by visualization of the fragment at the joint level on radiographs or by limited range of motion, the fragment must be removed from the joint and fixed to the medial condyle. Arthrography will confirm entrapment of the fragment.

A complete neurologic examination must be done for any elbow injury since the ulnar nerve is often injured. Areas of paresthesia or small sensory deficits should be observed. Usually, they resolve, but if there are motor deficits, with or without sensory loss, surgical exploration is warranted. The ulnar nerve may be entrapped in the joint or in the fracture. In these cases, the medial epicondyle is reattached and ulnar nerve neurolysis, with transposition, is performed.

Surgical treatment is also recommended if the displaced medial epicondyle results in valgus instability in an athlete. Significant valgus elbow instability can be detrimental to high-level throwing athletes.[5] Woods and Tullos have described the gravity stress test radiograph of the elbow as a means of determining valgus instability.[5] With the patient supine and the shoulder externally rotated, the elbow is flexed 15° to 20°. Significant medial opening with movement of the fragment indicates medial instability. This anteroposterior stress radiograph is compared with the normal anteroposterior radiograph. If the fragment has moved, surgical treatment is indicated. The investigators found that athletes with medial instability are disabled unless the fracture is surgically repaired.

If surgical treatment is needed, it must be performed as an open procedure, adhering to principles of rigid anatomic internal fixation. This is important so that range of motion exercises can be started early, as soon as the pain is tolerable (as early as 1 week). The splint is removed 3 weeks postoperatively. Strengthening is started when full range of motion is attained. Return to throwing is started at the 6- to 8-week point, with a regimented program beginning with short distances.

CORONOID FRACTURES

Another fracture that can be specific to athletes, the coronoid fracture, is often associated with elbow dislocations, radial head fractures, and medial ligament disruptions. When a "contact athlete" exhibits these findings, the physician must consider the possibility of a spontaneously reduced elbow dislocation. In both contact and noncontact athletes, the coronoid fracture is caused by violent contraction of the brachialis muscle. This occurs when the elbow is forced into extension while the brachialis is contracting to prevent extension.

The diagnosis is best made from a good history that describes the mechanism of injury and from a thorough physical examination. The history suggests the area of concentration for the physical examination. As mentioned previously, a complete neurovascular and stability examination is necessary when an elbow dislocation occurs. An isolated coronoid fracture is recognized by anterior elbow swelling and tenderness with pain on extension.

The radiographic examination consists of anteroposterior, lateral, and oblique views. If these do not reveal the fracture, a radial head-capitellum view may be needed. Coronoid fractures are classified according to the percentage of the coronoid involved: Type I, less than 25%; Type II, 25 to 50%; and Type III, more than 50%.

Treatment

If a Type II or Type III coronoid fracture is associated with an elbow dislocation or multiple fractures, open reduction and internal fixation is indicated. Anatomic reduction of large coronoid fractures is necessary because they create elbow instability.

Type I coronoid fractures, small chip avulsion fractures, are treated nonoperatively. No elbow instability is involved. The elbow is immobilized for 3 to 4 days; then, range of motion exercises are started. Progression of therapy and return to sports are dictated by the patient's symptoms. No protection is needed for sports.

OLECRANON FRACTURES

The olecranon process is a large, curved eminence that makes up the proximal and posterior portions of the ulna. Its subcutaneous position makes it especially vulnerable to direct trauma. Injury can occur in one of three ways: direct violence to the olecranon, like a fall on the point of the elbow; indirect violence, like a fall on the outstretched hand with the elbow in flexion accompanied by a strong contraction of the triceps; or a combination of direct and indirect forces. This type of injury usually results in effusion, which causes swelling and pain over the olecranon. The most important sign is inability to extend the elbow actively against gravity, which indicates discontinuity of the triceps mechanism. A true lateral view is needed to detect the fractures, and an anteroposterior view can help delineate the fracture line in the sagittal plane.

Fractures of the olecranon are generally classified as displaced and nondisplaced (i.e., less than 2 mm displacement, no increase in minimal degree of separation with 90° of flexion, and ability of the patient to extend the elbow actively against gravity). Nondisplaced fractures can be treated with immobilization in a long arm cast with the elbow in 45° to 90° of flexion. Movement can usually be started after 3 weeks, but flexion past 90° should be avoided until bone healing is complete (6 to 8 weeks). Displaced fractures require open reduction and internal fixation or primary excision.

RADIAL HEAD FRACTURES

Radial head fractures are not specific to athletes, but such fractures can have serious consequences for throwing athletes because of the force transmission through the radiocapitellar joint and the contribution of the radial head to valgus elbow instability.[6,7] Radial head fractures are caused either by a direct blow or by a fall on an outstretched upper extremity. They can also occur during elbow dislocation.

Mason has given the most widely used classification of radial head fractures (Fig. 51–3)[8]: Type I, marginal fracture without displacement; Type II, marginal fracture with displacement; and Type III, comminuted entire head fracture. Johnston added a Type IV: any radial head fracture associated with elbow dislocation.[9]

When radial head fractures occur, pain is usually on the lateral side of the elbow; however, swelling can be global because of joint hemarthrosis. There is tenderness over the radial head and pain on palpation. Full range of motion may be limited because of the pain, swelling, or loose bodies from the radial head fracture. For patient comfort and to aid in diagnosis, any hemarthrosis should be aspirated and a local anesthetic injected into the joint. If anesthesia does not allow full range of motion, a loose body should be suspected. If the fracture is Type II, III, or IV, the athlete's wrist must be examined for a possible radioulnar disassociation, which signifies a greater degree of injury.

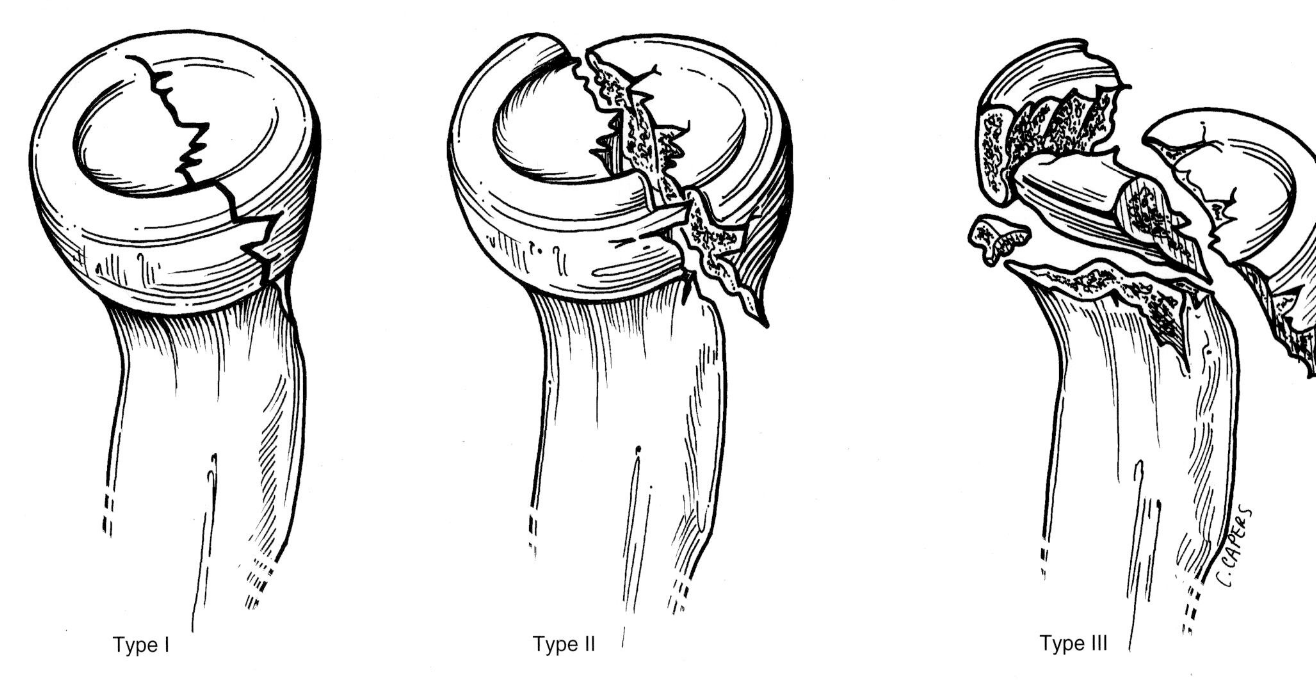

Fig. 51–3. **Classification of radial head fractures. Type I, marginal fracture without displacement; Type II, marginal fracture with displacement; Type III, comminuted entire head fracture.**

Radiographic assessment is made with anteroposterior and lateral views. If no fracture is seen and a posterior fat pad sign is evident, a radiocapitellar view is needed. A wrist series is required if there is wrist pain. Computed axial tomography in two planes can be used to further delineate the fracture and for use in treatment planning.

Treatment

Type I fractures, marginal nondisplaced ones, require treatment of symptoms and early range of motion. Aspiration of any hemarthrosis and injection of local anesthetic provides good pain relief. The arm is placed in a sling for 2 or 3 days; then, flexion and extension are started. Pronation and supination are added later. Full range of motion must be attained early because an athlete's throwing will be affected by failure to achieve full extension. Full athletic participation is allowed when the patient has achieved a full painless range of motion (usually 2 to 3 months). No protective equipment is required.

Type II and III fractures require operative fixation, depending on the fracture pattern. In the Type II fracture, if there is 2 mm or less displacement, closed treatment as described for Type I is indicated. If there is no comminution and more than 2 mm displacement, open reduction, and internal fixation is indicated. If operative fixation is performed it must be stable, to allow early range of motion. All efforts should be made to fix and retain the radial head, unless it is a comminuted fracture, because of the importance of the radial head for valgus stability. Internal fixation can be performed with mini-AO screws or Herbert screws. If the comminution is too great to allow fixation, a silicone prosthesis may be needed as a temporary spacer, to prevent proximal migration of the radius if there has been disruption of the interosseous membrane.

If the fracture fragment is less than 25 to 30% of the radial head and there is a mechanical block, the fragment should be excised. If there is no mechanical block, the forearm is splinted in full supination for 2 to 3 weeks. This allows the interosseous membrane to heal.

In Types I and II fractures and some Type IIIs, the fragment can be excised arthroscopically. If there are other related injuries, such as elbow dislocation or medial instability, arthroscopy should not be performed.

SUMMARY

Elbow injuries in an athlete, especially a thrower, can end a career. The type of injury may preclude further athletic participation, regardless of treatment. But every effort should be made to get the athlete back to the playing field. A full range of motion with a stable elbow is most important; with a less than perfect result, the athlete's career may be over.

REFERENCES

1. Smith, F. M.: Medial epicondyle injuries. J.A.M.A. *142*:396, 1950.
2. Gray, H.: Anatomy of the Human Body. 30th American Edition. Edited by C. D. Clemente. Philadelphia, Lea & Febiger, 1985.
3. Bernstein, S. M., King, J. D., and Sanderson, R. A.: Fractures of the medial epicondyle of the humerus. Contemp. Orthop. *3*:637, 1981.

4. Wilson, N. I. L., Ingram, R., Rymaszewski, L., and Miller, J. H.: Treatment of fractures of the medial epicondyle of the humerus. Injury *19*:342, 1988.
5. Woods, G. W., and Tullos, H. S.: Elbow instability and medial epicondyle fractures. Am. J. Sports Med. *5*:23, 1977.
6. Morrey, B. F., and An, K. N.: Articular and ligamentous contributions to the stability of the elbow joint. Am. J. Sports Med. *11*:315, 1983.
7. Morrey, B. F., An, K. N., and Stormont, T. J.: Force transmission through the radial head. J. Bone Joint Surg. *70A*:250, 1988.
8. Mason, M. L.: Some observations on fractures of the head of the radius with a review of one hundred cases. Br. J. Surg. *42*:123, 1954.
9. Johnston, G. W.: A follow-up of one hundred cases of fracture of the head of the radius with a review of the literature. Ulster Med. J. *31*:51, 1962.

52 Hugh S. Tullos and Gerard T. Gabel

Elbow Instability

Elbow instability is an uncommon clinical concern in sports medicine, except for throwing athletes.[1,2] Acute elbow instability (dislocations and fracture-dislocations) may occur in any sport as a result of accidental loading of the upper extremity, but it is more common in sports that, by their nature, impose upper extremity stress (e.g., gymnastics, wrestling). Even if spontaneous reduction occurs, acute instability is usually easily recognized; the management of elbow instability, however, may be controversial, especially in younger athletes.[3] Historically, evaluation of chronic ligamentous laxity has focused on deficiency of the medial collateral ligamentous complex,[1,4] but awareness of post-traumatic posterolateral instability is essential when evaluating the injured elbow.[2,5] Recognizing symptomatic elbow instability may be difficult because of concomitant (or independent) medial or lateral epicondylitis,[1] intra-articular abnormalities, or referred pain from a cervical spine or shoulder level injury. Even with an accurate diagnosis, management of athletes with elbow instability is difficult because of the over-riding goal of return to maximum competitive function as quickly as possible.[1]

ANATOMY

The ligamentous and osseous anatomy of the elbow provide discrete passive stability while allowing the elbow, in concert with the shoulder and forearm, to position the hand in space. Active stabilization is an important additional protective mechanism.[6] By increasing the joint reactive force, active stabilization enhances the osseous contribution to elbow stability. If the active and passive constraints are compromised, clinical instability can occur.

Valgus instability, whether from an acute or a chronic process, is caused wholly or partially by compromise of the medial collateral ligamentous complex. The essential functional element of this complex is the anterior oblique component.[2] Because of its origin on the inferior aspect of the medial epicondyle and its insertion onto the medial aspect of the coronoid process, the anterior oblique ligament is the centric portion of the medial ligament complex. Thus, the ligament is taut when the elbow is flexed and when it is extended, so it imparts valgus stability throughout the flexion-extension arc of the joint.[2]

The posterior bundle of the medial collateral ligament complex has a similar origin, but its insertion lies farther posterior on the olecranon. An eccentric ligament, it contributes principally to flexion. Because of its origin and insertion on the medial aspect of the olecranon, the transverse ligament, which is at times quite vestigial, serves no apparent role in elbow stability and may be of purely phylogenetic interest.[6,7] An accessory anterior medial collateral ligament has recently been described. Like its posterior counterpart, it is an eccentric ligament;[8] however, because of its origin on the anterior aspect of the medial epicondyle and its insertion on the anterior aspect of the coronoid, the accessory anterior medial collateral ligament plays a role in valgus stability only in positions of extension. This accessory anterior medial collateral ligament is a weak one as compared with the anterior oblique ligament, though mechanically it is a consistent valgus stabilizer in the absence of the medial collateral ligament proper.

The ligamentous complex on the lateral aspect of the joint is less well developed because varus load to the human elbow is less common. The annular ligament is involved in stabilization of the proximal radioulnar joint, and the radial collateral ligament, which has an origin on the lateral epicondyle and insertion into the annular ligament, is a varus stabilizer. The lateral ulnar collateral ligament has recently been demonstrated to be the primary stabilizer during forearm supination.[5] It originates on the inferior aspect of the lateral epicondyle and inserts on the supinator crest of the lateral ulna. Although this ligament is a discrete varus stabilizer, no clinical varus instability has been noted to be associated with compromise to the ligament. The primary clinical importance of this structure is related to posterolateral rotatory instability, when the proximal radius and ulna rotate as a unit in a transverse plane around the axis of the medial collateral ligament. This results in subluxation or dislocation of the radial head and, to a lesser degree, of the proximal ulna when the arm is in a position of near extension and a valgus-supination load is applied to the elbow and forearm.[2,5] Unlike valgus instability, which has been noted after both acute and chronic events, posterolateral rotatory instability has been noted only after acute trauma, although it is rarely appreciated at the time of the trauma.

INSTABILITY

Acute Dislocation

Acute instability of the elbow (i.e., dislocation or fracture-dislocation) usually results from a fall on the outstretched arm, direct trauma, or a motor vehicle accident. Valgus, supination, and hyperextension stresses are applied to the elbow, resulting in posterior dislocation of the ulna relative to the distal humerus.[9–13] This may result in posteromedial or posterolateral dislocation; however, the mechanisms, as well as the pathologic anatomy, are similar. Anterior dislocation, a rare injury, is usually associated with a proximal olecranon fracture, whereas the even less common divergent dislocation results from compromise of the annular ligament and interosseous membrane.

Physical examination demonstrates a swollen, disfigured extremity and, in 2% to 4% of cases, neurovascular deficits. Although ulnar nerve lesions are most common, median nerve, anterior interosseous nerve, and brachial artery injuries have been reported. Associated injuries, including fractures at the level of the elbow, shoulder, or wrist, are seen in as many as 10% of cases.[9] Open injuries are uncommon.

Radiographic examination of the elbow defines the type of dislocation and any associated fractures, although in cases of spontaneous reduction of a dislocated elbow joint, radiographs may demonstrate only soft tissue swelling. Radiographic examination of associated injuries is mandatory because failure to recognize these may result in longterm dysfunction.[14] If a spontaneously reduced dislocation is suspected, radiographic verification of instability can be confirmed by use of valgus gravity stress testing (Fig. 52–1).[2,4] Medial joint widening greater than 1 to 2 mm or valgus angulation exceeding 7° of the contralateral side indicates probable dislocation, and the elbow should be evaluated and the injury managed as a dislocation.

TREATMENT

Management of a dislocated elbow requires early reduction and treatment of associated conditions, including fractures, arterial injuries, and compartment syndromes. The reduction can sometimes be performed in the emergency room with intravenous sedation; however, when associated neurovascular injuries are present or when treatment of associated injuries requires general anesthesia, reduction should be performed in the operating room. The method of reduction is similar in either case. Longitudinal traction is applied to the forearm and wrist while the elbow is held in a slightly flexed position. Posterolateral or posteromedial dislocations are reduced by manual translation. Gentle traction is applied to unlock the coronoid from the olecranon fossa. In some cases this requires posterior translation of the proximal forearm relative to the distal humerus by an assistant. Reduction of the elbow joint is usually easily appreciated as the sigmoid notch snaps onto the trochlea. Repeat radiographic and physical examinations are essential after reduction as documentation of a congruous reduction is required and, on rare occasions, reduction may be associated with neural injuries. Incongruous reduction may be caused by interposition of fracture fragments, ligamentous tissue, or the median or the ulnar nerve. Each of these situations requires open management to obtain congruous reduction.

Once congruous reduction of a simple dislocation has been obtained, the extremity should be put through a range of motion to test joint stability. If the joint is stable, the elbow is splinted for a few days for pain control and then the patient starts early active range of motion exercises.[12,13] Restoration of motion is generally prompt; however, flexion contractures can occur if immobilization is prolonged.[12] Because of this, early

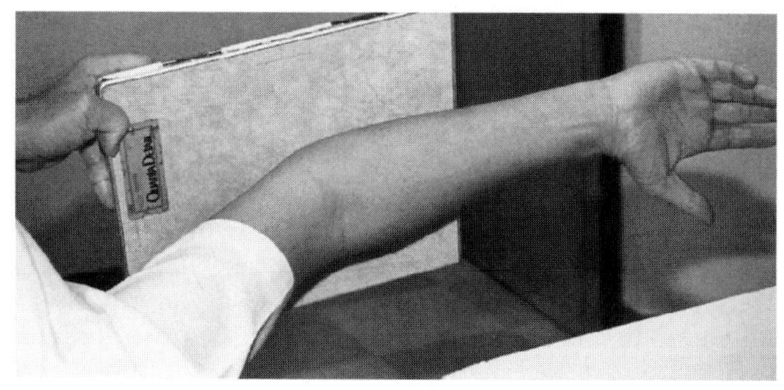

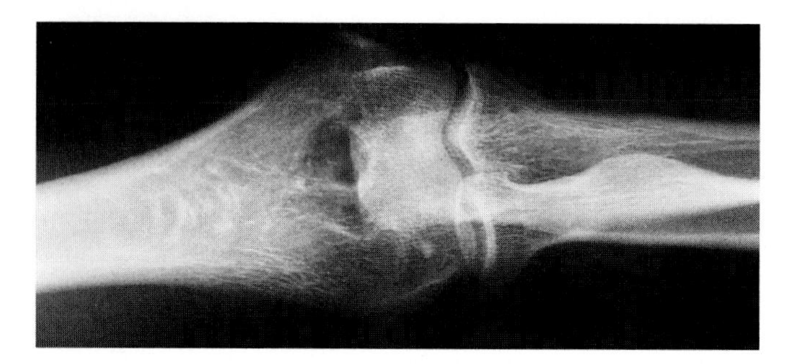

Fig. 52–1. Gravity stress testing can be used to detect spontaneous dislocation of the elbow.

mobilization is required. Children are more likely to develop chronic instability and may be immobilized longer.[3] If the elbow remains unstable in extension after reduction, an extension block splint may be used initially, followed by sequential decrease of the extension block over a 2- to 3-week period.

Concomitant fractures of the lateral column require either internal fixation or prosthetic replacement, and they present the most difficult situation in acute elbow instability. Concomitant fractures of the wrist should be treated aggressively, to allow early range of motion of the elbow and to minimize the period of immobilization as the rate of recurrent dislocations and poor outcomes associated with this combination of injuries may approach 50%.[9]

Primary open management, including medial collateral ligament repair or reconstruction or repair of the flexor-pronator mass, plays no role in a simple dislocation with a congruous reduction.[11,12] Open management may be required if the dislocation is more than 3 weeks old; reduction by closed means is usually impossible after that point.[9] Associated nerve injuries, if not caused by interposition of the nerve in the joint, are managed expectantly. Associated arterial injuries (specifically brachial artery thrombosis) require thrombectomy or arterial reconstruction.

Postreduction management of these simple dislocations includes an active range of motion exercise program, usually begun within the first week. Range of motion is generally restored quickly as swelling subsides and the range should approach an 80° to 100° arc within 2 weeks. There should be no limit placed on flexion; extension is limited at first only when instability is noted at terminal extension. Should restoration of motion be slower than expected, an active assisted program can be instituted 2 weeks after initiation of range of motion. It should be stressed that early passive range of motion programs are to be avoided since they exacerbate tissue trauma and may result in heterotopic ossification. Antiedema methods at the level of the elbow may prove helpful for early restoration of motion. If, at 4 to 6 weeks, a flexion contracture is still evident, an extension orthosis is useful to restore full extension. A strengthening program can be initiated at 6 to 8 weeks, but loading of the elbow, either in contact or noncontact sports (including valgus loading, as in throwing sports), is delayed until strength has been restored and range of motion has been restored to within 30° of preinjury capability. This usually requires a minimum of 2 to 3 months. At this point in time, the medial collateral ligament is functionally reconstituted so that it withstands valgus loading. The return to competition at the preinjury level depends on the athlete's clinical course. With a generally favorable prognosis, the athlete can expect to return to competition by 3 to 6 months.

Chronic Posterolateral Instability

Posterolateral rotatory instability represents a chronic instability pattern that follows an acute injury.[3,5] It is probably the most common form of chronic instability secondary to acute elbow dislocation. The patient's history reveals an injury—either frank dislocation or near dislocation. After a period of recovery from the initial trauma, recurrent instability is manifested by apprehension and posterolateral elbow pain while the elbow bears valgus axial load and the forearm is in supination. Findings on physical examination are normal except for apprehension on the posterolateral pivot shift test.[5] This test, best performed with general anesthesia, consists of hyperflexion of the shoulder, to lock the shoulder girdle, followed by application of a valgus, supination, and axial compression load to the elbow (Fig. 52–2). With the elbow in extension, subluxation or dislocation of the radius and of the proximal ulna (as evidenced by prominence of the radial head and a sulcus sign) is seen. The elbow is then flexed, and a palpable or audible "clunk" is appreciated as the radial head reduces on the capitellum.

In the office this confirmatory test is usually negative because of patient apprehension, and a high index of suspicion is required to diagnose this disorder. Radiographic examination of the elbow is usually negative, except for occasional evidence of avulsion fractures of the lateral epicondyle.

Management of posterolateral rotatory instability, if documented in the office or detected very early after the injury, when some potential for healing is possible, includes an extension block orthosis applied with the forearm in pronation. No such lesion reported to date—and none in our experience—has been diagnosed early enough after injury to validate this method. The subsequent course is similar to that outlined later in this chapter in the postoperative course. If the diagnosis is confirmed under general anesthesia in a patient who has chronic symptoms, surgical reconstruction is required. No effective nonoperative management is

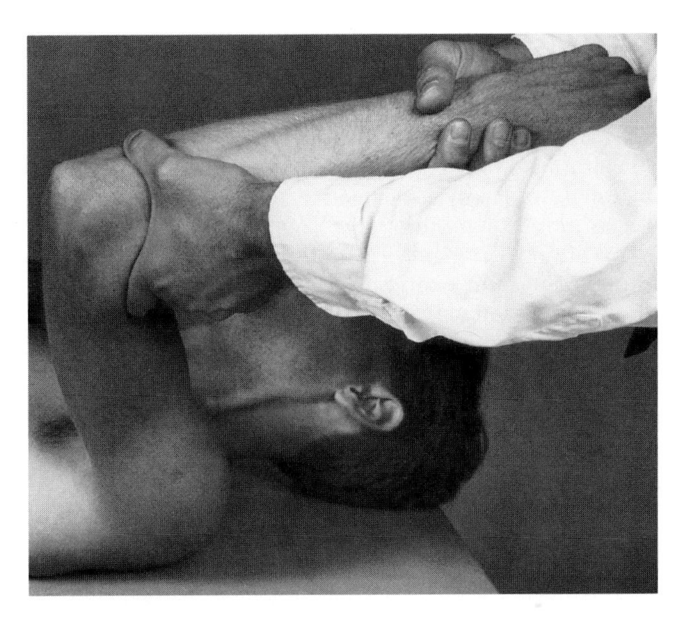

Fig. 52–2. The posterolateral pivot shift test for posterolateral rotatory instability.

available, and episodes of recurrent instability are difficult, if not impossible, to prevent with activities of daily living. It is in these cases that surgical reconstruction is necessary, and the majority of patients have a successful outcome.

SURGICAL TECHNIQUE

Surgical treatment of posterolateral rotatory instability consists of repair of an avulsed lateral ulnar collateral ligament or reconstruction in the more common circumstance when the ligament is irreparable. The elbow is approached laterally in the interval between the common extensor and the anconeus muscle. Elevation of the extensor carpi radialis brevis and the common extensor of the anterior and inferior aspect off the lateral epicondyle affords visualization of the origin of the lateral ulnar collateral ligament. The anconeus and the triceps are reflected posteriorly. The interval is developed distally between the extensor carpi ulnaris and the anconeus, allowing visualization of the supinator crest on the lateral proximal ulna. If an avulsed but functionally intact ligament is identified, a Bunnell's suture is placed. For reconstruction of an irreparable ligament, the origin and insertion of the lateral ulnar collateral ligament on the humerus and ulna are identified. Plication of the lateral ulnar humeral capsule and the anterior elbow capsule is performed. Reconstruction using the palmaris longus tendon is accomplished by direct suturing to drill holes at the isometric point of the lateral epicondyle or by suture anchors. The isometric point is determined by creation of the ulnar insertion point initially. This is located just posterior to the supinator crest, at the level of the radial neck. Sutures are tied with the elbow at 30° of flexion and in full pronation. To evaluate the efficacy of the repair, the lateral pivot shift test should be performed, with minimum axial load to avoid pullout of the repair.

Postoperatively, the extremity is placed in a long arm cast with the elbow at 90° flexion and the forearm fully pronated. The cast is worn for 4 weeks, after which a hinged cast with an extension block of 30° is worn 6 weeks more. The extension block is removed at that time if the patient has no evidence of ligamentous laxity, although younger patients or those with generalized ligamentous laxity may need extension block splinting for as long as 6 months. Use of a splint is continued for a minimum of 3 months postoperatively, after which range of motion exercises are allowed in forearm rotation. No loaded activities are allowed for a minimum of 6 months postoperatively, and extension past neutral is avoided.

The results of reconstruction, as reported by Nestor and coworkers, are gratifying, especially if no previous operative procedure has been performed on the elbow.[3]

Chronic Medial Instability

Chronic medial elbow instability is a common condition in athletes whose sport places repetitive valgus stress on the elbow. These include javelin throw and football, among others; however, the most common sports setting is baseball pitching.[1] The athlete's history reveals medial elbow pain after repeated throwing. Occasionally, an acute episode associated with sharp pain may be reported, but a chronic progressive process is more typical. The pain is most severe in the cocking and acceleration phases of throwing since this is the period of maximum valgus stress. Lateral elbow pain may be evident as well, especially in younger athletes, since compromise of the medial stabilizers results in overload of the lateral stabilizer (i.e., the radiocapitellar joint). Ulnar neuropathy at the elbow is evidenced by paresthesia in the ulnar distribution of the hand. Additionally, forced palmar flexion of the wrist and forearm rotation during the acceleration phase of pitching frequently overload the flexor-pronator mass and result in a concomitant medial epicondylitis.[1]

Physical examination is directed at determining the status of the passive and active valgus stabilizers of the elbow. Evaluation of the medial collateral ligament involves application of a valgus stress with the elbow in 25° flexion, to unlock the olecranon from its fossa and isolate stress to the medial collateral ligament (Fig. 52–3). This is performed most easily with the patient's hand and wrist held in the examiner's axilla, against the trunk with the upper arm. The examiner's hands are cupped at the level of the elbow, with one thumb on the inferior margin of the medial epicondyle along the medial collateral ligament. The examiner's other hand applies valgus stress to the elbow. Pain with this maneuver, with or without gross laxity, confirms clinical dysfunction in the medial collateral ligament. This test should be performed with the forearm pronated to prevent a false-positive finding that represents medial epicondylitis. Because of the combined function of the flexor-pronator mass and the medial epicondyle in val-

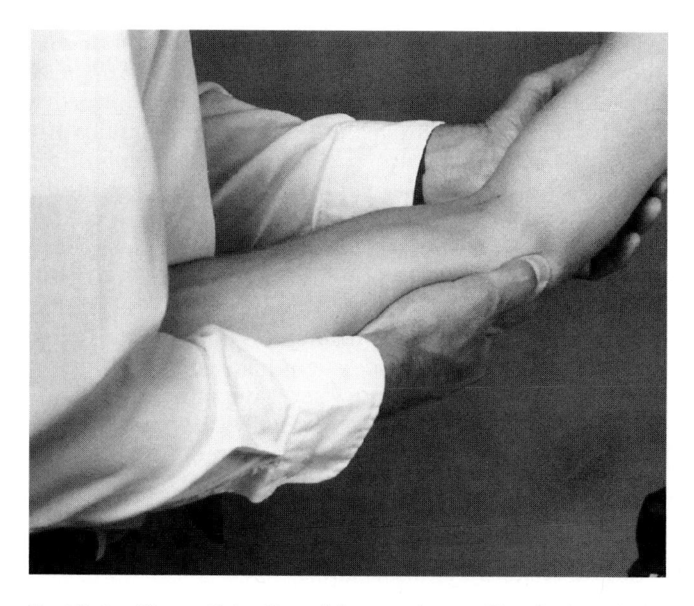

Fig. 52–3. The medial collateral ligament is tested by placing valgus stress on the elbow with the joint in 25° of flexion, to unlock the olecranon from its fossa.

gus stability of the elbow, it is not uncommon for these conditions to coexist. Evaluation of the ulnar nerve with Tinel's nerve percussion test and the elbow flexion test is performed to assess for ulnar neuropathy at the elbow.[14] Additionally, two-point discrimination and hand intrinsic muscle strength are determined.

Radiographic examination is performed to assess articular dysfunction, including osteochondritis or osteochondrosis of the radial head or capitellum, loose bodies, and marginal osteophytes. Radiographs using gravity stress testing or with loads applied may verify gross laxity of the ligament. Electrodiagnostic studies may be used, if necessary, to evaluate dysfunction of the ulnar nerve.

Initially, nonoperative management should be attempted in the majority of cases.[9] Conservative management is likely to be successful for mild cases or those in which the symptom history is relatively brief. Conservative management consists of rest and avoidance of valgus and pronation stress. Oral anti-inflammatory medication is given. A stretching program for the flexor-pronator mass may be started as pain subsides. Pronation and wrist palmar flexion strengthening programs should be performed on an incremental basis, and throwing activity is gradually resumed after several weeks' rest. If there is no recurrence of pain, a pitching program, with increasing speed and duration, and return to full level of activity can be instituted. Recurrence of pain is an indication for slowing down the rehabilitation process. Counterforce bracing for the medial epicondylitis may be useful. Corticosteroid injections for medial epicondylitis, though useful in a nonathletic patient, may predispose an athlete to acute rupture of the flexor-pronator mass and, so, should be avoided. Injection of corticosteroid preparations into the medial collateral ligament proper is contraindicated.

Though modification of activity with avoidance of valgus stress almost invariably alleviates the symptoms, most affected athletes have the therapeutic goal of return to competitive sports. If an extended period of conservative management fails to restore the elbow to preinjury status, surgical reconstruction of the medial collateral ligament may be indicated.[1]

SURGICAL TECHNIQUE

Preoperative evaluation determines whether surgical decompression of the ulnar nerve is necessary. Ulnar nerve transposition is usually required for these patients because the cubital tunnel is compromised. The approach to the medial collateral ligament can be either through the flexor-pronator mass or along the flexor-pronator-medial collateral ligament interval.[1,15] This interval consistently allows discrete identification of both the origin and the insertion of the medial collateral ligament with limited violation of the flexor-pronator mass. The medial collateral ligament is usually attenuated and requires reconstruction using the palmaris longus tendon graft, or, if necessary, a tendon graft from the foot or ankle. The elbow capsule, anterior to the ligament, is identified, and an arthrotomy is performed and the joint inspected. A valgus stress with slight elbow flexion allows intraoperative assessment of the medial collateral ligament insufficiency. If an avulsion of the origin or insertion of the ligament is identified and the ligament can be salvaged, it is mobilized and attached with Bunnell-type sutures. If repair is not possible, the ligament remnant is resected or reflected and a palmaris longus tendon graft is performed. This can be done either through drill holes or using suture anchors. Either way, a figure-of-eight orientation or doubling of the graft is created across the elbow joint (Fig. 52–4). The graft is sutured with the elbow in 30° to 40° flexion. Varus stress is applied while suturing is performed to close the medial opening. Range of motion is evaluated to ascertain joint isometricity, as well as to assess abrasion of the undersurface of the graft on the ulnar humeral joint. A repair, as necessary, of the flexor-pronator mass is performed and a long arm cast with the elbow at 90° and the forearm pronated 30° is applied.

Postoperatively, immobilization is maintained for 2 weeks. A digital active range of motion program is started immediately postoperatively. Active elbow range of motion is started at 2 weeks. A digital- and forearm-strengthening program can be started at 4 to 6 weeks. Elbow strengthening is avoided until 8 weeks postoperatively, and it should be performed in a manner that precludes valgus stress (i.e., avoiding active internal rotation of the shoulder and passive external rotation of the shoulder).

A return to a pitching program is begun, as outlined by Jobe.[1] At 4 months, pitching is started—without windup, for distances of 30 to 40 feet, and for brief periods. Ice is used after activity, to limit inflammation and edema. The distance, frequency, and duration of these activities are gradually increased postoperatively, up to the seventh to eighth month. Reintegration of body mechanics, including the windup, starts at 7 to 8 months. Velocities are limited to 50% of maximal during this time, but they may increase to 70% at approximately 9 months postoperatively. During the 9-month to 1-year period, attention is required to shoulder and torso mechanics, for restoration of proper throwing mechanism. Competitive pitching is resumed, at the earliest, at 1 year postoperatively, but only if the patient's progress has been optimal. In many cases, continuation of an incremental integration program is necessary for 18 months to regain the preoperative competitive level.

Even with this carefully supervised program, restoration of the preinjury level of activity is possible for only two thirds of high-demand athletes. This fact must be reviewed with the athlete before embarking on the surgical procedure and the extended rehabilitation program that follows.

SUMMARY

Elbow instability in an athlete can take two distinct clinical forms. The first, acute elbow instability, as in the case of simple dislocations, ultimately has a very good

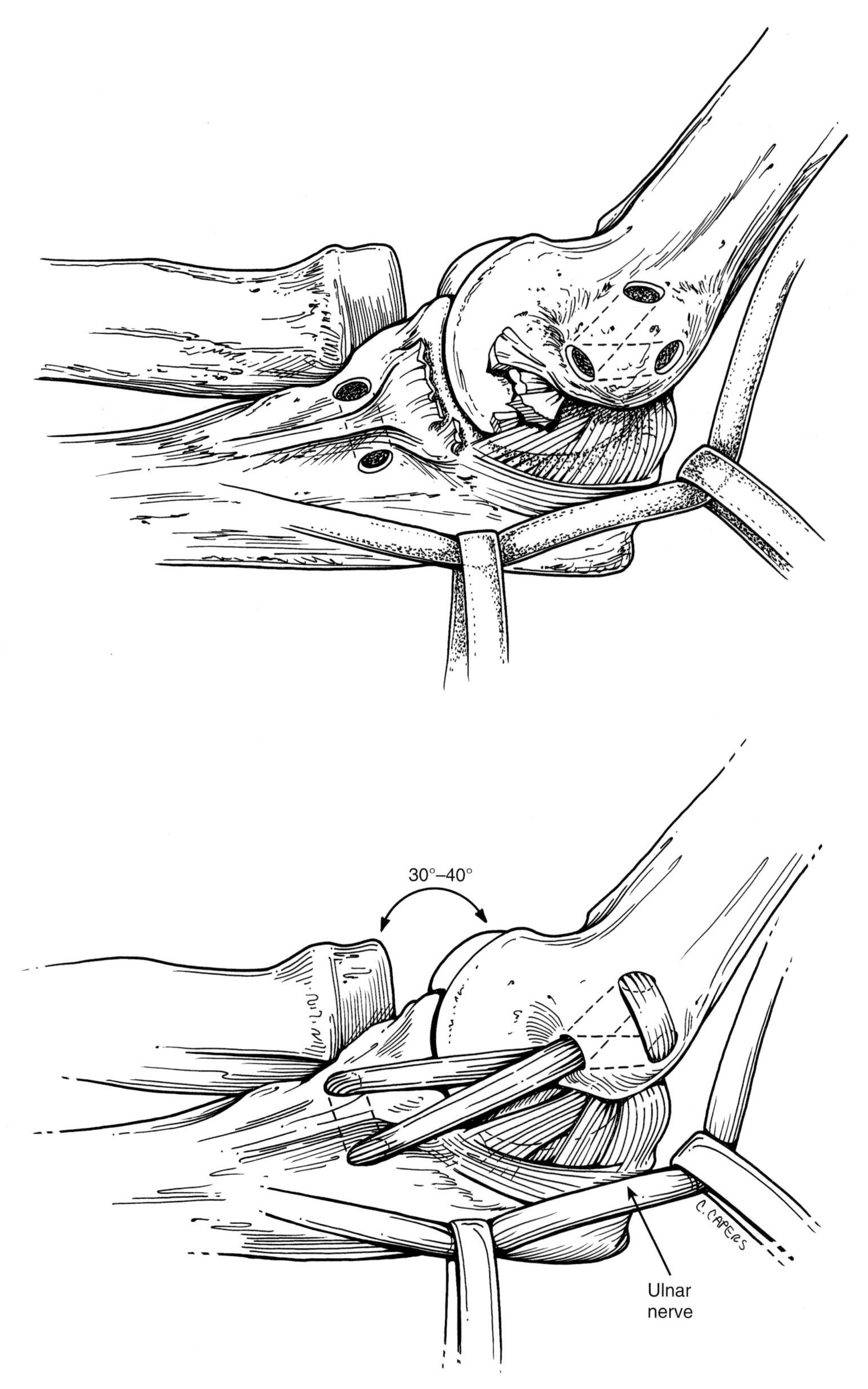

Fig. 52–4. The medial collateral ligament is reconstructed with palmaris longus tendon graft through drill holes. The graft is sutured with the elbow in 30° to 40° of flexion in a figure-of-eight pattern, doubling the graft across the joint.

prognosis for return to the preinjury activity level. Fracture-dislocations have a less favorable prognosis, depending on the nature of the associated fracture. Unlike chronic instability, a recovery period of as little as 6 months can be anticipated after dislocations, at which time full activity of the elbow can be resumed. Chronic instability, including chronic valgus and chronic posterolateral instability, usually requires surgical reconstruction and has a poorer prognosis and a longer recovery period as compared with acute instability. The decision to treat valgus instability with surgical reconstruction depends on the patient's career expectations. Should the patient have a longterm goal of extending his or her career over years, and should he or she be willing to undergo the 1- to 2-year period of healing and rehabilitation, valgus reconstruction is a reasonable option.

Unfortunately, elbow instability, even when it is managed optimally, often is a career-altering or career-ending injury. Although acute instability may be avoided by proper supervision during practice sessions and competition, prevention of chronic instability requires a carefully supervised program to prevent the athlete from performing repetitive motions that may cause injury. This includes preactivity stretching and a strengthening program to maximize active stabilizers of the elbow. Additionally, use of ice after activity, and alteration of activity early on in the process, may prevent a reversible condition from becoming a "surgical condition." If these tenets are observed, the maintenance of a symptom-free competitive athlete can be anticipated in the majority of cases.

REFERENCES

1. Gabel, G. T., and Morrey, B.: Medial epicondylitis: Surgical management and influence of concomitant ulnar neuropathy at the elbow. J. Bone Joint Surg. (In press).
2. Schwab, G. H., Bennett, J. B., Woods, G. W., and Tullos, H. S.: Biomechanics of elbow instability. The role of the medial collateral ligament. Clin. Orthop. *146*:42, 1980.
3. Nestor, B. J., O'Driscoll, S. W., and Morrey, B. F.: Ligamentous reconstruction for posterolateral rotatory instability of the elbow. J. Bone Joint Surg. *74A*:1235, 1992.
4. Al-Habbal, G., et al.: Clinical and radiographic evaluation of the gravity stress valgus test of the elbow.
5. O'Driscoll, S. W., Bell, D. F., and Morrey, B. F.: Posterolateral rotatory instability of the elbow. J. Bone Joint Surg. *73A*:440, 1991.
6. Morrey, B. F., Tanaka, S., and An, K. N.: Valgus stability of the elbow. Clin. Orthop. *265*:187, 1991.
7. Morrey, B. F., and An, K. N.: Functional anatomy of the ligaments of the elbow. Clin. Orthop. *201*:84, 1985.
8. Al-Habbal, G. A.: Anatomical and mechanical evaluation of the accessory anterior band of the elbow medial collateral ligament. Presented at the Annual Meeting of the American Academy of Orthopaedic Surgeons, New Orleans, 1994.
9. Gabel, G. T., Chang, W., Coonrad, R., and Morrey, B. F.: Concomitant ipsilateral elbow dislocation and distal radius fractures. J. Bone Joint Surg. (In preparation).
10. Josefsson, P. O., Johnell, O., and Gentz, C. F.: Long-term sequelae of simple dislocation of the elbow. J. Bone Joint Surg. *66A*:927, 1984.
11. Josefsson, P. O., Gentz, C. F., Johnell, O., and Wendeberg, B.: Surgical versus non-surgical treatment of ligamentous injuries following dislocation of the elbow joint. A prospective randomized study. J. Bone Joint Surg. *69A*:605, 1987.
12. Mehlhoff, T. L., Noble, P. C., Bennett, J. B., and Tullos, H. S.: Simple dislocation of the elbow in the adult. J. Bone Joint Surg. *70A*:244, 1988.
13. Protzman, R. R.: Dislocation of the elbow joint. J. Bone Joint Surg. *60A*:539, 1978.
14. Gabel, G. T.: Clinical and surgical significance of the elbow flexion test in ulnar neuropathy at the elbow. American Association for Hand Surgery, 1993, Cancun, Mexico, and the Annual Meeting of the American Academy of Orthopaedic Surgens, New Orleans, 1994.
15. Gabel, G. T., and Al-Habbal, G.: The Flexor Pronator-Medial Collateral Ligament Interval. (In preparation).

53 *William G. Carson, Jr.*

Overuse Injuries of the Elbow in the Throwing Athlete

Throwing athletes often sustain elbow injuries. These injuries are particularly common in baseball pitchers because tremendous forces are applied to the elbow during the throwing act.[1] It is also estimated that the rate of motion of the elbow exceeds 300 degrees per second during sports.[2]

Many throwing athletes experience minor discomfort about the elbow after throwing; however, persistent elbow pain in the throwing athlete with a history of repetitive activities may indicate more significant overuse problems. This overuse phenomenon occurs when the body's physiologic ability to heal the injured areas falls behind the microtrauma that occurs with repetitive throwing.[1] Early diagnosis, treatment, and rehabilitation of these injuries can reverse the damage in most instances. However, with continued stress to the elbow, more irreversible changes could occur, such as calcium deposits, restriction of motion, and the development of scar tissue within ligamentous structures. More serious elbow problems could develop, such as degenerative bony changes, loose bodies, and, possibly, ligament failure.

THROWING INJURIES OF THE MEDIAL ELBOW

Flexor-Pronator Strain

Flexor pronator muscle strains are among the most commonly encountered elbow injuries in the throwing athlete. Repeated valgus stress in throwing may lead to inflammation or even microtearing of the flexor muscles at their attachment to the medial humeral epicondyle. Large forces are applied to the medial aspect of the elbow during the cocking and acceleration phases of throwing (Fig. 53–1). These stresses continue during ball release as the medial elbow muscles contract to flex and pronate the wrist. Repetitive trauma to a chronically fatigued muscle can lead to microscopic tearing and pain. Complete ruptures of the flexor musculature are rare.[1]

Throwing athletes with flexor-pronator strain usually complain of pain or tenderness and possibly swelling over the medial aspect of the elbow, usually after a workout or throwing. The pain occurs over the flexor-pronator muscle group, a broader and more distal area than that affected by medial humeral epicondylitis[3] or ulnar collateral ligament problems.[1] There may be loss of full extension of the elbow, and active resisted flexion of the wrist or pronation of the forearm may produce medial elbow pain.

The treatment of a flexor-pronator strain depends on the intensity and duration of symptoms. Symptoms that occur only after throwing and are of short duration are usually treated with ice, nonsteroidal anti-inflammatory medications, and rest from painful activities. Occasionally heat will be added to the regimen after approximately 36 hours. Other modalities such as phonophoresis and galvanic stimulation may also be helpful. The throwing athlete should not be allowed to "throw through" the pain and should not return to throwing if activity-related pain is present.

Once the diagnosis is made the athlete begins stretching the involved flexor-pronator muscles. These exercises consist of stretching the wrist flexors and pronators by fully extending the elbow and extending and supinating the wrist. Cortisone injections are rarely, if ever, indicated for flexor–pronator strains because of the deleterious effects of collagen inhibition, subcutaneous atrophy, and skin pigmentation changes.[4]

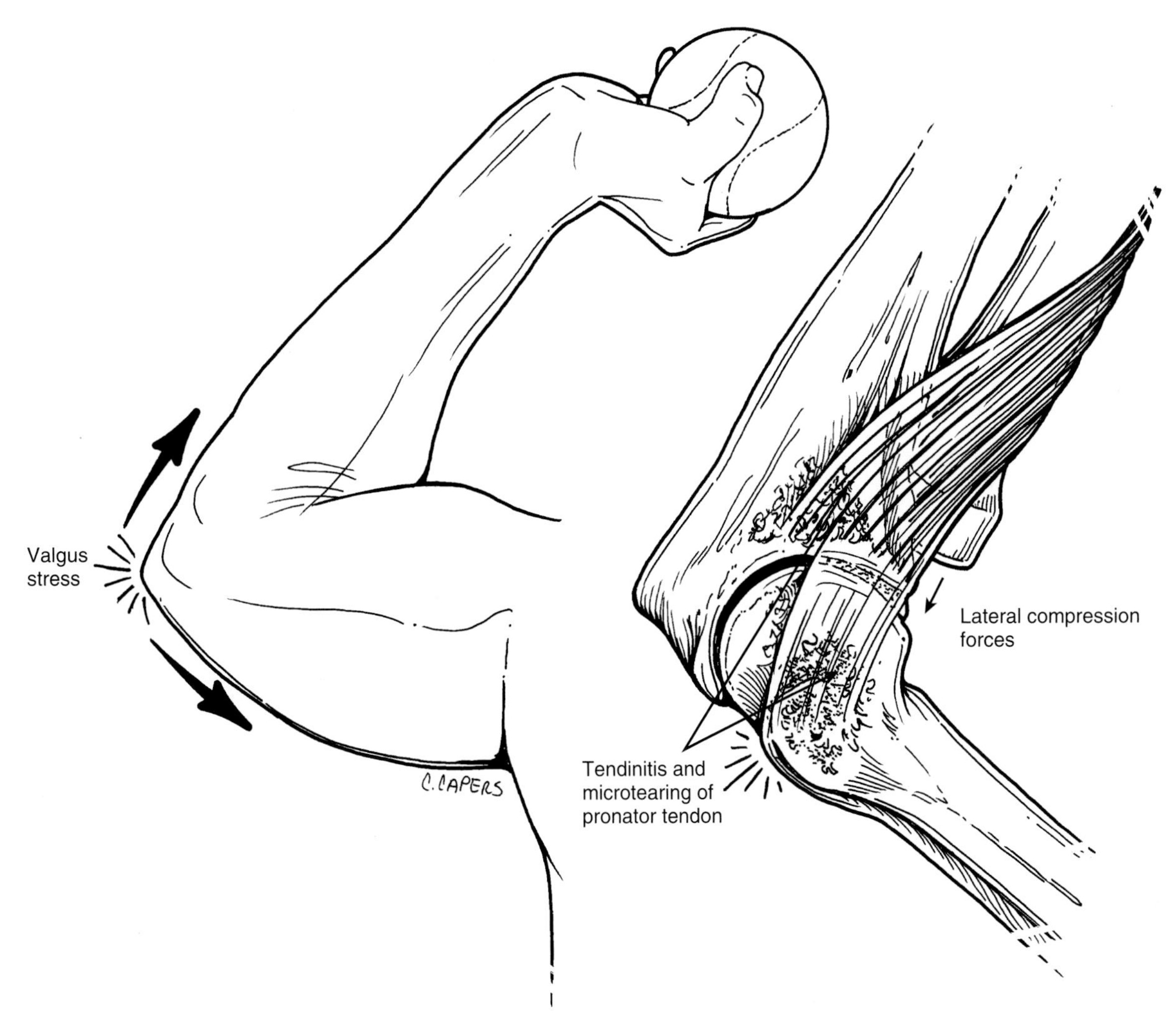

Fig. 53–1. During the act of throwing, medial tension and lateral compression forces are applied to the elbow. These can lead to microscopic tearing and pain.

Flexor-pronator strains may occasionally occur secondary to a force overload from faulty mechanics and improper pitching techniques. In more resistant cases of flexor-pronator strain, an evaluation of the throwing technique with video analysis or slow motion photography may be appropriate.

Medial Humeral Epicondylitis

In the throwing athlete, medial humeral epicondylitis or "medial" or "reverse tennis elbow" is more likely a variant of the more common flexor–pronator strain. However, with medial humeral epicondylitis the pain is more proximal and discretely localized, predominantly over the tip of the medial humeral epicondyle. Occasionally the tenderness may be more distal for approximately 1 inch along the pronator teres and flexor carpi radialis insertion.[3] Most of the pathologic changes are in the origin of the pronator teres, flexor carpi radialis, and palmaris longus, and secondarily they can involve the flexor carpi ulnaris and flexor sublimus. Resisted testing of the flexor pronator group may or may not cause medial elbow pain. Mild cases of medial humeral epicondylitis usually respond to ice, nonsteroidal anti-inflammatory medications, stretching, and strengthening. In addition, rest from painful activities and avoidance of further force overload are necessary. More advanced cases with greater pathologic changes will demonstrate angiofibroblastic changes, as can be seen with chronic tendinitis. Biologic healing must occur if pain is to be relieved.[3] It has been theorized that rehabilitation will stimulate healing of injured tissues as long as force overload is avoided.

Cortisone injections are occasionally indicated if other treatment modalities fail. A mixture of local anesthetic and a water-soluble cortisone preparation is injected into the area of maximum tenderness over the medial humeral epicondyle, taking care to avoid the ulnar nerve, which is located posterior to the epicondyle. Usually no more than three injections are given, one month apart, always in conjunction with rest and stretching and strengthening.

Surgery for chronic resistant medial humeral epicondylitis is uncommon and generally consists of excision of the focal degenerative tissue of the flexor-pronator insertion with reattachment of the muscle groups over decorticated bone.[5]

Ulnar Collateral Ligament Injury

The primary stabilizer of the medial aspect of the elbow is the anterior oblique band of the ulnar collateral ligament. Baseball pitchers, javelin throwers, and football quarterbacks are most at risk for injury to the ulnar collateral ligament.

The throwing athlete with an ulnar collateral ligament injury may present with medial elbow pain directly over the course of the anterior band of the ulnar collateral ligament and no history of significant trauma. These probable sprains can be treated with ice, nonsteroidal anti-inflammatory medications, and rest. If the physical examination reveals that the pain is associated with the ulnar collateral ligament rather than over the medial humeral epicondyle or flexor-pronator muscles, complete rest from throwing, possibly up to two to three weeks, may be appropriate. If pain is completely gone after this period of rest, the athlete is allowed gradually to return to throwing after completing a supervised program with proper stretching, warm-up, and attention to proper technique.

An acute rupture of the ulnar collateral ligament in a throwing athlete is a significant injury that can possibly interfere with future throwing abilities. The athlete may present with a history of a traumatic valgus thrust applied to the medial elbow that resulted in an audible pop. The athlete is unable to continue throwing because of acute medial elbow pain. There may also be associated ulnar nerve symptoms of paresthesia in the ring finger and little finger or a sensation of weakness of the hand. The physical examination demonstrates tenderness along the medial aspect of the elbow in the area of the ulnar collateral ligament, and there is usually swelling in that area.[6] Ecchymosis is usually present, but may be delayed up to 72 hours. Valgus stress of the elbow will produce medial pain and an abduction stress test should be performed. Radiographically a gravity stress test can demonstrate medial elbow opening.[7]

Other diagnostic techniques, such as magnetic resonance imaging (MRI), can be used to document ulnar collateral ligament ruptures (Fig. 53–2). In addition, computed tomography (CT) arthrograms may be helpful. An instrumented graded stress radiographic technique has recently been described to document laxity of the ulnar collateral ligament.[8] Arthroscopy of the elbow can also be used to detect ulnar collateral ligament insufficiency.[9]

If there is sufficient clinical and radiographic evidence of acute ulnar collateral ligament rupture, immediate exploration and ligament repair are indicated. At the time of surgical exploration, the surgeon may find the acutely torn ligament appears to be of poor substance, or is significantly frayed or degenerated. If so, a reconstruction of the ligament may be indicated in addition to simple repair.

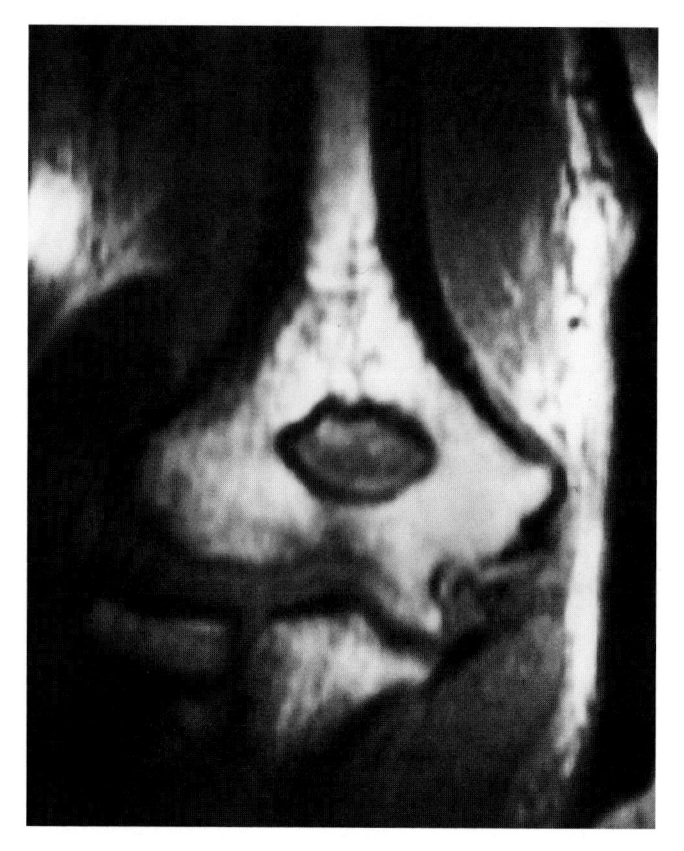

Fig. 53–2. MRI scan shows a partial rupture of the ulnar collateral ligament.

Repetitive throwing can lead to microscopic tearing of the ulnar collateral ligament. Jobe and Nuber[1] classified four stages of ulnar collateral ligament pathologic changes: Stage I, edema; Stage II, scarring and desiccation of ligament fibers; Stage III, calcification; and Stage IV, ossification. These changes weaken the ligament; stress risers occur that could lead to ligament rupture.

Throwing athletes with chronic ulnar collateral ligament insufficiency should have an initial course of conservative treatment consisting of elbow and wrist endurance strengthening (both concentrically and eccentrically), stretching, nonsteroidal anti-inflammatory medications, and occasional rest from normal activities. In addition, the athlete's pitching and throwing mechanics and techniques should be evaluated. Chronic overuse and fatigue could be produced by improper mechanics, as in the case of a pitcher who "opens up" too soon and allows the dominant extremity to trail behind the rotation of the trunk during pitching. If other conservative treatment measures fail and the athlete continues to have throwing-related pain or is unable to throw and wants to remain active with throwing, then reconstruction of the ulnar collateral ligament might be considered.[10] Some believe, however, that procedures such as traction spur removal or ulnar collateral ligament reconstruction should be performed only as a salvage procedure for limited future playing, possibly one or two further seasons.[6] Returning a player with chronic degenerative changes of the elbow to high levels of throwing after an elbow reconstruction may lead to recurrence of symptoms and further degenerative changes. If ulnar collateral ligament reconstruction is performed, the palmaris longus or a short toe extensor is usually used to reconstruct the ligament. Some surgeons prefer the short toe extensor because of its easy accessibility and length and the fact that no significant loss of function occurs. Also, approximately 10 to 20% of patients lack a palmaris longus.

After ulnar collateral ligament reconstruction, the throwing athlete may require 8 to 10 months—possibly up to a year—of rehabilitation to allow for proper graft revascularization and for strength and function to return.

THROWING INJURIES OF THE LATERAL ELBOW

Lateral Humeral Epicondylitis

Although less common in the throwing athlete than medial elbow injuries, lateral elbow problems occasionally result secondary to tensile stresses over the lateral epicondyle that produce inflammation or partial tearing of the extensor musculature. These stresses occur during extreme forearm pronation and wrist flexion that take place in the release and deceleration phases of throwing. This can cause lateral humeral epicondylitis, or "tennis elbow." In addition, lateral elbow inflammation is not infrequently caused by overuse in batting practice or associated with injuries sustained during weight training.

Patients with lateral humeral epicondylitis describe a history of weak grip and a gradual onset of pain over the lateral humeral epicondyle. The pain is usually just distal to the lateral humeral epicondyle and occurs at the origin of insertion of the extensor carpi radialis brevis. Pain can result from activities of daily living, such as carrying certain objects, shaking hands, or other activities that require the wrist to extend.

Distal palpation along the muscle belly of the extensor carpi radialis brevis may also demonstrate tenderness. Lateral elbow symptoms may be reproduced by extension of the wrist against resistance with the elbow slightly flexed, or with passive stretching of the extensor carpi radialis brevis by full elbow extension and wrist flexion. Swelling and ecchymoses are usually not prominent findings. Radiographs are usually normal; however, they may occasionally show soft tissue calcifications laterally.

The origin of lateral humeral epicondylitis appears to be overuse and poor muscle conditioning. Nirschl[3] and others feel that the term "tendinitis" should be abandoned in favor of "tendinosis" when describing lateral humeral epicondylitis or tennis elbow. "Tendinitis" implies acute inflammation, but the classic pathologic finding seen at surgery for resistant tennis elbow is angiofibroblastic tissue, with no acute inflammatory cells identified.[3] Thus, lateral humeral epicondylitis, or tendinosis, appears to be more of a degenerative process than an acute inflammatory process or one associated with a single-episode injury.

Treatment of lateral humeral epicondylitis consists of ice, nonsteroidal anti-inflammatory medications, relative rest from painful activities, and stretching and endurance strengthening of the wrist extensors. Counter force bracing of the extensor carpi radialis brevis may be helpful, as may such other modalities as phonophoresis and galvanic stimulation. Cortisone injections are given only as a last resort and are placed not in the musculotendinous area, but just under the aponeurosis, bathing the exterior tendinous area. A series of three injections is given over a 3- to 6-month period; the patient should be aware of the possible complications, such as subcutaneous atrophy and skin pigmentation changes. If the patient continues to complain of pain despite six months of conservative treatment, surgery might be indicated. Surgery consists of elevation of the extensor communis and extensor carpi radialis brevis from the lateral humeral epicondyle, débridement of the granulation tissue, roughing up of the bone, and reattachment of the musculotendinous origin to its normal resting length.

Osteochondritis Dissecans of the Capitellum

Osteochondritis dissecans of the capitellum is a lesion of bone and articular cartilage that occurs on the anterolateral surface of the capitellum. The articular cartilage and underlying subchondral bone undergo various stages of inflammation, swelling, fragmentation, and occasional loose body formation, as well as secondary degenerative changes throughout the elbow.

The origins of osteochondritis dissecans are unclear and both traumatic and familial theories have been proposed.[11–13] These changes may be caused by repetitive compression loads leading to fragmentation or disruption of the vascular supply in pitchers or gymnasts.

Clinically, patients with osteochondritis dissecans of the capitellum are usually teens experiencing pain, loss of motion (particularly extension), swelling, catching, and occasional locking. The symptoms may be insidious in onset and somewhat vague, and the athlete may present many years after the initial onset of symptoms.

Physical findings may reveal localized pain with palpation over the capitellum; decreased range of motion; swelling; and occasional crepitus, usually associated with attempts at full extension or forearm supination. Radiographs are very helpful to demonstrate fragmentation of the capitellum and associated loose bodies.[14] In younger patients, MRI can demonstrate involvement of the articular cartilage and possibly reveal the presence of stable or unstable osteochondral fragments.

Osteochondritis dissecans of the capitellum can be divided into three stages; the treatment is usually based on the stage at presentation and the amount of articular and bony fragmentation.[13] Stage I occurs in children up to the age of 13. Symptoms may be minimal—the diagnosis is sometimes made from incidental findings on radiographs. This condition is most likely the original classification of *Panner's disease,* or osteochondrosis and has a more favorable prognosis than osteochondritic dissecans. The lesion seldom fragments, and treatment is usually directed at decreasing the patient's activity level. Symptomatic adolescent throwing athletes with radiographic or MRI documentation of osteochondritis dissecans of the capitellum should not be allowed to throw and should rest the elbow completely. Rest might be prolonged, perhaps 6 months to a year, and some would argue that any throwing athlete with radiographic documentation of osteochondritis dissecans of the elbow should never throw again. Although there is controversy concerning continued throwing with osteochondritis dissecans, certainly any adolescent (having open epiphyses) with symptoms of pain, locking, and associated radiographic findings of osteochondritis dissecans should be kept from any further throwing.

Stage II lesions involve patients age 13 years to adult who may have a history of prolonged competition and repetitive throwing activities. The diagnosis is generally made with the help of radiographs or MRI scans and the treatment consists of decreasing the activity level. In the presence of sufficient symptoms of catching, pain, and loose bodies, arthroscopic surgery should be considered for débridement and loose body removal.[15–17] Arthroscopic surgery generally consists of removing loose bodies and débriding the degenerative areas of the capitellum, as well as occasional drilling of the osteochondritis dissecans crater. Reduction and pinning of displaced or significantly loosened osteochondritis dissecans fragments is technically difficult and has equivocal results.[13]

Stage III osteochondritis dissecans also occurs in adults. They have the poorest prognosis. In adults, symptoms have been present for many years, and there are often capitellar fragments, loose bodies, joint incongruity, and secondary degenerative changes. Treatment consists of decreased activity, non-steroidal anti-inflammatory medications, and occasional arthroscopic loose body removal and débridement of degenerative areas.

POSTERIOR ELBOW

Posterior elbow problems in the throwing athlete are relatively uncommon, but they can manifest as overuse syndromes, such as triceps tendinitis and posterior olecranon impingement syndrome. These posterior pathologic processes usually occur secondary to forced hyperextension or from direct trauma. Occasionally, minor triceps avulsion fractures can occur. If a throwing athlete (including the tennis player) presents with persistent posterior elbow pain on full elbow extension, radiographs—and occasionally bone scans—should be performed to rule out subtle avulsion or stress fractures of the olecranon.

Triceps tendinitis is treated with ice, non-steroidal anti-inflammatory medications, rest, stretching, and strengthening. Rupture of the triceps tendon from throwing is extremely rare.

ANTERIOR ELBOW

Throwing athletes occasionally sprain or actually avulse the insertion of the biceps brachialis tendon from the radius. Anterior capsular sprains can also occur, usually not from pitching, but from hyperextension of the elbow secondary to sliding into a base, lifting weights, or batting.[5]

Many baseball pitchers, especially at the professional level, have chronic flexion contractures of the elbow.[18] Some of these flexion contractures are entirely compatible with normal function and throwing. These contractures are probably multifactorial in origin and are combinations of thickening of the anterior capsule, fibrosis of the flexor-pronator group, enlargement of the trochlea, and secondary degenerative changes of the joint. Surgery for correcting chronic flexion contractures in the throwing athlete is generally unsuccessful and not usually indicated.

The treatment of anterior capsular strain or mild insertional biceps strain is rest, nonsteroidal anti-inflammatory medications, ice, and gentle stretching. Hyperextension of the elbow should be avoided whenever possible. Distal biceps tendon avulsions from the radius in the throwing athlete are unusual; if they do occur, they should be surgically repaired.

Valgus Extension Overload Syndrome

Valgus extension overload syndrome[18–21] is a throwing-related syndrome of the posterior and posteromedial elbow. Valgus and extension stresses to the elbow cause olecranon impingement that results in pain. This pain can occur during the acceleration phase of throwing; however, it most commonly occurs during the release and deceleration phases. The medial aspect of the olecranon impinges against the posteromedial aspect of the olecranon fossa as the elbow is extended (Fig. 53–3). Valgus laxity secondary to stretching of the ulnar collateral ligament alters throwing mechanics and can worsen this syndrome. Chondromalacia "kissing" lesions occur on the olecranon and olecranon fossa; if forces continue, osteophytes can develop over the posteromedial olecranon and hit the medial aspect of the olecranon fossa with the elbow fully extended. Advanced cases demonstrate degenerative changes and loose bodies.

A baseball pitcher with this syndrome usually has a history of pain in the elbow after pitching and reports a loss of control and onset of fatigue after two to three innings. In addition, pitches appear to "sail" or go high as the pitcher loses control. Most of the pain occurs as the pitcher attempts to "whip" the arm to gain maximum speed.

Physical examination reveals pain over the posterior aspect of the elbow with forced extension and valgus loading. Occasionally, pain on palpation may present posteriorly over the olecranon, and swelling may occur. More advanced cases may present with a history of lock-

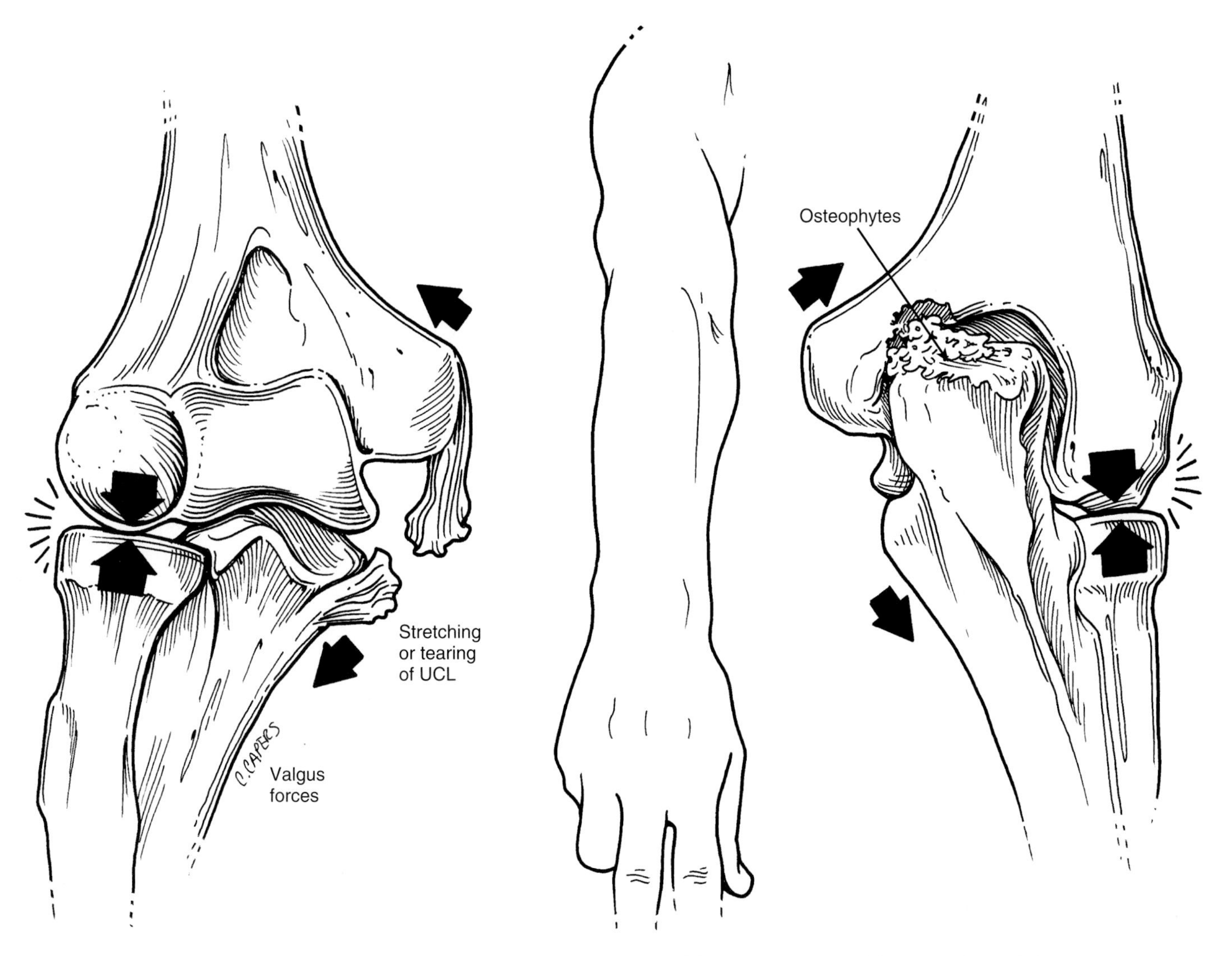

Fig. 53–3. Valgus extension overload usually occurs in the release and deceleration phases of throwing. The medial aspect of the olecranon impinges against the posteromedial aspect of the olecranon fossa as the elbow is brought into extension. Stretching or tearing of the ulnar collateral ligament (UCL) leads to valgus laxity and can worsen the problem.

ing and catching. In addition to the routine anteroposterior, lateral, and oblique views, a radiographic "olecranon" or axial view should be obtained to demonstrate osteophytes.

The initial treatment of valgus extension overload syndrome is conservative: ice, stretching, relative rest from throwing, non-steroidal anti-inflammatory medications, and other conservative modalities. If symptoms persist and the athlete wishes to continue throwing, surgical intervention could be warranted. Surgery consists of removing 1 cm of bone from the tip of the olecranon and curving the cut medially to remove the posteromedial osteophyte. The olecranon fossa is also débrided.

LITTLE LEAGUER'S ELBOW

The term *Little Leaguer's elbow* has been used to describe multiple pathologic processes in the adolescent throwing athlete's elbow. The medial tension–lateral compression forces placed on the elbow during throwing have been implicated as causative factors.

Adolescent baseball pitchers may present with a history of pain during or after throwing, as well as occasional loss of control. They also may complain of joint stiffness and loss of motion. The pain is nonspecific in nature because of the multifactorial nature of Little Leaguer's elbow. The physical examination may demonstrate diffuse tenderness, decreased range of motion secondary to soft tissue fibrosis, occasional swelling, and at times an increased valgus appearance of the elbow. Radiographs may reveal various findings, including medial humeral epicondyle overgrowth and fragmentation, osteochondritis dissecans of the capitellum, generalized trabecular and cortical thickening of the bony structures of the elbow, and possible loose bodies. Abnormal elbow radiographic findings may be present in both symptomatic and nonsymptomatic adolescent pitchers.[22]

Early detection is paramount in the treatment of Little Leaguer's elbow. The initial treatment for the adolescent pitcher with prolonged stiffness or pain associated with throwing consists of radiographic evaluation to determine associated bony or other damage. If radiographs are relatively normal, symptoms can be treated with rest, ice, and stretching. Adolescent pitchers should not be allowed to return to pitching until all of the symptoms have subsided. Symptomatic adolescent pitchers with radiographic documentation of changes about the elbow associated with throwing should not be allowed to continue throwing. Degenerative changes of the lateral compartment are associated with a poorer prognosis, and surgery for removal of loose bodies or débridement of osteochondritis dissecans is occasionally indicated.

Prevention is the best treatment for Little Leaguer's elbow; rules exist limiting the amount of pitching a child can perform during a game in a given week. However, there are no formal limitations on throwing at practice or at home. Educating coaches and parents regarding the early signs and symptoms of adolescent elbow problems associated with throwing is of prime importance, as is the use of proper throwing technique.

THROWING NEUROPATHIES OF THE ELBOW AND FOREARM

Ulnar Nerve

The most common elbow neuropathy seen in the throwing athlete involves the ulnar nerve. Because of its superficial location at the cubital tunnel or epicondylar groove, the ulnar nerve is particularly susceptible to injury. Injury to the ulnar nerve could result from (1) direct trauma; (2) repetitive traction injury secondary to cubitus valgus alignment or associated with ulnar collateral ligament laxity; (3) hypermobility of the nerve with recurrent subluxation or dislocation of the nerve; (4) calcification or ossification of the medial soft tissues; (5) acute ulnar collateral ligament tears; or (6) epicondylar fractures or separations. Most often, however, the thrower develops ulnar nerve symptoms from mechanical compromise of the nerve medially from traction, friction, or compression.[1]

Normally, the ulnar nerve is free to move in its groove in both a medial and longitudinal direction. If movement is restricted, the nerve might be compressed or tethered during the act of throwing (Fig. 53–4). With repeated trauma to the nerve, inflammation develops with possible adhesions and further restriction of the normal nerve movement in the cubital tunnel. Fibrosis and even vascular compromise to the nerve could result. In addition, any surgical procedure over the medial aspect of the elbow—such as an ulnar collateral ligament reconstruction or repair—might lead to a hostile scar environment for the nerve.

Clinically, the athlete with ulnar nerve neuritis or neuropathy may complain of posteromedial elbow pain associated with an occasional heavy feeling of the hand. There may also be tingling or paresthesia over the ulnar distribution to the ring finger and little finger. Initially, there are usually no complaints of motor weakness.

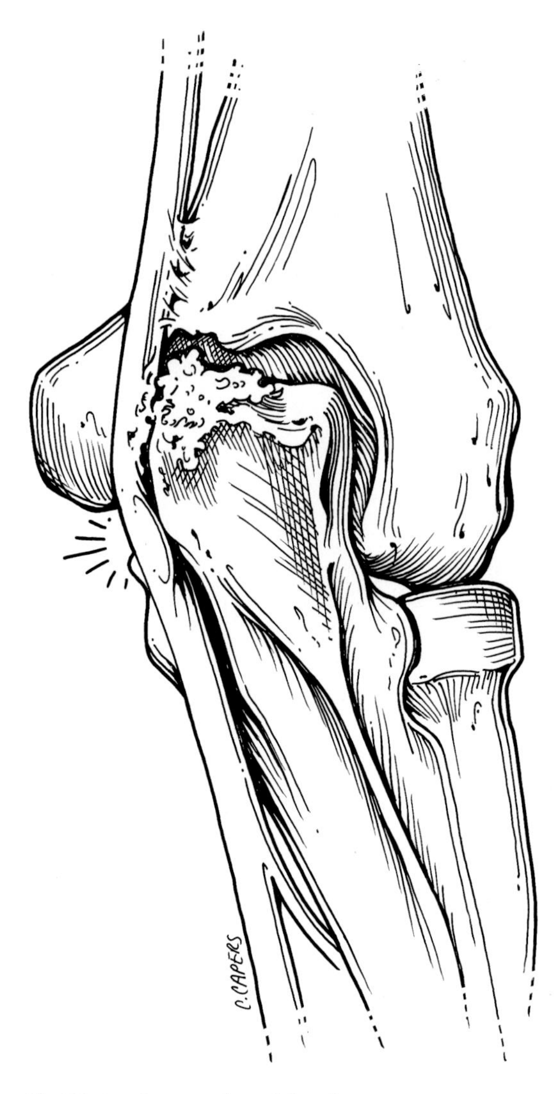

Fig. 53–4. Compression of the ulnar nerve.

Physical examination may reveal swelling and tenderness in the ulnar groove. Sensory deficits may be present in the ulnar half of the ring finger, the little finger, the palmar hypothenar area, and the dorsal ulnar aspect of the hand. A positive Tinel's sign may be present manifesting as paresthesia and tingling in the distribution of the nerve after percussion is applied. Nerve conduction studies may or may not be helpful; however, they will occasionally show decreased nerve conduction across the elbow.

If diagnosed early, ulnar neuropathies can be successfully treated with 2 to 3 weeks of rest, splinting, and the institution of nonsteroidal anti-inflammatory medications. When the player is asymptomatic, the return to throwing begins with emphasis on proper pitching technique and correction of any altered biomechanics that may have developed.

More resistant cases of ulnar neuropathy are usually treated by anterior transposition of the ulnar nerve. During this procedure the compressed or tethered nerve is transferred from its normal posterior position in the cubital tunnel to the less compressive, more mobile anterior aspect of the elbow.

Indications for anterior transposition of the ulnar nerve include those patients who have failed conservative treatment, who have prolonged symptoms, and who wish to continue to throw. In addition, anterior transposition is generally recommended if there is electromyographic evidence of neuropathy or clinical evidence of motor weakness. The ulnar nerve is also usually transferred anteriorly at the time of ulnar collateral ligament repair or reconstruction because of the potential for scar formation and because of the dissection required over the medial aspect of the elbow.

Median Nerve

Although not as common as ulnar neuropathy, median nerve symptoms are occasionally seen in throwing athletes. Injury can occur as a result of direct trauma or repetitive stress. The median nerve can be compressed in the proximal forearm and present as a pronator teres syndrome,[23,24] or be compressed more distally in the forearm and present as the anterior interosseous syndrome.[25]

Treatment of median nerve compression is conservative and includes stretching, correction of throwing technique, and correction of equipment, such as racquet size and grip. If symptoms are prolonged and disabling, it may be appropriate to explore the pronator teres, sublimis arch, and lacertus fibrosis, with appropriate release of impinging structures on the median nerve.

Radial Nerve

Although uncommon, radial nerve neuropathies occasionally exist in the throwing athlete, either secondary to direct trauma or secondary to muscular exertion during the throwing motion. There are four potential sites of compression of the radial nerve[26]: (1) fibrous bands coursing anterior to the radial head; (2) radial recurrent vessels anterior to the lateral epicondyle; (3) compression by extensor carpi radialis brevis; or (4) by the arcade of Frohse, which is a fibrous band at the proximal end of the supinator muscle. This last compression of the radial nerve is the most frequent compressive neuropathy of the radial nerve.

As for the other neuropathies, treatment is conservative initially, consisting of stretching, non-steroidal anti-inflammatory medications, and rest. Surgery is reserved for more resistant cases; it involves exploration of the radial tunnel and radial nerve with release of any impinging structures.

REFERENCES

1. Jobe, F. W., and Nuber, G.: Throwing injuries of the elbow. Clin. Sports Med. *5*:621, 1986.
2. Morrey, B. F., An, K. N., and Chao, E. Y. S.: Functional evaluation of the elbow. *In* The Elbow and Its Disorders. Edited by B. F. Morrey. Philadelphia, W. B. Saunders, 1985.
3. Nirschl, R. P.: Elbow tendinosis/tennis elbow. Clin. Sports Med. *11*:851, 1992.
4. Noyes, F. R., Grood, E. S., Nussbaum, N. S., and Cooper, S. M.: Effect of intra-articular corticosteroids on ligament properties. Clin. Orthop. *123*:197, 1977.
5. Cabrera, J. M., and McCue, F. C., III: Nonosseous athletic injuries of the elbow, forearm, and hand. Clin. Sports Med. *5*:681, 1986.
6. Berkeley, M. E., Bennett, J. B., and Woods, G. W.: Surgical management of acute and chronic elbow problems. *In* Injuries to the Throwing Arm. Edited by B. Zarins, J. R. Andrews, and W. G. Carson, Jr. Philadelphia, W. B. Saunders, 1985.
7. Woods, G. W., Tullos, H. S., and King, J. W.: The throwing arm: Elbow joint injuries. J. Sports Med. *1*(4):43, 1973.
8. Rijke, A. M., Goitz, H. T., McCue, F. C., and Andrews, J. R.: Stress radiography of the medial elbow ligaments. Presented at Annual Meeting, American Academy of Orthopaedic Surgeons, San Francisco, CA, 1993.
9. Timmerman, L. A., and Andrews, J. R.: The histologic and arthroscopic anatomy of the ulnar collateral ligament of the elbow. Presented at Annual Meeting, American Academy of Orthopaedic Surgeons, San Francisco, CA, 1993.
10. Conway, J. E., Jobe, F. W., Glousman, R. E., and Pink, M.: Medial instability of the elbow in throwing athletes. Treatment by repair or reconstruction of the ulnar collateral ligament. J. Bone Joint Surg. *74A*:67, 1992.
11. Singer, K. M., and Roy, S. P.: Osteochondrosis of the humeral capitellum. Am. J. Sports Med. *12*:351, 1984.
12. Mitsunaga, M. M., Adishian, D. A., and Bianco, A. J., Jr.: Osteochondritis dissecans of the capitellum. J. Trauma *22*:53, 1982.
13. Pappas, A. M., Osteochondrosis dissecans. Clin. Orthop. *158*:59, 1981.
14. Singer, K. M.: Radiographic evaluation of the throwing elbow. *In* Injuries to the Throwing Arm. Edited by B. Zarins, J. R. Andrews, and W. G. Carson, Jr. Philadelphia, W. B. Saunders, 1985.
15. Carson, W. G., Jr. and Andrews, J. R.: Arthroscopy of the elbow. *In* Injuries to the Throwing Arm. Edited by B. Zarins, J. R. Andrews, and W. G., Carson Jr. Philadelphia, W. B. Saunders, 1985.
16. Carson, W. G., Jr.: Arthroscopy of the elbow. Instr. Course Lect. *37*:195, 1988.
17. Carson, W. G., and Meyers, J. F.: Diagnostic Arthroscopy of the Elbow: Surgical Technique and Arthroscopic Portal Anatomy. *In* Operative Arthroscopy. Edited by J. B. McGinty. New York, Raven Press, 1993.
18. King, J., Brelsford, H. J., and Tullos, H. S.: Analysis of the pitching arm of the professional baseball pitcher. Clin. Orthop. *67*:116, 1969.
19. Indelicato, P. A., et al.: Correctable elbow lesions in professional baseball players: A review of 25 cases. Am. J. Sports Med. *7*:72, 1979.
20. Andrews, J. R., and Wilson, F.: Valgus extension overload in the pitching elbow. *In* Injuries to the Throwing Arm. Edited by B. Zarins, J. R. Andrews, and W. G. Carson, Jr. Philadelphia, W. B. Saunders, 1985.
21. Wilson, F. D., Andrews, J. R., Blackburn, T. A., and McCluskey, G.: Valgus extension overload in the pitching elbow. Am. J. Sports Med. *11*:83, 1983.
22. Larson, R. L., Singer, K. M., Bergstrom, R., and Thomas, S.: Little League survey: the Eugene study. Am. J. Sports Med. *4*:201, 1976.
23. Farber, J. S., and Bryan, R. S.: The anterior interosseous nerve syndrome. J. Bone Joint Surg. *50A*:521, 1968.
24. Spinner, M.: The anterior interosseous-nerve syndrome, with special attention to its variations. J. Bone Joint Surg. *52A*:84, 1970.
25. Posner, M. A.: Compressive neuropathies of the median and radial nerves at the elbow. Clin. Sports Med. *9*:343, 1990.
26. Roles, N. C., and Maudsley, R. H.: Radial tunnel syndrome: resistant tennis elbow as a nerve entrapment. J. Bone Joint Surg. *54B*:499, 1972.

54

Richard L. Angelo

Arthroscopy in the Treatment of Elbow Disorders

Arthroscopy of the elbow involves very precise and demanding technique. Because of the proximity of neurovascular structures to the recommended portals, a thorough knowledge of regional and intra-articular anatomy is essential. The high degree of congruity of the articular surfaces and the relatively small capsular volume make sound arthroscopic skills a necessity. With proper precautions, the technique is safe and can be used to obtain valuable diagnostic information and to perform selected procedures without the complications associated with arthrotomy. Minimal tissue dissection is necessary to establish the arthroscopic portals. Less scarring is produced, permitting more rapid rehabilitation and decreasing the possibility of a permanent restriction of motion. Compared with an arthrotomy, the arthroscope provides more universal access to the elbow. Consequently, the surgeon can perform a more thorough diagnostic evaluation and more easily treat problems in more than one location.

INDICATIONS AND CONTRAINDICATIONS

There are a number of indications for elbow arthroscopy:

1. Loose bodies of cartilage or bone can be retrieved from either the anterior or posterior compartments.
2. Osteochondritis dissecans lesions may be amenable to arthroscopic débridement,[1] abrasion, drilling, and occasionally internal fixation of larger unstable bony fragments.
3. Degenerative or post-traumatic arthritis often results in joint debris, which may be lavaged from the joint under arthroscopic visualization. In addition, osteophytes in some locations can be freed with an osteotome and removed with graspers. Andrews and Carson[2] have described the treatment of localized posteromedial ulnohumeral degenerative lesions secondary to repetitive extension overload in throwing athletes.
4. Post-traumatic adhesions and arthrofibrosis may be treated by arthroscopic débridement.
5. Lateral synovial plicas have been described, and successful treatment with arthroscopic resection has been reported in a small number of cases.[3,4]
6. Radial head fractures may lend themselves to arthroscopically assisted reduction and internal fixation.
7. A subtotal arthroscopic synovectomy is valuable in treating selected synovial disorders, e.g., rheumatoid arthritis and synovial chondromatosis.
8. Irrigation and drainage for septic arthritis can be performed arthroscopically.
9. Chronic elbow pain of undetermined origin may be evaluated with diagnostic arthroscopy. Significant chondral lesions, cartilaginous loose bodies, and synovial disorders are sometimes found.

Any significant distortion of normal anatomy, including bony deformity (congenital or post-traumatic), bony or fibrous ankylosis, and, in some cases, previous surgery (e.g., ulnar nerve transposition), is a contraindication to elbow arthroscopy. These disorders may place the neurovascular structures at substantially greater risk during the establishment of portals and make it difficult to safely and effectively introduce the arthroscope or manipulate it within the joint. Infection and reflex sympathetic dystrophy are also contraindications.

GENERAL SETUP AND INSTRUMENTATION

Patient Preparation

A general anesthetic is usually preferable and provides excellent relaxation. Although regional or local anesthesia can be used,[5] if the block is incomplete it will postpone accurate postoperative neurologic examination for several hours.

Two options exist for patient positioning. Andrews and Carson[6–8] have popularized the method of placing the patient in the supine position, while Hempfling[9] and Poehling and colleagues[5] have advocated the use of the prone position for the patient (Fig. 54–1). Either method works well, but if the majority of the surgical procedure involves the posterior compartment, the prone position may offer some advantages, as described below.

With the patient in the supine position, the shoulder of the affected arm is allowed to overhang slightly the edge of the operating table.[6] The shoulder is placed in 90° of abduction and in neutral rotation, with the elbow in 90° of flexion. This position affords access to all sides of the elbow joint and permits unrestricted pronation and supination of the forearm during the procedure. The forearm is suspended from the boom of an arthroscopic shoulder holder or similar device using a sterile stockinette with an attached strap and cord.

With the patient prone, the shoulder is abducted 90° and the upper arm is placed in a horizontal position supported by an armboard oriented parallel to the operating table. The elbow is flexed approximately 90° with the forearm directed toward the floor. This position minimizes the chance that gravity-directed fluid will leak from the posterior portals and produce fogging of the camera lens. An additional advantage is the ability to control easily the degree of elbow flexion by adjusting the table height.

The most commonly used portals in elbow arthroscopy include the anterolateral, anteromedial, posterior, and direct or straight lateral. A detailed knowledge of the anatomic relationships within the elbow joint is particularly important during arthroscopy, because the relatively small fields of view may show only a portion of several structures to use for orientation. Optimal visualization of either the medial or lateral portions of the anterior compartment is afforded by viewing from the opposite side.

The first step in the procedure is to use a centimeter ruler to map out the various portals. The "soft spot" is palpated at the confluence of the radial head, olecranon, and capitellum. An 18-gauge spinal needle is introduced at this site to instill 30 to 40 ml of saline. Joint distension plays an important role in displacing the neurovascular structures anteriorly and provides for safer portal placement.[6,10]

Portals

Anterolateral Portal. The anterolateral portal courses posterolaterally to the radial nerve. From this view, the coronoid process, trochlea, coronoid fossa, and medial capsule can be visualized. The intra-articular portion of the coronoid is the basic landmark. A view from this portal may reveal loose bodies that often rest in the coronoid fossa (Fig. 54–2). Osteophytes may also develop at this site, limiting full elbow flexion. Occasionally a capsular thickening is appreciated on the medial wall and represents the anterior bundle of the medial collateral ligament.

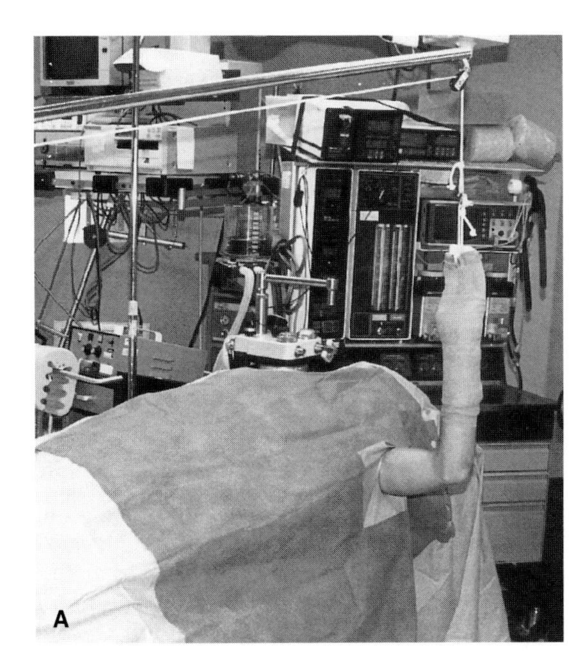

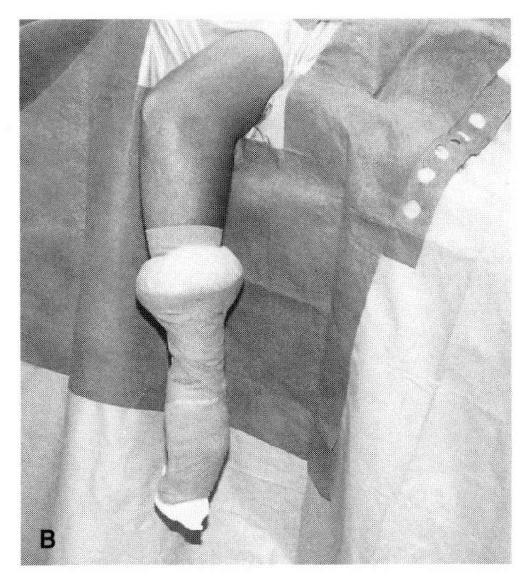

Fig. 54–1. ***(A)*** **Supine and** ***(B)*** **prone positioning of the patient for elbow arthroscopy.**

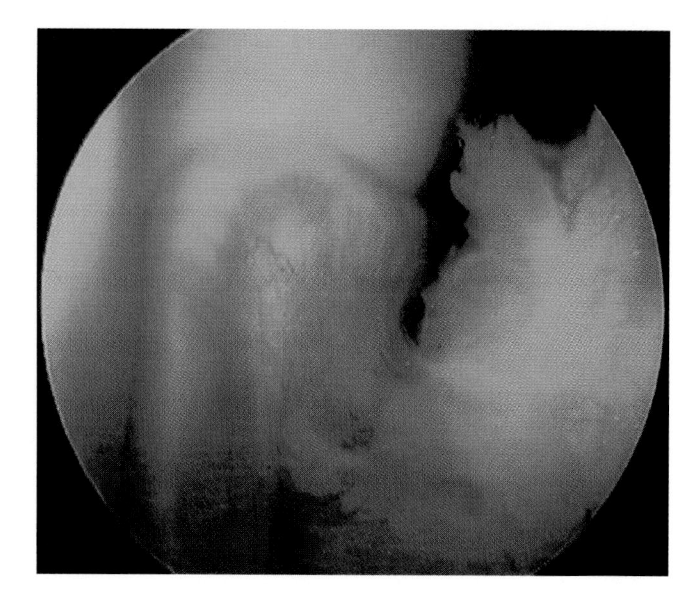

Fig. 54–2. View from the anterolateral portal.

Anteromedial Portal. Several anteromedial portals have been described, but all approach the elbow joint from the anterior aspect of the joint at the supracondylar level, then pass posteromedially to the median nerve and brachial artery. From the anteromedial portals, the radial head is the basic landmark; it is obvious as it rotates during pronation and supination. By distracting the radiocapitellar joint, a good view of the central articular depression of the head is possible for assessing degenerative changes or depressed fracture fragments. The anterosuperior portion of the capitellum is present in the field of view, as well as the bare radial fossa immediately proximal to the capitellum. Because the lateral ligamentous tissues are more lax than those on the medial side, a larger recess is present laterally and may harbor loose bodies.

Posterolateral Portal. The posterolateral portal is located proximal to the tip of the olecranon and just lateral to the triceps tendon. From the posterior arthroscopic portal, the articulation of the olecranon tip with the posterior trochlea is noted during flexion and extension of the elbow. Because of valgus extension overload forces related to throwing sports, osteophytes may form at the posteromedial aspect of the olecranon and trochlea. The large triangular olecranon fossa may also be the site of osteophyte formation or can harbor loose bodies (Fig. 54–3). Both the posteromedial and posterolateral gutters are generally well visualized.

Direct Lateral Portal. The direct lateral portal is located at the confluence of the capitellum, radial head, and olecranon. The direct lateral portal offers a much greater view of the capitellum and permits a more thorough evaluation of osteochondritis dissecans lesions. In addition, a more complete view of the radial head is present. The trochlear notch may be followed from distal to proximal, noting the normal transverse area devoid of articular cartilage that separates the proximal and distal facets.

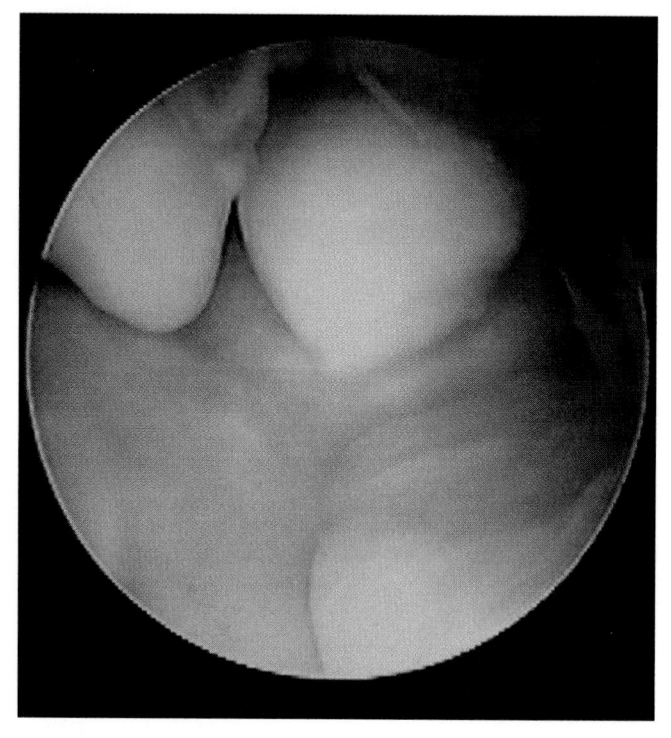

Fig. 54–3. View of olecranon fossa with loose bodies seen from a posterolateral portal.

THERAPEUTIC ELBOW ARTHROSCOPY

Once safe and efficient portals have been established, procedures performed within the elbow joint require the same skills used during arthroscopy of other joints. Loose bodies may be harbored in any of the recesses in the elbow, necessitating a meticulous diagnostic examination. Triangulation skills are essential because the bodies may have to be manipulated to a more favorable location for extraction. Occasionally larger fragments may have to be sectioned with an osteotome before removal.

Osteochondritis dissecans lesions are frequently found on the capitellum (Fig. 54–4). Jackson and colleagues[11] reported on 10 patients with osteochondritis who were examined with an arthroscope and then treated with arthrotomy for curettage and drilling. Ruch and Poehling[1] advocated performing the same procedure using arthroscopy alone. Through a second working portal adjacent to the direct lateral portal, débridement with a motorized bur and drilling with a Kirschner wire are possible. The relative success of the procedure is often determined by the extent of the articular damage.

Osteophytes can form in either the anterior or posterior elbow compartments, and their location will largely determine how amenable they are to arthroscopic resection. A quarter-inch curved osteotome is useful for releasing and dividing the osteophyte, which can then be removed with graspers. Spurs at the posteromedial aspect of the ulnohumeral joint are not uncommon in throwing athletes.[2,12] Débridement and osteophyte

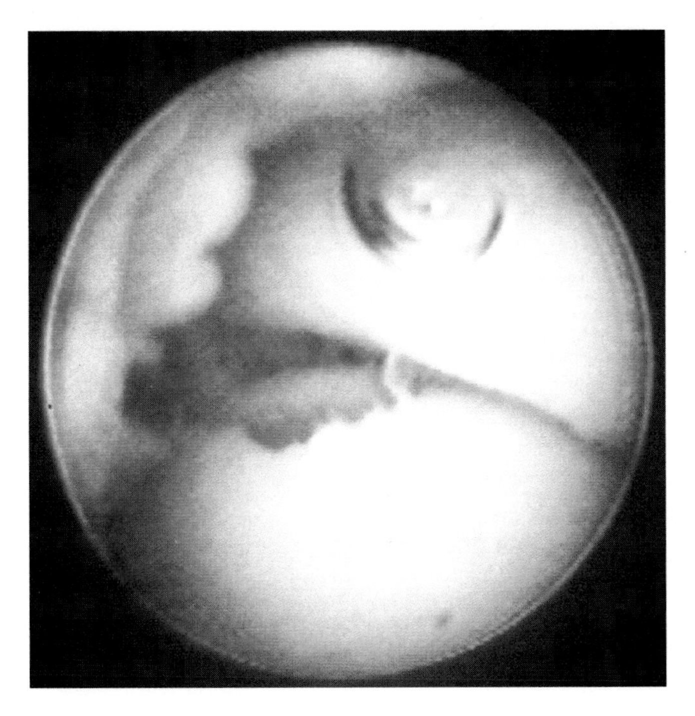

Fig. 54–4. Osteochondritis dissecans of the capitellum.

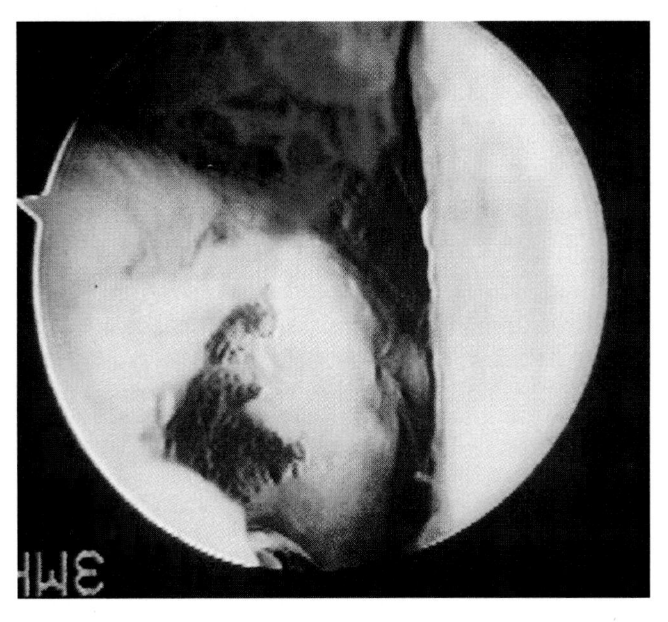

Fig. 54–5. Radial head fracture.

removal are often effective in relieving pain. However, care must be taken not to injure the ulnar nerve, which lies in the posteromedial gutter and is only separated from the bone by relatively thin layers of synovium, capsule, and ligamentous tissue.

Intra-articular adhesions are generally easily resected, but the soft tissue abnormalities limiting full elbow motion may be intra-articular or extra-articular, and arthroscopic débridement alone rarely restores full motion. Jones and Savoie[13] reported on 12 patients with elbow flexion contractures treated by arthroscopic partial anterior capsulectomy and débridement of the olecranon fossa. The mean flexion contracture improved from 38° to 3°. There was one serious complication involving the transection of the posterior interosseous nerve.

Several case reports[3,4] have described the findings of a lateral synovial plica and indicated that, in addition to lateral elbow pain, clicking and loose body symptoms were often present. Resection of the plica can result in the dramatic relief of symptoms.

Visualization of radial head fractures depends on the location and extent of the fracture (Fig. 54–5). Débridement of unstable fragments and, in some cases, arthroscopically assisted reduction and internal fixation of larger fragments may be accomplished.

Patients with chronic elbow pain of undetermined origin may be candidates for elbow arthroscopy if they have undergone a thorough nonoperative treatment program. Computed tomography arthrography scans are helpful in evaluating the extent of degenerative changes secondary to valgus extension overload and aiding in the diagnosis of ulnar collateral ligament injuries. Magnetic resonance imaging scans are particularly helpful in studying osteochondritis dissecans lesions, but synovial and more subtle chondral lesions may be difficult to diagnose without an arthroscopic evaluation.

Finally, in one of the largest reported series of elbow arthroscopic procedures, O'Driscoll and Morrey[14] reported that 64% of 56 patients who had diagnostic arthroscopy had benefitted from the procedure. Seventy percent of the 43 elbows in which a therapeutic procedure was done also benefitted. In addition to the indications listed above, posterolateral rotatory instability was diagnosed at arthroscopy in four of their 71 cases. Neither the preoperative history nor the physical examination suggested this diagnosis.

POSTOPERATIVE CARE AND REHABILITATION

A well-padded posterior plaster splint and a mildly compressive elastic bandage are placed on the elbow after surgery. A sling is provided for comfort, and the patient is discharged the day of surgery. The dressing is removed on the third postoperative day and rehabilitation exercises are begun.

The return to athletic activity must be individualized, but all patients should have minimal to no elbow pain, full or maximized range of motion, and near normal strength. In most cases in which the procedure has been limited to the removal of tissue (e.g., loose body removal or débridement), there is commonly a 6- to 8-week period before resumption of demanding activities. When tissue healing is expected (i.e., after fixation of a bony osteochondritis dissecans fragment or radial head fracture fragment), an additional 8-week period may be necessary.

COMPLICATIONS

The list of complications from elbow arthroscopy is similar to that of other arthroscopic procedures, but the reported incidence is most pronounced for neurologic deficits. Exact numbers of complications are not available, but case reports have included radial, posterior interosseous, median, and ulnar nerve palsies, or transections. Medial antebrachial cutaneous neuromas have also occurred.

In at least one instance, a forearm compartment syndrome developed secondary to fluid extravasation and required a fasciotomy.[15] Multiple capsular penetrations produce the greatest risk of this complication. Careful monitoring of the extent of fluid extravasation during the case is mandatory.

The chance of infection should be minimized by properly preparing and sterilizing the arthroscopic instruments; by carefully preparing, and draping, the arm and the forearm and obtaining secure seals; and by watching mindfully for possible contamination of cords and tubing.

Instrument breakage will remain a possible complication of any arthroscopic procedure. Levering against bony structures to gain access or exposure, careless handling of instruments between cases, and failure to routinely check proper working order will lead to more frequent tool breakage.

SUMMARY

In addition to its value as a diagnostic tool, the arthroscope is an effective aid in the treatment of certain elbow disorders. The greatest success rate has been with the management of mechanical derangements. Both the supine and prone patient positions have their advantages. The procedure demands a thorough knowledge of regional anatomy including the proximity of neurovascular structures to the recommended portals. Meticulous attention to detail must be paid when mapping bony landmarks and introducing cannulas. When the recommended techniques are employed, the morbidity of elbow arthroscopy should be very low.

REFERENCES

1. Ruch, D. S., and Poehling, G. G.: Arthroscopic treatment of Panner's disease. Clin. Sports Med. *10*:629, 1991.
2. Andrews, J. R., and Craven, W. M.: Lesions of the posterior compartment of the elbow. Clin. Sports Med. *10*:637, 1991.
3. Taillan, F. A., et al.: Plica synovialis (synovial fold) of the elbow. J. Sports Med. Phys. Fitness *28*:209, 1988.
4. Clarke, R. P.: Symptomatic, lateral synovial fringe (plica) of the elbow joint. Arthroscopy *4*:112, 1988.
5. Poehling, G. G., Whipple, T. L., Sisco, L., and Goldman, B. III: Elbow arthroscopy: A new technique. Arthroscopy *5*:222, 1989.
6. Andrews, J. R., and Carson, W. G.: Arthroscopy of the elbow. Arthroscopy *1*:97, 1985.
7. Andrews, J. R., and Carson, W. G., Jr.: Arthroscopy of the elbow. *In* Techniques in Orthopaedics: Arthroscopic Surgery Update. Edited by J. B. McGinty. Rockville, MD, Aspen Systems Corp., 1985.
8. Carson, W. G., Jr., and Andrews, J. R.: Arthroscopy of the elbow. *In* Injuries to the Throwing Arm. Edited by B. Zarins, J. R. Andrews, and W. G. Carson, Jr. Philadelphia, W. B. Saunders, 1985.
9. Hempfling, H.: Die endoskopische Untersuchyng des Ellenbogengelenkes vom dorso-radialen Zugang. Zeitschrift fur Orthopadie *121*:331, 1983.
10. Morrey, B. F.: Anatomy of the elbow joint. *In* The Elbow and Its Disorders. Edited by B. F. Morrey. Philadelphia, W. B. Saunders, 1985.
11. Jackson, D. W., Silvino, N., and Reiman, P.: Osteochondritis in the female gymnast's elbow. Arthroscopy *5*:129, 1989.
12. Wilson, F. D., Andrews, J. R., Blackburn, T. A., and McCluskey, G.: Valgus extension overload in the pitching elbow. Am. J. Sports Med. *11*:83, 1983.
13. Jones, G. S., and Savoie, F. H. III: Arthroscopic capsular release of flexion contractures (arthrofibrosis) of the elbow. Arthroscopy *9*:277, 1993.
14. O'Driscoll, S. W., and Morrey, B. F.: Arthroscopy of the elbow: diagnostic and therapeutic benefits and hazards. J. Bone Joint Surg. *74A*:84, 1992.
15. Andrews, J. R.: Personal communication.

55 *Anne Hollister*

Functional Anatomy of the Hand

The anatomy of the upper extremity is quite different from that of the lower extremity. The bones of the arms are entirely enveloped by muscles, unlike the tibia, with its broad subcutaneous medial face. Nerves (such as the axillary and radial nerves) and vessels wrap around the bones, so no approaches to the upper extremity skeleton are as benign as those for the lateral side of the femur. The tendon excursions for the finger- and the wrist-moving muscles are much longer than those in the foot, a factor that predisposes the hand and arm to stiffness after injury. Unlike the leg, the upper extremity is blessed with very extensive collateral circulation. The abundant soft tissue coverage and excellent circulation render the upper extremity less susceptible to infection and wound management easier than in the lower extremity. As a consequence of the anatomy and function of the upper extremity, surgical approaches, interventions, therapies, and the philosophies of treating injuries are different from those for the lower extremity.

THE FINGERS

The working parts of the hand, the fingers, are composed mostly of bone, tendon, and skin. There are no muscles distal to the metacarpophalangeal (MCP) joints. The main neurovascular structures lie on the lateral side of the fingers, out of harm's way. The dorsal skin is thin and very mobile, whereas the volar skin is padded with a thick dermis and fat globules, to protect the volar aspect of the hand that is most stressed during use. The volar skin is also densely innervated.

The interphalangeal (IP) joints are single-axis joints, the axis lying just volar to the origin of the collateral ligaments. The axes are parallel to the flexion and extension creases and pass just above the dorsal end of the flexion creases of the IP joints. The axes of rotation of the joints are in line with the midshaft of the bones on a lateral view of the finger. Except for those of the long finger, the IP joints all have carrying angles, which has something to do with the fact that the fingertips close in an arc to point at the volar carpal ligament.

The joints have an intercondylar groove on the proximal surface that articulates with an eminence on the distal joint surface and is perpendicular to the axis of rotation. This trochlea gives lateral and rotational stability when the joints are compressed by the flexors and extensors during use. There is a small dorsal lip, on which the central slip inserts, and a broader volar lip that attaches to the volar plate. The bony volar lip of the proximal interphalangeal (PIP) joint is very important in maintaining congruity when the joint is in the terminal part of extension.

Muscles

Since the IP joints are single-axis joints, they require only one agonist-antagonist pair to function. All of the muscles are either flexors or extensors of the joints. The interossei and the lumbricals are flexors of the MCP joint and extensors of the IP joints.

FLEXORS

There are two flexors of the PIP (flexor digitorum profundus and flexor digitorum superficialis) and one flexor of the distal interphalangeal (DIP) (flexor digitorum profundus) joints. This arrangement, with two flexors for the proximal joint and only one for the distal joint is necessary to prevent collapse of the finger with flexion of the DIP joint and extension of the PIP joint when load is applied to the fingertip. The tendency exhibited by fingers that have only a profundus tendon, as after a free tendon graft or repair of the flexor digitorum profundus alone, to develop distal joint flexion contractures is related to this imbalance. It is necessary to repair both digital flexors, if normal finger movement is to occur.

The finger flexor tendon paths are controlled by the fibro-osseous tunnel (Fig. 55–1), a structure that extends from the distal palm to the distal phalanx. Thickenings of the tunnel are referred to as pulleys—annular (A) and cruciate (C) pulleys. The A1, A3, and A5 pulleys extend from the accessory collateral ligaments and the volar plates of the MCP, PIP, and DIP joints, respectively, to encircle the flexor tendons. The stiff A2 and A4 pulleys have their origins on the shafts of the proximal and middle phalanges and are the strongest pulleys in the system. Cruciate pulleys are interposed between the A2, A3, A4, and A5 pulleys. The cruciate pulleys are more flexible and change shape as the joints flex and extend. They also show much variability in form from finger to finger. The pulleys prevent the finger flexors from pulling away from the bones as the joints flex. If the pulleys about the MCP joint are destroyed, the joint develops a flexion contracture, and the prominent cord of the flexors is easily palpated under the skin. The IP joints usually are fixed in extension since all of the flexor tendon excursion is used at the MCP joint. If the pulleys about the PIP joint are absent, that joint develops a flexion contracture, as the tight cord of the tendons tents the skin.

The flexor tendons are invested with synovial sheaths as they pass through the fibro-osseous sheath, insulating them from the skeleton. There is a good deal of excursion of the flexor tendons relative to the bones and to each other when the fingers move. Hand surgeons often debate the need to repair the flexor digitorum

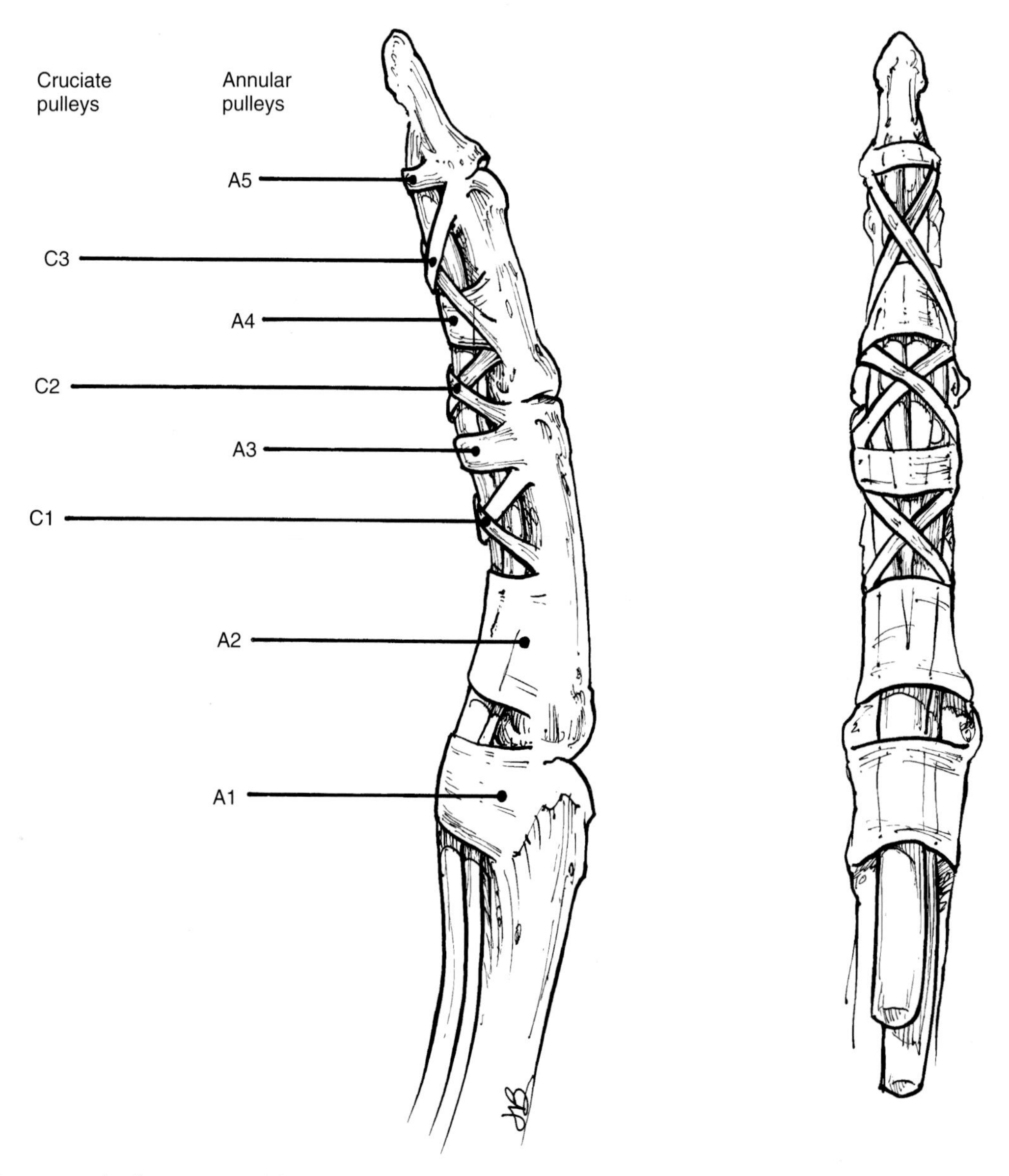

Fig. 55–1. The flexor system of the fingers is made up of the flexor digitorum profundus and the flexor digitorum superficialis. Their paths are controlled by the fibro-osseous tunnel, which has thickenings, the *annular* and *cruciate pulleys.*

superficialis when it is lacerated in the area where the flexor digitorum profundus and -sublimis move past each other in the sheath. Certainly, excision of the flexor digitorum superficialis makes it much easier to pass and repair the flexor digitorum profundus; however, the flexor digitorum superficialis is vital for normal finger function. Once the sublimis is gone, there is only one flexor for the last two joints of the finger. As the hand heals and is subjected to active use, the finger is bound to be required to oppose distal loading. Distal load always produces much greater torque force at the PIP than at the DIP joint. One tendon cannot, by itself, control two joints. If there is no flexor sublimis, there will not be enough flexor torque at the PIP joint. If more tension is added to the flexor digitorum profundus to balance that at the PIP joint, the PIP joint will go into extension and the DIP joint will flex. As time goes on, the imbalance of forces stretches the dorsal capsule of the distal joint, an effect often accompanied by stretching of the volar plate of the PIP joint. The deformity is more serious in very mobile fingers, but it develops more slowly in thicker, stiff fingers.

Extensor Mechanism

The extensor mechanism is one of the great marvels of the human hand. One structure with many contributors, it depends on normal function of all to work properly. For a single tendon to extend two joints smoothly is asking a lot. The extensor mechanism manages to do this easily.

The extensor mechanism is one structure distal to the MCP joint. At this level, the finger extensor tendon, the interossei, and the lumbrical come together to form one tendon (Fig. 55–2). Though, at any given time, the muscles have different mechanical advantages at the MCP joint, they have the same mechanical advantage at the IP joint. The second dorsal interosseous has the same extensor moment arm at the PIP joint as the extensor digitorum communis. It is not possible to identify individual muscle insertions at either IP joint.

The geometry of the bones is important for normal function of the extensor mechanism. The proximal phalanx is cone shaped in its proximal two thirds. As the extensor mechanism moves distally with IP joint flexion, it becomes narrower, and, therefore, longer. This allows for more IP joint motion for a given excursion of the muscles at the MCP joint.

There are two fixed insertion points in the system: the insertion on the distal phalanx and the central slip insertion on the middle phalanx. The fixed relationship with the flexion-extension axis of the PIP joint is maintained by the lateral retinacular ligaments. These ligaments also form a link between the flexor sheath and the extensor mechanism, which does not ordinarily restrain motion in the mechanism but can become a firm anchor in pathologic conditions.

Because of these fixed points in a system that controls two joints, the motion at one joint is linked to the position of the other. When the PIP joint is held in flexion, the extensor mechanism exerts no extensor torque on the DIP joint. If the PIP joint is in extension, the mechanism can exert strong DIP extensor torque, but the range of motion of the distal joint into flexion is limited. If the DIP joint is held in maximum flexion when the PIP joint is in flexion, the extensor mechanism can exert no extensor torque at the PIP joint.

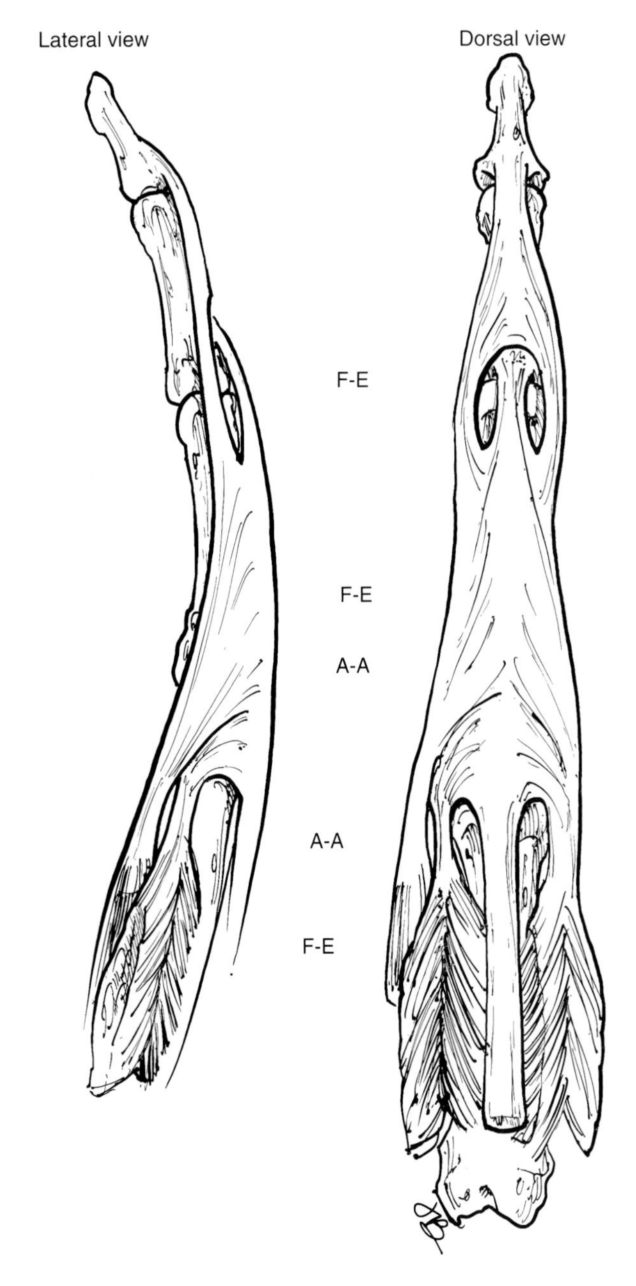

Fig. 55–2. The extensor mechanism is a single structure distal to the metacarpal joint. It has insertions at the distal phalanx and the middle phalanx (the central slip). (Key: F-E = flexion-extension axis; A-A = abduction-adduction axis.)

There is evidence that the oblique retinacular ligament is probably of little importance in normal hand function. Stack cut the ligament and observed no effect on finger mechanics. He points out that many fingers do not have a demonstrable ligament but function as those that do.

METACARPOPHALANGEAL JOINTS

The IP joints of the fingers are the terminal parts of a chain in which the MCP joint is key. Position of the finger, mechanisms of application and dissipation of load, and the mechanics of the muscles are all determined principally at the MCP joint.

The MCP joints have two axes of rotation, a flexion-extension axis that lies under the epicondyles and an abduction-adduction axis that moves with the metacarpals. The abduction-adduction axis forms an angle of about 60° with the proximal phalanx, so that the motion of the proximal phalanx describes a cone as it abducts and adducts. In this manner, abduction and pronation are linked, as are adduction and supination. The adduction-abduction axis passes just proximal to the volar beak on the proximal phalanx, through the volar plate.

Ligaments

The collateral ligaments at the MCP joint arise from the epicondyles of the metacarpals. The true collateral ligament inserts on the base of the proximal phalanx, and the larger accessory collateral ligament inserts on the volar plate with fibers joining the A1 pulley and the deep intermetacarpal ligament. The accessory collateral ligaments are slack when the finger is in extension, and they tighten as the finger flexes and the flexor tendons pull the sheath volad. The MCP joint has a shallow surface, and joint congruency depends on the integrity of the collateral ligaments. If they are lacerated or destroyed by a disease process such as rheumatoid arthritis, subluxation or dislocation of the joints occurs. Without the restraints of the ligaments, volar force of the flexor tendons pulls the proximal phalanx into the palm.

Muscles

Four muscle groups cross the MCP joints: the extensors, the flexors, the interossei, and the lumbricals. The extensors are pure extensors of the MCP joint and join the interossei and lumbrical at the MCP joint to form the extensor mechanism. The flexor digitorum profundus and–superficialis are pure MCP flexors. The interossei are very strong muscles with cross-sectional areas in the same range as that of the flexor digitorum superficialis. This large cross-sectional area means that the interossei contribute much more to MCP flexion and IP extension than do the tiny lumbricals. Their tendons cross the MCP joint just dorsal to the deep transverse intermetacarpal ligament, and they have small moment arms for MCP flexion but large moment arms for abduction and adduction. The first dorsal interosseous muscle, the largest and most prominent, has about three times the cross-sectional area of the other dorsal interossei and usually does not have any attachment to the index extensor mechanism. A very powerful MCP radial deviator, it balances the index finger and others against the ulnar deviating forces of pinch and power grasp. Removal of the first dorsal interosseous for use as a muscle flap can lead to ulnar drift of the fingers.

The lumbricals extend from the flexor digitorum profundus in the palm to the radial side of the extensor mechanism. They do not contribute to MCP flexion since their tension is a part of that produced by the flexor digitorum profundus, but they do act as weak MCP radial deviators and IP extensors. The lumbrical origin in the palm is of surgical significance because it often extends into the carpal tunnel and because the flexor digitorum profundus muscles of the ulnar three digits have lumbrical origins on both the radial and ulnar sides of their tendons. The lumbricals link the three tendons together, limiting their ability to move independently. They also limit proximal migration of the flexor digitorum profundus following laceration or avulsion in the fingers. If the profundus is not present in the finger, it will be found in the palm. This is in contrast to the independent flexor pollicis longus and flexor digitorum superficialis tendons, which after forceful division in the finger can retract into the proximal forearm.

CARPOMETACARPAL JOINTS

The thumb, and the third and fourth fingers, have very mobile carpometacarpal (CMC) joints. In the first, and especially the second finger, the same joints produce little motion. The CMC joints are saddle joints, and the motions occur about two offset hinges, a flexion-extension axis in the proximal bone and an abduction-adduction axis in the distal one. Whereas the contribution to thumb motion of the CMC joint is well appreciated, the third and fourth CMC joints are also important for normal hand function. Flexion of the fingers is accompanied by flexion of these CMC joints. They allow cupping of the palm as well as normal closure of the fingers. The joints are moved by the digital flexors, and especially by the ulnar nerve–innervated hypothenar muscles. An early sign of ulnar nerve palsy is weakness of the hypothenar muscles and inability to supinate the little finger while attempting thumb-to-little finger pinch.

THE THUMB

The thumb CMC is the most mobile of the CMC joints. Its flexion-extension axis is in the trapezium, and its abduction-adduction axis, in the metacarpal. The hinges are offset from the anatomic planes and are not at right angles with the bones or with each other. This allows the thumb metacarpal to pronate with abduction and supinate with adduction. These motions, combined with MCP abduction and adduction, produce opposition and the other motions of the thumb (Fig. 55–3).

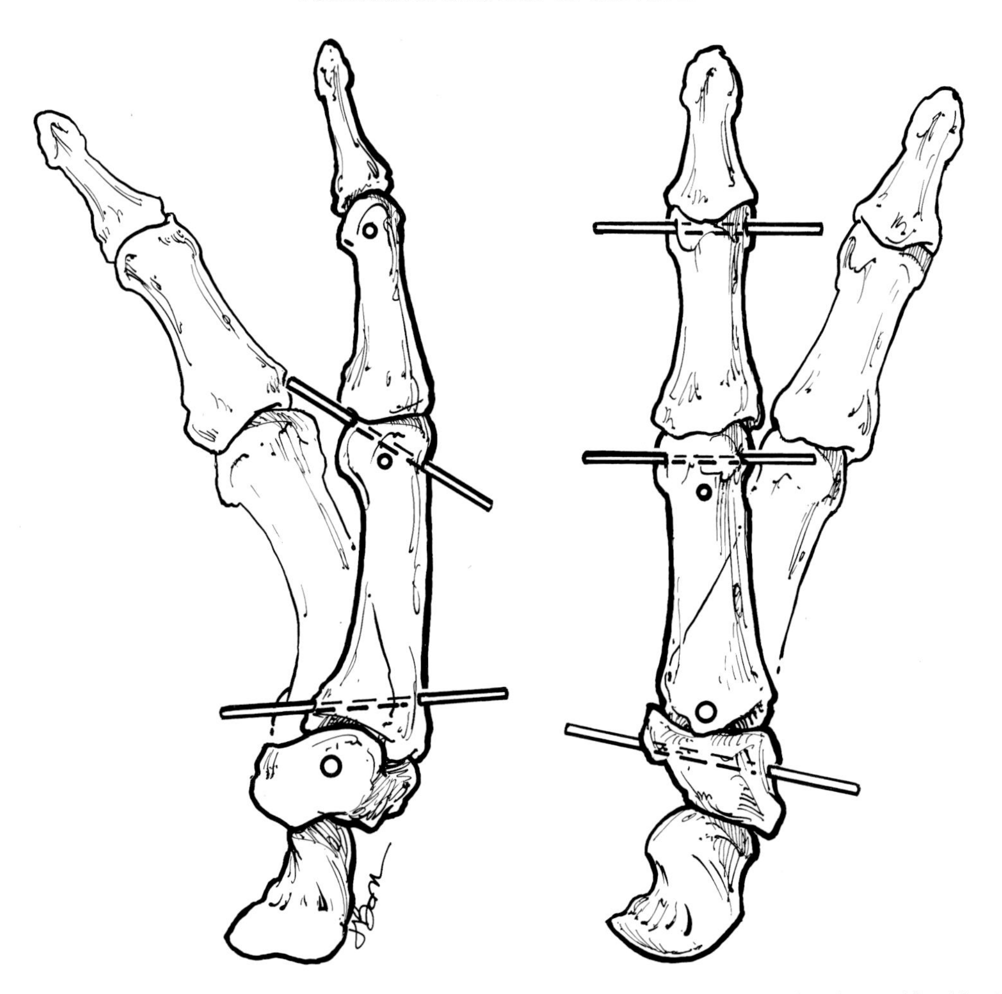

Fig. 55–3. The thumb CMC joint allows the thumb metacarpal to pronate with abduction and supinate with adduction because the flexion-extension axis in the trapezium and the abduction-adduction axis in the metacarpal are offset from the bones and each other.

The thumb muscles include the extrinsic and intrinsic flexors and extensors (Fig. 55–4). The extrinsic extensors are innervated by the posterior interosseous branch of the radial nerve and include the extensor pollicis longus, the extensor pollicis brevis, and the abductor pollicis longus. The flexor pollicis longus is innervated by the anterior interosseus branch of the median nerve. The intrinsic muscles include the median nerve-innervated abductor pollicis brevis, the opponens, and a variable portion of the short flexor. The rest of the short flexor, the adductor, and the first dorsal interosseous are "ulnar innervated." All of these muscles cross the CMC joint, and some, including the adductor pollicis and the abductor pollicis brevis, act across the IP joint. The mechanism of each of the muscles' actions can be understood if we examine the muscle's line of pull relative to the joint's axis of rotation.

The abductor pollicis brevis is an abductor of both the CMC and the MCP joints, having the largest moment arm of any muscle for abduction of both joints. The muscle is a flexor of the CMC joint. Its tendon moves as the MCP joint flexes and extends, being a weak flexor with MCP flexion and a weak extensor with MCP hyperextension. It inserts into the extensor mechanism and, thus, acts to extend the IP joint.

The opponens pollicis crosses only the CMC joint. It is a flexor and abductor, and the combination of these movements produces opposition of the metacarpal. The flexor pollicis brevis acts principally as a flexor of the CMC joint. Its fibers lie on both sides of the abduction-adduction axis at the CMC joint. It is also an MCP abductor since it inserts into the radial sesamoid and has a large moment arm for MCP flexion. The sesamoid gives the flexor pollicis brevis a larger moment arm than the flexor pollicis longus tendon for MCP flexion.

The adductor pollicis acts on all three thumb joints. It is a flexor and adductor of the CMC and MCP joints. The moment arm for adduction varies for each joint because of the muscle's wide origin and insertion, and it is quite large at the CMC joint. CMC adduction is performed by a combination of adductor pollicis, flexor pollicis longus, and some of the fibers of the flexor pollicis brevis. The adductor pollicis is the only adductor of the MCP joint, but its absence is often overlooked in patients with ulnar nerve palsy because the weakness in CMC adduction from the loss of the adductor pollicis

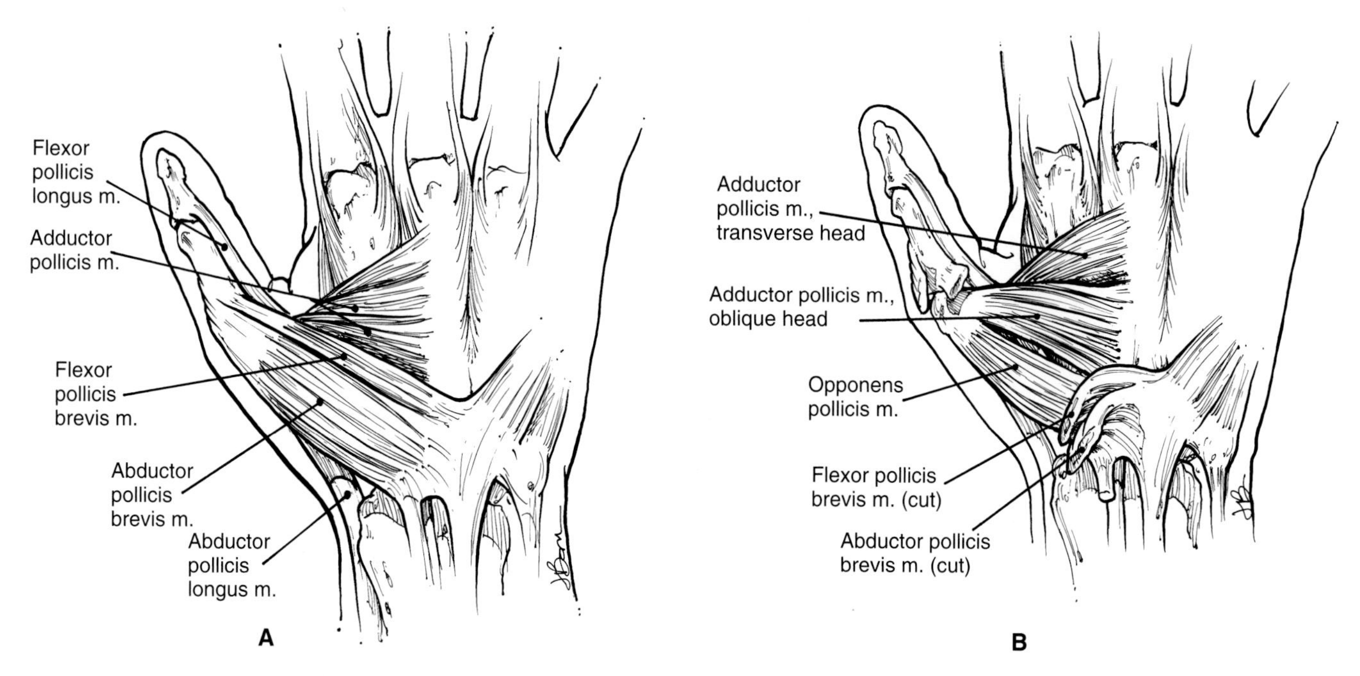

Fig. 55–4. *(A)* **Superficial dorsal thumb muscles.** *(B)* **Deep dorsal thumb muscles.**

and the flexor pollicis brevis prevents the use of the thumb in positions that abduct the MCP joint. The moment arm for most adductor pollicis fibers of MCP flexion is larger than that of the flexor pollicis longus because of the insertion onto the ulnar sesamoid. The insertion of some of its fibers into the extensor mechanism allows it to act as an IP extensor.

The first dorsal interosseous acts on the CMC joint of the thumb. Its direction of pull is nearly 90° to 120° from that of the adductor pollicis, and it acts to distract the CMC joint and to pull the metacarpal distally and ulnad. It has fibers on both sides of the abduction-adduction axis and lies nearly parallel to the flexion-extension axis, so it does little to move the joint. A very important stabilizer of the CMC joint, it acts against the dorsal radial subluxating forces of the adductor pollicis and the flexor pollicis brevis.

The extensor pollicis brevis and the abductor pollicis longus are extensors and abductors of the CMC joint. The abductor pollicis longus has a good moment arm for CMC abduction and is just dorsal to the flexion-extension axis. The extensor pollicis brevis is an extensor of the MCP joint but crosses the MCP's abduction-adduction axis, making it a pure MCP extensor.

The extensor pollicis longus extends all three thumb joints. It is ulnad to the center of both the MCP and the CMC joints and has a smaller moment arm for extension at both joints than does the extensor pollicis brevis. It is an adductor of both the MCP and CMC joints, and it slides farther ulnad at both joints with adduction, increasing its moment arm for adduction. This increased adduction moment arm at both joints is used by patients with intrinsic palsy in side pinch.

The flexor pollicis longus is a flexor of all three joints. It is the only IP joint flexor. It has a relatively small moment arm for MCP, and particularly for CMC flexion, as compared with the intrinsic muscles. It crosses the MCP abduction-adduction axis and is a pure MCP flexor, but it is a weak CMC adductor. Like the finger flexors, the flexor pollicis longus passes through a fibro-osseous tunnel between the MCP joint and its insertion. The A1 pulley is at the MCP joint; the A2 is at the distal joint; and the oblique pulley holds the tendon to the proximal phalanx. As in the fingers, the annular pulleys at the joints are attached to the volar plates. The oblique ligament extends from the ulnar side of the A1 to the radial side of the A2 pulley. Its presence can prevent bow-stringing of the flexor pollicis longus at either joint.

BLOOD SUPPLY AND INNERVATION OF THE HAND

The blood supply to the hand is very rich, and vascular anastomoses are numerous. Major arteries supplying the hand are the radial, ulnar, and anterior and posterior interosseous vessels. Frequently, a median artery is also present, and it can be a major vessel. There are two palmar arches: the more distal superficial arch is usually supplied primarily by the ulnar artery, and the more proximal deep arch is supplied mainly by the radial artery after it emerges from the arcade between the first and second metacarpals (Fig. 55–5).

The deep arch forms a series of anastomoses with the dorsum of the hand through the spaces between the bases of the metacarpals. Small arteries run from the deep arch on the volar surface of the metacarpals and form anastomoses with the digital vessel and the dorsum of the hand at the level of the MCP joints. The superficial arch gives off the common digital vessels that split into the proper digital vessels proximal to the MCP joints. These vessels continue into the fingers, lying between Grayson's fascia and Cleland's ligaments on the

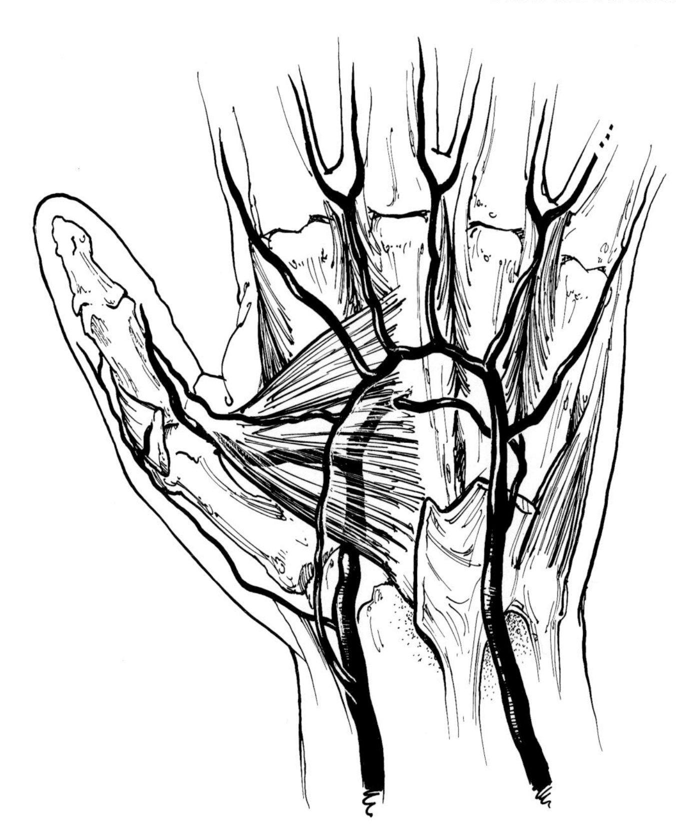

Fig. 55–5. The vascular supply of the human hand.

lateral sides of the fingers. A sizable dorsal branch is given off each digital artery just proximal to the PIP joint, and the artery passes dorsally with a dorsal branch of the nerve just distal to the PIP joint. Numerous other small dorsal and volar branches are present in the finger.

The major blood supply to the thumb comes from the princeps pollicis, the first branch off the deep arch that runs between the adductor pollicis and the first dorsal interosseous muscles. The thumb also receives a blood supply from branches of the superficial arch and from the volar branch of the radial artery. The second branch off the deep arch is the index radialis, and this artery's size, length, and position allow it to be used to resupply the thumb if the princeps pollicis cannot be repaired.

The veins that drain the fingers and the hand lie mainly on the dorsum of the hand. As with the arteries, there are many anastomoses in the venous system, and these tend to parallel those of the arteries. The veins of the hand should be respected and ligated only if it is absolutely necessary. An understanding and respect for the rich anastomotic network in the hand should be actively cultivated, particularly by trauma surgeons. I have seen many cases in which a flap or digit has survived on this collateral circulation alone, and I have also seen unfortunate cases in which a viable flap or digit was rendered avascular by an incision that disrupted the collateral flow.

Three nerves, the radial, median, and ulnar, provide the major sensory and motor innervation to the hand. The lateral and medial antebrachial cutaneous nerves can contribute to the sensory innervation of the proximal palm and the sides of the hand. There is a good deal of variation and overlap in the sensory and motor innervation of the hand. Anastomoses between nerves are common, and the surgeon must appreciate the entire spectrum of neural anatomy rather than a single picture.

The radial nerve supplies the motor innervation for the wrist, finger, and thumb extensors and the long abductors in the forearm, and occasionally to the extensor digitorum manus. It supplies the dorsum of the radial aspect of the hand and thumb. The sensory area extends on the fingers to the PIP joints and on the thumb can include the radial side of the pulp. The radial nerve innervation of all of the extensors is very constant, but the sensory distribution can overlap with that of the lateral antebrachial cutaneous, ulnar, and median nerves. The radial sensory branch can form anastomoses with the dorsal sensory branch of the ulnar nerve in the hand.

The median nerve passes through the volar radial side of the carpal canal after giving off the palmar cutaneous nerve. It lies volad to the finger flexor tendons. With wrist flexion, the transverse carpal ligament becomes a pulley that resists volar bow-stringing of the flexor tendons. Sectioning the carpal ligament should be avoided during flexor repair, and the carpal ligament should be repaired to prevent bow-stringing of the flexor tendons when postoperatively the wrist must be held in volar flexion. The median nerve lies between the flexor tendons and the ligament and can be squeezed by tension in the tendons associated with volar flexion of the wrist. For this reason, volar flexion of the wrist should be avoided in the treatment of fractures.

The median nerve gives off one or more recurrent motor branches and splits into the common digital branches, in or just distal to the carpal tunnel. The recurrent branches usually loop over the distal end of the transverse carpal ligament, but some penetrate the ligament instead, and these variants can be lacerated by the unwary surgeon during carpal tunnel surgery. The recurrent branch supplies the abductor pollicis brevis, opponens pollicis, and a portion of the short flexor. The common digital nerves split into proper digital nerves at the level of the superficial arch. In about 80% of hands, a median-to-ulnar nerve anastomosis also occurs at this level. The common digital nerves supply the lumbricals to the index and long fingers and the sensation in the distal palm, the volar side and the dorsum of the digits distal to the PIP joints of the index and long fingers, and to the radial side of the third finger. A common digital nerve to the thumb is also given off at the level of the superficial arch. This branch can split into proper digital nerves at any level between the takeoff from the nerve to the proximal phalanx.

The ulnar nerve supplies the flexor carpi ulnaris and a portion of the flexor digitorum profundus in the forearm. It gives off a dorsal sensory branch in the distal forearm, which passes under the flexor carpi ulnaris tendon and across the ulnar styloid to innervate the dorsum of the ulnar aspect of the hand and the fourth finger and the ulnar half of the third finger. In about 20% of hands, the ulnar nerve receives a branch from the median nerve—the Martin-Gruber anastomosis—in its course through the forearm. This branch can carry the sensory or motor innervation for the hand. The nerve continues distally and gives off sensory branches that supply the palm plus motor branches to the hypothenar muscles, before entering Guyon's canal. In Guyon's canal, the nerve splits into the motor branch and branches that supply the distal palm, the digital nerves to the fourth and to the ulnar side of the third finger, and the palmaris brevis. The motor branch dives through the opponens digiti mini to run along the volar surfaces of the metacarpal bases. It innervates the interossei, the ulnar lumbricals, and the adductor pollicis.

The ulnar nerve frequently is involved with compression neuropathy in the hand, either in conjunction with carpal tunnel syndrome, following trauma to the hamate or pisiform, or as a consequence of compression or repetitive trauma to Guyon's canal. These conditions can be differentiated from ulnar nerve compression at the elbow because sensation in the proximal palm and on the dorsum of the hand is preserved, whereas that in the digits is impaired if the compression is in Guyon's canal. Motor function of the flexor digitorum profundus, flexor carpi ulnaris, and the hypothenar muscles is spared, whereas that of the interossei and thumb adductor is not. If the compression is secondary to a lesion of the motor branch distal to Guyon's canal, as with a fracture of the hook of the hamate, motor involvement of the interossei and the thumb adductor can occur without any sensory changes.

SUMMARY

The hand is a complex structure. Understanding the mechanical basis of hand function makes possible appropriate preoperative planning in traumatic and reconstructive cases. The design is efficient, and all of the structures in the hand serve important purposes, so appropriate incisions and appreciation of the positions of all mechanical, neural, and vascular elements are vital for the surgeon's success. In the human hand, everything is close by.

SUGGESTED READINGS

Brand, P. W., and Hollister, A. M.: Clinical Mechanics of the Hand. 2nd Ed. St. Louis, C. V. Mosby, 1993.

Bunnell, S.: Surgery of the Hand. Philadelphia, J. B. Lippincott, 1944.

Kaplan, E. G.: Functional and Surgical Anatomy of the Hand. 2nd Ed. Philadelphia, J. B. Lippincott, 1965.

Landsmeer, J. M. F.: The coordination of finger-joint motions. J. Bone Joint Surg. *45A*:1654, 1963.

Sarrafian, S. K., et al.: Strain variation in the components of the extensor apparatus of the finger during flexion and extension. J. Bone Joint Surg. *52A*:980, 1970.

Spinner, M. K.: Nerve entrapment in the upper extremity. *In* Management of Peripheral Nerve Problems. Edited by G. E. Omer, Jr., and M. K. Spinner. Philadelphia, W. B. Saunders, 1980.

56

Hugh A. Frederick

Physical Examination and Ancillary Tests of the Wrist and Hand

Injuries to the hand and wrist are among the most common injuries incurred by athletes. In most sports, the hand and wrist are relatively unprotected and are used to divert or absorb impacts. Acute injuries are associated with fractures, dislocations, ligament injuries, and tendon avulsions. Chronic repetitive-type injuries also occur; they usually involve tenosynovitis, neurapraxia, and vascular injuries. Hand injuries are often thought to be trivial, labeled a "jammed finger" or a "sprained wrist." These nonspecific diagnoses can lead to inaccurate treatment and delayed recovery.

As with all medical problems, the first step in treating these injuries involves taking an accurate history, including the patient's hand dominance; it should also include the precise site and mechanism of injury. Correlating this information with the regional anatomy makes it possible to concentrate the physical examination on the specific area. Be sure to evaluate the bones, ligaments, tendons, nerves, and circulation. Always check the neurovascular status distal to the injury. Also, it is a good idea to compare the findings with the patient's opposite uninjured hand or wrist.

Radiographs can also add useful information. All too often the evaluating physician accepts inadequate views. Typically, for a digital or wrist injury, radiographs are taken of the entire hand, but these radiographs may not show subtle findings. Always obtain at least a true anteroposterior and lateral view of the specific part involved. Occasionally, a specific view or tomogram is needed to demonstrate a fracture. Other radiographic tests, including bone scans, arthrograms, and magnetic resonance imaging (MRI), can help in specific situations, but they are not routinely needed. These high-tech and expensive tests do not take the place of an adequate history and physical examination.

The primary goals of treatment involve restoring normal anatomy and function. To do so requires an accurate diagnosis, proper treatment, and rehabilitation. Fortunately, most hand and wrist injuries heal with conservative care. Do not sacrifice appropriate care to meet the desires of the player, coach, or public. Even simple injuries, if not treated properly, can cause chronic functional deficits both on and off the playing field.

PHYSICAL EXAMINATION OF THE WRIST

Knowledge of the topographic anatomy is critical to a good wrist examination (Fig. 56–1). The anatomic snuffbox, the "soft spot" just distal to the radial styloid, should always be palpated. Pain or swelling in this area may represent a scaphoid fracture. With practice, one can learn to palpate the scapholunate and lunotriquetral joints dorsally along the proximal carpal row. These joints can be tender and swollen in the presence of ligament injuries or fractures. The mid-carpal joint can also be directly palpated dorsally; however, less of the osseous structures are palpable on the volar side, mainly just the pisiform and pisotriquetral joint. The hook of the hamate can also be palpated just distal and radial to the pisiform in the ulnar palm. The distal pole of the scaphoid can also be palpated radially.

The Watson maneuver is a good clinical test for scaphoid instability. The patient should be sitting in a comfortable position with the elbow resting on his or her lap or on an examination table and with the forearm pronated. With one hand bring the patient's wrist into ulnar deviation. In this position, the scaphoid is longitudinal. Next, radially deviate the patient's wrist using your thumb to maintain pressure on the distal pole of the

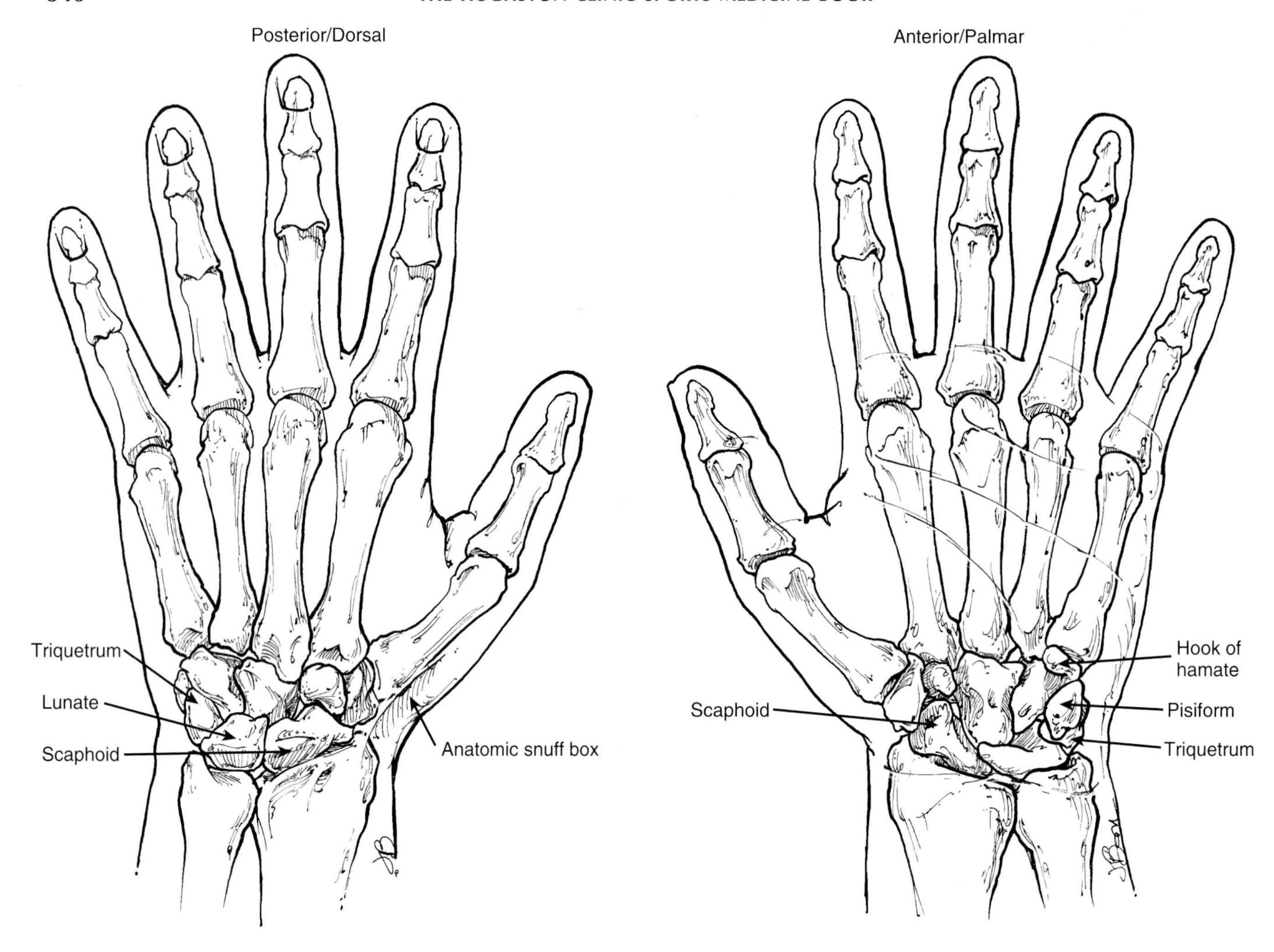

Fig. 56–1. Underlying structures related to topographic anatomy.

scaphoid to prevent its normal palmar flexion. An unstable scaphoid will subluxate dorsally and be painful. Sometimes there is a palpable or even audible clunk as the scaphoid subluxates. It is helpful to compare this maneuver with the same on the opposite wrist.

Axially loading the wrist will cause pain and apprehension in most patients with carpal instability. Pain with axial loading and ulnar deviation can be a sign of ulnar impaction or of a triangular fibrocartilage injury. Check the ulnar styloid and the surrounding soft tissue for tenderness. Check the distal radioulnar joint for stability and tenderness. Check range of motion, including flexion, extension, radial deviation, ulnar deviation, pronation, and supination, and compare with the opposite wrist. Also, to quantify accurately the strength, compare grip strengths using a grip meter. The dominant grip strength is usually 10 to 15% greater than the nondominant grip.

Evaluate the vascular status of the hand and wrist. With any injury, the radial pulse at the wrist and the capillary refill in the digits should be evaluated. If there is any doubt, perform an Allen test. The Allen test checks the patency of the radial and ulnar arteries and of the palmar arches. Instruct the patient to make a tight fist; apply digital pressure over the radial and ulnar arteries along the volar wrist. Have the patient relax his/her fist and open his/her hand, then remove pressure from the radial artery while maintaining pressure on the ulnar artery, watching for digital capillary refill distally. All digits should become pink and have good refill in two to three seconds. Then repeat the procedure, removing pressure from the ulnar artery while maintaining pressure on the radial artery. If the Allen test is abnormal, further vascular evaluation may be required. Noninvasive Doppler studies or even an arteriogram may be needed, depending on the clinical situation.

Most injuries involving an athlete's hands and wrist are closed injuries. If there is an open wound, control bleeding with direct pressure and elevation. Do not try to control bleeding with a blind grab of a hemostat. Doing so can result in crushing a nearby nerve. Remember, most major arteries in the hand and wrist run in close proximity to nerves.

Two-point discrimination sensibility testing can be performed quickly and adequately with only a paperclip (Fig. 56–2). This tests the patient's ability to distinguish

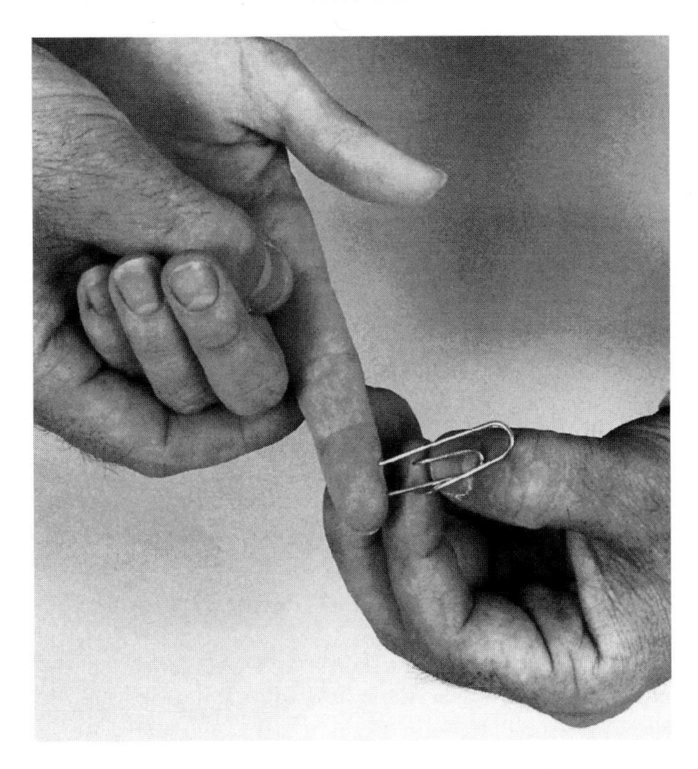

Fig. 56–2. The two-point discrimination test evaluates the patient's ability to distinguish between two points along the volar tip of the finger.

between two points along the volar tip of the finger. Perform the test by applying light pressure that just blanches the skin. Remember to position the paperclip linearly along the radial or ulnar aspect of the finger to isolate each digital nerve. Normal sensibility can distinguish two points when the ends of the paperclip are 5 mm apart. Two-point discrimination tests innervation density and is a good evaluation for nerve lacerations and acute neurapraxias. Compressive neuropathies, like carpal tunnel syndrome, maintain fairly normal innervation densities until there is severe compression. Threshold testing using Semmes-Weinstein monofilaments or tuning forks is much more sensitive to early nerve compression.

Signs of carpal tunnel syndrome and irritation of the median nerve at the wrist can be elicited with a Phalen's test. The patient holds both wrists in a flexed position. The test is positive for median nerve irritation if the patient experiences areas of paresthesia in the median nerve distribution. Also, direct percussion over the median nerve along the volar wrist can cause median nerve paresthesia, called a Tinel's sign; it is often positive in carpal tunnel syndrome. These same maneuvers can also be used to check for ulnar tunnel syndrome if the paresthesia is in an ulnar nerve distribution.

Motor function testing is also important if a nerve injury is suspected. The extrinsic muscles to the hand and wrist, including the wrist digital flexors and extensors, all receive innervation in the proximal forearm. Check all these muscles and compare with the opposite arm. Check the hypothenar muscles for strength with abduction of the little finger. Palpate the first dorsal interosseous and assess abduction strength of the index finger. Weakness or atrophy of the hypothenar or interossei muscles would point to an ulnar nerve injury. Also check the thenar muscles. Compare thumb opposition with that of the opposite hand. Weakness or atrophy of the thenar muscles would point to a median nerve injury.

Tenderness directly over a tendon sheath can be a sign of tendinitis, which can occur volarly over the flexor carpi radialis or flexor carpi ulnaris. Dorsally, the sixth extensor compartment can become inflamed. De Quervain's disease is a common tendinitis of the wrist involving the abductor pollicis longus and the extensor pollicis brevis of the first extensor compartment. Local tenderness and swelling and sometimes crepitance with thumb motion are present. Finkelstein's test is positive in de Quervain's disease. This maneuver re-quires the patient to make a fist with the thumb inside the fist. The examiner then passively moves the wrist into ulnar deviation. Pain along the first extensor compartment at the level of the radial styloid is considered a positive test.

After any wrist injury, it is important to monitor the status of the extensor pollicis longus. This tendon can rupture weeks to months after a distal radius fracture. These patients usually complain of pain and tenderness around Lister's tubercle and the third extensor compartment. The intrinsic thenar muscles of the thumb can extend the interphalangeal joint of the thumb because they insert into the extensor hood. Therefore, it is important to specifically check the continuity of the extensor pollicis longus. This test is best done with the patient's palm flat on the table. Ask the patient to lift his/her thumb off the table. This position isolates the extensor pollicis longus, which can easily be palpated back to Lister's tubercle.

ANCILLARY TESTS OF THE WRIST

Wrist radiographs often intimidate nonorthopedic physicians. The overlap of the eight carpal bones can be confusing, especially if poor quality radiographs are accepted by the physician. If the patient has had a recent injury, it is a good idea to get radiographs before the examination. However, an abnormal radiograph does not absolve the need for physical examination. Other soft tissue injuries may be present and the neurovascular status must be evaluated. Remember, carpal bone injuries are among the most frequently missed diagnoses of all emergent orthopedic problems.

The lateral radiograph is the most useful view in the diagnosis of carpal dislocations. The radiograph should be a true lateral, with the radial and ulnar styloid superimposed. The radius, lunate, and capitate should be colinear. Dorsal or volar tilt of the lunate can be a sign of ligament injury and carpal instability. If in doubt, it is easy to compare radiographs of the opposite uninjured wrist. Some patients do have "physiologic instability patterns" that are normal for them.

The posterior to anterior (PA) radiograph can also reveal fractures or instabilities. On a PA view, three carpal arcs should be visible along the proximal and midcarpal joint. A disruption in the continuity of these arcs implies abnormal carpal alignment. Radiographic signs of a scapholunate ligament injury and carpal instability are a widened scapholunate interval over 3 mm along with a volar flexed scaphoid, creating a "ring sign" and a triangular-shaped lunate (Fig. 56–3).

The radial and ulnar deviation views allow good visualization of the scaphoid in its dynamic relationship with the proximal and distal carpal rows. Carpal instabilities are defined as static when visualized on routine radiographs. They can also be dynamic and require provocative maneuvers to demonstrate the instability patterns. A clenched-fist view in supination causes compression across the carpus and may reveal more subtle instability. Sometimes a fluoroscopic evaluation is needed to show a dynamic instability.

Patients with carpal injuries can have normal radiographs. Scaphoid fractures sometimes do not show as obvious fractures until two weeks after the injury. Bone scans can be helpful in identifying occult fractures. Sometimes even with proper radiographs it is hard to determine the full extent of a carpal fracture (Fig. 56–4). Trispiral tomography can provide excellent detail of the bony anatomy in the carpus and is superior to computed tomography (CT) or MRI.

Hook of the hamate fractures are not well-visualized on anteroposterior or lateral projections. The carpal tunnel view or an oblique in 45° of supination can often show the fracture. CT is probably the best radiographic test to fully evaluate the hook of the hamate.

In cases of suspected ligamentous injuries arthrography may be helpful. For a thorough arthrographic study, the midcarpal, radiocarpal, and distal radioulnar joints must all be injected. MRI is becoming more useful in defining ligament injuries in the wrist.

Wrist injuries in gymnastics are common. A unique injury called *gymnast's wrist* is actually a distal radius physeal stress reaction. It only occurs in skeletally immature patients and is seen radiographically as a widened and irregular physis. Bone scans are not useful in this group of patients because of the superimposed activity of the physis.

PHYSICAL EXAMINATION OF THE HAND

As with the wrist, the physical examination of the hand should follow a systematic approach. Always check the neurovascular status of the digits distal to the injury, noting capillary refill and two-point discrimination. Most of the bony anatomy is palpable; suspect fracture with any area of significant point tenderness and swelling. Again, as with the wrist, it is a good idea to get

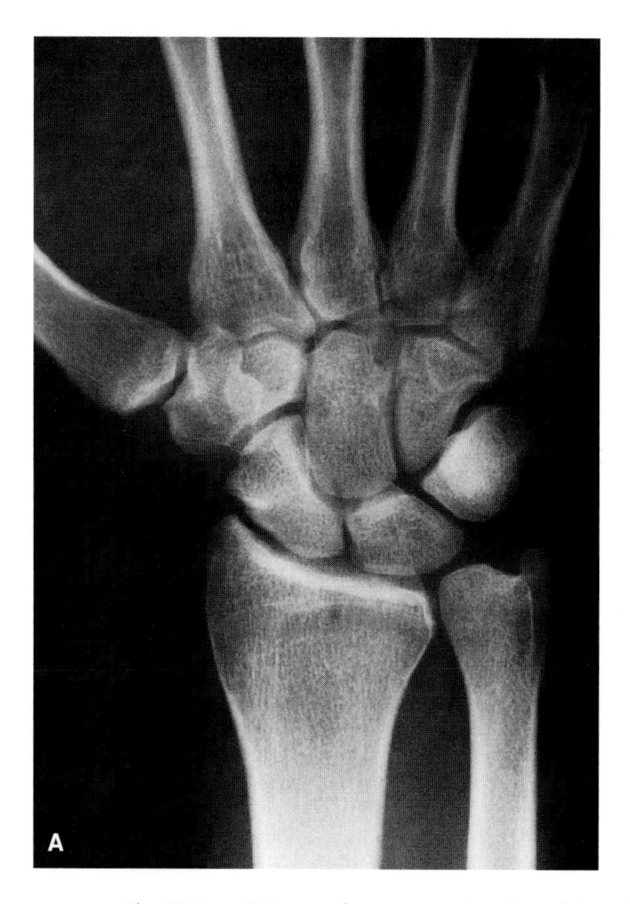

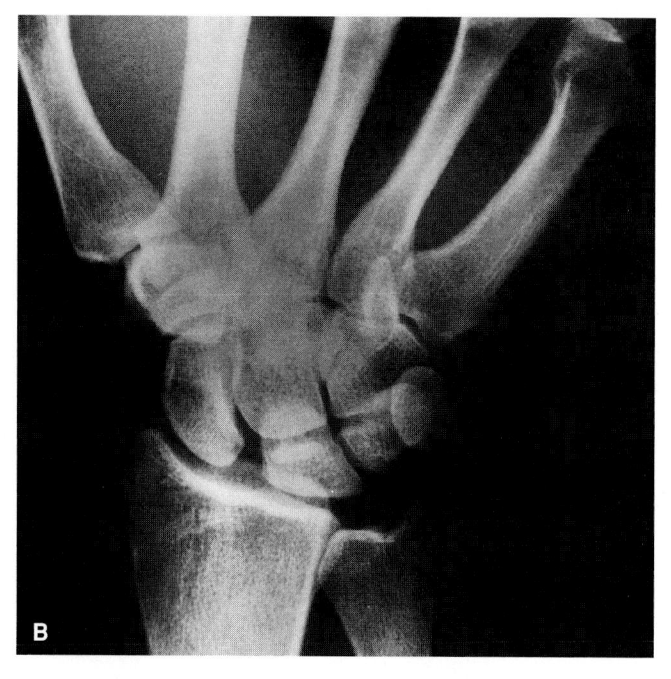

Fig. 56–3. *(A)* **A normal posteroanterior view of the wrist shows the three carpal arcs.** *(B)* **The widened scapholunate interval with a volar flexed scaphoid indicates scapholunate ligament injury.**

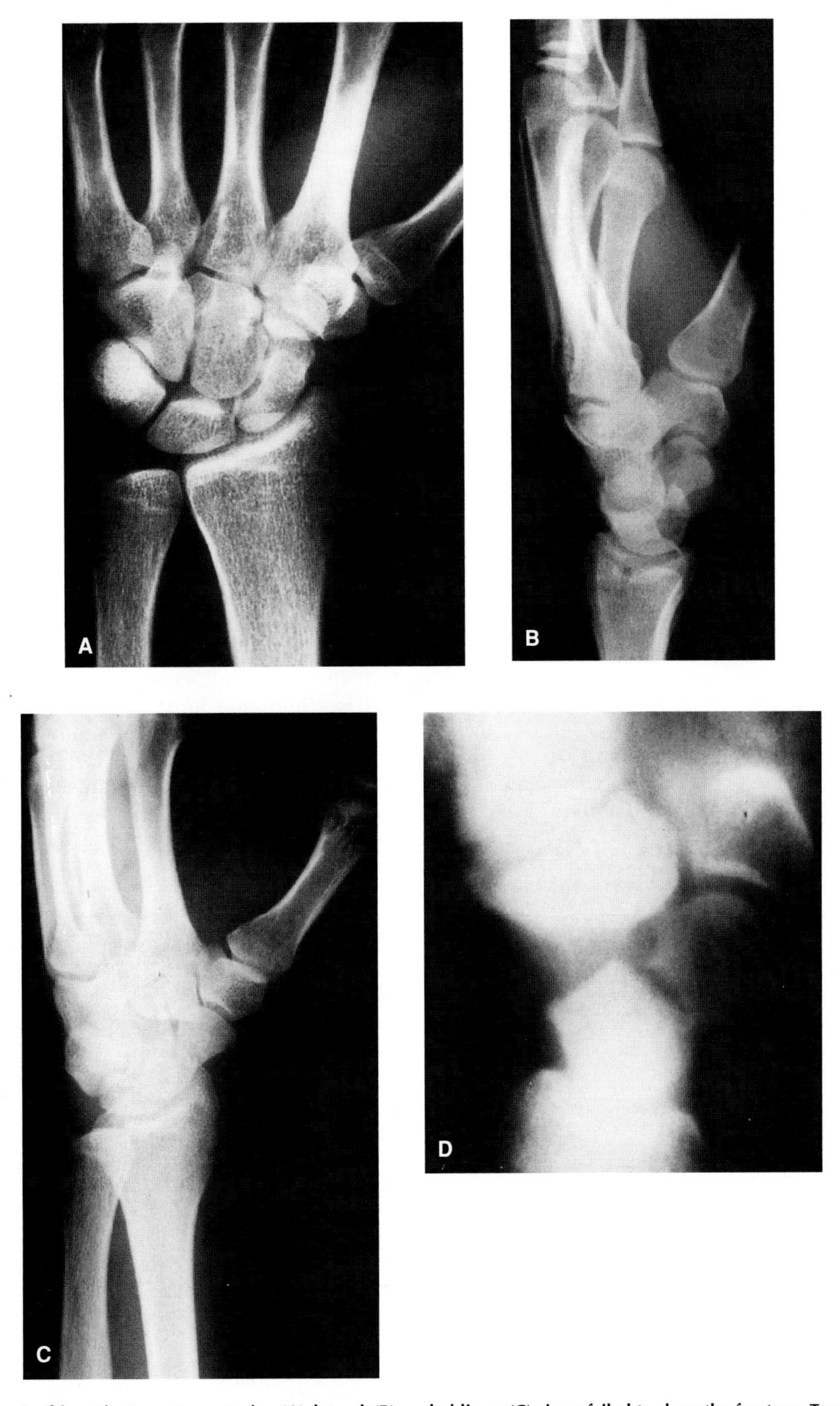

Fig. 56–4. In this patient, posteroanterior *(A)*, lateral *(B)*, and oblique *(C)* views failed to show the fracture. Tomography *(D)* showed the displacement, revealing the fracture.

radiographs of the injured area after an abbreviated physical examination (Handling too vigorously a nondisplaced fracture can cause displacement). Then specifically test the injured areas during the physical examination.

Fractures in the hand can involve either the metacarpals or the phalanges. A displaced fracture is usually obvious from clinical observation. Evaluate carefully any open wound, even a small puncture wound, in close proximity to the fracture. Such wounds can indicate an open fracture that needs thorough cleansing and débridement. The rotational alignment is also important to evaluate. As the patient gently makes a fist, the nails should stay parallel and the fingertips should all point to the scaphoid.

Begin evaluation of an injured thumb at the carpometacarpal (CMC) joint. The CMC joint can be palpated dorsally in the palm through the proximal aspect of the thenar muscles. The grind test is used to evaluate pain and instability in the CMC joint. Hold the distal aspect of the thumb metacarpal and apply pressure and rotation across the CMC joint. Use your opposite hand to palpate the CMC joint, feeling for crepitance or subluxation. The thumb metacarpophalangeal (MCP) joint is another area commonly injured. Check the collateral ligaments for stability by direct manipulation, applying varus and valgus stress to the joint. Check the volar plate by applying hyperextension stress to the joint. It can be helpful to compare stability with the opposite uninjured thumb. Palpate the sesamoids along the volar aspect of the thumb MP joint.

The "jammed finger" is probably one of the most common injuries sustained by an athlete. These patients usually present with a tender and swollen proximal interphalangeal (PIP) joint with limited motion. It is important to palpate carefully to localize the exact area of tenderness. Then stress the ligament in question and determine stability. Before stressing the ligament, check the radiograph for fracture or dislocation.

An examination under anesthesia is not always required, but it can be helpful; it is usually performed under a digital block or wrist block. It is then possible to perform a stress test to check for joint stability and to evaluate the status of the extrinsic flexor and extensor tendons. The active motion test can check for entrapped soft tissue in the injured joint. Ask the patient to make a fist gently and then extend the fingers. Loss of smooth flexion or extension usually indicates that part of a torn collateral ligament is caught in the joint. After a thorough examination an accurate diagnosis can be made. For example, a mild strain of the radial collateral ligament involving the index PIP joint is a much better diagnosis than a "jammed finger."

Ligament injuries to the metacarpophalangeal joint are less common than PIP injuries. The MCP collateral ligament should be checked for stability with the MCP joint flexed 90°. This puts the collateral ligament in tension by the cam-shaft effect of the metacarpal head and allows for more accurate diagnosis.

Dislocations in the hand are common. Often the patient presents with a history of a deformity at the time of injury that was "reduced on the field." Most PIP dislocations are dorsal or lateral. Carefully assess the status of the collateral ligaments and the volar plates. Also, check the central slip, the extensor tendon to the PIP joint. If PIP extension is weak or painful, the central slip might be injured, leading to a boutonnière deformity if not treated. MP dislocations in the thumb or fingers are less common. These can be complex dislocations requiring open reduction. Dislocations of the distal interphalangeal (DIP) joint are uncommon. They are associated with nail bed injuries and extensor tendon disruptions. Often they are open dislocations.

Examination of patients with hand injuries should include a thorough examination of the flexor and extensor tendons. With the wrist in extension and the uninjured hand at rest, the flexor muscle tone causes a "normal cascade." The fingers are progressively more flexed moving from the index to the small fingers. When a tendon is injured, the stance of the digit is altered, disrupting the cascade.

The flexor digitorum profundus and flexor pollicis may be examined by stabilizing all proximal joints and then asking the patient to flex the digital tip (Fig. 56–5A). Isolating the flexor sublimus function is more difficult. The sublimus muscle-tendon units are all independent. The profundus tendons to the small, ring, and long fingers have a common muscle belly, making them function together. By holding the adjacent fingers in full extension, the effect of the profundus is eliminated and PIP flexion is provided by the sublimus (Fig. 56–5B). The sublimus test is reliable for the long and ring fingers. The index finger has an independent profundus tendon, so the sublimus test is not reliable. The small finger often does not have an independent sublimus. When checking the small finger sublimus tendon, allow the patient to flex both the ring and small fingers.

Complete tendon lacerations are fairly easy to diagnose. Partial tendon injuries are more difficult. Partial tendon injuries are painful when the patient actively attempts to move the finger. The flexion cascade is often altered and flexion against resistance is weak.

Both flexor and extensor tendon injuries commonly occur in athletes without an open wound. These injuries are often initially missed because no complete physical examination was performed.

The most common closed flexor injury in an athlete is a rupture of the insertion of the flexor digitorum profundus tendon. The ring finger is the most commonly affected. Pain and swelling are usually present in the flexor sheath, and DIP flexion is absent. Sometimes a small fragment of bone is avulsed with the profundus insertion, and it can be seen on a lateral radiograph.

Closed extensor tendon injuries, especially mallet finger injuries, are very common in athletes. The mallet finger injury involves avulsion of the terminal insertion of the extensor tendon into the distal phalanx. These patients present with an extensor lag at the DIP joint and local tenderness. Radiographs sometimes reveal a bony avulsion from the distal phalanx.

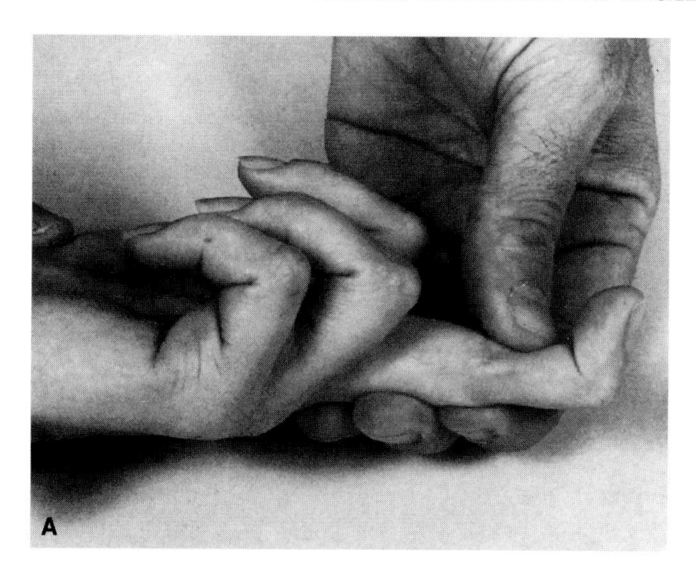
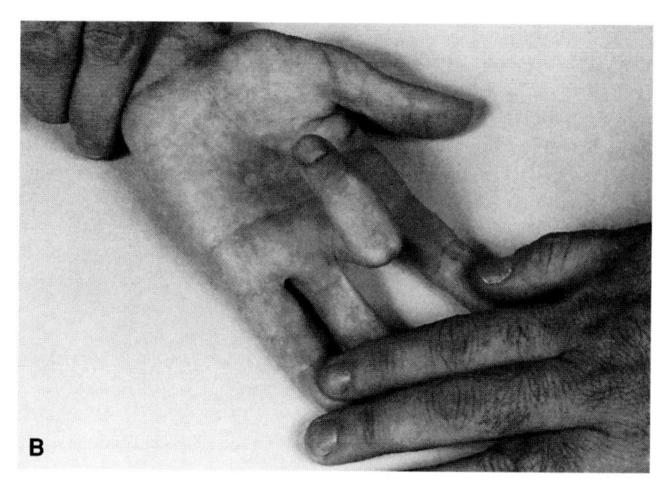

Fig. 56–5. *(A),* The flexor digitorum profundus test isolates the flexor profundus. *(B),* The flexor digitorum sublimus test is used to isolate the flexor sublimus.

A boutonnière deformity can occur with an open or closed injury to the extensor mechanism at the dorsum of the PIP joint. These patients present with a flexion contracture at the PIP joint and hyperextension of the DIP joint. Initially the deformity is mild and passively correctable. If allowed to progress, the deformity becomes more severe and quite disabling. Early diagnosis and splinting are usually preventative.

Stenosing tenosynovitis is a common problem seen in athletes who use their hands. The patients present with pain and stiffness in the involved fingers, centering around the A1 pulley of the flexor sheath in the distal palm. Often there is a tender nodule on the flexor tendon that moves with flexion and extension of the finger. The patient may have a history of triggering as the nodule moves proximal and distal to the A1 pulley causing a painful clicking sensation.

ANCILLARY TESTS OF THE HAND

Radiographs are needed with hand injuries when a fracture or dislocation is suspected. A true anteroposterior and a lateral view of the area in question are necessary. If dealing with a finger injury, an anteroposterior and lateral of the finger in question must be obtained. A

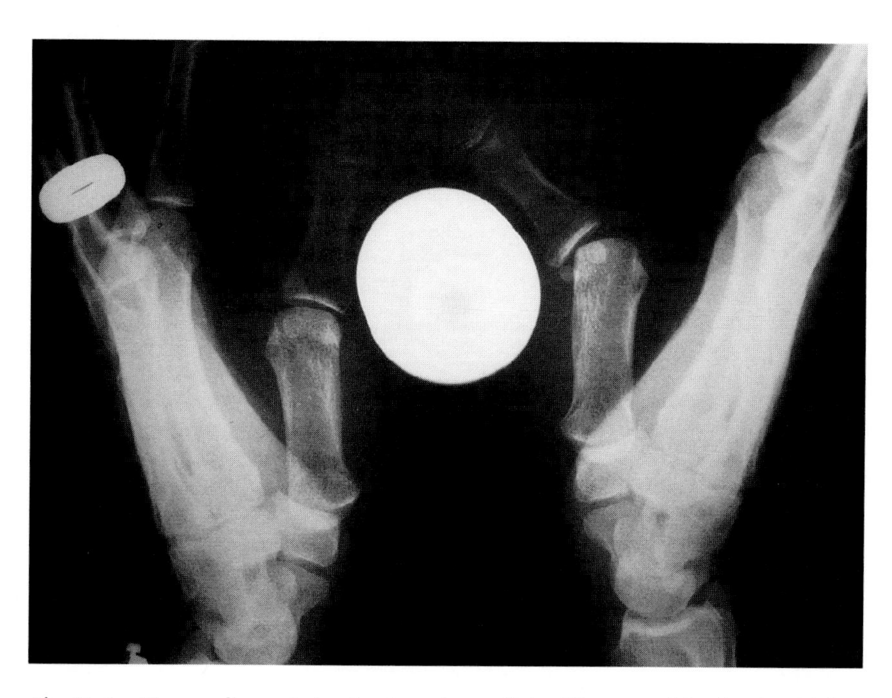

Fig. 56–6. Stress radiograph showing torn ulnar collateral ligament of the thumb MP joint.

radiograph of the entire hand will often miss a subtle finding seen on an isolated view of the finger.

The MP joints of the hand overlap on the lateral radiograph and are difficult to isolate. An oblique view of the hand can help in evaluating MP joints. For the same reason, the CMC joints are hard to evasluate on a lateral radiograph. The fourth and fifth CMC joints can be visualized by pronating the hand 20° from the true lateral view.

Stress views can be helpful with ligament injuries about the hand. These are best performed under local anesthesia. Stress is applied across the joint and the radiograph obtained. This technique is most commonly used in evaluating the ulnar collateral ligament of the thumb MP joint. Significant widening along the ulnar side of the joint indicates a ligament injury (Fig. 56–6).

57

Andrew A. Brooks

Ligamentous Injuries and Fractures of the Wrist

The functions of the wrist are to position the hand in space and to transmit forces to and from the hand and forearm. Few athletic endeavors do not require these functions. The elegant anatomic arrangement of the wrist makes it peculiarly vulnerable to many modes of injury.

Previously, unless an obvious abnormality was evident, many wrist injuries were simply dismissed as "strains" or "sprains" and treated symptomatically with rest or immobilization. Today, the "sprained wrist" has changed from a diagnostic wastebasket to a very specific diagnosis, arrived at only after other entities have been ruled out by thorough clinical, radiographic, and special examinations.

Improvements in noninvasive diagnostic testing have provided greater understanding of the pathologic anatomy of wrist injuries and a better appreciation of their nature. They include provocative stress tests, fluoroscopy, stress radiographs, and minimally invasive studies such as arthrography and bone scans.

ANATOMY

Osseous Anatomy

The carpus is made up of eight bones, arranged into two rows (Fig. 57–1). The scaphoid bridges the proximal and distal rows and is a part of each. Thus, any break in the scaphoid can render the wrist unstable with compression forces. The proximal row is made up of the scaphoid, lunate, triquetrum, and pisiform (some consider the pisiform a sesamoid and not a true carpal bone). The distal row consists of the hamate, capitate, trapezoid, and trapezium.

As the wrist moves, there is not only intercarpal motion (between the rows), but also intracarpal motion (within the rows).[1] Almost all wrist motion is initiated by muscles that insert proximal and distal to the wrist, making the carpus an intercalated segment.[2]

It is partly this unique anatomic arrangement that has made understanding wrist injuries a significant challenge.

Ligamentous Anatomy

The ligaments of the wrist are generally classified as extrinsic, coursing between the carpal bones and the radius or the metacarpals; and intrinsic, originating and inserting on the carpal bones.[3] Among the extrinsic ligaments there are two layers of volar ligaments, superficial and deep. The strong deep volar radiocarpal ligaments are the radiocapitate ligament, the radiolunate ligament, and the deep radioscapholunate ligament. The radiocapitate and radioscapholunate tether the proximal pole of the scaphoid to the volar margin of the radius and act as the main stabilizer of the proximal pole of the scaphoid. Dorsal rotatory subluxation of the scaphoid cannot occur if these ligaments are intact.[3] The dorsal and ulnar corner of the radius is bound strongly to the volar carpus by the ulnocarpal meniscus and the triangular fibrocartilage-ulnolunate ligament complex while the volar and radial corner of the radius is connected to the carpus by the deep radiocarpal volar ligaments. Thus, the carpus is entirely suspended from the radius. The head of the ulna is not a part of the wrist joint, only of the radioulnar joint.[3]

The dorsal ligaments of the wrist are weak compared with the volar ligaments. The dorsal radiocarpal liga-

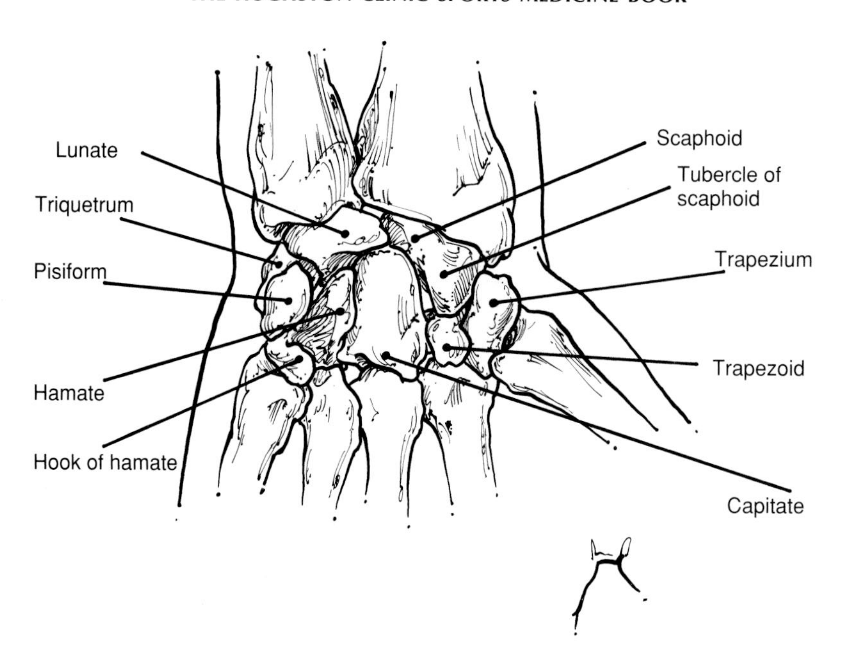

Fig. 57–1. The carpal bones of the wrist.

ment originates from the radius and inserts into the lunate and the triquetrum. On the radial side of the wrist, the radial collateral ligament originates from the volar margin of the radial styloid; it has a strong attachment to the tuberosity of the scaphoid and inserts into the walls of the tunnel for the flexor carpi radialis tendon. The ulnar collateral ligament is poorly developed and is actually a thickening of the joint capsule. It adds little support to the wrist.

The intrinsic ligaments of the wrist originate and insert on the carpal bones. The volar ligaments are thicker and stronger than the dorsal ligaments.[3] The short intrinsic ligaments (volar, dorsal, and interosseous) bind the four bones of the distal carpal row into a single functional unit. There are two long intrinsic ligaments: the dorsal and the volar. The volar ligament stabilizes the capitate by attaching the capitate to the scaphoid and triquetrum. The three intermediate intrinsic ligaments are the scaphoid-trapezium, the lunate-triquetrum, and the scaphoid-lunate.

OVERVIEW OF WRIST BIOMECHANICS

Several different theories have been proposed to explain the complex pattern of motion that exists in the wrist. In 1935, Navarro proposed his theory of the "columnar carpus," noting that the wrist is made up of three individual longitudinal columns as opposed to transverse articulations.[4]

Taleisnik modified and incorporated Navarro's theory to help explain patterns of carpal instability.[5] The scaphoid is the mobile lateral column, the triquetrum is the rotary medial column, and the lunate and entire distal carpal row function as a flexion-extension column.

Lichtman and coworkers proposed an "oval ring" theory, conceptualizing the carpus as a dynamic ring with links between the proximal and distal carpal rows that allow motion with radial and ulnar deviation.[6] Any break in this ring, through either bone or ligament, would result in destabilization and abnormal motion.

In 1984, Weber introduced a slightly different concept, dividing the carpus into two longitudinal columns.[7] The distal radius, the proximal two thirds of the scaphoid, the trapezoid, and the bases of the second and third metacarpals make up the force-bearing column. The distal ulna, the triangular fibrocartilage, the triquetrum, the hamate, and the bases of the fourth and fifth metacarpals make up the control column. The forces generated by the hand are ultimately directed radially via bony and ligamentous anatomy, first toward the scaphoid and lunate and then to the distal radius.

In summary, although each of those models differ in their explanations of wrist mechanics, they all serve to increase our conceptual understanding of wrist motion, which in turn aids in understanding carpal injury patterns.

CARPAL INJURIES

Carpal injuries present a spectrum of bone and ligamentous damage resulting from loading of the wrist in extreme hyperextension. The resulting injury can range from a minor sprain to a complete fracture-dislocation.

The most widely accepted classification of ligamentous injury to the wrist was put forth by Mayfield and coworkers.[8] Their classification is based on cadaveric experiments in which wrists were loaded in extension, ulnar deviation, and intercarpal supination to produce sequential carpal dislocation. This method allowed quantification of the degree of ligamentous damage and provided an understanding of the logical sequence of injury. The authors described a perilunate pattern of injury to the wrist that is broken into four stages: Stage 1 is a scapholunate dissociation; Stage 2 progresses to include dislocation of the capitate-lunate joint; Stage 3 includes triquetrum dislocation; and Stage 4 corresponds to a complete lunate dislocation.

Recently, Cooney and coworkers proposed a two-part classification system consisting of (1) carpal instability dissociative (CID); and (2) carpal instability nondissociative (CIND).[9] CID applied to all instability patterns involving complete ligamentous disruptions with instability within the proximal carpal row, including scapholunate and lunotriquetral dissociation. Conversely, CIND applies to collapse patterns that occur despite continued integrity of the intrinsic ligaments. CIND patterns tend to result from malunions and malalignments of the distal radial fractures and from disruptions or attenuation of the extrinsic palmar ligaments.

Scapholunate Instability

Scapholunate is the most commonly identified carpal instability. This instability results from loss of support of the proximal pole of the scaphoid through rupture of its ligamentous restraints. Delay in diagnosis is the most significant problem with these injuries.[10] It is critical to have a high index of suspicion to make the diagnosis promptly so that appropriate early treatment can be undertaken.

DIAGNOSIS

The history will generally involve a fall onto an outstretched wrist leading to a hyperextension, ulnar deviation, and supination force applied to the wrist. Pain, swelling, and tenderness over the dorsoradial aspect of the wrist on clinical examination should certainly increase one's suspicion that injury has occurred at the scapholunate complex. Watson's test (Fig. 57–2) can be used to assess dynamic instability; pain is the hallmark of a positive test.

The most important diagnostic study to be performed in these patients is radiographic examination of the wrist. The classic radiographic sign is a gap between the scaphoid and lunate greater than 2 mm; this is often referred to as the "Terry Thomas" sign.[11] Other radi-

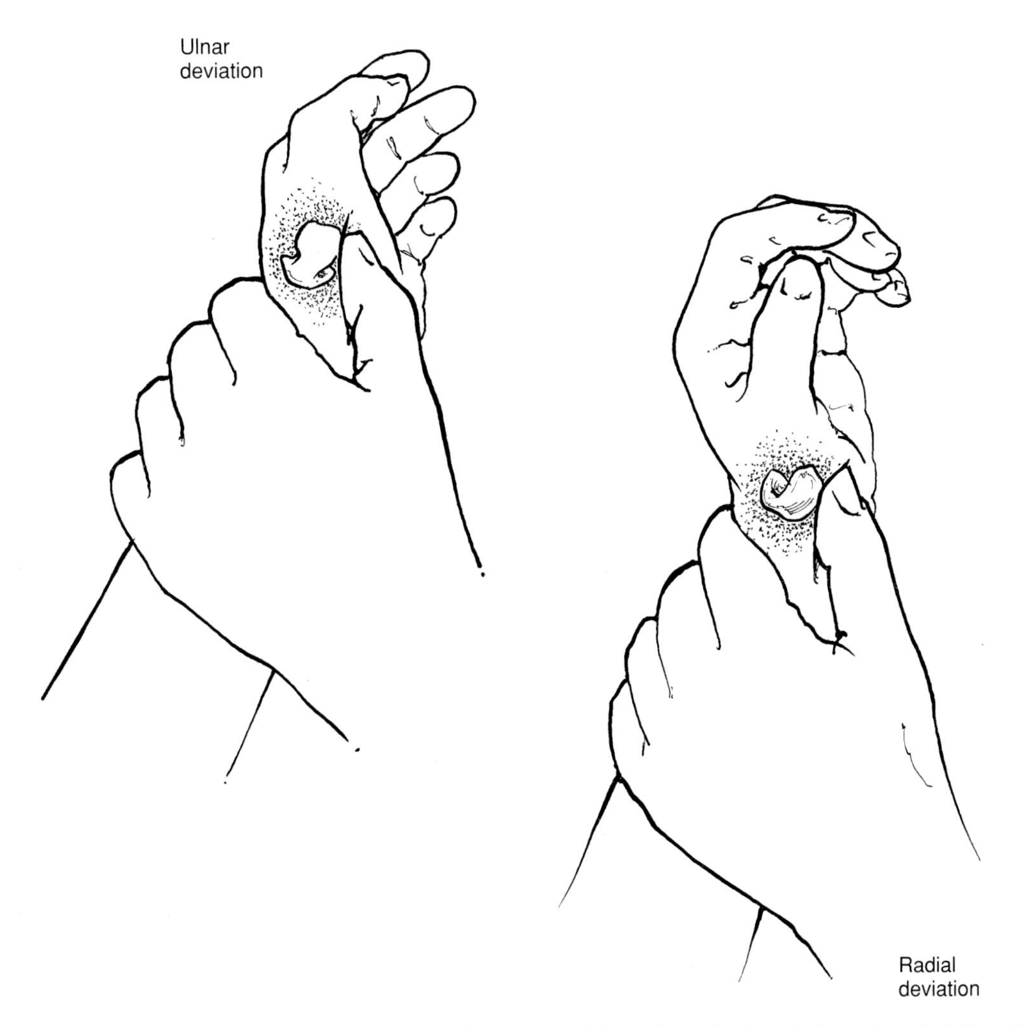

Fig. 57–2. In Watson's test for scaphoid instability, the examiner brings the patient's wrist into ulnar deviation. Then the patient's wrist is radially deviated while the examiner maintains pressure on the distal pole of the scaphoid. An unstable scaphoid will subluxate dorsally and be painful.

ographic findings include the cortical "ring" sign, seen because the distal pole of the perpendicular scaphoid is viewed on end. The lateral projection may reveal a dorsiflexion instability pattern with the scaphoid in a vertical position and corresponding scapholunate angle of greater than 65° to 70°.[12]

TREATMENT

Treatment of acute scapholunate dissociation is surgical. Most hand surgeons do not believe that cast treatment alone can be effective. In terms of operative management of acute injuries, there are essentially two schools of thought. Some believe an adequate repair can be made with percutaneous pin fixation under radiographic control;[13, 14] others believe the best chance at a good result is with open repair of the torn ligaments.[15]

Management of chronic scapholunate dislocations is controversial and considered to be one of the most difficult problems in hand surgery. Current options for treatment include direct ligament reconstruction of the scapholunate interosseus ligament,[16] dorsal capsulodesis as described by Blatt,[17] and intercarpal arthrodesis.[18] Selecting which procedure to use is important and is based on the patient's age, level of symptoms, and avocational demands on the wrist.

Generally, with both acute and chronic scapholunate dislocations, treatment will usually require an athlete to remain out of competition for four to eight weeks. Upon returning to play, the wrist should be protected with an orthosis, such as a silicone cast, for four to six months; at this time, most athletes will have maximum range of motion and strength and the orthosis can usually be discontinued.

Medial Carpal Instabilities

Medial carpal instabilities involve the ligaments attached to the ulnar side of the wrist. As in any ligament injury, a spectrum of injury can be seen, ranging from mild sprains to complete ligament disruptions with static volar intercalated instability deformities.[14] In the past decade, our understanding of these injuries has advanced significantly.

TRIQUETROHAMATE INSTABILITY

This is the most common medial carpal instability. Most of these patients are able to describe a specific injury to the wrist. The mechanism of injury is usually dorsiflexion. This instability is thought to be a result of disruption of the capitotriquetral arm of the arcuate ligament.[19]

Diagnosis. The clinical tipoff of triquetrohamate instability is an audible, palpable, and often painful "clunk" as the wrist is moved from radial to ulnar deviation. Point tenderness is usually noted with palpation over the triquetrohamate interspace. Plain radiographs may show either a dorsiflexion instability or a volarflexion instability pattern, depending on wrist position at the time of the radiograph. The volarflexion instability pattern is more common (Fig. 57–3). Cineradiography can be very helpful to confirm the diagnosis.

TRIQUETROLUNATE INSTABILITY

Again, most patients describe a dorsiflexion injury to the wrist. The major presenting complaint is usually wrist pain on the ulnar side of the wrist.

Diagnosis. The most important physical finding is point tenderness over the triquetrolunate joint. The other important clinical test is the ballottement test (Fig. 57–4). Routine radiographs taken acutely are generally normal. In the chronic injury, a volarflexion instability pattern can occasionally be identified. Arthrography can be very helpful in assessing these injuries. A tear of the lunotriquetral interosseus ligament will be demonstrated by the presence of an abnormal communication of dye between the radiocarpal and midcarpal joints.[19] In the future, arthroscopy may have an increased role in an evaluation of these lesions.

Treatment. An acute ulnar carpal ligamentous injury generally warrants a trial of nonoperative treatment consisting of immobilization in an above-elbow cast and anti-inflammatory nonsteroidal medications. A well-defined, acute ligamentous tear can also be treated with percutaneous pinning under fluoroscopy, followed by cast immo-

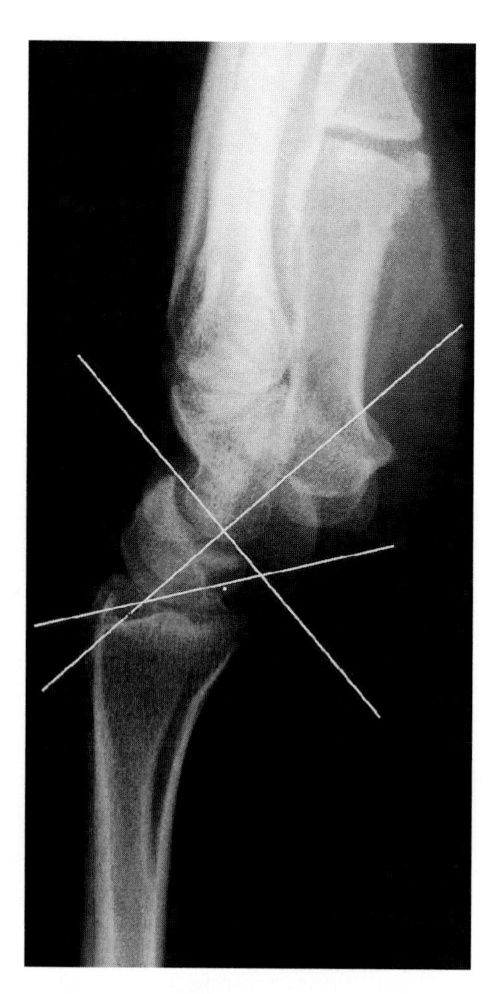

Fig. 57–3. Radiograph showing volar flexion instability pattern.

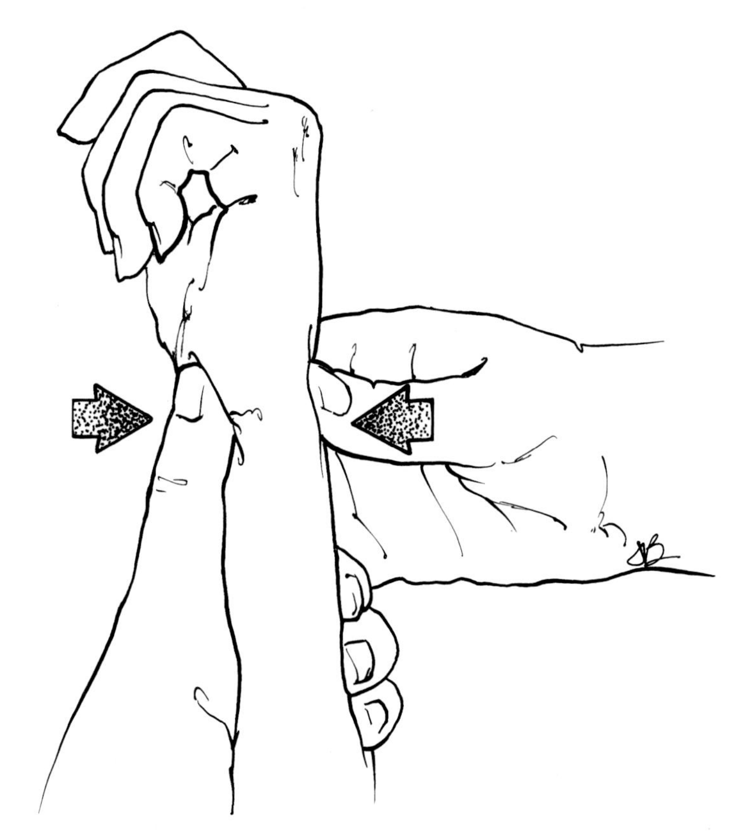

Fig. 57–4. With the ballottement test, the examiner stabilizes the lunate while attempting to displace the triquetrum dorsally.

bilization for six to eight weeks. In chronic cases, most authors recommend triquetrohamate or triquetrolunate arthrodesis as indicated. Ligamentous reconstructions of these joints have proven to be unpredictable. Patients will lose wrist motion after arthrodesis, which can have serious implications for the throwing athlete.

Triquetrolunate arthrodesis has been shown to produce less alteration of preoperative motion. This is most likely because there is less physiologic motion at the triquetrolunate joint in comparison with the triquetrohamate.

In general, the athlete may return to competition after strength and range of motion are demonstrated in a supervised rehabilitation program. This will usually take 6 to 12 weeks. The wrist should be protected with a removable orthosis for 6 months after the initial injury.

FRACTURES OF THE CARPAL BONES

Scaphoid Fractures

Because of the scaphoid's anatomic position in the wrist, scaphoid fractures are the most common carpal fracture.[20] Experimental studies have shown that for a fracture to occur, the wrist must be dorsiflexed a minimum of 95°, with the force applied primarily to the radial aspect of the palm.[21] The most significant problem with these injuries is the high incidence of nonunion and, more importantly, the development of avascular necrosis (AVN). In addition to the bone's precarious blood supply, a major cause of the nonunion and AVN is failure to recognize the fracture soon after the injury. It is not uncommon for an athlete to dismiss a significant injury as a sprain and continue to play the rest of the season, only to discover that a nonunion has developed. A significant percentage of patients with nonunions will go on to develop degenerative arthritis within five to ten years.[22]

CLINICAL EVALUATION

A scaphoid fracture should be suspected in an athlete complaining of wrist pain with associated tenderness over the dorsal snuffbox or directly over the scaphoid. The injury must be confirmed radiographically; it is best seen on posteroanterior and posterior oblique views with the wrist in ulnar deviation. Repeat radiographs at 1 and 3 weeks are essential if the patient is still symptomatic and a fracture is not confirmed. During this time the wrist should be treated as if it were fractured and kept immobilized. Occasionally, it is important to make an early diagnosis; if so, order a technetium bone scan 3 to 5 days after injury.[23] If the scan is negative, a fracture is ruled out.

TREATMENT

The majority of acute nondisplaced scaphoid fractures will heal if immobilized properly and for a long enough period of time. If a fracture is considered stable (i.e., with minimal displacement and angulation), it can be treated in a short arm-thumb spica cast. The cast should be changed every 4 weeks to assure a good fit. Serial radiographs should be obtained to follow healing and maintenance of reduction. The average duration of immobilization is 12 to 16 weeks. After initial immobilization and healing, the wrist should continue to be immobilized and protected from impact loading for an additional three months. Immobilization can easily be achieved with a rigid removable splint.

For the athlete with an acute scaphoid fracture, return to competition should be individualized based on many variables. These include fracture pattern, type of sport, level and degree of competition, and understanding and acceptance of added risk. Football players with acute scaphoid fractures have been successfully treated with rigid Silastic casts that allow continued participation during treatment.[24]

Fractures considered unstable are those with displacement greater than 1 mm or angulation with an abnormal carpal alignment. Treatment of these injuries depends on several individual factors, such as degree of instability and late presentation. Some of these injuries can be treated with closed reduction, followed by long arm-thumb spica casting for 6 weeks and conversion to short arm-thumb spica for an additional 6 weeks. Others require open reduction and internal fixation with either Kirschner wires, Herbert screws, or cancellous screws. Both open and closed types of treatment require immobilization for at least 8 to 12 weeks. Again, after initial immobilization and healing, the wrist should be protected from impact loading with a removable rigid splint for an additional 3 months.

Hamate Fractures

Fractures of the hook of the hamate generally occur as a result of direct trauma to the hypothenar region of the hand. These injuries are seen frequently in racquet and club sports, especially golf, baseball, tennis, and racquetball.

CLINICAL EVALUATION AND TREATMENT

The difficulty with these injuries is making the diagnosis. Often, this fracture is misdiagnosed as a sprain or tendinitis. Generally, the diagnosis should be considered in athletes who complain of persistent pain on the ulnar side of the wrist and proximal palm. These athletes will usually be affected more by activities that require making a forceful grip to hold a racquet or club. Activities of daily living are less affected.

Palpation over the end of the hamate hook in the hypothenar eminence is usually tender. Routine radiographs will not show the fracture. Obtain special radiographs consisting of a carpal tunnel view (Fig. 57–5) and a supination oblique view of the wrist.[25] This latter film shows the hamate hook in profile. If these special views do not show a fracture and a hamate hook fracture is still clinically suspected, further imaging with tomography, computed tomography (CT) scan, or technetium bone scanning is indicated.

Treatment of fractures of the hook of the hamate is best accomplished by excision of the bony process.[26] The patient can resume racquet sports when the pain and tenderness have subsided, usually 6 to 8 weeks.

Capitate Fractures

Fractures of the capitate make up only 1% of all carpal fractures. These fractures have been produced experimentally by applying to the wrist extreme flexion or extension forces combined with axial loading. The proximal pole of the capitate has weak ligamentous attachments that are often disrupted by excessive rotation when the capitate neck is fractured. This soft tissue disruption makes displaced fractures highly susceptible to avascular necrosis.[27]

CLINICAL EVALUATION AND TREATMENT

Patients typically present with swelling, point tenderness, pain, and loss of motion. A careful neurovascular assessment should be performed. Plain radiographs are usually sufficient to show the fracture. Occasionally, oblique radiographs are useful to define the fracture plane. It is important to assess the wrist for associated injuries. Nondisplaced fractures are treated by cast immobilization for 6 weeks. Displaced fractures usually require open reduction and internal fixation with Kirschner wires. Inadequate reduction of a capitate frac-

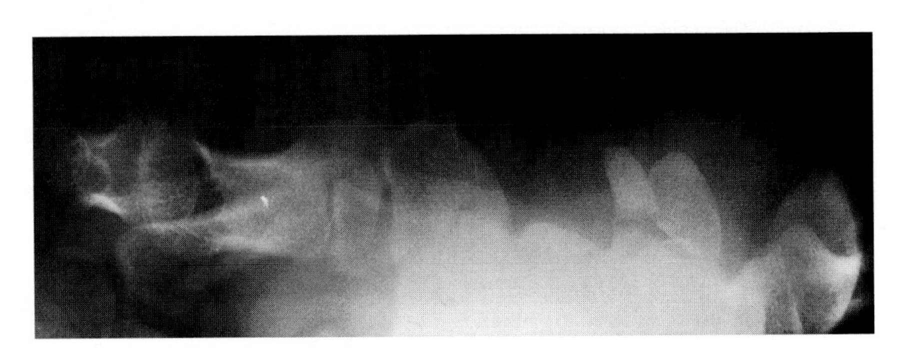

Fig. 57–5. Carpal tunnel view showing a hook of hamate fracture.

ture can result in post-traumatic midcarpal arthritis, which may require treatment with midcarpal fusion.

Lunate Fractures

Compression fractures of the lunate from repetitive trauma have been implicated as a cause of avascular necrosis of the lunate or Kienböck's disease. These fractures are difficult to detect by plain films and may require diagnosis with bone scan, CT, or magnetic resonance imaging (MRI). Acute lunate fractures should be immobilized for 8 weeks. Treatment of avascular necrosis of the lunate is controversial, but basically should include either attempts to unload the lunate in early cases or intercarpal fusion in advanced cases.

Pisiform Fractures

The pisiform is a sesamoid within the flexor carpi ulnaris tendon that forms the pisotriquetral joint by articulating with the triquetrum. Pisiform fractures usually occur as a result of direct trauma to the hypothenar eminence. Acute fractures are treated with short arm casting for 4 to 6 weeks. Pisotriquetral arthritis is best treated with pisiform excision. Generally, athletes can resume sports 8 weeks after surgery.[26]

Trapezium Fractures

Trapezial fractures occur when the trapezial body is compressed with radial deviation between the first metacarpal and the radial styloid. Nondisplaced fractures can be treated with casting for 6 weeks. Displaced fractures require closed reduction and pinning or open reduction with internal fixation.

Triquetrum Fractures

The triquetrum is the third most commonly injured carpal bone.[28] These fractures are rarely a significant problem to the injured athlete, because they are usually chip or avulsion fractures. Treatment of these injuries usually requires splinting for 4 to 6 weeks. Occasionally, these chip fractures do not unite properly, causing persistent pain. This is easily treated with excision of the fragment.

ARTHROSCOPY OF THE WRIST

Wrist arthroscopy has had an increasing role in the diagnosis and treatment of acute and chronic wrist injuries. Arthroscopy is a minimally invasive operative procedure that is generally well tolerated. The sites of entry are dorsal through the thin dorsal capsule and ligaments.

Radiocarpal and midcarpal arthroscopy permit examination of the extrinsic and intrinsic ligaments as well as any cartilaginous and bony abnormalities. Arthroscopy is particularly valuable for defining partial ligamentous injuries that may not be well visualized by other studies; it may be the most effective way to evaluate the triangular fibrocartilage complex (TFCC).

Initially, wrist arthroscopy was primarily used as a diagnostic and evaluational tool. Recently, its role as a method for treatment of wrist problems has increased significantly. Wrist arthroscopy has been used to assist in treatment of distal radius fractures, scaphoid fractures, removal of loose bodies, and repair of the TFCC.[29]

For the athletic patient, the most significant benefit of wrist arthroscopy is its minimal invasiveness, which reduces recovery time and facilitates earlier return to competition.

REFERENCES

1. Ruby, L. K., et al.: Relative motion of selected carpal bones: Kinematic analysis of the normal wrist. J. Hand Surg. *13A*:1, 1988.
2. Landsmeer, J. M. F.: Studies in the anatomy of articulation. Acta Morphol. Neerl. Scand. *3*:287, 1961.
3. Taleisnik, J.: The ligaments of the wrist. J. Hand Surg. *1*:110, 1976.
4. Navarro, A.: Anatomia y fisiologia del carpo, An Inst Clin Quir Cir Exp. 1935, Montevideo.
5. Taleisnik, J.: Wrist: Anatomy, function and injury. Instr. Course Lect. *27*:61, 1978.
6. Lichtman, D. M., Schneider, J. R., Swafford, A. R., and Mack, G. R.: Ulnar midcarpal instability—Clinical and laboratory analysis. J. Hand Surg. *6*:515, 1981.
7. Weber, E. R.: Concepts governing the rotational shift of the intercalated segment of the carpus. Orthop. Clin. North Am. *15*:193, 1984.
8. Mayfield, J. K., Johnson, R. P., and Kilcoyne, R. K.: Carpal dislocations: Pathomechanics and progressive perilunar instability. J. Hand Surg. *5*:226, 1980.
9. Cooney, W. P., Garcia-Elias, M., Dobyns, J. H., and Linsheid, R. L.: Anatomy and mechanics of carpal instability. Surg. Rounds Orthop. *3*(9):15, 1989.
10. Jones, W. A.: Beware the sprained wrist: the incidence and diagnosis of scapholunate instability, J. Bone Joint Surg. *70B*:293, 1988.
11. Frankel, V. H.: The Terry-Thomas Sign. Clin. Orthop. 129:321, 1977.
12. Linscheid, R. L., Dobyns, J. H., Beabout, J. W., and Bryan, R. S.: Traumatic instability of the wrist: Diagnosis, classification, and pathomechanics, J. Bone Joint Surg. *54A*:1612, 1972.
13. Taleisnik, J.: Scapholunate dissociation. *In* Difficult Problems in Hand Surgery. Edited by J. W. Strickland and J. B. Steichen. St. Louis, C. V. Mosby, 1982.
14. Linscheid, R. L., and Dobyns, J. H.: Athletic injuries of the wrist. Clin. Orthop. *198*:141, 1985.
15. O'Brien, E. T.: Acute fractures and dislocations of the carpus. Orthop. Clin. North Am. *15*:237, 1984.
16. Goldner, J. L.: Treatment of carpal instability without joint fusion-current assessment. (editorial) J. Hand Surg. *7*:325, 1982.
17. Blatt, G.: Capsulodesis in reconstructive hand surgery. Dorsal capsulodesis for the unstable scaphoid and volar capsulodesis following excision of the distal ulna. Hand Clin. *3*:81, 1987.
18. Watson, H. K., and Hempton, R. F.: Limited wrist arthrodesis. I. The triscaphoid joint. J. Hand Surg. *5*:320, 1980.
19. Alexander, C. E., and Lichtman, D. M.: Ulnar carpal instabilities. Orthop. Clin. North Am. *15*:307, 1984.
20. Cooney, W. P., Dobyns, J. H., and Linscheid, R. L.: Fractures of the scaphoid: a rational approach to management. Clin. Orthop. *149*:90, 1980.
21. Weber, E. R., and Chao, E. Y.: An experimental approach to the mechanism of scaphoid waist fractures. J. Hand Surg. *3*:142, 1978.

22. Mack, G. R., Bosse, M. J., Gelberman, R. H., and Yu, E.: The natural history of scaphoid non-union. J. Bone Joint Surg. *66A*:504, 1984.
23. Nielsen, P. T., Hedeboe, J., and Thommesen, P.: Bone scintigraphy in the evaluation of fracture of the carpal scaphoid bone. Acta Orthop. Scand. *54*:303, 1983.
24. Bergfeld, J. A., Weiker, G. G., Andrish, J. T., and Hall, R.: Soft playing splint for protection of significant hand and wrist injuries in sports. Am. J. Sports Med. *10*:293, 1982.
25. Zemel, N. P., and Stark, H. H.: Fractures and dislocations of the carpal bones. Clin. Sports Med. *5*:709, 1986.
26. Stark, H. H., et al.: Fracture of the hook of the hamate in athletes, J. Bone Joint Surg. *59A*:575, 1977.
27. Gelberman, R. H., Panagis, J. S., Taleisnik, J. and Baumgaertner, M.: The arterial anatomy of the human carpus. I. The extraosseus vascularity. J. Hand Surg. *8*:367, 1983.
28. Bryan, R. S., and Dobyns, J. H.: Fractures of the carpal bones other than lunate and navicular. Clin. Orthop. *149*:107, 1980.
29. Whipple, T. L.: The role of arthroscopy in the treatment of wrist injuries in the athlete. Clin. Sports Med. *11*:227, 1992.

58

Frank C. McCue III and Robert S. Franco

Hand Injuries in Athletes

The hand is susceptible to injury in nearly all popular sports activities, particularly those that involve ball handling or heavy physical contact. A wide variety of injuries can occur to the distal interphalangeal (DIP), proximal interphalangeal (PIP), and metacarpophalangeal (MCP) joints, as well as to the phalangeal shafts, that initially appear minor in nature, but subsequently result in longterm disability. In addition, although nerve compression injuries in the hand are not as common as musculoskeletal injuries, they are potentially serious and, for competitive athletes can be career threatening.

Athletic support personnel often minimize the severity and importance of these injuries because initial functional loss may not incapacitate the athlete. However, failure to recognize the significance of articular injuries can result in subsequent disabilities such as "coach's finger," a stiff, painful, deformed joint that often interferes with athletic performance.[1] This condition usually presents 2 to 3 months after injury, at which time restoration of normal function may be difficult, if not impossible. If nerve compression persists for an extended period, even at low levels, irreversible damage, with loss of axons and nerve fibrosis, will occur.

Thus, even the most insignificant-looking hand injury should be properly evaluated so that an accurate diagnosis can be made and appropriate treatment applied. Most injuries can be treated nonsurgically, with appropriate rehabilitation and adequate protection upon return to activity allowing for minimal loss of time from competition. Certain articular fractures and ligament injuries, however, are best treated surgically. In addition, different injury patterns may require different types of immobilization and varying periods of abstinence from participation. The following guidelines will help prevent potentially devastating longterm complications and disabilities frequently associated with undertreated hand injuries.

INJURY TO THE DISTAL PHALANX

A frequently seen injury is a crushed fingertip with resultant fracture of the distal phalanx. In most cases, these fractures are not displaced and there is no intra-articular involvement, but radiographs should be taken to rule out associated injuries. For a nondisplaced fracture, a compressive dressing should be applied and the finger splinted to provide protection and relieve the pain.

If a subungual hematoma is present, it should be drained (as by piercing the nail with a heated paper clip) to alleviate the pressure and pain. If the fracture is displaced, the nail and the matrix may be disrupted, especially at the base. To permit proper healing and prevent nail deformity, the nail matrix must be replaced and repaired anatomically. Nonunion is unusual in this area, but if it does occur, reconstruction may be necessary.

INJURIES TO THE DISTAL INTERPHALANGEAL JOINT

Mallet Finger

The term *mallet finger* is used to describe an avulsion of the extensor tendon, which occurs when the DIP joint is forcibly hyperflexed (Fig. 58–1). This injury, common in baseball catchers and football receivers, occurs when the tip of the finger is struck by a ball. The mechanism of injury is a longitudinal force at the tip of the finger that transfers a sudden acute flexion force across the DIP joint. Avulsion of the extensor tendon may occur with or without concomitant avulsion of a small fragment of bone from its insertion on the distal phalanx.

The athlete presents with a characteristically dropped finger and is unable to fully extend the distal phalanx

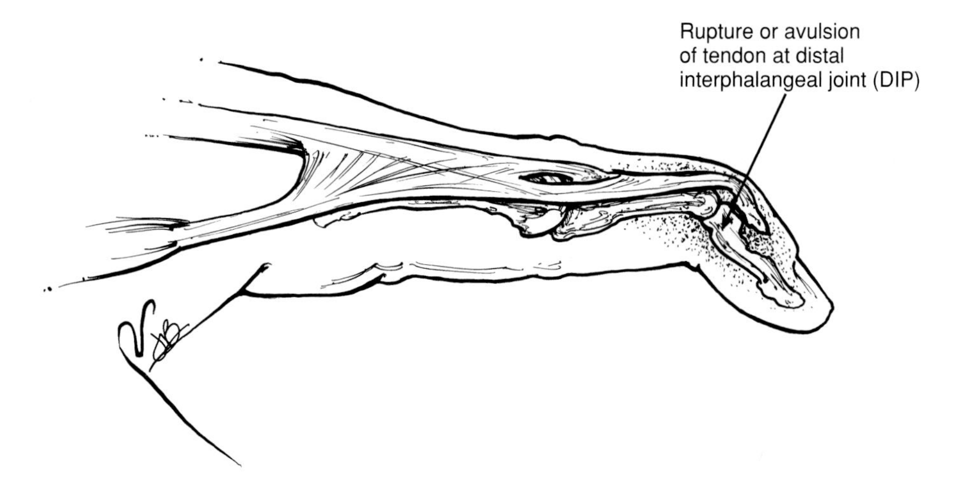

Fig. 58–1. Mallet finger describes an avulsion of the extensor tendon that occurs with the DIP joint is forcibly hyperflexed.

(though full passive extension usually is possible). There is local swelling and tenderness over the dorsal aspect of the DIP joint. During examination, the PIP joint should be carefully assessed to rule out associated injury. Radiographs should be taken to rule out a fracture. In addition, whenever an avulsion fracture is present it is important to determine if subluxation of the joint has occurred.

If there is only avulsion of the extensor tendon, the finger is treated by dorsal splinting with the DIP joint in full extension or hyperextension and the PIP joint in 60° of flexion for approximately 6 weeks. If in 6 weeks the patient does not regain the ability to actively extend the DIP joint, the splint should be maintained for another 2 or 3 weeks. It should also be emphasized to the patient that the splint should not be removed at any time during this period. Excellent results have been achieved with conservative treatment. Although incomplete extension is not always associated with disability, surgical intervention may be necessary in some cases.

If there is concomitant avulsion of a large bone fragment or if joint subluxation is present, the injury must be treated by open reduction and internal fixation. If the bone chip is small or does not involve the articular surface, the injury can often be treated as one would treat an isolated tendon avulsion.

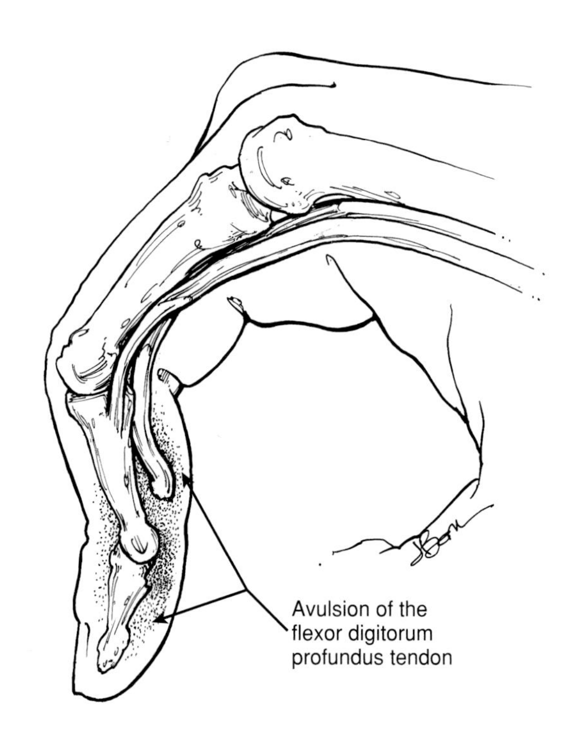

Fig. 58–2. Avulsion of the flexor digitorum profundus tendon of the DIP joint.

Avulsion of the Flexor Digitorum Profundus Tendon

Avulsion of the flexor digitorum profundus tendon occurs when a hyperextension force is applied to an actively flexed DIP joint, causing rupture of the flexor digitorum profundus tendon at its insertion (Fig. 58–2). The injury is commonly referred to as *sweater finger* and is frequently seen in football and rugby players when a finger (most often the third finger) catches on an opposing player's jersey. During examination, the entire volar aspect of the patient's hand should be palpated, as a tender mass may be felt in the palm of the proximal finger where the avulsed flexor digitorum profundus tendon is retracted. Loss of flexion of the DIP joint may not be noticed initially by the athlete or physician because of partial compensation from an intact flexor digitorum superficialis tendon. Thus, it is important to isolate the flexor digitorum profundus when testing flexor strength.

In addition, the correct diagnosis may be delayed when the loss of DIP joint flexion is attributed to pain or soft tissue swelling. The extent of soft tissue reaction and the degree of retraction of the flexor digitorum profundus tendon vary from patient to patient; however, even when pain or swelling is present, the patient should almost always be able to flex the DIP joint at least 10° if the flexor digitorum profundus tendon is intact.

If the diagnosis is made early (within 3 weeks), the tendon can be surgically repaired in most cases. After 6 weeks, however, the tendon becomes fibrotic and soft tissue contracture makes surgical repair impossible. Depending on the status of the PIP joint and the functional demands of the athlete, DIP fusion or reconstruction with a tendon graft can be attempted in these cases; however, the results are not as satisfactory as those of primary repair.

Distal Interphalangeal Joint Dislocation

Dislocation of the DIP joint is rare. When it does occur, it is almost always dorsally, and often open. The extensor and flexor tendons usually are not anatomically interrupted. Normally, reduction is easily accomplished and is done on the field by a trainer or the person who has initial contact with the patient. Applying adequate traction and getting the bones out to length usually ensures a good and stable reduction. The joint should be immobilized for about 3 weeks and then protected during sports participation for 2 to 3 weeks more.

INJURIES TO THE PROXIMAL INTERPHALANGEAL JOINT

The PIP joints of the fingers are the most commonly injured joints in the hand. The PIP joints have only one degree of freedom and must withstand substantial angular stresses produced by the long lever arm of the finger. Loss of PIP motion after injury to the joint is common and may even occur in uninjured joints that have been immobilized for other reasons. Any fixed deformity of the PIP joint, either in flexion or extension, can result in considerable disability for the athlete.

The "Jammed" Finger

A jammed finger occurs when a longitudinally directed force is applied to the extended PIP joint. Localized tenderness is the best clue to determining the injury site; however, jammed finger is a diagnosis of exclusion in which intra-articular fractures, dislocations, and disruptions of the extensor mechanism, volar plate, and collateral ligaments need to be ruled out.

Anteroposterior (AP) and lateral radiographs are necessary to rule out bone injury. Rupture of the central extensor tendon at its insertion into the base of the middle phalanx can be assessed by having the patient extend the finger against resistance. Integrity of the volar plate can be tested by hyperextending the PIP joint and comparing its extension to that of an adjacent normal PIP joint. Integrity of the collateral ligaments can be determined by stressing the extended joint in a mediolateral direction.

After the acute phase of inflammation, warm soaks and buddy taping to an adjacent normal finger are the treatment. Pain and swelling associated with this injury may persist for 3 to 6 months. Buddy taping should be employed during athletic participation as long as the joint is sore.

Articular Fractures

Fractures of the articular surface of the PIP joint can involve either the condyles of the proximal phalanx or the articular base of the middle phalanx. Condylar fractures often are not displaced when seen initially but frequently become displaced and shorten during healing, resulting in joint angulation and impingement on adjacent fingers during grip (Fig. 58–3).

All nondisplaced or minimally displaced fractures (i.e., less than 2 mm displacement) should first be treated conservatively. The PIP joint is splinted in no more than 30° of flexion. It is often advisable to also immobilize the MCP joint of the injured finger and an adjacent finger in the splint, especially if rotational and angulatory instability are possible. Radiographs should be taken weekly during the first 2 weeks to ensure that reduction is being maintained. Unless the fracture pattern is clearly stable, the athlete should refrain from participating in sports activities during this time. Three to

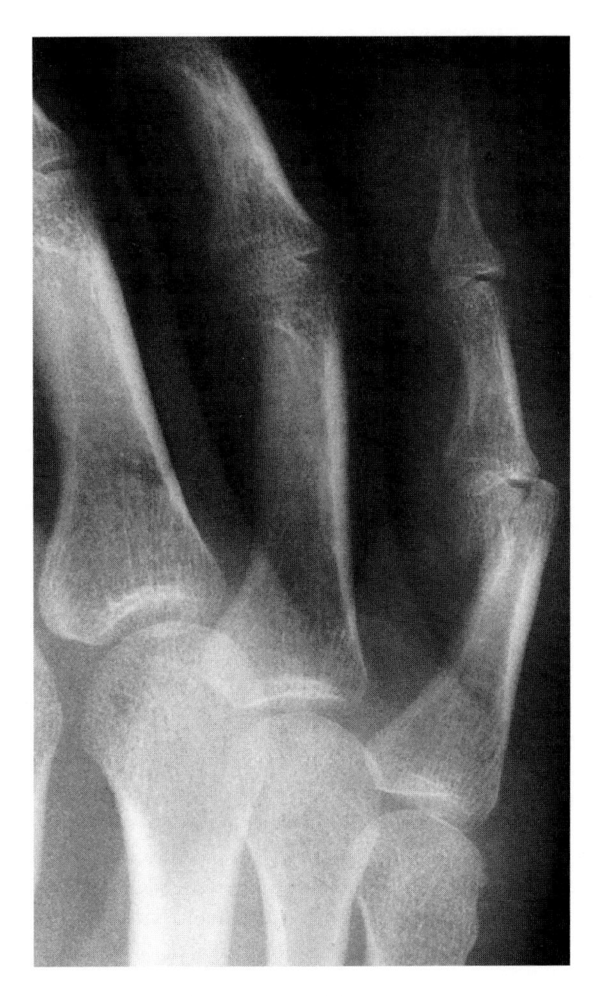

Fig. 58–3. Condylar fracture of the PIP joint.

four weeks' healing is usually necessary to minimize the risk of displacement and subsequent disability.

Fractures with considerable comminution or very small fragments are best treated by closed reduction and splinting. Joint motion exercises are initiated within 2 to 3 weeks. Surgery is indicated for displaced fractures if the fragments are large enough to be secured with Kirschner wires.

Forcible hyperextension or acute flexion against resistance usually causes avulsion fractures of the base of the middle phalanx. Dorsal fractures are splinted with the PIP joint in full extension, whereas volar fractures are splinted with the PIP joint in approximately 25° of flexion. Surgery is indicated when the fracture involves more than one third of the articular surface, displacement is greater than 3 mm, or there is subluxation of the PIP joint.

Rehabilitation is normally started well before the fracture is completely healed. Two to three weeks after the injury or surgery, the splint should be removed and the finger protectively exercised several times a day. At 4 weeks, passive mobilization is added to the rehabilitation program. If the athlete's sport permits the use of protective splints and buddy taping, early return to participation is possible.

Fracture-Dislocations

The most common fracture-dislocation pattern of the PIP joint is a dorsal dislocation with a small volar plate avulsion fracture (Fig. 58–4). The mechanism of injury is the same as that of a jammed finger: a longitudinally directed force applied to the extended PIP joint. The clinical picture is also the same as that for the jammed finger, and too often the diagnosis is delayed. Fracture of the volar lip of the middle phalanx with concomitant dorsal dislocation of the middle phalanx will be seen on a lateral radiograph. Collateral ligament avulsion fractures are also seen occasionally.

Reduction of the dislocation, frequently by the athletic trainer or coach, is relatively easy and is accomplished by applying longitudinal traction to the finger. Ideally, initial closed reduction should be performed under local or regional anesthesia, so that joint stability and ligament integrity can be assessed. If the joint is stable, further treatment depends on the fracture pattern because the ability to achieve and maintain the reduction depends on the amount of congruity of the remaining intact articular surface of the middle phalanx with the head of the proximal phalanx. If the collateral ligament is lax, immediate surgical repair of the ligament provides better results than closed treatment or delayed repair.[2–4]

With a dorsal fracture-dislocation that is stable after reduction, the PIP joint is initially splinted in approximately 60° of flexion to maintain the reduction. This may be followed by extension block splinting, whereby each week the joint is extended approximately 15° until full extension is possible, usually within 4 to 6 weeks.[5] This permits early motion without risk of subluxation or repeat dislocation. For athletic participation, buddy taping of the affected finger is continued 2 to 3 weeks more.

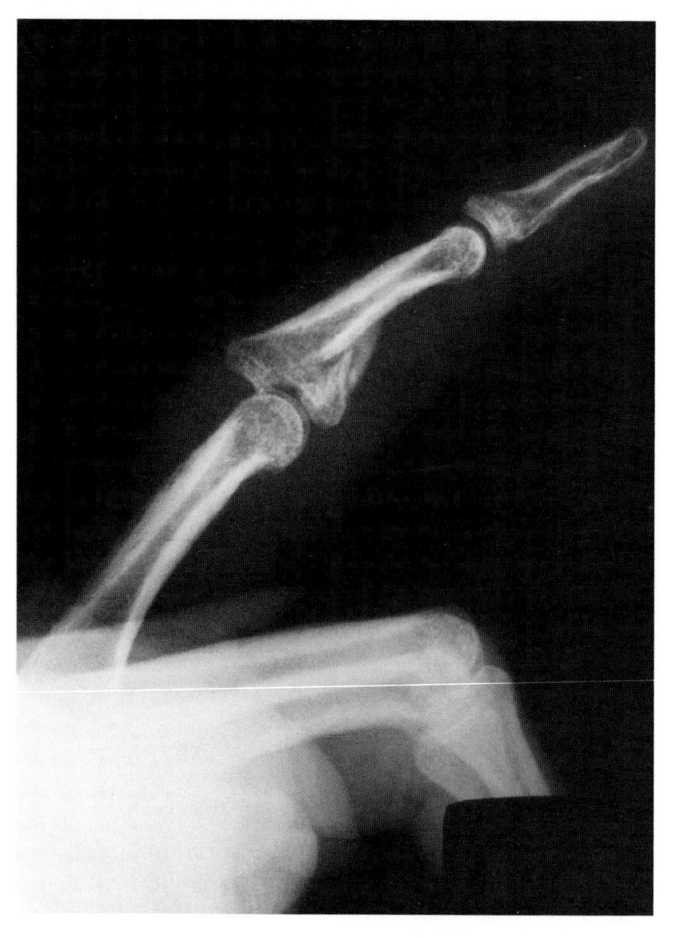

Fig. 58–4. Dorsal fracture-dislocation of the PIP joint.

Surgery is indicated if the fracture is comminuted or if the injury involves more than 35 to 40% of the articular surface, which places the joint at greater risk of dorsal subluxation. After surgery, the finger is splinted at about 25° of flexion for 2 to 3 weeks, after which gentle active exercises are started. Full extension is not permitted until 4 weeks after surgery. During the interim, extension block splinting may be used.

Proximal Interphalangeal Joint Dislocations

Dislocation of the PIP joint, which may be dorsal, lateral, or volar, is the most common ligamentous injury in the hand. Dorsal dislocations, the most common ones, are usually caused by hyperextension of the joint (Fig. 58–5). In a dorsal dislocation, the volar plate is disrupted and the accessory collateral ligaments tear, but the collateral ligaments themselves often are not affected.

It is important to obtain radiographs to rule out associated fractures. If there are no coexisting fractures, the dislocated PIP joint is reduced by accentuating the

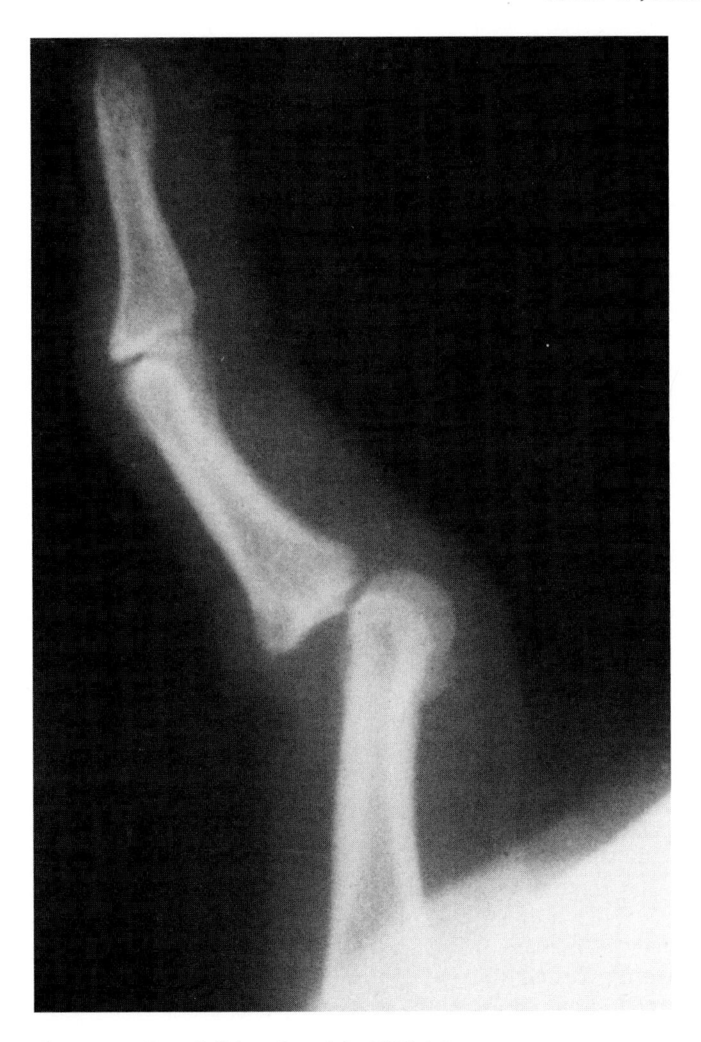

Fig. 58–5. Dorsal dislocation of the PIP joint.

deformity and then applying traction to the finger while flexing it. Postreduction radiographs are then taken, to ensure that the joint is in proper position. The collateral ligaments are then tested for stability by stressing the finger in neutral extension and in slight flexion.

For uncomplicated dorsal dislocations without collateral ligament damage, the finger is splinted with the PIP joint at 25° to 30° of flexion, which allows for early participation in most sports. The finger is kept splinted 2 to 3 weeks; then gentle range of motion exercises are in order. Buddy taping is used until full painless motion is possible. Generally, these patients are permitted to return to sports when the joint is felt to be stable.

Dorsal dislocations with collateral ligament injury and lateral dislocation of the PIP joint (where a single collateral ligament ruptures) should be treated surgically.[2–4] The rare volar disruption of the PIP joint always represents a severe soft tissue injury that, if left untreated, results in a chronic boutonnière deformity with collateral ligament laxity. Thus, surgery is also indicated for this injury. Because some flexion of the joint is invariably lost after this severe injury, aggressive therapy is recommended as soon as possible.

Injuries to the Collateral Ligament

Isolated injury to the collateral ligaments can occur in the absence of dislocation of the joint or injury to the volar plate. The typical "sprained finger" is usually a collateral ligament or volar plate injury. Partial tears, or those that show only mild laxity with a good end point, are splinted in slight flexion until the pain has abated. Buddy taping or protective splinting is then used during activity until full painless motion has been returned. The athlete should be told that tenderness and swelling of the joint may persist several months.

All complete tears of the collateral ligaments should be surgically repaired. This approach reduces lost time from competition and minimizes postinjury problems commonly associated with conservative treatment (e.g., recurrent or residual instability, pain with stress or motion due to chronic instability, and locking of the joint).[2] After surgery, the finger is splinted in slight flexion for 3 weeks, after which motion exercises are initiated.

Boutonnière Deformity

The mechanism of injury of a boutonnière deformity is either a severe flexion force to the PIP joint or a direct blow to the dorsal aspect of the PIP joint. The deformity presents as fixed flexion of the PIP joint with fixed hyperextension of the DIP joint (Fig. 58–6). It most often develops after failure to diagnose and correctly treat an avulsion or fracture of the central slip on the middle phalanx. The diagnosis is confirmed by the patient's inability to extend the PIP joint. It is important to obtain radiographs to rule out a fracture.

The injured finger must be splinted with the PIP joint in full extension to allow for proper healing. If the

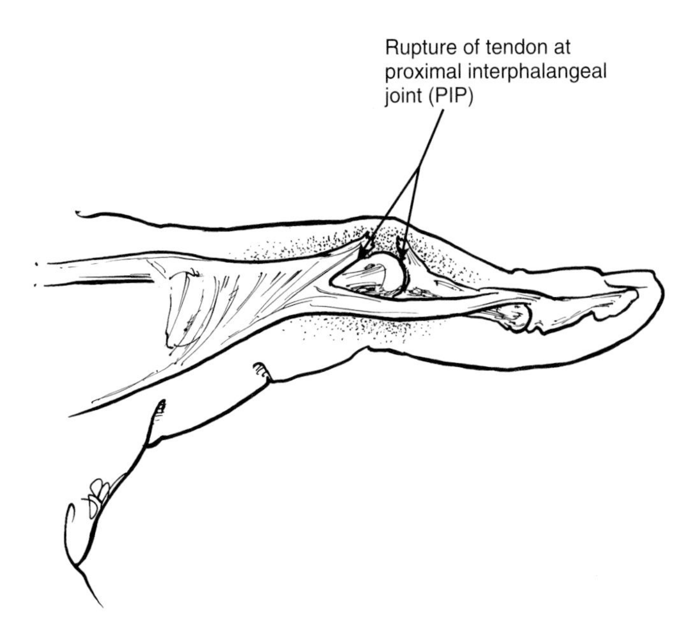

Fig. 58–6. Classic boutonnière deformity: fixed flexion of the PIP joint with fixed hyperextension of the DIP joint.

injured joint is splinted in slight flexion, the deformity is most likely to occur. Signs of impending fixed deformity often are manifested about 3 weeks after injury. If the joints are still flexible, conservative therapy may be instituted to prevent the deformity from progressing. Three months or more of splinting may be necessary to obtain correction. After this, additional night splinting and splinting during competition for another 2 months is recommended. For chronic boutonnière deformity, several surgical options are available.[6]

Pseudoboutonnière Deformity

This slowly progressive condition follows hyperextension injury to the PIP joint and occurs in response to rupture of the volar plate. Unlike boutonnière deformity, the central slip is not injured. The deformity presents as flexion contracture of the PIP joint with slight hyperextension of the DIP joint that is not fixed, which permits active flexion.[7] The ulnar digits are more often involved. Calcification at the proximal attachment of the PIP volar plate can be seen on radiographs. The deformity seems to occur only in adults.

It is important to differentiate this condition from true boutonnière deformity because the causes differ and the DIP joint contracture is less significant. Mild deformities (i.e., flexion contracture less than 40° at the PIP joint) can be treated nonsurgically with a dynamic extension or "safety pin" splint to passively improve extension at the PIP joint. Surgery is usually reserved for cases in which flexion contracture is greater than 40°. The finger is maintained in extension for 3 weeks following surgery.

Injuries to the Volar Plate

Hyperextension injuries to the PIP joint may cause disruption of the volar plate without resulting in frank dorsal dislocation of the joint. Clinically, a patient with a volar plate injury has a swollen PIP joint and tenderness over the palmar aspect of the joint. Normally, the finger is slightly flexed. Because of pain, swelling, and guarding, it may be difficult to demonstrate acute hyperextension.

The joint should be immobilized in slight flexion for 2 to 3 weeks. After that, active exercises are started, with interim protective splinting. If full extension is slow to return, passive stretching may be initiated at four weeks.

Left untreated, distal disruptions result in hyperextension laxity of the PIP joint with subsequent formation of swan-neck deformity; proximal disruptions result in early flexion deformity, which may develop into a pseudoboutonnière deformity. Swan-neck deformity normally requires surgical correction.

Another injury that causes swelling and tenderness on the volar aspect of the finger and is similar to a volar plate injury is acute rupture of the A2 pulley, usually in the third finger of the dominant hand.[8] This injury is extremely common in rock climbers; the pulley is apparently ruptured during a "crimping" maneuver while trying to obtain a handhold on a very narrow ridge. Conservative treatment is usually adequate.

INJURIES TO THE METACARPOPHALANGEAL JOINTS

An injured MCP joint should always be splinted in at least 45° of flexion, and preferably in about 70°. As flexion increases, the collateral ligaments tighten, bony contact of the joint surfaces increases, and the MCP joint becomes more stable. If the joint is immobilized in extension, the supporting structures contract during healing and seriously limit flexion when movement is initiated. It is much easier to correct an extension deficit than to restore lost flexion.

Dislocations

Forced hyperextension of the fingers can cause dorsal dislocation of the MCP joint, the border digits being affected most often (Fig. 58–7). Normally, the volar plate ruptures proximally and remains attached to the proximal phalanx.

With an incomplete, or "simple," dislocation, the volar plate does not become interposed in the joint, and the MCP joint is usually fixed in hyperextension. It is very important not to apply longitudinal traction to a simple dislocation lest it be converted to a complex, irreducible dislocation, with the volar plate becoming interposed in the joint.[9] Instead, the dislocation should be reduced by holding the joint surfaces in contact while accentuating the deformity, flexing the wrist to reduce tension on the flexor tendons, and gently manipulating the joint into place.

Complex dislocations of the MCP joint can be recognized by a characteristic dimple in the palm, the fact that the joint is not fixed in a grossly hyperextended position, and the presence of ulnar deviation in the injured finger. Closed reduction usually is not successful, and open reduction most often is necessary.

Injuries to the Collateral Ligament

Lateral deviation of the MCP joint while in flexion with the collateral ligaments under tension can cause injury to the radial collateral ligaments of the joint. This injury can usually be treated conservatively with buddy taping until symptoms resolve. Surgery is rarely necessary. Radiographs should be taken to make sure that an avulsion fracture from the metacarpal head is not entrapped in the MCP joint. In chronic cases, the ligament ends may become interposed in the joint, resulting in irritation and chronic pain. Surgical intervention may be required to correct the problem.

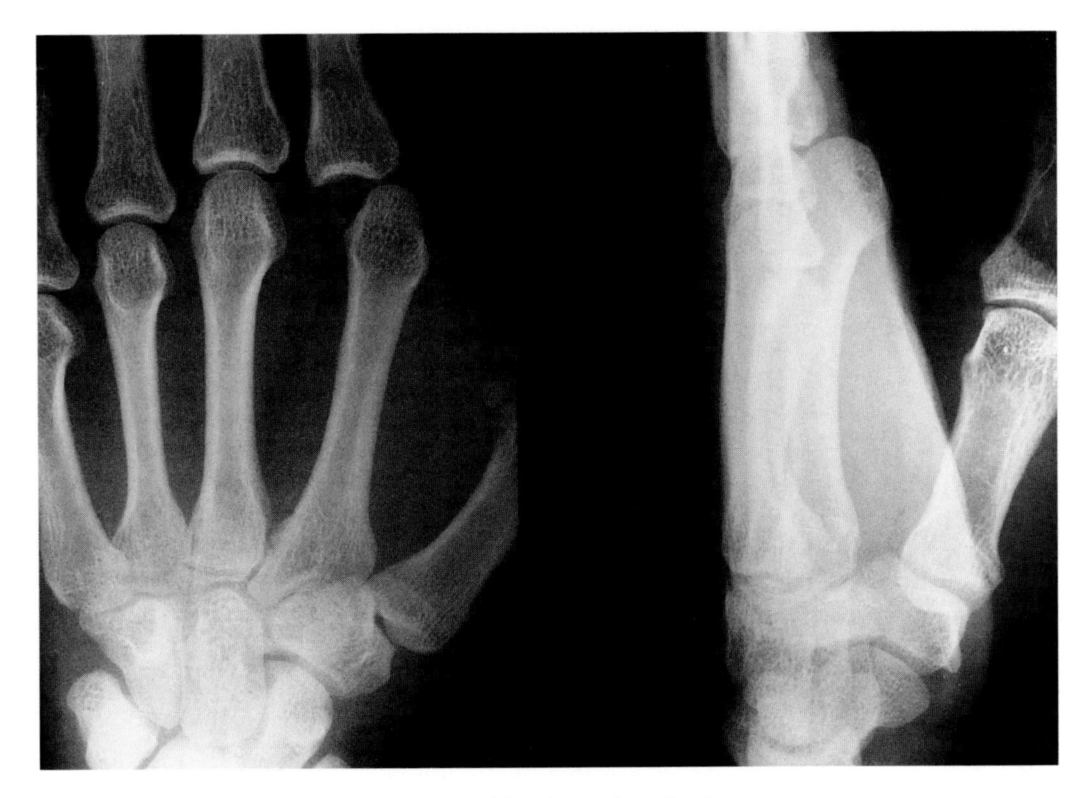

Fig. 58–7. Dislocation of the MCP joint.

Rupture of the Extensor Hood

Rupture of the extensor hood permits the extensor tendon to subluxate into the sulcus between adjacent metacarpal heads, resulting in extensor lag at the MCP joint with loss of strength. When this injury is sports related, the radial fibers of the MCP joint of the long finger are most often involved. The injury can be treated nonsurgically, but the required prolonged splinting of the joint in extension increases the risk of loss of flexion. Thus, acute ruptures are best managed surgically.

Fractures Involving the Metacarpophalangeal Joint

Fractures involving the MCP joints are treated like those of the PIP joints. Whether management is closed or open reduction, the primary goal is maintenance of normal motion and function.

INJURIES TO THE THUMB

Injuries to the Interphalangeal Joint

Soft tissue injuries and fractures to the IP joint of the thumb (which is analogous to the PIP joints of the fingers) are treated like those of the fingers. If there is hyperextension laxity and a suspected volar plate injury, rupture of the flexor- or extensor pollicis longus tendon needs to be ruled out because both would require surgical repair. Patients generally tolerate mild stiffness of the IP joint well.

Dislocations of the Metacarpophalangeal Joint

Dorsal dislocation of the MCP joint of the thumb is similar to that of the MCP joints of the fingers. The volar plate may tear proximally, as in the fingers, or distally, through the sesamoids or the insertion on the proximal phalanx. Although closed reduction by gentle manipulation is possible more often than with similar dislocations of finger MCP joints, open reduction is frequently required to ensure stability.

Injuries to the Ulnar Collateral Ligament of the Metacarpophalangeal Joint

The ulnar collateral ligament can be torn when abduction stress is applied to the thumb while the MCP joint is near full extension (Fig. 58–8).[10] It is important to look for associated injuries such as injuries to the dorsal capsule or the ulnar aspect of the volar plate, a rent in the adductor aponeurosis, or avulsion fracture of the collateral insertion on the volar base of the proximal phalanx.

This injury is frequently seen in football players and in skiers who fall and catch the web of the thumb in the strap of the ski pole. Skeletally mature athletes can dis-

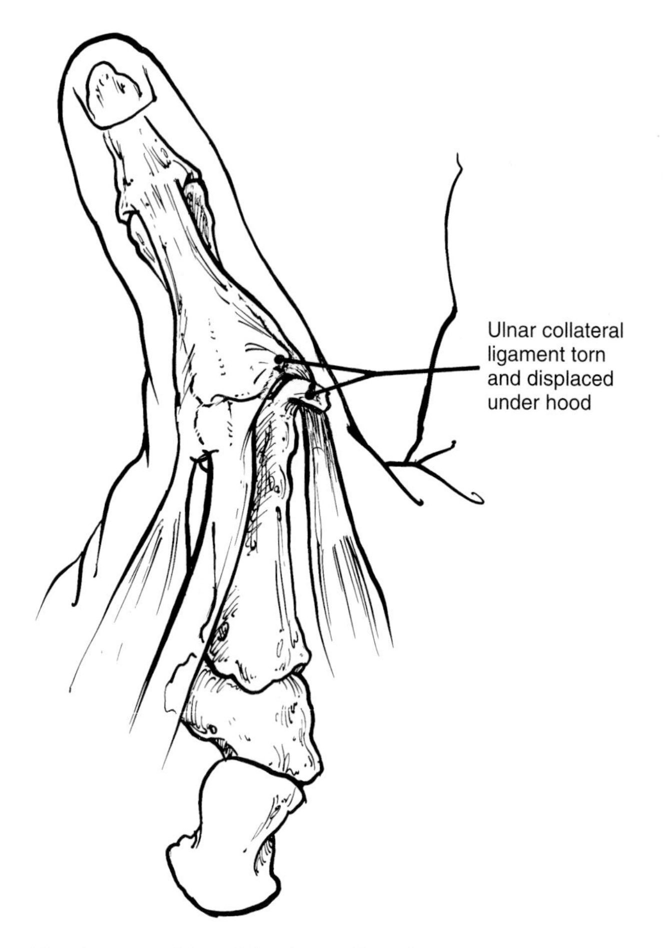

Fig. 58–8. Avulsion of the ulnar collateral ligament.

rupt the ulnar collateral ligament (gamekeeper's thumb), whereas skeletally immature athletes often fracture the proximal phalanx. Various types of epiphyseal fractures can occur; a Salter III or IV injury suggests a concomitant tear of the ulnar collateral ligament.

Because a bone fragment can be displaced as a result of stress, it is important to obtain radiographs before stressing the joint during examination. Plain radiographs may reveal a collateral ligament avulsion off the ulnar aspect of the proximal phalanx. If the radiographs are "negative," the integrity of the ulnar collateral ligament should be assessed. Because there is significant variation from person to person in MCP range of motion and stability, it is important to compare the injured thumb with the uninjured one.

The integrity of the ulnar collateral ligament is tested by stressing the MCP joint in full extension and in 30° flexion (in the latter position the stabilizing effect of the volar plate is overcome); (Fig. 58–9). If radial deviation is greater than 25° to 30°, at least a partial tear of the ligament most likely is present. Lack of a firm end point, particularly in full extension, indicates a complete ligament tear. The thumb displays hyperextension laxity if the volar plate and accessory collateral ligaments have also been injured. Stress radiographs can be helpful in documenting instability in abduction (again, comparison should be made with the uninjured thumb).

Patients often suffer chronic laxity of the MCP joint after an injury to the ulnar collateral ligament when interposition of the adductor aponeurosis between the distal avulsed ligament and its insertion into the base of the proximal phalanx hinders proper healing (Stener's lesion). Because adductor aponeurosis interposition normally cannot occur in partial ruptures, it is associated with complete rupture of the ulnar collateral ligament. The resultant loss of stability can be very disabling, particularly when the dominant hand is affected.

Complete ligament tears require surgical repair. In most cases, acute rupture of the ulnar collateral ligament should be treated surgically, to prevent chronic laxity. Hyperextension laxity and marked laxity in full extension are general indications for surgical intervention since these signs indicate coexisting injury to the volar plate. Partial tears of the ligament, however, do not require surgery and can be treated by immobilization in a thumb spica cast. If in a younger athlete with an epiphyseal fracture the bone fragment is undisplaced or minimally displaced, the lesion may be managed effectively by immobilization.

Rehabilitation is the same, regardless of the treatment. The thumb is immobilized in 20° of flexion in a spica cast for 3 weeks. The IP joint is left free, to permit active motion and prevent scarring of the extensor mechanism. Three to four weeks later, a removable splint is employed and active exercises are performed several times a day. After 5 to 6 weeks, the splint may be removed and the patient is allowed to perform routine activities. For sports activities, the thumb should be protected for about 3 months, either by buddy taping it in adduction to the index finger or by using a silicone cast during sports participation.

Injuries to the Radial Collateral Ligament of the Metacarpophalangeal Joint

The radial collateral ligament is less likely than the ulnar collateral ligament to be injured; however, when injuries do occur, they are generally treated in the same manner. Indications for conservative and surgical treatment are the same. Injuries to the radial collateral ligament tend toward volar subluxation of the proximal phalanx, and treatment is directed at preventing further volar subluxation or laxity of the radial side of the joint.

Injuries to the Carpometacarpal Joint of the Thumb

BENNETT'S FRACTURE

Forcible abduction on the thumb can result in an oblique intra-articular fracture involving the base of the carpometacarpal (CMC) joint of the thumb and transecting the proximal articular surface. Resulting instability causes subluxation of the shaft and the remaining articular surface.

If the fracture-dislocation is not properly reduced, the patient's normal range of abduction and CMC joint

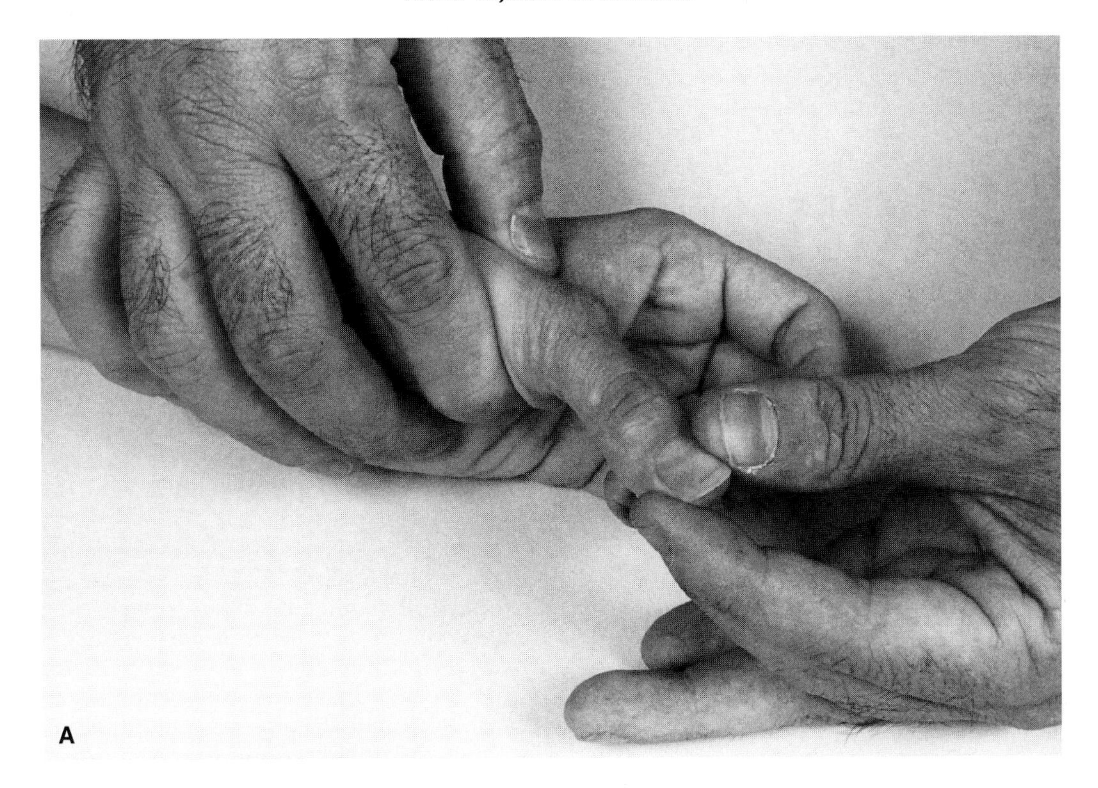

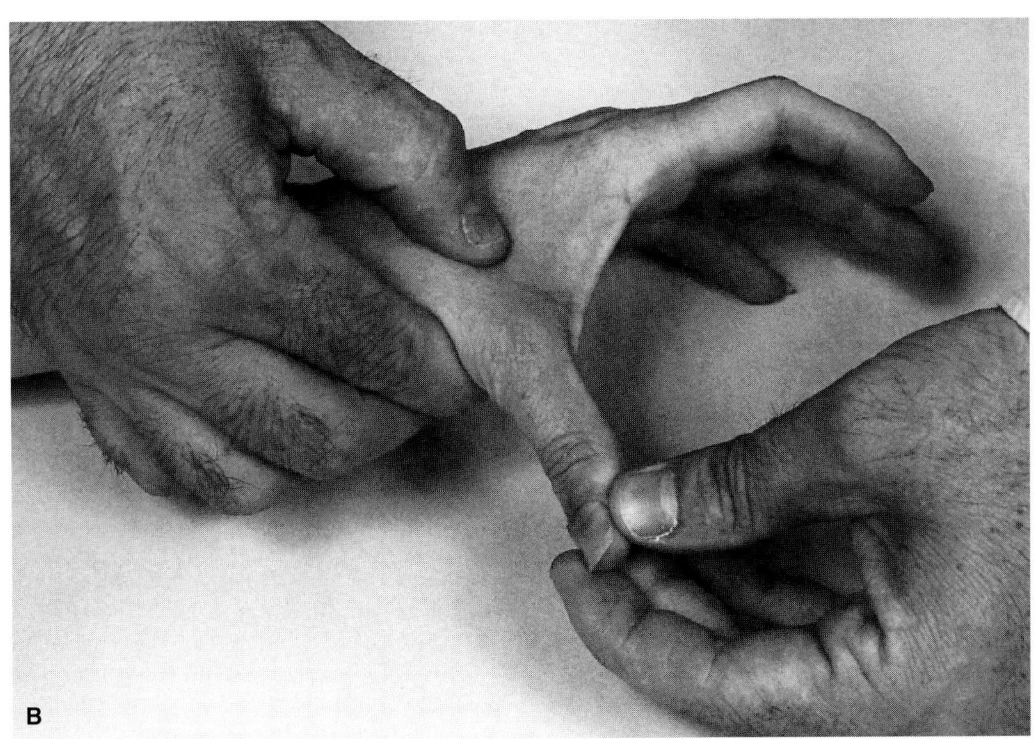

Fig. 58–9. Stress testing of the ulnar collateral ligament with the thumb in slight flexion *(A)* and in full extension *(B)*.

motion will be compromised. In cases of nondisplaced or minimally displaced fractures, closed reduction may be effective. If displacement prevails, closed reduction and external fixation of the CMC joint may maintain reduction. If this is not adequate, open reduction and internal fixation is indicated.

FRACTURE-DISLOCATION OF THE CARPOMETACARPAL JOINT

Fracture-dislocation of the CMC joint is rare but may occur when severe force is exerted against a hyperextended hand. If possible, this type of injury should be treated by closed reduction; however, if there is associated interposition of soft tissue and tendons, open reduction and internal fixation will be necessary.

DISLOCATION OF THE CARPOMETACARPAL JOINT

Complete dislocation of the CMC joint of the thumb without concomitant fracture is relatively rare. The injury is most often caused by a fall on the outstretched hand in which hyperabduction or hyperextension forces are directed across the volar aspect of the metacarpal bone. Axial forces, which usually cause the more common Bennett's fracture-dislocation of this joint, may be a factor, as may cyclical forces, especially with chronic instability. When treating this dislocation, it is important that ligament stability be maintained to prevent disabling chronic instability and subsequent degenerative joint changes.

Acute dislocations are easily reduced in most cases. The joint is then immobilized in either a long- or short-arm thumb spica cast for 3 weeks, followed by 3 more weeks in a short-arm thumb spica cast. If joint stability is questionable, the joint may be stabilized with a Kirschner wire placed under fluoroscopic guidance. Six weeks after immobilization, an active exercise program is started. In cases of chronic instability or subluxation, open reduction and repair of the volar ligament is indicated.

FRACTURES TO THE SHAFTS OF THE FINGERS

Phalangeal Fractures

An undisplaced fracture of a phalangeal shaft should be splinted with the MCP joint of the finger in 70° of flexion and the IP joints in slight flexion. If the fracture is displaced, it should first be manipulated into position and then immobilized like an undisplaced fracture.

Metacarpal Fractures

Metacarpal fractures result from direct trauma, as when the athlete's hand is struck against an object or another person (usually affecting the neck of the fourth and fifth metacarpals) or in crushing injuries. Various types of fracture patterns can occur, including intra-articular fracture of the metacarpal head, impacted fracture of the metacarpal neck (boxer's fracture), transverse or short oblique fracture of the shaft, spiral fracture of the shaft, and proximal fracture-dislocation of the fifth metacarpal.

Because local swelling at the fracture site can minimize the degree of anterior angulation of the metacarpal head, the actual degree of angulation can be determined only by radiography. Rotational deformity of a metacarpal fracture is assessed clinically by individually flexing each finger into the palm. Normally, they point to the scaphoid. Any deviation from this indicates rotational deformity of the finger or its metacarpal shaft.

An acute metacarpal neck fracture is treated by closed reduction, making sure that any rotational deformity is corrected. The finger is then splinted with the MCP and IP joints in 45° of flexion and with the tip of the finger pointing toward the scaphoid. Oblique or spiral fractures can usually be managed simply by anterior splinting for 2 to 3 weeks. With anterior angulated fractures of the second and third metacarpals that do not have CMC joint mobility, it is important to protect against anterior angulation, lest the patient's grasping ability subsequently be compromised. Multiple fractures of metacarpal shafts may require open reduction and internal fixation.

NEUROCOMPRESSIVE INJURIES TO THE HAND

Most nerve injuries in athletes are neurapraxias—conduction blocks along a nerve where all nerve elements, axons, and connective tissue remain in continuity.[11] This is the mildest form of nerve injury, and the prognosis for full recovery is good if the compression is not sustained. An axonotmesis is a more acute injury that consists of axonal injury and distal axon degeneration without disruption of the supporting connective tissue sleeve. Prognosis is good, but the injury often requires prolonged rehabilitation. Complete nerve disruption, neurotmesis, is rare in athletes and is usually caused by high-energy fractures, dislocations, or lacerations.

The most common mechanism of compressive neuropathies in athletes is persistent, repetitive, controlled stress. Because onset is usually insidious, the correct diagnosis may be delayed, which can lead to irreversible sequelae. Compressive nerve injuries may be either acute or chronic.

Acute injuries, which may be mechanical or secondary to ischemic insult, are common in athletes and occur when any powerful force compresses a nerve against an unyielding structure. The injury is normally isolated and transitory and is often seen in young or untrained athletes, when, during a single outing, the stress at one anatomic site exceeds the threshold for injury. Most compressive neuropathies of athletes are chronic and occur at predictable anatomic sites. Nerve compression may affect either the median nerve in the carpal tunnel or the ulnar nerve in Guyon's canal.

Compression of the median nerve can cause paresthesia in the thumb, index, or long finger, and subsequent atrophy of the thenar muscle. Symptoms can often be elicited by tapping over the median nerve (Tinel's sign) at the wrist or by prolonged flexion of the wrist (Phalen's sign). Gymnasts often develop symptoms of carpal tunnel syndrome secondary to overuse flexor tenosynovitis. In archery, a grip-intensive activity, the median nerve may be compressed at the carpal tunnel or more proximally by the flexor digitorum superficialis of the third and the long fingers. Conservative treatment (rest and nonsteroidal anti-inflammatory drugs) provides relief in most cases. Surgical intervention is reserved for cases that do not respond to these measures.

Compression of the ulnar nerve can be secondary to fractures of the pisiform or the hamate or scarring in Guyon's canal following blunt trauma to the heel of the palm. Treatment consists of correcting the underlying cause. Ulnar neuropathy is commonly seen in cyclists because of their grip on the handlebars and constant pressure on the ulnar nerve. Padded gloves and handlebars and changing hand position alleviate this condition. Perineural fibrosis of the ulnar digital nerve of the thumb (bowler's thumb) is caused by repetitive direct, external force. Most of the time, there is a painful mass at the base of the thumb and possible distal sensory changes. Changing the depth and location of finger holes may prevent recurrence.

REFERENCES

1. McCue, F. C., et al.: The coach's finger. J. Sports Med. *2*:270, 1974.
2. McCue, F. C., et al.: Athletic injuries of the proximal interphalangeal joint requiring surgical treatment. J. Bone Joint Surg. *52A*:937, 1970.
3. Redler, I., and Williams, J. T.: Rupture of a collateral ligament of the proximal interphalangeal joint of the finger. Analysis of 18 cases. J. Bone Joint Surg. *49A*:322, 1967.
4. Rodriguez, A. L.: Injuries to the collateral ligaments of the proximal interphalangeal joints. Hand *5*:66, 1990.
5. McElfresh, E. C., Dobyns, J. H., and O'Brien, E. T.: Management of fracture dislocation of the proximal interphalangeal joints by extension block splinting. J. Bone Joint Surg. *54A*:1705, 1972.
6. Spinner, M., and Choi, B. Y.: Anterior dislocation of the proximal interphalangeal joint. J. Bone Joint Surg. *52A*:1329, 1970.
7. McCue, F. C., et al.: A pseudoboutonniere deformity. J. Br. Soc. Surg. Hand *7*:166, 1975.
8. Bollen, S. R.: Injury to the A2 pulley in rock climbers. J. Hand Surg. *15B*:268, 1990.
9. Kahler, D. M., and McCue, F. C. III: Metacarpophalangeal and proximal interphalangeal joint injuries of the hand, including the thumb. Clin. Sports Med. *11*:57, 1992.
10. McCue, F. C., et al.: Ulnar collateral ligament injuries of the thumb in athletes. J. Sports Med. *2*:70, 1974.
11. Terzis, J. K., and Smith, K. L.: The Peripheral Nerve: Structure, Function, and Reconstruction. New York, Raven Press, 1990.

59

Paula R. Tisdale

Rehabilitation of the Elbow, Wrist, and Hand

For some athletes, success depends on the status of the elbow, wrist, and hand. For this reason, it is important to be knowledgeable about the various injuries that can occur to the elbow, wrist, and hand, as well as the most effective treatment to assist the healing process. As with any injury, the faster the recovery the better. Oftentimes, an injury is overlooked because the athlete is not completely disabled. However, the longterm effect on the athlete should not be taken for granted and the injury should be treated as if the competition depends on the elbow, wrist, or hand. For many of these injuries, the treatment needed may be just a splint or taping for protection while healing occurs.

THE ELBOW

Lateral Epicondylitis

Goals of rehabilitation for lateral epicondylitis are to reduce pain and tenderness and restore strength, endurance, and flexibility of the wrist extensors at the elbow.[1]

On initial evaluation of the patient with lateral epicondylitis, the elbow is assessed by how recently the injury occurred. Active range of motion, grip strength, manual muscle test, and points of tenderness are recorded. The athlete is issued a counterforce brace and instructed on its use. This brace is used to create pressure over the muscle bellies and dissipate the impact load through the muscles, taking stress off the inflamed tendons.[2] The brace is worn about 1 inch distal to the elbow, and the patient should be able to fully flex the joint. The brace is to be worn at all times except while sleeping and bathing.

In the more acute stages, the athlete may be instructed to wear the brace, complete exercises without weights, and try to rest the elbow. Once acute symptoms subside, stretching and strengthening exercises are begun. Instructions should be given to the athlete to always use smooth controlled movements during exercises and not to move too quickly.

The athlete is instructed on the "Super 7" exercises, which consist of grip strength, stretching extensors, wrist curls, reverse wrist curls, neutral wrist curls, pronation, and supination.

Grip strengthening can be done by having the patient squeeze Theraputty or a racquetball. The athlete should work on grip-strengthening exercises for 3 to 5 minutes three times a day, gradually increasing the exercise time. Stretching the extensors is done with the arm held out in front, palm facing the ground, and the elbow extended. The patient pulls the hand of the affected side with the unaffected hand so that the wrist flexes (Fig. 59–1). The patient holds this position for five counts; the complete exercise is repeated three times a day at 10 repetitions for each set.

For wrist curls and rotation exercises, the patient's forearm should be supported with the wrist free to allow full range of motion (Fig. 59–2). A hammer may be used for neutral wrist curl, pronation, and supination exercises (Fig. 59–3). The position of the hand on the shaft of the hammer will determine the amount of weight that is being used. The athlete is instructed to begin with a one- to two-pound weight, holding the position for five counts at 10 repetitions three times a day to build muscular endurance. When the athlete has reached 30 repetitions and is doing well, the weight is increased by 1 pound, and the repetitions decrease to 10. The progression is begun again.

Deep friction massage can be beneficial to patients with lateral epicondylitis. This is often a natural response to the pain; the athlete will rub the painful

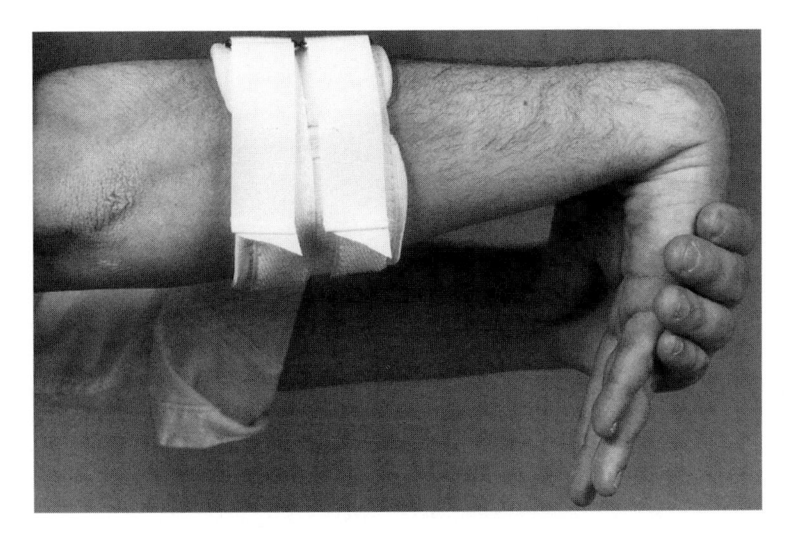

Fig. 59–1. Stretching the extensors is done with the arm held out in front, palm facing the ground, and the elbow extended. The patient uses the unaffected hand to pull the hand of the affected side so that the wrist flexes.

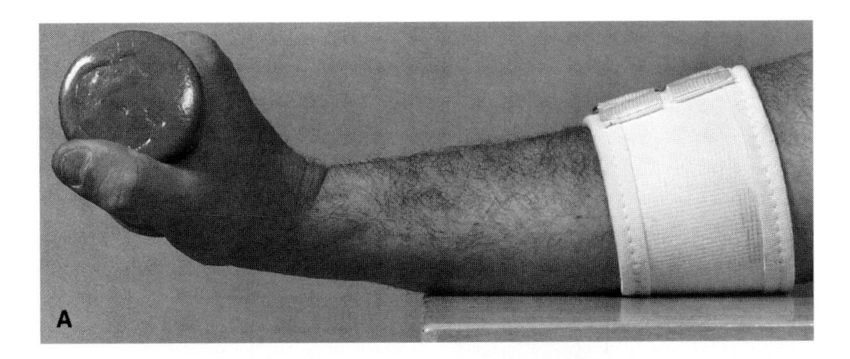

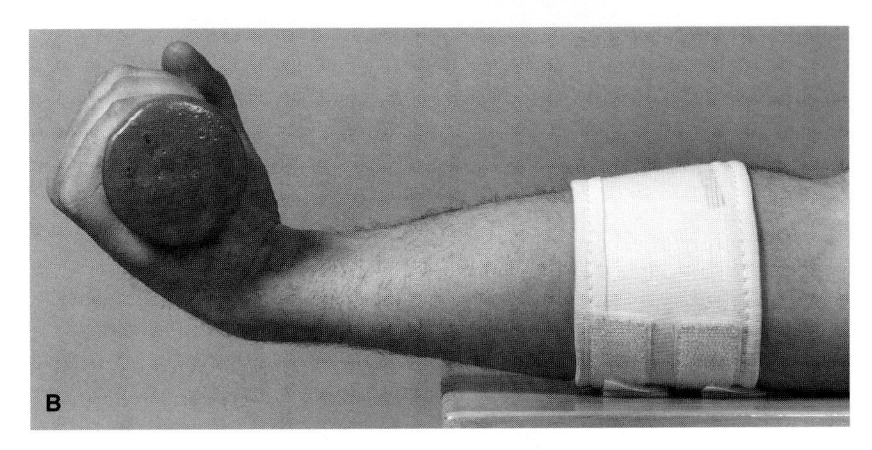

Fig. 59–2. Wrist curls are done with the forearm supported leaving the wrist free to have full motion. *(A)* Flexors; *(B)* Extensors.

area to help relieve symptoms. This can be done three times a day for 3 to 5 minutes.

Therapeutic modalities are often used in the treatment of lateral epicondylitis, e.g., moist heat, ice, iontophoresis, or phonophoresis. Moist heat should be used before exercise for relaxation, and ice can be used to relieve the intensity of the pain after exercise. Iontophoresis can be used for one single visit, or the procedure may be used for four to six treatments in conjunction with exercises and bracing. Iontophoresis is used with the drug dexamethasone, and the current is based on the patient's tolerance to the sensation when activated (a base setting is 2.0 mA). Depending on the dose, the treatment may take 15 to 20 minutes. The skin area where the medicated and ground pads are placed must be wiped clean with alcohol. The medicated pad,

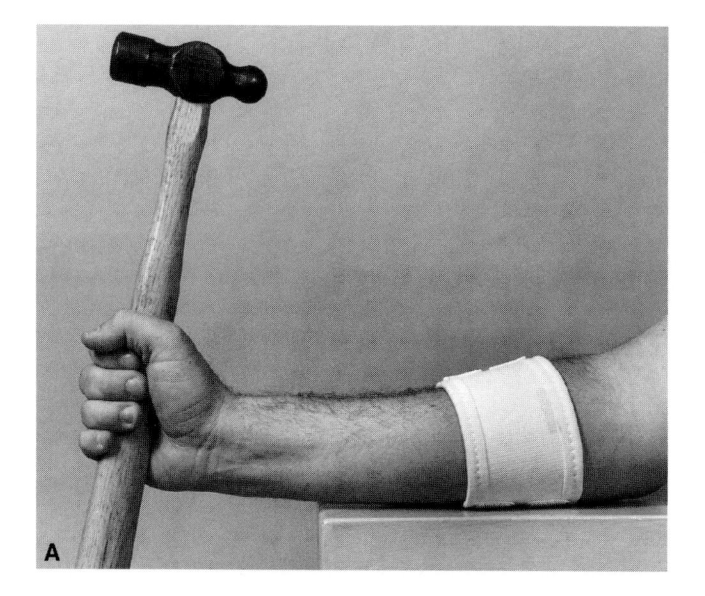

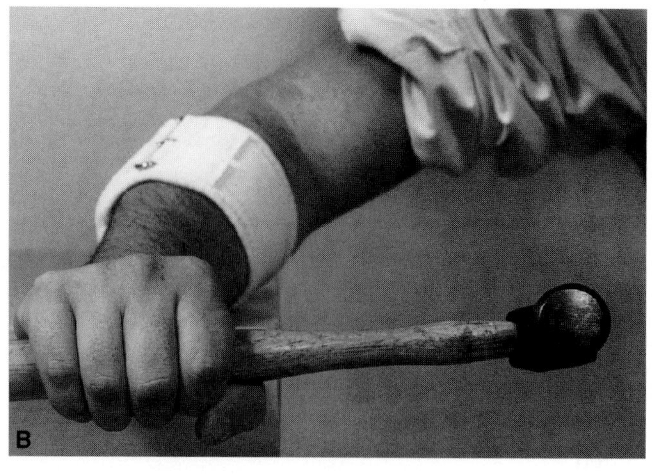

Fig. 59–3. *(A)* Neutral wrist curls, *(B)* pronation, and *(C)* supination.

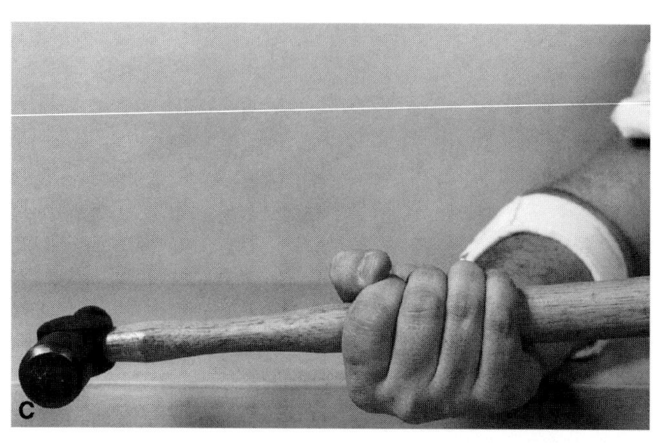

depending on the machine used, is usually saturated with 1 ml of dexamethasone. The patient should feel a mild tingling sensation once the treatment has begun. If the sensation becomes too intense, there is a chance of burning the skin: The current should be reduced.

Through the use of the counterforce brace, stretching and strengthening exercises, modalities, and anti-inflammatory medications, the athlete may expect to return to play within 2 to 3 weeks. During this time, the therapist should intermittently check the patient's progress and make sure weights are being used properly.[1]

It is best for the athlete to continue stretching before and after competition; icing can also be continued after activity and stretching. If the elbow is directly involved with the activity, it may be necessary to gradually increase playing time so that the movements can be pain-free.

Sometimes, if the conservative method is not successful, surgery is needed to treat the problem. After surgery, the patient may be placed in a long arm splint at 90° of flexion for 1 week and may then begin gentle stretch exercises and active wrist range of motion.[3] The patient may begin active range of motion exercises to the elbow after 2 to 3 weeks. At 3 weeks after surgery, stretching and strengthening exercises may begin.[4] Exercises are continued until full strength returns, usually 4 to 5 months. Return to competition may be possible with a modified sport technique 6 weeks after surgery.[4]

Dislocations

After the dislocated elbow has been reduced, the arm is placed in a posterior long arm splint at 90° of flexion for 2 to 3 days. The athlete is instructed to begin active range of motion exercises in a pain-free range in an anti-gravity position for 2 weeks.[5] Methods to reduce edema include icing, elevation, compressive wrap (tubigrip), and electrogalvanic stimulation at the elbow. The splint may be discontinued in a week or two if the elbow is stable. If not, the elbow may be splinted for 4 weeks and the splint adjusted for more extension as the athlete tolerates and stability permits.[5]

Depending on the stability, the elbow may be placed in a hinged splint that allows free motion in a protected range. The hinge can be used laterally or medially or on both sides, depending on the condition of the elbow. The splint allows the athlete to return to light activities of daily living. It is worn for 4 weeks and then taken off to allow full motion, but the splint is still used to give support during activities.[1]

Isometric exercises may be started while the splint is being worn. Strengthening exercises may begin after full, active range of motion is achieved. Strengthening exercises include wrist curls, supination and pronation, biceps and triceps curls, and grip strength. If there are any signs of heterotopic calcifications during the rehabilitation, all strengthening exercises should be stopped and only active range of motion continued.

Loss of extension is common after an elbow dislocation. Some athletes may have a seemingly straight arm on clinic examination, but they have lost their normal hyperextension. In this case, the focus should be on the triceps for strengthening to resist elbow flexion during forced extension activities, e.g., the gymnast who needs to "lock out" the elbows during a drill.[5]

Scotchwrap (3M) can be used for splinting the elbow for return to play after an elbow dislocation. The splinting material, along with strapping material to be attached to the splint, can be used to prevent hyperextension of the elbow but otherwise allow full motion. For full return to play, the athlete should have full, pain-free, and stable range of motion.

Radial Head Fractures

If an athlete has a nondisplaced radial head fracture, it is necessary to begin early mobilization 1 week after injury. The athlete is instructed to resume activities of daily living as tolerated.

Moist heat applied to the elbow before exercise helps relax the tissues and promote better active range of motion. Exercises can be completed in an anti-gravity position actively or through the use of a constant passive motion machine (CPM). The CPM machine can be sent home with the athlete on a rental basis.

At times, the elbow may be placed in a hinged elbow splint to give added support as the athlete completes the exercises and activities of daily living.

Sprains

The protocol for treating elbow sprains is to use ice and to attain normal range of motion. When normal range of motion returns, progressive resistance exercises begin, but return to play is gradual. Protective taping should be used to guard the elbow against hyperextension and medial stresses when the athlete returns to play.

Contusions

Contusions about the elbow are best treated with rest and ice to the elbow. If bursitis develops, it can be treated with compression of the inflamed bursa for several days and avoidance of aggravating activities. Myositis ossificans can develop after a direct blow to the brachialis muscle; it can be treated by protecting the injured arm and beginning early active range of motion.

THE WRIST

Fractures of the Distal Radius

Fractures of the distal radius require casting. After the cast is removed with physician's approval, the patient begins active and passive range of motion exercises of the wrist. Modalities to be used in treatment may included fluidotherapy, hydrocollators, and paraffin. It is important to warm the joint for 15 to 20 minutes before exercise. Exercises assigned to the athlete for the home exercise program include all active wrist motions, as well as digital range of motion. Once range of motion is achieved, strengthening exercises may be started.

The athlete may return to play 6 to 8 weeks after the fracture, but he or she needs to be fitted with a playing splint and exercises need to be continued for range of motion and strengthening.

Scaphoid Fractures

Most often wrist injuries occur from a compressive loading on the wrist, such as falling on the hand with the wrist in extension. This may result in a scaphoid fracture, the most common fracture of the carpal bones. The athlete may need to be casted 2 to 4 months. Depending on the severity of the fracture, the athlete may return to play with a playing splint in as little as 2 weeks.[8] If surgery is indicated, the athlete may return to play 3 to 6 weeks after the surgery with a playing splint.

When it is time for rehabilitation, active range of motion and the use of modalities are necessary. In two months, resistive exercises may begin. For return to play, adequate healing must have occurred, and the athlete must use a protective splint.[7]

THE HAND

Metacarpal Fractures

Metacarpal fractures are classified by the location of the fracture: head, neck, shaft, or base. These fractures are generally more stable because of the surrounding structures in the hand. Generally, the fracture is casted, but with certain fractures a Galveston Metacarpal Brace may be used. The Galveston brace is used as a three-point pressure reduction to the fracture; it allows motion at the joints, i.e., the wrist, metacarpophalangeal (MCP), and interphalangeal (IP) joints (Fig. 59–4).

The brace can only be applied to metacarpals II through V, but it can fit any size hand because it comes in small, medium, large, and extra large. It is possible to take a radiograph with the brace on the hand to check

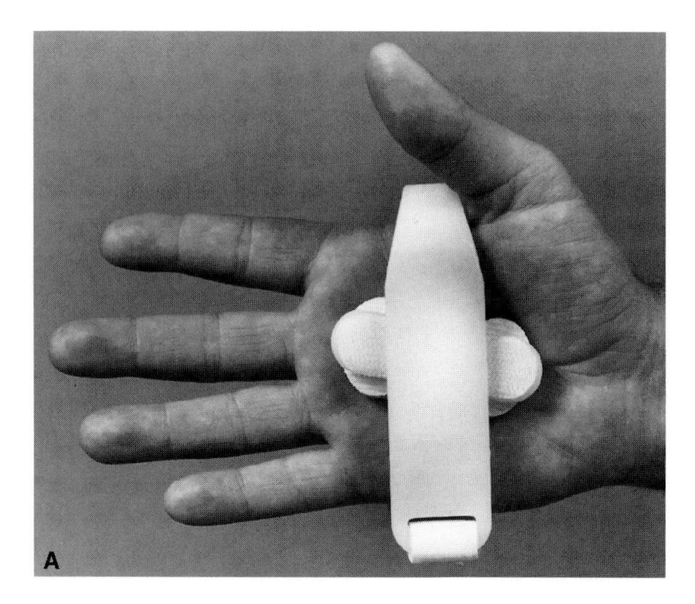

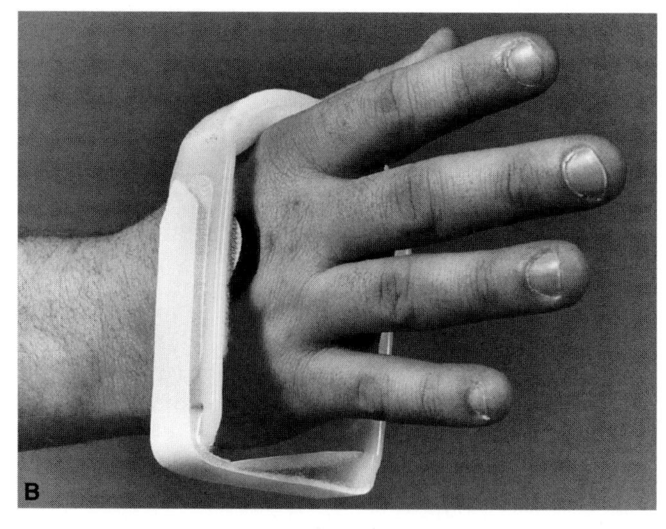

Fig. 59–4. The Galveston Metacarpal Brace to reduce metacarpal fractures. ***(A)*** **Volar view.** ***(B)*** **Dorsal view.**

the alignment of the fracture. If the Galveston brace is inappropriate initially, the situation can be re-assessed in 2 to 3 weeks.

The Galveston brace is a U-shaped plastic brace with an adjustable strap for closure. Inside the U-brace are three foam pads with Velcro attachments. The larger, two-toned pad is placed on the dorsum transversely over the apex of the fracture. The crossbar with the two smaller pads is aligned with the long axis of the fractured metacarpal, with one pad proximal and one distal to the fracture. Pressure on closure is monitored by the dorsal pad; the two tones of the dorsal pad must be visible after reduction and the pressure must be fairly comfortable to the athlete. The athlete is given instructions for wear and care of the brace, e.g., draw an outline of the pads before removing the brace to maintain proper position. The brace also comes with an extra set of pads for replacements.

Return to play depends on the type of metacarpal fracture and the physician's plan of treatment; the athlete may return to play with a protective playing splint as symptoms permit.[6]

Mallet Finger

A mallet finger occurs when a force hits an extended fingertip and forces flexion of the distal interphalangeal (DIP) joint. This forced flexion renders the athlete unable to fully extend the DIP joint. This can be treated in a dorsal aluminum foam or volar splint (a Stack splint) with the DIP joint in full extension (0°) or near extension initially and later, as edema decreases, the extension is increased. Whatever the splint, the goal is to keep the DIP joint in extension and the other joints free. The joint should be splinted for 6 to 9 weeks before active flexion exercises are begun. The splint may be continued if the DIP joint cannot be actively extended. The athlete may continue playing with the splint in place after injury. Mallet fingers may need to be splinted for 12 weeks. If there is an avulsion fracture, surgery may be necessary.

Avulsion of the Flexor Digitorum Profundus

Also known as the "jersey finger," avulsion of the flexor digitorum profundus (FDP) is commonly found in the ring finger. It is the result of forced hyperextension to an actively flexed DIP joint. It usually occurs when a football player gets his finger caught in the opponent's jersey.

Surgery is indicated for this injury. After surgery, a dorsal splint is worn for 3 weeks with the wrist slightly flexed, MCP joint flexed at 60° to 70°, and IP joint in extension. After the 3 weeks, active range of motion exercises (blocking and composite) are begun and completed throughout the day. Up until the fifth week, all exercises are completed in a protected position and the splint is only taken off for exercises. Light activities of daily living are initiated when the splint is discontinued. More strenuous exercises should begin at 8 weeks.[7] With medical clearance, the player could return to play as early as 3 weeks with a protective silicone playing splint shaped like a boxing glove. This protection should be continued until full mobility has been restored.

Boutonnière Deformity

A boutonnière deformity is usually created by a direct force to the dorsum of the proximal interphalangeal PIP joint or by a force to the end of an extended finger forcing flexion against a tight extensor mechanism of the proximal interphalangeal joint.[8] The PIP is splinted in extension for at least 6 to 8 weeks; the DIP can be left to actively flex and extend. After 6 to 8 weeks, active range of motion may begin, with the patient continuing to wear the splint at night. Buddy taping may be used to assist in active range of motion and should be continued as long as the joint is sore. The athlete may continue in competition as long as the digit is protected. Pain and swelling may persist for 3 to 6 months.

Dislocation of the Proximal Interphalangeal Joint

There are two types of dislocations of the proximal interphalangeal joint: dorsal and volar. After the reduction of a dorsal dislocation, the digit needs to be splinted at 30° of flexion to prevent full extension for 3 to 4 weeks. For return to play, the athlete will need to be instructed to buddy tape the injured and adjacent digits and to use a padded splint to protect the digit. In volar dislocations, the extensor mechanism may be disrupted. This will need to be surgically repaired. The PIP joint is splinted at 0° of extension for 6 weeks. The athlete may return to play as symptoms permit, keeping the digit splinted.[6]

THE THUMB

Gamekeeper's or skier's thumb is caused by a direct force to the thumb causing a partial or complete tear of the ulnar collateral ligament of the MCP joint.[9] There are three classifications for gamekeeper's thumb. Treatment for a Grade I gamekeeper's thumb consists of a splint for immobilization for 3 weeks, followed by active and passive range of motion, edema control, and cryotherapy. For Grade II, the splint should be worn an extra 2 weeks. A hand-based thumb spica can be fabricated to prevent ulnar and radial deviation of the joint. Return to play can be expected at 4 to 6 weeks if the dominant hand is injured, or 1 to 2 weeks if the nondominant hand is injured. With a Grade III tear, the thumb should be immobilized for 4 to 6 weeks and the MCP joint should be protected until range of motion and strength return. If surgery is necessary, the athlete wears a cast for 4 weeks after surgery, followed by active and passive range of motion, edema control, and a taping program to decrease stiffness. At 6 weeks, strengthening exercises can begin for the thumb. Depending on the physician's treatment plan, the athlete may return to play wearing a splint 2 to 9 weeks after surgery.[9]

SPLINTS FOR RETURNING TO COMPETITION

Often, the physician may allow the athlete to return to play after an injury to the hand or wrist. However, the hand or wrist may need extra support and protection during game time. These splints are specialized so that re-injury is prevented; they are lightweight, compact, and cause minimal interference with the playing skills of the athlete.[10] The National Collegiate Athletic Association (NCAA) and most high schools set rules regarding what the player can wear during a game. The NCAA has ruled that splints below the elbow cannot be made from unyielding material.[11] The GE RTV-11 silicone splint or the 3M Scotchwrap (a less rigid fiberglass) splint may be used to protect the injured player. It is important to clarify to the injured player that both of these devices are splints, rather than casts, in case he or she is questioned by a referee (splints are allowed in play, but casts are not).

The 3M Scotchwrap is applied like a fiberglass cast, but applying the GE RTV-11 is more like icing a cake with thin icing. The procedure for applying the GE RTV-11 is as follows:

1. Use pre-wrap around the area to be splinted, followed by Kerlex gauze (3/4 to one roll).
2. Place the catalyst in silicone and stir with a tongue depressor.
3. Begin pouring and spreading the RTV-11 over the Kerlex; use about half the can.
4. Place another half a roll of Kerlex around the hand and finish applying the RTV-11.
5. Place a large ziplock bag or plastic wrap around the silicone followed by an elastic bandage.
6. After the splint is dry (3 to 4 hours), remove it by cutting along the ulnar side of hand. (The elastic bandage and plastic should be removed before cutting the splint.) The splint can then be applied before a game or practice to protect the hand.

The goal of rehabilitation of the elbow, wrist, and hand is to return the injured athlete to the field of competition as soon as possible. Through the evaluation and diagnosis of the physician, the treatment by the therapist, and the motivation of the participant, the end result cannot be anything less than success.

REFERENCES

1. Curwin, S., and Stanish, W. D.: Tendinitis: Its Etiology and Treatment. Lexington, MA, D. C. Heath & Co., 1984.
2. Kamien, M.: A rational management of tennis elbow. Sports Med. *9*:173, 1990.
3. Wright, C. S.: Tendon injuries in the hand and wrist. *In* Current Therapy in Sports Medicine, 2. Edited by J. S. Torg, R. P. Welsh, and R. J. Shephard. Philadelphia, B. C. Decker, 1990.
4. Nirschl, R. P.: Soft-tissue injuries about the elbow. Clin. Sports Med. *5*:637, 1986.
5. Garrick, J. G., and Webb, D. R.: Sports Injuries: Diagnosis and Management. Philadelphia, W. B. Saunders Co., 1990.
6. Rettig, A. C.: Current concepts in management of football injuries of the hand and wrist. J. Hand Ther. *4*:42, 1991.
7. McCue, F. C. III, and Mayer, V.: Rehabilitation of common athletic injuries of the hand and wrist. Clin. Sports Med. *8*:731, 1989.
8. Culver, J. E.: Office management of athletic injuries of the hand and wrist. Instr. Course Lect. *38*:473, 1989.
9. Wright, H. H.: Hand therapists set the pace in sports medicine. J. Hand Ther. *4*:37, 1991.
10. Hilfrank, B. C.: Protecting the injured hand for sports. J. Hand Ther. *4*:51, 1991.
11. Zemel, N. P., and Stark, H. H.: Fractures and dislocations of the carpal bones. Clin. Sports Med. *5*:709, 1986.

60

William R. Sutton

Functional Anatomy of the Pelvis and Hip

Functional anatomy of the pelvis and hip reflects the task of weight transfer between the trunk and lower extremity and the sites of origin of muscles, ligaments, and articulations that affect almost every aspect of sport. The pelvis and hip are the site of strong biomechanical forces that predispose humans to many sports-related injuries.

OSTEOLOGY

The pelvis consists of three paired bones (ilium, ischium, and pubis) that interconnect and form the innominate bones, or os coxae, meeting in the midline at the pubic symphysis anteriorly and the sacrum posteriorly. These osseous structures are all present at birth and fuse approximately at age 15 years.[1] Pelvic apophysis sites (iliac crests and spines, ischial tuberosities, and pubic rami) appear at age 8 to 16 years and fuse in the mid-20s.[1]

The junction of the ilium, ischium, and pubis is the triradiate cartilage, which makes up the acetabular cup and fuses by approximately 16 years of age. The femur is visible radiographically at birth, but the head becomes completely ossified during the first few months after birth. The greater and lesser trochanters appear at age 5 to 9 years and fuse in the mid-teens.[1]

The ilium forms the superior element of the pelvis, with the iliac crest serving as the site of multiple muscle origins and insertions. The crest lies at the L4 vertebral level when a person is standing. Because the iliac crest ossifies from the peripheral edge toward the center during adolescence, it provides a radiographic estimate of skeletal development (Risser's Stages 0 through 4), which is especially useful in estimating curve progression among scoliosis patients. The ilium connects to the sacrum by tight ligamentous attachments that can become symptomatic in the patient with a sacroiliac dysfunction (see Chapter 38).

Anteriorly, the ilium descends to the pubis via the arcuate line to the iliopubic eminence (Fig. 60–1). The pubis forms the anterior coxal bone and the anterior portion of the obturator foramen. The pubic symphysis serves as the junction site of the two innominate bones, which are attached by strong fibrous and ligamentous attachments. The inferior ramus of the pubis also runs posteriorly and downward to the ischiopubic region. The ischia extend downward and backward to form the ischial tuberosities (on which we sit), which are just medial to the sciatic notch. Posteriorly, the sacrum interconnects with the ilium via a small synovial joint cavity and extremely strong ligamentous attachments.

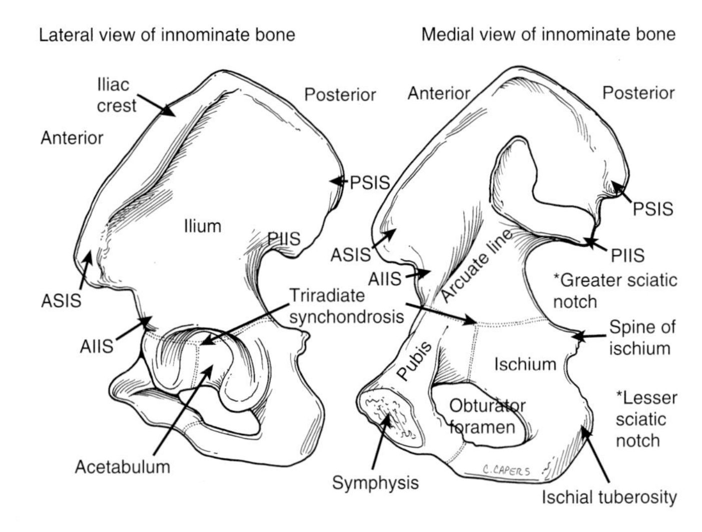

Fig. 60–1. ***(A)*** **Lateral and** ***(B)*** **medial view of innominate bone. Key: ASIS, anterior superior iliac spine; AIIS, anterior inferior iliac spine; PSIS, posterior superior iliac spine; PIIS, posterior inferior iliac spine.**

These consist of the iliolumbar, sacrotuberous, sacrospinous, and anterior and posterior sacroiliac ligaments, which resist downward and forward forces from the lumbar spine and upward forces from the hip joint. Sashin asserts that the sacroiliac joint rotates a maximum of only 4° because of this tight ligament complex.[2]

The hip joint consists of the acetabulum and the proximal femur, a ball-and-socket joint that is reinforced by a strong fibrocartilaginous labral rim and capsule-ligamentous complex, as well as the inferior transverse ligament of the acetabulum. Hip stability depends principally on the tight ligamentous-capsular complex formed by the iliofemoral, pubofemoral, and ischiofemoral ligaments. The iliofemoral ligament runs anteriorly from the anterior inferior iliac spine, spiraling mediad to the intertrochanteric line to make the "inverted Y ligament of Bigelow." Tight on internal rotation and lax on external rotation, it resists hip hyperextension and helps maintain the human's erect posture without constant muscle action (Fig. 60–2A). The pubofemoral ligament runs from the pubic body and rami anteriorly and inferiorly to blend with the iliofemoral ligament going to the femoral neck. It resists excessive abduction and extension. The ischiofemoral ligament runs transversely from the ischial rim to the femoral neck, to resist excessive extension (Fig. 60–2B).

The proximal femur consists of the femoral head and neck, the greater and lesser trochanters, and the proximal femoral shaft (Fig. 60–3). Femoral anteversion gradually lessens, from approximately 30° at birth to 14° at maturity; the average neck shaft angle is approximately 120°.[3] Ward, who studied the forces across this area, divided them into four zones.[4] The strongest trabecular regions are seen medially in the *primary compressive zone* between the femoral calcar and the neck. Thinner bone is seen laterally along the tensile area of the superior neck and greater trochanter. The female pelvis is broader than the male's with a wider abduction angle, which is thought to be related to a higher prevalence of trochanteric bursitis.[5]

Average hip motion consists of 45° of external rotation and internal rotation, 45° of abduction, 20° of adduction, flexion of 135°, and extension of 30°. The hip joint is subject to great biomechanical forces during sports and in daily living, which are transmitted principally by the hip abductors. Studies show that standing on one leg creates a force of 2.5 times body weight, and running forces of 4.5 to 5 times body weight.[6]

MYOLOGY

The pelvis bears the origins and insertions of many muscles along the pelvic rim. Potential sites for avulsion include the anterior inferior iliac spine (rectus femoris), anterior superior iliac spine (sartorius), ischial tuberosity (biceps femoris, or hamstrings, also known as hurdler's fracture), or the lesser trochanter (iliopsoas, seen when a placekicker's cleats catch in the turf).

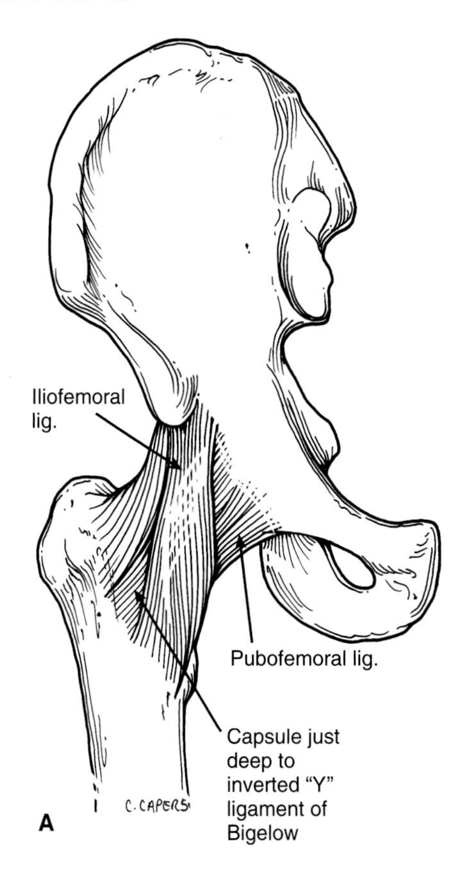

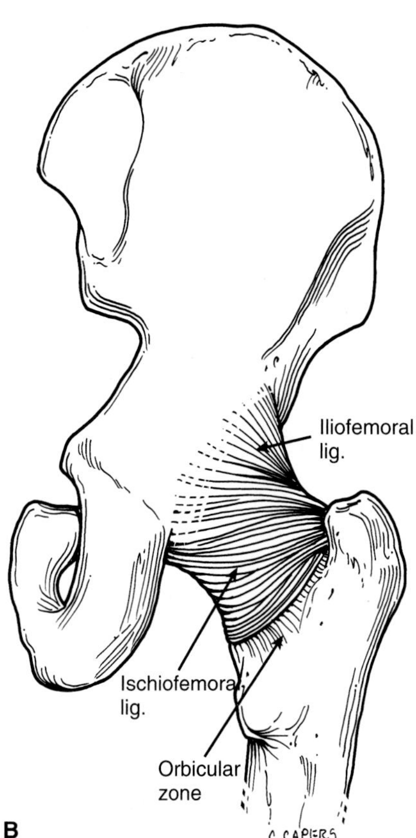

Fig. 60–2. ***(A)*** **Anterior and** ***(B)*** **posterior view of the ligaments of the hip.**

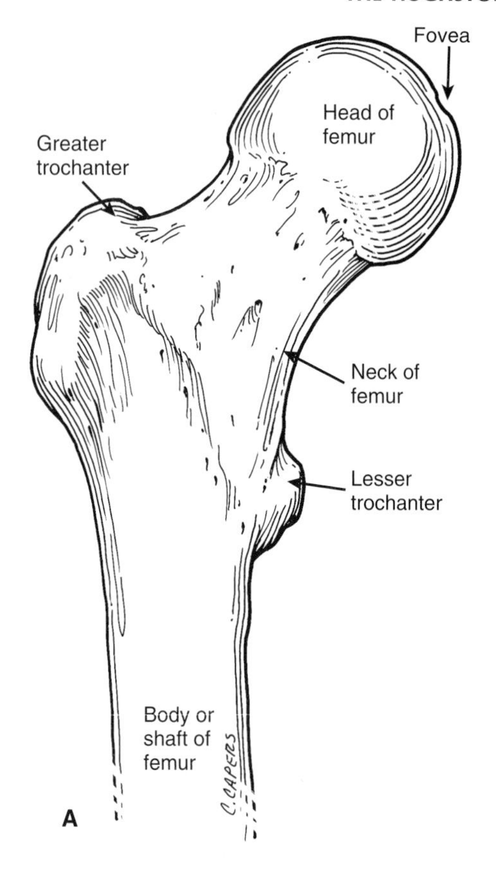

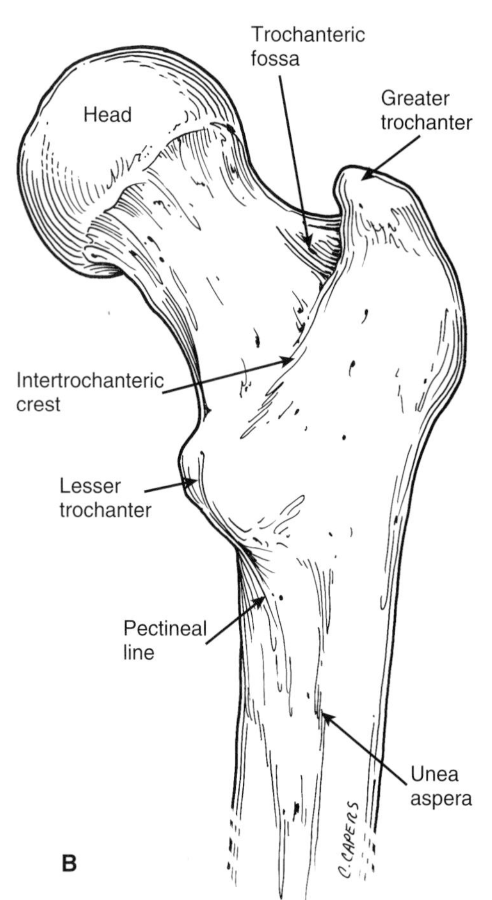

Fig. 60–3. ***(A)*** **Lateral and** ***(B)*** **medial view of the head of the femur.**

Muscles affecting the hip joint act to flex, extend, adduct, abduct, and externally and internally rotate the leg. The primary hip extensors consist of the gluteus maximus (innervated by the inferior gluteal nerve) and the ischial portion of the adductor magnus; the secondary hip extensors are the hamstrings (Fig. 60–4A). The primary hip flexor is the iliopsoas (innervated by the femoral nerve), which inserts into the lesser tuberosity, with the secondary hip flexors being the rectus femoris, pectineus, tensor fascia lata, and sartorius. Hip abduction is performed principally by the gluteus medius and -minimus (innervated by the superior gluteal nerve), which insert into the greater tuberosity, and secondarily by the tensor fascia lata (Fig. 60–4B). Weakness of these muscles is evidenced by Trendelenburg gait and stance. Adduction is performed primarily by the adductor longus (innervated by the obturator nerve), which runs into the medial femoral shaft with secondary adduction power supplied by the adductor brevis and -magnus, as well as the pectineus muscle (Fig. 60–4C). The hip is externally rotated by the short rotators (piriformis, obturator internus and externus, superior and inferior gemelli, and the quadratus femoris) that insert into the posterolateral portion of the greater trochanter (Fig. 60–4D). Internal rotation is relatively weak and supplied by portions of the semitendinosus, semimembranosus, adductor magnus, gracilis, and gluteus medius and minimus.

NEUROLOGY

The nerve supply to the pelvis and hip is through the lumbar sacral plexus by the femoral, obturator, and sciatic nerve roots. The femoral nerve branches off the L2-4 nerve roots and ascends through the pelvis over the iliopsoas and the pectineus muscle, laterally out through the femoral triangle, and terminates into the motor branches that supply the anterior muscles of the thigh. The femoral nerve supplies the sensory distribution of the anterior thigh as well (Fig. 60–5A). The obturator nerve arises from the L2-4 lumbar plexus, descends within the iliopsoas muscle, laterally to the ureter and internal iliac vessels, out the obturator canal, obturator foramen, splitting into an anterior and posterior branch (relative to the obturator externus muscle). It supplies the hip adductors and provides sensory distribution for a small area in the distal medial thigh. Last, the sciatic nerve arises from the L4-S3 lumbar sacral plexus posteriorly, passing out of the pelvis through the sciatic notch, lateral to the ischial tuberosity and deep to the piriformis muscle, where it can sometimes be symptomatically compressed (one cause of sciatica) (Fig. 60–5B). In the proximal thigh it divides into a common peroneal nerve (laterally) and the tibial nerve to supply the hip flexors and muscles of the lower leg. It also provides sensory distribution along the posterior thigh by the posterior femoral cutaneous branch. It should be noted that the hip joint and capsule have sensory innervation from branches of the femoral, obturator, superior gluteal, and sciatic nerves.

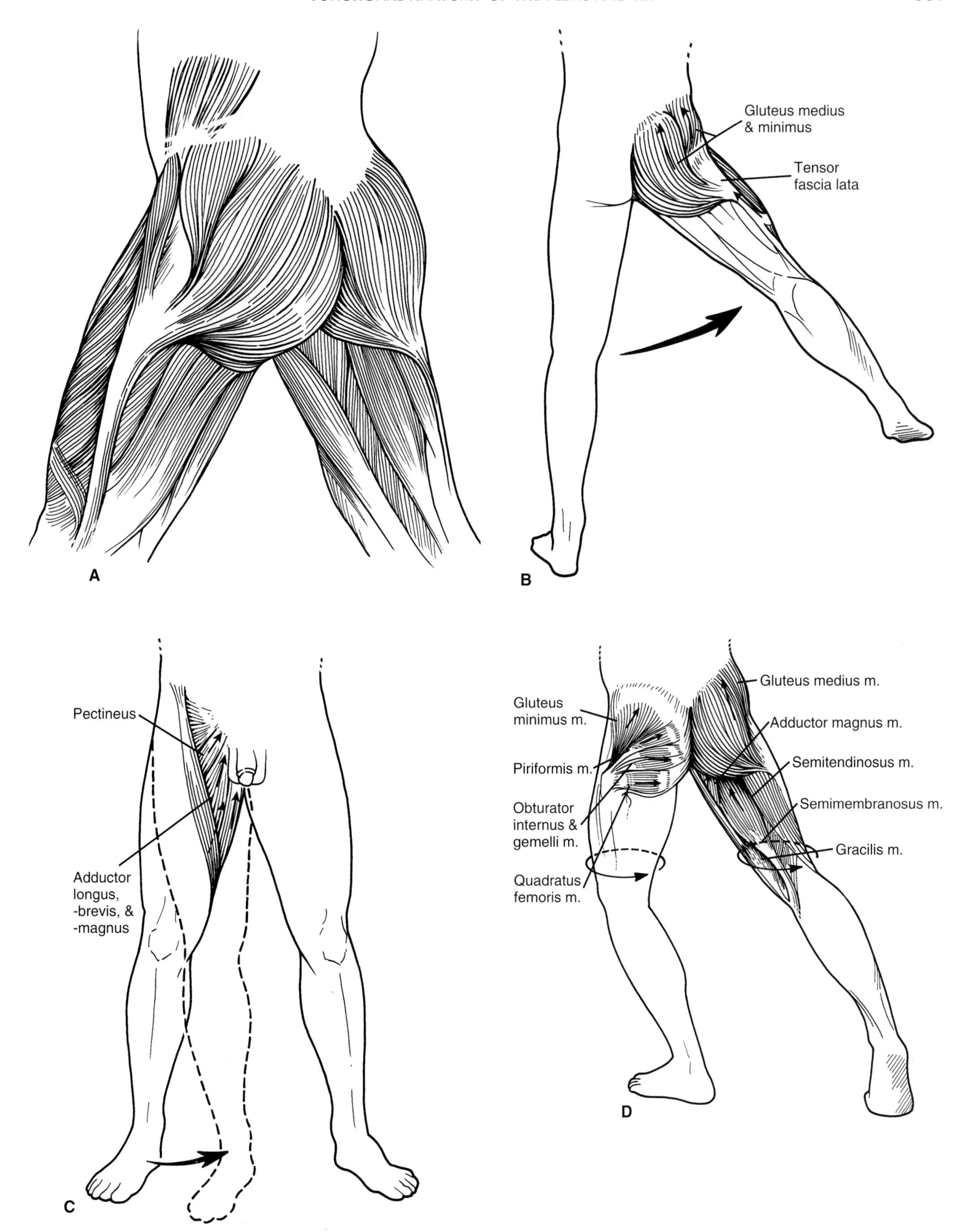

Fig. 60–4. *(A)* Primary extensors and flexors of the hip. *(B)* Abductors of the hip. *(C)* Adductors of the hip. *(D)* Primary external and internal rotators.

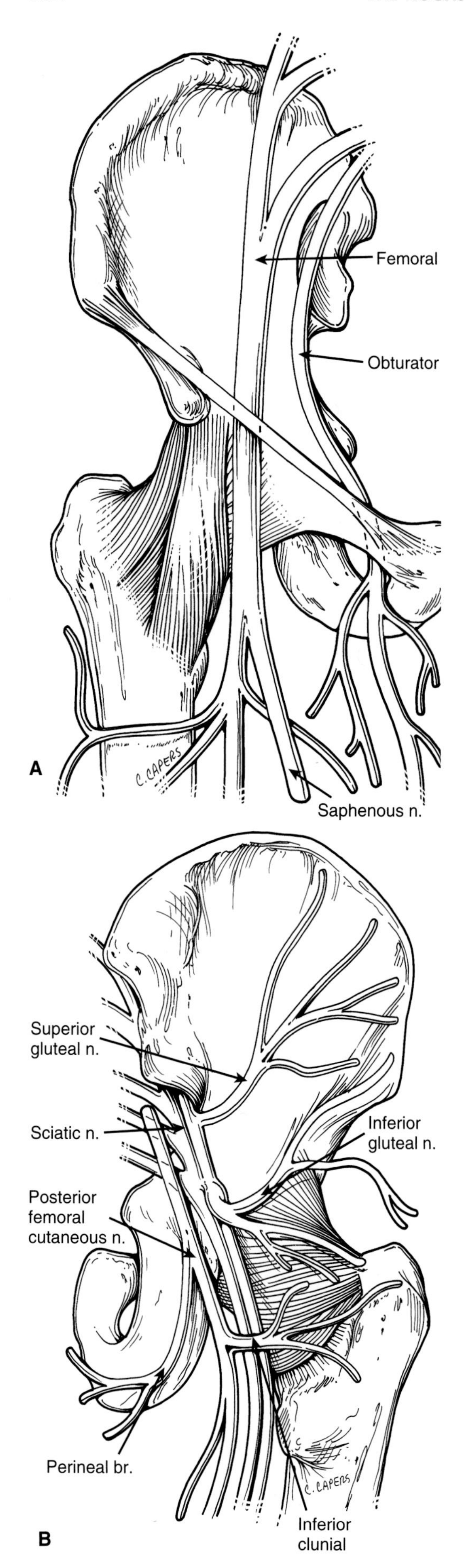

Fig. 60–5. *(A)* Posterior and *(B)* anterior view of the nerves of the hip.

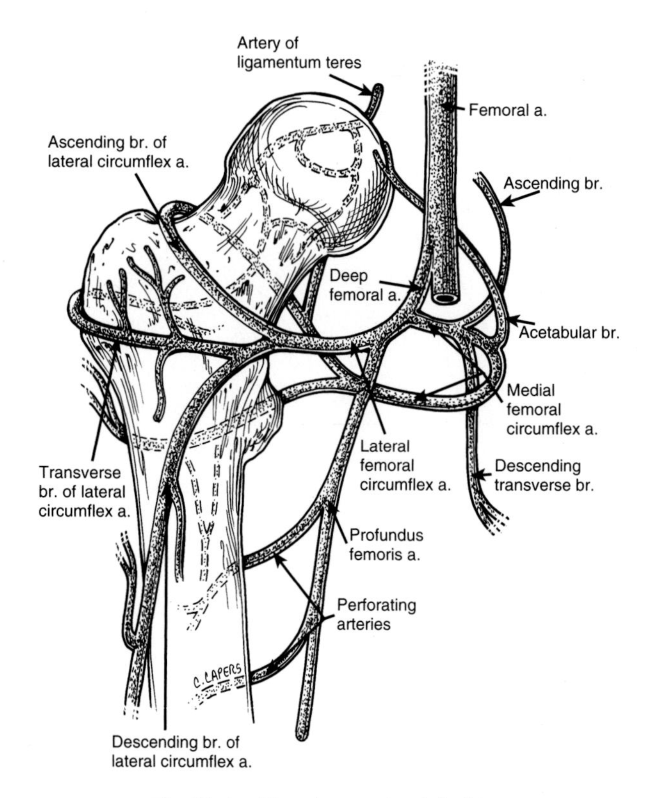

Fig. 60–6. Vascular supply of the hip.

VASCULATURE

Last, the rich pelvic blood supply is provided by the internal and external iliac arteries and the collateral circulation from the inferior aorta. The hip vascular supply has been studied extensively with the primary component being from the femoral artery, which is a continuation of the external iliac artery (Fig. 60–6). The profundus artery branches off the femoral artery just beyond the femoral triangle to supply the anterior thigh. The proximal femur has an anterior branch of the lateral femoral circumflex and posterior branch from the medial femoral circumflex to supply the retinacular vessels of the hip capsule. The artery of ligamentum teres is a residual branch from the obturator artery and is thought to contribute a small amount into the femoral head, which decreases as the patient ages.

REFERENCES

1. Camp, J. D., and Cilley, E. I. L.: Diagrammatic chart showing time and appearance of the various centers of ossification and period of union. Am. J. Roentgenol. Radium Ther. *26*:905, 1931.
2. Sashin, D.: A critical analysis of the anatomy and the pathologic changes of the sacro-iliac joints. J. Bone Joint Surg. *12*:891, 1930.
3. Pick, J. W., Stack, J. K., and Anson, B. J.: Measurements on human femur: Lengths, diameters, and angles. Q. Bull. Northwestern Univ. Med. School *15*:281, 1941.
4. Ward, F. O.: Outlines of Human Osteology. London, Renshaw, 1838.
5. Sim, F. H., and Scott, S. G.: Pelvis and hip. *In* The Lower Extremity and Spine in Sports Medicine. Edited by J. E. Nicholas and E. B. Hershman. St. Louis, C. V. Mosby, 1986.
6. Rydell, N.: Biomechanics of the hip joint. Clin. Orthop. *92*:6, 1973.

61

Carl G. Savory

Evaluation of the Hip Joint

The hip joint, an enarthrodial (ball-and-socket) joint, is one of the largest joints in the body. Unlike the shoulder, where through evolution stability has been sacrificed for mobility, the hip remains perhaps the most stable and mobile of all human articulations.

The basic anatomic configuration of the hip places the femoral head deep within the acetabulum, where it is surrounded by some of the body's most powerful muscles and strongest ligaments. The acetabulum is a relatively deep spherical confluence of three bones: the ilium, the ischium, and the pubis. The acetabulum is deepened further by the presence of a circumferential "gasketlike" structure, the fibrocartilaginous labrum. The general orientation of the acetabulum is lateral, anterior, and inferior.

The femoral head is roughly two thirds of a sphere and, along with the femoral neck, is normally oriented anterior to the coronal plane (anteverted). The angle that the neck makes with the femoral shaft varies from individual to individual and, in adults, generally measures between 120° and 130°.

The hip becomes maximally congruous with loading and is subject to significant forces with the normal activities of daily living, such as walking, arising from a sitting position, and climbing. With athletic activities, these forces are significantly increased. Examples of forces generated at the hip include these:

Double limb stance: ⅓ body weight.
Single limb stance: 1½ to 2 times body weight.
Normal walking: 1½ to 2 times body weight.
Climbing: 2 to 3 times body weight.
Running and jumping: 3 to 5 times body weight.

In general, significant injuries or diseases of the hip usually manifest themselves in some sort of gait abnormality or restriction of motion, but frequent exceptions make the evaluation of the hip quite challenging. Because of the overlap of symptoms related to the lower spine and the pelvis, a complete examination of the hip demands a thorough evaluation of these structures. Knowledge of anatomy is extremely important in evaluating the hip because of the relationship the hip joint has with the overlying muscles and soft tissue. As for any evaluation, a systematic approach to the examination is likely to be the most rewarding. This chapter is organized to describe such an approach. This sequence can maximize efficiency and completeness of the evaluation for the examiner and can reduce the amount of effort required of the patient.

HISTORY

As always, the first step in evaluation is an appropriate, complete history. The *what, how, when,* and *where* of the injury are the essential elements that merely need to be expanded. In addition to the normal medical history, specific information about the hip should be obtained to help direct the physical examination and further diagnostic testing.

The first series of questions should explore the *what,* as the chief complaint is carefully explored. While pain may be the most common complaint, it is usually the most nonspecific. Other frequently encountered complaints are clicking, catching, a feeling of instability, restriction of motion, weakness, and limping. Often a combination of these complaints is the reason for the consultation. With athletes, a very nonspecific feeling of change in performance attributed to the hip may be the presenting complaint. The examiner proceeds to determine whether the problem is acute or chronic. Any trauma should be investigated, particularly the mechanism of injury. Changes from normal activities or athletic endeavors should be determined. Other questions are relevant: Are the symptoms increasing or decreasing? Are the symptoms activity related? Is there anything the patient can do that diminishes or increases the symptoms? Are the symptoms localized? Do the symptoms occur at certain times other than during activity (i.e., day, night, or rest pain)? Has the patient ever had a similar problem, and if so how was it treated and what was the outcome?

PHYSICAL EXAMINATION

A complete physical examination of the hip and pelvis is difficult to perform without having the patient undress. Obviously the location where the examination takes place will dictate this to a great degree, but generally a patient should wear underclothing, athletic shorts, or an examination gown. As previously noted, an examination of the spine and the pelvis is usually necessary for complete evaluation of the hip.

Observation is the first order, and the examiner should watch as the patient moves about the examination room and undresses. Any abnormalities in gait or restriction of motion should be noted. The examiner should then observe the patient in the standing position from the front, side, and back for general posture, particularly any asymmetry; pelvic obliquity and scoliosis; abnormal hip, knee, or foot position; lower extremity rotation; muscle atrophy; and skin changes (e.g., color, scars, wounds). Swelling in and around the hip is difficult to detect by observation, but occasionally it can be seen. The examiner should always compare one side of the body to the other, noting any differences.

With the patient standing in front of and facing away from the examiner, the examiner should observe the patient in alternate single-limb stance by having the patient flex first one hip and then the other to approximately 90°. The willingness and the ability to do this should be noted, as well as the patient's ability to maintain balance. This is Trendelenburg's test. It evaluates the strength of the abductor muscles, principally the gluteus medius. Normally, when the patient stands with weight distributed equally on both lower extremities, the gluteal folds are seen at the same level as the dimples over the posterior superior iliac spines. When the patient is asked to stand erect on one leg, the gluteus medius muscle on the supported side should contract as soon as the opposite leg is lifted off of the ground. This should elevate the pelvis on the unsupported side. If this elevation occurs, the gluteus medius muscle on the supported side is functioning normally. This is a negative Trendelenburg's sign (Fig. 61–1A). If the pelvis on the unsupported side drops or stays in position, the gluteus medius muscle on the supported side is either weak or nonfunctional. This represents a positive Trendelenburg's sign (Fig. 61–1B).

Numerous conditions can cause weakness in the abductor muscles, including congenital abnormalities, osteoarthrosis, coxa vara, fractures of the greater trochanter, slipped capital femoral epiphysis, peripheral nerve root lesion, and other neuromuscular problems. A positive Trendelenburg's test should alert the examiner to the possibility of significant underlying hip problems.

At this point, the iliac spine and the iliac crest should be palpated. Along with observation of the posterior superior iliac spine dimples, palpation should reveal the pelvis to be level (i.e., symmetry of the iliac crests and spines). If there is a discrepancy, it is due either to pelvic obliquity or limb length inequality. If asymmetry is present, the pelvis can be leveled with a series of blocks under the foot of the short limb. This is one method of measuring limb length; it is quite accurate and simple to perform with either Plexiglas or wooden blocks of varying thickness, beginning with ¼ inch and adding ¼-inch increments up to 3 inches. Other methods of measuring limb length should be performed after the patient is lying on the examination table.

After noting any limb length inequality and measuring it with the blocks, posterior and lateral palpation should be performed in an attempt to elicit tenderness in specific anatomic areas (i.e., iliac crest, posterior superior iliac spine, sacroiliac joint, greater sciatic notch, ischial tuberosity, and greater trochanter). This palpation can be done sequentially in a very rapid fashion; any tenderness is noted.

Next, gait is examined. The patient is asked to walk in a normal fashion while being observed from front and back (i.e., walking toward and away from the examiner). The entire lower extremity is involved in ambulation and weight bearing. Pathologic conditions in any part of the extremity often manifest themselves clearly during walking or running. This part of the physical examination should be included, no matter which part of the lower extremity or spine is being evaluated. To perform the most effective evaluation, the examiner must be aware of normal and abnormal gait patterns.

Normal walking involves two phases of gait: the stance phase, where the body is supported by the extremity being examined, and the swing phase when this same extremity is moving forward. Approximately 60% of the normal cycle of gait is spent in the stance phase and 40% in the swing phase. Each phase is in turn subdivided into smaller components: heel strike, foot flat, midstance, and push-off occur during the stance phase and acceleration, midswing, and deceleration during the swing phase.

The function of the hip with a normal gait is to extend the thigh in the stance phase and to flex the thigh during the swing phase. If some hip mobility is lost, compensatory mechanisms include increased mobility of the knee on the ipsilateral side and of the hip on the contralateral side. In addition, the lumbar spine is subjected to more force and increased movement. Hip extensors and flexors work phasically in the initiation of gait. They also work eccentrically as the hip flexors function to help slow extension and the hip extensors help slow flexion. The abductor muscles are critical in providing stability during the single-limb support phase of gait.

Normal gait is an efficient function designed to propel the body forward with minimal displacement of the center of gravity. The center of gravity normally oscillates vertically approximately 5 cm and shifts laterally

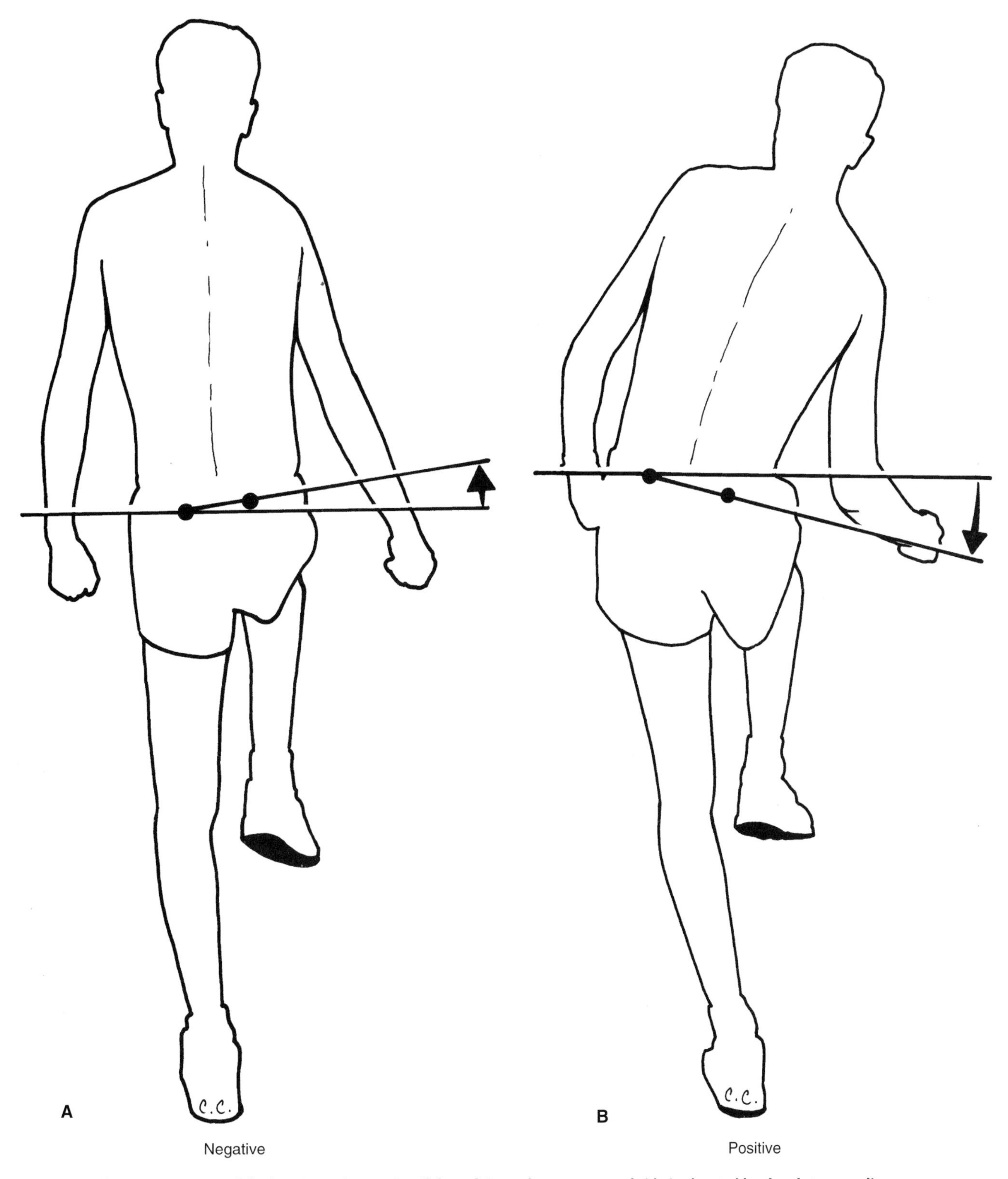

Fig. 61–1. ***(A)*** **Trendelenburg's test is negative if the pelvis on the unsupported side is elevated by the gluteus medius muscle.** ***(B)*** **In a positive test, the pelvis on the unsupported side drops or stays in position.**

about 2.5 cm. The reciprocal pattern of heel strike to toe-off reflects all of the elements of the stance phase. The normal base between the feet is 10 to 20 cm and the normal step length is approximately 38 cm. During the swing phase, the pelvis rotates approximately 40°, anteriorly around the hip of the supported extremity.

Pathologic conditions can be recognized by abnormalities in the gait such as an increase in the vertical motion of the body's center of gravity, an increase in the lateral shift of the trunk and pelvis, a decrease in stride length or cadence, or decreased ability to rotate normally on a hip that is either stiff or painful.

Abnormal gait patterns are particularly important when examining the hip. An antalgic or painful limp usually manifests itself as a very slow, deliberate gait with a decreased stride length and a very short stance phase. While the patient may have pain in all phases of gait, in general, effort is directed to spending as little time as possible in the stance phase. This gives the appearance of a slight hop, as the patient attempts to unload the painful extremity rapidly.

Patients with an extensor or gluteus maximus lurch often have weakness of the gluteus maximus muscle. In this type of gait, the patient thrusts the thorax posteriorly in initiation of the stance phase, in an attempt to maintain hip extension and stability.

A gluteus medius or abductor lurch (Trendelenburg gait) is perhaps the most specific gait abnormality for underlying hip problems. During this gait pattern, the functionally or physiologically weakened gluteus medius forces the patient to lurch or shift the thorax toward the involved side (Fig. 61–2), in an effort to place the center of gravity over the supported hip. This abnormal gait is usually accompanied by a positive Trendelenburg's sign, described previously. If there is bilateral weakness of the gluteus medius, the patient walks with a gait frequently described as a waddle, an accentuated side to side movement.

A patient with leg length inequality or a significant deformity in the extremity exhibits a gait pattern in which a lateral shift to the affected side is noted. In addition, the pelvis tilts down on the involved side, creating the short-leg limp.

Active range of motion of the hip can be rapidly evaluated to determine if there are any gross restrictions. Abduction can be checked by asking the patient to stand and spread the lower extremities apart as far as possible. The patient should be able to abduct each lower extremity between 40° and 45° from the midline. Adduction is observed by having the patient bring the lower extremities together, alternately crossing one in front of the other. The patient should be able to achieve at least 20° to 30° of adduction.

After analysis of the gait pattern and gross active range of motion, the patient is asked to perform certain movements, such as squatting, hopping on the affected extremity, and climbing a step or stairs. Some functions can be evaluated by observing the patient get up on the examination table.

Once the patient is seated on the edge of the examination table, further active range of motion can be checked. The patient is asked to alternately cross one thigh over the other to demonstrate flexion and adduction. Then the patient flexes, abducts, and externally rotates each hip by placing the lateral aspect of the foot on the contralateral knee. Patients with unrestricted hip motion should be able to accomplish this with relative ease; inability to do so or any complaint of pain brought on by this maneuver should be noted.

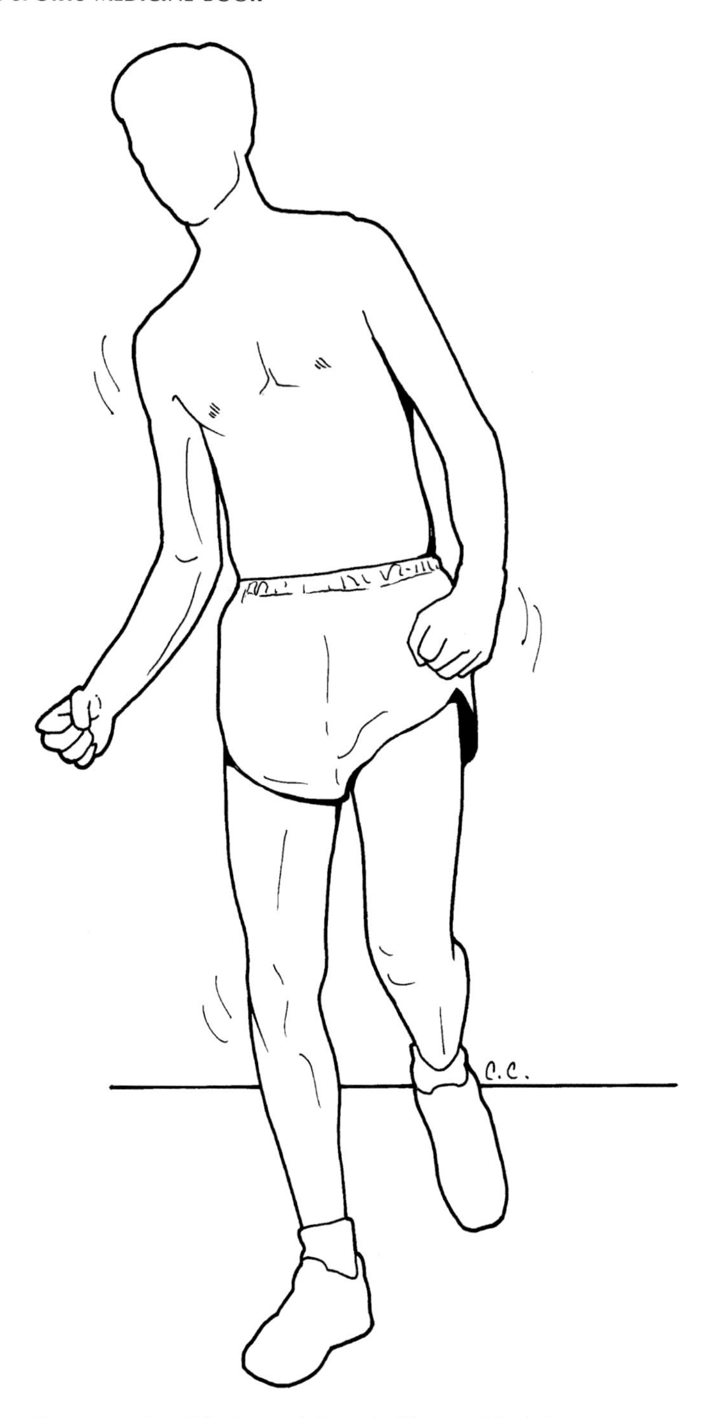

Fig. 61–2. Trendelenburg gait is marked by "waddle"; that is, accentuated side-to-side movement.

Generalized muscle testing can be performed according to function with regard to hip motion (i.e., flexion, extension, adduction, abduction). As a general rule, individual muscles are not tested at this point. By testing the muscles in functional groups, gross evaluation of their innervation is possible.

Initial muscle evaluation begins with the examiner standing in front of the patient, who is seated at the edge of the examination table. The patient is then asked to flex the uninvolved hip by raising the thigh up off the table while the examiner places resistance over the distal thigh; maximum resistance is determined. The maneuver is then performed on the involved side. If the patient is lifting the pelvis, the examiner may need to stabilize the pelvis by placing a hand over the iliac crest. Abductor strength can initially be tested with the patient seated by having the patient spread the thighs apart while resisting forces are applied from the lateral aspects of the knees. The same type of test can be used to test adductor strength by having the patient bring the knees together while the examiner attempts to keep the thighs apart.

If there is any suspicion of neurologic dysfunction, reflexes and sensation should be checked at this point. Before having the patient move to the supine position, active and passive internal and external rotation with the hip in the flexed position can rapidly be performed by moving the ankle and leg laterally and medially. The patient is then asked to lie supine on the examination table, and the remainder of the assessment is completed. The examiner should ensure that the patient is lying flat on the table with the pelvis level and as "square" to the trunk as possible. Range of motion of the hip is evaluated first. If the patient has been able to perform Trendelenburg's test, active flexion can be checked in the supine position by asking the patient to flex the hip and bring the knee toward the chest as far as possible without lifting the back from the table. The patient should be able to bring the knee almost to the chest, which represents approximately 130° to 140° flexion. For most of the range of motion examination, the pelvis must be stabilized.

Although Thomas' test is a specific test to evaluate hip flexion contractures, it can also be used to determine passive flexion. The examiner places a hand under the lumbar spine and flexes the uninvolved hip, bringing the thigh toward the trunk as far as possible. As flexion occurs, the lordosis in the lumbar spine is flattened and the pelvis is thus stabilized. Any further flexion can then be attributed to the hip joint alone.

The examiner then brings the involved hip into the same maximally flexed position. The patient is asked to hold one thigh in a maximally flexed position and to return the other thigh to a flat position on the table. If this is not possible (i.e., if the patient cannot fully extend the hip), a hip flexion contracture is present (Fig. 61–3). The degree of the contracture can be measured by observing the patient from the side and measuring the angle between the thigh and the table at the point of maximal extension. This maneuver is repeated for the unaffected side. If there is any uncertainty, this test can be easily and rapidly repeated.

With a hip flexion contracture, attempts to extend the thigh often cause the thoracic spine to arch, to reconstitute the normal lumbar lordosis that has been reduced by the maneuver. Many times, flexion contractures are not isolated but are associated with adduction or external rotation contracture, or both. This may have to be taken into consideration when performing these maneuvers. Knee flexion contractures can also influence this part of the examination and should be noted.

With the examiner still at the patient's side, passive abduction can be measured. The normal range is between 40° and 50°. During this examination it is necessary to stabilize the pelvis, which can be accomplished by the examiner extending a forearm across the abdomen and placing a hand on the opposite anterior iliac spine. By holding on to the patient's ankle or leg, the examiner can gently abduct the lower extremity as far as possible. When the examiner feels the pelvis move, maximum abduction has been achieved. The degree of motion is recorded as an angle of the thigh measured from the midline. It should be noted that, with a pathologic hip, abduction is usually more limited than adduction.

Adduction can be checked in the same manner as abduction. Normal adduction is between 25° and 35°. The examiner holds the patient's ankle or leg and moves the lower extremity across the midline of the body and over the opposite extremity. The pelvis moves at the end point of adduction. Again, this measurement is recorded as an angle from the midline.

The Patrick, or FABER, test can be performed at this time to evaluate both the hip and the sacroiliac joint. The patient is still in the supine position and the involved foot is placed on the contralateral knee, anteri-

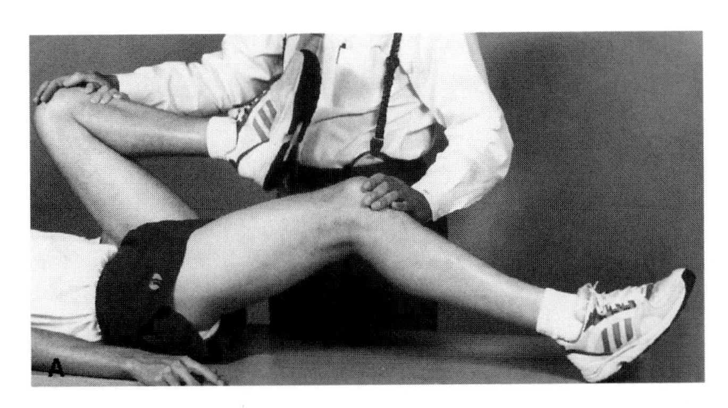

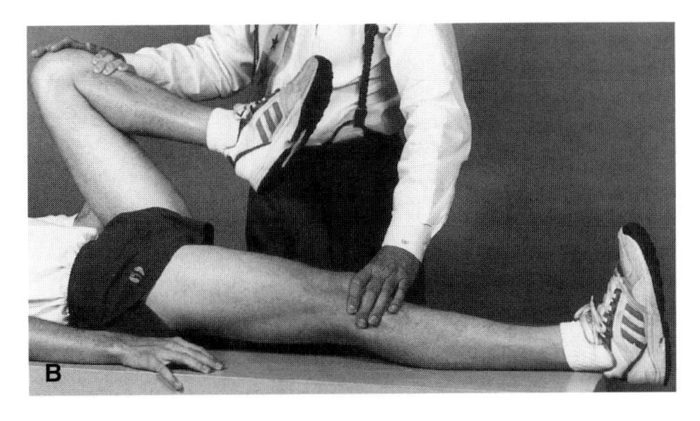

Fig. 61–3. *(A)* **A positive Thomas' test demonstrates hip flexion contracture. The patient holds one thigh maximally flexed and attempts to let the other thigh down flat on the table. If this is not possible, the result is positive.** *(B)* **A negative Thomas' test result.**

orly. The hip is now *f*lexed, *ab*ducted and *e*xternally *r*otated (FABER). Any complaint of pain or discomfort and the site are noted. Inguinal pain may indicate a hip problem. To test for pain at the point of maximum flexion abduction and external rotation, the examiner fixes the pelvis with his or her hand on the contralateral anterior iliac spine and applies outwardly directed stress at the level of the knee. Again, the patient's complaints of increased pain and the site of the pain are recorded.

With the patient's thigh and hip in this position, palpation of the soft tissue of the femoral triangle and the anterior pelvis is facilitated. The femoral triangle should be palpated and inspected for an inguinal or femoral hernia, which can occasionally cause hip pain. The femoral artery is readily palpated with the thigh in this position. To the lateral side of the femoral artery lies the femoral nerve and to the medial side, the femoral vein. The femoral nerve and vein are not normally palpable. Any inguinal adenopathy should be noted. Enlargements may be related to infection of the lower extremities or localized pelvic conditions. Palpation of the anterior soft tissues may detect detachment of the rectus femoris from its insertions, and this area should be palpated for tenderness. The direct head of the rectus femoris originates from the anterior inferior iliac spine, and the indirect head from the anterior superior hip capsule. The direct head is injured more often, and detachment of the head can result in an avulsion fracture. Often, such avulsion injuries are sports related. Palpation of the iliac crest as well as the anterior superior and -inferior iliac spines is completed.

The patient's extremity can now be returned to the normal supine position on the examination table. At this point, the determination of apparent true limb lengths can be made. With the patient supine, the lower limbs are placed in neutral position. The true leg length is measured from the anterior superior iliac spine to the base of the medial malleolus. This is done on both sides, and the measurements are compared. Any difference in measurement confirms that one leg is shorter than the other.

Once the true leg length has been measured, apparent limb length can be determined. The patient remains with the lower extremities in as neutral a position as possible. The measurement is taken from the umbilicus to the base of the medial malleolus of the ankle. Discrepancies between the two sides present an apparent leg length inequality. Apparent shortening may be the result of pelvic obliquity or various contractures about the hip joint itself.

At this point the patient is asked to move to the lateral decubitus position with the affected hip in the superior position. The examiner stands behind the patient, and, once again, specific areas can be rapidly palpated in an attempt to elicit tenderness. In the greater trochanteric area, the trochanter itself is usually readily palpable. Trochanteric bursitis is a frequent cause of hip pain. On palpation of the greater trochanteric region, patients with trochanteric bursitis may have exquisite tenderness, and possibly some induration. In this condition, abduction against resistance also causes localized trochanteric pain as well as referred knee discomfort laterally.

The greater sciatic notch, through which the sciatic nerve passes, is located roughly halfway between the greater trochanter and the ischial tuberosity. Tenderness in this area may be due to nerve root irritation caused by pathologic conditions in the lumbar spine. The piriformis muscle, one of the hip external rotators, has a tendinous attachment just at the posterior portion of the greater trochanter. The sciatic nerve normally lies close to the muscle belly itself, and the insertion on the superior posterior aspect of the greater trochanter should be palpated and complaints of tenderness recorded. At this point, the ischial tuberosity should also be palpated as a bursa in this area can become inflamed and cause localized pain. Palpation of the sciatic nerve area, as well as the ischial tuberosity, should be done with the hip in both the extended position and flexed to approximately 70°.

With the patient still in the lateral decubitus position, testing of abductor strength can be completed. The pelvis is stabilized by the examiner placing a hand on the iliac crest. The patient is instructed to abduct the lower extremity by extending the hip and pointing the toes. Once the patient has abducted the extremity, the examiner applies downward force to the lateral thigh, attempting to adduct the leg while the patient resists.

While the patient is still in the same position, Ober's test for contracture of the iliotibial tract and band can be performed. The lower extremity is abducted as far as possible while the pelvis is still stabilized in a vertical position (i.e., perpendicular to the examination table). The examiner passively flexes the patient's knee to 90°, keeping the hip joint in neutral position to relax the iliotibial tract. The examiner then releases the abducted lower extremity. If the iliotibial tract is normal, the thigh should drop to an adducted position; if there is a contracture, the thigh remains abducted when the leg is released.

The patient now moves to the prone position. The gluteus maximus muscle is tested for strength by having the patient flex the knee to relax the hamstring muscles. The examiner's forearm is placed over the posterior iliac crests, and the patient is instructed to lift the thigh off of the examination table. The examiner resists this motion by pushing down on the posterior aspect of the thigh at the level of the knee joint. This procedure is repeated for both sides.

While the patient is prone, Ely's test can be performed to determine the presence or absence of a tight rectus femoris muscle. The examiner passively flexes the knee to approximately 90°. If the patient's hip on the same side spontaneously flexes, the rectus femoris muscle is tight on that side and the finding is considered positive. Again, both sides should be tested and findings compared. Thus, a complete and thorough examination is performed that "economizes" on time as well as the efforts of the patient and the examiner.

In evaluating complaints of hip problems, laboratory data are rarely helpful. If there is suspicion of infection, laboratory data should include a complete blood count with a differential count, sedimentation rate, and cultures of hip synovial fluid. If some sort of inflammatory arthritis is suspected, a rheumatoid serology panel including antinuclear antigen, rheumatoid arthritis screen, and HLA B27 may be indicated. A sedimentation rate can also be helpful in both instances, but an elevated result is quite nonspecific.

IMAGING OF THE PELVIS AND HIP JOINT

In general, an orthopedic evaluation is hardly considered complete without some sort of imaging. The hip is not an exception, and, in fact, may be the rule because pathologic conditions in the hip and pelvis are not always definable by observation, palpation, or other standard clinical examination techniques that have previously been described.

If any imaging is contemplated, standard radiographs are essential. This includes an anteroposterior view of the pelvis with some sort of lateral view of the involved side (Figs. 61–4 and 61–5; either a true Smith-Petersen lateral or a frog-leg lateral). Internal and external oblique views should be obtained if there are specific questions about anterior or posterior acetabular structures. These "Judet views" are normally most helpful when acetabular fracture results from significant trauma. The advantage of standard radiographs is that they are probably the most readily obtainable images, radiation for the patient is minimal, they are relatively inexpensive, and, if abnormal, they can be extremely helpful and may obviate more expensive and time-consuming diagnostic imaging. The disadvantages of standard radiographs are that they evaluate essentially only the bony structures around the hip and pelvis. Standard radiographs do not always detect early stress fractures or stress reactions, early stages of osteonecrosis, soft tissue abnormalities, or subtle changes of the cartilage early in a neoplastic process.

Standard tomography can be helpful, but the indications are limited to detecting entities such as delayed union or nonunion of a fracture or an osteoid osteoma. The examination requires special equipment, is moderately expensive, and subjects the patient to relatively large doses of radiation. Standard tomography is used infrequently in routine evaluation of hip conditions and has been supplanted in large part by more sophisticated computed tomography (CT).

CT has become more readily available and is only moderately expensive. Again, CT is most valuable when dealing with osseous abnormalities, unless it is combined with arthrography. One advantage of CT is that both hips can be scanned simultaneously for comparison. CT can define fractures, articular loose bodies, joint incongruity, certain osseous neoplasms, and early osteonecrosis (Fig. 61–6). Its ability to adequately image most of the soft tissues in and around the hip is limited. Arthrography can be combined with CT to detect intra-articular, labral, and capsular abnormalities. CT is used

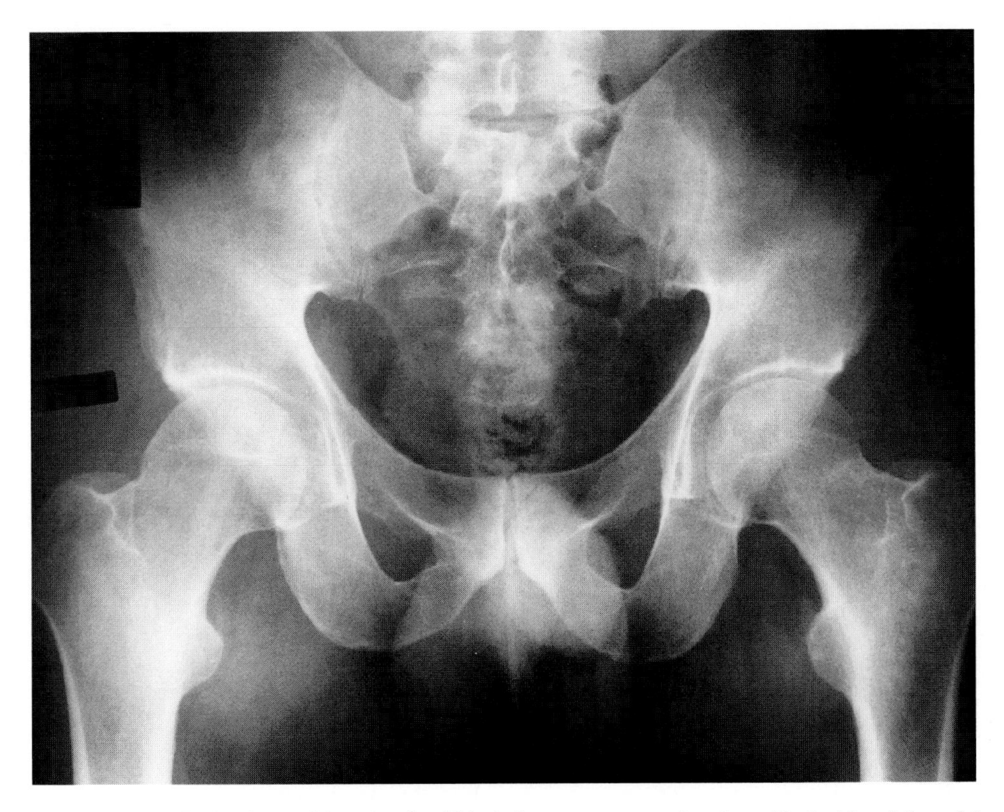

Fig. 61–4. A standard radiographic series should include an anteroposterior view of both sides of the pelvis.

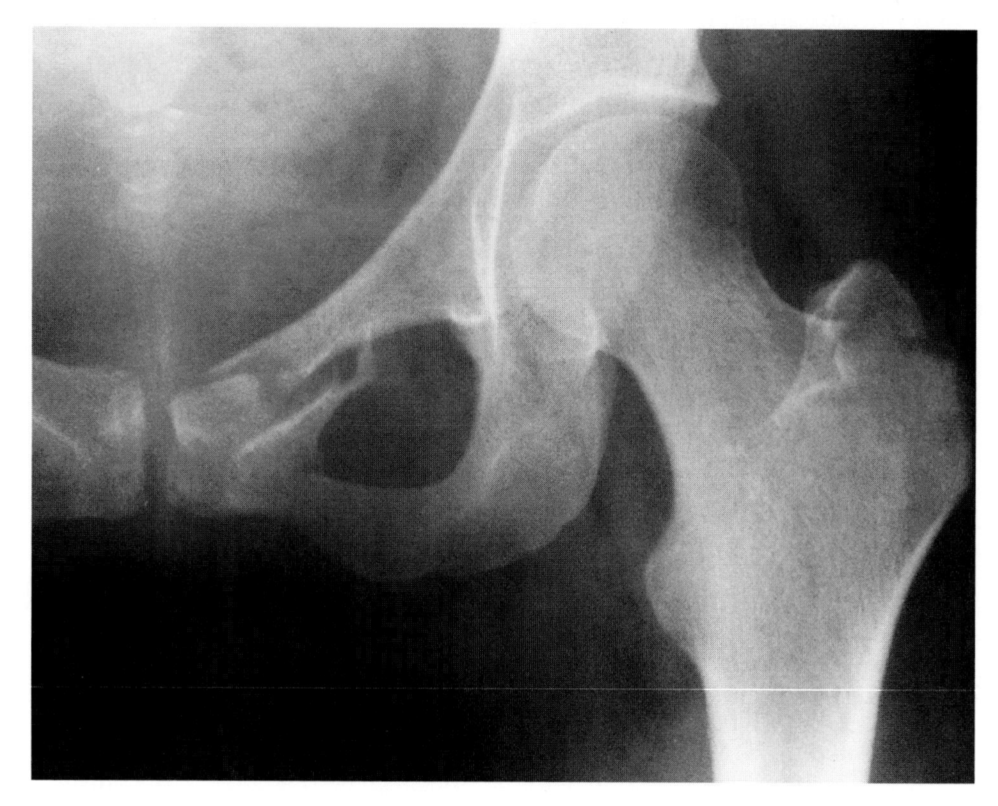

Fig. 61–5. An anteroposterior radiograph can be used to detect a greater trochanter fracture.

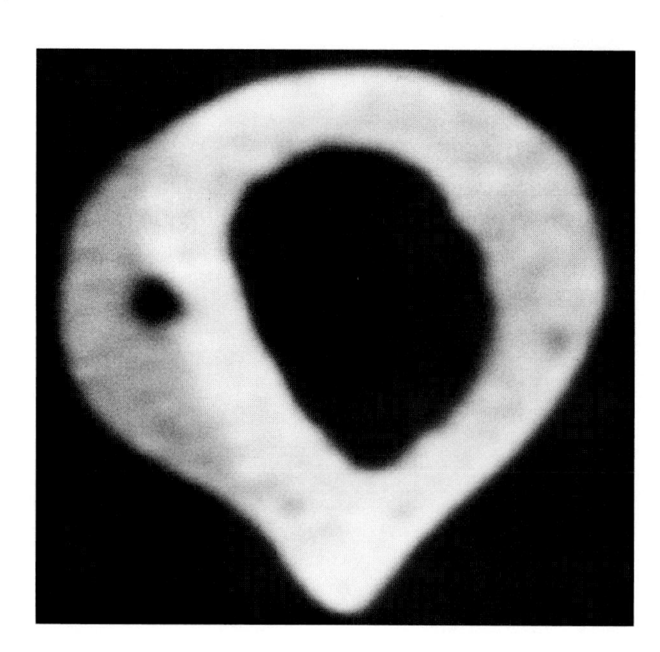

Fig. 61–6. CT shows osteoid osteoma.

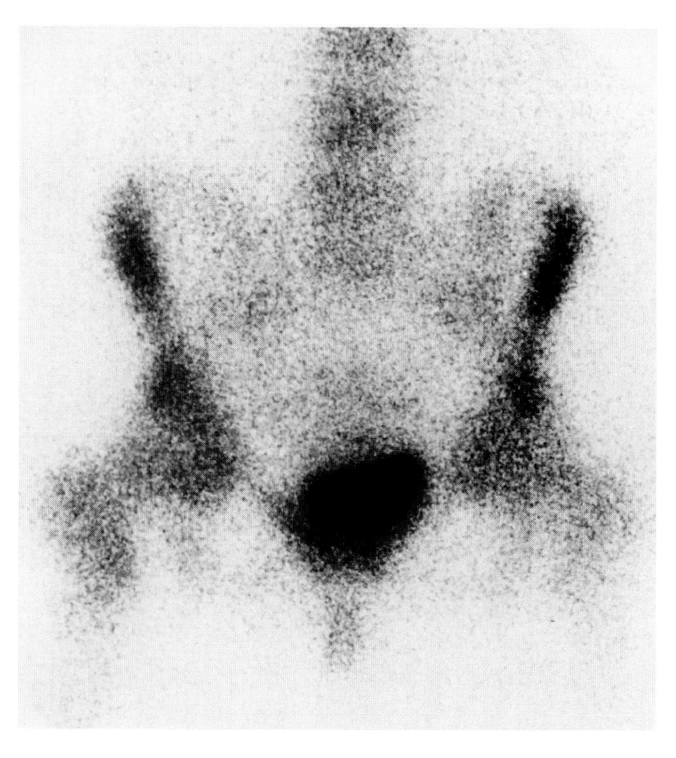

Fig. 61–7. A bone scan can detect osteonecrosis or stress fracture of the pelvis.

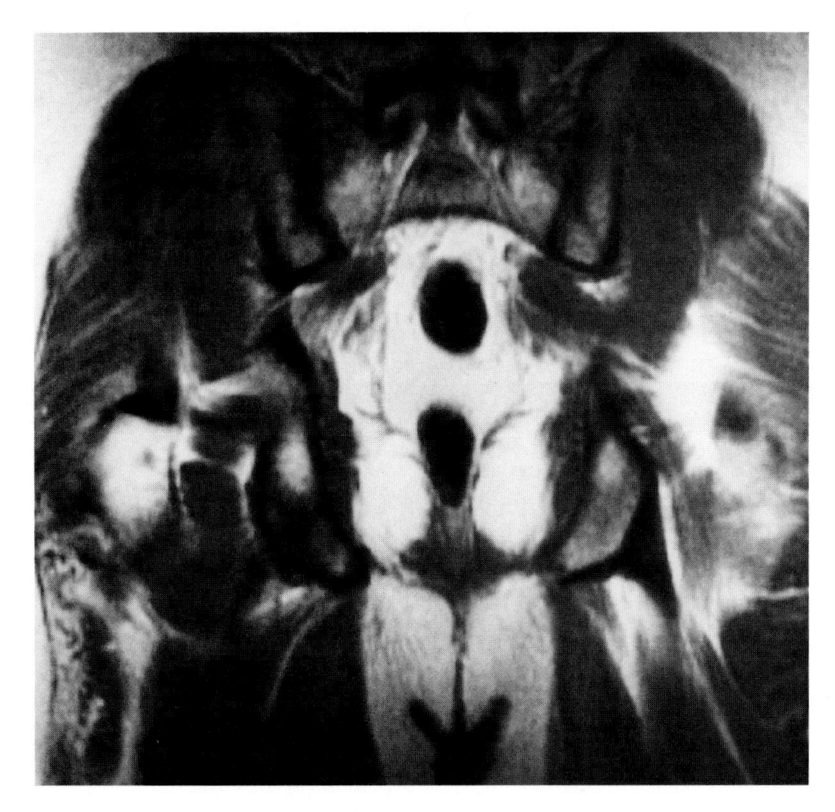

Fig. 61–8. MRI of the pelvis shows a hamstring avulsion.

most frequently when significant trauma to the hip or pelvis has occurred or when the diagnosis is obscure.

Aspiration arthrography, although it is occasionally useful, is rarely used because of its limitations. Intra-articular loose bodies and other abnormalities are frequently defined better by either CT or magnetic resonance imaging (MRI). Arthrography requires fluoroscopy and a skilled radiologist. The advantage of an aspiration arthrogram is that joint fluid can be sampled, and it is the definitive procedure for suspected intra-articular infection or when analysis of the synovial fluid of the hip is essential. Aspiration of the hip joint can be performed without fluoroscopy, but it is difficult, particularly if no joint fluid is obtained. An arthrogram can confirm that the aspiration needle is in the correct intra-articular position. Aspiration arthrography is a moderately expensive procedure that exposes the patient to a small dose of radiation.

Bone scans are generally available at moderate cost, and they expose the patient to minimal radiation. The advantage of a bone scan is that it normally images the entire skeletal system. Technetium bone scanning, the most common type, can define early stress reactions and stress fractures, osteonecrosis, osseous neoplasms, and infection (Fig. 61–7). Other types of bone-scanning techniques that are specific for infection include indium and gallium scintigraphy. They are normally used in conjunction with a technetium scan to help define intraosseous or intra-articular septic processes.

MRI is becoming a very popular diagnostic tool. At present, its major disadvantage is its very high cost and, in some places, limited availability. MRI is extremely sensitive and can define intraosseous and soft tissue abnormalities around the hip (Fig. 61–8). It can image the capsular structures, the labrum, fluid-filled bursas, articular surfaces, muscles, and tendons. It is the definitive test for evaluation of osteonecrosis and has the highest degree of specificity and sensitivity. It can also be extremely useful in defining stress reactions, stress fractures, and neoplasms. Other advantages are the absence of ionizing radiation and the fact that both hips are normally imaged simultaneously. Interpretation of MRI is becoming much more reliable as radiologists become more familiar with the technique.

62 *Jack H. Henry and David M. Kahler*

Traumatic Injuries to the Hip

Fractures and Dislocations of the Hip

Jack H. Henry

Even though injuries of the hip are not as common in athletes as injuries of other major lower extremity joints, their diagnosis and treatment can be perplexing at times. Severe traumatic injuries can occur, and, when they do, they are among the most urgent problems in sports medicine. Therefore, the diagnosis and treatment of these injuries are of utmost importance to sports medicine physicians.

FRACTURES OF THE PELVIS

It is important to remember that the pelvis is a ring completed by the ilium, ischium, and pubis. The posterior part of the ring is involved in weight transmission. The principal function of the anterior portion of the ring is protection. Fractures that break the continuity of the pelvic ring require a force of great magnitude. This obviously produces more bleeding and may require massive blood replacement.[1] Fractures of the pelvis are rare athletic injuries; horseback riding and motorcross have produced most of the pelvic fractures I have seen.

Fractures of the Ilium

Fractures of the ilium are usually caused by a backward fall.[1] Even though this is a weight-bearing part of the ring, the ring's integrity may be preserved. Damage to the pelvic viscera and retroperitoneal hemorrhage can occur. After fracture to the ilium, there is immediate pain that usually prohibits ambulation. Tenderness over the pelvis, swelling of the hip posteriorly, and ecchymosis all occur. Adequate radiographs are necessary to evaluate the bone injury, and the patient should be observed carefully in the hospital, to rule out visceral damage. These fractures usually do not require surgery; conservative treatment is successful. Simple bed rest is the treatment of choice until the acute pain subsides. Protected weight bearing with crutches is usually necessary for 2 to 3 weeks. The athlete's activity is restricted until pain decreases. Support or taping may help as activities are resumed. Active athletic participation is not recommended for 3 to 4 months.

Fractures of the Sacrum

Fractures of the sacrum are usually caused by a fall in the sitting position or a direct blow. The distal fragment angulates forward and becomes impacted. At the time of injury pain is severe. Examination reveals tenderness over the sacrum, and rectal examination pinpoints the tenderness anteriorly. Displacement can injure the sacral nerve roots, and paralysis of the bladder can occur, which requires surgery. Radiography and magnetic resonance imaging (MRI) identify the lesion. Treatment is usually bed rest followed by protected weight bearing. Surgical treatment is necessary only if the fracture fragments are much displaced.

Fractures of the Coccyx

Sports injuries to the coccyx are not uncommon. The mechanism of injury is a fall in the sitting position. The fracture may occur at the sacrococcygeal junction or in the body of the coccyx.

Marked pain occurs at the time of injury and sudden movements accentuate the pain. Likewise, sitting is almost impossible, especially sitting in a position other than erect with the weight on the ischial tuberosities. Tenderness is present over the coccyx, and rectal examination reveals tenderness and painful motion of the coccyx. Radiographs in the lateral projection reveal the lesion (Fig. 62–1).

Treatment is directed at pain relief. Sitting increases the pain if the patient is allowed to "sit back" on the coccyx. Sitting forward with the weight distributed on the ischial tuberosities is recommended. This can be accomplished by sitting on a firm surface, such as a book, or a firm chair and allowing the coccyx to be free of pressure posteriorly. Tight clothing can irritate the anal cleft and should be avoided. Lying supine obviously relieves pressure on the bone and is comfortable. Pain and tenderness may persist, but the athlete is usually not disabled. The coccyx may remain chronically painful, and excision of the bone has been described, though I do not recommend it. Return to athletics is permitted as soon as comfort allows.

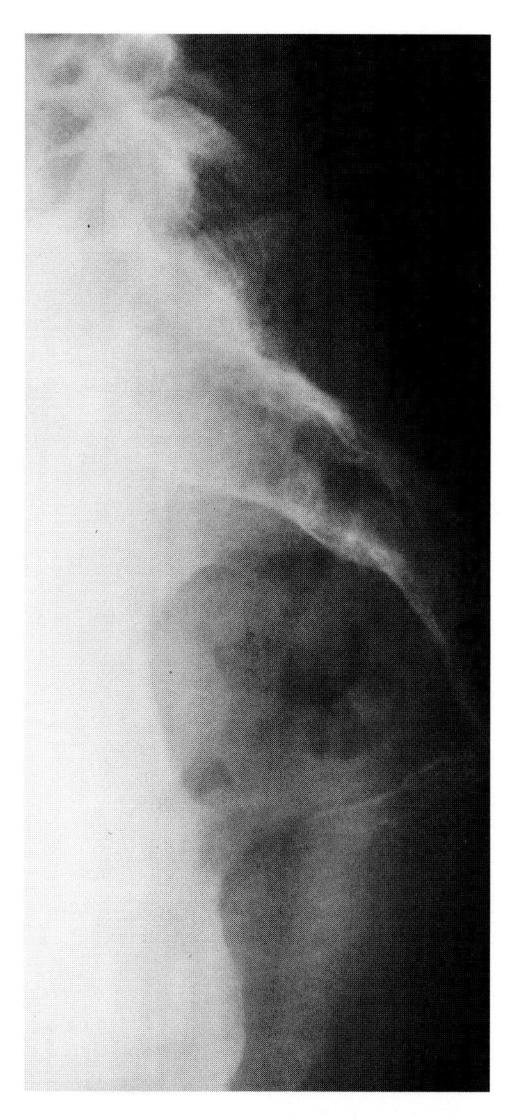

Fig. 62–1. Lateral projection of the sacrum shows a fracture at the sacrococcygeal junction sustained playing rugby. (Henry, J. H.: The Hip. *In* Principles of Sports Medicine. Edited by W. N. Scott. Baltimore, Williams & Wilkins, 1984.)

Fractures of the Acetabulum

Fractures of the acetabulum are even more rare than fractures of the pelvic ring. Severe trauma is implicated in this injury. The mechanism is usually a direct violent force that passes through the femoral neck into the acetabulum. High jumping and motorcross are two of the sports that have been implicated, in my experience. Immediate pain and the inability to walk on the leg are common symptoms. Examination reveals pain with passive or active range of motion of the hip. Central displacement of the acetabulum produces shortening of the extremity. Treatment depends on good radiographic evaluation. Skeletal traction may be necessary to reduce a displaced fracture, or possibly open reduction and internal fixation; however, this has not occurred in my experience. Until pain subsides and early healing occurs, bed rest, followed by range of motion, is indicated for both displaced and undisplaced fractures. Protected weight bearing with crutches allows the acetabulum to heal. Even with the best treatment, osteoarthritis of the hip is a common complication.

TRAUMATIC DISLOCATIONS OF THE HIP

In athletes, the bone is usually strong, and the hip is more likely to dislocate than to break in persons of the "athletic age group."[(2)] Dislocations are seen almost exclusively in young adults or those in the middle years, but they can occur in children. Dislocation of the hip is a very serious insult;[(3)] it is a true medical emergency. Circulation to the femoral head is compromised, and avascular necrosis can result. Early reduction is important to prevent avascular necrosis.[(4)] In my opinion, no attempt at reduction should be made on the field, lest further damage to the blood supply of the femoral head result from repeated manipulation.

Traumatic dislocation of the hip of a child requires less forceful trauma, and soft tissue interposition can occur on reduction. If radiographs taken after reduction reveal an increased medial joint space, soft tissue interposition should be suspected.[(5)]

Dislocation of the hip can be anterior, posterior, or central (Fig. 62–2).[(6)] Central dislocation, protrusion of the femoral head into the fractured acetabulum, may be treated like fractures of the acetabulum.

Posterior Dislocations

Posterior dislocations are the most common type of dislocation I have seen in athletes, probably because of

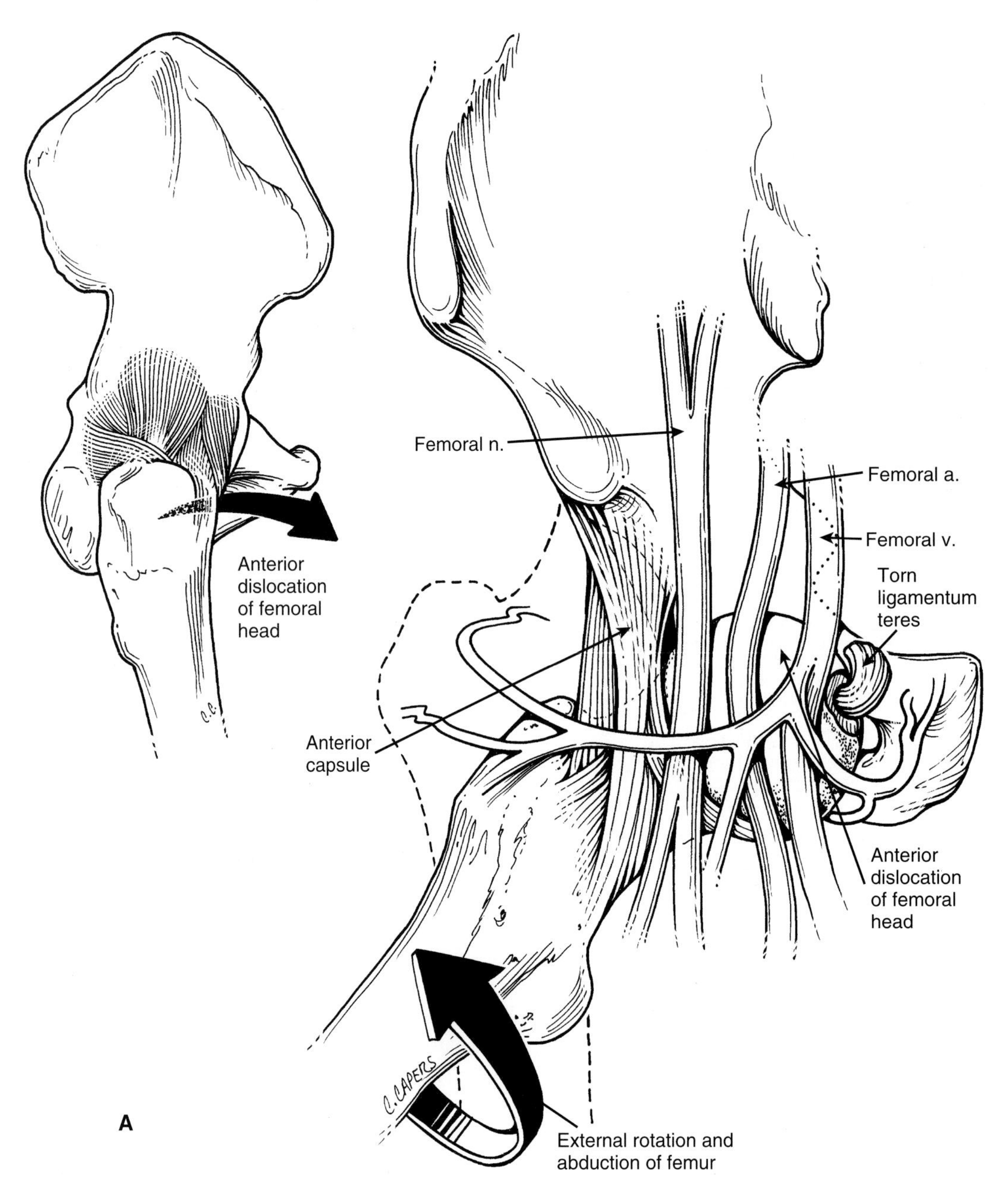

Fig. 62–2A. Diagram of an anterior dislocation of the hip.

the greater strength of the anterior capsule of the joint and because the mechanism of injury occurs more commonly in athletes. Posterior dislocations can occur in football, rugby, or soccer. The impact forces the femoral head posteriorly, tearing the ligamentum teres and the posterior capsule. Fractures of the posterior acetabular rim can also occur. The vascular supply to the femoral head is stretched and torn as the posterior displacement increases, and the sciatic nerve may be injured.

Pain is the most striking symptom. During examination, the limb is held in internal rotation as the hip is flexed and adducted. Diagnosis may be made by inspection alone; however, one should have the patient dorsiflex the foot (to evaluate the peroneal division of the sciatic nerve) and plantar flex and invert the foot (to evaluate the tibial portion of the sciatic nerve). On-field evaluation of the nerve is essential. If function does not return with reduction of the hip, surgical exploration might be indicated.

The patient should be transferred immediately to a facility where radiographs can be taken and the diagnosis can be confirmed. Reduction usually requires adequate analgesia or general anesthesia. After reduction, posterior stability of the hip should be tested since a fracture of the acetabulum may allow redislocation; if this does occur, open reduction may be necessary. After reduction, the limb is placed in traction suspension. Range of motion exercises are started early, to nourish the articular cartilage. The patient is allowed up on crutches approximately 2 weeks after injury. Protected weight bearing is continued for 2 to 6 months, depending on the surgeon's school of thought.

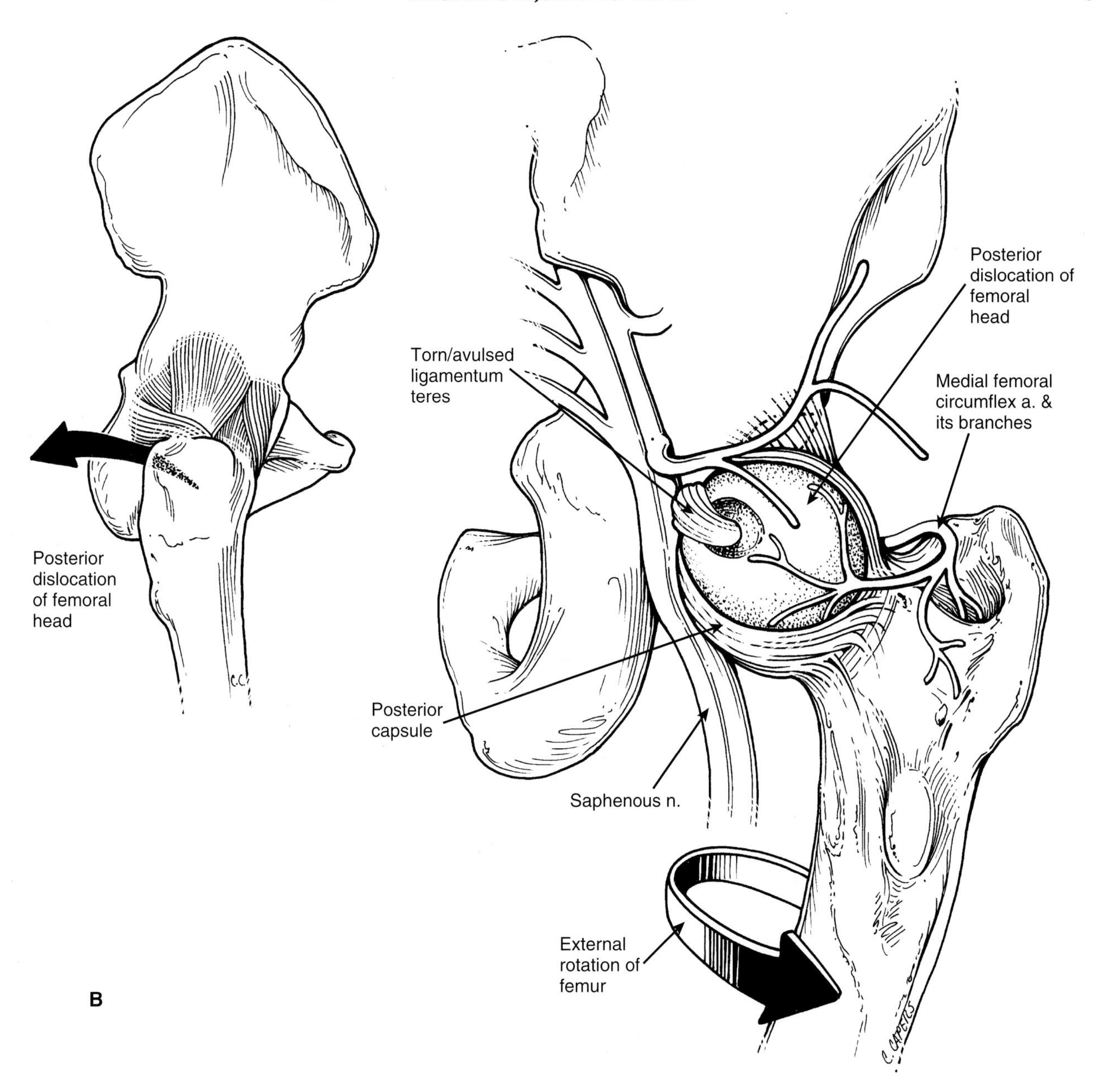

Fig. 62–2B. Diagram of a posterior dislocation of the hip.

If surgical fixation of the posterior capsule or acetabular rim is necessary, a period of 6 weeks' protection is recommended to allow adequate healing. Return to athletics should not be allowed for a minimum of 3 months after the dislocation. Complications of posterior dislocation include permanent sciatic nerve injury, avascular necrosis of the femoral head, osteoarthritis, and chondrolysis. Early detection of chondrolysis is possible by bone scintigraphy.[7] Decreased activity in the greater trochanter on the bone scan is thought to predict chondrolysis and indicates early fusion of the greater trochanteric epiphysis. Traumatic posterior subluxation of the hip resulting in a case of avascular necrosis and chondrolysis has been described in a professional football player.[8] The diagnosis of chondrolysis is very difficult in the early stages and, unfortunately, is usually made retrospectively. Likewise, slipped capital femoral epiphysis can produce chondrolysis. If internal fixation of a slipped capital femoral epiphysis is necessary, the incidence of chondrolysis increases.[2] One should remember that technetium bone scans are better than radiographs for evaluating early avascular necrosis.

Anterior Dislocations

Anterior dislocations comprise only about 5% of all dislocations of the hip.[3] The mechanism of injury is forceful abduction and external rotation. This can occur in football, rugby, and soccer.

The symptoms include immediate pain, and the limb is usually abducted and externally rotated. Inspection may reveal a palpable mass in the groin. The displaced femoral head can compress the femoral vein and produce a thrombus.

As in posterior dislocation, treatment is urgent. Reduction is preceded by adequate radiographic evaluation to rule out a fracture of the femur. Reduction is usually accomplished under general anesthesia with longitudinal traction and internal rotation of the extremity. Open reduction is rarely required. If manipulation is delayed, pulmonary embolism can occur because of thrombus formation.

SLIPPED CAPITAL FEMORAL EPIPHYSIS

Slipped capital femoral epiphysis can occur in a growing athlete who is nearing skeletal maturity. Growth hormones and sex hormones, which are stimulated later than the growth hormones by anterior pituitary gonadotropin, coexist during adolescence.[3] Either decreased levels of gonadotropins (Fröhlich's syndrome) or an increased level of growth hormone upsets the normal hormone balance. The effect of the imbalance is a high level of growth hormone that causes the layer of hypertrophic cartilage cells in the epiphyseal line to widen. Harris found that fractures of the epiphyseal plate pass through this zone.[9]

This lesion is more common in boys than in girls, and it usually occurs between age 11 and 15 years. It is rare in girls after the onset of menses. Short, heavy boys are more commonly affected.[10]

A mechanism of injury is not always identifiable since the weakened growth plate is subject to fracture from the normal stresses across the hip. Pain is common but it cannot always be used as a basis for diagnosis. Pain is often referred to the knee; it is not uncommon to see a coach have a small, heavy boy with mild knee pain try to "run it out" when the patient actually has a slipped capital femoral epiphysis.

The most common early sign of the condition is a limp, usually a gluteus medius limp. This occurs because the femoral head of the epiphysis slips posteriorly and medially and the athlete has no fulcrum on which to walk (Fig. 62–3). As the force on the displaced epiphysis increases, displacement increases, and the other hip is likewise at risk.[11]

There are two rates of slipping of the upper femoral epiphysis: fast, or acute, and slow, or chronic. The two rates can coexist. In other words, a patient may have a chronic undiagnosed slipped capital femoral epiphysis and as the rate of slipping increases the head falls off farther and the pain increases. The diagnosis is made by the radiographic appearance of the femoral neck. Patients with chronic slips tend to have fewer symptoms.

This injury requires immediate evaluation by an orthopedist. Radiographs of the hip may appear normal if the examiner does not expect the lesion (Fig. 62–4A). Widening and irregularity of the epiphyseal line or other early signs can be missed. A frog-leg lateral radiograph may reveal a slip when the anteroposterior view appears normal (Fig. 62–4B).

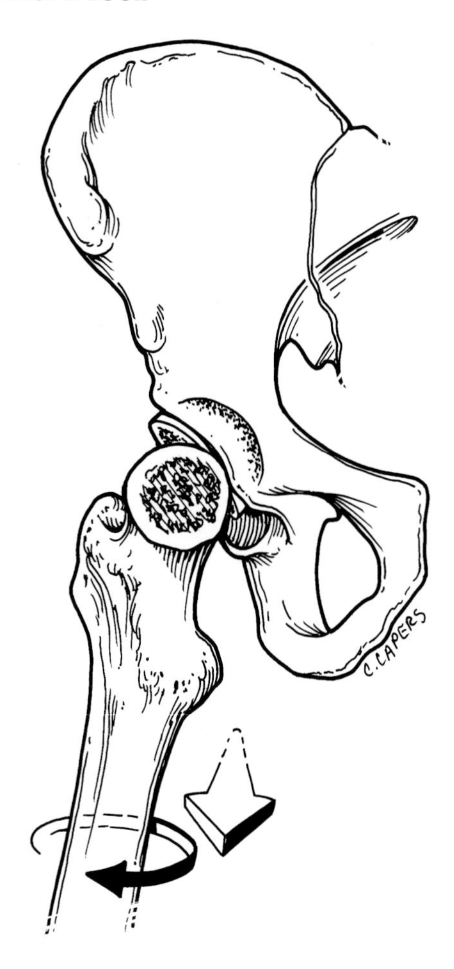

Fig. 62–3. In slipped capital femoral epiphysis, the femoral neck rotates anterior and laterad, while the head goes posterior and mediad.

Treatment depends on the type and degree of slip. Reduction and internal fixation are the treatment of choice and should be undertaken as soon as possible to prevent further displacement and risk of avascular necrosis. Although there is some controversy about the long-term results of operative treatment, internal fixation prevents further slipping and subsequent deformity.

FRACTURES OF THE FEMUR

The strength of the femur of adolescents and young adults is extremely good; however, this is the group who are most frequently involved in athletics. Fracture of the proximal femur itself is a rare athletic injury, but it does occur.[12] Severe trauma usually causes the injury. With the increased popularity of skiing, fractures of the hip and of the proximal femur have been seen in cross-country skiers.[13]

Fractures of the proximal femur are divided into extracapsular and intracapsular lesions.[14] Intracapsular fractures may be caused by indirect force such as a shear force on the angulated femoral neck.[15] Symptoms include immediate pain at time of injury and inability to walk. If the fracture is displaced, the leg may be short-

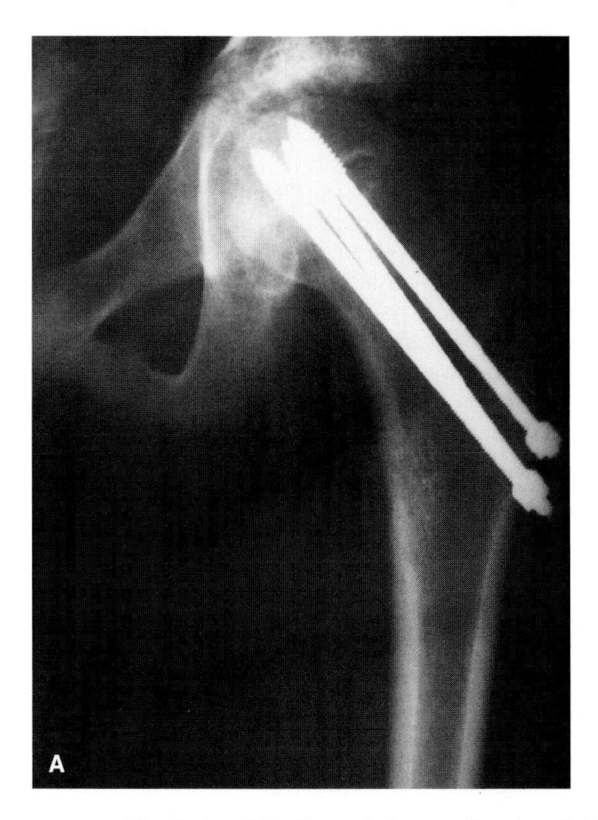

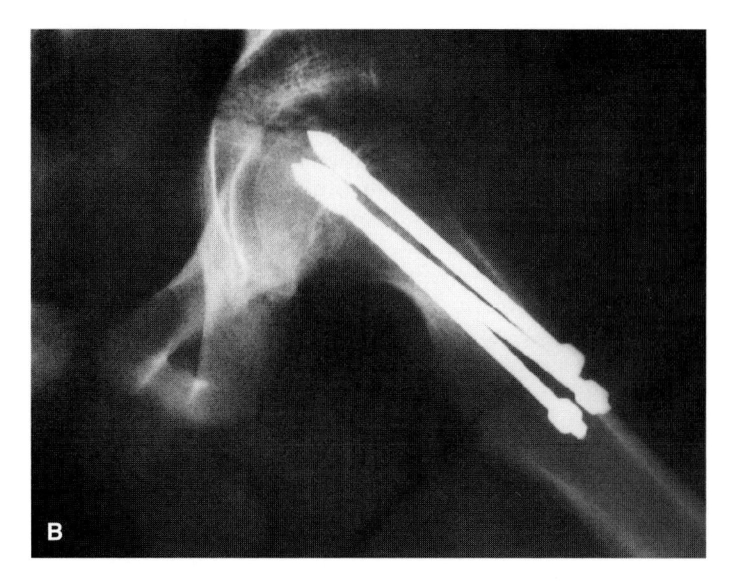

Fig. 62–4. *(A)* Radiograph shows a slipped capital femoral epiphysis that has been internally fixed. This anteroposterior view shows little deformity. *(B)* The frogleg x-ray projection of the patient in Figure 62–4A shows the minimal slip. (Henry, J. H.: The Hip. *In* Principles of Sports Medicine. Edited by W. N. Scott. Baltimore, Williams & Wilkins, 1984.)

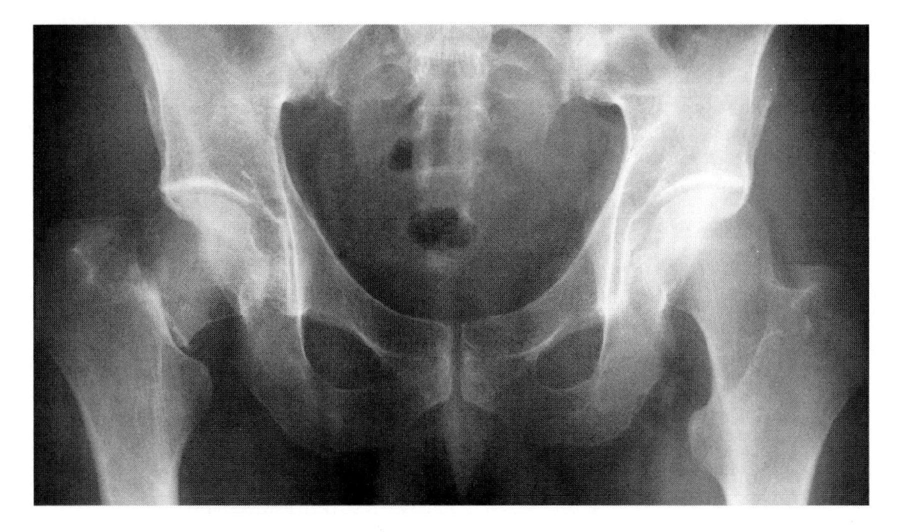

Fig. 62–5. Radiograph shows extracapsular fracture of the femur sustained in motorcross racing. (Henry, J. H.: The Hip. *In* Principles of Sports Medicine. Edited by W. N. Scott. Baltimore, Williams & Wilkins, 1984.)

ened and lying in external rotation. The fracture can be impacted or nondisplaced, and deformity of the leg is minimal. Pain on range of motion is the most consistent sign. Treatment is obviously immediate referral to an orthopedic surgeon because internal fixation is the treatment of choice.

Extracapsular fractures (Fig. 62–5) of the femur can occur with direct violence to the hip. In many cases, the fracture line is comminuted and blood loss is significant. As with the intracapsular variety, immediate pain and inability to walk on the hip are common. External rotation and shortening of the leg are usually more marked with extracapsular fractures. The treatment is open reduction and internal fixation. Traction applied to the extremity relieves the pain while the patient is being transferred.

Determination of the type of proximal femoral fracture is not important in an on-field examination. Rapid transfer of the patient is critical, however, since complications increase with delay in treatment. Radiographic evaluation is necessary before surgical treatment can be undertaken.

I would re-emphasize that fractures and dislocations of the hip are infrequent in athletes; however, early diagnosis is critical since delay of treatment can have devastating results. In most cases, a relatively conclusive diagnosis can be based on history and physical examination alone. However, early radiography at a facility within a short distance of the athletic field is of utmost importance since delay of treatment (e.g., for transfer) can affect the best surgical treatment.

REFERENCES

1. Cave, E. F., Burke, J. F., and Boyd, R. J.: Trauma Management. Chicago, Year Book, 1974.
2. O'Donoghue, D. H.: Treatment of Injuries to Athletes. 3rd Ed. Philadelphia, W. B. Saunders, 1976.
3. Strange, F. G. St. C.: The Hip. London, William Heinemann, 1965.
4. Rosenthal, R. E., and Coker, W. L.: Posterior fracture-dislocation of the hip: An epidemiologic review. J Trauma *19*:572, 1979.
5. Offierski, C. M.: Traumatic dislocation of the hip in children. J. Bone Joint Surg. *63B*:194, 1981.
6. Rockwood, C. A., and Green, D. P.: Fractures. Philadelphia, J. B. Lippincott, 1975.
7. Mandell, G. A., Keret, D., Harcke, T., and Bowen, J. R.: Chondrolysis: detection by bone scintigraphy. J. Pediatr. Orthop. *12*:80, 1992.
8. Cooper, D. E., Warren, R. F., and Barnes, R.: Traumatic subluxation of the hip resulting in aseptic necrosis and chondrolysis in a professional football player. Am. J. Sports Med. *19*:322, 1991.
9. Harris, W. R.: The endocrine basis for slipping of the upper femoral epiphysis. J. Bone Joint Surg. *32B*:5, 1950.
10. Scott, J. C.: Displacement of the upper epiphysis of the femur. *In* Platt, H.: Modern Trends in Orthopedics, Series 2. London, Butterworths, 1956.
11. Tachdjian, M. O.: Pediatric Orthopaedics. Philadelphia, W. B. Saunders, 1972.
12. Hachenbruch, V. W.: Schenkelhalsfraktur und pertrochantere Fraktur des Skifahrers. Fortschr. Med. *96*:123, 1978.
13. Frost, A., and Bauer, M.: Skier's hip—a new clinical entity? J. Orthop. Trauma *5*:47, 1991.
14. Watson-Jones, R.: *In* Wilson, J. N.: Fractures and joint injuries. 5th Ed. Vol. 2. New York, Churchill Livingstone, 1976.
15. McLaughlin, H. L.: Trauma. Philadelphia, W. B. Saunders, 1960.

Overuse Injuries of the Hip

David M. Kahler

The complaint of vague hip or groin pain is exceedingly common among athletes. It has been reported that 28% of soccer players have a history of a groin injury, and that 5% of all soccer injuries involve the hip or groin region.[1,2] Athletes who participate in cutting sports or in repetitive cyclic loading are at risk for overuse injuries, owing to the great stresses generated in the muscles and skeletal structures surrounding the hip joint.

The perceived location of pain is paramount in evaluating hip pain in an athlete. Most athletes think that lateral hip pain in the region of the greater trochanter is coming from the hip joint. In reality, lateral pain is usually caused by muscle strains or trochanteric bursitis. Pain from the hip joint itself usually radiates to the groin or the anterior thigh. Groin pain is often caused by routine sprains or strains, but it can be a manifestation of a potentially serious condition such as stress fracture, inguinal hernia, or slipped capital femoral epiphysis. Though initially, lateral pain can be treated symptomatically, the athlete with groin pain must be evaluated aggressively to determine the source of pain. Early appropriate treatment of the more serious conditions much reduces the risk of prolonged disability from an overuse injury.

The patient's age and history often direct the clinician to a tentative diagnosis. Growing athletes are prone to bony apophyseal avulsions following strenuous activity or repetitive stress, while skeletally mature athletes most often strain muscles or musculotendinous junctions. Stress fractures are nearly always preceded by an unaccustomed increase in training; this might include an increase in running mileage while training for a marathon or the strenuous first week in boot camp. Careful questioning can help to eliminate referred pain from the back or the genitourinary system as the source of a hip complaint. It should be kept in mind that a young athlete with vague knee pain may actually be describing referred pain from the hip, and this complaint should always prompt a hip examination.

STRESS FRACTURES

Stress Fractures of the Femoral Neck

Stress fracture of the femoral neck is perhaps the most commonly missed serious overuse injury involving the hip. This injury appears to be most common in distance runners. In a large series of stress fractures in military recruits, only nine of 257 fractures involved the femoral neck.[3] In the absence of underlying bone disease (such as osteoporosis), a history of an increase or change in training is always present. A simple stress fracture, if left untreated, may progress to a displaced femoral neck fracture; this disastrous consequence of a delay in diagnosis requires surgical treatment and may result in loss of the hip joint due to avascular necrosis. When detected and treated early, these injuries usually follow a benign course.

The symptoms of stress fracture of the femoral neck are often vague, and the athlete may not seek treatment until training is impossible, because of pain. The pain is achy and is usually localized to the anterior groin or thigh. Symptoms are most prominent upon arising in the morning and are often relieved by moderate activity. The athlete may not notice significant hip pain until the middle of a training run.

Physical examination of a patient with stress fracture of the femoral neck may reveal only subtle loss of motion and pain at the extremes of flexion and internal rotation. Tenderness to direct palpation is not prominent because of the thick pelvic girdle musculature surrounding the hip joint. Radiographic studies of the hip

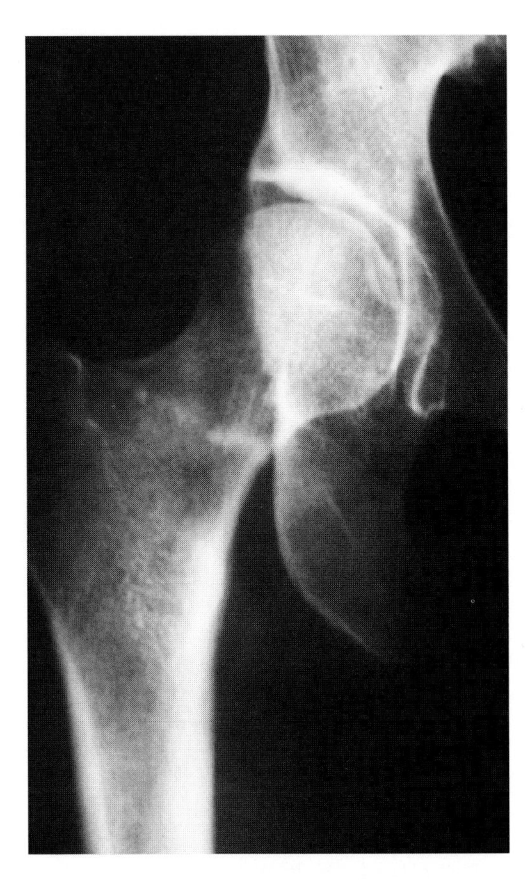

Fig. 62–6. This medial compression type stress fracture of the femoral neck demonstrates the typical sclerosis and endosteal callus seen 2 to 4 weeks after onset of symptoms.

are usually normal at the time of initial presentation and do not show the characteristic sclerosis and subtle fracture line until several weeks after the onset of symptoms (Fig. 62–6). For this reason, a high index of suspicion is necessary, and sophisticated imaging techniques are often required to confirm the diagnosis.

Radioisotope bone scanning has become the standard diagnostic test for the evaluation of suspected stress fractures. Bone scintigraphy typically shows positive findings well before radiographic changes become evident (Fig. 62–7). When the bone scan is positive but no fracture or healing response is identified radiographically, the injury is more properly referred to as a *stress reaction*. A case has been reported in which a patient who was later found to have a stress fracture had a negative bone scan 12 days after onset of symptoms.[4] When stress fracture is suspected but radiographs and bone scans are negative, magnetic resonance imaging (MRI) can be used to confirm the diagnosis (Fig. 62–8). As the cost of MRI decreases, it may become the diagnostic procedure of choice.

The radiographic appearance of a stress fracture of the femoral neck is important in determining the course of treatment. The fracture usually appears on radiographs as an area of increased density or "endosteal callus" in the medial aspect of the femoral neck, just proximal to the lesser trochanter.[5] This becomes more pronounced in the following 2 weeks. Less commonly, a fracture line is seen in the superior femoral neck. These tension-side stress fractures are more likely to progress and become displaced than the

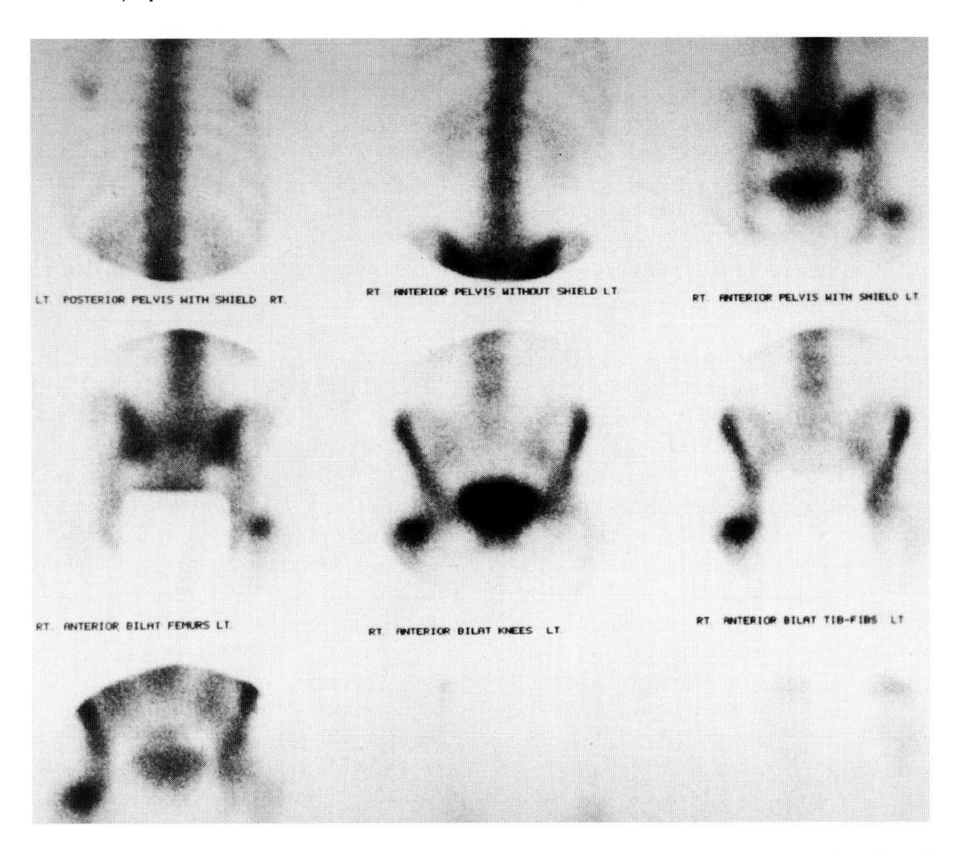

Fig. 62–7. The late phase of a technetium bone scan reveals increased uptake in the right femoral neck, indicating a healing stress fracture.

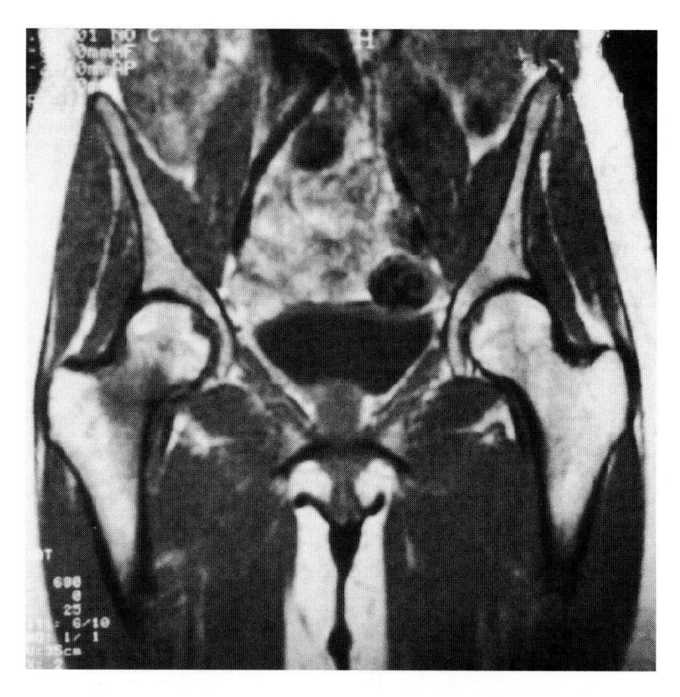

Fig. 62–8. MRI reveals marrow edema and bony sclerosis *(dark area)* typical of a stress fracture of the medial right femoral neck.

more common compression-side stress fracture.[6] It is rare for a stress fracture of the femoral neck to present as a complete or displaced fracture unless diagnosis has been delayed.

Treatment of a stress fracture of the femoral neck is relatively straightforward if the diagnosis is made in a timely fashion. Stress reactions and medial compression-side stress injuries are treated with protected weight bearing until morning pain is eliminated and painless ambulation is possible. Water exercises and stationary cycling may be used to maintain aerobic capacity during the healing process. Pain-free activity is gradually increased until repetitive loading is possible without pain. Six to eight weeks of restricted activity often is necessary, and activity must be curtailed if there is any recurrence of pain. Intermittent radiographs should be obtained to document that there has been no progression of the fracture line. Although there is a low complication rate in this population, full recovery may take 2 years or longer.[7] In a longterm followup of stress fractures of the femoral neck, all elite athletes in the series had to end their careers as a result of their injuries; in most of these cases, diagnosis had been significantly delayed.[8]

Tension-side stress fractures are usually treated surgically, to prevent the disastrous complication of fracture displacement. Cannulated screws are placed percutaneously across the femoral neck under fluoroscopic guidance. Athletic activity is interdicted until radiographs show healing of the fracture. Displaced fractures of the femoral neck are treated by closed or open reduction and fixation with cannulated screws or a sliding compression screw. The prognosis for displaced fractures is poor. In one series, six of ten athletes with a displaced femoral neck stress fracture had serious complications after treatment, including avascular necrosis, nonunion, and refracture; all required repeat surgery, and two underwent total hip replacement. The average delay in diagnosis in this group was 11 weeks. The authors of this series speculate that early use of bone scintigraphy when a runner presents with exertional groin pain could prevent the high complication rate seen in this series, although they noted that this was often a sports career–ending injury, even when properly treated.[8]

Other Stress Fractures

In distance runners, the inferior pubic ramus is at risk for stress fracture. This injury is much more common in women and usually occurs in experienced runners after a marathon or a sudden increase in training distance.[5] Tensile stresses generated in the hamstring muscle origins are responsible for pubic ramus stress fractures, and bilateral lesions or subsequent development of a contralateral fracture are common. Despite the frequent radiographic appearance of nonunion, these injuries heal eventually if painful activity is restricted sufficiently.[9] The amenorrheic female distance runner who presents with this condition should have a bone density study and endocrine evaluation to determine whether adjunctive treatment of the underlying abnormality is indicated.

Stress fractures of the femoral shaft can occur in the medial subtrochanteric region, where great compressive stresses are generated. Thickening of the medial cortex of the femur is seen, and occasionally a fracture line becomes evident. An athlete who has radiographic evidence of focal cortical thickening but fails to respond to restriction of activity should be evaluated by CT, to rule out the possibility of osteoid osteoma. This benign tumor of bone causes chronic pain and reactive cortical changes, and a characteristic central nidus is usually well demonstrated by CT. Similarly, any patient with a persistent fracture line after treatment should be evaluated with routine laboratory testing for metabolic bone disease.

PAIN AT MUSCLE ORIGINS

Strain of the proximal adductor musculature is the most common painful overuse injury about the hip in adult athletes. The abductor musculature may be similarly involved, and tendinitis of the gluteus medius origin near the iliac crest can cause painful disability. After the initial pain has subsided, application of heat or ultrasound, gentle stretching, nonsteroidal anti-inflammatory drugs, and progressive resistance exercises may hasten a return to full activity.

The growing athlete more commonly injures the apophyses where the pelvic girdle musculature originates rather than the muscles or tendons themselves (Fig. 62–9). The apophyses appear between the ages of 11 and 15 years and account for circumferential growth of the pelvis and trochanters. The cartilaginous growth

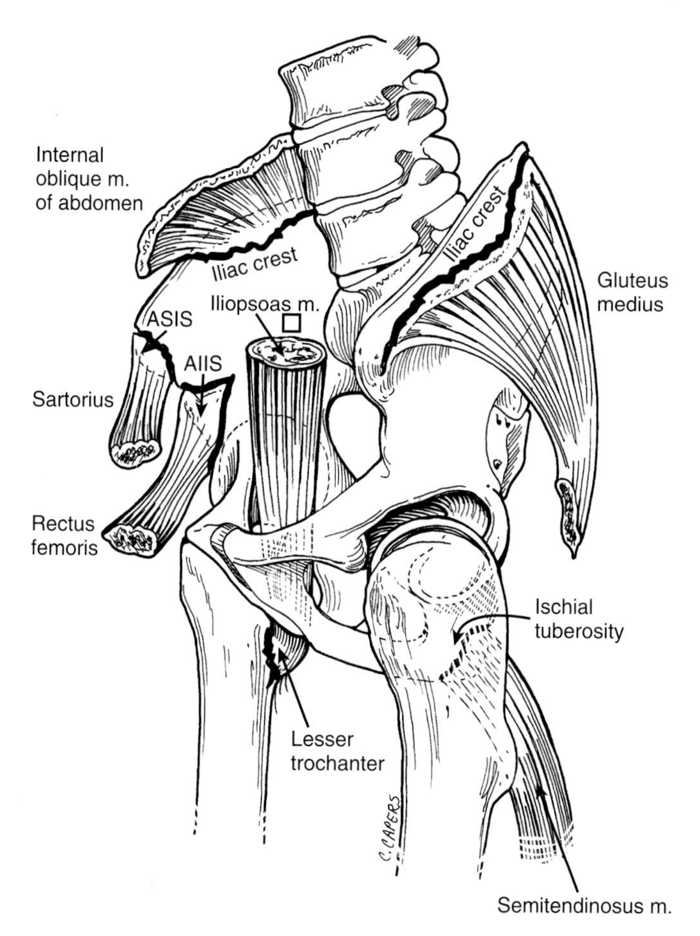

Fig. 62–9. Common sites of avulsion injuries of the hip in adolescents.

plates are the weakest point in the continuum from bone to muscle and may fail with sudden muscle loading or more gradually, with repetitive stress.[10] Gradual failure of muscle attachments to the growing skeleton is termed *apophysitis,* since it is the bony apophysis that becomes displaced. These injuries are readily demonstrated on routine radiographs and often heal with exuberant bone formation. Local tenderness can be used to direct the radiographic examination, and views of the contralateral side are helpful for comparison because of the great variability in the ossification of the apophyses. The diagnosis is based on history, physical examination, and characteristic radiographic changes.

Treatment of apophysitis includes protecting the apophysis from loading during the healing process, usually by protected weight bearing with crutches. It is not necessary to surgically replace the displaced apophysis. Gradual return to activity is allowed, as dictated by pain, and careful attention is given to stretching the involved muscle groups to prevent excessive tension on the apophysis. Radiographs should be obtained before full return to activity, to document healing. In rare cases, it may be necessary to remove the displaced apophysis or the mass of ectopic bone that forms during the healing process. The temptation to take a biopsy specimen of these lesions should be resisted because on microscopic examination the repair process is easily mistaken for osteogenic sarcoma.[5] In the growing athlete, a "hip pointer" is usually an avulsion of the iliac apophysis from the pelvis by strong contraction of the abdominal musculature or a direct blow. Padding the apophysis to prevent reinjury should be considered when the athlete returns to contact sports. In all cases, full return to competition is restricted until flexibility and strength are reestablished.

BURSITIS AND THE SNAPPING HIP

Two large bursas adjacent to the hip are responsible for a significant proportion of athletic hip and groin pain. The generic term *trochanteric bursitis* refers to chronic inflammation of the bursa between the gluteus maximus–tensor fascia lata muscles and the greater trochanter of the femur. Bursitis in this region is easily diagnosed by direct palpation, and sometimes by diagnostic injection of local anesthetic. Treatment of this condition consists of eliminating the activity that causes pain and by stretching the iliotibial band, both in flexion and in extension. Oral nonsteroidal anti- inflammatory agents or local injections of corticosteroids may hasten recovery. Chronic bursitis or fibrosis of the gluteus maximus can cause a syndrome known as *the snapping hip,* or more properly *external snapping hip.*[11,12]

The iliopsoas bursa lies beneath the muscle bellies of the iliac and psoas muscles as they pass over the pelvic brim and the anterior hip capsule. This largest of all of the synovial bursas in the human body communicates directly with the hip joint in 15% of all persons.[13] Bursitis of the iliopsoas bursa can cause groin pain in athletes. Although this primary condition is rarely diagnosed, secondary tendinitis and chronic bursitis can cause "internal snapping hip."

External snapping hip, first described in 1884,[14] causes a sensation of clunking or subluxation in the hip while the athlete is walking, running, or pivoting. The patient may insist that the hip is "coming out of joint." The symptomatic snap may be elicited by extending the knee and hip in adduction and then flexing the hip. The patient usually demonstrates the snapping while standing with the hip in extension and forcibly internally rotating it. This condition is often alleviated by treating the underlying bursitis. Resistant cases with fibrosis of the overlying structures may be treated surgically by Z-plasty of the iliotibial band or by excision of the portion of the iliotibial band overlying the greater trochanter.[12,15]

Internal snapping hip is less common and is caused by the iliopsoas tendon snapping over the iliopectineal eminence where it crosses the pelvic brim. This condition usually occurs as the patient extends the hip from a flexed, abducted, and externally rotated position. The snapping sensation is associated with pain in the deep anterior groin. Although this maneuver may be diagnostic, iliopsoas bursography may be performed when the diagnosis is in question. Most patients respond to stretching of the hip flexor musculature. The rare resistant case may be amenable to surgical lengthening of the iliopsoas tendon.[16]

INGUINAL HERNIA

Inguinal hernia represents extrusion of a portion of the abdominal contents through a defect in the abdominal wall and typically causes pain in the anterior groin. Although a frank inguinal hernia is easily demonstrated on physical examination, occult weakness of the abdominal muscular insertions has been demonstrated to be a cause of groin pain in athletes. A series of nine athletes who underwent herniorrhaphy for groin pain revealed two patients who had no physical evidence of hernia preoperatively. At surgery one was found to have an inguinal hernia; the other had an abnormality of the internal oblique muscle insertion at the pubic tubercle. The authors of this series noted that athletes reliably returned to sporting activity within 3 months after the surgical procedure.[17]

CONCLUSION

Chronic hip pain may be a manifestation of a serious underlying condition in athletes. Knowledge of the various overuse conditions and their associated findings allows rapid diagnosis and may prevent a period of prolonged disability or permanent damage to the hip joint. Although stress fracture of the femoral neck is the most important injury to be ruled out, the clinician should be wary of the other less common diagnoses that may cause hip or groin pain in athletes.

REFERENCES

1. Renstrom, P., and Peterson, L.: Groin injuries in athletes. Br. J. Sports Med. *14*:30, 1980.
2. Smodlaka, V. N.: Groin pain in soccer players. Physician Sportsmed. *8*:57, 1980.
3. Volpin, G., et al.: Stress fractures of the femoral neck following strenuous activity. J. Orthop. Trauma *4*:394, 1990.
4. Keene, J. S., and Lash, E. G.: Negative bone scan in a femoral neck stress fracture: A case report. Am. J. Sports Med. *20*:234, 1992.
5. Pavlov, H.: Roentgen examination of groin and hip pain in the athlete. Clin. Sports Med. 6:829, 1987.
6. Blickenstaff, L. D., and Morris, J. M.: Fatigue fracture of the femoral neck. J. Bone Joint Surg. *48A*:1031, 1966.
7. Fullerton, L. R., Jr., and Snowdy, H. A.: Femoral neck stress fractures. Am. J. Sports Med. *16*:365, 1988.
8. Johansson, C., et al.: Stress fractures of the femoral neck in athletes: The consequence of a delay in diagnosis. Am. J. Sports Med. *18*:524, 1990.
9. Pavlov, H., Nelson, T. L., and Warren, R. F.: Stress fractures of the pubic ramus. A report of twelve cases. J. Bone Joint Surg. *64A*:1020, 1982.
10. Waters, P. M., and Millis, M. B.: Hip and pelvic injuries in the young athlete. Clin. Sports Med. *7*:513, 1988.
11. Brignall, C. G., Brown, R. M., and Stainsby, G. D.: Fibrosis of the gluteus maximus as a cause of snapping hip. J. Bone Joint Surg. *75A*:909, 1993.
12. Brignall, C. G., and Stainsby, G. D.: The snapping hip. J. Bone Joint Surg. *73B*:253, 1991.
13. Michele, A. A.: Iliopsoas. Springfield, IL, Charles C Thomas, 1962.
14. Gibney, V. P.: The hip and its diseases. New York/London, Bermingham and Co., 1884.
15. Zoltan, D. J., Clancy, W. G., Jr., and Keene, J. S.: A new operative approach to snapping hip and refractory trochanteric bursitis in athletes. Am. J. Sports Med. *14*:201, 1986.
16. Jacobson, T., and Allen, W. C.: Surgical correction of the snapping iliopsoas tendon. Am. J. Sports Med. *18*:470, 1990.
17. Taylor, D. C., et al.: Abdominal musculature abnormalities as a cause of groin pain in athletes; inguinal hernias and pubalgia. Am. J. Sports Med. *19*:239, 1991.

63 *Geoffrey Vaupel and Scott Dye*

Functional Knee Anatomy

The knee is uniquely vulnerable to injury because of its precarious location midway between the hip and the ankle and because of the tremendous forces transmitted from the ground through the knee to the hip. Menschik and Dye have compared the knee to a "stepless transmission," in which the ligaments act as the linkage and the menisci and articular cartilage as the bearings.[1, 2] This analogy is useful in explaining to patients the nature of their injuries; however, understanding and describing the complex interplay between the numerous anatomic components of this living transmission is a never-ending challenge.

FEMOROTIBIAL JOINT

Osseous Anatomy

The medial knee compartment is more constrained than the lateral one because of the osseous, meniscal, and ligamentous morphology. This may explain the greater prevalence of medial knee injuries. The medial femoral condyle is smaller in anteroposterior diameter than the lateral condyle, and the lateral condyle is broader in the transverse plane. The width of the medial femoral condyle is nearly constant, but the lateral condyle is narrower on its posterior surface. The wider portion is in contact with the tibia during knee extension (Fig. 63–1).

The medial tibial plateau is concave and, combined with the deepening of the medial meniscus, provides a more constrained articulation for the medial femoral condyle. The lateral tibial plateau is slightly convex, which appears to be incongruous with the shape of the femoral condyle, but this convex surface allows greater "roll-back" of the lateral femoral condyle with flexion.[3] Both the convexity of the lateral tibial plateau and the larger surface area of the lateral femoral condyle contribute to the screw-home mechanism, that is, internal rotation of the femur with terminal extension.

The tibial surface slopes posteriorly about 10°.[4] Since the knee is flexed during running and cutting, this angulation brings the tibial plateau almost parallel with the weight-bearing surface. Without this natural posterior slope, the plateau would slope anteriorly in functional positions, which would compromise functional stability.

The spaces between the medial and lateral femoral condyles and the joint capsule are called the medial and lateral gutters. If scarring occurs within the gutters, range of motion can be severely restricted. Therefore, surgical dissection in these areas must be undertaken with great care.

Menisci

The menisci are fibrocartilaginous wedges that lie between the femoral condyles and the tibial plateaus (Fig. 63–2). The medial meniscus has been described as being more C shaped than the nearly circular lateral meniscus. The lateral meniscus covers a larger surface area of the tibial plateau (approximately two thirds) than the medial meniscus. The concave superior surface of each meniscus conforms to the shape of the femoral condyles, whereas the inferior surface is flat as it sits on the tibial plateau. The periphery of each meniscus is convex and thicker than the concave, thin inner margin. The menisci are divided into thirds for descriptive purposes: the anterior horn, the body, and the posterior horn. The posterior horn is usually thicker than the body and the anterior horn. The anterior horn of each meniscus is connected to the other by the intermeniscal or transverse ligament.

The medial meniscus has a continuous and less compliant peripheral attachment than the lateral meniscus.

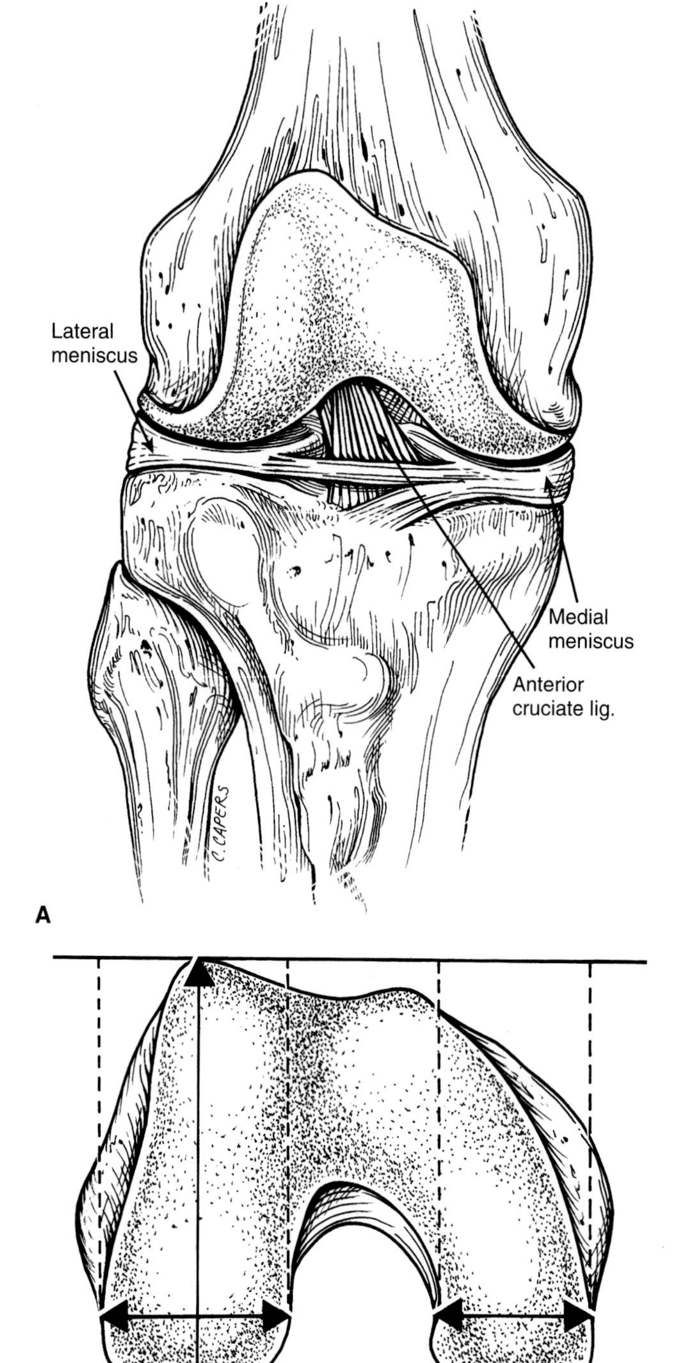

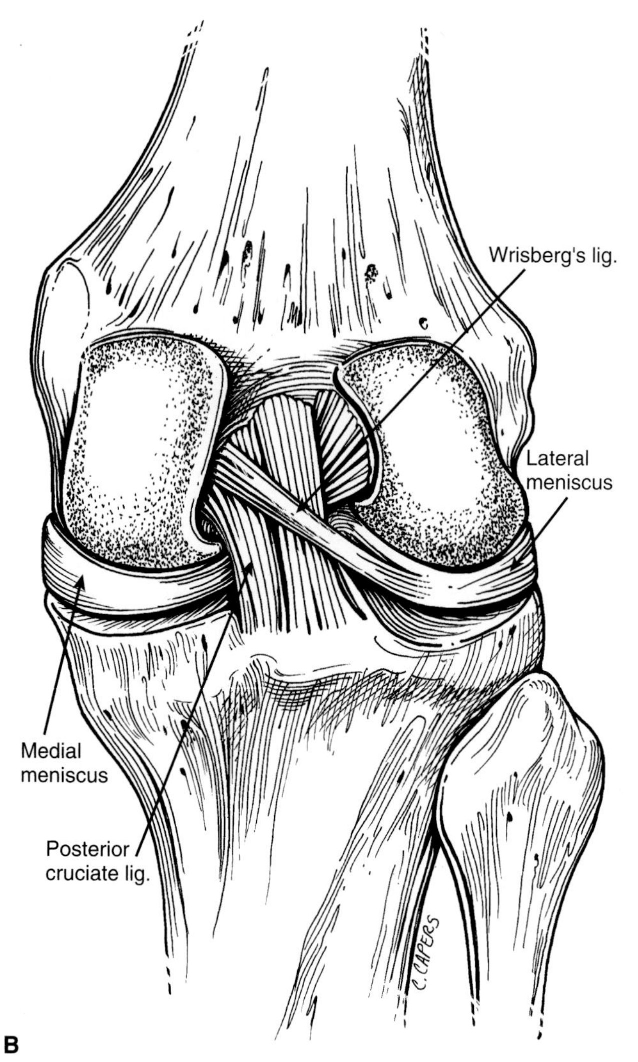

Fig. 63–1. ***(A)*** **Anterior and** ***(B)*** **posterior views of the knee show the osseous morphology, the menisci, and the orientation of the cruciate ligaments.** ***(C)*** **A comparison of the medial and lateral femoral condyles shows that the lateral condyle is broader in the transverse plane.**

There is an interruption in the peripheral attachment of the lateral meniscus where the popliteus tendon passes through a hiatus in the posterolateral aspect. The posterior horn of the lateral meniscus has attachments to the posterior cruciate ligament and the medial femoral condyle through the ligaments of Wrisberg and Humphry.[5]

Both menisci passively follow the femur posteriorly with knee flexion. The lateral meniscus travels approximately twice as far posteriorly as the medial one (11 mm versus 5 mm, respectively) as documented by cine–magnetic resonance imaging (cine-MRI).[6] The increased motion of the lateral meniscus necessitates a more compliant meniscotibial ligament attachment. The more adherent medial meniscus anchor may explain the greater incidence of medial meniscus tears. The contribution of the popliteus and the semimembranosus to active retraction, respectively, of the lateral and medial meniscus, is unknown.

Many functions have been attributed to the menisci, including load transmission, shock absorption, stress reduction, joint stability, limiting extremes of flexion and extension, and joint lubrication and nutrition.[7] The menisci also deepen the tibial plateau, making the femoral articulation comparable to a shallow ball-and-socket arrangement.[4]

Intercondylar Anatomy

The intercondylar region consists of the femoral intercondylar notch, the tibial intercondylar eminence

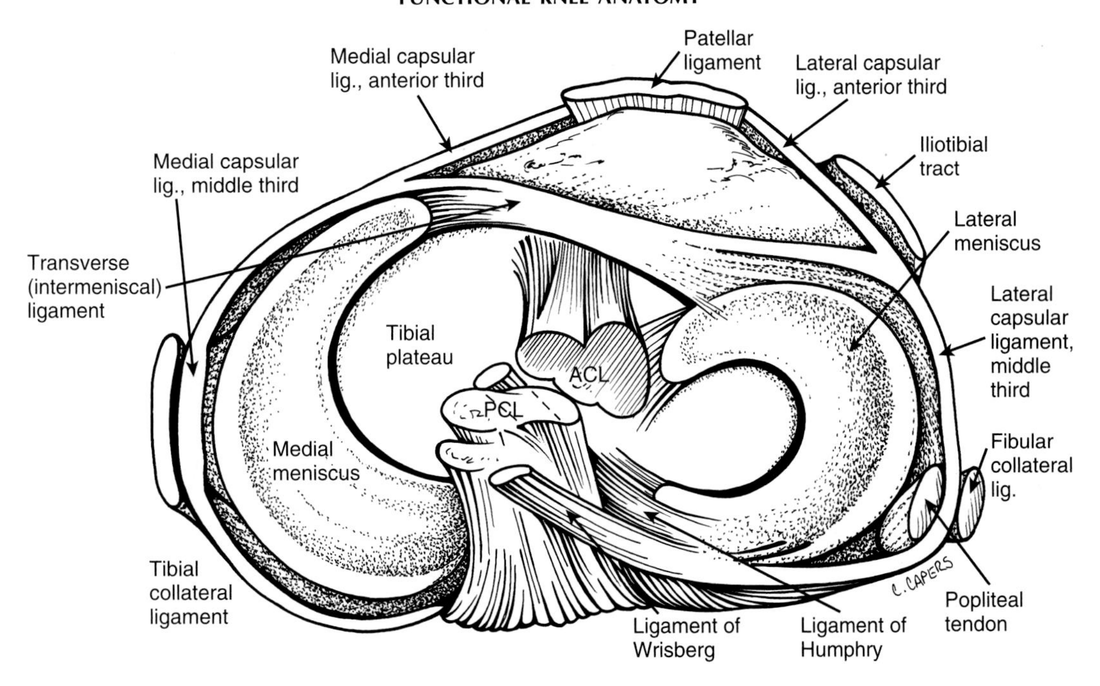

Fig. 63–2. An overhead view of the menisci shows the ligamentous attachment by the transverse ligament and the ligaments of Humphry and Wrisberg.

or spine, both cruciate ligaments, and the anterior and posterior horn attachments of the menisci. This area, situated at the center of axial rotation in the knee, is termed the *central pivot.*[8] The intercondylar eminence functions as the base of the central pivot. It helps guide and stabilize the femur through the flexion arc. This is accomplished in two ways: (1) The anterior and posterior horns of the menisci are anchored at the tibial eminence and, so, serve as checkreins to rotation and translation of the femur. (2) The intercondylar articular surface of the femur articulates with the tibial eminence, sharing the compressive weight-bearing forces with the menisci and the tibial plateau. Thus, the tibial eminence guides the femur much as a monorail guides a train. This is especially significant in the middle range of flexion, when axial loads are great and the peripheral ligaments relatively lax. It also explains the typical position of osteochondritis dissecans, which may be thought of more accurately as an osteochondral fracture rather than an avascular event.

Posterior Cruciate Ligament

Most authors consider the posterior cruciate ligament the principal ligamentous contribution to the central pivot.[8–11] Evidence to support this lies in its greater thickness [12] and strength as compared with the anterior cruciate ligament.[13] Furthermore, its position most closely approximates the axis of knee rotation.[14]

The posterior cruciate ligament is divided into the posteromedial and anterolateral bundles vis à vis the site of femoral attachment. Only the posteromedial fibers are taut in knee extension. During flexion, the anterolateral fibers are progressively tensed (Fig. 63–3A). At full knee flexion all fibers are equally taut. The posterior cruciate ligament assumes a nearly vertical orientation in full flexion and is more horizontal with knee extension. With full flexion, the posterior cruciate ligament is in contact with the roof of the posterior intercondylar notch.[15]

The tibial attachment of the posterior cruciate ligament is in the tibial fovea, just anterior to the posterior tibial condyles and extending at least 1 cm distal to the joint line. The femoral attachment, however, extends well anterior and ends just posterior to the articular surface of the intercondylar surface of the medial femoral condyle. The "tibial footprint" is almost square, whereas that of the femur is more oblong and rectangular because the posterior cruciate ligament fans out as it approaches the femur.

Simple point-to-point kinematics cannot explain the function of either the posterior or the anterior cruciate ligament. These structures must be thought of as a continuum of thousands of collagen fibers acting in concert through the flexion arc. Thinking in these terms, one can understand the frustration in trying to interpret isometric measurements.

Two meniscofemoral ligaments commonly are associated with the posterior cruciate ligament, the ligament of Humphry anteriorly and the ligament of Wrisberg posteriorly (*see* Fig. 63–2). They vary in size and are sometimes absent entirely. One of the meniscofemoral ligaments is found in nearly every knee, but rarely are both found in the same knee, and even more rarely are both ligaments found in both knees.[16] The ligament of Wrisberg may be as large as half the diameter of the posterior cruciate ligament, whereas the ligament of Humphry is no larger than one-third the diameter of the posterior cruciate ligament.[17]

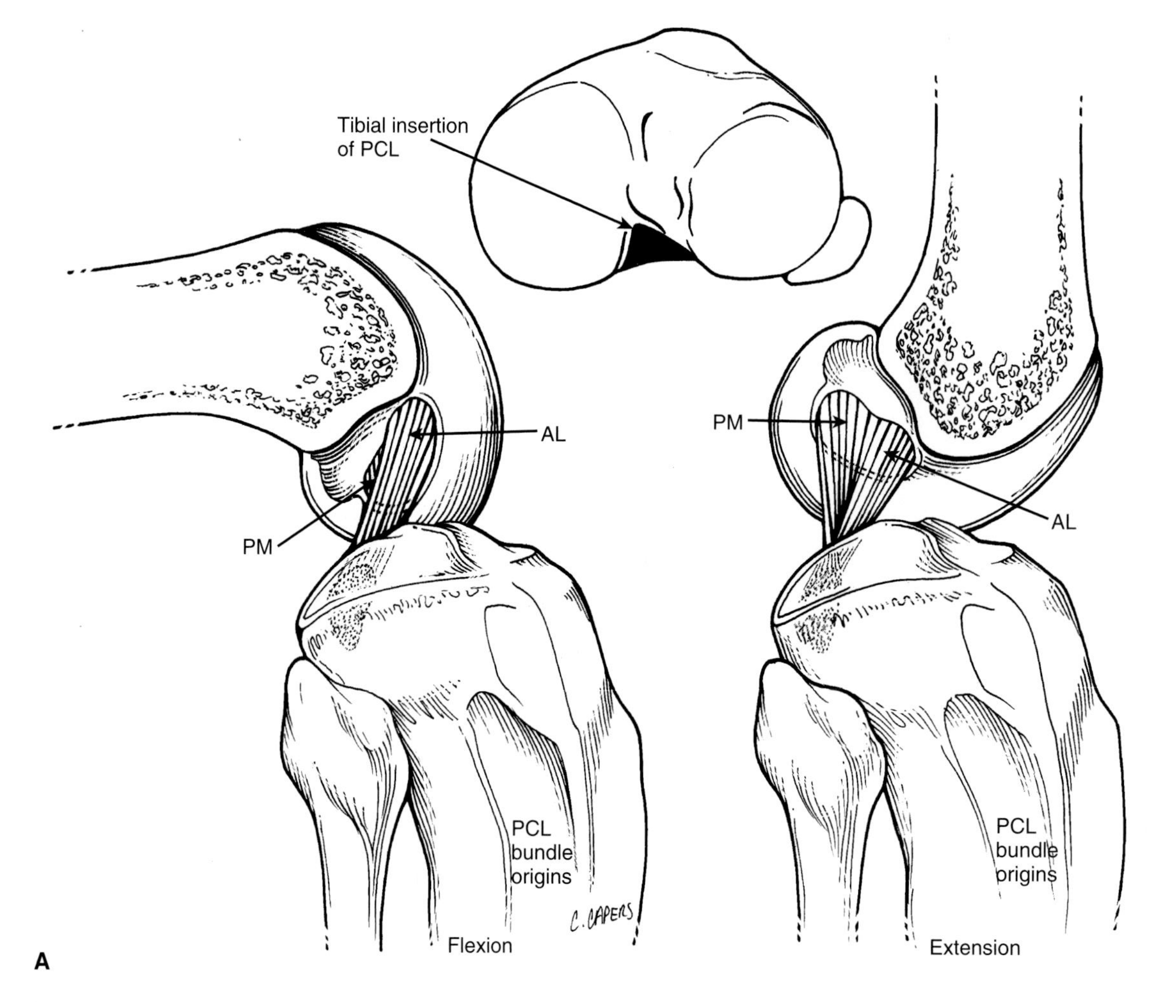

Fig. 63–3. ***(A)*** **Attachment sites of the posteromedial (PM) and anterolateral (AL) bundles of the posterior cruciate ligament (PCL). During knee flexion, the anterolateral fibers are progressively tensed.** ***(B)*** **The anterior cruciate ligament is divided into three bundles based on the tibial attachment: the anteromedial (AM), the intermediate (I), and the posterolateral (PL). With knee flexion, the posterior fibers loosen and the anteromedial fibers coil around the posterolateral ones.**

The ligament of Wrisberg is variably attached to the posterior lateral meniscus, the tibia, or the posterior capsule. It then runs proximally and obliquely across the posterior aspect of the posterior cruciate ligament and attaches to the medial femoral condyle at the posterior cruciate ligament attachment.

The ligament of Humphry arises from the posterior horn of the lateral meniscus, runs anterior to the posterior cruciate ligament, and attaches to the medial femoral condyle with the anterolateral bundle.

The ligament of Humphry is taut in flexion, and the ligament of Wrisberg is taut in extension. Both ligaments tighten with internal rotation of the tibia and can confound the posterior drawer test. Thus, the posterior drawer test must also be done with the tibia in neutral position and in external rotation.[18]

Anterior Cruciate Ligament

The anterior cruciate ligament, like the posterior cruciate ligament, is an intracapsular but extrasynovial structure. It is covered by a synovial sheath that protects it from the synovial fluid. The anterior cruciate ligament, like the posterior cruciate, has been divided into bundles, but, instead of two bundles defined by the femoral attachments, the anterior cruciate ligament has three bundles defined by the tibial attachments [19]: the anteromedial, the intermediate, and the posterolateral bundles (Fig. 63–3B). In many knees, these bundles are difficult to discern on gross inspection. The purpose in describing them is to help readers conceptualize the different behavior displayed by the anterior and posterior fibers throughout the flexion arc.

In terminal knee extension, all fibers of the anterior cruciate ligament are taut. The anterior fibers abut the intercondylar roof; though with progressive knee flexion, the posterior fibers loosen and the anteromedial fibers coil around the posterolateral ones. The anterior fibers remain taut throughout the flexion arc and are the most isometric. Therefore, the anterior edge of the anterior cruciate ligament serves as the rotational axis of the ligament during knee motion.[15] The anterior cruciate ligament is the principal restraint to anterior

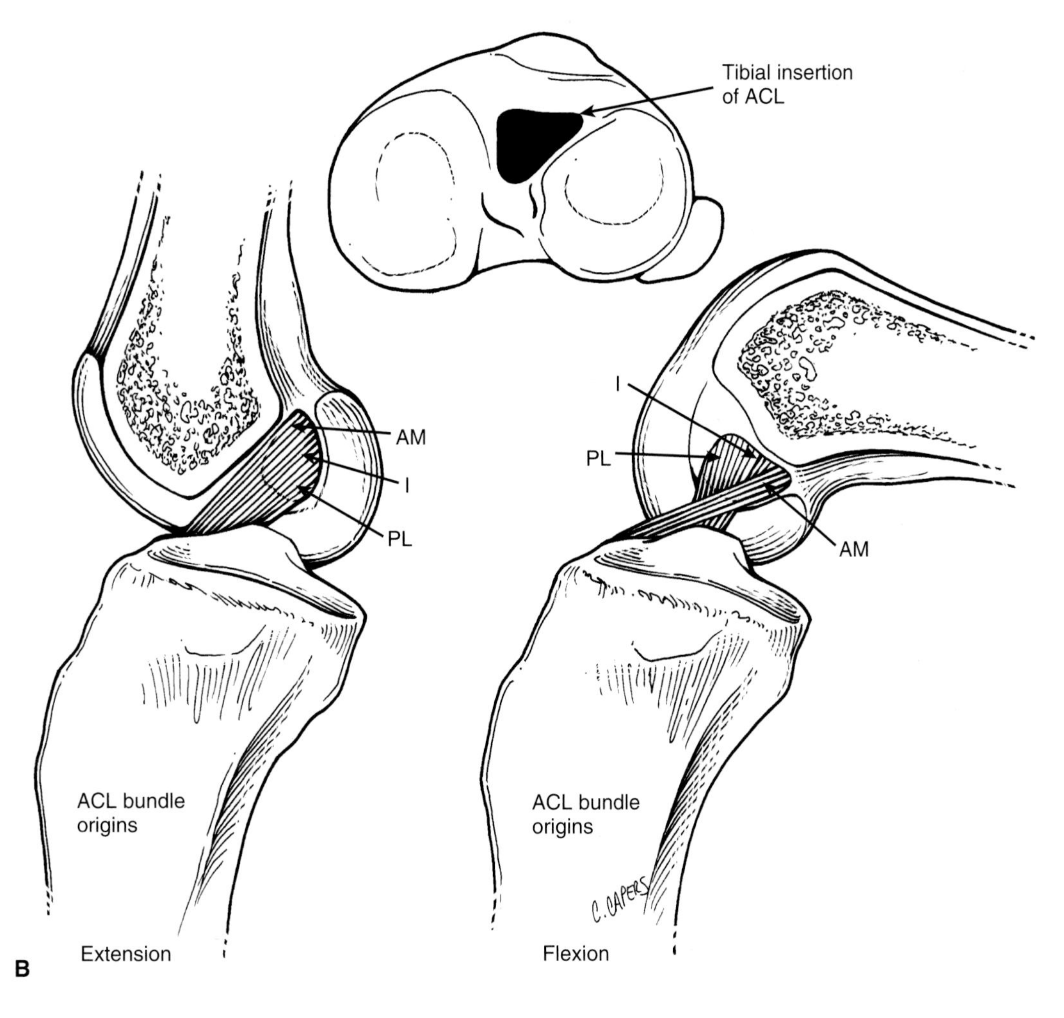

Fig. 63–3. *(Continued)*

tibial translation and is a secondary restraint to varus and valgus forces.[20]

PATELLOFEMORAL JOINT

The function of the patellofemoral joint is to increase the force of quadriceps pull by increasing the lever arm of the extensor mechanism. The thickness of the patella displaces the patellar tendon away from the femorotibial contact point.[21] The patella has three facets, medial, lateral, and odd. The medial and lateral facets are separated by a longitudinal ridge called the median ridge. The odd facet is smaller in area than the medial and lateral facets and lies at the extreme medial border of the patellar articular surface. The articular cartilage on the undersurface of the patella is the thickest of any of the human diarthrodial joints. It is thickest in cross section at its midportion and relatively thinner near the proximal and distal poles.[22]

The trochlea is that portion of the anterior femur that articulates with the patella. Its two facets, medial and lateral, unite in the midline to form a groove. The median ridge of the patella rides in this groove, whereas the medial and lateral facets of the patella contact the corresponding trochlear facets. The lateral facet projects farther anterior and proximal than the medial facet, adding to patellar stability.

The area of contact between the patella and the femur varies with the position of the knee (Fig. 63–4).[23] With the knee in full extension, the patella lies superior and lateral to the trochlea and rests in the supratrochlear pulvinar (Latin "a cushioned seat"), or fat pad.[2] The distal patellar surface contacts the proximal trochlea in 20° of flexion. As the knee flexes, the patella becomes centralized within the femoral trochlea, and by 10° to 20° of flexion any patellar tilt or subluxation should be corrected. By 30° of flexion, the patella sits farthest anterior, giving the extensor mechanism its greatest lever arm. By 45° to 60° of flexion, the midportion of the patella articulates with the midportion of the trochlea. Further flexion creates maximum centralization of the patella at 80°, which is maintained throughout the remainder of flexion. At 90° of flexion, the proximal patella contacts the distal trochlea, and at full flexion (at least 135°) only the supralateral patella and the odd facet articulate with the femur distal to the trochlea on the lateral femoral condyle and lateral surface of the medial femoral condyle.[22]

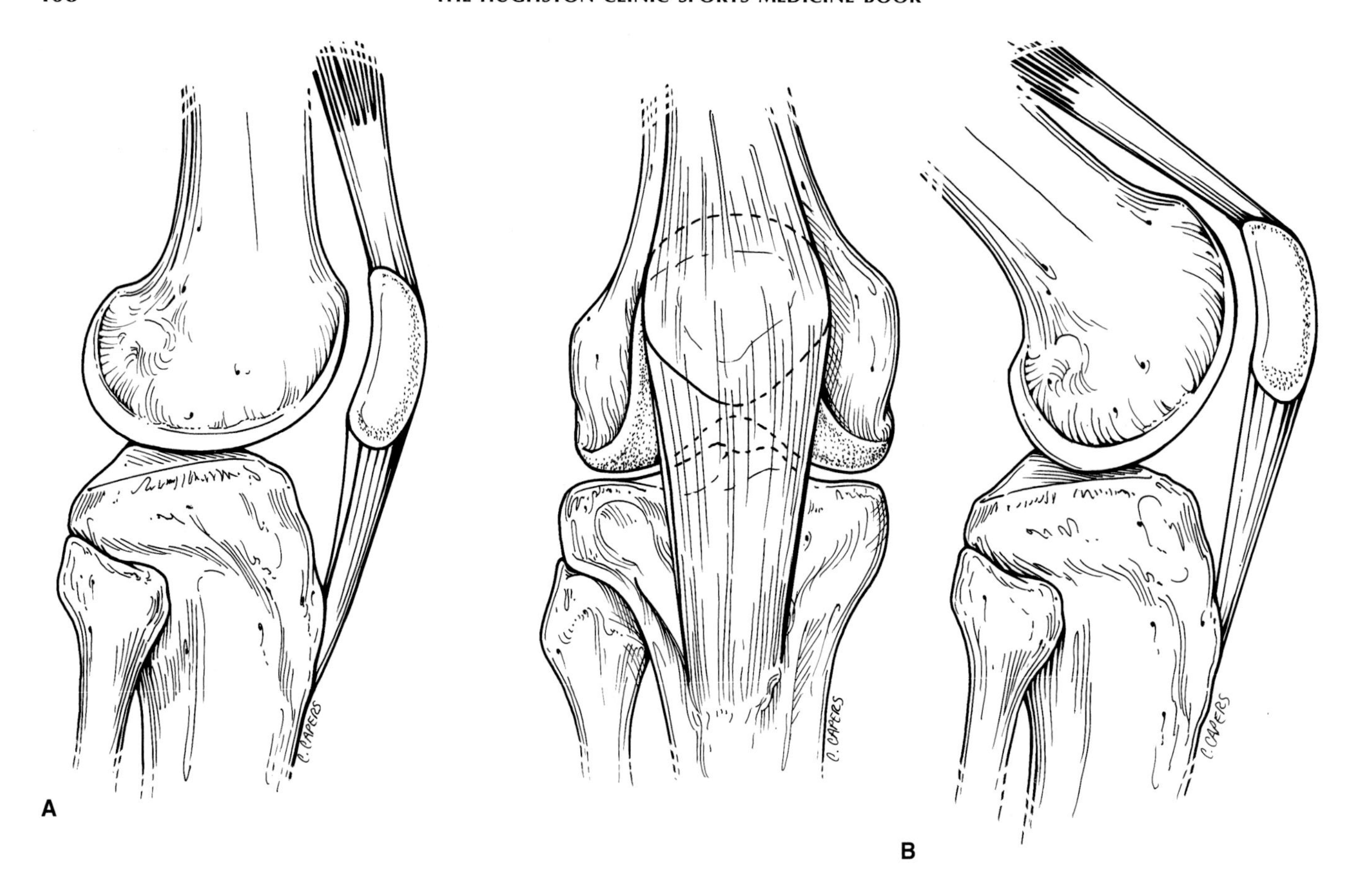

Fig. 63–4. ***(A)*** **With the knee in extension, the patella is superior and lateral to the trochlea.** ***(B)*** **At 30° of flexion, the patella sits most anteriorly, giving the extensor mechanism its greatest lever arm.**

The Q angle is the angle between the quadriceps mechanism and the patellar tendon. It is measured with the knee in full extension and the quadriceps contracted or with the patient seated and the knee in 90° of flexion. Normal values for these two measurements are 10° or less with the knee in extension and 0° with the knee in flexion.[24]

The screw-home mechanism has a profound influence on patellofemoral kinematics. As the knee extends, the tibia rotates externally, causing an increase in the Q angle. This creates a lateral, or valgus, vector on the patella, which is resisted principally by the vastus medialis obliquus and the medial retinaculum.[22]

The infrapatellar fat pad rests in the cavity posterior to the patellar tendon and sends a frenulum, called the *infrapatellar plica* or *ligamentum mucosum,* to the roof of the anterior intercondylar notch. The fat pad is well-vascularized and, if damaged, may form a hematoma with subsequent fibrosis, scar contracture, and possible development of patella baja.[4]

KNEE CAPSULE

The knee capsule extends proximally from the femoral trochlea, on average 4 to 5 cm, and is termed the *suprapatellar pouch.*[22] This rather voluminous cavity is commonly interrupted by a transverse fibrous band called the *suprapatellar plica,* a vestigial rest that once divided the embryonic knee into two cavities.[25] The adult expression of this structure is variable in that it may be a complete septum separating the knee joint cavity from the suprapatellar bursa or one of several variations of an incomplete septum.[26]

The superomedial portion of the suprapatellar plica blends with the medial patellar plica, which runs distally in the medial gutter and attaches to the infrapatellar fat pad. The medial patellar plica occasionally becomes inflamed when pinched between the medial facet of the patella and the medial femoral condyle or when it snaps over that condyle. Because of the horseshoe shape of this inter-related complex and its close association with the articularis genus muscle, it is thought that the plica constitutes a "synovial type of tendon aponeurosis of the articularis genus muscle" (Fig. 63–5).[4]

EXTRA-ARTICULAR LIGAMENTS

Anterior

The patellar tendon is the terminal extension of the extensor mechanism. Some authors refer to this as the *patellar ligament* since its fibers run from patella to tibia, as any ligament runs from bone to bone. However, tendinous fibers from the vastus medialis, vastus later-

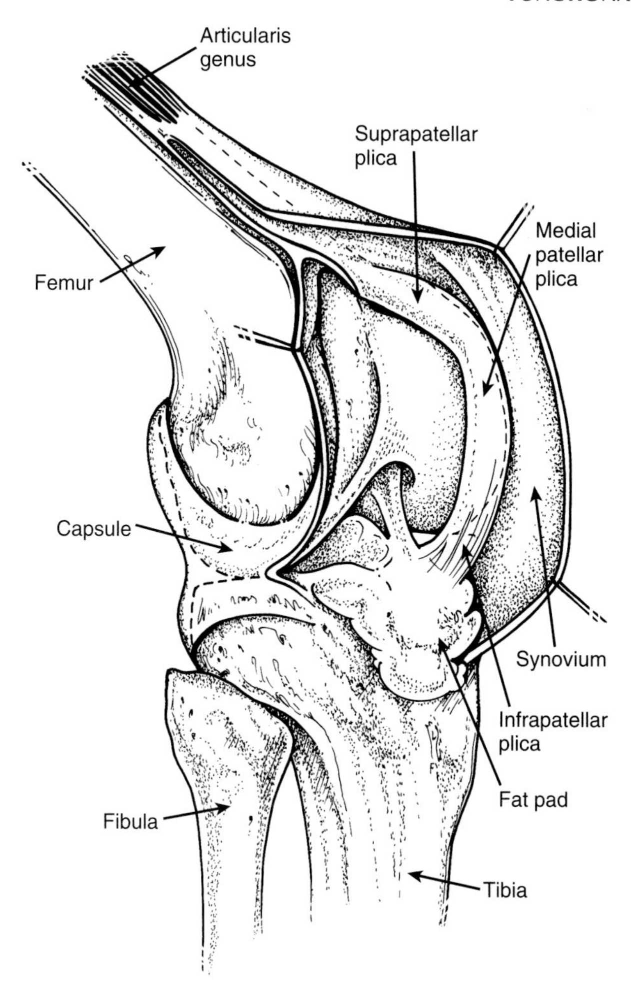

Fig. 63–5. The plica is thought to act as a synovial-type tendon aponeurosis for the articularis genus muscle. (Adapted from Hughston, J. C. Knee Ligaments: Injury and Repair. St. Louis, Mosby-Year Book, 1993, pp. 35.)

alis, and rectus femoris form an intermediate layer within the quadriceps tendon, which attaches to the superior pole of the patella. These fibers continue over the anterior patella and then distally, as the patellar tendon, to the insertion at the tibial tuberosity. In this sense, the patellar tendon behaves as a direct extension of the quadriceps muscle group and its function is thus more consistent with that of a tendon.

The anterior capsule lies medial and lateral to the patellar tendon. It is a relatively weak tissue, except where its fibers condense to form the medial and lateral patellofemoral and patellotibial ligaments.[27]

Medial

The tibial collateral ligament is a long, well-defined structure that lies superficial to the medial capsule and capsular ligaments. Its origin is the medial femoral epicondyle, and it inserts 4 to 7 cm distal to the joint line on the posterior half of the tibial metaphysis, deep to the pes anserinus tendons. The tibial collateral ligament is the principal restraint to valgus force.[28]

Deep to the tibial collateral ligament are the capsular or coronary ligaments, which have been divided into the anterior, middle, and posterior thirds (Fig. 63–6). A small bursa separates the tibial collateral ligament from the capsular ligaments.[29] The middle third medial capsular ligament is sometimes termed the *deep medial collateral ligament* because it acts as a strong secondary restraint to valgus force. These capsular ligaments, both medially and laterally, are also referred to as *meniscofemoral* and *meniscotibial ligaments* because they act as peripheral attachments for the menisci to the femur and tibia. They also act as secondary restraints to valgus and varus forces.[20]

Directly posterior to the tibial collateral ligament is the posterior oblique ligament (POL), which has its femoral attachment at the adductor tubercle. The POL has been described as having three arms, the superficial, tibial, and capsular arms. The POL contributes to dynamic stability of the knee in flexion through its capsular arm by confluence of its fibers with the semimembranosus.[30]

Lateral

The static structures of the lateral knee are lax in flexion. Only when the dynamic lateral muscle groups contract do the ligaments become taut in flexion. The iliotibial band is the distal extension of the tensor fascia lata. The posterior half of the iliotibial band is called the iliotibial tract. The iliotibial band sends an attachment (the iliopatellar ligament) obliquely toward the patella. The iliotibial band inserts at the anterior half of the lateral tibial tubercle, and the iliotibial tract inserts at the posterior half of the lateral tibial tubercle (Fig. 63–7).[4] The iliotibial band acts as a knee extensor in 0° to 30° of flexion and as a flexor in 40° to 145° of flexion.[8] It also acts as a static stabilizer of the knee through its attachment to the intermuscular septum and the iliopatellar ligament. The iliopatellar ligament provides further stability by its condensation with the lateral patellotibial and patellofemoral ligaments.

The fibular collateral ligament has been described as a "cordlike" ligament attaching on the lateral epicondyle of the femur and distally on the tip of the fibular head. These descriptions have been proven misleading by dissection in vivo: fibers from the arcuate ligament and the fascia of the lateral head of the gastrocnemius envelop the fibular collateral ligament. Furthermore, distal expansions of the fibular collateral ligament envelop the fibular head, blending with the biceps femoris and sending fibers to the fascia overlying the anterior muscle compartment of the leg. Regardless, the fibular collateral ligament functions principally as a static restraint against varus force.[20]

Posterior

The arcuate ligament is a condensation of the posterolateral capsule that covers the posterolateral femoral

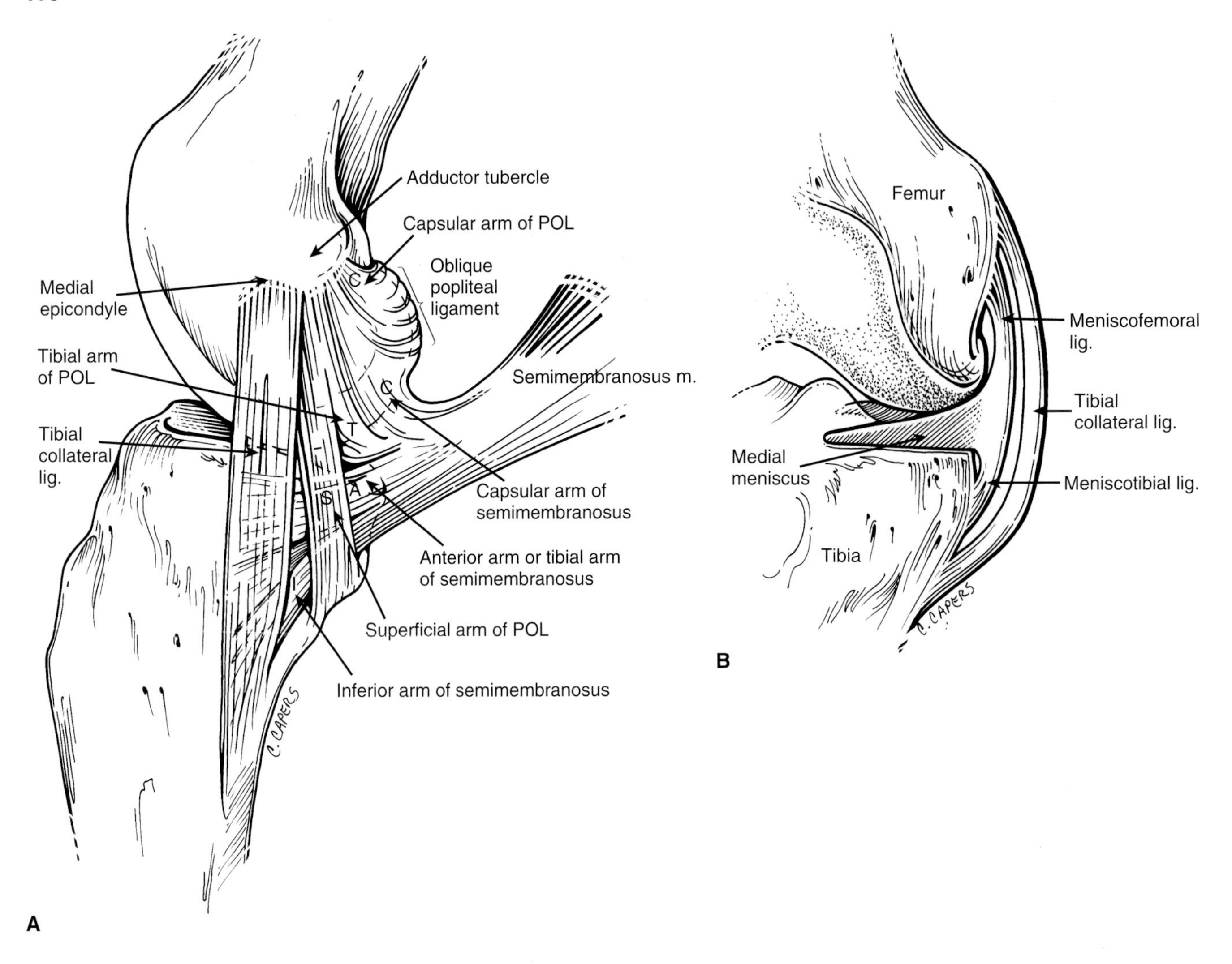

Fig. 63–6. The medial ligaments of the knee: (A) medial view, (B) anteroposterior view.

condyle. Its proximal attachment is just beneath the origin of the lateral head of the gastrocnemius, where its fibers are enmeshed with the gastrocnemius tendon. The distal expansion of the arcuate ligament becomes the posterior third of the meniscotibial ligament where it blends with the popliteus. This is the immediate area of attachment for the capsular arm of the popliteus to the posterior horn lateral meniscus. The arcuate also sends attachments to the posterior fibular head. The arcuate acts as a restraint to posterior and posterolateral forces.

The oblique popliteal ligament is the expansion of the semimembranosus, running from the semimembranosus insertion at the posteromedial tibia obliquely, proximally, and laterally toward the origin of the lateral head of the gastrocnemius on the posterolateral femur. The oblique popliteal ligament acts as a secondary restraint to posterior instability.

MUSCLE ANATOMY

The quadriceps comprises four separate muscles: the rectus femoris, the vastus intermedius, the vastus lateralis, and the vastus medialis. These four muscles condense in the quadriceps tendon to a common attachment on the superior pole of the patella (Fig. 63–8). The vastus lateralis and vastus medialis have oblique arms that insert into the patella as well. The angles of insertion in the sagittal plane vary between each of these arms: 15° to 18° for the vastus medialis, 50° to 55° for the vastus medialis obliquus, 12° to 15° for the vastus lateralis, and 38° to 48° for the vastus lateralis obliquus.[27, 31]

These muscles act in concert to extend the knee with a concentric contraction. An eccentric contraction of the quadriceps acts as a decelerator of the knee.[32] During knee extension and deceleration, a balance must be attained between these muscles to dynamically stabilize the patella. If there is an imbalance between the vastus lateralis and the vastus medialis, the result is subluxation of the patella to the "stronger" side. Of course, the static restraints also play an important role in stabilizing the patella.

The articularis genus muscle (the "fifth quadriceps muscle") is a small muscle deep to the vastus intermedius. Its origin is on the anterior surface of the distal

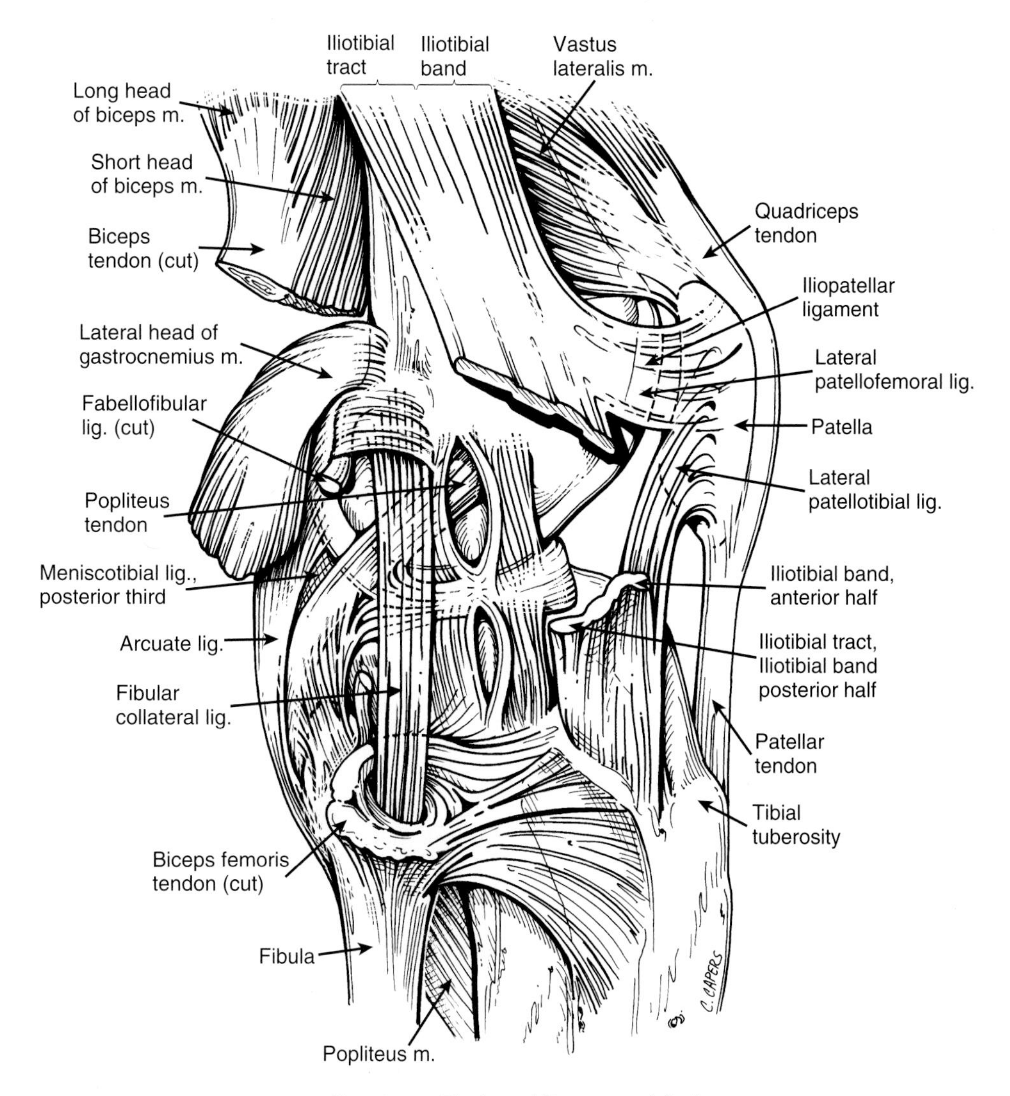

Fig. 63–7. The lateral ligaments of the knee.

femur, and its insertion into the proximal knee joint capsule. Its function is felt to be proximal retraction of the suprapatellar pouch with quadriceps contraction.[4]

The quadriceps acts synergistically with the posterior cruciate ligament to stabilize the knee against posterior subluxation. Conversely, the hamstrings (specifically the semimembranosus and biceps femoris) act in concert with the anterior cruciate ligament to prevent anterior subluxation.[33]

The hamstrings act as knee flexors and comprise the semitendinosus, semimembranosus, and biceps femoris. The pes anserinus is the combined insertion of the tendinous expansion of the sartorius, gracilis, and semitendinosus (Fig. 63–9). The pes anserinus is thought to act as an internal rotator and flexor of the tibia; thus it stabilizes the knee against anteromedial rotatory instability.[4]

The semimembranosus has a five-fingered insertion into the posteromedial aspect of the knee: (1) the oblique popliteal ligament, (2) the posterior capsule and posterior horn of the medial meniscus, (3) the anterior or deep arm, (4) the direct arm, and (5) the inferior arm. This complex insertion pattern serves several functions, including tightening the posterior oblique ligament and oblique popliteal ligament and thereby dynamically stabilizing the knee in flexion. It also retracts the posterior horn of the medial meniscus posteriorly in flexion, preventing a compression injury to the meniscus between the posterior femoral condyle and the tibial plateau.[4]

The biceps femoris has a long and a short head of insertion. The long head is more superficial and attaches to the fibular head as well as sending investing fibers around the fibular head and extending distally to the proximal tibia. The deeper fibers also coalesce with the fibular collateral ligament. The short head of the biceps femoris arises from the lateral and medial linea aspera on the posterior femur and inserts into the long head of the biceps femoris, as well as into the posterolateral capsule.

The function of the biceps femoris is to actively flex the knee and to retract the posterior horn of the lateral meniscus posteriorly with knee flexion, similar to the function of the semimembranosus medially.

The popliteus muscle has a tripartite attachment proximally and extends obliquely, distally, and medially to attach on the posterior tibia. The tripartite attachment is divided between the lateral femoral condyle, the

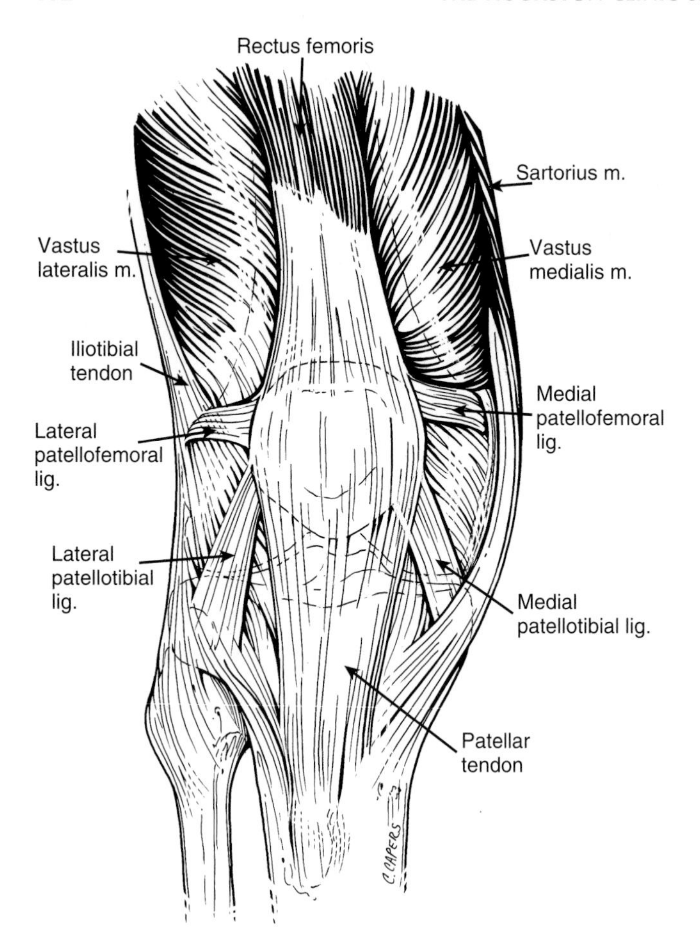

Fig. 63–8. Muscular anatomy of the anterior aspect of the knee.

posterior horn of the lateral meniscus, and the fibular head. The fascicular attachments from the popliteus tendon have been demonstrated in detail by Stäubli and Birrer.[34] Through this complex scheme of bony anchors, the popliteus is thought to act both dynamically and statically. The dynamic function is to produce internal rotation of the tibia and retraction of the posterior horn of the lateral meniscus. Its static function is as a secondary restraint to posterolateral rotation, varus, and hyperextension forces. It also helps maintain hoop tension in the lateral meniscus.

The gastrocnemius muscle has a medial and a lateral head, which originate from the popliteal surface of the femur above the medial femoral condyle and the lateral aspect of the lateral femoral condyle, respectively. The two heads join in the posterior aspect of the Achilles tendon to insert on the posterior calcaneus. The gastrocnemius, because of its origin proximal to the knee, assists in knee flexion, though its primary function is plantar flexion of the foot.

The soleus muscle originates from the soleal line on the posterior proximal tibia and fibula. It then joins with the gastrocnemius on the anterior surface of the Achilles tendon.

The plantaris muscle is a feeble plantar flexor of the foot and an accessory knee flexor as it accompanies the gastrocnemius. Its origin is the lateral supracondylar ridge of the femur, and it extends obliquely to its insertion on the medial border of the Achilles tendon.

VASCULATURE

The popliteal artery is the principal blood supply to the knee. It is commonly injured with knee dislocation and fractures because it is securely fixed proximally at the adductor hiatus and distally under the soleus muscle. Damage is usually incurred by stretching of the vessel away from the point of firm attachment with a knee dislocation or by direct puncture from a bone fragment.

The medial and lateral superior genicular arteries branch off the popliteal artery proximal to the posterior joint space. The medial and lateral inferior genicular arteries branch off the popliteal artery distal to the joint space. The lateral inferior genicular artery runs along the lateral joint line, making it susceptible to injury during lateral meniscus surgery. All four vessels pass forward to form an anastomosis called the rete articulare genus (Fig. 63–10).[8]

The middle genicular artery arises directly from the anterior aspect of the popliteal artery and pierces the posterior capsule, supplying the cruciate ligaments and the posterior capsule. It has two branches that run anteriorly along the periphery of the medial and lateral menisci to form anastomoses at the anterior meniscal horns. The anterior tibial recurrent artery arises from the anterior tibial artery and exits the anterior muscle compartment laterally to form an anastomosis with the medial inferior genicular artery anteriorly.

Two areas of the knee deserve special mention with regard to vascular supply, the patella and the menisci. There has been increasing concern about patellar avascular necrosis secondary to iatrogenic injury. The principal blood supply is from an anterior anastomotic ring supplied by the medial and lateral superior– and the medial and lateral inferior genicular arteries. There is also a small contribution from an infrapatellar anastomosis in the fat pad.[35] If medial and lateral capsular incisions are made (as is common for total knee arthroplasty), the patella is at great risk of developing avascular necrosis.[36]

The meniscal blood supply is well-documented. A perimeniscal capsular plexus within the synovium and capsule supplies blood to the peripheral 10 to 30% of the menisci, except for the area immediately adjacent to the popliteus tendon, which is completely avascular.[37] This suggests that meniscal healing is more predictable in the peripheral vascular zones. For their nutrition the inner portions of the menisci depend on diffusion.

NEUROANATOMY

Motor Innervation

The femoral nerve, tibial nerve, and common peroneal nerve are the primary motor nerves to the knee. The femoral nerve divides into anterior and posterior

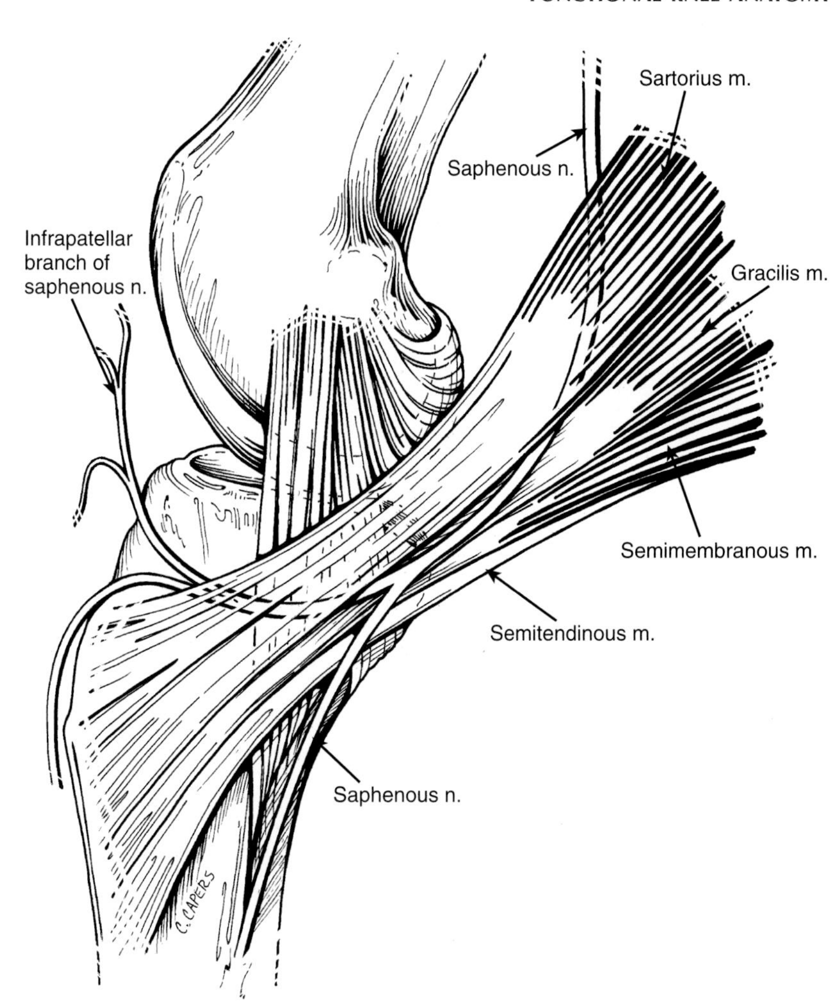

Fig. 63–9. The pes anserinus is the insertion of the tendinous expansions of the sartorius, the gracilis, and the semimembranosus muscles.

divisions approximately 4 cm distal to the inguinal ligament. The anterior division gives off two cutaneous (medial femoral cutaneous nerve and intermediate femoral cutaneous nerve) and two muscular branches (sartorius and pectineus). The posterior division gives off one cutaneous branch (saphenous nerve) and all the muscular branches to the quadriceps muscles.

The tibial nerve arises in the lower one third of the posterior thigh, passes through the popliteal fossa, and enters the posterior compartment beneath the soleus muscle. It supplies the gastrocnemius, soleus, popliteus, semimembranosus, semitendinosus, and long head of the biceps femoris.

The common peroneal nerve enters the popliteal fossa on the lateral side of the tibial nerve and follows closely the medial border of the biceps femoris muscle. It then leaves the fossa by crossing superficially the lateral head of the gastrocnemius, passes behind the head of the fibula, and then crosses the fibular neck before piercing the peroneus longus muscle. The muscle branch to the short head of biceps femoris is given off proximally in the popliteal fossa. The peroneal nerve is vulnerable to injury because it lies just under the skin at the fibular neck.

Sensory Innervation

The femoral nerve supplies sensation to the proximal medial quadrant of the knee. The medial femoral cutaneous branches descend with the vastus medialis muscle and then pass laterally across the midline above the joint space.

The saphenous nerve gives sensation along the medial aspect of the leg. The infrapatellar branch of the saphenous nerve is commonly injured with medial meniscus repair because it emerges between the tendons of the sartorius and gracilis muscles.[38] The infrapatellar branch crosses the midline to supply the skin, subcutis, knee capsule, infrapatellar fat pad, and iliotibial tract. The lateral aspect of the knee has a cutaneous nerve supply, from the lateral femoral cutaneous nerve proximally and the lateral sural cutaneous branch distally.

The knee joint itself has sensory contributions from the obturator nerve with its terminal branches, the tibial, peroneal, and saphenous nerves, and branches from the vastus lateralis, vastus intermedius, and vastus medialis muscles.

The medial articular nerve should be identified and protected when dissecting near the proximal tibial col-

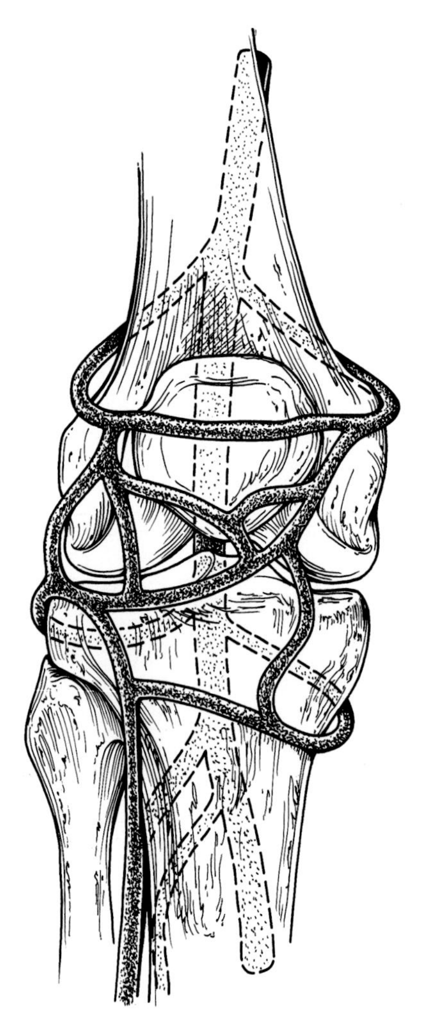

Fig. 63–10. Vasculature of the knee shows popliteal arteries and genicular arteries.

lateral ligament.[8] This nerve descends across the adductor tubercle close to the femoral attachment of the tibial collateral ligament. It then passes into the joint capsule, to the fat pad, and below the patellar tendon to the lateral knee.

REFERENCES

1. Menschik, A.: Personal communication, 1991.
2. Dye, S. F.: Patellofemoral anatomy. *In* The Patellofemoral Joint. Edited by J. M. Fox and W. Del Pizzo. New York, McGraw-Hill, 1993.
3. Dye, S. F., et al.: Quantitative assessment of functional knee morphology by means of cine computed tomography. Am. J. Sports Med. *15*:387, 1987.
4. Hughston, J. C.: Knee Ligaments: Injury and Repair. St. Louis, Mosby-Year Book, 1993.
5. Brantigan, O. C., and Voshell, A. F.: Ligaments of the knee joint: The relationship of the ligament of Humphry to the ligament of Wrisberg. J. Bone Joint Surg. *28*:66, 1946.
6. Thompson, W. O., Thaete, F. L., Fu, F. H., and Dye, S. F.: Tibial meniscal dynamics using three-dimensional reconstruction of magnetic resonance images. Am. J. Sports Med. *19*:210, 1991.
7. Renström, P., and Johnson, R. J.: Anatomy and biomechanics of the menisci. Clin. Sports Med. *9*:523, 1990.
8. Muller, W.: The Knee: Form, Function, and Ligament Reconstruction. New York, Springer-Verlag, 1983.
9. Abbott, L. C., Saunders, J. B., Bost, F. C., and Anderson, C. E.: Injuries to the ligaments of the knee joint. J. Bone Joint Surg. *26A*:503, 1944.
10. Hughston, J. C., Andrews, J. R., Cross, M. J., and Moschi, A.: Classification of knee ligament instabilities: Part I. The medial compartment and cruciate ligaments. J. Bone Joint Surg. *58A*:159, 1976.
11. Kennedy, J. C., and Grainger, R. W.: The posterior cruciate ligament. J. Trauma *7*:367, 1967.
12. Girgis, F. G., Marshall, J. L., and Al-Monajem, A. R. S.: The cruciate ligaments of the knee joint: Anatomical, functional, and experimental analysis. Clin. Orthop. *106*:216, 1975.
13. Kennedy, J. C., Hawkins, R. J., Willis, R. B., and Danylchuk, K. D.: Tension study of the human knee ligaments. Yield point, ultimate failure, and disruption of the cruciate and tibial collateral ligaments. J. Bone Joint Surg. *58A*:350, 1976.
14. Wang, C. J., and Walker, P. S.: Rotatory laxity of the human knee joint. J. Bone Joint Surg. *56A*:161, 1974.
15. O'Brien, W. R., Friederich, N. F., Muller, W., and Henning, C. E.: Functional anatomy of the cruciate ligaments. American Academy of Orthopaedic Surgeons Instructional Videotape. Park Ridge, IL, AAOS, 1991.
16. Van Dommelen, B. A., and Fowler, P. J.: Anatomy of the posterior cruciate ligament: A review. Am. J. Sports Med *17*:24, 1989.
17. Heller, L., and Langmen, J.: The menisco-femoral ligaments of the human knee. J. Bone Joint Surg. *46B*:307, 1964.
18. Clancy, W. G., Jr., et al.: Treatment of knee joint instability secondary to rupture of the posterior cruciate ligament: Report of a new procedure. J. Bone Joint Surg. *65A*:310, 1983.
19. Norwood, L. A., and Cross, M. J.: Anterior cruciate ligament: Functional anatomy of its bundles in rotatory instabilities. Am. J. Sports Med. *7*:23, 1979.
20. Noyes, F. R., Grood, E. S., Butler, D. L., and Paulos, L. E.: Clinical biomechanics of the knee-ligament restraints and functional stability. *In* American Academy of Orthopaedic Surgeons Symposium on The Athlete's Knee: Surgical Repair and Reconstruction. St. Louis, C. V. Mosby, 1980.
21. Aglietti, P., Buzzi, R., and Insall, J. N.: Disorders of the patellofemoral joint. *In* Surgery of the Knee. 2nd Ed. Edited by J. N. Insall et al. New York, Churchill Livingstone, 1993.
22. Fulkerson, J. P., and Hungerford, D.S.: Normal anatomy. *In* Disorders of The Patellofemoral Joint. 2nd Ed. Baltimore, Williams & Wilkins, 1990.
23. Hungerford, D. S., and Barry, M.: Biomechanics of the patellofemoral joint. Clin. Orthop. *144*:9, 1979.
24. Hughston, J. C., Walsh, W. M., and Puddu, G.: Diagnosis. *In* Patellar Subluxation and Dislocation. Philadelphia, W. B. Saunders, 1984.
25. Zidorn, T.: Classification of the suprapatellar septum considering ontogenetic development. Arthroscopy *8*:459, 1992.
26. Dandy, D. J.: Anatomy of the medial suprapatellar plica and medial synovial shelf. Arthroscopy *6*:79, 1990.
27. Terry, G. C.: The anatomy of the extensor mechanism. Clin. Sports Med. *8*:163, 1989.
28. Warren, L. A., Marshall, J. L., and Girgis, F.: The prime static stabilizer of the medial side of the knee. J. Bone Joint Surg. *56A*:665, 1974.
29. Brantigan, O. C., and Voshell, A. F.: The tibial collateral ligament: its function, its bursae, and its relation to the medial meniscus. J. Bone Joint Surg. *25A*:121, 1943.
30. Hughston, J. C., and Eilers, A. F.: The role of the posterior oblique ligament in repairs of acute medial (collateral) ligament tears of the knee. J. Bone Joint Surg. *55A*:923, 1973.
31. Hallisey, M. J., Doherty, N., Bennett, W. F., and Fulkerson, J. P.: Anatomy of the junction of the vastus lateralis tendon and the patella. J. Bone Joint Surg. *69A*:545, 1987.
32. Hughston, J. C., Walsh, W. M., and Puddu, G.: Functional anatomy of the extensor (decelerator) mechanism. *In* Patellar Subluxation and Dislocation. Philadelphia, W. B. Saunders, 1984.

33. More, R. C., et al.: Hamstrings—an anterior cruciate ligament protagonist: An in vitro study, Am. J. Sports Med. *21*:231, 1993.
34. Stäubli, H.-U., and Birrer, S.: The popliteus tendon and its fascicles at the popliteal hiatus: Gross anatomy and functional arthroscopic evaluation with and without anterior cruciate ligament deficiency. Arthroscopy *6*:209, 1990.
35. Scapinelli, R.: Blood supply of the human patella: Its relation to ischemic necrosis after fracture. J. Bone Joint Surg. *49B*:563, 1967.
36. McMahon, M. S., et al.: Scintigraphic determination of patellar viability after excision of infrapatellar fat pad and/or lateral retinacular release in total knee arthroplasty. Clin. Orthop. *260*:10, 1990.
37. Arnoczky, S. P., and Warren, F.: Microvasculature of the human meniscus. Am. J. Sports Med. *10*:90, 1982.
38. Arthornthurasook, A., Gaew-Im, K.: The sartorial nerve: Its relationship to the medial aspect of the knee. Am. J. Sports Med. *18*:41, 1990.

64

Patrick A. Smith

Physical Examination of the Knee

The key to accurate knee examination is a thorough, systematic, and repetitive routine, to ensure that nothing is missed. The goal of the examination should always be to arrive at a definitive diagnosis. I believe the physical examination should be comprehensive and accurate enough so that the examiner can avoid the temptation to reflexively order magnetic resonance imaging (MRI) or consider diagnostic arthroscopy. Obviously, the particular format one chooses for the knee examination can vary, but it should incorporate the basics in terms of history, physical examination, and standard radiographic studies.

HISTORY

As in most areas of clinical medicine, taking a good history is essential because in many cases this provides clues to the diagnosis. It is essential that the examiner have a solid knowledge of knee anatomy as this much facilitates accurate diagnosis. To provide a framework for comprehensive knee examination, I have found it helpful always to think in terms of three basic injury sites: patellofemoral, meniscal, and ligamentous.

Mechanism of Injury

The examination starts with the basic question, What was the mechanism of injury? I am always amazed at how accurately an athlete recalls an injury in terms of knee position at the time and the stresses incurred as a result. Whether the athlete incurred a twisting, noncontact injury or a direct blow to the knee is important. Also, knee position at the time of injury can provide clues to the exact injury pattern.

In my experience, the anterior cruciate ligament is more likely to be torn by significant varus stress than significant valgus stress. An anterior hyperextension force can tear the anterior cruciate ligament or the posterolateral corner. A fall on a flexed knee with a direct blow to the proximal tibia is a well-known mechanism for tearing the posterior cruciate ligament, and a "dashboard injury" can do the same thing. In terms of hyperflexion injuries, those without contact are a good way to tear a meniscus and those with contact, usually from a fall, can tear the anterior cruciate ligament because of distraction stress.

Swelling

Besides mechanism of injury, knee swelling is a key point of the history. The first question is whether joint swelling occurred within the first couple of hours after injury and whether it was significant. Early significant swelling indicates bleeding into the joint and hemarthrosis. The most likely diagnosis in that case is a tear of the anterior cruciate ligament; studies have shown hemarthrosis to be associated with anterior cruciate ligament tears in more than 80% of such cases. Patellar dislocation is the next likely condition to cause hemarthrosis, followed by peripheral meniscus tears and osteochondral fractures.

If an athlete's knee swelling is less pronounced and develops 24 hours after injury, this indicates a reactive effusion, which is frequently caused by a meniscus tear. I would emphasize that, though an effusion is most often related to ligament instability or a meniscus tear, patellofemoral inflammation with a pathologic plica *can* occasionally result in true joint swelling. I attribute this to a synovial irritation–type reaction. In addition, I have seen many cases when an articular cartilage breakdown lesion resulted in an effusion, presumably owing to the inflammatory effect of articular cartilage debris free in the joint. Also, patients who are asked about swelling may report that the knee swells, but if pinned down about where and how much, what they are really describing is a sensation of "tightness," which in my mind usually signifies a patellofemoral problem.

The question of joint aspiration always comes up. Usually I do not find it to be necessary after a thorough history, physical examination, and routine radiograph series, but I would not hesitate to perform aspiration in a difficult case. I employ strict sterile technique for aspiration. A helpful hint to facilitate ligament re-examination after aspiration is to inject some local anesthetic into the joint for pain relief.

Pain

Another important question during history taking concerns the location and type of pain experienced after the injury. If the athletes complain of intermittent, sharp pain that is well localized toward either the medial or lateral joint line, I think of a meniscal tear or perhaps an anterior cruciate ligament tear, particularly if they also describe giving way occurring at the time of the pain. If the patient complains of constant, aching discomfort about the patella, the patellofemoral joint is frequently implicated as the origin of the difficulty. If a patient experiences severe knee pain that seems out of proportion to the injury, I worry about an occult fracture involving the joint.

Mechanical Symptoms

The last area related to history concerns what I term *mechanical symptoms*. It is well-known that many patients who tear the anterior cruciate ligament feel or hear a "pop" at the time of injury. But patients who incur a medial ligament tear also frequently feel a pop, as do patients who subluxate their patella. The history of a pop is not helpful. It usually is a fairly nonspecific symptom related to patellofemoral chondromalacia or the plica, and in many cases it does not actually cause pain. It should be kept in mind, however, that some patients with a meniscal tear experience popping, but the big difference is that they experience pain related to the popping.

The mechanical symptom of giving way can mean something totally different to a patient and to the examiner. Classic giving way indicates a ligament problem with joint instability, but giving way caused by reflex quadriceps inhibition from patellofemoral problems such as a pathologic plica or patellar chondromalacia is just as common. Patellar subluxation also usually causes the knee to give way; and in some instances a torn meniscus caught in the joint causes sharp pain and the feeling of the knee buckling. To understand exactly what giving way means for a patient what I find helpful is first to ask what circumstances result in the giving way: does it occur more with twisting, pivoting, or cutting-type activity? Giving way associated with twisting, pivoting, or cutting is more likely to reflect an anterior cruciate ligament deficiency caused by the rotational pivot shift phenomenon. If giving way is related to stair climbing, or particularly *descending* stairs, it is more likely caused by patellofemoral dysfunction and quadriceps inhibition. Second, I ask patients if they actually fall when the knee gives way. Falling indicates giving way from ligamentous injury, whereas giving way that does not produce a fall is more commonly associated with a patellofemoral disorder.

The last two mechanical symptoms I always inquire about are catching and locking. Again, the examiner can be fooled if the patient is not asked precisely what the response to the question means. Specifically, many patients say the knee locks and the immediate thought of the examiner is that this is due to a meniscal tear, but on closer questioning, the patient relates that the locking episodes only last a few seconds and that the knee is in extension and not flexed. In my mind, that is not "true" locking from a meniscal tear but rather the "sensation" of locking from the patellofemoral joint because of a plica or chondromalacia. A bucket-handle tear of the medial meniscus causes locking when the knee is flexed. This locking usually requires some sort of manipulation, either on the patient's part or on the part of another person, to twist or flex the knee to unlock it, at which point the patient typically feels a pop and full motion is restored. Thus, when questioning a patient about locking, I ask if it occurs in extension or flexion and whether it is transient or lasts several seconds. True meniscal locking generally lasts at least several seconds.

One other consideration is that some patients with a loose body or joint "noise" also describe locking of the joint, but it is usually more transient. If asked, they often describe feeling something moving about loose in the knee, especially in the suprapatellar area. This greatly helps to differentiate the presence of a loose body from other problems.

I think it is also appropriate to describe a fairly common clinical presentation, what I term *pseudolocking*. A common scenario is an athlete, typically a high school girl, who injures her knee playing basketball and presents with an acute flexion contracture and posterior knee discomfort. On examination, a joint effusion is usually present and the patient is very irritated by attempts to extend the knee, which cause posterior pain. In this setting, the lack of knee extension is most commonly due to a tear of the anterior cruciate ligament, as opposed to the meniscus. I believe the pathophysiology relates to the innervation of the anterior cruciate ligament being from the posterior capsular area, and with an anterior cruciate ligament tear protective hamstring spasm accounts for the pseudolocking. Generally, with time and quadriceps exercises, the flexion contracture resolves, so urgent arthroscopic intervention, which would be needed for a locked meniscal tear, is not indicated.

The symptom of catching can be either meniscal or patellofemoral in origin. I find that a patient with a meniscal tear who describes a catch usually points to the medial or lateral joint line as the site of this mechanical sensation. However, one pathologic condition that can mimic a meniscal tear, in terms of catching, is a chondromalacia-type lesion of either the medial or lateral femoral condyle with a loose flap of articular surface. This loose flap can create a mechanical catch that causes localized joint line pain and thus may be similar to the presentation of a meniscal tear, but this is a much less common entity. Besides a tear of the meniscus, the other common source of catching is the patellofemoral joint, either from a thick plica impinging on the rim of the medial femoral condyle or an area of chondromalacia of the patella or trochlear groove causing a mechanical catch with knee flexion secondary to joint surface incongruity.

PHYSICAL EXAMINATION

To complement a good history, an examiner needs to perform a thorough physical examination to arrive at an accurate diagnosis. One cannot overstate the importance of a solid knowledge of knee anatomy for clinical proficiency. My approach during the examination process is to try and instinctively correlate the physical findings with the potential pathologic anatomy. I believe the ideal physical examination is a thorough and methodical one that includes *gentle* stress testing. Side-to-side comparison should always be used—and repeated frequently if there is any question of articular damage. As with the history, the primary goal of the physical examination is to establish the exact diagnosis and thus avoid MRI or "diagnostic" arthroscopy. Again, I find it helpful as I go through the examination to think of the basic knee injury sites: patellofemoral, meniscal, and ligamentous.

Inspection

The physical examination can be divided into three parts: inspection, palpation, and physical testing. Beginning with inspection, I watch the patient walk either down the hall or into the examination room, to look for antalgic gait associated with either a flexed or extended knee. Before examining the knee itself, I have the patient stand so I can assess the alignment of the lower extremity from the hip to the foot for any obvious rotational problem with the hip, in terms of patellar position. Also, I check to see whether genu valgum or genu varum is present with leg alignment and check the feet for pes cavus or pes planus. Next, I have the patient sit on the examination table, to afford optimal inspection of the patellofemoral joint, specifically for patella alta with the knee flexed 90° or vastus medialis obliquus dysplasia, which is best appreciated as the patient actively extends the knee. As the knee moves from flexion to extension, the examiner should also assess whether patellar tracking is abnormal, particularly laterally. Next, the Q angle should be measured, with the knee both extended and at 90° of flexion. Inspection continues by looking for swelling from either a true joint effusion, prepatellar bursa, or soft tissue swelling with associated ecchymoses from a significant ligament or capsule injury. Also, I look for any muscle atrophy, particularly with the quadriceps or gastrocnemius, the two muscle groups most evident visually for lower extremity atrophy. Finally, I check for any scars that could be a clue to some type of surgery.

Palpation

Palpation should be systematic and should include the patellofemoral joint, ligamentous structures, and the menisci. First, I palpate for the plica. Every patient has a medial plica band that can be palpated along the rim of the medial femoral condyle (Fig. 64–1); it may be thick or thin, tender or not. I also palpate for a lateral plica, which is not distinctly present in all patients. Next, I manipulate the patella with the knee in full extension and assess whether this causes pain or crepitation. By placing a hand on top of the patella and asking the patient to move the knee from flexion to extension I feel for crepitation or a pop and also determine if that motion is painful. The fat pad should be palpated medially and laterally for tenderness or induration. At the same time, I can see if patellar mobility is normal or restricted by entrapment from scar tissue, which typically can occur from the fat pad.

Palpation continues along the quadriceps tendon, where it inserts along the superior pole of the patella;

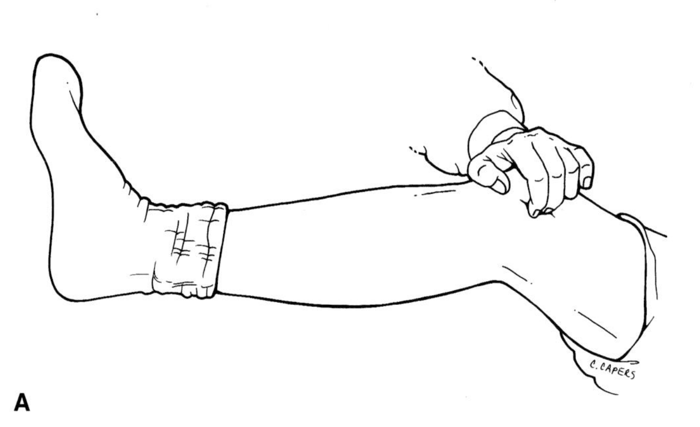

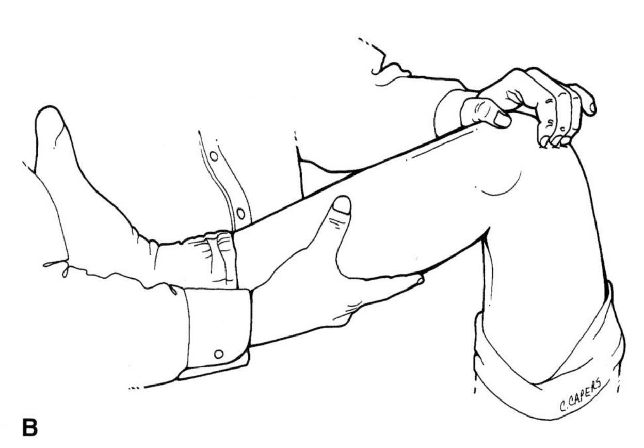

Fig. 64–1. The medial plica can be palpated along the rim of the medial femoral condyle: *(A)* extension, *(B)* flexion.

any tenderness, swelling, or crepitation should be noted. Similarly, I palpate the patellar tendon from the inferior pole down toward the tibial tubercle for tenderness, edema, and crepitation, followed by the tibial tubercle itself for tenderness or enlargement consistent with Osgood-Schlatter calcification. One should also always palpate the quadriceps muscle for tone and test the hamstrings for tightness by flexing the hip to 90° and then extending the knee.

The examination of ligamentous structures by palpation is not as limited as one might think, considering that the cruciate ligaments obviously are not accessible to palpation. Specifically, I can palpate very nicely along the course of the capsular ligaments and correlate tenderness and swelling with injury. First, I position the patient's knee in the figure-of-four position (Fig. 64–2) and begin palpating along the medial joint line. This palpation begins at the prominent medial epicondyle of the femur, at the tibial collateral ligament origin. Then, picturing the anatomy in my mind, I palpate down over the meniscus and tibia, covering the course of the middle third of the capsular ligament and ending at the proximal tibial insertion of the tibial collateral ligament. Next, I move posteriorly and palpate over the course of the posterior oblique ligament from the femur to the tibia, appreciating any tenderness, obvious edema, or ecchymoses. Again, this allows me to determine where the medial ligament complex is torn, which is important when it comes to treatment decisions.

Palpation of the lateral ligamentous structures is also done with the knee flexed, beginning with the middle third capsular ligament from the femur to the tibia. Moving slightly posterior, I palpate the fibular collateral ligament, which is particularly prominent with the knee in the figure-of-four position. Then I continue to palpate posteriorly over the arcuate ligament and the lateral head of the gastrocnemius; I also check the iliotibial tract, both at the lateral epicondyle, where tenderness would indicate iliotibial band tendinitis, and along the deep tract fibers, which can be tender with an acute anterior cruciate ligament injury.

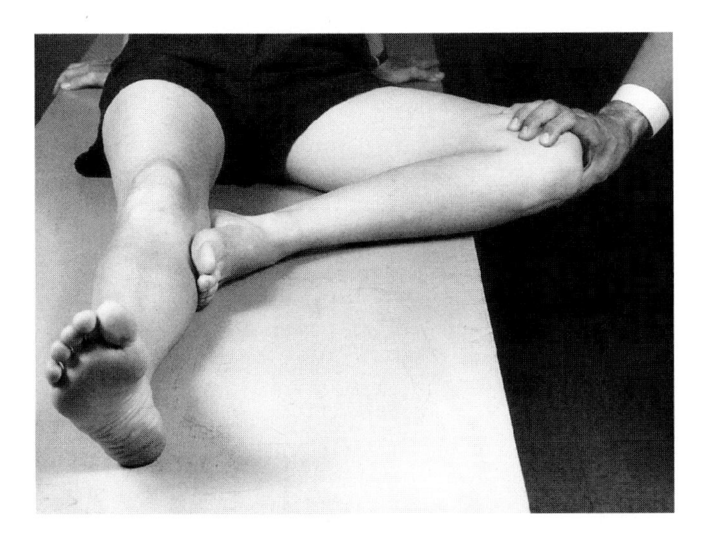

Fig. 64–2. Figure-of-four position.

Finally, palpation can also be very helpful in examining the meniscus. I begin by palpating directly over the medial joint line from anterior to posterior, where localized tenderness can be fairly specific for meniscal lesions. I find this to be especially true with tenderness directly over the posterior medial joint line, in contrast to tenderness along the medial meniscus in the middle third area, which frequently is related to plica irritation. Laterally, the meniscus is nicely palpated from anterior to posterior with the knee in the figure-of-four position. The examiner should be aware of any focal joint line swelling that could indicate a meniscal cyst and of bone spurs that might be palpable.

Physical Tests

An especially important part of the physical examination is based on physical tests. In keeping with the theme of the injury sites, I usually begin with the patellofemoral joint and assess for possible plica involvement with two entrapment maneuvers. I call the first plica maneuver the *trap test,* which consists of having the patient actively perform a quadriceps set while in the supine position with the examiner's hand pressed firmly above the superior pole of the patella. As in many cases with acute plica or synovial irritation, the patient feels pain, or even a pop, with this stress. It should be emphasized, however, that a positive "trap test" is not totally specific for the plica. Patients with patellar chondromalacia also seem to have pain with the trap test, though why they feel discomfort is more difficult to explain, since, unlike the plica, which is innervated synovial tissue, the articular surface does not have nerve endings. A more specific plica test is to palpate with three fingers along the medial femoral condylar rim and to take the knee into flexion and then extend it with rotation. Sometimes the plica pops right beneath my fingers over the rim of the medial femoral condyle, especially when it is thick and fibrotic.

Next, the examiner tests for patellar stability. The optimal position for assessing such stability is with the knee flexed 45°. This is best done with the examiner seated on the table and the patient supine and in a relaxed position with the knee over the examiner's thigh. With firm but gentle pressure along the medial border of the patella, the examiner stresses the patella laterally (Fig. 64–3); true patellar subluxation is indicated if *both* lateral hypermobility out of the trochlear groove and apprehension on the patient's part are observed. Care must be taken when doing this test to avoid palpating directly over the plica or medial retinaculum because that can elicit pain (and falsely mimic apprehension). I check for medial patellar subluxation with associated apprehension in the same position by just reversing the stress. This is a primary concern if a patient previously underwent operation for lateral release, which can lead to medial patellar subluxation.

The next test for patellar stability is done with the patient supine and the knee positioned toward exten-

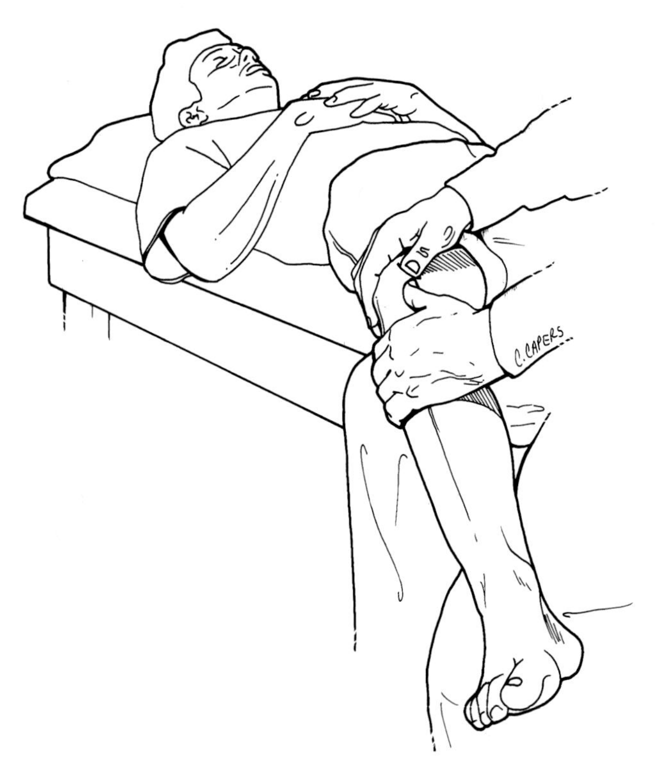

Fig. 64–3. To examine for patellar stability, the patient's knee is placed over the examiner's thigh and lateral pressure is applied to the patella.

sion. I place my thumb at the inferior pole of the right patella and take the knee through a range of motion from flexion to extension, applying first lateral and then medial stress on the patella, to see whether it subluxates excessively in extension. The patella is normally more hypermobile with the knee in extension because the retinaculum is lax in this position; although with abnormal lateral subluxation lateral movement of the patella is accentuated and associated with apprehension. In patients who have had lateral release, pathologic medial subluxation in extension can commonly be appreciated with this test.

There are several maneuvers that I term *provocative* for meniscal injury. First, I like to flex the knee as fully as possible, placing my index finger along one joint line and my thumb around the other so that I can palpate for a click. I then rotate the tibia by the ankle. Even if a click is not appreciated, I note whether this flexion and rotation maneuver causes discomfort and, if so, whether the pain is medial or lateral. Next I perform a variation of the McMurray test (Fig. 64–4), applying varus stress to the joint in flexion to load the medial compartment and then externally rotating the tibia with the other hand at the ankle as the knee is extended. While performing this maneuver, I again palpate one joint line with the index finger and the other with the thumb, feeling for a pop and noting whether this provocative maneuver causes pain. Next, I repeat the test with varus stress and internal rotation. To assess the lateral meniscus, I apply valgus stress to the knee, to load the lateral compartment, beginning in flexion, and I do the same, first with internal rotation and then with external rotation, extending the knee while palpating both joint lines to see if there is a pop or pain. The other physical test that is helpful for diagnosing a meniscal tear is the classic Apley's maneuver. This test is done with the patient prone and the knee flexed 90°, palpating the joint line both medially and laterally. The examiner then applies compression to the heel while rotating the tibia with the opposite hand and feeling for a pop over either joint line. Again, noting if the patient experiences pain with this provocative maneuver is helpful in making a diagnosis, even if a pop is not appreciated.

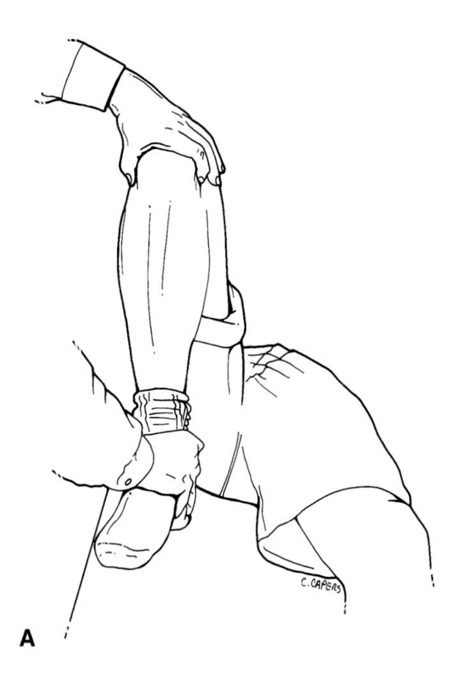

A

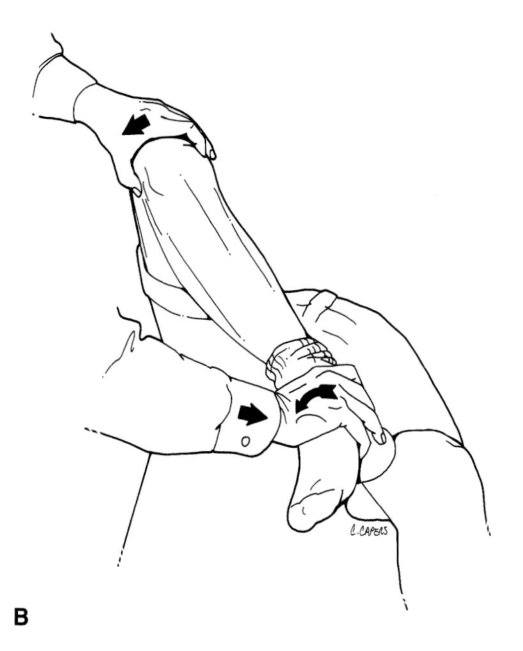

B

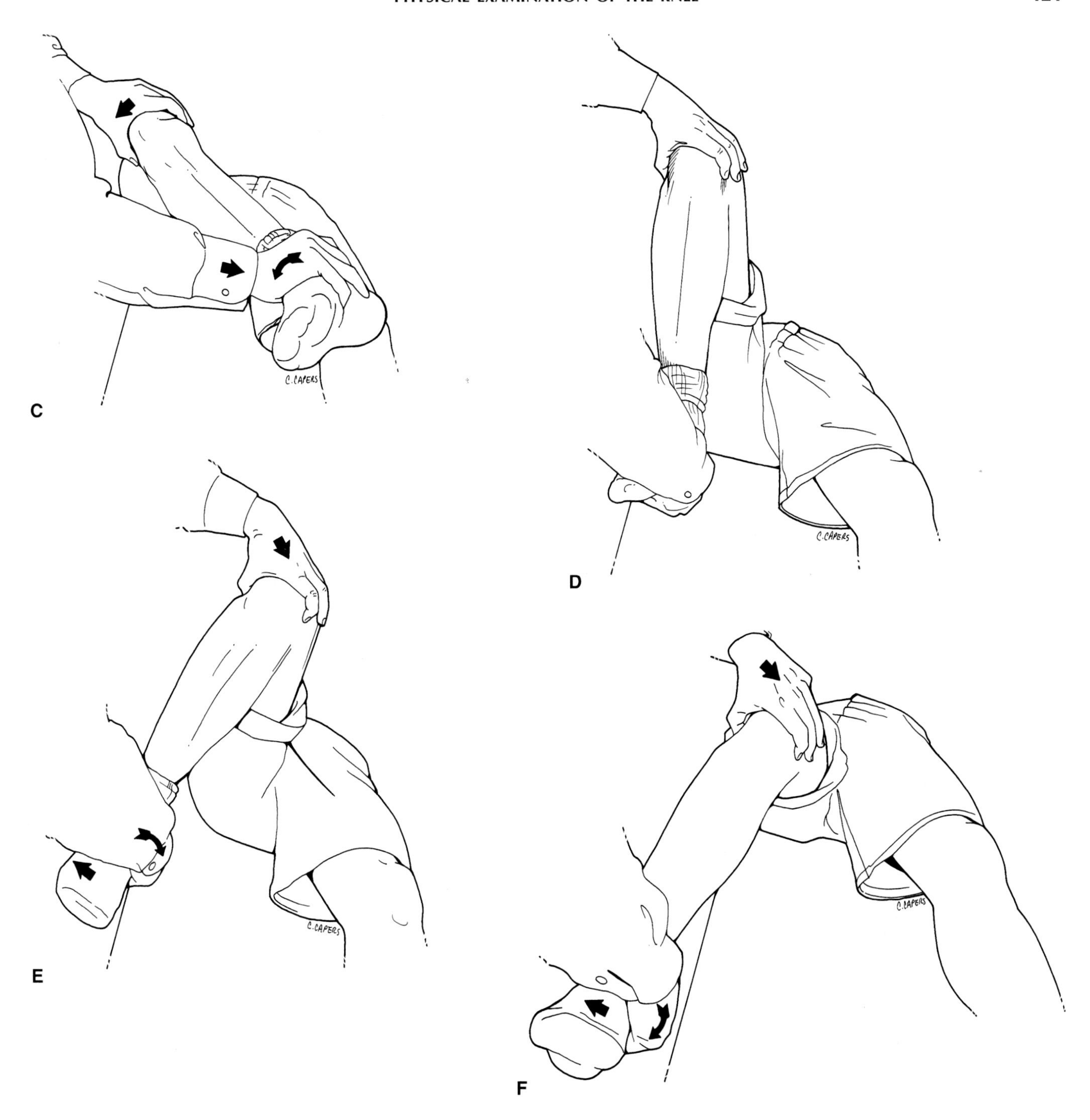

Fig. 64–4. Variation of the McMurray test. ***(A)*** **The examiner positions the hand to palpate one joint line with the index finger and the other with the thumb.** ***(B)*** **Varus stress is applied to the flexed knee joint while the tibia is externally rotated.** ***(C)*** **The varus stress and external rotation continue as the knee is brought into extension.** ***(D–F)*** **The maneuver is repeated with valgus stress and internal rotation.**

When using physical tests to grade ligament injuries, I first establish an appropriate grading system to quantitate the subjective translation appreciated with the various tests. I arbitrarily use a system by which, if I feel the subjective translation is 3 mm I grade it trace, 3 to 5 mm is graded 1+, 5 to 10 mm is graded 2+, and greater than 10 mm translation is graded 3+. Obviously, this varies from examiner to examiner, depending on how forcefully one performs the test. There can also be variability in the patient's degree of relaxation, because muscle guarding serves to mitigate the degree of translation. Nonetheless, these grading criteria are fairly well accepted. It should be emphasized that it is very important always to check the uninjured knee, too. I routinely do this *first* whenever I examine a patient, because many people have physiologic laxity, for them, and a trace to 1+ grade is normal. This fact obviously needs to be appreciated so that similar laxity is not misinterpreted on the injured side.

The basic approach to the ligamentous structures is to assess the state of the anterior cruciate ligament, the posterior cruciate ligament, the medial ligament complex, and then the lateral ligament complex, especially the posterolateral corner. The most sensitive and specific test for an anterior cruciate ligament tear is Lachman's test, which actually was first described by Ritchey (Fig. 64–5). This test is done with the knee at 15° to 20° of flexion. The examiner stabilizes the femur with one hand and then applies an anterior translation stress to the tibia with the other hand. Even with an acute knee injury that results in significant pain and swelling, the patient is generally relaxed enough for this test in this position. If there is excessive translation as compared with the opposite side, particularly with loss of a good end point, that is considered a positive result.

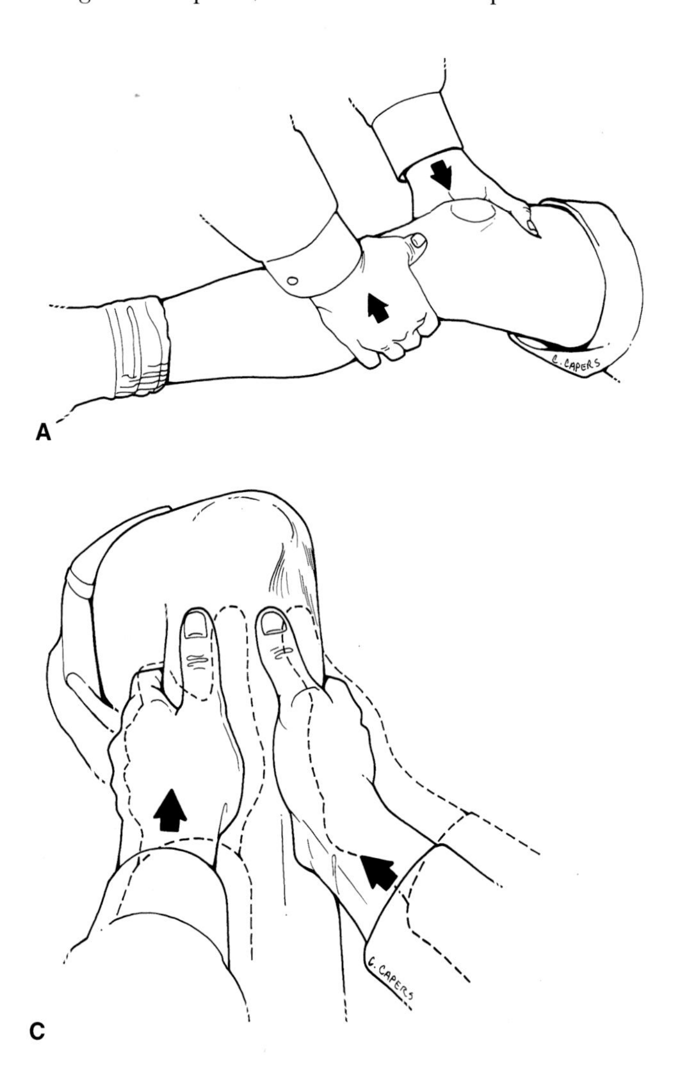

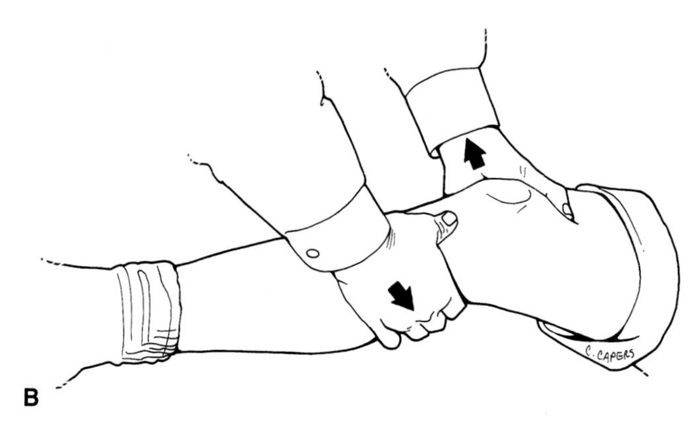

Fig. 64–5. ***(A)*** **Lachman's test is most sensitive for an anterior cruciate ligament tear. The femur is stabilized in 15° to 20° of flexion while the examiner applies anterior translation force to the tibia. If there is excessive translation as compared with the opposite side, the test is positive.** ***(B)*** **The posterior Lachman's test is done at 30° of flexion, reversing the stress on the tibia posteriorly.** ***(C)*** **The posterolateral stress test is done at 30°, applying posterolateral rotatory stress to the tibia.**

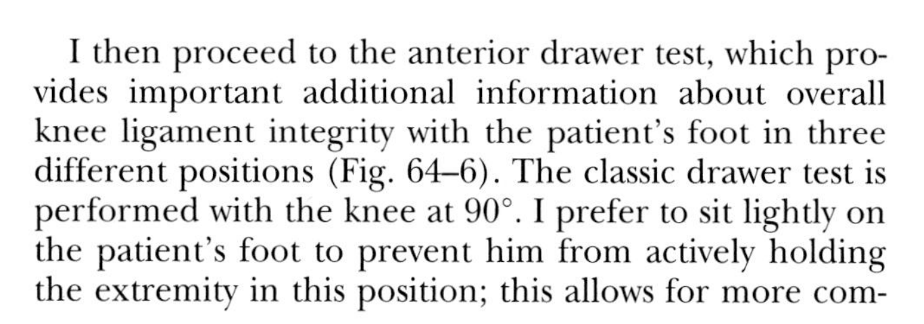

I then proceed to the anterior drawer test, which provides important additional information about overall knee ligament integrity with the patient's foot in three different positions (Fig. 64–6). The classic drawer test is performed with the knee at 90°. I prefer to sit lightly on the patient's foot to prevent him from actively holding the extremity in this position; this allows for more complete relaxation. I palpate the hamstrings to be sure the patient is thoroughly relaxed before testing. The test begins with the patient's foot in neutral position. I pull the tibia forward. Excessive anterior translation of the tibia as compared with the opposite knee, either with both the lateral and medial sides coming forward equally or the lateral side only coming forward, indicates anterior cruciate ligament laxity. The test is then performed with the foot externally rotated. If the tibia comes forward excessively, this usually indicates a medial ligament injury, because of the stress applied to the medial side. It is significant to point out that results of the anterior drawer test in external rotation can be positive with a medial ligament disruption and an *intact* anterior cruciate ligament. On the other hand, if the anterior drawer test is negative in external rotation, that

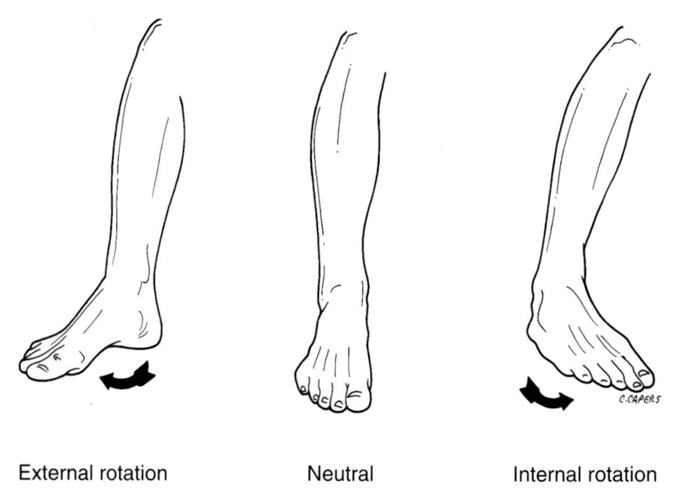

Fig. 64–6. The anterior and posterior drawer tests are done with the knee flexed to 90°. Both are performed with the patient's foot in three different positions: external rotation, neutral, and internal rotation.

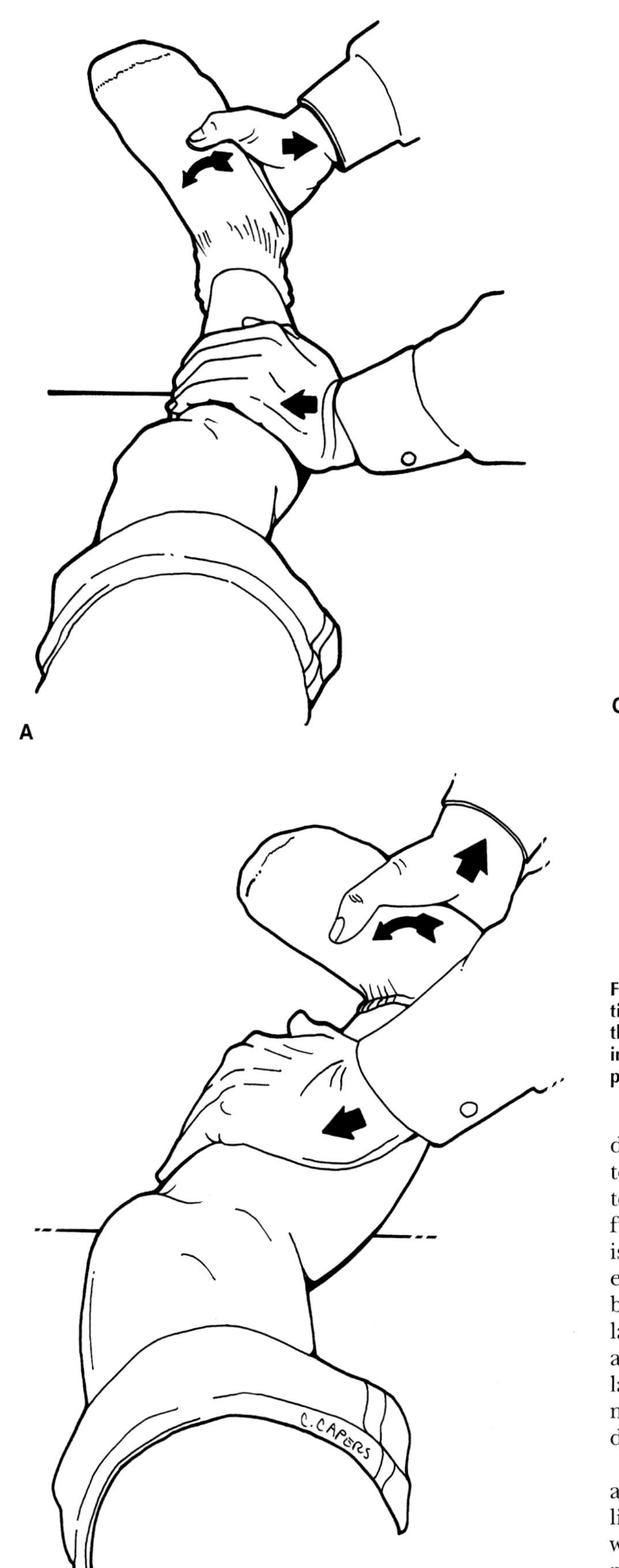

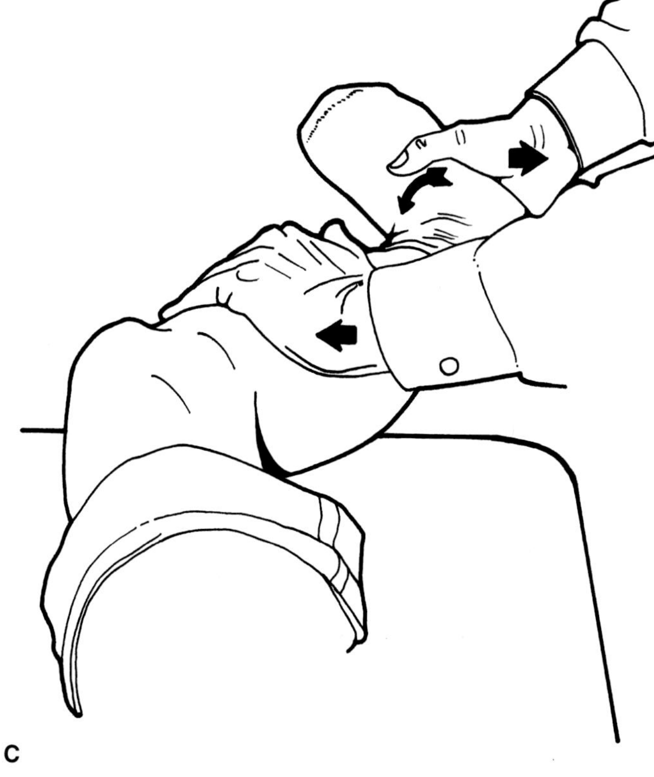

Fig. 64–7. The pivot shift test starts with the knee in extension. The tibia is rotated internally, and valgus stress is applied *(A)*. The knee is then flexed, which causes the tibia to rotate excessively anteriorly and internally *(B)*. At about 30°, the tibia forcefully reduces from its position of subluxation *(C)*.

does not mean the anterior cruciate ligament is not torn, it means only that the medial side is intact. The test is performed a third time with the patient's foot in full internal rotation. If the posterior cruciate ligament is intact there is no anterior translation in this position, even with a complete anterior cruciate ligament tear, because the posterior cruciate ligament and the posterolateral capsule tighten in internal rotation. This negates any anterior translation from anterior cruciate ligament laxity, even in the loosest case of anterior cruciate ligament deficiency with a 3+ Lachman's and the anterior drawer 3+ in neutral position.

The third test that is critical, especially when trying to ascertain functional disability from an anterior cruciate ligament tear, is the pivot shift maneuver (Fig. 64–7), which can be done in several ways. The pivot shift is a rotational phenomenon that reproduces the giving way that can occur with anterior cruciate ligament insufficiency. Unfortunately, it is a difficult test to perform with an acute injury because of patient guarding, but it is obviously done easily in a patient under anesthesia and is tolerated fairly well by patients with an injury of long standing. There are several different ways to perform the pivot shift. I prefer the original one described by McIntosh, starting with the knee in full extension. The tibia is rotated internally while applying a valgus-type stress at the same time, and then the knee is flexed, which initially causes the tibia to rotate excessively anteriorly and internally at about 10°. Then, as the knee is flexed farther, at about 30° the tibia forcefully reduces from its subluxated position because of the shape of the femoral condyle and tightening of the iliotibial tract. This action creates the shift.

Dr. Hughston described the "jerk test," which denotes rapid acceleration. It is performed from flexion to extension with exactly the same stresses as the pivot shift. Variations of the test have been described by Slocum and Losee and Noyes with the flexion-rotation drawer, and these can all be done, depending on the examiner's preference.

For assessment of the posterior cruciate ligament, I first like to perform what is termed the *90° sag test,* or *Godfrey's maneuver* (Fig. 64–8). The knee and the hip are both flexed to 90°, and the leg is held in this position by the examiner so that the quadriceps muscle relaxes. If the posterior ligament is torn, the tibia subluxates posteriorly. This can be compared easily with the normal side held in this same position to check for any visible difference. The examiner can palpate the medial tibial plateau, which generally should be 1 cm or so prominent from the flare of the medial femoral condyle, according to Clancy. If the normal step-off is not present here, posterior cruciate laxity is indicated.

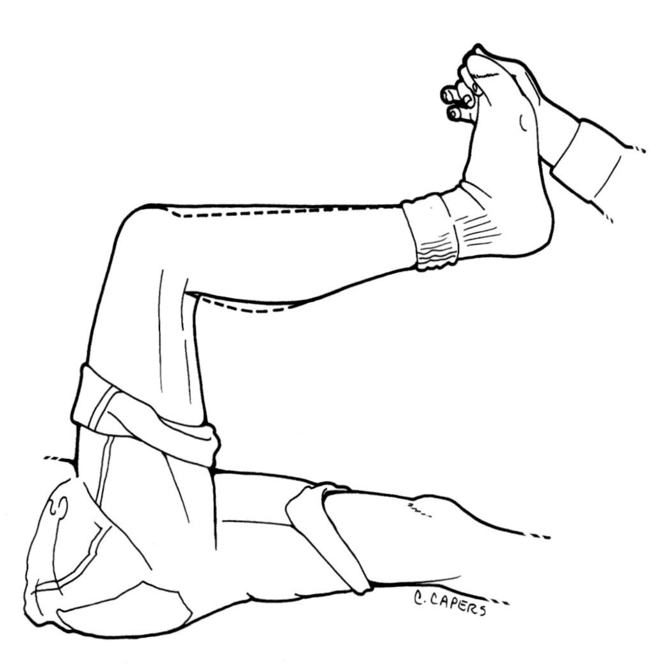

Fig. 64–8. The 90° sag test indicates the presence of a posterior cruciate ligament injury. With the knee and hip flexed 90°, the tibia subluxates posteriorly if the posterior cruciate ligament is ruptured.

Next, I perform the posterior drawer test at 90°. As with the anterior drawer test, it is easier for the patient to avoid contracting the muscles if the examiner sits lightly on the foot while the tibia is pushed posteriorly. This test is also done in three positions: neutral, which is best to determine the extent of posterior cruciate laxity; external rotation, which also helps determine the status of the posterolateral corner; and internal rotation, which is important because, if the posterior drawer sign is elicited in this position, the posterior cruciate ligament is lax, even if the excessive tibial movement on posterior drawer seems greater in the anterior than in the posterior orientation, which is sometimes the case because of the effect of gravity and an equivocal starting point. When both the anterior cruciate and the posterior cruciate ligaments are torn, it can be especially difficult to assess the starting point for drawer testing, but, again, a positive drawer test in internal rotation signifies that the posterior cruciate ligament is definitely involved. If there is a question of combined anterior and posterior cruciate injury, the best test is the pivot shift, which of course is specific for anterior cruciate ligament instability.

The last test I use for checking the posterior cruciate is the "posterior Lachman," which is done with a bit more flexion—at approximately 30° as opposed to 15° to 20° for the anterior Lachman's test. The concept is the same, but the force is reversed; the examiner stabilizes the femur with one hand and applies posterior stress to the tibia, feeling for laxity.

In terms of the medial ligament complex, the two diagnostic tests performed are the abduction stress test and the anterior drawer in external rotation (Fig. 64–9). The abduction, or valgus, stress test is done at both 0° and 30° of flexion. Applying abduction stress in full extension actually tests not only the medial side but also the posterior cruciate ligament and posterior capsule. This test will be negative unless there is disruption both posteriorly and medially. At 30° of flexion, the abduction stress test is sensitive for medial ligament laxity. The examiner should palpate the medial joint line at the time of stress testing, to feel for "gapping." It is also critical to feel whether the meniscus is popping, which could indicate either a true peripheral tear or a meniscus rendered unstable by a meniscotibial ligament tear. As previously described, the anterior drawer sign in external rotation is positive in the presence of a significant medial ligament injury. This is especially the case when the meniscus is torn peripherally or torn through the meniscotibial ligament, because the normal buttress effect of the posterior horn of the meniscus on the back of the medial femoral condyle is lost, and the tibia shows excessive anterior translation. Also, it should be remembered that a patient with an intact anterior cruciate ligament can still show a positive anterior drawer test in external rotation if the medial side is torn.

For the lateral side, the test comparable to the abduction stress test is the adduction, or varus, stress test, which again is done at 0° first, to determine posterior capsule and posterior cruciate integrity, and then at 30° of

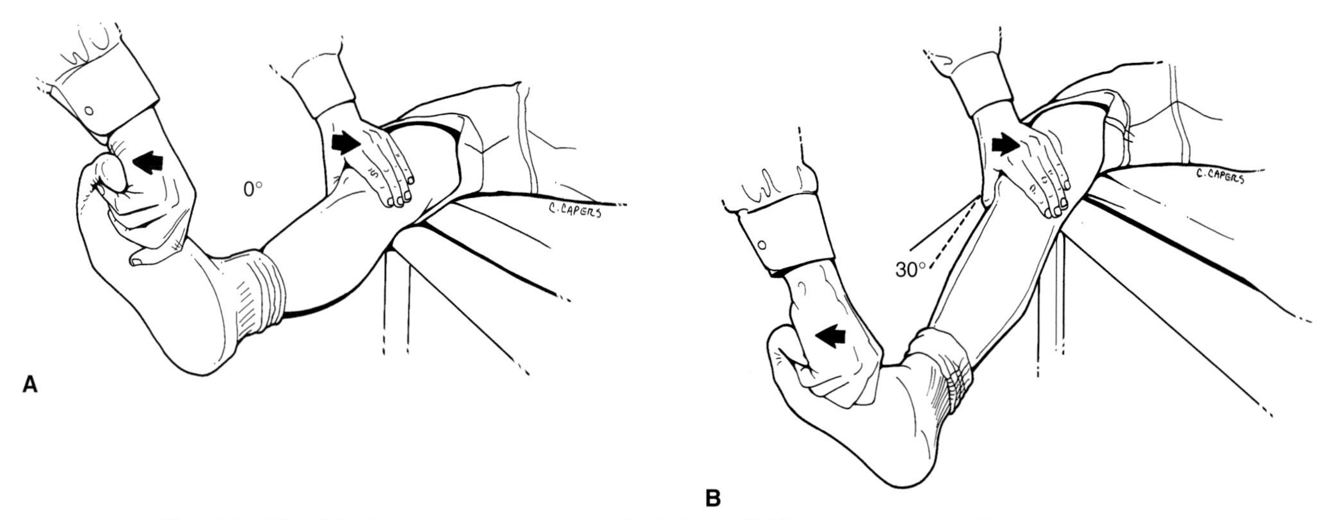

Fig. 64–9. The abduction stress test at 0° *(A)* tests both the medial ligament structures and the posterior cruciate ligament. In 30° of flexion *(B),* the abduction stress test is very sensitive to the medial ligaments.

flexion. The difference on the lateral side is that some degree of adduction laxity is usually present because of the normal valgus posture at the knee joint. The initial adduction stress corrects only for this valgus, but, again, it is important to compare it to the uninjured side. Anterior drawer testing really does not come into play, in terms of assessing lateral side stability, as it does on the medial side, even though internal rotation of the tibia tends to stress the lateral side; however, the posterior cruciate and posterior capsule also tighten, thus limiting anterior translation with an anterior drawer test.

The major difference on the lateral side is the importance of the posterolateral corner, which has to be checked specifically through a series of physical tests. The posterolateral stress test at 30° is basically very similar to the Lachman's test: one hand stabilizes the femur but, instead of translating the tibia anteriorly with the other, hand a posterolateral rotatory stress is applied to the tibia. I find that a positive Lachman's test can at times be difficult to differentiate from a positive posterolateral stress test. This may lead the examiner to think the Lachman's test is positive and the anterior cruciate ligament is torn when in fact the laxity is actually due to injury at the posterolateral corner. Also, the posterior drawer test at 90° with external rotation can indicate posterolateral corner injury and, so, can be confused for posterior cruciate laxity.

Two other essential tests for posterolateral instability include the external rotation recurvatum test and the reverse pivot shift. The external rotation recurvatum test is done by grasping the big toe with the patient relaxed and picking up the leg with the knee extended, looking for accentuated recurvatum (hyperextension) with associated external rotation of the tibia. This is best seen by watching the tibial tubercle, because when the test is positive the tibia rotates externally. This, of course, has to be compared to the normal side to determine if pathologic laxity exists. Patients who normally have hypermobile joints and excessive recurvatum may demonstrate hyperextension in this position; but they do not usually show the external rotation of the tibial tubercle because the posterolateral corner is still intact. Finally, the reverse pivot shift is done with the knee flexed and the tibia externally rotated. In this position, valgus stress is applied as the knee is extended, and the tibia goes from a subluxated posterolateral position to a reduced position. A "clunk" (as opposed to a jerk) is felt at the reduction point.

65 *Tarek O. Souryal*

Imaging of the Knee

RADIOGRAPHY

After a complete history and physical examination, plain radiographs of the knee are the main staple of diagnostic evaluation of the bones for acute knee injuries. Anteroposterior, lateral, sunrise patellar, and notch views are the minimum necessary to fully evaluate the bony anatomy of the knee. These views should show the distal third of the femur and the proximal third of the tibia. The anteroposterior and lateral views are essential for detecting fractures and dislocations of the femoral articulation with the tibia. The overlying patellar shadow may also indicate fracture or dislocation of that structure. Standing views are used in elders to demonstrate compartmental collapse. The patellar sunrise view is used to inspect patellar tilt and patellar fracture. Small avulsion fractures that may occur with patellar dislocation may be seen on this view. The tunnel view of the intercondylar notch is used to detect loose bodies that may be entrapped in the notch, avulsion fractures of the anterior cruciate ligament, or intercondylar notch stenosis. Standard radiology texts, such as V. Merrill's *Atlas of Roentgenographic Positions* (St. Louis, C. V. Mosby, 1967), are an excellent source for proper positioning for these views.

Proper interpretation of radiographs can also suggest injuries that may not be seen directly on the films themselves. A lateral capsular sign is associated with an anterior cruciate ligament injury or a lateral loose body may be suggestive of patellar dislocation. The notch width index has been used to evaluate intercondylar notch stenosis (Fig. 65–1), which has been associated with anterior cruciate ligament injury in athletes. This simple to compute parameter is a ratio of the intercondylar notch width to the width of the distal femur at the level of the popliteus on a tunnel view. The notch width index is not unlike Torg's ratio for assessing cervical spine stenosis in athletes.

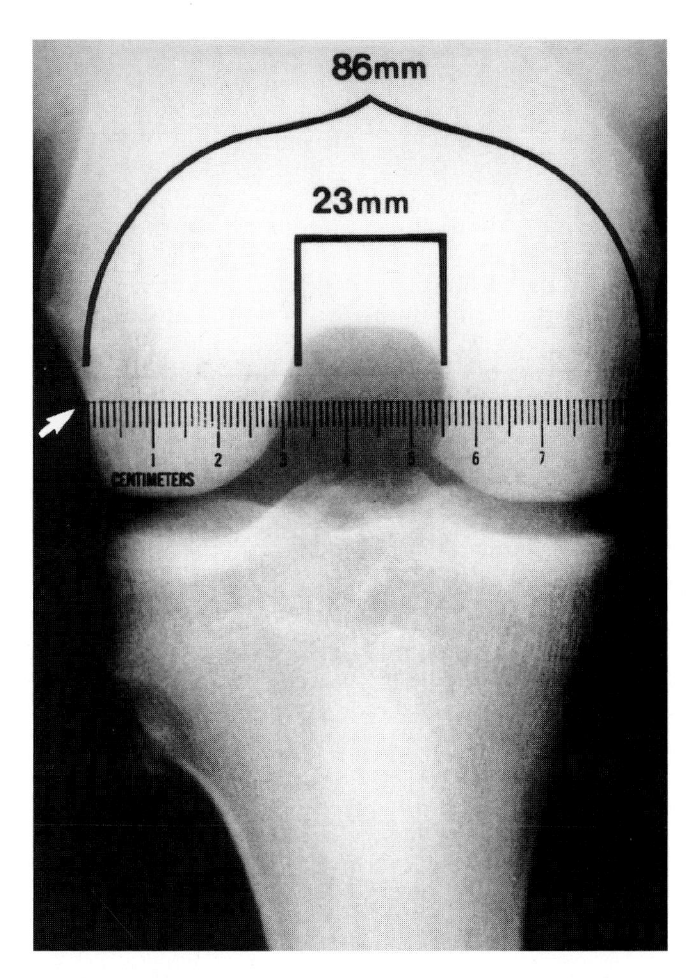

Fig. 65–1. To derive the notch width index, a line is drawn parallel to the joint line at the level of the popliteus groove. The notch and the distal femur are measured, and a ratio is calculated. (Reprinted from Souryal, T. O. et al.: Bilaterality in anterior cruciate ligament injuries. Am. J. Sports Med. *16*:449, 1988.)

ARTHROGRAPHY

Arthrography is similar to plain radiography in that x-ray beams are used to study the articular anatomy; however, radiopaque dyes are used to outline soft tissue structures that otherwise would not be seen. Arthrography of the knee is used to evaluate meniscal tears. Medial meniscal tears are more readily seen with this method than lateral ones. This method of evaluation has fallen out of favor in recent years, partly because it is considered an "invasive" procedure and not as accurate as magnetic resonance imaging (MRI). It can be helpful in determining the size of popliteal cysts and may be used if a patient cannot or will not undergo MRI.

TOMOGRAPHY AND COMPUTED TOMOGRAPHY

Tomography and computed tomography (CT) have a limited but vital role in knee evaluation. Both methods use single-plane x-ray beams. Tomography delineates the bony anatomy in great detail. It can show areas of suspected fractures that otherwise are not clearly visualized on plain films, such as depressed lateral tibial plateau fractures. CT has limited use in evaluations for athletic injuries to the knee, except when better visualization of a fracture is necessary. CT of the knee yields valuable information on bone tumors about the knee. Both methods are useful for assessing osteochondritis dissecans and tibial plateau fractures (Fig. 65–2). The spiral scanning mode of the CT scan has decreased scanning time, improved reconstruction capability, and afforded better resolution.

NUCLEAR IMAGING

Osseous scintigraphy (radionuclide bone scanning) is an indirect test of the biologic activity of bone. This test is often used in sports medicine to look for occult stress fractures about the knee. Osseous scintigraphy is also useful in detecting infection or reflex sympathetic dystrophy. In this test, a small amount of radioisotope (technetium 99^{m}) is injected intravenously. The isotope, which has an affinity for bone, is rapidly incorporated into new bone. The radioisotope is allowed to circulate for a time, then the affected area is scanned to see in which areas it has localized.

Repeated scanning at various intervals (phases) yields information about the vascularity of the area and the bones' metabolic activity. Diffuse uptake in the early blood pool phase is a sign of increased vascularity, as in reflex sympathetic dystrophy. Intense focal uptake in the later bone phase is a sign of rapid bone remodeling, as in a stress fracture (Fig. 65–3).

Single proton–emission CT (SPECT), the latest advance in nuclear medicine, produces tomographic

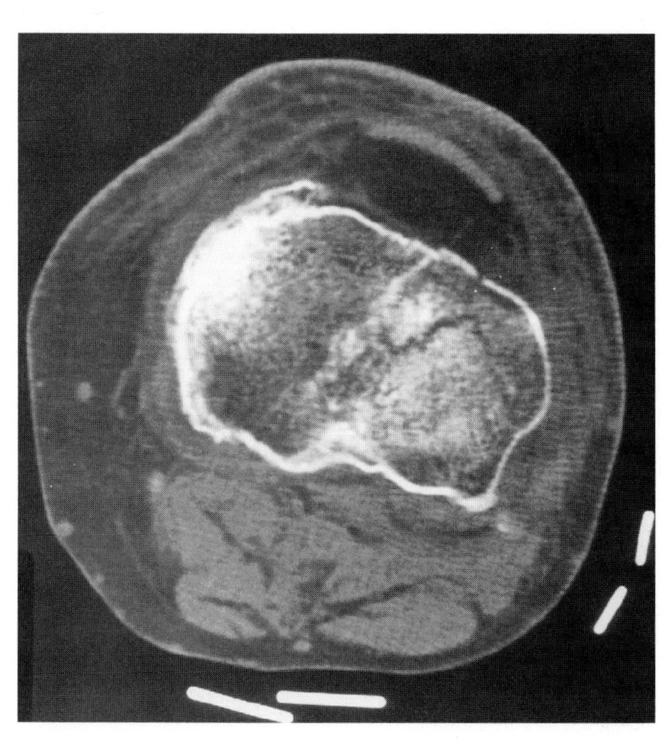

Fig. 65–2. CT of the knee shows tibial plateau fracture.

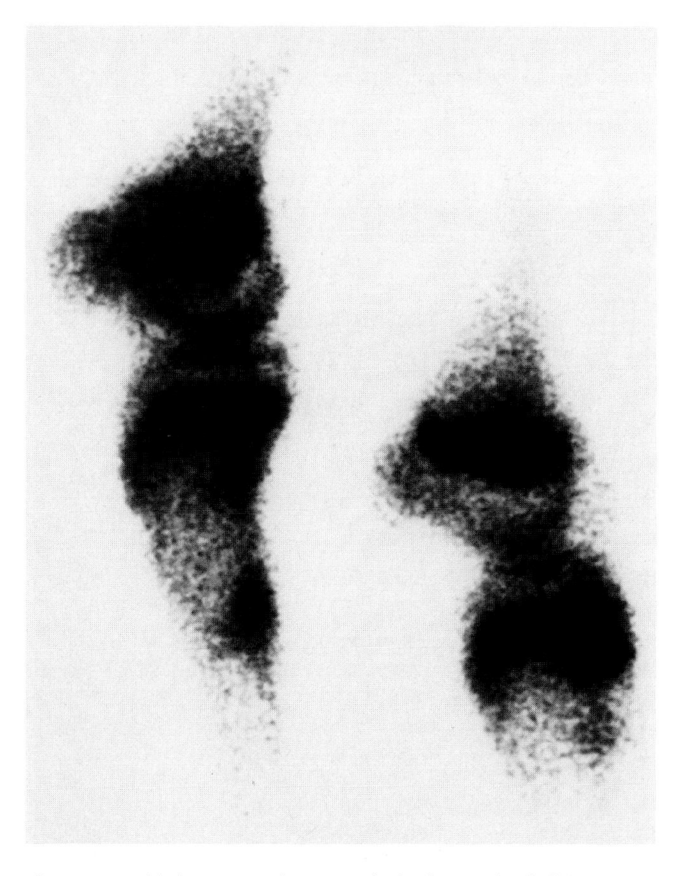

Fig. 65–3. This bone scan shows uptake in the proximal tibia, indicating a stress fracture.

"cuts" of the study area that are more sensitive and therefore more accurate in anatomically complex regions of the body.

MAGNETIC RESONANCE IMAGING

MRI is a remarkable tool that uses resonance and magnetic fields to differentiate between adjacent body tissues. Simply stated, the large magnetic field aligns the protons in the tissues in a uniform orientation. Radiofrequency waves are then used to excite the protons. As the radio waves are turned off, the protons relax into their previous orientation. The relaxation times are then processed to yield an image. Different tissue types have different proton-relaxation times. Varying the frequency of the radio waves gives different relaxation times, and, therefore, different images of the same group of tissues (T1, T2, and 3D). Three-dimensional reconstruction of the images has provided markedly improved diagnostic capabilities.

In sports medicine, MRI is used to make or confirm a soft tissue diagnosis. Meniscal lesions, muscle tears, tendinitis, bursitis, articular cartilage lesions, and ligament injuries are clearly identified by MRI (Fig. 65–4). If the diagnosis is in doubt or the patient is difficult to examine and there is a strong possibility that surgery may not be necessary, MRI is indicated. Likewise, if the diagnosis is clear and surgery is imminent, MRI may not be indicated.

Indications in sports medicine include acute knee injuries with hemarthrosis, an ill-defined meniscal or articular cartilage lesion, or a suspected anterior cruciate ligament injury in a knee that is difficult to evaluate. MRI is used to supplement the knee examination and should not be used in place of an accurate physical examination. The quality of the scanner and the training of the radiologist are important factors in accuracy and cost effectiveness of MRI.

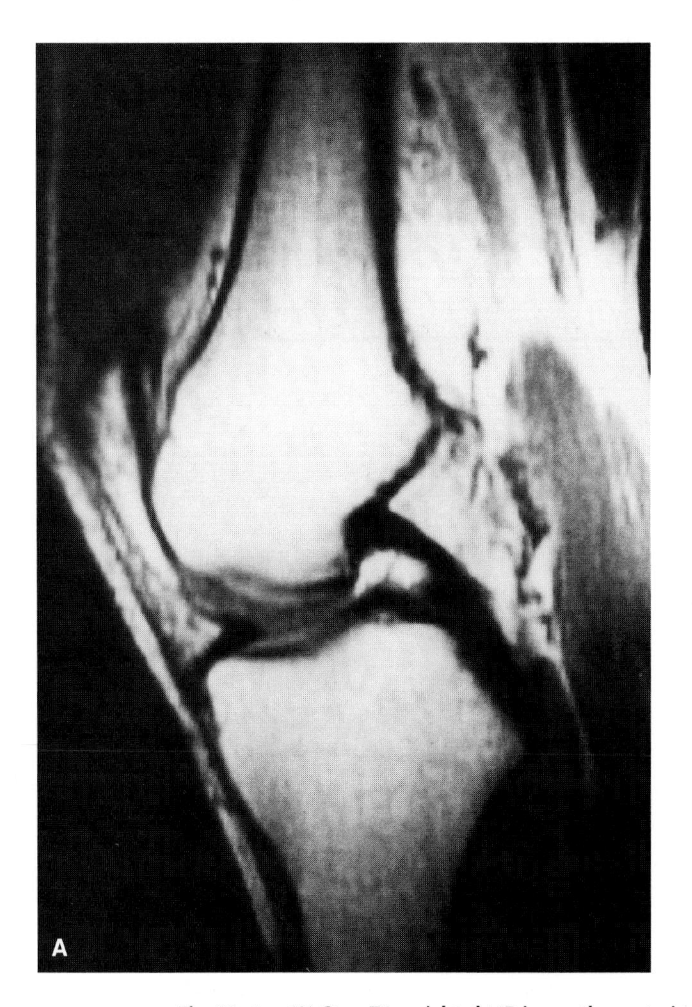

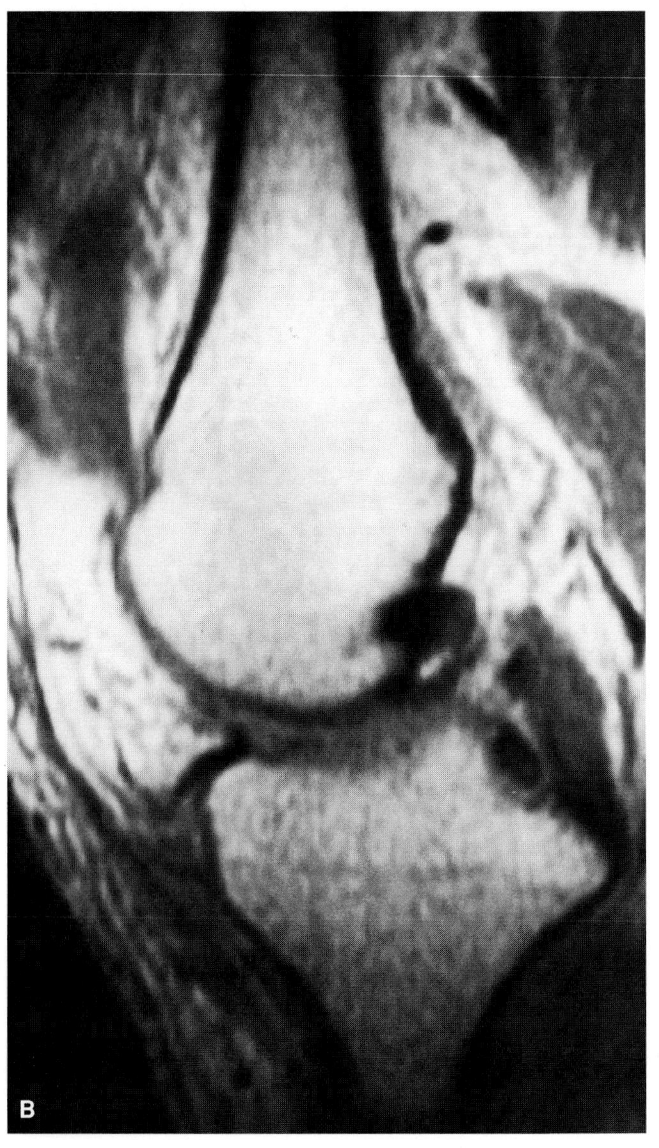

Fig. 65–4. ***(A)*** **On a T1-weighted MR image the posterior cruciate ligament shows as a dark band.** ***(B)*** **MRI shows disruption of the posterior cruciate ligament.**

66

Giancarlo Puddu, Vittorio Franco, Alberto Selvanetti, Massimo Cipolla

Jumper's Knee and Other Forms of Tendinitis About the Knee

JUMPER'S KNEE

Jumper's knee is an insertional tendinitis of mechanical origin caused by overuse. It usually affects athletes who expose their knees to continuous stresses and eccentric efforts that exceed the intrinsic tensile resistance of the extensor apparatus structures (i.e., those involved in basketball, football, soccer, track and field, volleyball, fencing, cycling, dancing, skiing, rugby, handball, weight lifting, and gymnastics). The prevalence is almost the same for men and women, and it increases after age 15 years.[1]

The term *jumper's knee* refers to insertional tendinopathies of both the quadriceps and the patellar tendon.[2] Quadriceps tendinitis is more frequent in patients older than 40 and is located at the upper pole of the patella (apex). Patellar tendinitis is the most frequent tendinitis about the knee (80% according to Curwin and Stanish[3]) and generally affects patients between 20 and 40 years old. It is localized to the lower pole of the patella (base).

Causes

The sudden and repeated overload of the knee extensor mechanism, sometimes aggravated by a lack of balance of this apparatus, weakens the tendon structures. Overload occurs when the athlete lands on the leg with the knee in semiflexion (as in volleyball, basketball, soccer); when the foot leaves the ground after the eccentric contraction phase of the quadriceps (sprinting, jumping) or in acceleration, deceleration, stopping, or cutting movements (rugby, football, soccer, basketball, throwing).

This sudden and repeated overload can start a traction lesion of the quadriceps or of the patellar tendon. The lesion begins with microtearing and fraying of the fibers, followed by focal degeneration, and sometimes calcification. It usually involves the deep central fibers near the insertion, because they are less elastic and are subjected to a higher elongation rate when the knee is flexed. It is not certain whether training sessions with specific plyometric or isotonic exercises represent a risk factor for these types of tendinitis. A risk condition observed in dancers and basketball and volleyball players is pronounced adduction of the knee during jumping, both in the lifting and in the landing moment. This situation causes the highest stresses to the tendon, especially in the eccentric phases.[4]

External factors can also contribute to this injury.

Playing surfaces: Hard, inelastic surfaces (cement, asphalt) are more harmful than elastic ones (linoleum, parquet).

Years of play: Among volleyball players, the incidence of patellar tendinitis is highest in those who have played 3 to 6 years. After this, the incidence decreases, probably because by this time the structures are strengthened.

Commitments per week: Tendinitis is more frequent in volleyball players who play more than four times a week.

On the other hand, we have found that intrinsic factors (lower limb morphology, high-riding patella, malalignment of the extensor mechanism, joint laxity or flexibility, and altered plantar support) do not seem to be associated with the incidence of this injury.

History and Physical Examination

The main symptom reported with jumper's knee is pain in the anterior region of the knee (the infrapatellar or, less often, suprapatellar area). The pain begins insidiously, almost always without trauma, and progressively increases. The pain is exacerbated by physical activity or when the patient remains sitting with the knee flexed for long periods ("movie sign"). The pain is more often located at the tendinous insertion on the lower pole of the patella (65 to 82% of the cases) rather than on the upper patellar pole (quadriceps tendon) or the distal insertion of the patellar tendon to the tibial tuberosity.[1, 5–7]

Blazina described four clinical stages of jumper's knee, which are distinguished by the subjective symptoms and the relative levels of functional motion[2,8]:

Stage 1: Pain after sports activity
Stage 2: Pain at the beginning of sports activity that disappears with warm-up and sometimes reappears with fatigue
Stage 3: Pain at rest and during activity, inability to participate in sports
Stage 4: Rupture of the tendon.

Curwin and Stanish proposed a more complete classification of six levels[9]:

Level 1: No pain
Level 2: Pain with extreme exertion only
Level 3: Pain with exertion and 1 to 2 hours afterward
Level 4: Pain during any athletic activity and 4 to 6 hours after, performance level decreased
Level 5: Pain immediately after beginning sports activity, withdrawal from activity
Level 6: Pain during daily activities, inability to participate in any sports.

In patients with this tendinitis, pain can be elicited by palpation over the tendinous insertion on the lower or upper pole of the patella or, less frequently, over the tendon belly or the tibial tuberosity. Sometimes the examiner can feel mild swelling of the tendon belly (peritendinitis), which is sensitive to finger pressure. The pain is also aggravated by sudden contraction of the quadriceps, passive flexion of the leg past 120°, squatting exercises, and resisted extension of the leg. Another clinical sign of jumper's knee is the rising of the apex when the patella is pushed downward with the knee in full extension (Fig. 66–1). Quadriceps atrophy, dysplasia of the vastus medialis obliquus (VMO), and functional insufficiency of the flexors dorsalis of the ankle could be more or less evident. Joint swelling is never present, and meniscal tests are always negative.

Rupture of the quadriceps or patellar tendon is rare; it is, however, more common in elderly athletes. The rupture can be induced in younger athletes by local infiltration of corticosteroids into the tendon. Very uncommonly, a direct blow on the proximal epiphysis of the tibia can produce a complete tear of the healthy tendon.[9]

Instrumented Examination

The clinical diagnosis can be supported by instrumented examinations—traditional radiography to more sophisticated magnetic resonance imaging (MRI) and

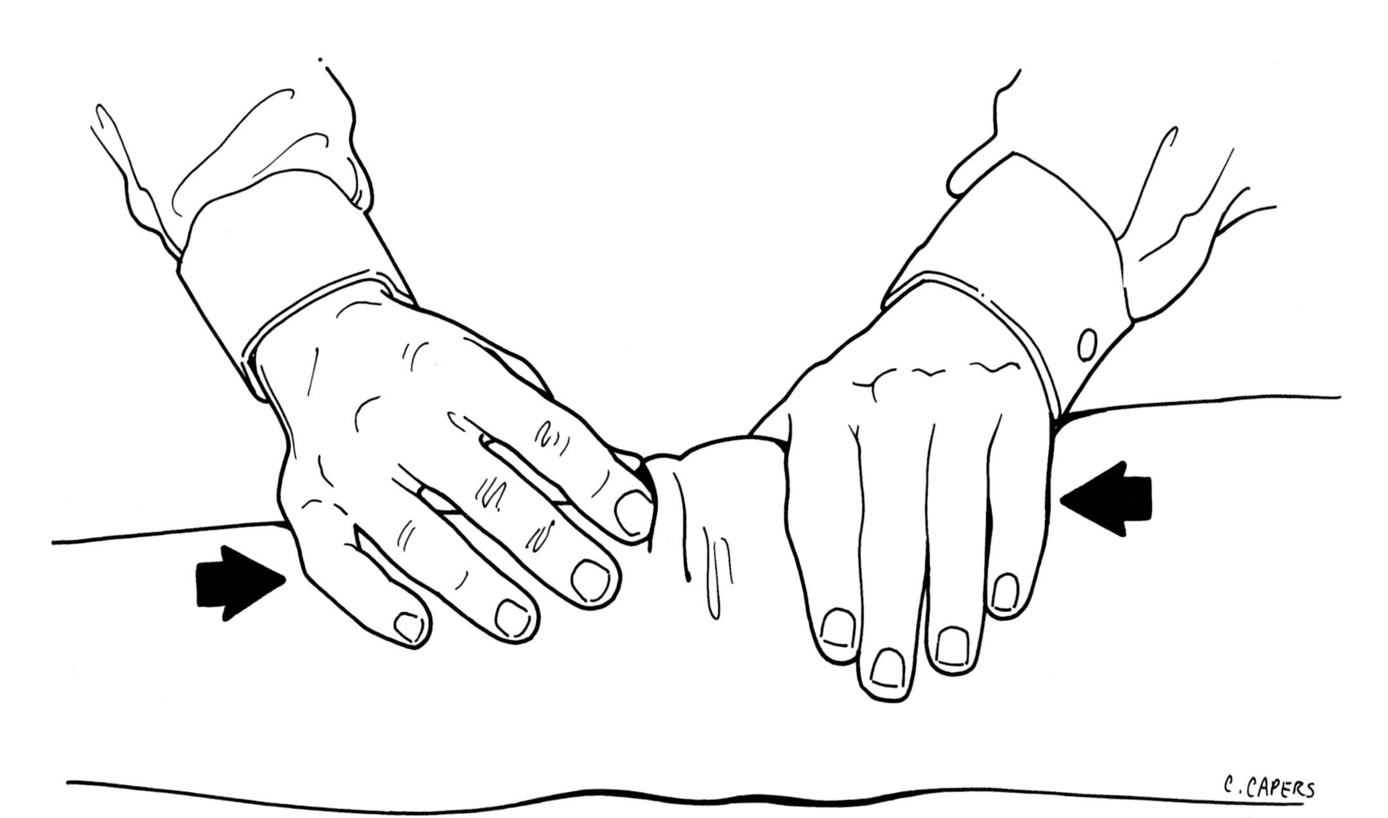

Fig. 66–1. With the knee in extension, the patella is forced distally, which slightly elevates the distal pole. The distal pole is then palpated for tenderness.

computed tomography (CT). Radiographic examination is meaningful only in a chronic case that involves the whole tendon. A lateral radiograph using soft tissue techniques shows a tendon belly that is thicker than normal, evidence of degeneration, and occasionally elongations or irregularities of the distal pole of the patella. Ossicles may be observed in the tendon as well.

Ultrasonography allows periodic evaluation and noninvasive examination of the evolution of the disease, which Fritschy divided into three stages, as follows[9]:

Stage 1 (pure inflammation): Edema of tendon fibers
Stage 2 (irreversible anatomic lesions): The tendon has a heterogeneous appearance, with hypoechoic and hyperechoic areas, with or without edema
Stage 3 (final evolution): The tendon sheath is irregularly thickened, tendon fibers appear heterogeneous, and swelling is no longer present.

CT and MRI can help to assess the stage of disease and to localize the site and the extent of the involved areas.

In case of a complete rupture of the tendon, radiographic examination shows the patella dislocated proximally or distally, and occasionally bone fragments at the origin of the patellar tendon or at the insertion of the quadriceps tendon. The rupture has to be confirmed by other investigations, such as ultrasonography, CT, or MRI.

Differential Diagnosis

Other conditions that can be associated with jumper's knee must be recognized and distinguished. Synovial infrapatellar plica can provoke locking sensations in extension and pain in the superomedial or superolateral quadrant of the knee. Meniscal lesions can cause actual locking episodes, sharp pain at the joint line, and joint effusion. Patellofemoral arthrosis and chondromalacia cause anterior knee pain during squatting or jumping, but there is no point tenderness and the "grinding" sign is often present. Bursitis of the four bursas around the knee (suprapatellar, prepatellar, subcutaneous, and deep infrapatellar), especially deep infrapatellar bursitis, can mimic jumper's knee, but one must remember that pain localized at the tibial tubercle (as in deep infrapatellar bursitis) is uncommon in tendinitis beyond adolescence. Fat pad inflammation (Hoffa's disease) is distinguished by swelling and pain when the fat pad is squeezed. Osgood-Schlatter disease and Sinding-Larsen-Johansson disease have to be considered as peculiar types of traction tendinitis in adolescents. They are characterized by pain localized at the tibial tubercle or at the lower pole of the patella (very rarely at the upper pole).

Treatment

In the first two stages, according to Blazina's classification (or Curwin and Stanish's first five levels) conservative treatment is the best choice. Rest is important, but the athlete can continue activity within the limits of symptoms to maintain physical fitness and to preserve athletic conditioning. Nonsteroidal anti-inflammatory drugs (NSAIDs) and cryotherapy are also part of the nonoperative treatment. When necessary, other physical therapy modalities can be used to control pain and swelling: ultrasound therapy, iontophoresis, and diadynamic currents. Intratendinous injection of corticosteroidal drugs should be avoided because there is a high risk of rupture. Massage therapy is a safe alternative of moderate efficacy.

The whole treatment is based on functional rehabilitation of the muscles. Athletes are instructed in correct warm-up techniques for the hamstrings, quadriceps, triceps surae, and hip flexors and extensors. During the first few days, isometric exercises of the quadriceps can be done (starting in full extension and then also with various degrees of flexion). The athlete progresses to isotonic exercises to strengthen the hamstrings and quadriceps. The strengthening sessions should also include exercises for the hip muscles. It is very important to start early concentric and eccentric exercise of the tibialis anterior muscle, which promotes infrapatellar stretching and improves the biomechanics of jumping, both in the lifting and the landing phases.[10] The range of motion of each exercise must be completely painless.

During the early period of rehabilitation, the jumping athlete works in a swimming pool, beginning with slow movements in deep water using flotation devices (cycling, jogging, and straight-leg hip flexion and extension motions). The athlete can then progress to more difficult exercises in shallow water.

Curwin and Stanish proposed the "drop and stop" method of working.[8, 11] After a warm-up phase and static or proprioceptive neuromuscular facilitation stretching of the quadriceps and hamstrings, the athlete progressively increases semisquat exercises, starting with larger and faster squats and progressing to weights. The session is concluded by recovery exercises (stretching) and local application of ice.

We recommend the use of an orthotic device (the infrapatellar strap) to reduce the stress on the tendon insertion (Fig. 66–2). For patients in the third stage of Blazina or the sixth level of Curwin and Stanish, we propose the same conservative treatment indicated above, but we recommend a longer period of abstinence from any activity that produces pain. After 4 to 6 months' conservative treatment without any appreciable result we advise surgical therapy or that athletes end their sports career.

Surgical Treatment

Surgical treatment for jumper's knee consists of accurate curettage of the tendon insertion. When possible, the pathologic tissue should be removed with a triangular incision of the tendon. We complete the surgery by bone drilling the insertional area and scarring the tendon parallel to its fibers. At the same time, it is advisable to perform arthroscopic examination of the joint, to evaluate and treat any associated articular injuries of the knee.

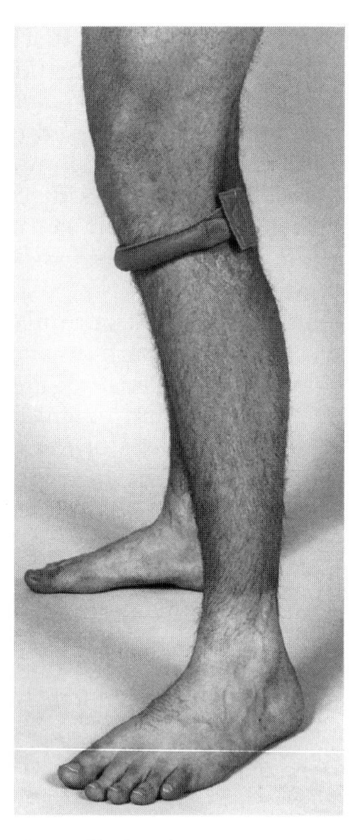

Fig. 66–2. The infrapatellar band can be worn to reduce stress on the tendon insertion.

Complete rupture or avulsion of the tendons (Stage 4 of Blazina) requires surgical treatment. An interstitial lesion of the quadriceps tendon can be repaired with end-to-end suture augmented by a polydioxanone suture (PDS) band or reinforced with a flap of healthy tendon tissue turned over the lesion.

An avulsion of the tendon from the proximal pole of the patella must be reinserted with transosseous stitches, reconstructing the osseotendinous junction. It is necessary to reinforce the suture with an augmentation of absorbable material (PDS band), which transmits part of the tensile stress from the quadriceps to the bone, bypassing the rupture site.

A complete interstitial rupture of the patellar tendon, a rare lesion, must be treated in the way described above for quadriceps injuries. When the avulsion involves the distal insertion of the patellar tendon with a large bone fragment from the tibial tuberosity, we advise open reduction and fixation of the fragment with a malleolar screw.

Prevention

All athletes who practice sports that place much stress on the extensor mechanism of the knee must be informed of the importance of general warming up and stretching of the lower limb muscles, before and after their agonistic performances *and* simple training sessions. From the first stages of the agonistic season, training sessions have to include essential exercises dedicated to concentric-eccentric work for the quadriceps. Plyometric exercises and strengthening of the VMO muscle are also important.

Among the prophylactic measures are observing and correcting techniques in sports performance, ensuring a proper playing surface, regulating the number and frequency of training sessions, and, of course, encouraging the use of shoes with better shock absorption.

OSGOOD-SCHLATTER DISEASE

Osgood-Schlatter disease is apophysitis of the tibial tubercle at the insertion of the patellar tendon. It generally appears in young athletes and adolescents between 10 and 15 years old,[(12)] very often at the beginning of pubertal growth. It is more frequent among young boys, especially those who practice sports with high functional stress on the extensor mechanism of the knee.

This affliction could be considered nonarticular osteochondritis or traction apophysitis caused by trauma or, more often, functional overload secondary to repetitive stresses of the patellar tendon at the insertion on the tibial tuberosity. Almost always, the disease is self-limiting, and it ends with complete ossification and fusion of the tuberosity to the tibial metaphysis.

History and Physical Examination

A young athlete with Osgood-Schlatter disease complains of pain during and after physical efforts, especially activities that demand vigorous contraction of the quadriceps (jumping, running, or going up and down stairs) or after direct trauma to the tibial tuberosity. Rarely are the symptoms so severe as to worry the patient or the parents and trainers, and sometimes the disease goes undiagnosed for months.

At the physical examination, the tibial tuberosity and the surrounding area are painful when palpated, and they are more prominent, edematous, and often warm. The patient's active range of motion is complete, but passive flexion and resisted extension cause pain. Flexibility of the quadriceps and the hamstrings is compromised; in chronic cases the quadriceps is atrophic. Associated biomechanic alterations are rather frequent: valgus knee, pronated foot, and excessive tibial external rotation.[(13,14)]

The radiographic examination must be performed with soft tissue technique, taking a lateral view with slight internal rotation of the tibia. Radiographic examination may not be necessary to make the diagnosis, especially when the history is characteristic, but it is useful to follow the patient's progress until complete ossification and fusion of the tuberosity.

Positive radiographs show the fragmentation of the tibial tuberosity (Fig. 66–3), a thickened patellar tendon, and a dishomogeneous space corresponding to the infrapatellar fat pad with the obliteration of the lower corner.[(15,16)]

Woolfrey and Chandler distinguished three classes of radiographic manifestations in the late stages of the disease[(15)]:

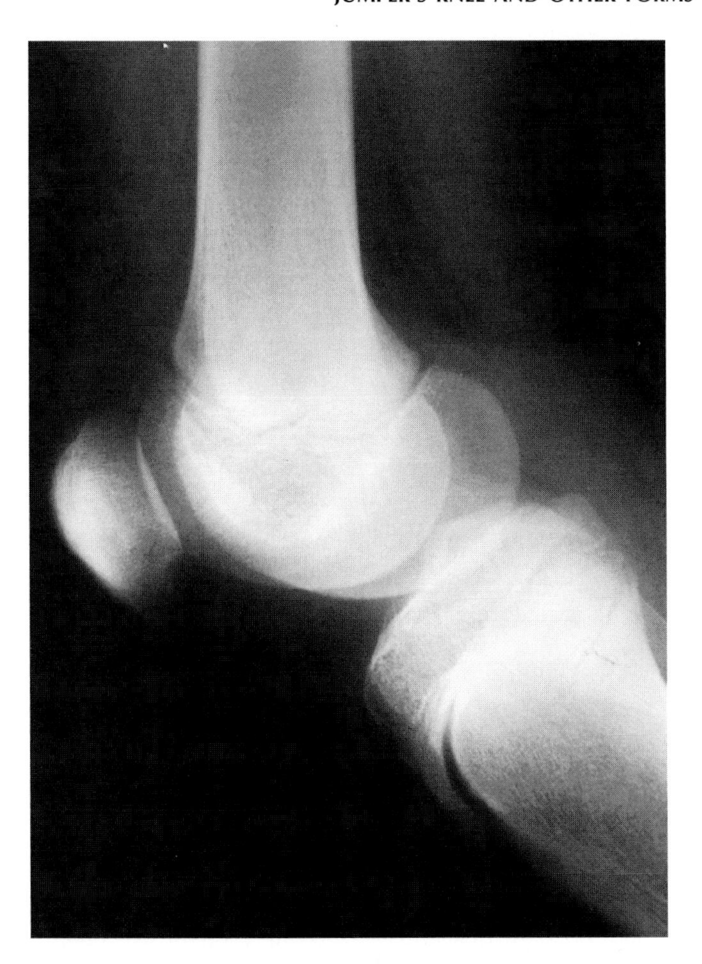

Fig. 66–3. A positive radiograph for Osgood-Schlatter disease shows fragmentation of the tibial tuberosity.

Type 1: The tibial tuberosity is prominent and irregular.
Type 2: The tibial tuberosity is prominent and irregular, but in addition there is a small, free ossicle located anterior and superior to the tuberosity.
Type 3: There is an anterosuperior ossicle, but the tuberosity appears otherwise normal. Probably, these free particles of bone are not lifted from the tibial tubercle but rather are the result of heterotopic bone formation in the deep surface of the patellar tendon.[17]

Ultrasonography shows the hypoechoic area at the level of the lower third of the infrapatellar fat pad, loss of definition between the posterior profile of the tendon and the fat pad, increased thickness of the distal segment of the patellar tendon with a hypoechogenic and dishomogeneous structure, edema of the soft tissues surrounding the tibial tuberosity, small retrotendinous hypoechoic areas (reactive bursitis), and fragmentation of the anterior tibial ossification nucleus.

Treatment

The main course of therapy is abstinence from any sport or playing activity (3 to 6 months or more). The aim of rest is to avoid the repetitive stresses that can injure the ossification nucleus, causing isolation of bony fragments that remain independent from the rest of the tuberosity. The isolated fragments can become ossicles responsible for some of the frequent painful sequelae of Osgood-Schlatter disease.

Rest has to be understood not only as cessation from sports activity but avoidance of any activity that causes the pain. Athletes who ignore these restrictions in the early phases may suffer avulsion of the tuberosity (a very rare complication) or the extension of the symptoms, leading to chronic disease. In cases that require particularly severe functional limitations, the joint may need to be immobilized with a femoromalleolar brace for 1 to 2 weeks.

Generally, the pain is well controlled by cryotherapy (packages and massages) and NSAIDs. We do not advise local infiltrations of corticosteroids, and ultrasound therapy must be avoided in patients who are still growing.

After the acute stage, the functional rehabilitation program can be started: stretching exercises of the quadriceps and the hamstrings integrated with strengthening exercises. (We begin with isometric contractions, gradually progressing to the isotonic work.) Concentric exercises are begun in the second phase, and only the last part of the program is dedicated to the eccentric work.

The athlete can return to sports when the physical examination, radiographs, and sonograms are nearly normal. The tuberosity must not be painful to palpation, and the quadriceps and hamstrings must be fully recovered, especially for athletes involved in high-risk contact sports. Athletes in high risk sports can wear a padded brace to protect the tuberosity against direct blows.

Complications

If Osgood-Schlatter disease is misdiagnosed or not properly treated, some sequelae can affect the patient after skeletal growth ends: (1) high-riding patella,[18] (2) tibial tuberosity hypertrophy, which often is only an aesthetic deformity but sometimes can cause local bursitis and pain, and (3) genu recurvatum.

SINDING-LARSEN-JOHANSSON DISEASE

Sinding-Larsen-Johansson disease is traction osteochondritis secondary to functional overload of the proximal origin of the patellar tendon on the lower pole of the patella.[19, 20] This self-limiting condition generally involves young athletes (10 to 14 years old) and can be associated with Osgood-Schlatter or Sever-Blanke disease.

History and Physical Examination

The first symptom is anterior knee pain that is increased by running activities, going up and down stairs, and kneeling. At the physical examination, we find tenderness in the area of the lower pole of the patella; resisted extension of the knee causes pain as well.

From the radiographic point of view, the disease evolves through four stages[21]:

Stage 1: Normal appearance
Stage 2: Irregular calcifications of the lower pole of the patella
Stage 3: Partial fusion of the calcifications
Stage 4A: Complete fusion of the calcifications, again with a normal appearance, or sometimes, with a teardrop shape
Stage 4B: Presence of a separated ossicle in the context of the patellar tendon.

Treatment

Treatment is oriented toward control of the symptoms and demands temporary interruption of all activities that cause pain. In acute cases or in severe chronic cases, pain control requires a short period of immobilization of the joint.

Often, when a patient is first seen, he or she has what appears to be a Stage 1 radiographic classification but is really Stage 4A. In this case, complete healing takes 9 to 12 months. The athlete may return to sports activity sooner after following a rehabilitation program similar to that used for patients with Osgood-Schlatter disease, when he or she does not complain of local pain anymore.

PES ANSERINUS TENDINITIS

Pes anserinus tendinitis is an insertional tendinitis that is rather frequent, especially among athletes who practice sports involving running, pivoting, jumping, and sudden decelerations. How an athlete runs can be a causative factor. Athletes who train on a short and banked track, such as those of indoor game fields, must drive off hard on the outside foot, causing the muscles on the inner aspect of the leg to contract tightly.

The athlete complains of pain in the medial compartment of the knee when running, cutting, or kicking the ball. The pain can be reproduced by palpating the tibial insertion area of the pes anserinus tendons. Passive external rotation and resisted internal rotation during the flexion-extension movements of the knee can also reproduce the pain. When the tendinitis is associated with symptomatic bursitis, local swelling with crepitation can be palpated by the examiner.

Treatment consists of rest from athletic activity, local applications of ice, functional taping, NSAIDs, and, if necessary, infiltration of the bursa with corticosteroids. When the pain ceases to afflict the athlete, sports activity can be started gradually again. The athlete must be trained in adequate stretching and strengthening of the hamstring muscles.

Sometimes an orthosis may be indicated to control external rotation and pronation of the foot of the involved limb, and the athlete is instructed to alternate frequently the direction of running on the track.

SEMIMEMBRANOSUS TENDINITIS

Semimembranosus tendinitis, an insertional tendinitis especially frequent in runners and cyclists, can be a primary lesion or secondary to intra-articular derangements of the knee (patellar or femoral chondromalacia, medial meniscal tears, plica syndrome) that cause functional overload of the muscle-tendon unit.[22] The predisposing factors of primary cases are insufficient flexibility of the hamstrings, extensor apparatus malalignment, and training errors.

The main symptom is posteromedial pain of the knee, during or after long distance running, jumping, repetitive movements of flexion and extension (e.g., weight lifting), or protracted walking. Physical examination with the knee flexed demonstrates tenderness localized at the posteromedial corner, just below the joint line, on the tendon or at the tibial insertion. In the presence of cystic degeneration, local swelling can be palpated following the tendon (pars directa) to its insertion to the tibia.

When clinical onset of the affliction is recent, conservative treatment is the first choice: rest, local ice, NSAIDs, ultrasound, laser, interferential currents, local infiltrations of corticosteroids (if necessary), and hamstring stretching. If the pain persists after a proper period of conservative treatment, bone scintigraphy might be advisable, as when positive, it shows uptake of the marker in the area corresponding to the posteromedial corner of the proximal tibia. In this case, the only other possible diagnosis is osteonecrosis of the medial tibial plateau, which is not always evident on the radiographic examination.[23]

For chronic cases that do not respond to any therapy, arthroscopy seems useful to find and treat articular changes. In chronic cases complicated by cystic degeneration, the tendon should be debrided and the degenerated or necrotic areas excised. The remaining tendon can be scarified, following the direction of the fibers. Sometimes it may be necessary to detach the tendon at the tibial insertion and then to move the insertion proximally to the posterior edge of the tibial collateral ligament.[24]

ILIOTIBIAL BAND SYNDROME

The iliotibial band syndrome is relatively common among long distance runners (30 to 40 km weekly). Other athletes can also develop this problem: football, tennis, and soccer players, skiers, weight lifters, throwers, aerobic exercisers, and cyclists.[25] This tendinitis is more frequent in men than in women, perhaps because more male runners train at longer distances than women or because women more often have genu valgus, less prominent lateral femoral epicondyles, and more evident subcutaneous fat tissue.

The syndrome is caused by overuse related to repetitive movements of the knee in flexion and extension that provoke swelling in the structures underlying the iliotibial band (i.e., the bursal mucosa, the periosteum of the lateral femoral epicondyle) and the band itself.[26,27] The reason is the impingement phenomenon due to the friction caused by movement of the iliotibial band over the epicondyle during walking or running. Sometimes, direct blows can start the syndrome, producing acute hemorrhagic bursitis (e.g., as when a goalkeeper throws himself to one side to catch the ball).

The predisposing factors include these:

A sudden exaggerated increase in quality and quantity of training sessions
Improper warm-up and stretching, especially when flexibility of thigh muscles is poor
Too much downhill work during training sessions
Worn out or wrong shoes: usually a good running shoe loses more than 40% of its shock-absorbing capability after being used for 300 to 400 km.[28]
The habit of always running on one side of a cambered road or in the same direction on a banked track
Using a crossover gait during walking—and especially during running.

We are not completely sure how much the following anatomic factors may predispose the athlete to this injury:

Leg length discrepancy
The pronated foot could exaggerate internal rotation of the knee, producing tension stress of the lateral structures
Excessive dynamic pronation of the foot during the stance phase of running (with the same consequences on the lateral structures of the knee as above)
Genu varus and tibia vara
A prominent lateral epicondyle
Insufficiency of the quadriceps muscle: the quadriceps and the iliotibial band cooperate to extend the knee when the hip is internally rotated.

Knee pain on the lateral side, sometimes radiating toward the tibia or over the fascia lata, is the main symptom. The onset of pain is progressive: the pain appears after the athlete has already run or cycled many kilometers. It is promoted by repetitive movements of the knee and is exacerbated by some particular efforts, such as sprint attempts, running with speed acceleration, and running down stairs more than up stairs. An interruption in training leads to immediate disappearance of the pain, but the symptoms start again as soon as the athlete returns to running or cycling. When the inflammatory process is quite advanced, pain is also present during simple walking, compelling the athlete to limp.

At physical examination, tenderness, and sometimes crepitus, is appreciable when palpating the lateral femoral epicondyle 2 to 4 cm above the joint line and the tubercle of Gerdy. When the injury is in an advanced stage, the whole lateral compartment is painful, even if the two areas just mentioned remain the most sensitive.

Some maneuvers can elicit pain on the lateral femoral epicondyle, helping confirm the diagnosis. When the athlete lies supine and performs active flexion and extension of the knee while the examiner maintains compression on the focal point, pain should be greatest at about 30° to 40° of flexion. If the athlete lies in a lateral decubitus position on the noninvolved side with the

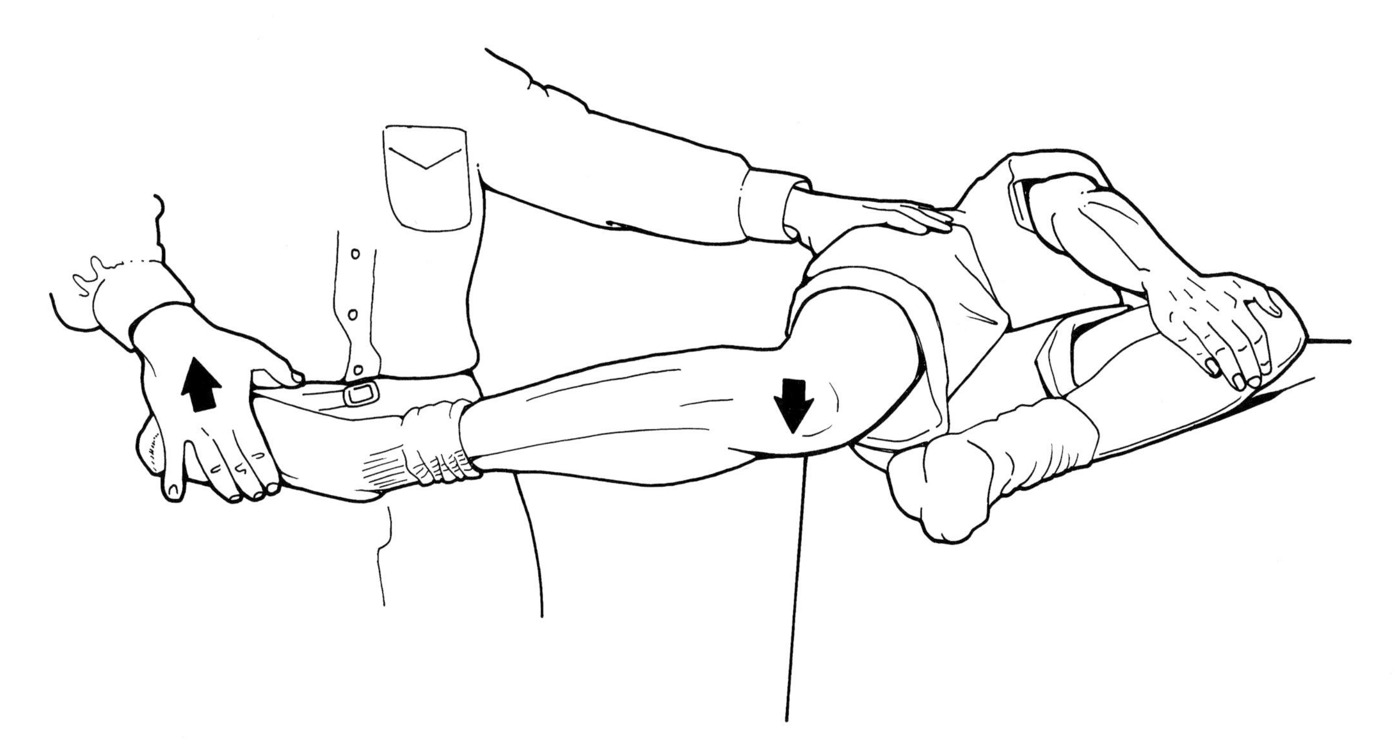

Fig. 66–4. Technique of assessing the flexibility of the iliotibial band (Ober's test). The athlete lies on the uninjured side, and the examiner stabilizes the pelvis with one hand and controls the limb with the other. The hip is first abducted and extended and then adducted toward the table. Tightness of the iliotibial band is demonstrated if the hip remains passively abducted.

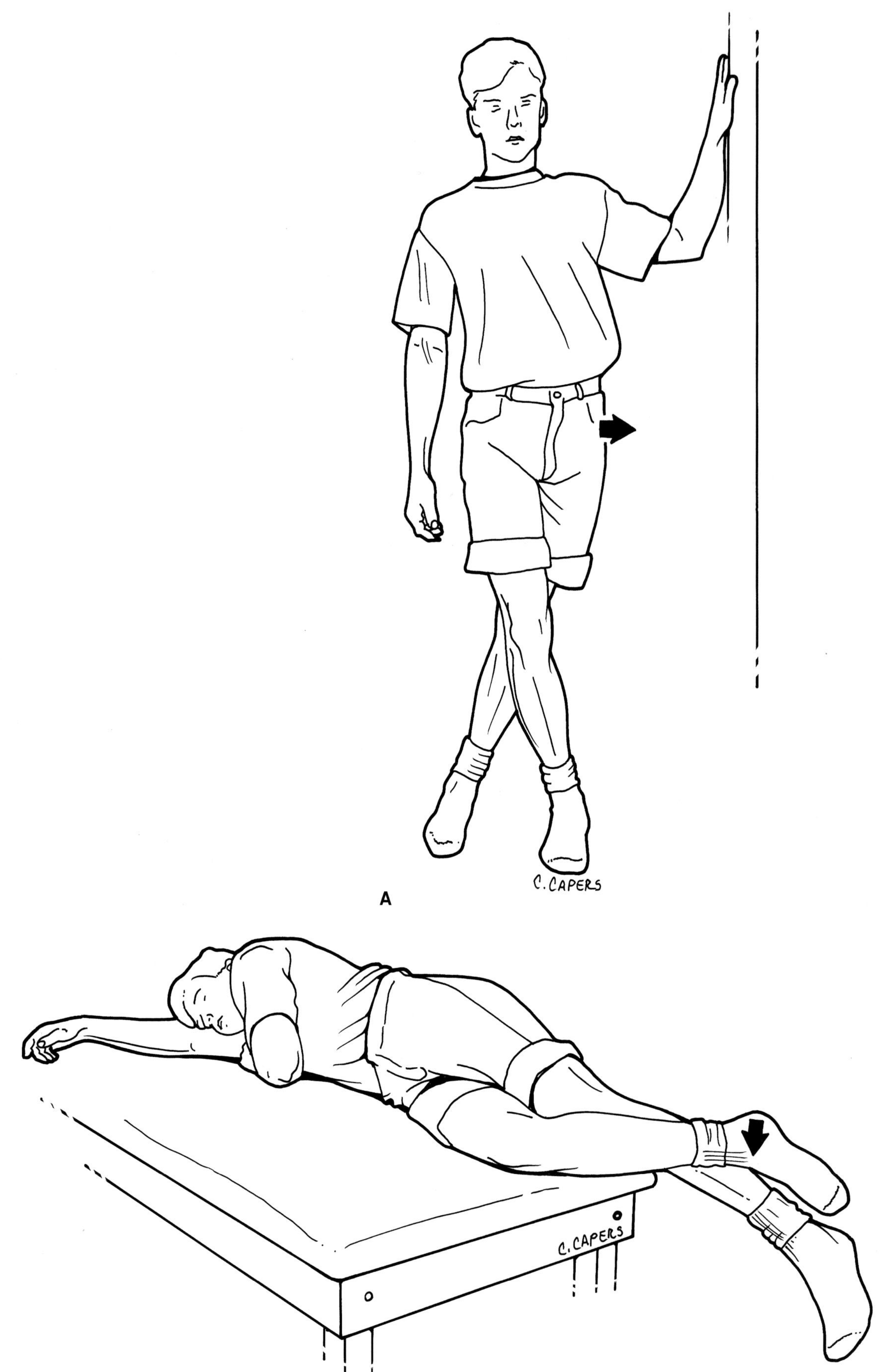
C. CAPERS
A
C. CAPERS
B

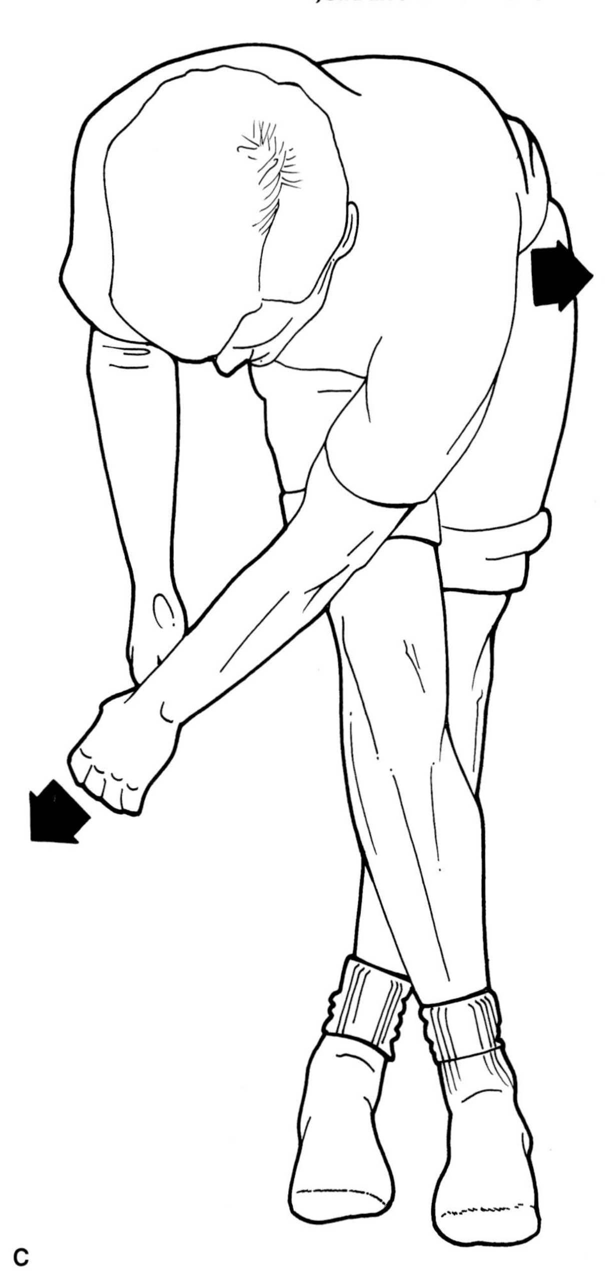

Fig. 66–5. ***(A)*** **Stretching exercise for the (left) iliotibial band in the standing position.** ***(B)*** **Stretching exercise for the** ***(left)*** **iliotibial band using the opposite foot to assist stabilization and maximize the stretch.** ***(C)*** **Stretching exercise for the (left) iliotibial band; the patient may rotate at the waist away from the affected side.**

hip abducted, pain is produced when the examiner applies varus stress. Standing on the involved limb with the knee flexed at 30° to 40° is painful. This test becomes more meaningful when the patient is requested to hop from this knee-flexed position.[29]

Ober's test (Fig. 66–4) is used to assess the flexibility of the iliotibial band.[30] The patient lies on the uninjured side and the examiner stabilizes the pelvis with one hand and controls the limb with the other. The hip is first abducted and extended and then adducted toward the table. Tightness of the iliotibial band is demonstrated if the hip remains passively abducted.

Radiographic findings are always negative. Ultrasonography can show a hypoechoic area corresponding to the femoral epicondyle, just under the iliotibial band. Traumatic events are normally missing from the history of iliotibial band syndrome. The knee is not swollen. There is no pain when the lateral joint line is palpated. The popliteus tendon and lateral collateral ligament are painless, and the meniscal and laxity tests are negative.

Treatment

In the acute stages, relative rest must be maintained for 3 to 4 days. (In the most severe cases it is convenient to immobilize the joint with a "Secure All" brace and to forbid weight bearing.) During the same first days, ice (local applications and massages), NSAIDs, ultrasound, microwaves, massage therapy, and laser therapy are very useful. Sometimes, local infiltration with corticosteroids in the bursa underlying the iliotibial band is necessary.

As soon as possible, a prudent program of stretching exercises must be started. The exercises involve the iliotibial band (Fig. 66–5), the tensor fascia lata,[31,32] the external rotator muscles of the hip, and the hamstrings. These exercises have to be continued throughout the rehabilitation period. Proprioceptive neuromuscular facilitation (PNF) techniques of stretching become very important in the advanced phase, when the brace has already been abandoned.

The patient does not start running again until the pain on the lateral femoral epicondyle disappears. If the lateral pain comes back, it is necessary to stop running.

When the athlete resumes the agonistic activity, he or she must correct the predisposing factors. Endurance runners may need to reduce their mileage. Runners who run on a short track or banked road need to choose a new running surface or change the running side of the road and direction frequently during the training session. All athletes need to use suitable running shoes, and those with anatomic factors may need special orthoses to control excessive pronation of a valgus foot or genu varus and asymmetry of the lower limbs.

If the conservative treatment fails, surgical therapy remains the last resort. We perform distal release of the iliotibial band by means of a cruciform incision of the band at the level of the femoral epicondyle, removing a small square of fibrotic tissue, to obtain full decompression of the underlying structures. We always excise the bursa.

POPLITEUS TENDINITIS

Popliteus tendinitis is an overuse lesion that occurs almost exclusively in endurance runners, though it can affect hikers and backpackers. It is nearly always caused by the same factors discussed under iliotibial band syndrome: worn or wrong shoes, excessive mileage, downhill running, or running on beaches or other banked surfaces. Anatomic factors (pronated foot, overstriding) or functional ones (insufficiency of the quadriceps, through either injury or fatigue) can be considered.[33]

The popliteus muscle, among its many functions, dynamically stabilizes the knee in flexion, checking anterior translation of the femur over the tibia together with the quadriceps muscle and the posterior cruciate ligament (e.g., during the deceleration phase of running, especially on the downhill slope).

The functional overload of the tendon can be explained with the already mentioned check action of the popliteus muscle on the anterior sliding of the femur on the tibia and the internal rotation of the tibia.

History and Physical Examination

The athlete complains of posterolateral pain in the knee whose unexpected onset occurred while going downstairs or running downhill. The pain appears after the physical activity has already started, typically after running for some distance. It could be so severe that the athlete is forced to interrupt the training. The patient gains immediate relief of the symptoms with a brief rest or by running uphill. The pain coincides with the stance phase of gait, when the knee is flexed about 20° to 30°; it is *reduced* by walking with the knee in full extension.

Physical examination by palpation over the lateral compartment reveals pain corresponding to the popliteus tendon, just anterior or posterior to the femoral origin of the lateral collateral ligament above the joint space, where the tendon crosses the ligament. The examination is facilitated by having the patient lie supine with the hip flexed, abducted, and externally rotated and the knee flexed in a figure-of-four position. Pain is also present over the medial margin of the tibia, above the insertion of the popliteus muscle, or anterior to the medial gastrocnemius. Sometimes, popliteus bursitis is present that is indistinguishable from the tendinitis itself.

The maneuvers that can evoke pain, helping confirm the diagnosis, are resisted internal rotation of the leg with the knee flexed 90° or fully extended, resisted flexion of the knee with the leg externally rotated, and passive stretching of the popliteus muscle with complete external rotation of the flexed leg.[34]

The differential diagnosis of popliteus tendinitis consists of these conditions: tendinitis of the biceps femoris (no tenderness of the biceps tendon and no pain with resisted flexion of the knee in the neutral position), iliotibial band syndrome (no tenderness of the iliotibial band and no pain with resisted abduction of the hip), lateral meniscal lesions, arthritis of the tibiofemoral joint, lateral collateral ligament tears, and anterior knee pain caused by overload of the lateral articular facet of the patella.

Treatment

When symptoms first appear we advise relative rest, ice (local applications and massages), NSAIDs, and ultrasound. If, in spite of such therapies, pain persists, local infiltration of corticosteroids could be useful for treatment or to determine the diagnosis. The injection must be directed at the most painful area, generally at the femoral origin; the needle must not be placed within the tendon fibers.

Treatment continues with stretching and strengthening exercises for the quadriceps and the popliteus, hamstring stretching, and correction of training errors. Exercise continues with progressive normalization of the training session, leaving downhill work for the final phase of the rehabilitation program.

BICEPS FEMORIS TENDINITIS

Biceps femoris tendinitis is an overuse problem that is rather common among track and field athletes. Traumatic tears of the muscle are much more frequent than isolated tendinitis; in our practice, we often see the consequences of poor warm-up before competition and, rather less frequently, pure tendinitis at the distal insertion of the tendon.

The main symptom is posterolateral knee pain, which is progressively aggravated according to the level of the physical effort. The onset of the symptoms can be very insidious. At the clinical examination, palpation of the tendinous insertion to the fibular head causes pain; functionally, the same pain can be evoked simply by resisting active forced knee flexion.

As usual, we first consider conservative treatment when symptoms appear: rest from athletic activities, local application of ice, functional taping of the knee, and NSAIDs. Before returning to athletic activity, the patient has to observe an adequate cycle of stretching (including proprioceptive neuromuscular facilitation techniques) and strengthening exercises for hamstring muscles through a program of isometric and isotonic exercises, and finally eccentric exercises.

REFERENCES

1. Ferretti, A., Puddu, G., Mariani, P. P., and Neri, M.: Jumper's knee: An epidemiological study of volley players. Physician Sportsmed. *12*(10):97, 1984.
2. Blazina, M. E., et al.: Jumper's knee. Orthop. Clin. North Am. *4*:665, 1973.
3. Curwin, S., and Stanish, W. D.: Tendinitis: Its Etiology and Treatment. Lexington, MA, Collamore Press, 1984.
4. Sommer, H. M.: Patellar chondropathy and apicitis, and muscle imbalances of the lower extremities in competitive sports. Sports Med. *5*:386, 1988.
5. Ferretti, A., Papandrea, P., and Conteduca, F.: Knee injuries in volleyball. Sports Med. *10*:132, 1990.
6. Ferretti, A., Puddu, G., Mariani, P. and Neri, M.: The natural history of jumper's knee. Int. Orthop. *8*:239, 1985.
7. Martens, M., Wouters, P., Burssens, A., and Mulier, J. C.: Patellar tendinitis: Pathology and results of treatment. Acta Orthop. Scand. *53*:445, 1982.

8. Roels, J., Martens, M., Muller, J. C., and Burssens, A.: Patellar tendinitis (jumper's knee). Am. J. Sports Med. *6*:362, 1978.
9. Fritschy, D., and deGautard, R.: Jumper's knee and ultrasonography. Am. J. Sports Med. *16*:637, 1988.
10. Black, J. E., and Alten, S. R.: How I manage infrapatellar tendinitis. Physician Sportsmed. *12*(10):86, 1984.
11. Stanish, W. D., Rubinovich, R. M., and Curwin, S.: Eccentric exercise in chronic tendinitis. Clin. Orthop. *208*:65, 1986.
12. Beovich, R., and Fricker, P.: Osgood-Schlatter's disease: A review of the literature and an Australian series. Austr. J. Sci. Med. Sport *20*:11, 1988.
13. Willner, P.: Osgood-Schlatter's disease: Etiology and treatment. Clin. Orthop. *62*:178, 1969.
14. Turner, M. S., and Smillie, I. S.: The effect of tibial torsion on the pathology of the knee. J. Bone Joint Surg. *63B*:396, 1981.
15. Woolfrey, B. F., and Chandler, E. F.: Manifestations of Osgood-Schlatter's disease in late teen age and early adulthood. J. Bone Joint Surg. *42A*:327, 1960.
16. Scotti, D. M., Sadhu, V. K., Heimberg, F., and O'Hara, A. E.: Osgood-Schlatter's disease: An emphasis on soft tissue changes in roentgen diagnosis. Skeletal Radiol. *4*:21, 1979.
17. Holstein, A., Lewis, G. B., and Schulze, E. R.: Heterotopic ossification of patellar tendon. J. Bone Joint Surg. *45A*:656, 1963.
18. Blackburne, J. S., and Peel, T. E.: A new method of measuring patellar height. J. Bone Joint Surg. *59B*:241, 1977.
19. Johansson, S.: En forut icke beskriven sjukdom i patella. Hygiea *84*:161, 1922.
20. Sinding-Larsen, M. F.: A hitherto unknown affection of the patella in children. Acta Radiol. *1*:171, 1921.
21. Medlar, R. C., and Lyne, E. D.: Sinding-Larsen-Johansson disease: Its etiology and natural history. J. Bone Joint Surg. *60A*:1113, 1978.
22. Ray, J. M., Clancy, W. G. Jr., and Lemon, R. A.: Semimembranosus tendinitis: An overlooked cause of medial knee pain. Am. J. Sports Med. *16*:347, 1988.
23. Lotke, P. A., and Ecker, M. L.: Osteonecrosis of the medial tibial plateau. Contemp. Orthop. *10*(2):47, 1985.
24. Slocum, D. B., Larson, R. L., and James, S. L.: Late reconstruction of ligamentous injuries of the medial compartment of the knee. Clin. Orthop. *100*:23, 1974.
25. Holmes, J. C., Pruitt, A. L., and Whalen, N. J.: Iliotibial band syndrome in cyclists. Am. J. Sports Med. *21*:419, 1993.
26. Orava, S.: The iliotibial tract friction syndrome in athletes. Br. J. Sports Med. *12*:69, 1978.
27. Smillie, I. S.: Injuries of the Knee Joint. 4th Ed. London, Churchill Livingston, 1973.
28. Cook, S. D., Kester, M. A., Brunet, M. E., and Haddal, R. J. Jr.: Biomechanics of running shoe performance. Clin. Sports Med. *4*:619, 1985.
29. Renne, J. W.: The iliotibial band friction syndrome. J. Bone Joint Surg. *57A*:1110, 1975.
30. Ober, F. R.: The role of the iliotibial band and fascia lata as a factor in the causation of low back disabilities and sciatica. J. Bone Joint Surg. *18*:105, 1936.
32. Cox, J. S.: Patellofemoral problems in runners. Clin. Sports Med. *4*:699, 1985.
33. Mayfield, G. W.: Popliteus tendon tenosynovitis. Am. J. Sports Med. *5*:31, 1977.
34. Allen, M. E., and Ray, G.: Popliteus tendinitis: A new perspective. Sports Training Med. Rehabil. *1*:219, 1989.

67 *Michael E. Brunet and Gregory W. Stewart*

Musculotendinous Injuries About the Knee

MUSCLE STRAINS

The musculoskeletal system can be viewed as a series of components specialized for force production and transmission. One would then expect adaptations and mechanical failure to occur within the various components of the system as well as at the interfaces between components; this translates into injuries. The appropriate place to start a discussion of musculotendinous injuries about the knee is with the muscles.

When loaded to failure, normal muscles fail at or near myotendinous junctions,[1] sites of force transmission between muscle and tendon. Though some muscle fiber tearing does occur near the myotendinous junctions, no tears are reported in the muscle midbelly or within the tendon. The musculotendinous junction disruption, therefore, is not clean, because the avulsed tendon almost always carries with it a small amount of muscle fiber.[1] It appears that the distal myotendinous junction is the weakest point in the entire myotendinous unit (Fig. 67–1).[2]

The most common cause of myotendinous junction disruption or muscle strain is a forcefully contracting muscle subjected to a strong passive force in the opposite direction.[3] Rapid stretching of an active muscle beyond its optimal length either disrupts or permanently weakens parts of the myotendinous junction.[4] Anatomic factors can predispose a person to muscle injury: inadequate flexibility, strength imbalance from one leg to the other, strength ratio imbalance between two groups of muscles in the same leg, previous injury, or muscle weakness. Muscles that cross two joints, such as the rectus femoris and hamstrings, are strained more often than muscles that cross only one joint, such as the vasti group. More important, the joints involved are acted on by other muscle groups; thus, the motion at each joint is not controlled by a single musculotendinous unit.[5]

Classification of Injury

With a Grade I strain, the pathologic changes in the muscle are primarily a low-grade inflammatory response and structural damage is minimal. Persons with Grade I muscle strains may complain of soreness or a tight feeling in the injured area (i.e., in the posterior thigh with hamstring strains and in the anterior portion of the thigh with quadriceps strains). With hamstring strains the athlete may complain of tightness during the extreme range of hip flexion, but resisted knee flexion is generally free of pain. Manually resisted knee extension may cause mild discomfort in patients with quadriceps strains, but loss of strength is minimal.

Generally with these injuries, there is no pain on palpation and no swelling or change in thigh girth. The gait cycle is unchanged and hip range of motion is normal. Athletes suspected to have a quadriceps strain should be tested for range of motion in the prone position with the hip fully extended. Range of motion should exceed 90°. Those with Grade I strains usually do not miss any competition or practice time, but they must be monitored closely and must undertake a rehabilitation program.

Grade II strains reflect actual tissue damage. With Grade II hamstring strains, the athlete generally reports feeling or hearing a "pop" in the posterior thigh region during activity. Swelling is often noted, and with both quadriceps and hamstring strains thigh circumference is increased. A defect in the muscle may be palpable, and the palpation may produce pain. The damage compro-

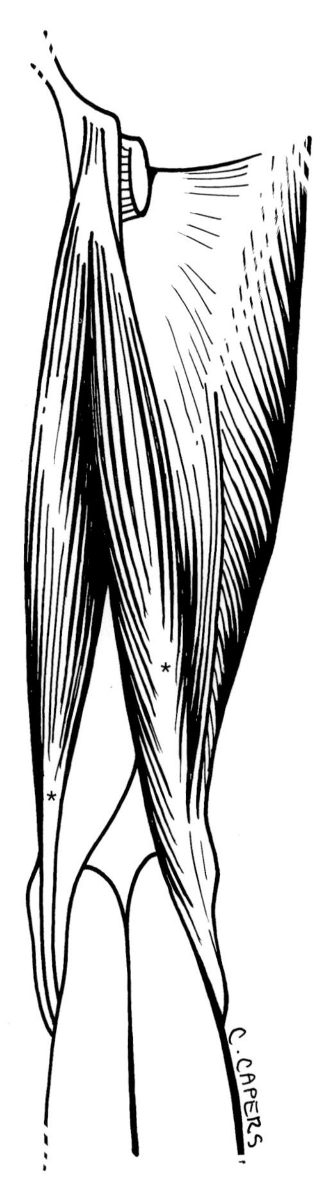

Fig. 67–1. A musculotendinous unit, showing tendon of origin and tendon of insertion.

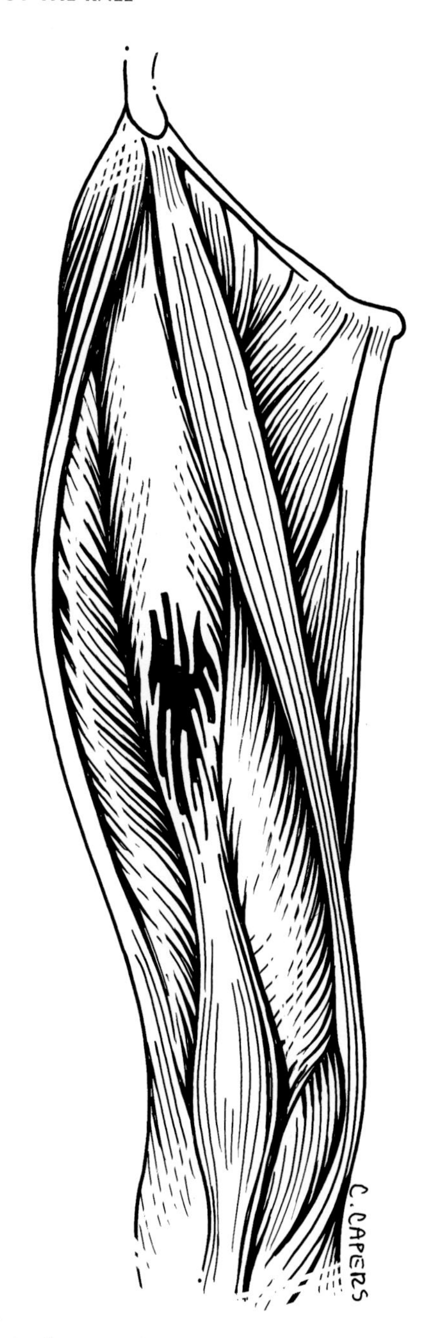

Fig. 67–2. Grade III muscle strain, showing complete disruption of some portion but not complete rupture.

mises the strength of the musculotendinous unit in quadriceps strains.

Pain may cause the athlete with a Grade II strain to have an abnormal gait. Quadriceps strains are associated with reluctance to flex the knee when walking. At times, the athlete uses the hip adductors to pull the leg through the swing phase of gait, causing the leg to rotate externally at the hip. Resisted knee extension may also produce pain. Likewise, an athlete with a hamstring strain walks with the knee flexed to prevent the pain of full extension because hip flexion with knee extension stretches the hamstrings. Hip flexion may be limited even with the knee flexed, which causes shortening of the hamstring muscles. Hamstring weakness is occasionally present, but often it is masked by pain. Athletes with Grade II strains may miss 1 to 3 weeks of competition.

A Grade III strain results in complete disruption of some portion of the musculotendinous unit but falls short of complete rupture (Fig. 67–2). The athlete complains of severe pain, and those with hamstring strains almost always report hearing or feeling a "pop" in the posterior thigh region. Swelling and a significant increase in thigh circumference are noted. Palpable muscle defects or masses almost always are present. Athletes with Grade III strains generally require crutches for ambulation. Decreased strength is common, but, again, this is difficult to test because of pain. Passive hip flexion or knee extension generally causes pain in athletes with hamstring strains. A Grade III strain can cost an athlete anything from 3 weeks to 3 months of competition.

Muscle strains generally become classifiable after 48 hours. This classification gives us information on the extent of the injury, the type and extent of treatment, and the anticipated time loss. Once the injury is classified, treatment is progressed according to the severity of the injury. The more common Grade I strain is usually evident within the first 48 hours, but it may take up to a week to identify Grade II and III strains, especially if the strain is near the tendon of origin.

Avulsion injuries of the hamstring muscles from the ischial tuberosity have also been described.[6,7] This injury causes pain of sudden onset in the buttock and difficulty on standing. A palpable defect and tenderness distal to the ischial tuberosity can be found. Weakness in flexing the knee and loss of normal outlining of the hamstring muscles are also noted. If the bone fragment is displaced 1 cm or more, we feel that surgical repair is warranted. If this degree of avulsion injury is allowed to heal without surgery, the callus will be large and uncomfortable—during activity and while sitting.

Treatment

The treatment and rehabilitation of muscle strains always begins with *r*est, *i*ce, *c*ompression, and *e*levation (RICE) for the first 48 hours. Rest ranges from temporary cessation of sports to avoidance of weight bearing with crutches. Crushed ice in a bag easily conforms to the injured area and can be held in place with a compression dressing. Ice should be used two to three times daily for 15 to 20 minutes per session. Treatment of acute injuries also includes nonsteroidal anti-inflammatory drugs to reduce swelling and pain.

The progression of treatment beyond this initial stage depends on the amount of pain and the patient's ability to perform functional activities. Daily evaluation of the injured area is imperative. In our experience, quadriceps reinjury is more of a problem than hamstring reinjury. Very close attention should be paid to the amount of pain, thigh girth, serial palpation of the injury site, the pain-free arc of knee motion, and muscle testing during the daily evaluations.

HAMSTRINGS

Daily evaluations determine the speed at which the exercises are progressed. Our philosophy on exercise progression is similar for both hamstring and quadriceps strains because both muscle groups have a preponderance of Type II muscle fibers. Our overall treatment program begins with isometric exercises. For the hamstrings this consists of contracting the hamstring muscle *without* moving the hip or the knee joint. Isometric exercises are performed with the knee joint positioned at multiple angles within the pain-free range. The knee angle is changed in 20° increments. When the athlete is able to perform isometric exercises without any pain, isotonic exercises are undertaken.

Patients with hamstring strains do isotonic exercises in the prone position, flexing the knee against gravity. Initially, only the weight of the leg is used for one or two sets of 10 repetitions. When the athlete can do this relatively pain free and without experiencing a real increase in symptoms the next day, isotonics are continued and progressed while isometrics are decreased, and ultimately discontinued. The number of sets of 10 repetitions is increased until the athlete can perform three sets per treatment session, no more often than three times daily. With pain as the guide, the amount of weight is increased in 2- to 3-pound increments no more often than every 2 days. Each time the weight is increased, the number of sets is decreased and then gradually increased as pain permits. When the athlete can perform isotonic exercises lifting 15 pounds for three sets of 10 repetitions three times daily, isokinetic exercises can be initiated.

Isokinetic exercises are performed on a Biodex type of machine. Isokinetic equipment controls the speed of motion, which is usually performed in a concentric or muscle-shortening contraction mode. We start with the concentric mode at 240° per second and have the athlete perform three sets of ten. The speed is then increased to 300° per second and the athlete performs two sets of thirty. As progression allows, speed is decreased and three sets of ten repetitions are added to the treatment regimen. If access to isokinetic equipment is not available, walking or running backward can be done. Once concentric training can be performed without difficulty, eccentric, or muscle-lengthening, contraction exercises can be added. With eccentric work, the speed should be started at 30° per second and advanced to faster speeds. Forward running can be used in place of eccentric training of the hamstrings.

QUADRICEPS

Straight leg raises are the first isotonic exercise for quadriceps strains. Other exercises are performed with the patient seated and the thigh resting on the treatment table and the heel resting on a variable height stool, to keep the knee within the pain-free range. This allows terminal knee extension exercises to be performed. The weight is increased up to 20 pounds in 2- to 3-pound increments no more often than every 2 days. Quadriceps isometric and isotonic exercises are performed in this position and progressed in a fashion similar to hamstring exercises. Isokinetic exercises are also performed in a fashion similar to hamstring exercises; however, with the quadriceps, concentric training is similar to forward running, and eccentric training is similar to backward running. Stretching of the quadriceps is performed with the athlete in the prone position, and self-stretching is recommended to prevent further injury. Because quadriceps injuries seem to be more sensitive to stretching injury than hamstring injuries, we recommend a very cautious approach. General conditioning, in the form of swimming and upper body workouts, should be initiated 2 to 3 days after injury. Biking should not be used as a general conditioning exercise until 100° of active knee motion has been obtained, and then the bicycle seat should be raised or lowered to accommodate the decreased range of motion.

Return to Sports

Since the primary goal is to return the athlete safely to sports participation as soon as possible, it should be understood that recurrence of the injury is considered a failure. Equal flexibility and endurance should be restored. We think that isokinetic testing should reveal function to be within 10% of that in the uninvolved limb. If isokinetic equipment is not available, functional testing becomes even more critical. After appropriate stretching and warm-up, the athlete is required to sprint 50 yards three times and run three 15-yard figure of eights. If all of this can be done at full speed with no discomfort, the athlete is considered fit to return to competition. No single strict treatment plan is successful for all athletes' muscle strains. Flexibility within the protocol, which is determined by daily evaluations and good judgment, has been successful in our hands.

QUADRICEPS CONTUSION

A quadriceps contusion or hematoma is the result of blunt trauma to the anterior aspect of the thigh that causes bleeding deep within the muscle and between muscle planes. The blunt trauma causes a compression wave within the quadriceps. This compression wave generally travels through the superficial musculature but cannot be transmitted through the incompressible bone. This causes the vastus intermedius to be crushed against the femur (Fig. 67–3).

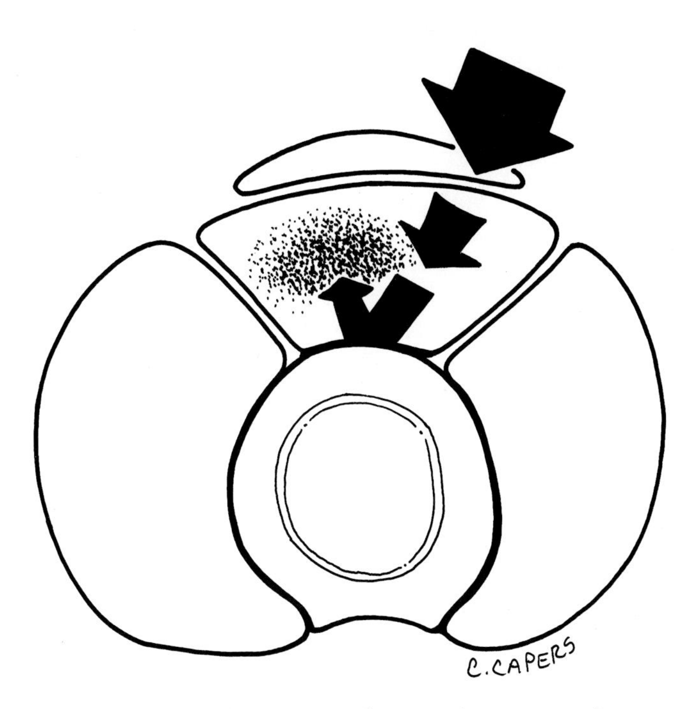

Fig. 67–3. Drawing shows motion of compression wave, causing quadriceps contusion.

The easiest way to distinguish such a contusion from a muscle strain or rupture is the history of direct trauma to the muscle group. The traditional presentation of a quadriceps hematoma consists of swelling and pain, a decreased range of knee motion, and knee stiffness.[8,9] Several authors advocate classifying the extent of the contusion according to the active range of knee motion a determined 12 to 24 hours after the injury[8,9]: patients with mild contusions have more than 90° of active knee motion; those with moderate contusions have between 45° and 90°; and those with severe contusions less than 45°. Classification is useful primarily for predicting return to play; treatment for the different grades is the same.

Treatment

Initial treatment of quadriceps contusions, regardless of the grade, consists of ice bags and compression wraps with the athlete's knee immobilized in maximal flexion. Distal vascular and neurologic examinations are performed regularly during the first 48 hours. Thigh girth is measured at intervals, to monitor any progression in the bleeding in the quadriceps.

If we evaluate the athlete within the first 8 hours, we aspirate the hematoma and inject the area with 1% xylocaine, steroid, and hyaluronidase, 150 USP units. Once the thigh girth has stabilized, the patient progresses to the next stage of treatment, which involves restoration of knee motion. Knee pain and range of motion must be evaluated daily, to guide the rehabilitation program. Weight bearing is allowed as tolerated, and crutches are discarded when there is greater than 90° of motion. Heat, whirlpool, and ultrasound have been advocated by some for treatment during this stage[9]; however, we feel these modalities increase the risk of rebleeding and of setback for the athlete. As a result, we never use heat during any phase of treatment for quadriceps contusions. We continue to use ice massage with gravity-assisted motion in both flexion and extension.

Treatment continues until pain-free active knee flexion exceeds 120°. At this point, the athlete progresses to the next stage of rehabilitation, dealing primarily with functional rehabilitation and return to competition. Sport-specific activities and agility drills such as running, cutting, and jumping are performed with increasing speed. When full range of motion of the knee and successful completion of functional tests have been performed, the athlete is allowed to return to competition with adequate protection about the thigh. For added protection of the contused area, the authors have used extra-large thigh pads or doughnut pads held in place with neoprene sleeves or elastic wraps (Fig. 67–4).

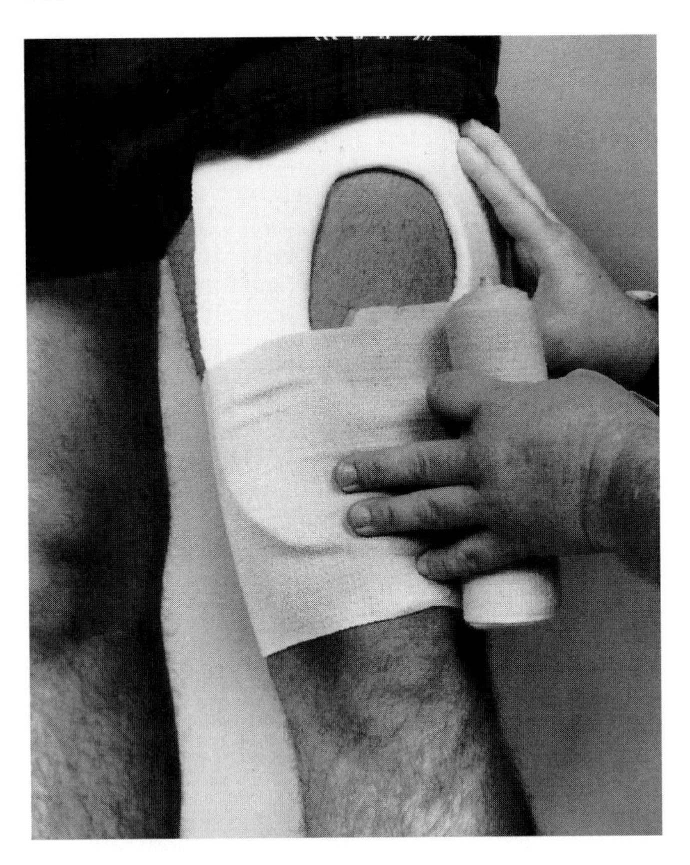

Fig. 67–4. Thigh pads or doughnut pads are used to protect a quadriceps contusion.

ACUTE COMPARTMENT SYNDROME

An occasional complication of moderate to severe quadriceps contusions, acute compartment syndrome in the thigh constitutes a true medical emergency. Compartment syndrome occurs when the contusion causes such severe swelling that the pressure in an unyielding fascial sheath causes vascular compromise. In the thigh, this occurs because of the fascia lata and the medial and lateral intermuscular septa. The result of this elevated pressure is reduced capillary blood flow and neuromuscular compromise. The primary sign of these elevated pressures is pain that appears to be out of proportion to the injury.[10]

Delayed diagnosis of compartment syndrome can result in permanent loss of function, and possibly amputation of the involved extremity.[11] The diagnosis is suspected from the clinical presentation and confirmed by intracompartmental pressure measurements. Clinical symptoms can appear if the patient is seen late: weak knee extension, pain on passive knee flexion, and altered sensation over the knee and medial aspect of the leg and foot. These findings occur because the anterior compartment contains (1) the femoral nerve, which supplies the quadriceps, and (2) branches to the saphenous nerve, which provides sensation over the knee, the medial aspect of the leg, and the foot. These findings are often absent, however, even in the presence of high intracompartmental pressures.

Intracompartmental pressure can be measured by the Whitesides' technique, the wick catheter, the slit catheter, or the infusion method.[11–14] An anterior thigh intracompartment pressure of 30 mm Hg or higher indicates the need for prompt surgical treatment.[13,15] Other authors have defined the critical pressure as 10 to 30 mm Hg less than the diastolic blood pressure.[16] Laboratory studies for suspected thigh compartment syndrome include hemoglobin, hematocrit, and electrolytes. Prothrombin time, partial thromboplastin time, and platelet count are obtained, to rule out a bleeding dyscrasia. Rapid drops in hemoglobin and hematocrit values imply arterial disruption, and arteriography may be required to determine the extent of vascular compromise. Regardless of the method, once the diagnosis is made, this condition is a surgical emergency. Irreversible injury can occur within 5 to 6 hours of onset of ischemia.[17–19] These time frames are important to keep in mind since compartment syndromes can develop as early as a few hours after injury or as long as 64 hours later.

Treatment of acute thigh compartment syndrome consists of fasciotomy. The thick fascia that surrounds the musculature is incised to relieve the elevated pressures and prevent cell death.

Postoperative rehabilitation of the patient with compartment syndrome varies, depending on the size of the fasciotomy wound and the amount of necrosis. The rate of exercise progression is determined by the surgeon. Generally, rehabilitation begins immediately postoperatively, with passive range of motion activities and partial weight-bearing exercises. These exercises help reduce the edema associated with compartment syndrome. As the wound heals and tolerance of weight bearing improves, progressive resistance training can be initiated. Range of motion, strengthening, and light jogging are added, as tolerated, up to the point where functional athletic activities are added to the rehabilitation process. Most athletes can return to sports participation with additional protection as described previously in 8 to 12 weeks. Return to play depends more on the initial contusion and the severity of the compartment damage than on whether fasciotomy has been successfully performed.

MYOSITIS OSSIFICANS TRAUMATICA

In patients who develop a quadriceps contusion, symptoms generally begin to respond to local conservative treatment within the first several days. If local pain, swelling, and tenderness do not respond within 4 to 5 days of the initial trauma, the early stages of myositis ossificans traumatica should be suspected.[20] Active myositis ossificans is very probable if local symptoms have not improved significantly in the first 2 weeks, if symptoms intensify during this early period, or particularly if the induration becomes more pronounced.[21]

Myositis ossificans has been identified as a benign, localized formation of heterotopic non-neoplastic bone that results from physical trauma usually occurring in muscles close to bone.[22] Severe compression of the muscles and other soft tissues against the bone results in disruption of muscle fibers, connective tissue, blood vessels, and probably periosteum.

Radiographically, the evolution of myositis ossificans parallels the histologic pattern of maturation (Fig. 67–5). Initially there is no radiographic evidence of myositis ossificans. By the third to the fourth week, flocculent densities arise within the muscle and a periosteal reaction may be present in the underlying bone. By 6 to 8 weeks, a sharply circumscribed lacy pattern of new bone is visible about the edges of the mass. The central core of the mass does not show evidence of ossification at this time. As the lesion matures, it becomes more dense, and occasionally a direct attachment to the bony shaft is demonstrated. By approximately 6 months after injury, the lesion has reached its maximum size and then can be observed to shrink in size over a period of several months.

The three-phase bone scan can be used to determine the presence of early myositis ossificans.[23, 24] Arteriography has also been used to differentiate traumatic myositis ossificans from malignant tumors, since, during its active phase, myositis ossificans exhibits hypervascularity without arteriovenous shunting or pooling.[25,26]

Computed tomography (CT) can be used to determine the size, density, and anatomic site of the myositis lesion. Because myositis ossificans characteristically does not invade surrounding tissue, CT can also be used to differentiate it from malignant tumors.[27] Other authors have found ultrasonography to provide, quickly and noninvasively, an image of soft tissue changes associated with myositis ossificans.[28] With magnetic resonance imaging (MRI), mature myositis ossificans demonstrates fat marrow signal intensity on T1-weighted images.

The acute-phase management of myositis ossificans is similar to that of a moderate to severe quadriceps contusion: rest, ice, compression, elevation, immobilization, and limited weight bearing. The thigh and the hematoma are examined daily. Aspiration of the hematoma and injection with 1% xylocaine, steroid, and lysosomal enzymes (hyaluronidase, 150 USP units) has also been recommended. Aspiration and injection should be done once immediately after injury. We believe that waiting beyond the first 8 to 12 hours diminishes the positive results of aspiration and of subsequent injections.

Once myositis ossificans traumatica is identified, we treat the lesion with oral indomethacin, 50 mg t.i.d. The rehabilitation protocol outlined for quadriceps

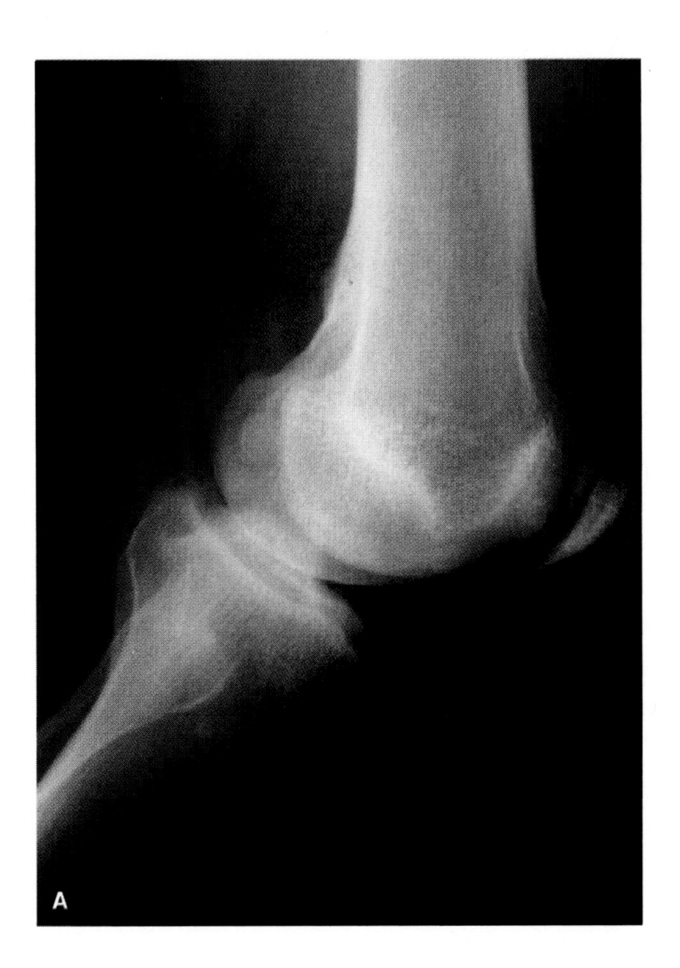

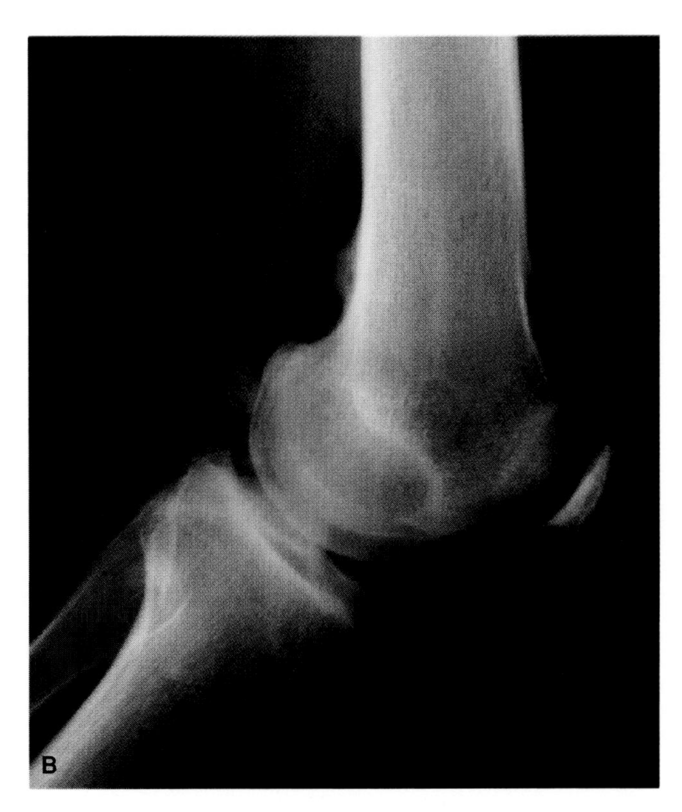

Fig. 67–5. Radiographs of early- and late-stage myositis ossificans.

contusion is followed, using pain and range of motion as guidelines for progression and return to competition.

Return to play criteria are the same as for quadriceps contusion: the athlete is allowed to return to competition when full painless range of motion is restored. The involved area must be protected from repeated trauma because this also appears to be a risk factor in the development of myositis ossificans traumatica. Oftentimes the commercially available protective pads provide adequate protection. If these pads are not large enough, doughnut pads can be made in an attempt to bridge the injured area.

Surgical removal of the lesion may be indicated if there is persistent local pain or muscle dysfunction, or if adjacent joint range of motion is limited to the extent of constituting functional disability. Surgical intervention should never be considered until at least 6 months after the injury, to ensure maturity of the lesion. If surgery is performed before maturity, ectopic ossification may not be completely removed and may return postoperatively.

QUADRICEPS TENDON RUPTURE

In normal, healthy persons, muscle-tendon unit disruption does not occur.[3] Thus, tendon ruptures are thought to be secondary to age-related degenerative changes. The mechanism of injury is generally a sudden violent contraction of the quadriceps, usually in a fall. Almost 90% of quadriceps tendon ruptures occur in patients older than 40 years.[29]

Patients frequently report hearing a loud "pop" and complain of immediate inability to extend the leg or to bear weight. The two diagnostic criteria for complete quadriceps tendon rupture are loss of the ability to maintain the knee in full extension against gravity and a palpable soft tissue defect proximal to the superior pole of the patella.[30] It therefore becomes imperative that a physician evaluating a knee should test the integrity of the extensor mechanism.

Most often, microscopic partial tears of the quadriceps tendon are secondary to excessive use of the muscle in the weight room, as with squats. If the offending forces are discontinued, rapid healing occurs in otherwise healthy young athletes. There should be no fear of progression to complete rupture of the tendon. In persons older than 40 years or ones who have a predisposing illness, a partial tear may progress to complete rupture.

Imaging diagnosis of rupture of the quadriceps tendon can often be made with plain radiographs. On the lateral view of the knee, loss of normal quadriceps outline is noted, plus a soft tissue mass with calcification representing the retracted quadriceps tendon.[31] In a separate study, diagnostic criteria on plain radiographs included poorly defined suprapatellar mass, obliterated quadriceps tendon, calcifications, patella baja, joint effusion, and spurring of the patella. Almost all knees evaluated showed more than three of these abnormalities and 50% showed more than four of them.[32]

Early diagnosis is important in the management of complete quadriceps tendon ruptures since primary surgical repair is necessary within the first 48 to 72 hours to preserve the extensor mechanism of the knee. CT and ultrasound can demonstrate the quadriceps tendon; however, surrounding hematoma or edema can degrade soft tissue contrast. Although arthrography shows extravasation of contrast agent from the suprapatellar pouch, this invasive modality has defined risks, such as infection.

MRI shows a corrugated appearance in the patellar tendon, patella baja, or the transected tendons.[32] MRI usually is not necessary for the diagnosis of complete quadriceps tendon rupture because history, physical findings, and plain radiographs are sufficient to make the diagnosis, but it can be beneficial for very early diagnosis.[32]

Patients who are treated conservatively for quadriceps tendon rupture do poorly. Surgical repair should be performed as soon as possible after injury, to obtain the best results.[33] The key to successful surgical repair of ruptured quadriceps tendons is reapproximation of the tendon ends without tension, postoperative immobilization, and appropriate rehabilitation after the period of immobilization.[34] Results of surgery are variable; however, satisfactory results can be expected in at least 80% of the cases.[34] Residual problems often exist—patellar pain, loss of quadriceps strength, residual extension lag, and myositis ossificans of the quadriceps tendon.

RUPTURE OF THE PATELLAR TENDON

Ruptures of the infrapatellar tendon can be detected by a consistent history and the finding of a palpable defect in the region of the patellar tendon plus patella alta. To detect the gap in the tendon or patella alta, tension must be placed on the tendon: the knee must be flexed to 90°. If there is a gap of more than one fingerbreadth between the inferior pole of the patella and the joint line, patella alta exists and rupture of the infrapatellar tendon must be suspected. Plain radiography may help in the diagnosis by outlining a patella alta. Ultrasound may also be helpful in detecting complete or partial ruptures of the infrapatellar ligament.

When the patellar tendon ruptures, the forces are generally sufficient to cause additional damage about the knee. Extracapsular structures that prevent anterior translation of the tibia on the femur can be damaged. The anterior cruciate ligament is almost always damaged to some extent. Medial or lateral stabilizing structures may also be damaged, depending on whether the leg is in internal or external rotation at the time of injury. The leg is generally in external rotation, so medial structures such as the medial collateral ligament are more apt to be damaged. It is therefore important to thoroughly evaluate the knee with a ruptured patellar tendon. These are usually "noncontact" injuries (from pivoting, twisting, or deceleration) rather than the result of direct trauma.

Early diagnosis and treatment are essential in the

management of the ruptured infrapatellar tendon. In patients with patellar tendon ruptures that are not detected for 2 weeks or more, significant proximal retraction of the patella may develop, with quadriceps contractures and adhesion.[33] Once the diagnosis is made, surgery is recommended. Subsequent rehabilitation, as outlined by the surgeon, and daily evaluations are imperative.

REFERENCES

1. Garrett, W. E., Jr., et al.: The effect of muscle architecture on the biomechanical failure properties of skeletal muscle under passive extension. Am. J. Sports Med. *16*:7, 1988.
2. Nikolaou, P. et al.: The effect of architecture on the anatomical failure site of skeletal muscle. Trans. Orthop. Res. Soc. *11*:228, 1986.
3. McMaster, P. E.: Tendon and muscle ruptures: Clinical and experimental studies on the causes and location of subcutaneous ruptures. J. Bone Joint Surg. *15*:705, 1933.
4. Katz, B.: The relation between force and speed in muscular contraction. J. Physiol. *96*:45, 1939.
5. Brewer, B. J.: Mechanism of injury to the musculotendinous unit. AAOS Instr. Course Lect. *17*:354, 1960.
6. Blasier, R. B., and Morawa, L. G.: Complete rupture of the hamstring origin from a water skiing injury. Am. J. Sports Med. *18*:435, 1990.
7. Ishikawa, K., Kai, K., and Mizuta, H.: Avulsion of the hamstring muscles from the ischial tuberosity: A report of two cases. Clin. Orthop. *232*:153, 1988.
8. Ryan, J. B., et al.: Quadriceps contusions—West Point update. Am. J. Sports Med. *19*:299, 1991.
9. Jackson, D. W., and Feagin, J. A.: Quadriceps contusions in young athletes—relation of severity of injury to treatment and prognosis. J. Bone Joint Surg. *55A*:95, 1973.
10. Martinez, S. F., Steingard, M. A., and Steingard, P. M.: Thigh compartment syndrome—a limb-threatening emergency. Physician Sportsmed. *21*(3):94, 1993.
11. Whitesides, T. E. Jr., Haney, T. C., Morimoto, K., and Harada, H.: Tissue pressure measurements as a determinant for the need of fasciotomy. Clin. Orthop. *113*:43, 1975.
12. Matsen, F. A. III, and Clawson, D. K.: The deep posterior compartmental syndrome of the leg. J. Bone Joint Surg. *57A*:34, 1975.
13. Mubarak, S. J., et al.: Acute compartment syndromes: Diagnosis and treatment with the aid of the wick catheter. J. Bone Joint Surg. *60A*:1091, 1978.
14. Shakespeare, D. T., Henderson, N. J., and Clough, G.: The slit catheter: A comparison with the wick catheter in the measurement of compartment pressure. Injury *13*:404, 1982.
15. An, H. S., Simpson, J. M., Gale, S., and Jackson, W. T.: Acute anterior compartment syndrome in the thigh: A case report and review of the literature. J. Orthop. Trauma *1*:180, 1987.
16. Rorabeck, C. H., and Armstrong, R. D.: Compartment syndromes: How to avert uncorrectable deformities. J. Musculoskel. Med. *2*:(9)54, 1985.
17. Skully, R. E., Shannon, J. M., and Dickersin, G. R.: Factors involved in recovery from experimental skeletal muscle ischemia produced in dogs: Histologic and histochemical pattern of ischemic muscle. Am. J. Pathol. *39*:721, 1961.
18. Walker, J. W., Paletta, F. X., and Cooper, T.: The relationship of post-ischemic histopathological changes to muscle and subcuticular temperature patterns in the canine extremity. Surg. Forum *10*:836, 1959.
19. Whitesides, T. E., Jr., Hirada, H., and Morimoto, K.: The response of skeletal muscle to temporary ischemia: An experimental study. J. Bone Joint Surg. *53A*:1027, 1971.
20. Thorndike, A. Jr.: Myositis ossificans traumatica. J. Bone Joint Surg. *22*:315, 1940.
21. Campbell, E. R.: Traumatic myositis ossificans. South. Med. J. *27*:763, 1934.
22. Gilmer, W. S., and Anderson, L. D.: Reactions of soft somatic tissue which may progress to bone formation: Circumscribed (traumatic) myositis ossificans. South. Med. J. *52*:1432, 1959.
23. Rupani, H. D., Holder, L. E., Espinola, D. A., and Engin, S. I.: Three-phase radionuclide bone imaging in sports medicine. Radiology *156*:187, 1985.
24. Drane, W. E.: Myositis ossificans and the three-phase bone scan. Am. J. Roentgenol. *142*:179, 1984.
25. Yaghmai, I.: Myositis ossificans: Diagnostic value of arteriography. Am. J. Roentgenol. *128*:811, 1977.
26. Hutcheson, J., Klatte, E. C., and Kremp, R.: The angiographic appearance of myositis ossificans circumscripta: A case report. Radiology *102*:57, 1972.
27. Zeanah, W. R., and Hudson, T. M.: Myositis ossificans: Radiologic evaluation of two cases with diagnostic computed tomograms. Clin. Orthop. *168*:187, 1982.
28. Kirkpatrick, J. S., Koman, L. A., and Rovere, G. D.: The role of ultrasound in the early diagnosis of myositis ossificans. Am. J. Sports Med. *15*:179, 1987.
29. Siwek, C. W., and Rao, J. P.: Ruptures of the extensor mechanism of the knee joint. J. Bone Joint Surg. *63A*:932, 1981.
30. Ramsey, R. H., Muller, G. E.: Quadriceps tendon rupture: A diagnostic trap. Clin. Orthop. *70*:161, 1970.
31. Newberg, A., and Wales, L.: Radiographic diagnosis of quadriceps tendon rupture. Radiology. *125*:367, 1977.
32. Kaneko, K., DeMouy, E. H., Brunet, M. E., and Benzian, J.: Radiographic diagnosis of quadriceps tendon rupture: analysis of diagnostic failure. J. Emerg. Med. *12*:225, 1994.
33. Haas, S. B., and Callaway, H.: Disruptions of the extensor mechanism. Orthop. Clin. North Am. *23*:687, 1992.
34. Kuivila, T. E., and Brems, J. J.: Diagnosis of acute rupture of the quadriceps tendon by magnetic resonance imaging: A case report. Clin. Orthop. *262*:236, 1991.

68

W. Michael Walsh

Extensor Mechanism Problems

Extensor mechanism problems are the most common knee disorders seen by physicians. These problems are almost universally caused by numerous anatomic and physiologic abnormalities in the lower extremities. Beyond these statements, there is almost no agreement among clinicians and researchers as to how these factors produce the clinical syndromes we see. Furthermore, the nomenclature for such problems is a jumble of terms and various authors often use them idiosyncratically. *Chondromalacia patellae* is the historical term that has been applied to painful conditions of the extensor mechanism. Today that designation is not appropriate for referring to pain syndromes and should be reserved only for the objective articular cartilage disease that can occur as a result of mechanical patellar problems. Even leaving chondromalacia patellae aside, we are left with such labels as anterior knee pain, patellofemoral pain syndrome, excessive lateral pressure syndrome, extensor mechanism malalignment, patellofemoral malalignment, patellar subluxation, and patellar dislocation, all terms that have been devised to describe the same clinical syndrome or some part of it.

Extensor mechanism malalignment (EMM) is the umbrella term I prefer to indicate the physical predisposition to patellar problems. This predisposition includes a myriad of anatomic findings, in both bone and muscle, extending from the pelvic region to the foot. Bony abnormalities of the lower extremity such as femoral anteversion, genu valgum, and external tibial torsion can increase the angle of quadriceps pull. Patella alta, shallow lateral femoral condyles, and the shape of the patella are other bone factors that can affect extensor mechanism (EM) function. Tightness in the rectus femoris, iliotibial band, hamstrings, gastrocnemius, soleus, or peripatellar retinaculum all may accentuate EM dysfunction.

Many of these findings are extremely common in the general population. One has only to screen junior high and high school athletes in a preseason examination to realize exactly how common they are. Thus it becomes obvious that a person may exhibit the physical findings typically associated with symptomatic problems yet be asymptomatic. This becomes even more obvious when a patient presents with precisely the same anatomic structure in both lower extremities but symptoms in only one knee. In many instances, trauma has served as a trigger for the onset of symptoms where previously there was only an asymptomatic predisposition. How, exactly, this trigger works is not known. Traumatic triggers can apparently be both overuse mechanisms and single episodes of specific injury. Once the cycle of symptom-producing events is set in motion, it can be extremely hard to stop. In this chapter I attempt to deal with this confusing group of problems that seem to be linked to EM mechanics.

TYPES OF PROBLEMS

Simply put, EM problems can be divided into those that are characterized primarily by symptoms of instability and those that are characterized primarily by pain without instability. In truth, many lesions fall into the middle range, producing some mix of instability and pain.

On one extreme of the instability category is patellar dislocation. In this case, the athlete has experienced at least one episode in which the patella was completely dislodged from the femoral trochlea and came to rest for some time against the lateral side of the femoral condyle. Recurrences may follow the first acute dislocation.

Somewhat lesser episodes of instability may take the form of patellar subluxation. In this instance, the athlete has definite, clearly describable symptoms: the patella slips out of its normal location briefly but then spontaneously—and momentarily—reduces. These patients have never experienced the prolonged loss of normal position characteristic of patellar dislocation. Of course, some patients who suffer acute dislocation may subsequently experience only symptoms of subluxation. It is also conceivable that a patient with a history of subluxation only may at some point in the future experience a more dramatic complete dislocation.

On the other end of the spectrum are patients who have no instability symptoms whatsoever but present for evaluation because of pain. Overall, a larger percentage of patients are seen for this problem. The majority of them experience gradual onset and development of their pain syndrome owing to overuse; however, occasionally the pain syndrome begins with some type of trauma, often blunt trauma to the anterior aspect of the knee.

DIAGNOSIS

Taking a History

Taking an accurate history is critically important. In dealing with suspected patellar instability, it is important to determine how it originally occurred. Most often, it results from a twisting, "noncontact" mechanism. Less frequently, it may result from a blow, usually to the lateral side of the knee, that forces the knee into valgus position. With the initial injury, some patients may report that they actually saw the patella dislocate over the lateral aspect of the knee. The knee usually collapses and the patient falls to the ground. The patella usually remains dislocated until the knee is fully extended—by the patient or by another player or coach seeking to help. It is important to ask about the feeling of something popping back into place associated with relief of pain at the time the knee was fully extended. Such a history is virtually diagnostic of acute patellar dislocation, particularly if the onset of swelling is noted in the knee shortly afterward.

In episodes of patellar subluxation, athletes usually feel the slipping as they attempt to pivot, twist, cut, turn, or otherwise apply rotational stress to the knee. Certainly, these symptoms may be confused with instability secondary to a ligamentous injury, but most patients with patellar subluxation can clearly state that it is the kneecap that they feel momentarily slipping out of place. This can later be distinguished through physical examination.

Patients who have pain symptoms alone, complain of pain over the anterior aspect of the knee. Typically the pain is aggravated, not only by activity, but by prolonged periods of knee flexion, especially when the patient is forced to sit in a tight seat, as in a theater or a small car. Pain on stairs is also typical, especially on descending them. Swelling usually is not a prominent feature if there are no episodes of instability, though, the patient may report mild puffiness associated with excessive use of the knees. Popping, grinding, or other crepitation around the anterior aspect of the knee is also quite common. Though locking episodes are more typical of meniscus problems, mild momentary catching episodes may occur from the EM. In contrast to meniscal locking, which usually occurs with the knee in slight flexion, EM episodes occur with the knee in extension, so that the knee does not seem to bend quite normally until the patella assumes its normal position.

Physical Examination

The EM is usually examined in the context of a complete knee examination. Indeed, important factors relating to the EM can be seen all the way from the pelvis to the foot. These findings can best be seen by evaluating the patient in the upright position, the sitting position, *and* the supine position.

The examiner should observe while the patient stands and walks. Excessive angular deformities of the lower extremities, either varus or valgus, can be associated with extensor mechanism problems. A functionally short leg can also place abnormal mechanical stress on the extensor mechanism. Viewing the patient from the side, the examiner can see any hyperextension or recurvatum of the knee. Excessive recurvatum goes along with generalized joint laxity, which may also be contributing to patellar instability. The examiner should pay particular attention to the action of the patellas as the patient walks. Stepping up onto and down from a low examination stool is another helpful dynamic activity.

With the patient seated, the knees are held flexed at 90°. The examiner should observe for abnormal patellar position. Tibial torsion can also be assessed by viewing the knee from above and estimating the transmalleolar axis of the ankle. Although the quadriceps angle (Q angle) is more commonly assessed in the supine position, it can also be assessed as the patient sits (Fig. 68–1A). Also called the *tubercle sulcus angle,* a residual lateral deviation of the patellar tendon with the knee flexed to 90° is considered abnormal distal EM alignment.[1] The patient should actively extend and flex the knee while sitting. Crepitation is often palpable in the anterior portion of the knee with this maneuver. The examiner also observes the tracking of the patella, which ordinarily describes a gentle C-shaped curve as the knee is extended.

By having the patient hold both knees actively at about 45° of flexion, one can assess the muscle forces acting on the patella. One of the prime causative factors in all EM disorders is a relative lack of the medial supporting forces of the vastus medialis obliquus (VMO), as opposed to the laterally deviating forces of the vastus lateralis.

Next the patient lies supine on the examination table. Patellofemoral tenderness and crepitation can be assessed by compression of the patellofemoral joint, both transversely and longitudinally. It must be remembered that, with the knee fully extended, many patellas lie above the trochlea of the femur, and such tenderness and crepitation can come from the patellas' rubbing against the supratrochlear soft tissues. The knee can

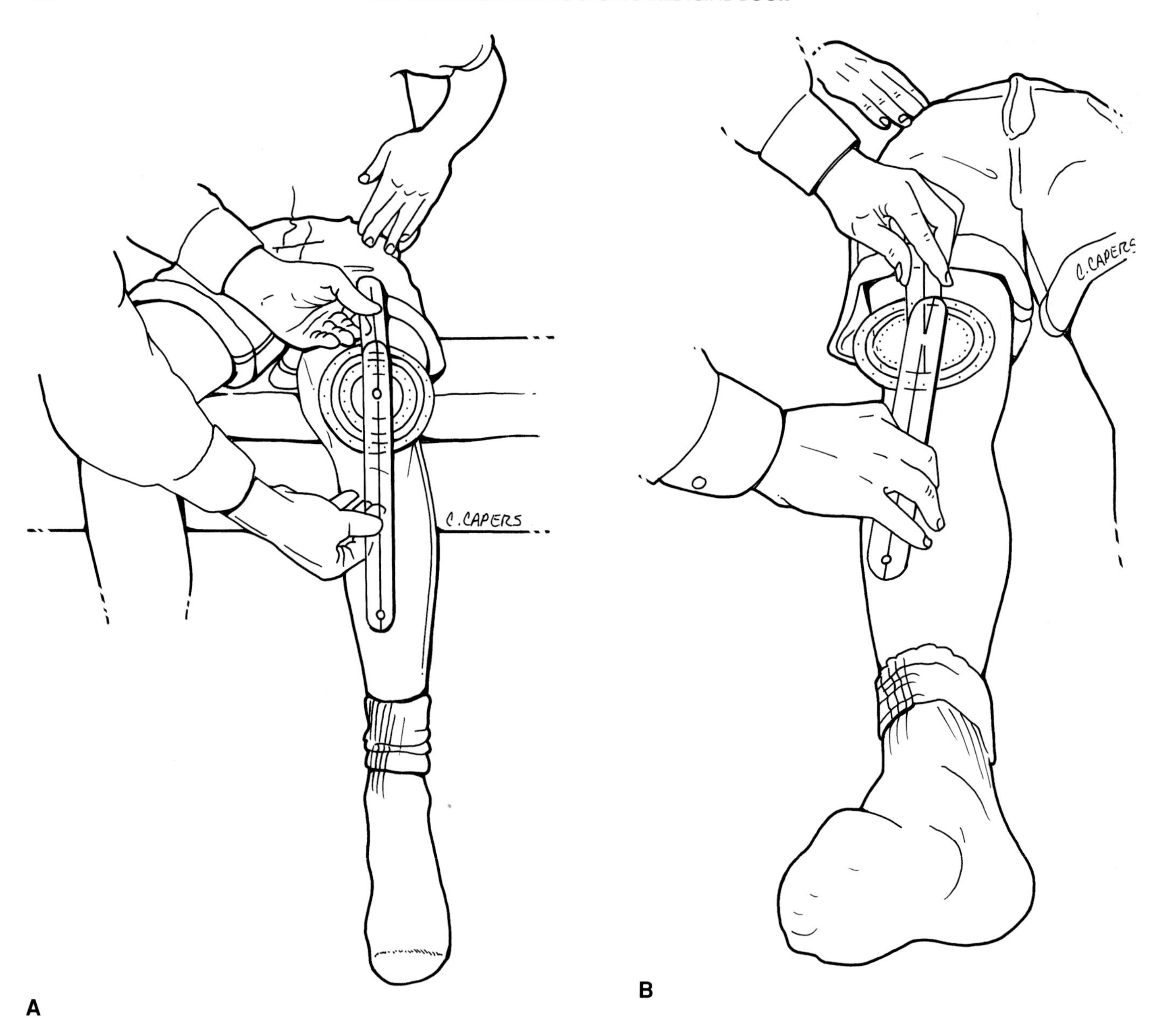

Fig. 68–1. The Q angle can be measured with the patient seated *(A)* or supine *(B)*. A goniometer is placed with the pivot point at the center of the patella. The proximal arm is directed toward the anterior superior iliac spine and the distal arm along the patellar tendon to the tibial tuberosity.

also be bent to about 30°, engaging the patella in the trochlea, and tenderness and crepitation are sought once again. Effusion in the knee should be assessed along with range of motion. One can now measure the Q angle in the more traditional fashion. With the knee fully extended and quadriceps tightened, a goniometer is placed with the pivot point at the center of the patella. The proximal arm is directed toward the palpated anterior superior iliac spine and the distal arm along the patellar tendon to the tibial tuberosity (Fig. 68–1B). Measured in this fashion, a quadriceps angle of 10° or less is thought to be normal. In women, the normal Q angle may extend up to 15°.

Other areas of tenderness around the anterior knee, such as the attachment of the patellar tendon to the inferior patellar pole, should be sought through palpation. A medial synovial plica may be found by passively flexing and extending the knee with the fingers over the medial patellofemoral region. Hip range of motion, especially internal and external rotation, is important to assess because of the role of rotational deformities in the femur in aggravating patellar problems. Evaluation of hamstring and heel cord tightness is also critically important.

Finally, in the supine position, patellar mobility can be assessed. This is done by sitting on the side of the examination table and flexing the patient's knee 20° to 30° over the examiner's leg. Both thumbs are then used to exert force along the medial edge of the patella, displacing it as far laterally as possible (Fig. 68–2). This can result in a feeling of hypermobility as compared with that in the opposite knee or in other patients' knees. It

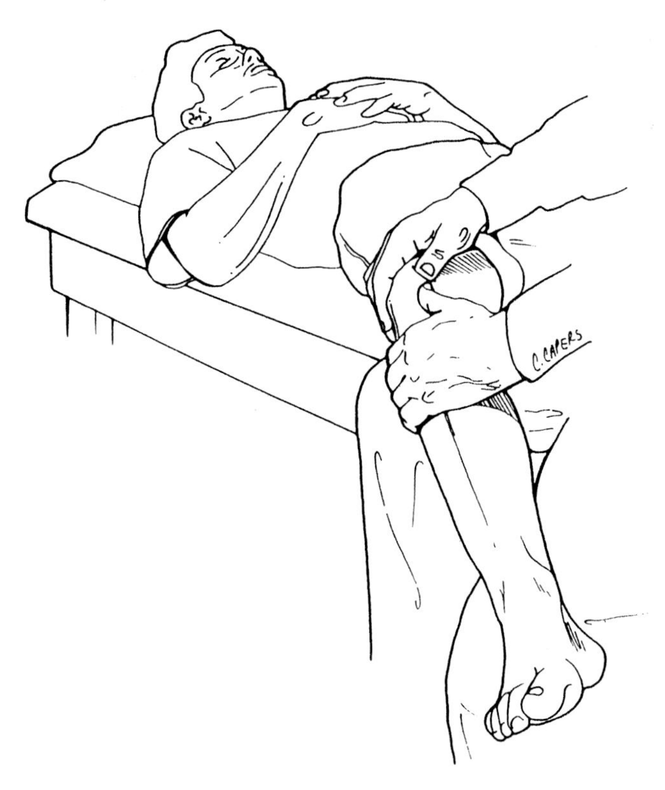

Fig. 68–2. Patellar instability is tested with the patient's knee flexed 20° to 30°. The examiner applies a force along the medial edge of the patella, displacing it as far laterally as possible. Hypermobility compared with the opposite knee is a positive finding.

can also produce certain degrees of apprehension as the patients report feeling that the patella is going to subluxate or dislocate. In this case, it is extremely important to ask whether this is the instability feeling they associate with the ongoing knee problem. Not only lateral hypermobility, but also increased medial mobility, should be assessed. Some patellas are extremely loose in all directions, seemingly demonstrating "multidirectional instability."

Radiographic Evaluation

By this point in the evaluation, the examiner should have an extremely accurate impression of whether this patient's problem is related to the EM. If this impression is not formed through careful history taking and physical examination, radiographs may be of some help. However, the diagnosis of extensor mechanism disorders is most often a clinical diagnosis and not a radiographic one. Radiographs in this situation can mislead just as easily as they can help.

The standard anteroposterior and lateral radiographs usually offer very little specific information about the patellofemoral joint. The major benefit of these views is to rule out other confounding factors such as osteoarthritis or osteochondritis dissecans.

The major emphasis in radiography of patellofemoral disorders is the infrapatellar radiograph. Many different techniques have been described for obtaining this view.[2,3] Regardless of which technique the clinician chooses, the single most important factor is to obtain a radiograph of the patellofemoral joint with the knee in nearly full extension rather than flexed 90° or more. In the traditional sunrise, or skyline, view, the knee is flexed acutely, forcing the patella to seat in the more distal part of the femoral trochlea and thereby providing little or no useful information. Hughston was one of the first to advocate routine clinical use of a patellofemoral view made with the knee in less than 90° flexion.[4] His technique, still a model of simplicity, can be done in any office by having the patient lie prone with an x-ray cassette under the distal femurs. The x-ray tube is angled 45° cephalad and the toes are propped on the x-ray machine. With feet and knees held together, the x-ray beam is directed along the line of the anterior tibias to the cassette under the patellofemoral joints (Fig. 68–3). The major criticism of this technique is that, because the plate is not perpendicular to the x-ray beam, some distortion is produced in the appearance of the patellofemoral area. When one becomes accustomed to this view, however, it can certainly be helpful and simple to obtain.

Other techniques have been described with the patient supine that allow the x-ray beam to be directed perpendicular to the plate. The cassette can be positioned either proximal or distal to the knee. In addition to lack of distortion, the major benefit of this method generally is that it allows visualization of patellofemoral alignment with the knee closer to full extension.

Various measurements and indices have been developed to assess the patellofemoral radiograph.[2,3] The critical points to evaluate include the overall development of the trochlear groove, lateral tilting of the patella (indicating tightness in the lateral supporting structures), lateral (or rarely medial) abnormal displacement of the patella out of the middle of the trochlear groove, and other miscellaneous bone abnormalities. These miscellaneous findings may include accessory ossification centers along the lateral edge of the patella, avulsion fractures or calcification along the medial edge, or osteochondritis dissecans of the patella itself.

More sophisticated techniques of radiographic evaluation of the patellofemoral joint have been described. The one most commonly used, computed tomography (CT),[5–7] allows visualization of the patellofemoral joint with the knee in full extension. Indices have been developed to indicate abnormal patellofemoral alignment.[7] Magnetic resonance imaging (MRI) has been described not only to assess the articular surface but also to give a somewhat dynamic picture of patellofemoral tracking through linking together multiple position exposures.[8] Scintigraphic techniques have been used to show the metabolic component of patellofemoral disease.[9]

Arthroscopic Examination

In certain instances, the full story of a patient's patellofemoral problem cannot be known without diag-

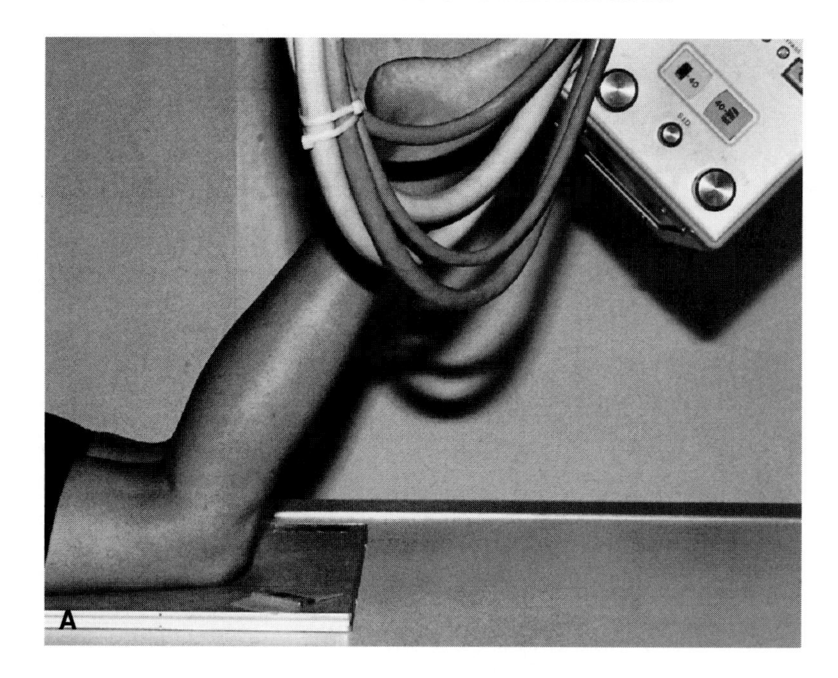

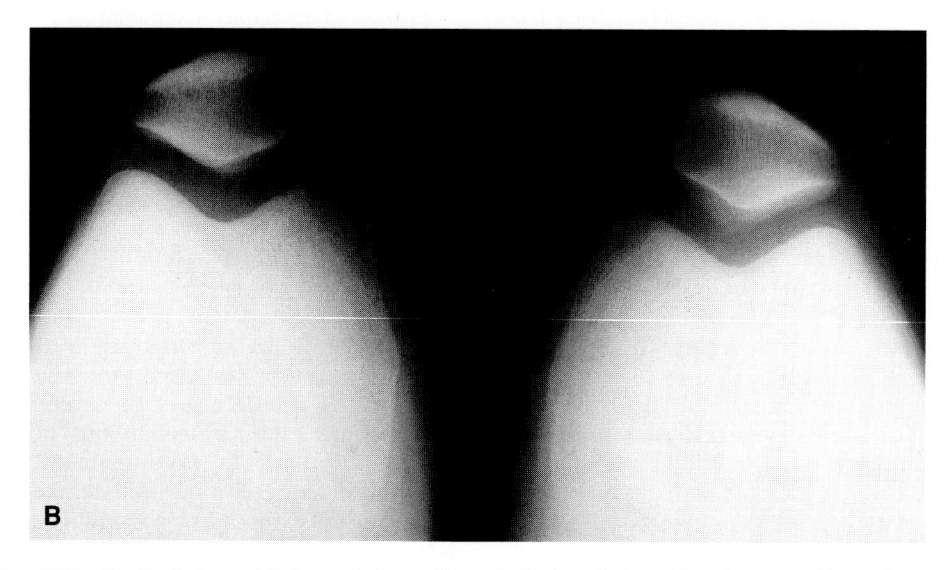

Fig. 68–3. *(A)* **For the Hughston patellofemoral view radiograph the knee is flexed less than 90°. This can be accomplished by having the patient lie prone with an x-ray cassette under the distal femurs. This view, as opposed to the view with the knee flexed, does not show the patella forced to the more distal part of the femoral trochlea** *(B).*

nostic arthroscopy. This usually takes place only when the program of conservative care has failed and the disability warrants surgical treatment.

The arthroscope allows full assessment of the patellofemoral area. The most helpful approach is through one of the proximal portals. Viewing from above, the arthroscopist can see the entire panorama of the patellofemoral joint and assess problems fully. Chondromalacia of the patella or the trochlea can easily be seen (Fig. 68–4). A large medial or suprapatellar plica can be detected. One can occasionally see extreme hypertrophy of the infrapatellar fat pad with obvious entrapment of the fat pad between the patella and femur on full knee extension. Excessive lateral tilt of the patella is quite easily seen, as is unusual lateral displacement in full extension, resulting in marked overhang of the lateral facet over the edge of the trochlea. While the patella is viewed from above, the knee can be passively flexed, in some measure to assess the tracking of the patella in the trochlea. Admittedly, this is a passive maneuver rather than the dynamic situation when the patient's muscles are contracting; nevertheless it still seems to have some value. Normal patellar alignment has been described as contact of the medial patellar facet against the medial trochlea by 40° of knee flexion.[10]

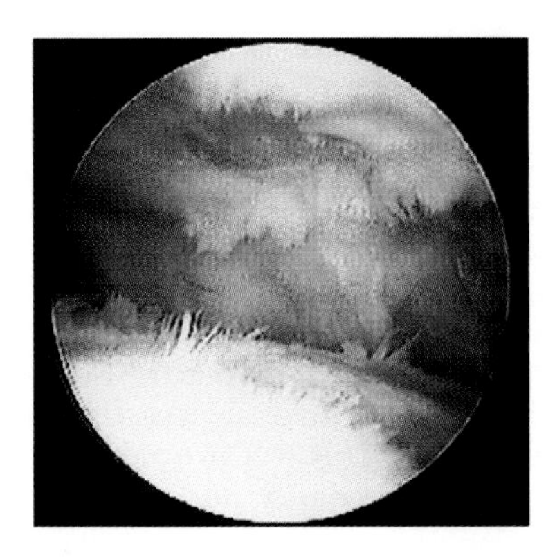

Fig. 68–4. Arthroscopic view of chondromalacia of the patella and trochlea.

TREATMENT

Nonsurgical Treatment

Therapeutic exercise is the cornerstone of treatment for all patellofemoral disorders. This is necessary not only to get the patient over any immediate problem but also to allow him or her to continue to lead an active life style in the future. It is critically important to communicate this to the patient early in the course of treatment. Patients must understand that they have a problem closely linked to their inherent anatomy and muscle function and that there is no "quick fix" for patellofemoral disorders. They must accept the fact that, with or without surgery, certain types of physical therapy concepts will probably always be important to them and that symptoms may wax and wane as life goes on.

The first concept is that of controlling patellar tracking through muscle activity in the quadriceps. To do this, one must strengthen the VMO selectively.[11] Exercises to accomplish this include straight leg raises with external twisting of the leg, simultaneous bilateral heel lifts while squeezing a rubber ball or pillow between the distal thighs to create hip adduction, or the use of side-lying hip adduction techniques with the VMO maintaining an antigravity position.

Most recently, thinking has arisen that challenges the traditional concept of any muscle-strengthening for patellofemoral disorders. McConnell has pointed out that the deficit is in areas such as timing of muscle firing and muscle fiber recruitment.[12] She therefore developed a method for both assessing and rehabilitating the lower extremity musculature that has gained widespread popularity (see Chapter 69).

In addition to muscle control over the patella, flexibility exercises are also extremely important. Probably the single most important one is to maintain flexibility in the hamstring muscles. There seems to be a direct relationship between hamstring tightness and patellofemoral symptoms, possibly because working against the posterior tightness in the functional setting requires generation of excessive force within the patellofemoral joint. For whatever reason, hamstring stretching must be done if any tightness is present. Flexibility of the gastrocsoleus group should also be maintained since the gastrocnemius muscles also cross the back of the knee joint. Quadriceps muscle flexibility is perhaps less important, but it should also be assessed and improved if the patient is extremely tight. Iliotibial band tightness also seems to increase lateral forces on the patella. Iliotibial band stretching can occasionally play a key role in relieving symptoms.

As with all lower extremity rehabilitation, agility and coordination are important, though more advanced, techniques. This objective can be achieved with a variety of balancing exercises. Various devices are marketed that allow exercising to improve proprioceptive function.

Finally, patients who accomplish the basic goals set for strengthening, flexibility, and coordination need to work through a progressive running program to return to most sporting activities. This should begin with brisk walking, followed by alternating straight-ahead walking and jogging, followed by running straight ahead for increasing distances. Depending on the sport, this could be followed by shorter-distance sprinting and cutting with various techniques in different directions.

Probably the most commonly used adjunctive treatment for patellofemoral disorders is anti-inflammatory medication. Presumably, the pain of patellofemoral malalignment has an inflammatory origin; so, even though swelling is usually not a prominent feature, most physicians prescribe nonsteroidal anti-inflammatory drugs. These can be helpful by allowing the patient to make progress through the more important therapeutic exercises. Occasionally, especially with patellar tendinitis, delivery of steroids to an inflamed area is accomplished through the technique of phonophoresis, using ultrasound and 10% hydrocortisone cream. Cortisone injections are to be avoided for patellofemoral problems in athletes, who are usually young people with no pre-existing degenerative disease in their knee. For them, intra-articular injection could actually be harmful in the long run. Injection into an inflamed patellar tendon may carry the risk of precipitating patellar tendon rupture. Some authors have described local infiltration of a synovial plica. It is hard to imagine that one could actually know that this injection is directed into the substance of a plica and not simply into the knee joint itself.

The next, and possibly more helpful, adjunctive treatment is external support. Bracing has traditionally been a part of treating patellofemoral problems. We still use a variety of bracing techniques, ranging from simple neoprene sleeves with lateral buttresses to the Palumbo brace,[13] which provides more dynamic lateral support to the extensor mechanism. With the advent of the McConnell techniques, however, use of braces has become somewhat less prevalent. This is because McConnell has described the use of specific and custom-made taping techniques for each individual patient, in an attempt to passively reposition the patella in the proper place to most immediately decrease symptoms and to allow the patient to effectively work on exercises.[12]

The next most frequently used adjunctive method is orthotics for pronated feet. Occasionally a physician struggles with a patient having patellar problems only to find that the addition of orthotics is the ultimate key to resolution of symptoms. Certainly, arch supports are not a panacea and do not need to be used in every patient; however, in the case of resistant problems, the physician should carefully assess foot posture in both weight-bearing and non–weight-bearing situations and try, at least, a set of temporary orthotics if excessive foot malalignment is observed.

What is the role of immobilization? Generally we are moving away from the use of prolonged immobilization, even for acute patellar dislocation. Certainly for patients with pain syndromes, the potential benefit of immobilization is usually vastly offset by the deleterious effect of immobilization on muscle and joint function. A patient with extremely acute patellar tendinitis might need immobilization for a day or two but certainly nothing more than this. For an acute instability episode, even a first time complete dislocation, we now use immobilization in a limited fashion, allowing resolution of swelling and pain but then moving almost immediately to functional rehabilitation techniques. The routine use of 6 weeks' cast immobilization for patellar dislocation has proven to have very little beneficial effect on the natural history of patellofemoral disease.[3]

Surgical Treatment

The major thrust of this chapter is the importance of nonsurgical treatment of patellofemoral disorders. Nonsurgical treatment should be successful in 80 to 90% of patients. Admittedly *successful* may mean reaching a steady state in which the patient has some intermittent problems or some mild limitations in life style that, by themselves, are not sufficient to warrant surgery. When a patient has tried a thorough program of nonsurgical treatment and continues to have significant functional disability, surgery may be considered.

I have already mentioned the role of diagnostic arthroscopy in confirming the diagnosis or discovering some unsuspected injury such as a meniscal tear. At the same time diagnostic arthroscopy is done, arthroscopic surgical techniques can be used to débride chondromalacia of the articular surfaces or remove loose bodies. If a significant thickened and fibrotic synovial plica is found, it can be removed through partial synovectomy. The problem with this is that many knees demonstrate some degree of plica formation that is not pathologic and not relevant to symptoms. The arthroscopic appearance of synovial plica should be put together with the typical clinical syndrome of popping and catching, discomfort with the knee flexed accompanied by a distinct pop when the knee is extended, and a palpable tender synovial fold on physical examination.

A hypertrophic infrapatellar fat pad can likewise be débrided arthroscopically. Again, the problem is in distinguishing an abnormal fat pad that is producing symptoms from one that is not. The former type looks irritated or inflamed and should be hypertrophic enough to clearly become impinged between the joint structures. These findings should be put together with clinical symptoms of infrapatellar pain and puffiness, perhaps resembling refractory patellar tendinitis. Distal tilting of the patella on quadriceps contraction has also been described by McConnell as a potential mechanism for impingement of the fat pad.

The most controversial area in arthroscopic treatment of the patellofemoral joint concerns the use of lateral retinacular release.[3] This is a procedure that, perhaps owing to its early popularity and simplicity, may well have been overused. Complications, such as medial subluxation of the patella and quadriceps tendon rupture, can occur.[14,15] This procedure certainly does not help every patient with patellofemoral problems. It appears to stand a better chance of helping those with a pure pain syndrome rather than those with patellar instability. Certain radiographic parameters have been described to indicate the need for lateral release.[16,17]

We currently use an arthroscopic technique of lateral release for patients with the abnormal arthroscopic findings noted above, which are consistent with tightness in the lateral retinaculum and abnormal tracking. In our estimation, this relatively minimal attempt at realigning the patellofemoral joint is successful in approximately 60 to 70% of patients who feel the need to resort to surgery; however, it must be undertaken with a great deal of caution and a thorough explanation to the patient of reasonable expectations. It should also be remembered that lateral release is the arthroscopic procedure associated with the highest rate of complications.[18,19] The most frequently reported complication from lateral release is that of postoperative hemarthrosis, sometimes to the point that repeat arthroscopy is necessary for drainage. Patients should also be warned that, even without major complications, an arthroscopic lateral release is neither a quick fix nor a substitute for rehabilitative exercises. In our experience, recovery from lateral release requires at least 3 months.

Even in the case of acute first-time patellar dislocation, the role of direct open surgical repair has been extremely limited. Direct surgical repair has been applied no more often for patellar dislocation than it has for other joint dislocations. Perhaps it should be done more often. By identifying specific problems that could be remedied through direct repair, one might affect the natural history of patellar problems and decrease the rate of recurrent symptoms. Some authors have suggested this.[20,21] However, oftentimes in the acute setting, the specific pathologic condition is less than obvious. Surgeons may therefore find themselves using standard reconstructive techniques rather than direct repair, so one may question why reconstructive techniques should be used early in the course of dealing with this injury rather than later, after the patient has tried controlling problems through conservative means.

Open extensor mechanism reconstruction has been described since at least the early 20th century. The techniques used today are in many ways very similar to those described originally. Basically, they include alteration of muscle forces on the patella and a change in patellar position. Most commonly, this includes release of the lateral side of the extensor mechanism, advancement of the vastus medialis obliquus and associated structures medially, and transfer of the patellar tendon insertion on the tibia. These surgical techniques have resulted in a reasonable rate of success.[22–24] Once again, however, they are usually reserved for patients who fail to control their problem through nonsurgical means. Like arthroscopic treatment, open extensor mechanism reconstruction does not eliminate the need for dealing with the extensor mechanism through exercise or other adjunctive means in the future.

REFERENCES

1. Kolowich, P. A., Paulos, L. E., Rosenberg, T. D., and Farnsworth, S.: Lateral release of the patella: Indications and contraindications. Am. J. Sports Med. *18*:359, 1990.
2. Minkoff, J., and Fein, L.: The role of radiography in the evaluation and treatment of common anarthrotic disorders of the patellofemoral joint. Clin. Sports Med. *8*:203, 1989.
3. Walsh, W. M.: The patellofemoral joint. *In* Orthopaedic Sports Medicine: Principles and Practice. Edited by J. C. DeLee and D. Drez. Philadelphia, W.B. Saunders, 1994.
4. Hughston, J. C.: Subluxation of the patella. J. Bone Joint Surg. *50A*:1003, 1968.
5. Galland, O., Walch, G., Dejour, H., and Carret, J. P.: An anatomical and radiological study of the femoropatellar articulation. Surg. Radiol. Anat. *12*:119, 1990.
6. Inoue, M., et al.: Subluxation of the patella. Computed tomography analysis of patellofemoral congruence. J. Bone Joint Surg. *70A*:1331, 1988.
7. Schutzer, S. F., Ramsby, G. R., and Fulkerson, J. P.: Computed tomographic classification of patellofemoral pain patients. Orthop. Clin. North Am. *17*:235, 1986.
8. Shellock, F. G., Mink, J. H., and Fox, J. M.: Patellofemoral joint: Kinematic MR imaging to assess tracking abnormalities. Radiology *168*:551, 1988.
9. Dye, S. F., and Boll, D. A.: Radionuclide imaging of the patellofemoral joint in young adults with anterior knee pain. Orthop. Clin. North Am. *17*:249, 1986.
10. Sojbjerg, J. O., Lauritzen, J., Hvid, I., and Boe, S.: Arthroscopic determination of patellofemoral malalignment. Clin. Orthop. *215*:243, 1987.
11. Shelton, G. L., and Thigpen, L. K.: Rehabilitation of patellofemoral dysfunction: A review of the literature. J. Orthop. Sports Phys. Ther. *14*:243, 1991.
12. McConnell, J.: The management of chondromalacia patellae: A long term solution. Austr. J. Physiother. *2*:215, 1986.
13. Palumbo, P. M.: Dynamic patellar brace: A new orthosis in the management of patellofemoral disorders. Am. J. Sports Med. *9*:45, 1981.
14. Hughston, J. C., and Deese, M.: Medial subluxation of the patella as a complication of lateral retinacular release. Am. J. Sports Med. *16*:383, 1988.
15. Blasier, R. B., and Ciullo, J. V.: Rupture of the quadriceps tendon after arthroscopic lateral release. Arthroscopy *2*:262, 1986.
16. Fulkerson, J. P., Schutzer, S. F., Ramsby, G. R., and Bernstein, R. A.: Computerized tomography of the patellofemoral joint before and after lateral release or realignment. Arthroscopy *3*:19, 1987.
17. Fulkerson, J. P., and Schutzer, S. F.: After failure of conservative treatment for painful patellofemoral malalignment: Lateral release or realignment? Orthop. Clin. North Am. *17*:283, 1986.
18. DeLee, J. C.: Complications of arthroscopy and arthroscopic surgery: Results of a national survey. Arthroscopy *1*:214, 1985.
19. Small, N. C.: Complications in arthroscopy: The knee and other joints. Arthroscopy *2*:253, 1986.
20. Boring, T. H., and O'Donoghue, D. H.: Acute patellar dislocation: Results of immediate surgical repair. Clin. Orthop. *136*:182, 1978.
21. Vainionpaa, S., et al.: Acute dislocation of the patella. A prospective review of operative treatment. J. Bone Joint Surg. *72B*:366, 1990.
22. Hughston, J. C., and Walsh, W. M.: Proximal and distal reconstruction of the extensor mechanism for patellar subluxation. Clin. Orthop. *144*:36, 1979.
23. Hughston, J. C., Walsh, W. M., and Puddu, G.: Patellar Subluxation and Dislocation. Philadelphia, W. B. Saunders, 1984.
24. Turba, J. E., Walsh, W. M., and McLeod, W. D.: Long-term results of extensor mechanism reconstruction. A standard for evaluation. Am. J. Sports Med. *7*:91, 1979.

69 *Dianne Bazor Olszak*

Rehabilitation of the Extensor Mechanism

The osseous components of the extensor mechanism (EM) are the femoral condyles, the trochlear groove, the patella, and the tibial tuberosity. Structurally, they form the patellofemoral joint. This articulation is controlled by the soft tissue components of the EM: the quadriceps muscle, quadriceps tendon, the patellar tendon, the synovial lining, and the extensive peripatellar retinaculum. Other structures included in the EM are the suprapatellar and the prepatellar bursas and the infrapatellar fat pad.

Anatomically, the extensor mechanism is at risk for injuries. It has relatively poor protection from external forces as well as the noncontact forces of pivoting, cutting, and twisting that occur during sports. Structurally, only the medial and lateral retinaculum and the quadriceps tendon offer support to this area. Many times, patellofemoral joint problems and injuries are overlooked during evaluation of athletes. Perhaps this is because of the mind set that says injuries to the knee usually affect the ligaments or the menisci. Also, the symptoms of patellofemoral joint dysfunction may closely mimic these injuries. Clicking, popping, giving way, and persistent pain in the knee all may be associated with both entities. Hughston's review of patients in the late 1960s has shown that patellofemoral joint dysfunction affects the athletic population as well as overweight adolescent girls.[1]

BIOMECHANICAL PRINCIPLES

To devise a successful rehabilitation program it is necessary to understand the biomechanics of the patellofemoral joint. The main function of the patella is to increase the mechanical advantage of the quadriceps muscle.[2] The compression between the patella and the femur is known as the patellofemoral joint reaction force (PFJRF). This force is 0° with the leg in full extension and increases with increasing knee flexion because of muscle tension as the patella enters the trochlear groove, around 20°. The contact area of the patella increases with knee flexion in squatting. Thus, more surface area of the patella is available to disperse compressive loads. The reverse is true in open-chain flexion-to-extension exercises; the PFJRF increases as the area decreases, applying undue stress to a smaller area on the undersurface of the patella.[3] This principle is ignored in many therapeutic rehabilitation programs and may lead to further irritation and hyaline cartilage breakdown around the patellofemoral joint.

VASTUS MEDIALIS OBLIQUUS STRENGTHENING

A tenuous balance exists between the medial and lateral stabilizers of the patellofemoral joint. Any imbalance, either static or dynamic, leads to "maltracking" of the patella. The function of the vastus medialis obliquus is to provide dynamic medial pull to align the patella in the femoral groove. In normal subjects, the vastus medialis obliquus fires before the vastus lateralis when tested by the patellar tendon reflex tap. Patients with EM dysfunction tend to show a reversal of this firing pattern.[4] Rehabilitation programs must aim to train the vastus medialis obliquus in its most optimal position, encouraging it to fire before the vastus lateralis for proper patella positioning.

It was originally thought that the vastus medialis obliquus was most active during the final degrees of knee extension. Lieb and Perry have shown that it is active through the entire range of motion.[5] However, the fact that terminal knee extension exercises work to strengthen the vastus medialis obliquus shows that its function is to realign the patella, not to extend the knee. It should be remembered that end-range exercises such as short arc quadriceps sets, terminal knee extension, and quadriceps sets recruit not only the vastus medialis obliquus but also the vastus lateralis. Some believe these exercises at end range may actually increase firing of the vastus lateralis, contributing to tracking problems in persons with EM dysfunction.[6,7]

Controversy surrounds the theory of using hip adduction to increase the firing pattern of the vastus medialis obliquus. Some studies have shown that straight leg raises combined with adduction show no increase in vastus medialis obliquus activity as compared with regular straight leg raises[8,9]; however, McConnell emphasizes the importance of limb position and the fact that the vastus medialis obliquus is not a knee extensor but a medial stabilizer.[10] She also advocates the use of isometric adduction in weight-bearing stance to facilitate vastus medialis obliquus activity. Hodges and Richardson have also shown vastus medialis obliquus activity increased relative to that of the vastus lateralis with the use of 20% of a maximal adduction contraction in a weight-bearing position.[11]

The vastus medialis obliquus is easily inhibited by pain and effusion. Spencer and coworkers have shown it takes only 20 to 30 ml of saline to inhibit the vastus medialis obliquus.[12] Therefore, even a slight knee effusion may alter its firing, contributing to EM dysfunction. In the postoperative knee, rehabilitation must emphasize decreasing swelling to prevent quadriceps atrophy and patellar tracking problems.

TYPES OF EXERCISE

The ultimate goal for any athlete with EM dysfunction is to return to sport asymptomatically. Most athletes respond to a conservative exercise program. Once a correct diagnosis is made, rest from sport or other activities, therapeutic modalities, and exercises usually relieve the athlete of symptoms. If the rehabilitation program is not sufficient for the athlete, who places more demand on the knee than a sedentary individual, return to sport will only cause the symptoms to reappear. Athletes may repeat this pattern several times, frustrating both athlete and therapist and leading to chronic patellofemoral joint irritation.

Isometric exercise, in the form of quadriceps sets and straight leg raises, are frequently begun during the initial stages of EM dysfunction. It has been shown by electromyographic testing that a quadriceps set produces greater quadriceps activity than a straight leg raise.[13] Initially, quadriceps sets help alleviate knee effusion and are normally tolerated by patients with acute patellofemoral joint injuries (Fig. 69–1). Attention should be paid to the vastus medialis obliquus during instruction of active quadriceps setting to gain maximal benefits.

True quadriceps isolation is a simple yet important concept that is often not addressed in exercise instruction. It is much easier for the patient with a painful knee to contract using the hamstrings and hip extensors. Palpation of the quadriceps muscle proximally can be deceiving. Placing a finger on the patellar tendon and feeling for tension during active contraction is a reliable way to ensure quadriceps activity. Many times, downward pressure applied to the patella facilitates isolation of the quadriceps. Also, having the patient sit inhibits the action of the hip extensors and helps promote quadriceps isolation.

Open-chain exercise, in which the proximal segment is fixed and the distal segment moves, causes both concentric shortening and eccentric lengthening of the muscle fibers. This type of exercise produces maximal motor unit activity and is prescribed frequently for athletes with EM dysfunction. Flexion to extension exercises increase PFJRF by decreasing the contact area. Exercises in this range may further irritate the joint by applying nonphysiologic compressive loads to the articular cartilage of the patella. Many times, increased PFJRF from open-chain exercises are ill-tolerated by the patient.

Closed-chain exercise with a fixed foot, causing the proximal segment to move, is a more functional type of exercise. The quadriceps functions as a decelerator and should be trained in this manner.[14] PFJRF is increased with increasing knee flexion; however, more of the patellar surface is able to disperse patellofemoral forces evenly.

Some clinicians use isokinetics in the treatment of EM dysfunction. This type of exercise allows the athlete to work at high exercise speeds against varying resistance. Some report that high-speed exercises of this nature reduce the PFJRF and closely mimic activities of the quadriceps during sport. Biomechanical principles of open-chain exercise should be adhered to in the use of isokinetics, to avoid further irritating the patellofemoral joint.[15,16]

Isometric, concentric, and eccentric components are combined in weight-bearing exercises. Athletes can progress from isometrics in standing to functional exercises such as step-ups, squats, lunges, slideboard, and other activities that mimic their sport (Fig. 69–2). Pelvis, knee, and foot control are heavily emphasized in closed-chain exercises, improving proprioception and kinesthetic awareness.[17]

REHABILITATION OF SPECIFIC EXTENSOR MECHANISM DYSFUNCTIONS

Anterior Knee Pain

Many advances in the treatment of anterior knee pain have been made by Jenny McConnell, an Australian physiotherapist. The McConnell program is based on a thorough structural evaluation of the lower extremity, both statically and dynamically.[18] Close attention is paid to biomechanical features of the lower extremity

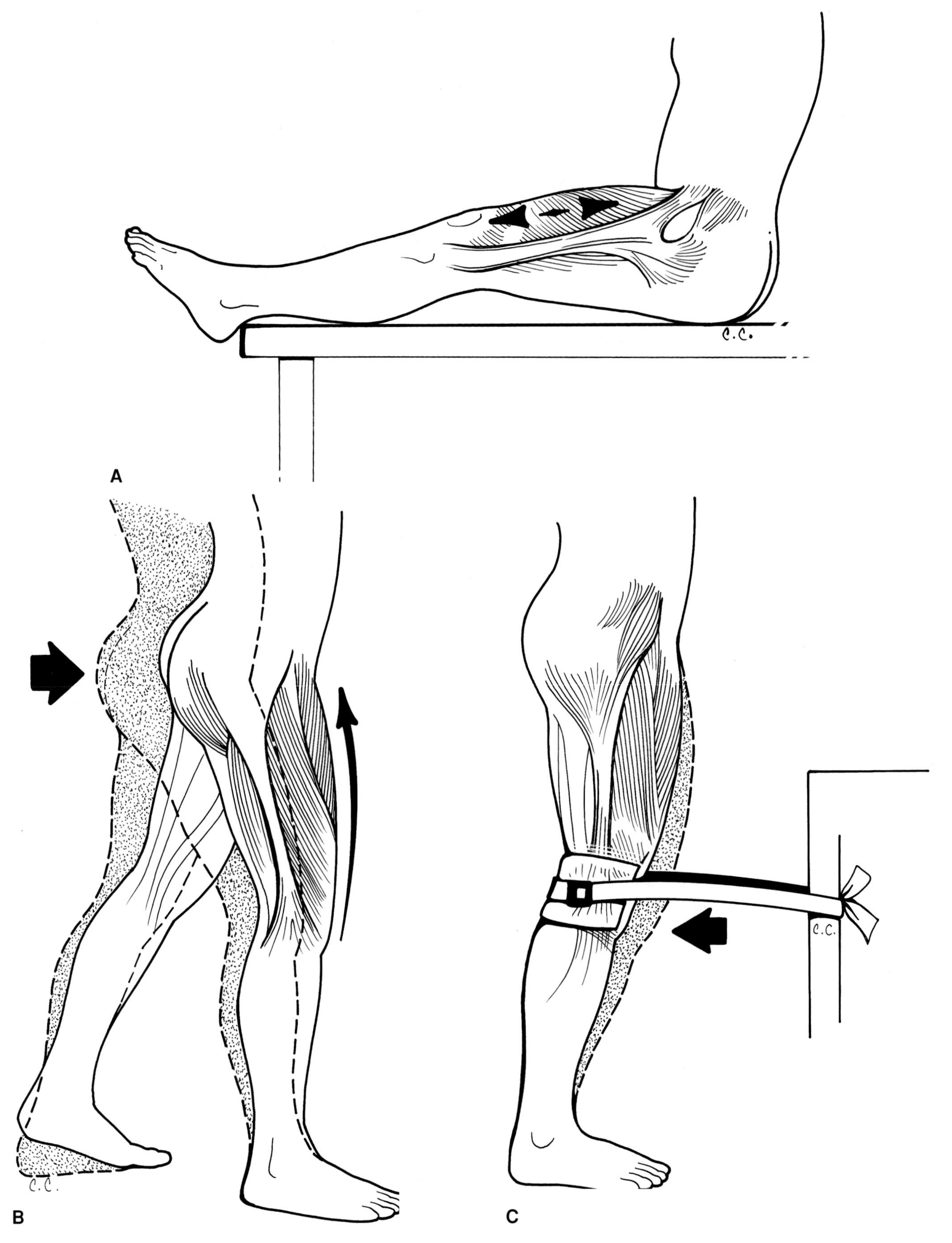

Fig. 69–1. Quadriceps sets: *(A)* seated, *(B)* stance, *(C)* standing set against resistance.

and their effect on the patellofemoral joint. The goals of this program are to gain optimal patellar position by taping and stretching tight soft tissue components and then functionally improving the firing pattern of the vastus medialis obliquus. Abnormal positioning of the patella is caused by retinacular shortening, structural laxity, or muscular imbalance. McConnell has defined four categories to describe these positions.[17] The first and most common is a glide, which is diagnosed by observation of marked lateral movement of the patella during an active quadriceps set. This is normally due to a late-firing vastus medialis obliquus and to tight lateral structures that promote a static lateral position of the patella.

The second type of abnormal patella position is the lateral tilt (Fig. 69–3), which is caused principally by deep lateral retinacular tightness or shortening. These deep retinacular transverse fibers run from the iliotibial band directly into the patella. Lateral positioning of the patella and tightness of the iliotibial band cause adaptive shortening of these fibers, causing the patella to be tilted laterally in relation to the femoral condyle. Fulkerson has shown damage to small nerves in the lateral retinaculum over time, implicating lateral patella positioning as a source of pain in patients with EM dysfunction who have lateral pain.[19]

The third position is rotational malalignment. In the McConnell scheme, this includes any deviation of the long axis of the patella from the axis of the femur.

The fourth position, anteroposterior, may cause fat pad irritation because the inferior pole of the patella is tilted posteriorly. This is most common in patients with genu recurvatum. The fat pad and surrounding synovium are richly innervated, causing stabbing and pinching pain. These patients normally have a hyperextension type gait pattern and pain with activation of the quadriceps as the inferior pole digs into the fat pad. Correction of this posterior tilting allows the patient to exercise pain free, thus strengthening the quadriceps while allowing the fat pad inflammation to calm down.

The McConnell program progresses from correction of patellar positioning with tape to improving lower extremity mechanics and control in sport. Correcting abnormal patellar positioning should allow the patient to exercise in a pain-free range, and it allows optimal function of the vastus medialis obliquus. Exercises begin in the nonweight-bearing position, using biofeedback to ensure proper firing of the vastus medialis obliquus. Next, the patient progresses to weight bearing, closed-chain exercises such as stance quadriceps activation, step-ups, step-downs, and 10° to 15° squats, all emphasizing pelvis, knee, and foot control. All exercises are performed in a pain-free range and progress as the athlete improves vastus medialis obliquus firing and lower extremity control. These closed-chain exercises are performed in combination with a stretching program for tightness in the gastrocnemius, hamstrings, iliotibial band, and lateral retinaculum. From this point the athlete's program is geared toward return to sport by functional training in his or her particular sport. The athlete is gradually weaned from the taping as vastus medialis obliquus firing improves, alleviating patellofemoral symptoms (Fig. 69–4).

Plica Irritation

The plica synovialis, a normal fold in the synovial lining of the knee joint, extends from the infrapatellar fat pad upward over the femoral condyles, crossing under the quadriceps tendon, and attaches to the lateral retinaculum.[20] The plica can be injured by trauma directly to the patella, since it is trapped between the patella and the femoral condyles. Plica tears have also been reported during athletic events.

Chronic plica irritation is usually caused by an underlying EM dysfunction.[21] Usually, the medial plica becomes inflamed and irritated because it receives abnormal pressure from a lateral-tracking patella. Tightness in the hamstrings contributes much to plica irritation by increasing the PFJRF. Prolonged aggravation leads to fibrotic thickening, and even calcification of the plica. Athletes who participate in cycling, swimming, and running, all sports that require repetitive knee flexion, may be more susceptible to plica irritation. Popping, giving way, and pain with prolonged sitting or walking down steps are all common complaints of plica irritation.

Swelling due to synovial irritation and tenderness over the plica medially are usually present with this condition. This effusion inhibits the action of the vastus medialis obliquus as well as the articularis genus, which is responsible for retracting the suprapatellar pouch, an extension of the plica, during quadriceps action. Failure of the articularis genus to retract these structures results in painful catching sensations as the patella impinges on the plica.

Treatment of an irritated plica is based on calming down the synovial irritation and proliferation by using modalities that decrease swelling. Emphasis is placed on increasing hamstring flexibility and quadriceps strengthening through isometrics, quadriceps sets, and straight leg raises because flexion to extension exercises aggravate the synovial lining. McConnell reports that a truly pathologic plica worsens in response to taping because excessive pressure is applied.[17] All patients diagnosed with plica syndrome should be carefully evaluated for patella tracking dysfunctions, which may be the source of irritation. Only when the athlete is free of pain and effusion should he or she progress to rehabilitation that increases PFJRF.

Patellar Instability

Any sport that produces torque about the knee, causing rotation of the femur on a planted foot, increases the athlete's risk of traumatic subluxation or dislocation of the patella. This, combined with anatomic deficits such as patella alta, vastus medialis obliquus dysplasia, irregular-shaped patella, or shallow lateral femoral condyle, predisposes the athlete to patellar stability problems.

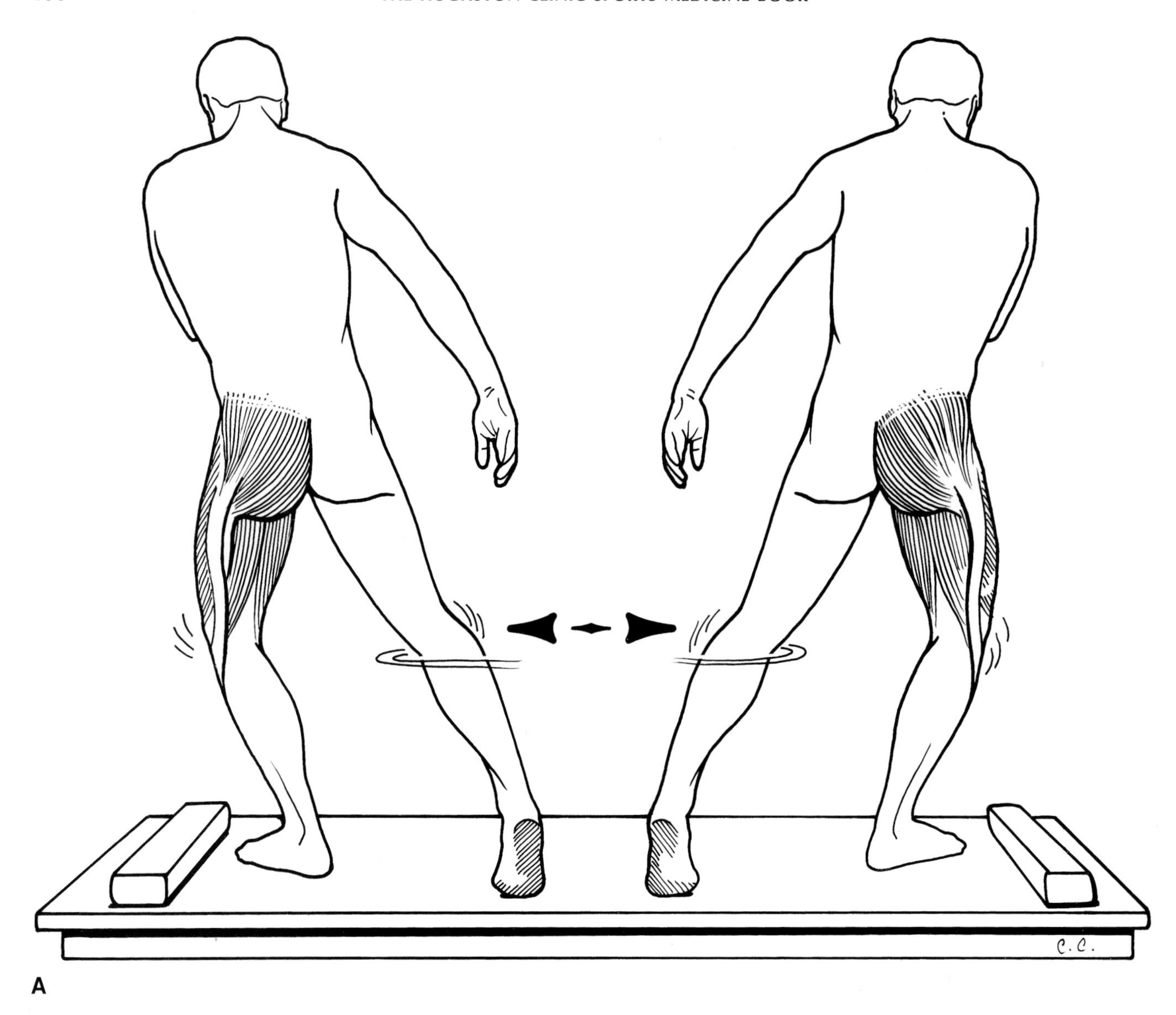

A

In acute patellar subluxation, ice, compression, and rest combined with isometric exercises calm the joint. Many times a knee sleeve or lateral felt pad with an Ace wrap is used for support for 3 to 5 days, to allow the medial tissues to heal. Electrical stimulation, biofeedback, and the McConnell taping program are begun as soon as possible to promote vastus medialis obliquus activation. Continued emphasis must be placed on training that muscle, to avoid chronic instability patterns that place undue stress on articular cartilage and synovium, which may lead to patellar dislocation.

Patellar Dislocations

Acute patellar dislocations occur when the athlete decelerates and simultaneously cuts or pivots on a planted foot. Valgus or varus stress may also force the patella laterally.[22] The majority of the time the knee gives way completely, causing the athlete to fall. Spontaneous reduction of the patella may occur, but medical attention should always be rendered in a timely manner.

The majority of acute patellar dislocations are managed conservatively, although some physicians recommend early surgical repair. Cash and Hughston reported good to excellent results with conservative treatment of primary acute traumatic dislocations[22]; however, prognosis in this series was worse if examination of the uninvolved knee showed predisposing congenital features.

Once the athlete has undergone a medical examination, the rehabilitation program begins. The program should be geared toward decreasing knee effusion, allowing the medial retinaculum to heal in a taut position, and activating the quadriceps muscle. The patient is fitted with a compressive dressing using a felt, lateral, C-shaped pad and is placed in a knee immobilizer. Active ankle pumps, quadriceps sets with vastus medialis obliquus emphasis, and straight leg raises are all initiated and performed in the immobilizer. The patient is also fitted with crutches and instructed in touch-down

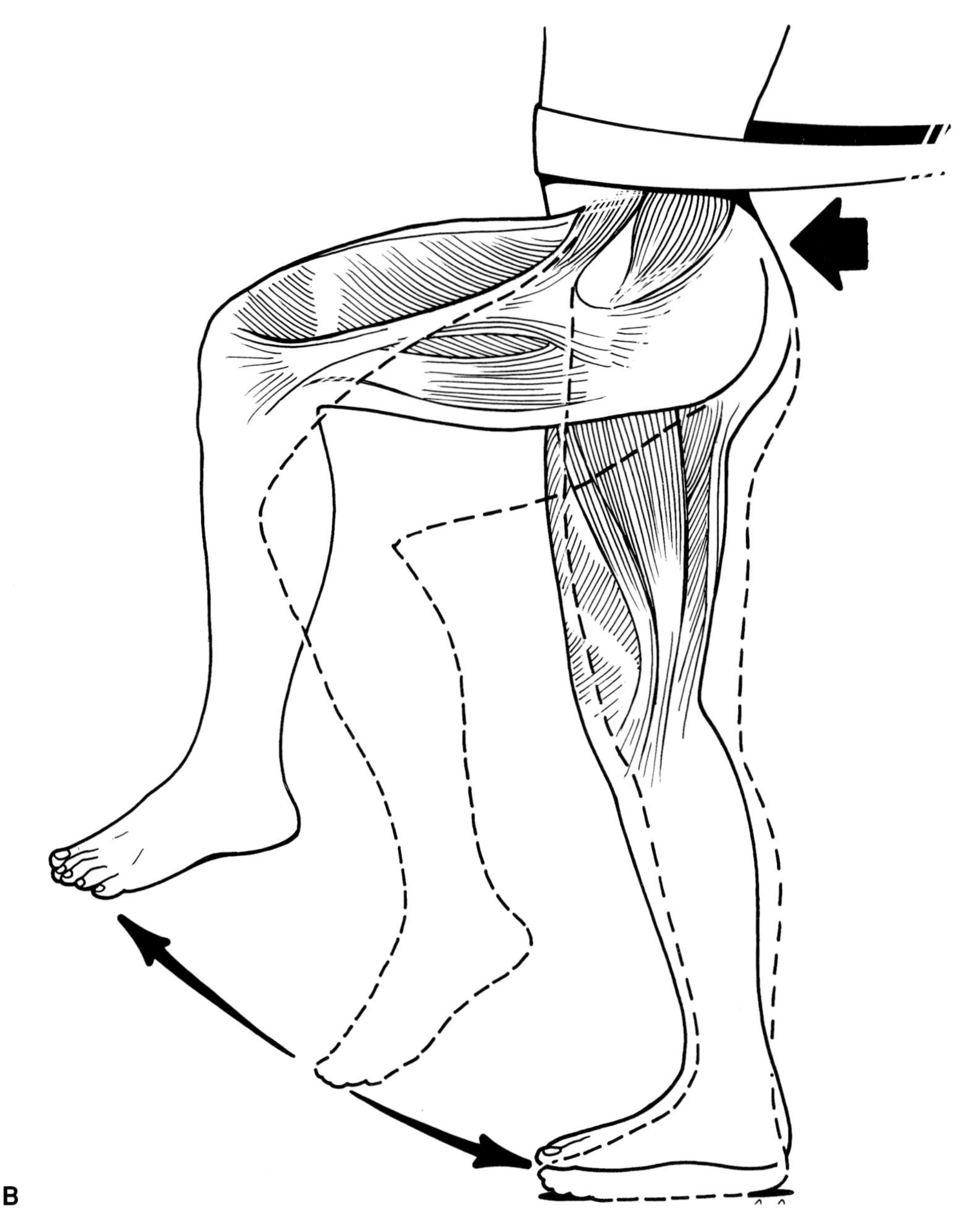

Fig. 69–2. Athletes progress to functional exercises that mimic motions used in sports, such as the slide board *(A)* and marching against resistance *(B)*.

weight bearing, which is continued for 2 to 3 weeks. After 2 to 3 weeks, the splint is removed and the patient is fitted with a neoprene sleeve or McConnell taping if the acutely injured knee allows. Modalities such as cryotherapy combined with electrical stimulation help reduce the swelling. Electrical stimulation and biofeedback are begun while concentrating on vastus medialis obliquus activity, and the patient progresses from bearing no weight to closed-chain exercises, as tolerated.

Since flexion is the position in which patients experience patellar dislocation, initially they are usually very apprehensive about working on knee flexion. Having the patient sit with the legs over the end of a table and using active resistive flexion against the therapist's or trainer's hand reflexively relaxes the quadriceps and allows the hamstring to flex the knee. This type of flexion is tolerated well by patients with acute knee injuries and those who have had surgery because quadriceps relaxation is the key to flexion in a painful knee. Prolonged periods of flexion tend to invite knee swelling so the patient is encouraged to work on flexion three or four times a day for short periods (5 to 7 minutes). Otherwise, the knee should remain in extension, to promote healing of the medial retinaculum in a shortened position.

The athlete is gradually weaned off crutches as quadriceps control in weight bearing improves. McConnell taping is beneficial, and as swelling decreases the patient progresses toward functional activities. The external support of the tape gives patients a feeling of security and

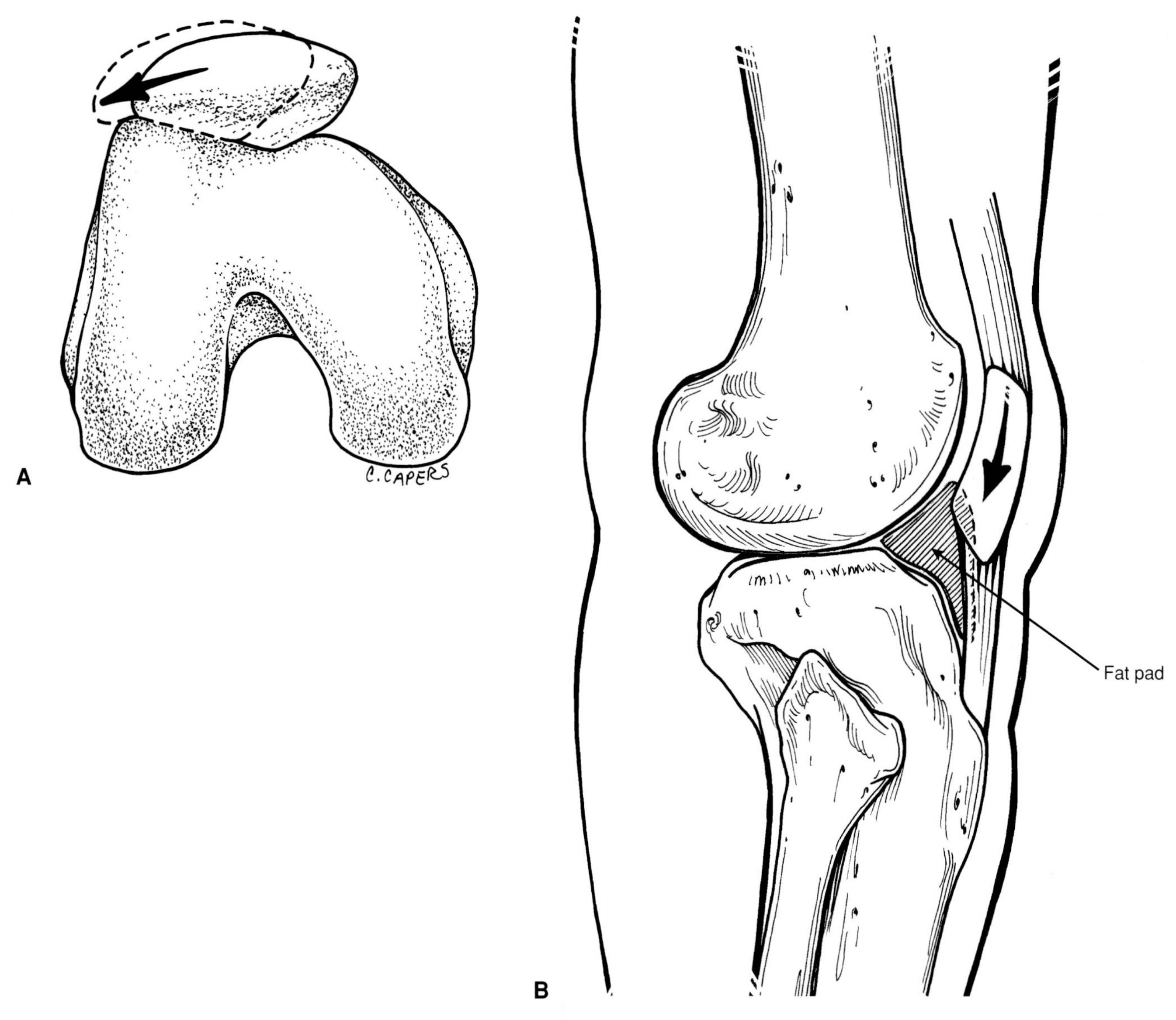

Fig. 69–3. Lateral tilt of the patella *(A)* and posterior tilt of the patella *(B)* are two of the abnormal positions that can cause patellofemoral symptoms.

gives proprioception to the vastus medialis obliquus during closed-chain exercises.

Patellar Tendinitis

Patellar tendinitis is frequently seen in sports requiring repetitive loading of the patellar tendon, such as volleyball, basketball, and running. This condition, also known as *jumper's knee,*[23] is an overuse syndrome of the patellar tendon at its insertion into the inferior pole of the patella. Diagnosis is rather straightforward: pinpoint tenderness is present at the bone-tendon interface on the inferior pole of the patella. The athlete may complain of exquisite pain in this area during activity or of a dull ache afterward. Careful evaluation of the EM must be performed so as not to overlook a patellar tracking problem that is causing fat pad irritation or impingement. Genu recurvatum, vastus medialis obliquus dysplasia, and an inferiorly tilted patella are commonly seen with fat pad irritation. McConnell taping alleviates the stabbing infrapatellar pain from fat pad irritation or injury. Patella alta and hamstring inflexibility are quite often associated with patellar tendinitis.

Initial treatment of patellar tendinitis begins with rest from sport; modalities such as ice, heat, deep massage, and iontophoresis; and a flexibility program for hamstrings, quadriceps, and heel cords. This is followed by an isometric quadriceps-strengthening program, progressing to weight-bearing closed-chain exercises. The benefits of eccentric exercises using isokinetics in the treatment of tendinitis are documented throughout the literature.[24] Curwin and Stanish describe eccentric programs designed to progressively strengthen the tensile

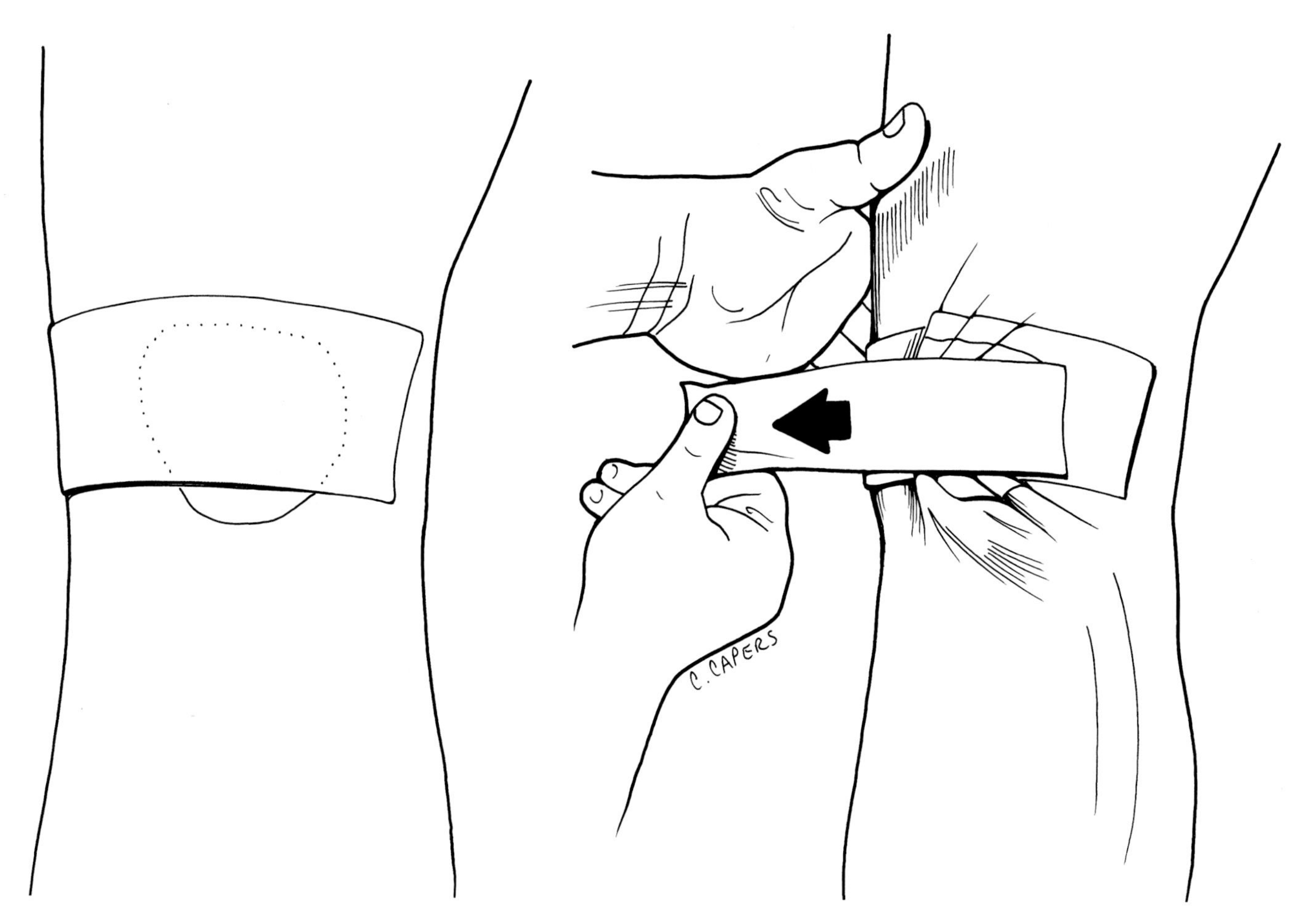

Fig. 69–4. An example of the McConnell taping program in which taping is used to correct patellar position and allow pain-free exercise.

components of the patellar tendon.[25] Closed–kinetic chain exercises encompass the eccentric action of the quadriceps and cause less PFJRF. Quick stretches, 15° to 20° single knee squats, side step-ups, and forward lunges are used to increase eccentric strength of the quadriceps. The athlete should be pain free before returning to sport. Knee sleeves are preferred by many athletes during rehabilitation as well as sporting events. Early intervention with a proper rehabilitation program shows much better results, as compared with athletes who suffer chronic patellar tendinitis. In later stages, the patellar tendon may show signs of necrosis and cystic degeneration, which may eventually result in patellar tendon rupture.

REFERENCES

1. Hughston, J. C.: Subluxation of the patella. J. Bone Joint Surg. *50A*:1003, 1968.
2. Blackburn, T. A., and Craig E.: Knee anatomy: A brief review. Phys. Ther. *60*:1556, 1980.
3. Hungerford, D. S., and Lennox, D. W.: Rehabilitation of the knee in disorders of the patellofemoral joint: Relevant biomechanics. Orthop. Clin. North Am. *14*:397, 1983.
4. Voight, M. L., and Wieder, D. L.: Comparative reflex response times of vastus medialis obliquus and vastus lateralis in normal subjects and subjects with extensor mechanism dysfunction. Am. J. Sports Med. *19*:131, 1991.
5. Lieb, F. J., and Perry, J.: Quadriceps function: An anatomical and mechanical study using amputated limbs. J. Bone Joint Surg. *50A*:1535, 1968.
6. Maviani, P. P., and Caruso, I.: An electromyographic investigation of subluxation of the patella. J. Bone Joint Surg. *61B*:169, 1979.
7. Grabiner, M. D., Koh, T. J., Miller, G. F., and DeLozier, G. S.: Fatigue patterns of vastus medialis oblique and vastus lateralis during short-arc quadriceps exercises. Sports Med. *5*:24, 1990.
8. Andriacchi, T. P., Andersson, G. B., Ortengren, R., and Mikosz, R. P.: A study of factors influencing muscle activity about the knee joint. J. Orthop. Res. *1*:266, 1984.
9. Karst, G. M., and Jewett, P. D.: Electromyographic analysis of exercises proposed for differential activation of medial and lateral quadriceps femoris muscle components. Phys. Ther. *73*:286, 1993.
10. McConnell, J.: The Advanced McConnell Patellofemoral Treatment Plan Course Notes. Jenny McConnell, 1991.
11. Hodges, P., and Richardson, C.: The influence of isometric hip adduction on quadriceps femoris activity. Scand. J. Rehabil. Med. *25*:57, 1993.
12. Spencer, J., Hayes, K., and Alexander, I.: Knee joint effusion and quadriceps reflex inhibition in man. Arch. Phys. Med. Rehabil. *65*:171, 1984.
13. Soderberg, G. L., and Cook, T. M.: An electromyographic analysis of quadriceps femoris muscle setting and straight leg raising. Phys. Ther. *63*:1434, 1983.
14. Hughston, J. C., Walsh, W. M., and Puddu, G.: Patellar Subluxation and Dislocation. Philadelphia, W. B. Saunders, 1984.
15. Case, W. S.: Minimizing patellofemoral joint compression during knee rehab. Phys. Ther. Forum *4*:1, 1985.

16. Daries, G. J.: A Compendium of Isokinetics in Clinical Usage. LaCrosse, WI, S&S, 1985.
17. McConnell, J.: McConnell Patellofemoral Treatment Plan. Course Notes. Jenny McConnell, 1990.
18. McConnell, J.: The management of chondromalacia patellae: A long-term solution. Austr. J. Physiother. *32*:215, 1986.
19. Fulkerson, J. P.: Evaluation of the peripatellar soft tissues and retinaculum in patients with patellofemoral pain. Clin. Sports Med. *8*:197, 1989.
20. Jacobson, K. E., and Flandry, F. C.: Diagnosis of anterior knee pain. Clin. Sports Med. *8*:179, 1989.
21. Walsh, M. W., and Helzer-Julin, M.: Patellar tracking problems in athletes. Sports Med.: Musculoskeletal Probl. *19*:303, 1992.
22. Cash, J. D., and Hughston, J. C.: Treatment of acute patellar dislocation. Am. J. Sports Med. *16*:244, 1988.
23. Blazina, M. E., et al.: Jumper's knee. Orthop. Clin. North Am. *4*:665, 1973.
24. Albert, M.: Eccentric Muscle Training in Sports and Orthopedics. New York, Churchill Livingston, 1991.
25. Curwin, S., and Stanish, W. D.: Tendinitis: Its Etiology and Treatment. Lexington, MA: Collamore Press, 1984.

70

Michael A. Oberlander and Julie A. Pryde

Meniscal Injuries

Meniscal lesions, the most common intra-articular injury in the knee, are most prevalent in contact and cutting sports such as football, soccer, and basketball. Medial meniscal lesions are most common. More than a third of all meniscal lesions are associated with an anterior cruciate ligament tear.[1] The intimate relationship between ligamentous lesions and meniscal tears demands a thorough understanding of the meniscal anatomy, biomechanics, clinical diagnosis, and surgical intervention, if the physician is to provide optimal treatment.

ANATOMY

The menisci are C-shaped fibrocartilaginous discs that lie between the condyles of the femur and the medial and lateral tibial plateaus. The menisci have a thick convex periphery and a thin concave central margin, giving them a wedgelike appearance in cross section.

The medial meniscus covers approximately 30% of the medial tibial plateau.[2] It is considerably wider at the posterior horn and narrows into the anterior horn, which is attached anterior to the tibial plateau by the meniscotibial (coronary) ligament. The anterior horn of the medial meniscus is attached to the transverse ligament, which inserts into the anterior horn of the lateral meniscus. The medial meniscus also is attached throughout its periphery to the joint capsule and at its midpoint to the deep fibers of the medial collateral ligament.[3] Through its attachment at the posteromedial corner of the capsule, the semimembranosus acts indirectly to retract the posterior horn of the medial meniscus, giving a dynamic action to the medial meniscus.[4]

The lateral meniscus covers approximately 50% of the lateral tibial plateau.[2] The anterior horn of the lateral meniscus attaches adjacent to the anterior cruciate ligament, whereas the posterior horn attaches to the posterior intercondylar region. Unlike the medial meniscus, it has no association with the collateral ligament. The posterior attachment of the lateral meniscus is weak and is interrupted by the popliteus tendon. The posterior border of the lateral meniscus often contains the meniscofemoral ligaments of Humphry (posterior) and of Wrisberg (anterior). One or both of these ligaments is present in 71% of knees, though considerable variation between specimens has been noted.[5] These structures travel through the intercondylar notch to insert on the medial femoral condyle along with the posterior cruciate ligament.

The structure and function of the menisci are dictated in part by the anatomy of the opposing joint surfaces of the knee. The medial tibial plateau is concave, oval, and longer in the anteroposterior direction, and the lateral tibial plateau is flatter, more circular, and convex centrally. Thus, because the horns of the medial meniscus are attached farther apart, its association with the medial capsular ligament and its position on a concave surface, the motion of the medial meniscus is minimal.[6,7] The lateral meniscus, in contrast, has an anteroposterior excursion of up to 11 mm because of the proximity of the attachments of its horns, the decrease in surface area of the capsular attachments, and the landscape of the lateral tibial plateau (Fig. 70–1).[8]

The vascular supply to the menisci originates from the lateral, middle, and medial genicular arteries. Branches of these vessels give rise to a perimeniscal capillary plexus originating within the synovial and capsular tissues of the knee joint. The superior and inferior surfaces of the menisci are nourished by diffusion from synovial fluid. The absence of a penetrating vessel in the posterolateral aspect of the lateral meniscus adjacent to the popliteal tendon is also a consistent finding. The anterior and posterior horns of both menisci are cov-

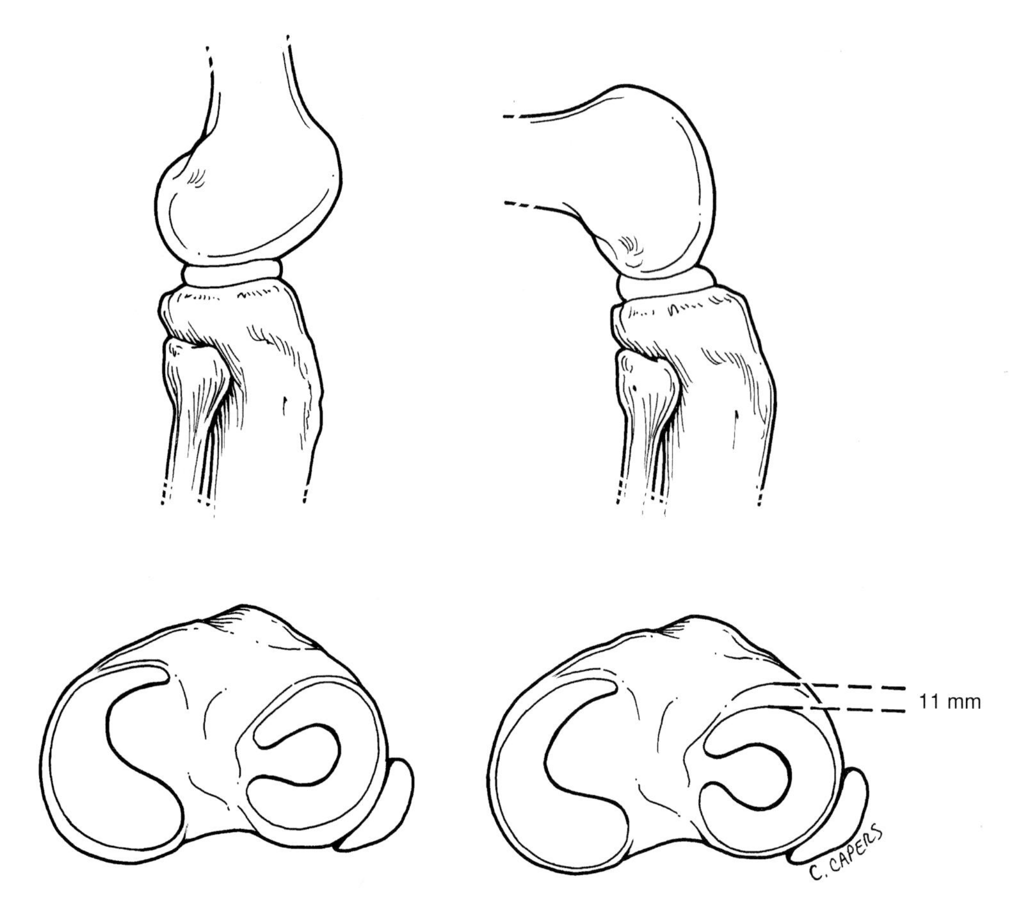

Fig. 70–1. **The fact that the horns of the medial meniscus are attached farther apart than the horns of the lateral meniscus, that it is firmly anchored by the medial capsular ligaments, and that the medial tibial plateau is more concave, all contribute to the medial meniscus' being relatively constrained. In contrast, the lateral meniscus has an excursion of as much as 11 mm because the horns are attached closer together, there are fewer capsular attachments, and the lateral tibial plateau is flatter.**

ered with vascular synovial tissue and have a particularly rich blood supply. It has been theorized that this may be due to their nonweightbearing status.[9]

FUNCTION

The menisci were once thought to be functionless vestigial remnants, but current thought holds that they are integral components of the complex biomechanics of the knee. They play a significant role in knee stability and load distribution. The overall importance of these structures cannot be overemphasized, as evidenced by the degenerative changes of the knee that follow meniscectomy.[10]

The menisci function as mechanical spacers that contribute to the stability of the joint. They serve to maintain proper position of the femur relative to the tibia by deepening the articular surfaces and filling the dead space at the periphery, thus allowing the joint to articulate congruently. The wedged shape, particularly the thicker posterior horn of the medial meniscus, and its firm attachment to the tibial plateau also assist the cruciate ligaments in maintaining anteroposterior stability.[11,12]

The menisci also serve to limit the extremes of flexion and extension. In the screw-home mechanism of the knee, the menisci are forced forward by the femoral condyles. The anterior horns of the menisci act to block further extension. In full flexion, the posterior horns are driven posteriorly and help block further flexion, as long as the capsular and ligamentous structures are intact.[2,13]

The menisci aid in joint lubrication by spreading synovial fluid over the articular surfaces, which decreases the coefficient of friction.

DIAGNOSIS

Mechanism of Injury

Meniscal injury, though quite common, often presents a difficult clinical diagnosis. Meniscal tears are caused either by an acute event or a degenerative process. Many involve either hyperflexion, hyperextension, or rotational (pivoting) forces and are primarily noncontact injuries. A twisting or cutting maneuver in which the meniscus is caught between the femoral condyle and the tibial plateau may cause a tear if the forces exceed the ultimate shear strength of the cartilage. Symptoms of a torn meniscus are typically caused by mechanical dysfunction or synovial irritation, as the meniscus itself is almost devoid of sensory nerves except at its periphery.[2]

History

The patient's age and history often give the clinician valuable insight into the nature of the problem. Younger patients tend to have injuries related to sports or trauma, whereas older patients tend to describe more insidious onset of symptoms. Often, the patient reports hearing or feeling a "pop" or "snap" with pain referred to the joint line. The patient may complain of increased pain with rotatory or flexion movements such as kneeling, squatting, or pivoting on the affected knee. Pain getting into or out of a car or difficulty participating in strenuous activity may also be reported. A feeling of insecurity or weakness about the knee and locking or giving way also are frequently noted. The feeling of giving way is thought to be caused by reflex inhibition of the quadriceps as the torn meniscus is displaced into the joint and causes a mechanical catching. The strength of the quadriceps has been shown to decrease as the size of the effusion increases.[14] True locking, which occurs at the time of injury or as the tear extends and gets trapped within the joint, typically prevents the terminal 20° to 30° of extension. Locking from a chronic tear tends to be more subtle and may constitute only a 5° loss of extension. A history of popping or the sensation that something unusual is in the joint may also be reported, and this must be differentiated from a chondral lesion or loose body. The severity of mechanical symptoms frequently depends on the morphology of the tear.

Many clinicians consider joint line pain to be one of the most reliable signs of meniscal injury. It is reportedly positive in as many as 77% of patients with meniscal injuries.[15] In injuries older than 2 weeks, quadriceps atrophy is a frequent sign of significant internal derangement. This should be evaluated at a distance from a fixed point. We prefer to take measurements at the joint line and 7 inches above the lateral joint line. Others prefer to measure from the superior pole of the patella. One must be certain when using the patella as a landmark that unilateral patella alta or -baja is not making the measurements inaccurate.

The presence of joint effusion may also aid in diagnosis, because it suggests internal derangement. Acute hemarthrosis is often associated with anterior cruciate ligament tears, osteochondral lesions, and peripheral meniscal lesions. This is in contrast to swelling that evolves hours after the injury or the next day, which is more suggestive of a loose body, meniscal tear, or chondral fracture. The effusion is caused in response to irritation of the synovial lining and, if aspirated, is typically straw colored. Swelling of the joint may be recurrent and associated with catching, locking, or increased activity.

With large effusions that present over time, especially in the presence of degenerative tears, an associated Baker's cyst may be identified. These cysts are collections of fluid secondary to herniations of the posterior capsule or swelling of the bursa in the region of the medial head of the gastrocnemius tendon. With this lesion, the patient typically complains of pain and fullness in the popliteal region. In many cases, treatment of the underlying problem in the joint causes the cyst to resolve. Younger patients who present with Baker's cyst may or may not have associated intra-articular abnormalities. In older patients, if swelling persists after treatment of the intra-articular lesion, the cyst can be aspirated and cortisone injected. If the cyst recurs and is symptomatic, excision may be required.

Manipulative tests are used to localize the pain to the joint line or to produce clicking due to abnormal meniscal mechanics. Tests such as McMurray's maneuver, however, are positive in only 58% of the cases and also positive *in 5% of normal knees.* Therefore, this test must be correlated with other positive clinical findings.[15,16] It is more commonly positive with large flap or bucket-handle tears. The modified McMurray's test is forced internal and external rotation of the tibia that accompanies flexion with the application of valgus and varus stress (Fig. 70–2). The classic sign is a painful "clunk." Other manipulative tests, such as Apley's, Steinmann's, and Anderson's can also be performed to identify meniscal lesions (see Chapter 64.) As with any of these tests, accuracy depends on the relaxation of the patient, the configuration of the tear, the presence of an effusion, and the experience of the examiner. Full passive extension frequently produces discomfort at the anteromedial or anterolateral joint line, which suggests a meniscal lesion. Pain with full flexion, with or without rotation, may correlate with a posterior horn lesion.

Classification

Several different types of meniscal tears can occur. The basic classification is based on the direction of the tear: vertical longitudinal, transverse, horizontal, and oblique (Fig. 70–3). The bucket-handle tear is the most common type of vertical longitudinal tear. Patients with this type of tear usually have the most dramatic history and classic findings on clinical examination (i.e., joint line pain, catching, giving way, frank locking, and limited range of motion). These tears can be displaced into the intercondylar notch. Once the knee unlocks, symptoms may resolve until the fragment is displaced again. Vertical tears usually occur in the posterior two thirds of the meniscus, and symptoms occur when the knee is brought from a flexed position to an extended position.

Transverse, or radial, tears are more common in the lateral meniscus and often occur in conjunction with other tears. The tear is usually located at the junction of the posterior and the middle third or at the posterior horn attachments. Horizontal tears frequently occur in the middle third of the meniscus. These patients pre-

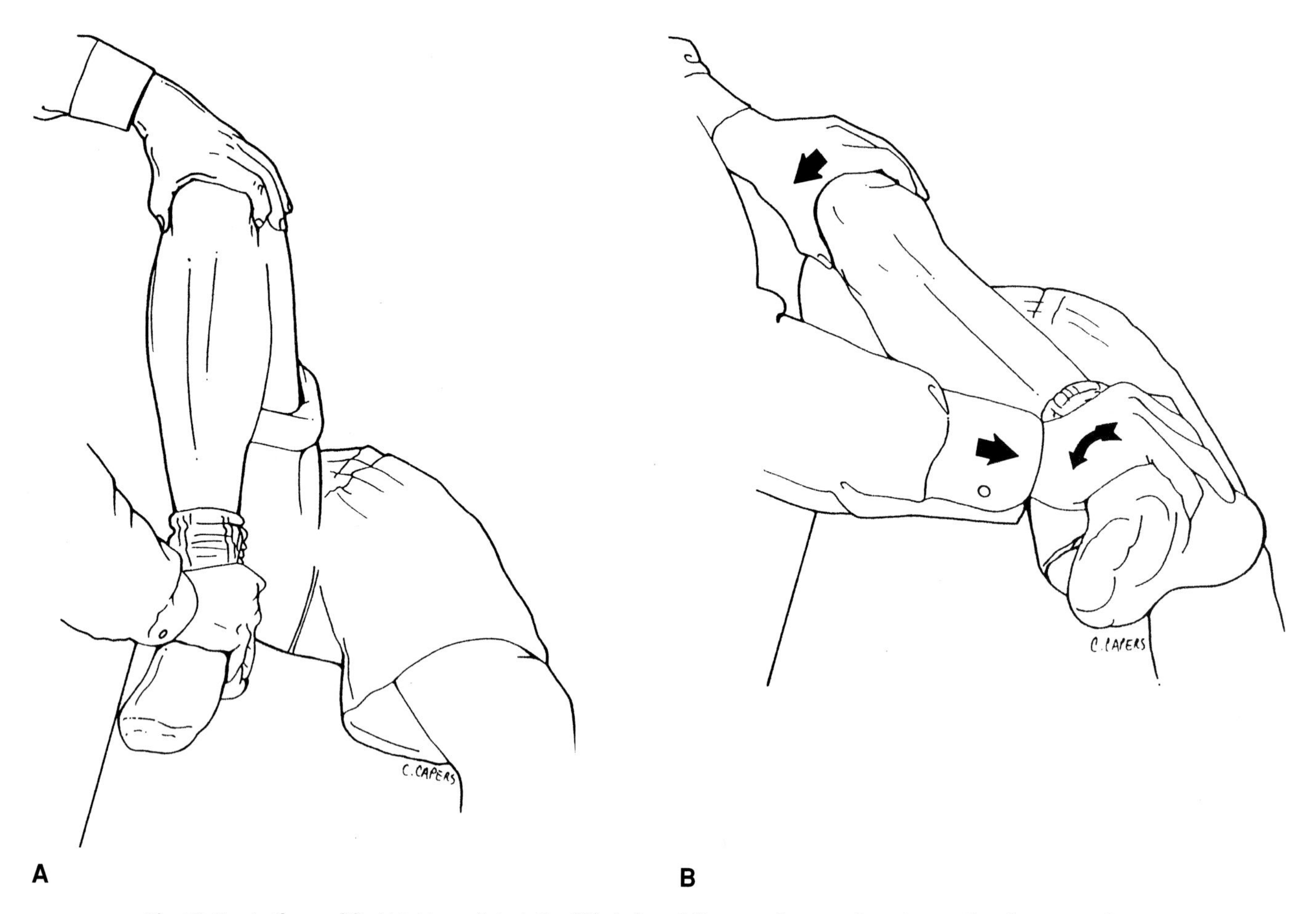

Fig. 70–2. In the modified McMurray's test, the tibia is forcefully rotated externally or internally whereas a valgus or varus stress is applied to the knee (depending on which side of the knee is being tested). The knee is started in a flexed position *(A)* and is moved to an extended position *(B)* while the examiner feels for a pop or clunk at the joint line.

sent with classic symptoms because the unstable portion of the meniscus is often displaced into the joint space.

The oblique tear (flap or parrot-beak tear) is the most common type. There are many variations, but tears at the junction of the middle and the posterior third of the medial meniscus are most common. These tears can cause catching and popping as the patient pivots or squats and the torn meniscus is displaced into the joint.

Degenerative tears usually present with insidious onset of pain and recurrent effusions. They may or may not be associated with mechanical symptoms of popping, catching, or giving way, depending on the severity of the tear. Radiographs typically demonstrate joint space narrowing and may also show flattening of the femoral condyles, sclerosis of the subchondral bone, or osteophyte formation.[10]

The incidence of certain meniscal tear types varies with age. Vertical longitudinal tears, including displaced bucket-handle tears, tend to occur in athletes in their 20s or 30s. Degenerative flap and horizontal cleavage tears tend to occur in people over 40 years old. Epidemiologic studies have shown that posterior horn tears are the most common tear associated with anterior cruciate ligament tears.[17,18]

Radiographic Evaluation

Plain radiographs are essential in the initial workup of a suspected meniscal tear. They are also helpful in ruling out other lesions that may mimic a meniscal tear, such as a loose body, fracture, osteochondritis dissecans, or degenerative arthritis. Pseudogout or chondrocalcinosis can also be diagnosed on plain radiographs. In this condition, calcification of the meniscus is noted secondary to deposition of calcium pyrophosphate crystals on the meniscus. Double-contrast arthrography is a very accurate means of diagnosing medial meniscus disease, though accuracy for the lateral meniscus is decreased because of the presence of dye around the popliteal tendon and hiatus.[19,20] This test has been largely replaced by magnetic resonance imaging (MRI) because of its great accuracy and noninvasiveness.

After multiple office visits, the diagnosis of meniscal tear is usually quite evident, and if questions remain as to whether a surgical lesion exists, MRI may be helpful. MRI is becoming an increasingly valuable tool in the diagnosis of meniscal injury. It should not, however, replace a careful history and thorough clinical examination; instead, it serves as an adjunct to the clinical

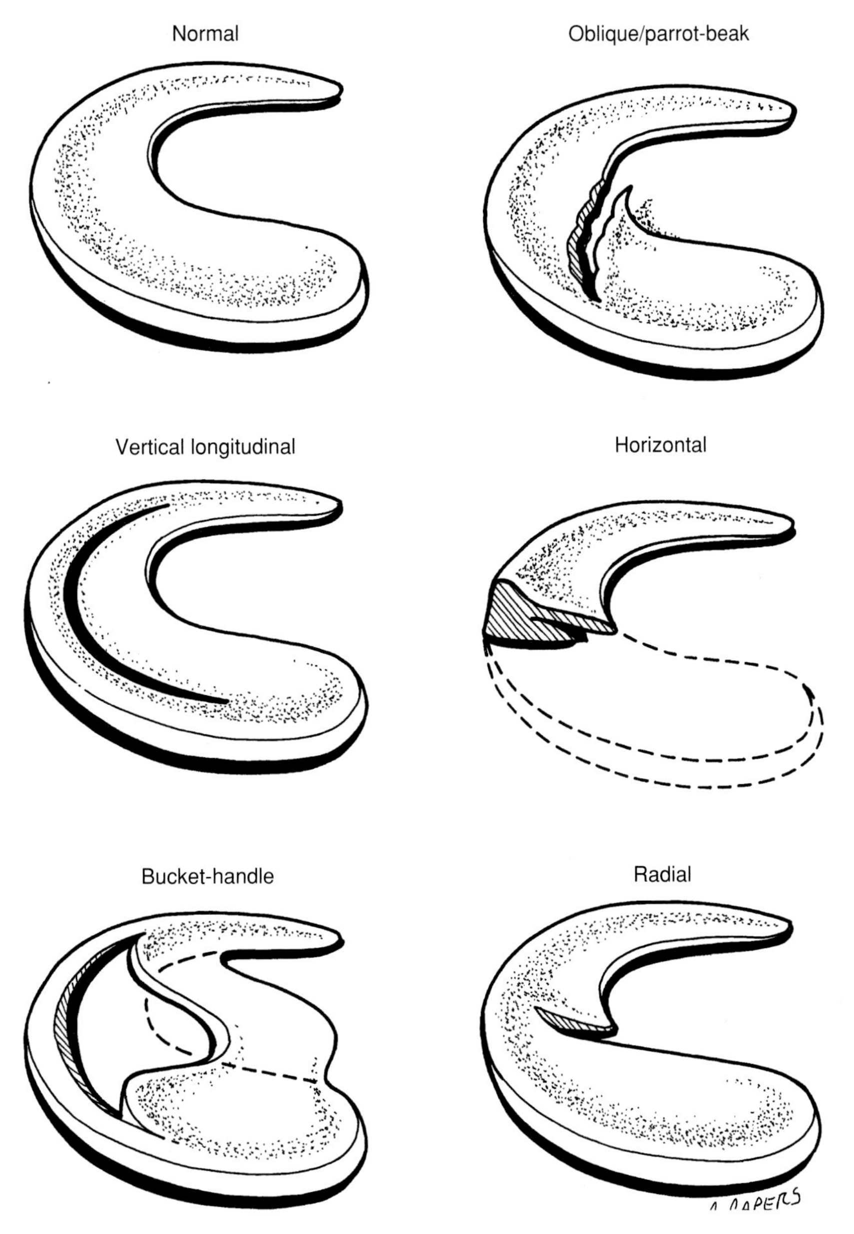

Fig. 70–3. Classification of meniscal tears.

workup. Some studies have shown nearly equal diagnostic accuracy using a good physical examination versus arthroscopy in the diagnosis of intra-articular lesions.[21] Because of the high cost of MRI, it should not be used routinely to make the diagnosis of meniscal tear. Instead, it should be reserved for cases with equivocal findings on physical examination and after failure of conservative treatment. Meniscal tears are identified by a higher signal intensity in a normal black meniscus. A significant tear demonstrates a white signal that communicates with the articular surface. MRI has been shown to be more useful in distinguishing medial meniscus tears than lateral meniscus tears.[22,23] False-positive findings are most common with posterior horn tears.[22–24]

TREATMENT OF MENISCAL TEARS

A trial of conservative treatment should be attempted in all but the most severe cases. The only patients who require urgent surgical treatment are the rare ones who present with a locked knee secondary to a displaced bucket-handle tear that cannot be reduced. In this case, arthroscopy and partial meniscectomy or meniscal repair is warranted, to allow the patient to ambulate and limit further injury to the meniscus or joint surface.

Conservative treatment consists of a good home exercise program and nonsteroidal anti-inflammatory drugs for significant swelling or joint irritation. When determining appropriate treatment, one must consider the amount and location of the associated injuries or degenerative changes, any previous injuries or surgeries, and the activity level and sport that the patient wishes to return to.

The early goals of physical therapy are to minimize the effusion, normalize gait, normalize pain-free range of motion, retard atrophy of the quadriceps, and maintain cardiovascular endurance. The most important factor in this treatment is that the knee be allowed to adapt to the changes in load-bearing capabilities and be given sufficient time for tissue healing to occur.

The intermediate phase of the program is to improve quadriceps strength and endurance as well as balance and proprioception by progressing from open-chain activities to controlled progressive loading through closed-chain exercises. The amount of swelling and pain dictate the appropriate pace of the program. To achieve an optimal result, the knee must be taken through a series of progressive activities, including an impact-loading series and an advancement of functional exercises specific to the demands of the individual sport or activity, to ensure safe return.

Degenerative tears are treated conservatively unless significant mechanical symptoms develop that are unresponsive to conservative treatment. If, despite conservative treatment, pain and swelling persist or if significant mechanical symptoms develop, arthroscopic débridement of the frayed and torn meniscus is helpful.[25]

If conservative treatment fails to resolve the symptoms so the patient can resume his occupation or sport, surgical treatment should be considered. Partial meniscectomy is the treatment of choice for the majority of meniscal tears. Approximately 85 to 90% of the tears are in the inner two thirds, or the avascular portion, of the meniscus. This portion does not have a direct blood supply and is better suited to partial meniscectomy than to meniscal repair. The arthroscopic procedure, an outpatient procedure, has decreased operative morbidity and improved visualization in the posterior horns and allows quicker rehabilitation of the knee.[26,27] This is now the standard of care for meniscal lesions.

When removing a tear, the surgeon should leave as much normal meniscus as possible. Creating a smooth transition between the torn meniscus and the normal adjacent cartilage is essential. This is called *balancing the meniscus.* A smooth transition is the key to a successful result and gives the patient the best chance for minimal residual symptoms. If the tear is removed and a good transition is not created, leaving an abnormal contour of the meniscus, residual symptoms may be similar to those of a meniscal tear. The surgeon must not leave any unstable meniscal remnant or residual tears in place, lest continued symptoms or further tearing occur postoperatively.

Repair is another option for treating meniscal lesions. Though some authors suggest that most tears can be repaired, most would recommend repair for tears that occur in the vascular region, are longer than 1 cm but shorter than 4 cm, and are unstable on arthroscopic probing.[28–30] The outer 10 to 30% of the meniscus is vascularized and thus has the ability to heal when repaired.[3,9] Whether done arthroscopically or open, meniscal repair in the vascular zone has yielded good or excellent results in 85 to 90% of patients.[29–32] These results with followup to 9 years appear not to diminish with time. Meniscal repair offers patients the best chance of restoring nearly normal kinematics of the knee and preventing degenerative arthritis.[30]

The principles of repair are the same whether the surgery is performed open or arthroscopically. The meniscal rim and body to be repaired are smoothed mechanically and the surface is abraded to stimulate a vascular response, which aids in healing.[30,31] A sufficient number of sutures must then be placed to stabilize the tear. The number and type of sutures depend on the size of the tear and the surgeon's preference.

The peripheral meniscus repair is normally used in patients with tears of the anterior cruciate ligament. When the meniscus is repaired without reconstruction of the anterior cruciate ligament, the failure rate for the repair is significantly increased.[30,33]

Recent research and development have addressed meniscal transplant.[34,35] The tissue is allograft from cadaver donors and thus carries the risk of transmission of communicable disease, depending on sterilization and preservation techniques. There have also been problems with appropriate sizing of the meniscus, shrinkage of the transplanted tissue once implanted, and restoring normal kinematics. Because only preliminary results are available, prevention of late degenerative arthritis has yet to be proven.[36] This alternative, despite its present shortfalls and unpredictable results, does hold promise for young patients with significant injury to the meniscus who require subtotal or total meniscectomy.

It appears that simple mechanical lavage of the joint decreases the amount of collagenase, prostaglandin, and degradative enzymes in the knee and that alone may be helpful in decreasing symptoms from degenerative or rheumatoid arthritis.[36,37] These irritants, as well as debris from deteriorated hyaline cartilage that accumulates from the arthritic process, incite the inflammatory processes. With significant chondromalacia or degenerative arthritis of the articular surface, however, as more meniscus is removed, more load is transferred to these already weakened structures. A frayed or torn meniscus may still be aiding some in the distribution of contact forces within the joint. If this structure is removed, more pain and limitation of motion may develop. Patients with this type of tear who undergo surgery should be forewarned of that possibility.

Poor prognosis has been noted in patients with existing chondromalacia or significant degenerative arthritis, work-related injuries, and prior knee surgeries.[38,39] Patients with horizontal cleavage tears, degenerative tears, and complex tears, as noted previously, also have a lower incidence of good and excellent results.[40]

Finally, misdiagnosis must be considered. Radiographs should be made in all cases, to rule out the unusual benign or malignant tumor as a cause of referred knee pain. Hip pain can also be referred to the knee. A child who presents with knee symptoms should always have the hips evaluated for possible hip problems such as slipped capital femoral epiphysis, Legg-Calve-Perthes' disease, or tumor.

The use of medical lasers has expanded into orthopaedics, most notably in conjunction with arthroscopy. Numerous reports describe use of the laser to treat intra-articular lesions of the knee. The lasers used in knee arthroscopy include the carbon dioxide (CO_2), holmium: yttrium-aluminum-garnet (Ho:YAG) and neodymium YAG (Nd:YAG) lasers. The Ho:YAG is a pulsed noncontact laser and the Nd:YAG a continuous-wave, contact laser. Both have been proven to be effective in débridement of chondromalacia and of meniscal tissue. Because of the small size of the probe (approximately 2 mm), they are especially helpful in removing posterior horn tears that would otherwise pose difficulty with access.[41,42]

MENISCAL CYSTS

Meniscal cysts of the knee joint are not uncommon. Most frequently they are seen in men in their 20s and 30s.[43,44] The cause of such cysts is controversial, but most patients do present with a history of trauma. The most frequently reported site is in the peripheral portion of the middle third of the lateral meniscus.[43] The cysts are directly attached to the meniscus; involvement of the cartilage itself is variable. Small cysts may be found within the meniscal tissue proper, whereas larger cysts protrude at the capsular border (Fig. 70–4). The cyst may remain within the capsule or expand outside it.

The size of the cyst is restricted on the lateral side by the lateral collateral ligament, the iliotibial band, and the biceps femoris tendon. In contrast, a much larger mass may present on the medial aspect of the knee because of its greater possibility for expansion secondary to the limited soft tissue restraints. These cysts are frequently asymptomatic, and the patient may ultimately see the clinician because of the associated pathologic changes or tears in the meniscus. The most common tear pattern associated with the meniscal cyst is the horizontal cleavage type.[45]

The classic clinical presentation of a patient with a cystic meniscus is pain and localized swelling at the joint line. The pain is often described as a dull, constant ache. Often, this cystic swelling is visible or palpable and is described as firm to semifluctuant. Larger cysts tend to be more fluctuant. The size of the cyst may vary with knee position, most cysts being evident at 20° to 30° of flexion. Seldom is there loss of motion, and quadriceps atrophy is rare unless associated with a meniscal tear. Tenderness is greatest after exercise, because the size of the cyst may increase after activity.[43] The diagnosis of this entity is primarily clinical, though computed tomography and MRI are helpful in confirming the cystic nature of the lesion and its relationship to the joint and meniscal tissue. Differential diagnosis includes popliteal cysts, ganglion cysts, inflamed bursas, arthritic spurs, loose bodies, and tumors.

Treatment of a symptomatic lesion without mechanical symptoms is aspiration of the cyst and injection of cortisone in an attempt to scar down the cyst wall. Partial meniscectomy and arthroscopic cystectomy are warranted for recurrent or symptomatic cysts with extension from a meniscal tear. Depending on the size and location of the cyst, open excision may be necessary.

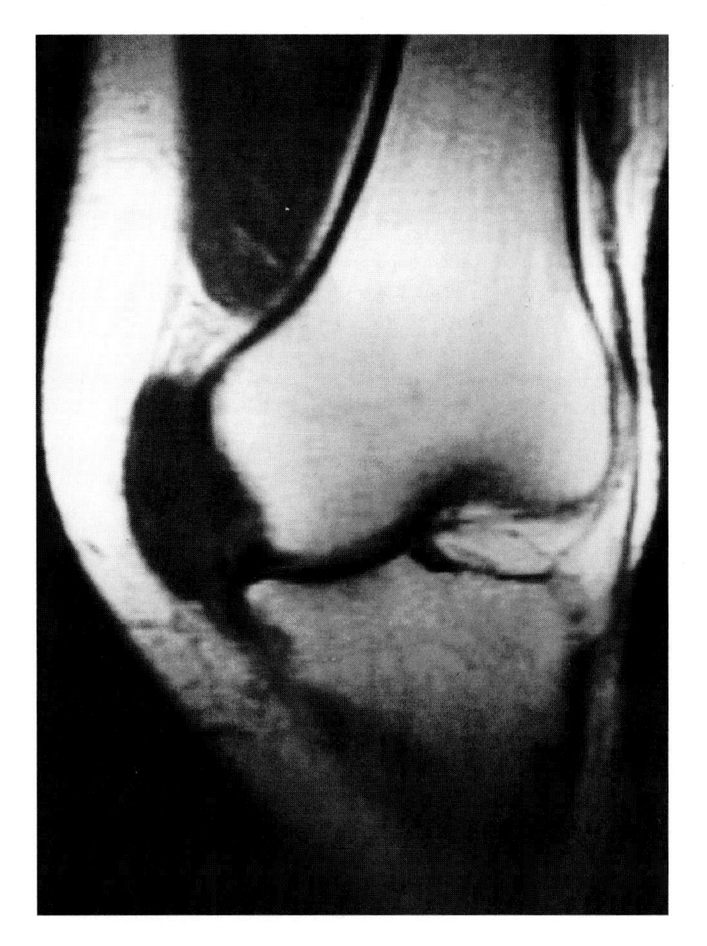

Fig. 70–4. MRI shows a meniscal cyst.

REFERENCES

1. Baker, B. E., et al.: Review of meniscal injury and associated sports. Am. J. Sports Med. *13*:1, 1985.
2. Renstrom, P., and Johnson, R. J.: Anatomy and biomechanics of the menisci. Clin. Sports Med. *9*:523, 1990.
3. Arnoczky, S., et al.: Meniscus. *In* Injury and Repair of the Musculoskeletal Soft Tissues. Edited by S. L. Woo and J. A. Buckwalter. Park Ridge, Ill., American Academy of Orthopedic Surgeons, 1988.
4. Hughston, J. C., and Eilers, A. F.: The role of the posterior oblique ligament in repairs of acute medial (collateral) ligament tears of the knee. J. Bone Joint Surg. *55A*:923, 1973.
5. Clancy, W. G., Jr., et al.: Treatment of knee joint instability secondary to rupture of the posterior cruciate ligament. J. Bone Joint Surg. *65A*:310, 1983.
6. Markolf, K. L., Mensch, J. S., and Amstutz, H. C.: Stiffness and laxity of the knee—the contributions of the supporting structures. J. Bone Joint Surg. *58A*:583, 1976.
7. Hughston, J. C., and Barrett, G. R.: Acute anteromedial rotatory instability: Long-term results of surgical repair. J. Bone Joint Surg. *65A*:145, 1983.
8. Brantigan, O. C., and Voshell, A. F.: The mechanics of the ligaments and menisci of the knee joint. J. Bone Joint Surg. *23*:44, 1941.

9. Arnoczky, S. P., and Warren, R. F.: Microvasculature of the human meniscus. Am J. Sports Med. *10*:90, 1982.
10. Fairbank, T. J.: Knee joint changes after meniscectomy. J. Bone Joint Surg. *30B*:664, 1948.
11. Markolf, K. L., et al.: The role of joint load in knee stability. J. Bone Joint Surg. *63A*:570, 1981.
12. Levy, I. M., Torzilli, P. A., and Warren, R. F.: The effect of medial meniscectomy on anterior-posterior motion of the knee. J. Bone Joint Surg. *64A*:883, 1982.
13. Brantigan, O. C., and Voshell, A. F.: The mechanics of the ligaments and the menisci of the knee joint. J. Bone Joint Surg. *23*:44, 1941.
14. Jensen, K., and Graf, B. K.: The effects of knee effusion on quadriceps strength and knee intraarticular pressure. Arthroscopy *9*:52, 1993.
15. Anderson, A. F., and Lipscomb, A. B.: Clinical diagnosis of meniscal tears-Description of a new manipulative test. Am. J. Sports Med. *14*:291, 1986.
16. McMurray, T. P.: The semilunar cartilages. Br. J. Surg. *29*:407, 1942.
17. Poehling, G. G., Ruch, D. S., and Chabon, S. J.: The landscape of meniscal injuries. Clin. Sports Med. *9*:539, 1990.
18. Childress, H. M.: Popliteal cysts associated with undiagnosed posterior lesions of the medial meniscus. J. Bone Joint Surg. *36A*:1233, 1954.
19. Selesnick, F. H., et al.: Internal derangement of the knee: Diagnosis by arthrography, arthroscopy, and arthrotomy. Clin. Orthop. *198*:26, 1985.
20. Ireland, J., et al.: Arthroscopy and arthrography of the knee: A critical review. J. Bone Joint Surg. *62B*:3, 1980.
21. Cerabona, F., et al.: Patterns of meniscal injury with acute anterior cruciate ligament tears. Am. J. Sports Med. *16*:603, 1988.
22. Fischer, S. P., et al.: Accuracy of diagnoses from magnetic imaging of the knee. A multi-center analysis of one thousand and fourteen patients. J. Bone Joint Surg. *73A*:2, 1991.
23. Raunest, J., et al.: The clinical value of magnetic resonance imaging in the evaluation of meniscal disorders. J. Bone Joint Surg. *73A*:11, 1991.
24. Oberlander, M. A., Shalvoy, R. M., and Hughston, J. C.: The accuracy of the clinical examination documented by arthroscopy. Am. J. Sports Med. *21*:773, 1993.
25. Noble, J., and Hamblen, D. L.: The pathology of the degenerate meniscus lesion. J. Bone Joint Surg. *57B*:180, 1975.
26. McGinty, J. B., Geuss, L. F., and Mavin, R. A.: Partial or total meniscectomy: A comparative analysis. J. Bone Joint Surg. *59A*:763, 1977.
27. Cox, J. S., and Cordell, L. D.: The degenerative effects of medial meniscus tears in dogs' knees. Clin. Orthop. *125*:236, 1977.
28. Scott, G. A., Jolly, B. L., and Henning, C. E.: Combined posterior incision and arthroscopic intra-articular repair of the meniscus. An examination of factors affecting healing. J. Bone Joint Surg. *68A*:847, 1986.
29. Cassidy, R. E., and Schaffer, A. J.: Repair of peripheral meniscus tears. Am. J. Sports Med. *9*:209, 1981.
30. DeHaven, K. E., Black, K. P., and Griffiths, H. J.: Open meniscus repair technique and two to nine year results. Am. J. Sports Med. *17*:788, 1989.
31. Henning, C. E., et al.: Use of the fascia sheath coverage and exogenous fibrin clot in the treatment of complex meniscal tears. Am. J. Sports Med. *19*:626, 1991.
32. Warren, R. F.: Arthroscopic meniscus repair. Arthroscopy *1*:170, 1985.
33. Johnson, R. J., et al.: Factors affecting late results after meniscectomy. J. Bone Joint Surg. *56A*:719, 1974.
34. Carpenter J. E., et al.: Preoperative sizing of meniscal allografts. Arthroscopy *9*:344, 1993.
35. Garrett, J. C., and Stevenson, R. N.: Meniscal transplantation in the human knee: A preliminary report. Arthroscopy *7*:57, 1991.
36. Jackson, R. W., Marans, H. J., and Silver, R. S.: The arthroscopic treatment of degenerative arthritis of the knee. J. Bone Joint Surg. *70B*:332, 1988.
37. Jackson, R. W.: Arthroscopic treatment of degenerative arthritis. *In* Operative Arthroscopy. Edited by J. B. McGinty. New York, Raven Press, 1991.
38. Wouters E., et al.: An algorithm for arthroscopy in the over 50 age group. Am. J. Sports Med. *20*:141, 1992.
39. Gross D. E., Brenner S. L., Esformes I., and Gross, M. L.: Arthroscopic treatment of degenerative joint disease of the knee. Orthopedics *14*:1317, 1991.
40. Ferkel, R. D., et al.: Arthroscopic partial medial meniscectomy: An analysis of unsatisfactory results. Arthroscopy *1*:44, 1985.
41. Sherk, H. H., Lane, G. J., and Black, J. D.: Laser arthroscopy. Orthop. Rev. *21*:1077, 1992.
42. Trauner, K., Nishioka, N., and Patel, D.: Pulsed holmium:yttrium-aluminum-garnet (Ho-YAG) laser ablation of fibrocartilage and articular cartilage. Am. J. Sports Med. *18*:316, 1990.
43. Lantz, B., and Singer, K. M.: Meniscal cysts. Clin. Sports Med. *9*:707, 1990.
44. Breck, L. W.: Cysts of the semilunar cartilages of the knee. Clin. Orthop. *3*:29, 1954.
45. Ferrer-Roca, O., and Vilalta, C.: Lesions of the meniscus. Part II: Horizontal cleavages and lateral cysts. Clin. Orthop. *146*:301, 1980.

71 *James R. Harris*

Chondral Lesions

Articular cartilage defects are common in athletic young persons. These defects result from various problems, including patellar malalignment, osteochondritis dissecans, avascular necrosis, congenital malformation, and trauma. They are usually characterized by focal involvement rather than diffuse involvement of articular surfaces like that seen in osteoarthritis.

Hyaline articular cartilage, which covers the ends of bones in synovial joints, is a highly specialized living tissue. It is well-suited to serve as a shock absorber, a weight-bearing surface, and a moveable joint. As compared with the other body tissues articular cartilage is isolated: it is aneural and alymphatic, and it has no vascular supply. It receives nutrition through synovial fluid that has to pass through its dense hyaline matrix to reach the imbedded chondrocytes (Fig. 71–1).[1] The full function of articular cartilage has not been completely explained. It protects the joint with its load-bearing quality and its ability to endure repetitive stress. Many times, despite the stress it must endure, it survives for a lifetime.

Damage to articular cartilage is the primary cause of pain and dysfunction in synovial joints. These lesions may be associated with other injuries, including instability patterns or meniscal damage, or they may be isolated articular surface defects. The lesions may remain relatively static or can be associated with further deterioration of the joint surface. Likewise, symptoms may become very incapacitating and progressive or the process can go on for many years with minimal disability.[2]

CARTILAGE RESPONSE TO INJURY

It is well-recognized that articular cartilage has a very limited capacity to repair itself.[3] At best, its response to injuries is to form a repair tissue that differs significantly in composition, organization of structure, and mechanical properties from normal articular cartilage.[4] Unfortunately, the mechanical properties of articular cartilage are believed to be vital to its function and survival while sustaining the great stresses of a weight-bearing joint.[5]

Several factors limit the capacity of articular cartilage to respond to injury. These include its avascularity, the absence of undifferentiated cells to repair injuries and lesions, and the fact that chondrocytes are encased and immobilized in a strong solid matrix and are not readily mobile. The lack of blood vessels prevents new cells from entering sites of injury. The lack of mesenchymal cells prevents initiation of the healing response that occurs in other tissues.[5]

Because of the low cell density and the inability of chondrocytes to migrate into a defect, repair of cartilage would require considerable proliferative effort in a tissue already compromised by lack of blood supply. However, when the lesion extends into subchondral bone, marrow cells and blood vessels have access to the defect. Some full-thickness defects undergo considerable repair, even without protection from weight bearing, although the repair tissue is not the same as normal articular cartilage.[2]

A substantial amount of research has been devoted to the search for valid repair procedures. In general, the repair procedures have had only limited success because of the problems of cartilage healing and regeneration.[5]

CHONDROMALACIA

Chondromalacia is in a separate subcategory of osteoarthritis. It primarily affects the articular cartilage of the patella and the femoral condyles in young persons. Cartilage changes consist of softening and mild arthritis, with fibrillation and surface irregularities predominating, without other changes consistent with osteoarthritis.[6]

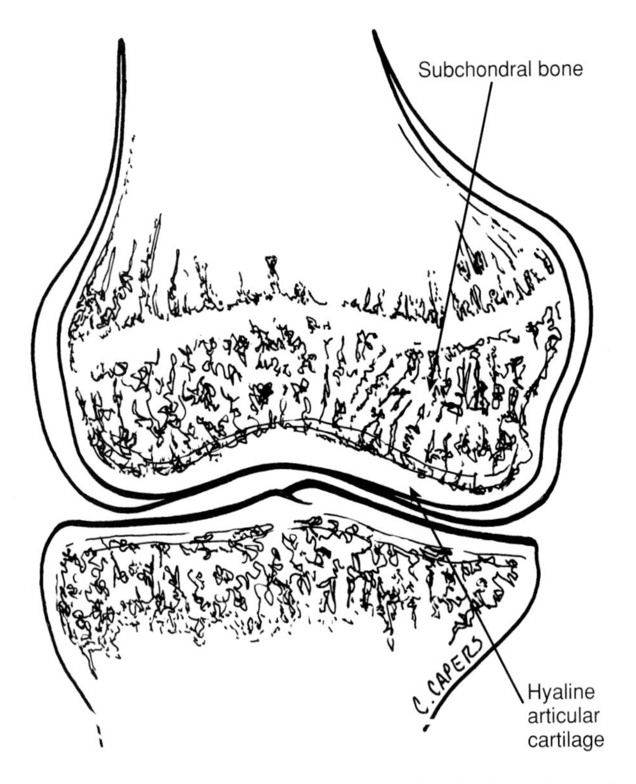

Fig. 71–1. Articular cartilage is aneural, alymphatic, and avascular. Its nutrition must come in the synovial fluid that passes through the dense hyaline matrix.

The many theories about the causes of chondromalacia can generally be grouped into three categories: trauma, nutritional disorders of the cartilage, and inborn errors of metabolism.

Trauma can be classified as either acute or chronic and cumulative. An example of an acute injury is patellofemoral chondral injury secondary to dashboard injury from a motor vehicle accident. Repetitive cumulative trauma can be secondary to alterations in functional conditions or mechanical malalignment. Degenerative changes are more common in mechanically deranged knees. Examples include accelerated degenerative changes caused by anterior cruciate ligament injuries, meniscectomies, or patellofemoral malalignment. Constant repetitive microtrauma in these joints exceeds the threshold for repair and is responsible for the degeneration.[7,8] Repetitive microtrauma can also result in a normal joint when normal activities are performed to excess, such as by prolonged long-distance running or other physical activity. In general, mechanical activities help diffuse synovial fluid by acting as a pump. Also, when there is a change in the quality of the synovial fluid or the pumping action, the nutrition of the articular cartilage can be jeopardized.

Other unfavorable conditions include excessive loading and prolonged standing, especially in overweight persons. This can cause excessive compression of the articular surface cartilage and can interfere with cartilage nutrition. Immobilization can also slow the diffusion of nutrients to the articular cartilage, causing chondral injury. Repeated intra-articular injection of corticosteroids can deplete the ground substance and cause the articular cartilage to become soft and fibrillated.[7,9]

Nontraumatic chondromalacia can be associated with nutritional disorders and inborn errors of metabolism. This type of chondromalacia, often associated with more extensive joint surface involvement, is thought to be caused by progressive depletion of ground substance. In longstanding disease, a similar lesion can develop on the opposing joint surface; this is called a *mirror lesion.*[7,10] By the time this occurs, radiographs often show narrowing of the joint space, osteophyte formation, or both.

Classification

Various staging classifications have been proposed for chondromalacia. Stage I chondromalacia has softening to palpation. The cartilage has a spongy consistency that on superficial inspection may appear normal. Stage II consists of blister formation. Stage III involves ulceration and fragmentation (Fig. 71–2). The articular surface often has a "crab meat" appearance. Stage IV chondromalacia is identified by crater formation and eburnation (Fig. 71–3). As the traumatic process continues, pieces of cartilage break off and complete loss of articular cartilage can occur. This exposes the bone in some areas, giving the damaged area the appearance of a crater surrounded by a rim of frayed cartilage.

History and Physical Examination

A thorough evaluation helps establish the diagnosis. A careful history may help reveal predisposing factors such as familial predisposition, obesity, a history of recent injury, change in physical activity, or a repetitive sporting activity. Physical findings in conjunction with the patient's history are often suggestive but not specific for chondromalacia. A patient may present with physical findings indicating patellofemoral malalignment or

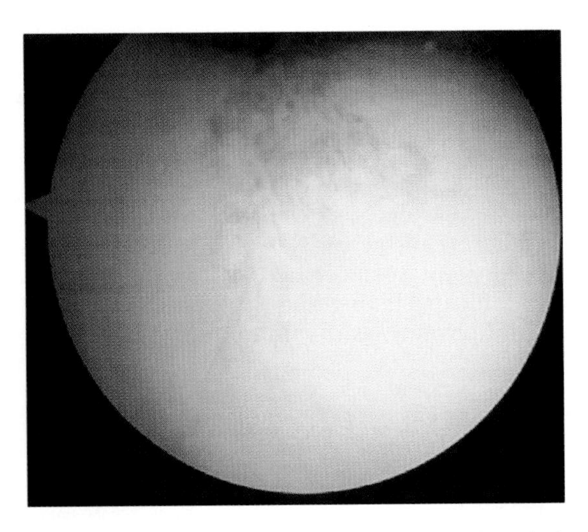

Fig. 71–2. Arthroscopic appearance of Stage III chondromalacia patellae.

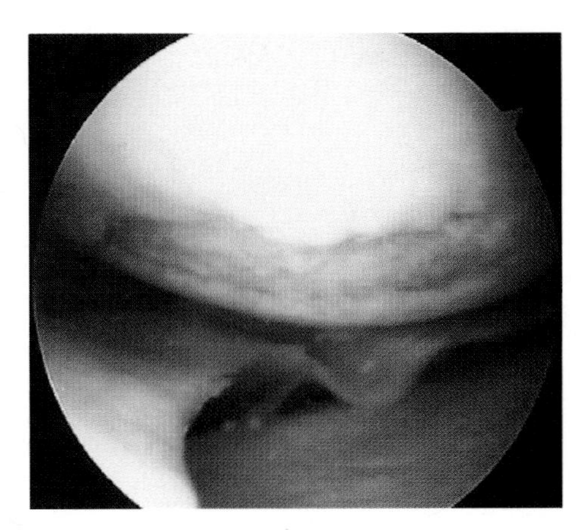

Fig. 71–3. Arthroscopic appearance of Stage IV chondromalacia patellae.

patellofemoral chondromalacia. Patients with tibial—or more commonly femoral—condylar chondromalacia often have mild quadriceps atrophy, joint line tenderness near the affected area, pain with McMurray's test, and pain with hyperflexion and hyperextension of the knee. An effusion is usually absent, except in the later stages of the disease. Ligamentous testing is negative for instability, except when chronic ligament instability is the underlying cause of the chondral problem.

Plain films are almost always negative and nondiagnostic. They may be helpful, however, in identifying axial or patellofemoral malalignment or an unsuspected cause of the patient's problem such as osteochondritis dissecans.

Treatment

Initial treatment of chondromalacia is conservative: rest, application of heat or ice, an isometric strengthening program, nonsteroidal anti-inflammatory medications, and avoidance of inciting activities. Impaction and stressful activities should be avoided, if possible.

If the patient fails to respond to an aggressive and complete trial of conservative measures, arthroscopic evaluation can be considered. Stage I chondromalacia should not be treated with surgical manipulation when it is identified arthroscopically. More severe involvement (Stage II to IV) may be treated with débridement of unstable cartilage, with or without drilling or abrasion chondroplasty.

OSTEOCHONDRITIS DISSECANS

The term *osteochondritis dissecans* is misleading because osteochondritis denotes a condition of inflammation. Osteochondritis dissecans is a condition in which a segment of bone and the overlying articular cartilage are separated from the underlying vascularized bone. It is most common in the knee, but it has also been reported in the elbow, the ankle, and the femoral head. The lesion is usually unilateral, but it may be bilateral. Osteochondritis dissecans is more common in men than in women. It is rare before age 10 years and after age 50 years.[11]

The exact cause of osteochondritis dissecans remains unknown.[11] Fairbank suggested that osteochondritis dissecans was caused by the anterior tibial spine impingeing against the lateral aspect of the medial femoral condyle during the last few degrees of extension.[12] Rosenberg elicited a history of significant trauma in 46% of patients.[13] He also thought that osteochondritis dissecans actually represents nonunion of an osteochondral or subchondral fracture. Many other authors have also reported the association of trauma with osteochondritis dissecans; however, the frequency of bilaterality is difficult to explain with the trauma theory.

A second popular theory is ischemia. Watson-Jones has suggested that osteochondritis in an adolescent is secondary to bone infarcts.[14] Mankin proposed that the primary cause of osteoarthritis was an ischemic event that resulted in a wedge-shaped segment of devascularized subchondral bone.[1,6] He suggested that there is an area of potentially impaired circulation at the end-artery arcades located in the epiphysis.

Diagnosis

The symptoms can often be vague and intermittent. The clinical history is not specific and consists of recurrent swelling, irritability, locking, and giving way. Physical findings are also nonspecific. There may be localized tenderness over the affected area. The patient may or may not have an effusion. Occasionally, a loose body may be palpable in the knee joint. There may be quadriceps atrophy, crepitation, and restriction of knee movement. One sign that is reported to be specific for osteochondritis dissecans is Wilson's sign, pain on extension of the knee and internal rotation of the tibia. This movement apparently abuts the medial tibial spine against the osteochondritic area.[11,15]

Plain radiographs are very helpful and usually show a well-circumscribed fragment of subchondral bone separated from the femoral condyle and of different density (Fig. 71–4A). As the fragment separates, a crater may be seen (71–4B). Bone scans, tomography, magnetic resonance imaging (MRI), and computed tomography (CT) may all be helpful in evaluating these lesions.[11]

CT can delineate osteochondritis dissecans; however, it may not provide sufficient resolution to evaluate whether a lesion is healing or to document the status of the articular cartilage. MRI has the potential to show articular cartilage, but its usefulness in the evaluation of this disorder is not confirmed.[16]

Cahill and colleagues concluded that bone scintigraphy is the most appropriate and the most sensitive diagnostic procedure for monitoring the clinical course of juvenile osteochondritis dissecans.[17] Arthroscopic evaluation is helpful for diagnostic confirmation and staging of the lesion. The most important advantage of arthroscopy, however, is that it can also be used to treat the disorder.[11]

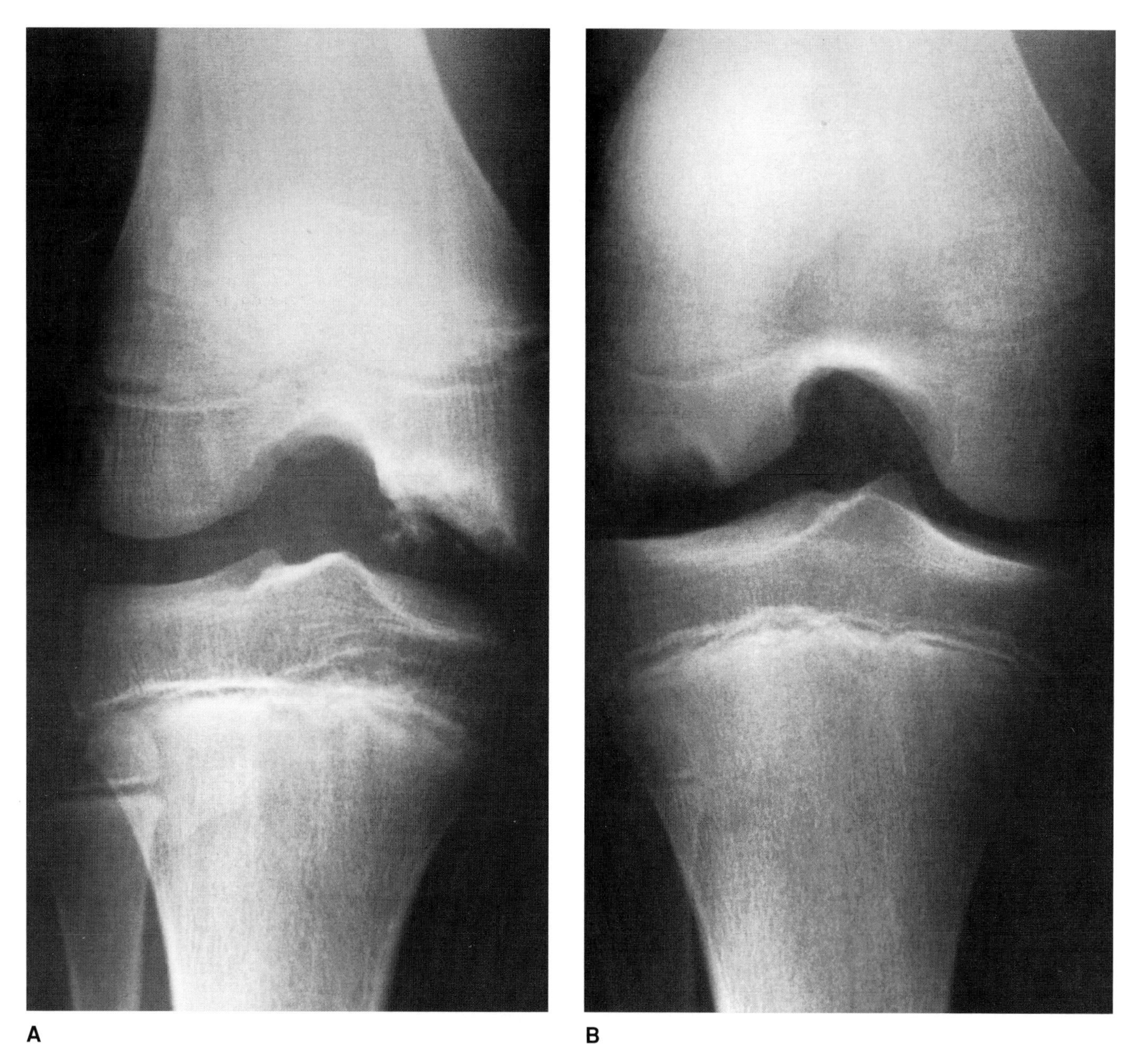

Fig. 71–4. *(A)* A well-circumscribed fragment of subchondral bone can be seen separated from the medial femoral condyle. *(B)* The crater seen on the lateral femoral condyle indicates osteochondritis dissecans.

Treatment

Before formulating a plan for treatment, the surgeon needs to assess the location of the lesion, its size, whether the weight-bearing surface is involved, the age of the patient, and the degree of separation of the bone fragment. Treatment differs, depending on the patient's age.

In a young person who is minimally symptomatic, a conservative trial may be all that it is needed to improve symptoms.[16] Spontaneous healing of juvenile osteochondritic lesions has been reported by various authors, though it is well-documented that not all lesions of juvenile osteochondritis dissecans heal spontaneously.[11, 17–21]

The management of juvenile osteochondritis dissecans is somewhat controversial. Although, at one time, prolonged immobilization was recommended, now it is generally believed that immobilization should be kept to a minimum and should be reserved for acute episodes.[11] The use of cast immobilization is rare. A hinged knee brace with limited motion is usually sufficient. Many authors recommend activity modification. Often a brief period of avoiding high-stress activity may be sufficient to relieve the symptoms.[17]

If symptoms do not subside within 8 to 10 weeks and bone scan or MRI shows no healing, arthroscopic assessment should be considered. Surgical treatments include drilling of the intact fragment, fixation with pins or screws, bone grafting, and excision of the unstable fragment, with or without curettage of the crater. A large fragment can be replaced if it is congruous with the defect. If a patient is treated conservatively and shows evidence of healing, activity can be resumed; however, full activity should be recommended with caution after surgical treatment.[11]

Linden reported on the natural history of adult-onset osteochondritis dissecans in 40 patients who were treated conservatively. Eighty percent of these patients had evidence of degenerative arthritis approximately 10 years earlier in life than controls. If the fracture does not heal spontaneously, the lack of support beneath the articular cartilage can cause the fragment to become detached and form a loose body. Fibrocartilage fills the crater when the fragment is loosening or hinging open, and eventually the osteochondritic segment separates completely from its origin.

If a patient is symptomatic, it is reasonable to restrict athletic activity. If symptoms persist despite appropriate conservative therapy, arthroscopy should be considered. If the fragment is stable on probing, it may either be left alone or drilled through the articular surface. Internal fixation usually is not required if the osteochondritic lesion is stable. Options include curettage of the lesion, drilling of the lesion, or replacement of the lesion and fixation if the opposing surfaces are congruent.[11] Fragments that have been separated from a crater longer than a few weeks should probably be removed. The typical histologic appearance of osteochondritis dissecans is usually consistent with ischemic necrosis of the subchondral bone.[11]

CHONDRAL FRACTURES

Although chondral injuries are frequently associated with other pathologic conditions, as isolated injuries they have received little attention in the literature.[22] Chondral fractures are a distinct entity and are different from the more frequently described osteochondral fractures.[23] The most common sites of chondral fractures are the lateral femoral condyle and the medial surface of the patella. Some authors believe that the chondral fractures of the medial femoral condyle are caused by the anterior tibial spine as it rotates into the medial femoral condyle, causing the fracture. They can occur independently or in association with meniscal injuries.

Chondral injuries can occur as a result of direct impact against the soft tissue overlying the articular surface. Chondral injuries more commonly occur in a skeletally mature patient, the fracture line occurring at the *tide mark,* a weak zone between the calcified and the uncalcified cartilage layers. Osteochondral fractures tend to occur in children and adolescents, whose tide mark has not yet developed. In these young persons the fracture line occurs in the weaker subchondral bone area.[24]

Bauer and Jackson divided femoral chondral lesions into six categories (Fig. 71–5).[25] The classification is based on the arthroscopic appearance of the chondral fractures. Type I is a linear crack; Type II, a stellate fracture; Type III, a chondral flap; and Type IV, a chondral crater. Type V has a fibrillar appearance, and Type VI is degraded. The authors think that Types I through IV are traumatic in origin and Types V and VI are degener-

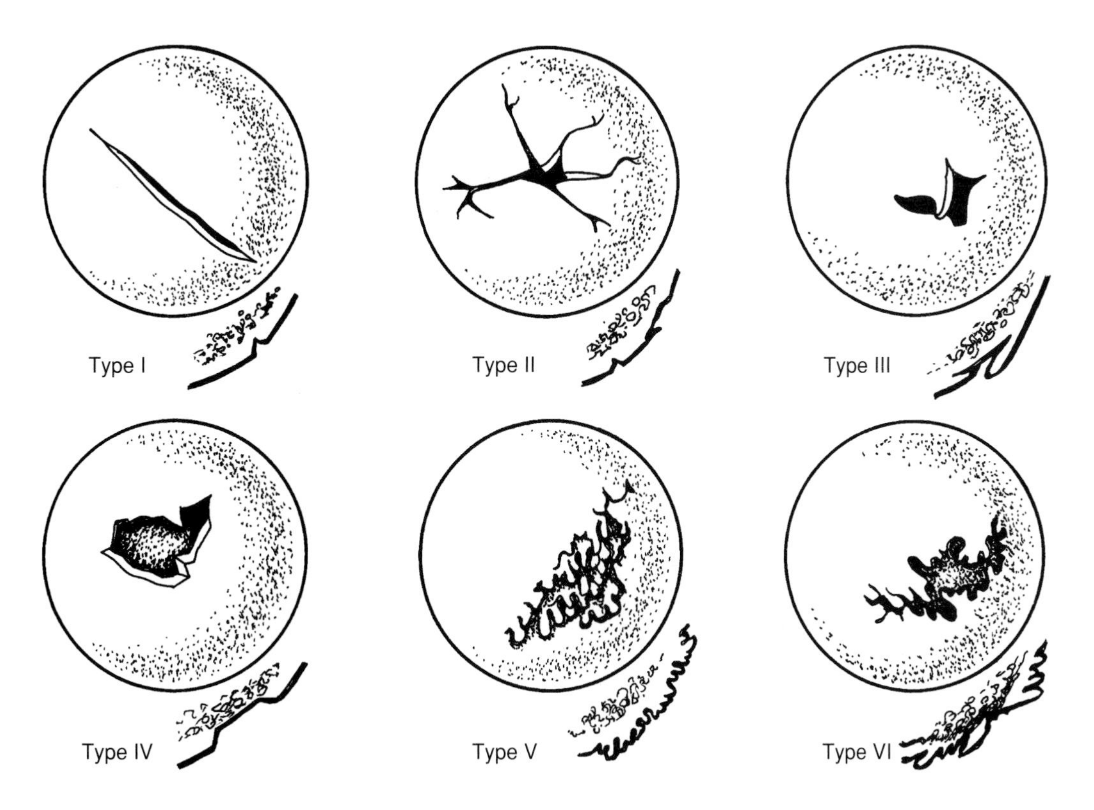

Fig. 71–5. Classification of chondral lesions.

ative. The disadvantage of this system is that it relies on the gross appearance of the cartilaginous lesion but does not address size, site, or prognosis.[24] Stellate fractures are the most common type; and flap- or crater-type lesions the next most common. The lesions are usually bordered by normal-looking articular cartilage, but on occasion there is chondromalacia on the borders.[22]

History and Physical Examination

Diagnosis of a joint surface defect can be difficult because there are no specific diagnostic signs.[2] Most often, patients present with symptoms suggesting meniscus problems. They often complain of locking, catching, and giving way. The patient usually reports a traumatic episode that occurred recently or several months earlier.[2] Most often, the injury occurs when the knee is flexed.[22] The patient often presents with a chronically painful joint.[2]

Historic findings often include some degree of morning stiffness and impairment in ambulation, either periodically or after vigorous exercise. Most patients exhibit impaired exercise tolerance and difficulty with stairs. With chondral fractures, ascending stairs appears to be more difficult than descending. Popping with flexion and extension of the knee is common.[22]

Physical findings also suggest meniscus involvement;[22] however, there may be few acute physical findings present, and those that are present usually are not specific. There may be mild quadriceps atrophy. A synovial effusion may be large, small, or entirely absent. Hemarthroses are uncommon. Joint line tenderness can usually be palpated near the chondral lesion.[2] Hyperflexion and hyperextension are often painful. Occasionally there is tenderness directly over the femoral condyle or pain with patellofemoral pressure.[2] Instability is not present unless the lesion is associated with a ligament injury.[24]

In the acute phase, joint aspiration can be performed. A bloody aspirate indicates possible osteoarticular damage with bleeding from the subchondral bone. An acute hemarthrosis may represent a tear of the anterior cruciate, or another ligament, of synovium, or of the peripheral meniscus. Fat in a hemarthrosis is strongly suggestive of an acute osteoarticular fracture. A synovial fluid white cell count helps distinguish a post-traumatic condition from an inflammatory disease such as rheumatoid arthritis. If clear synovial fluid is drawn, the exact nature of the injury cannot always be ascertained.

It is usually advisable to treat the patient with conservative measures and allow 6 to 8 weeks for the effusion to resolve. If, after 4 to 8 weeks, the patient becomes asymptomatic and is able to resume activity without difficulty, the effusion was probably secondary to a soft tissue contusion or sprain. On the other hand, if the effusion persists this probably indicates an intra-articular abnormality consistent with a chondral lesion or a meniscus problem. In more "chronic" lesions, a small effusion is often present.[24]

Standard radiographs are useless for pure chondral injuries, though they are quite helpful for osteochondral fractures.[24] These injuries usually are not well visualized with arthrography. Bone scintigraphy is often helpful in showing a focal area of joint damage. MRI may also be helpful. Further delineation usually requires arthroscopy.[24]

Terry and coworkers found that in 18 patients with isolated chondral fractures the preoperative diagnosis of chondral injury was uniformly missed. The usual preoperative diagnosis was a torn meniscus. They suggested that a negative arthroscopic meniscal examination in a patient with meniscus symptoms should alert the surgeon to the possibility of an isolated chondral fracture. They found in many cases that the lesion was located posteriorly and could not be seen unless the knee was flexed. Some patients have more than one chondral fracture.[22]

Arthroscopy is the most definitive method of diagnosing chondral fractures.[23] On arthroscopy an acute fracture appears as either a gouged-out defect, a flap, or a stellate pattern, depending on the mechanism of injury (Fig. 71–6).[22,23]

Treatment

Either surgical or nonsurgical treatment may be appropriate in the acute or the chronic phase of treatment.[2] Ultimately, however, treatment of most of these lesions is surgical. All loose pieces of cartilage should be removed until the hyaline rim is stable. The base of the lesion should be either drilled or abraded to stimulate the formation of fibrocartilage. A thorough search should be performed to find all loose pieces of articular cartilage.[24]

The patient should be informed that restoration to a preinjury level is unlikely; however, surgery frequently produces improvement. After surgical treatment, it usually is not advisable for patients to return to sports because this will diminish the chances of a longterm improvement. The goals of treatment are to preserve function, restore function, and alleviate pain. Surgery should not be regarded as a last resort but rather as

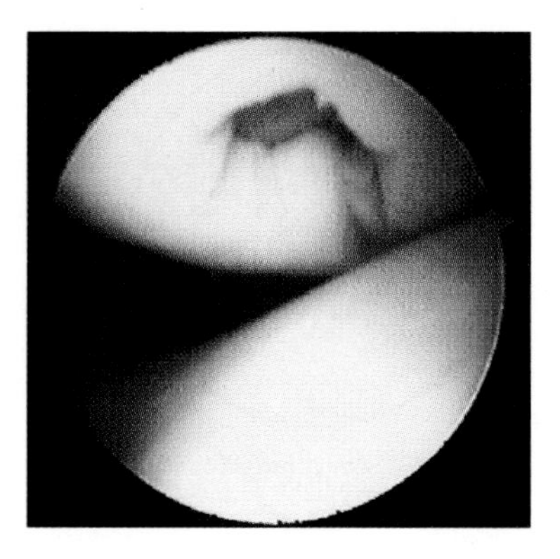

Fig. 71–6. Arthroscopic photograph of a chondral lesion.

adjunctive treatment.[2] Although chondral fractures are not common, a high index of suspicion is well-advised, as they are often difficult to diagnose.[23]

OSTEOCHONDRAL FRACTURES

Osteochondral fractures are fractures that occur through articular cartilage and also involve an attached piece of underlying subchondral bone. Osteochondral fractures may or may not be displaced. They usually occur in younger persons, before the tide mark appears in adult articular cartilage. Johnson-Nurse and Dandy postulated that, in younger persons, the chondral layer was so firmly attached to the subchondral bone that the fracture more commonly occurred in the subchondral bone than in the cartilage itself.[26]

Kennedy and Grainger divided these fractures into two groups.[27] Exogenous fractures occur when direct trauma is applied to articular cartilage. Endogenous fractures occur because of rotatory and compressive forces applied within the knee, and possibly from outside trauma. Sweeney reported that a review of the literature shows that the most common sites of osteocartilaginous fractures are the patella, the lateral femoral condyle, and the medial femoral condyle.[24] Lesions of the tibial plateau are rare.

In the Johnson-Nurse and Dandy study, all lesions occurred on an area of weight-bearing surface of the femoral condyle when the knee was fully extended.[26] The lesions were four times as likely to occur on the medial femoral condyle. It is common for patellar dislocations to result in osteochondral fractures of the patella and lateral femoral condyle.[28] Rorabeck and Bobechko reported that 5% of patellar dislocations resulted in osteocartilaginous fractures of the patella.[29]

Patients often give a history of an indirect force. This can be either a twisting valgus or varus injury on a straight or slightly flexed knee or patellar dislocation or subluxation. Occasionally, a direct force is the mechanism of injury. Patients often complain of a sudden pain and a snap in the knee. Chronic symptoms are similar to those of meniscus tears.

It is not uncommon for chondral or osteochondral fractures to occur in association with ligament injuries. Butler and Andrews reported that 11% of patients who presented with acute hemarthrosis of the knee were found to have osteochondral fractures at the time of arthroscopy.[30] These fractures were not evident on plain films.[24,30] The difference between the average age of patients with osteochondritis dissecans and that of those with osteochondral fractures suggests that the two are, indeed, separate entities.[31]

Radiographic examination of the injured joint should demonstrate an osteochondral fragment. Multiple views may be needed to demonstrate the fracture and its site of origin. The fragment often shows up as a very thin line on the radiograph that is a shell of subchondral bone. Sometimes the fracture is visible only when viewed end-on. Osteochondral patellar fractures are best seen on sunrise or Merchant views. Osteochondral fractures can be easily overlooked on MRI.[24,32]

If the lesion is acute and not displaced it can be treated conservatively with immobilization and avoidance of physical activity. If the fracture is displaced, surgical treatment is usually indicated. Arthroscopy is the best diagnostic procedure to determine the depth and extent of the lesion. If the fracture is acute, the configuration of the adjoining surfaces has not changed and the area of the fracture is accessible to arthroscopic positioning, the osteochondral fracture can be replaced arthroscopically. A loose osteochondral fragment can cause locking, abrade articular surfaces, and continue to grow within the joint. Pins, nails, and screws have all been used to transfix osteochondral fragments. All require enough bone to afford purchase for the hardware.[24]

The Herbert screw has the theoretical advantage of not having to be removed, since it is entirely buried. The differential pitch of the two screw threads causes compression between the loose fragment and the underlying bone.[33]

Old osteochondral fractures seldom require any treatment other than removing the loose fragment. Occasionally, the site of the loose fragment has healed so well that it is difficult to distinguish it from surrounding cartilage.[31]

REFERENCES

1. Mankin, H. J.: The reaction of articular cartilage to injury and osteoarthritis. Part I. N. Engl. J. Med. *291*:1285, 1974.
2. Rodrigo, J. J.: Biologic repair of joint surface defects in the young patient. *In* Operative Orthopaedics. 2nd Ed. Edited by M. Madison. Philadelphia, J. B. Lippincott, 1988.
3. Mankin, H. J., Dorfman, H., Lippiello, L., and Zarins, A.: Biomechanical and metabolic abnormalities in articular cartilage from osteo-arthritic human hips. II. Correlation of morphology with biochemical and metabolic data. J. Bone Joint Surg. *53A*:523, 1971.
4. Furukawa, T., Eyre, D. R., Koide, S., and Glimcher, M. J.: Biomechanical studies on repair cartilage resurfacing experimental effects in the rabbit knee. J. Bone Joint Surg. *62A*:79, 1980.
5. Mow, V. C., Ratcliffe, A., Rosenwasser, M. P., and Buckwalter, J. A.: Experimental studies on repair of large osteochondral defects at a high weight–bearing area of the knee joint: A tissue engineering study. J. Biomech. Eng. *113*:198, 1991.
6. Mankin, H. J.: The reaction of articular cartilage to injury and osteoarthritis. Part II. N. Engl. J. Med. *291*:1335, 1974.
7. Shahriaree, H. ed.: O'Connor's Textbook of Arthroscopic Surgery. Philadelphia, J.B. Lippincott, 1992.
8. Radin, E. L., Ehrlich, M. G., Chernack, R., et al.: Effect of repetitive impulsive loading on the knee joints of rabbits. Clin. Orthop. *131*:288, 1978.
9. Salter, R. B., Gross, A., and Hall, J. H.: Hydrocortisone arthropathy. Can. Med. Assoc. J. *97*:374, 1967.
10. Wiles, P., Andrews, P. S., and Devas, M. B.: Chondromalacia of the patella. J. Bone Joint Surg. *38B*:95, 1956.
11. Aichroth, P. M., and Dipak, V. P.: Osteochondritis dissecans of the knee: An overview. *In* Knee Surgery: Current Practice. Edited by P. M. Aichroth and W. D. Cannon. New York, Raven Press, 1992.
12. Fairbank, H. A. T.: Osteochondritis dissecans. Br. J. Surg. *21*:67, 1933.
13. Rosenberg, N. J.: Osteochondral fractures of the lateral femoral condyle. J. Bone Joint Surg. *46A*:1013, 1964.

14. Watson-Jones, R.: Fractures and Joint Injuries. Vol. 1. 4th Ed. London, E & S Livingstone, 1952.
15. Wilson, J. N.: A diagnostic sign in osteochondritis dissecans of the knee. J. Bone Joint Surg. *49A*:477, 1967.
16. Stone, J. W., and Guhl, J. F.: Osteochondritis dissecans. *In* Knee Surgery: Current Practice. Edited by P. M. Aichroth and W. D. Cannon. New York, Raven Press, 1992.
17. Cahill, B. R., Phillips, M. R., and Navarro, R.: The results of conservative management of juvenile osteochondritis dissecans using joint scintigraphy: A prospective study. Am. J. Sports Med. *17*:601, 1989.
18. Hughston, J. C., Hergenroeder, P. T., and Courtenay, B. G.: Osteochondritis dissecans of the femoral condyles. J. Bone Joint Surg. *66A*:1340, 1984.
19. Aichroth, P. M.: Osteochondritis dissecans of the knee: A clinical survey. J. Bone Joint Surg. *53B*:440, 1971.
20. Cahill, B. R., and Berg, B. C.: 99m-Technetium phosphate compound joint scintigraphy in the management of juvenile osteochondritis dissecans of the femoral condyles. Am. J. Sports Med. *11*:329, 1983.
21. Langer, F., and Percy, E. C.: Osteochondritis dissecans and anomalous centres of ossification: A review of 80 lesions in 61 patients. Can. J. Surg. *14*:208, 1971.
22. Terry, G. C., Flandry, F., VanManen, T. W., and Norwood, L. A.: Isolated chondral fractures of the knee. Clin. Orthop. *234*:170, 1988.
23. Gilley, J. S., et al.: Chondral fractures of the knee. Radiol. *138*:51, 1981.
24. Sweeney, H. J.: Chondral and osteochondral fractures of the knee. *In* Operative Arthroscopy. Edited by J. B. McGinty. New York, Raven Press, 1991.
25. Bauer, M., and Jackson, R. W.: Chondral lesions of the femoral condyles: A system of arthroscopic classifications. Arthroscopy *4*:97, 1988.
26. Johnson-Nurse, C., and Dandy, D. J.: Fracture-separation of articular cartilage in the adult knee. J. Bone Joint Surg. *67B*:42, 1985.
27. Kennedy, J. C., Grainger, R. W., and McGraw, R. W.: Osteochondral fractures of the femoral condyles. J. Bone Joint Surg. *48B*:436, 1966.
28. Morscher, E.: Cartilage-bone lesions of the knee joint following injury. Reconstr. Surg. Traumatol. *12*:2, 1971.
29. Rorabeck, C. H., and Bobechko, W. P.: Acute dislocation of the patella with osteochondral fracture. J. Bone Joint Surg. *56B*:237, 1976.
30. Butler, J. C., and Andrews, J. R.: The role of arthroscopic surgery in the evaluation of acute traumatic hemarthrosis of the knee. Clin. Orthop. *228*:150, 1988.
31. Dandy, D. J.: Chondral and osteochondral lesions of the femoral condyles. *In* Knee Surgery: Current Practice. Edited by P. M. Aichroth and W. D. Cannon. New York, Raven Press, 1992.
32. Mink, J. H., and Deutsch, A. L.: Occult cartilage and bone injuries of the knee: Detection, classification, and assessment with MR imaging. Radiology *170*:823, 1989.
33. Rae, P. S., and Khasawneh, Z. M.: Herbert screw fixation of osteochondral fractures of the patella. Injury. *19*:116, 1988.

72

Fred Flandry

A Classification of Knee Ligament Instability

The study of the literature on this subject leaves one bewildered.
—Brantigan and Voshell

THE ELEMENTS OF STABILITY

For the purpose of this discussion, the knee, a complex joint, can be divided into a tibiofemoral and a patellofemoral joint. In this chapter I address primarily disorders of tibiofemoral ligament stability. It is important to remember, in any such discussion, that the stability of the tibiofemoral joint results from an interplay of many static and dynamic elements.

Dynamic stability involves muscles acting on or across the knee joint. The quadriceps (Fig. 72–1A), as well as being the primary eccentric decelerator of the knee, act as a dynamic antagonist to an intact anterior cruciate ligament and can reduce posterior subluxation in the event of posterior cruciate ligament injury. The hamstrings function medially and laterally as antagonists to an intact posterior cruciate ligament (Fig. 72–1B) directly reducing anterior subluxation, but they can also tense the ligaments through their insertion into the capsular ligaments (Fig. 72–1C). This action eliminates any laxity that is present and increases the articular surface load as well. In this manner, muscles also augment the static mechanism of stability that will be described later. Similarly, the iliotibial band and gastrocnemius heads augment the stability derived from capsular ligaments.

The tibiofemoral ligaments provide static stability. They are assisted by the menisci, the topography of the articular surfaces, and the loads placed on these articular surfaces. Clearly, to attribute all stability of the knee to tibiofemoral ligaments is naive. However, it is important to be able to recognize and categorize patterns of ligament injury alone, so treatment algorithms can be created, tested, and applied to clinical practice. Constant awareness of all elements of stability serves to remind the physician that treatment of sprains succeeds or fails because of what is done to correct injury to the ligaments and the surrounding structures.

OVERVIEW OF THE CLASSIFICATION

With an injury such as a knee sprain that has many possible injury patterns and their respective appropriate treatments, for the physician to begin treatment without some categorization of the injury, anticipation of findings, and knowledge of expected outcome is to invite disaster.

What is the value of a classification system? The answer is twofold. In the area of research or business, classification allows us to identify cohorts or submit claims based on an injury pattern or diagnosis. Much more important, however, the classification scheme becomes a powerful clinical tool for communicating examination findings and for developing a specific treatment algorithm.

When ligament tests are performed, a specific pattern of test results corresponds with a discrete diagnostic classification. From previous research, the physician knows what surgical approach to use, what injuries to expect and to look for, and which operation is likely to correct this pattern of injuries. From a clinical standpoint, it is useless to classify sprains into 50 categories if only five basic treatment modalities exist.

A classification system should never be thought of as a substitute for careful documentation of injuries. All ligament disruptions, their severity, configuration, and loca-

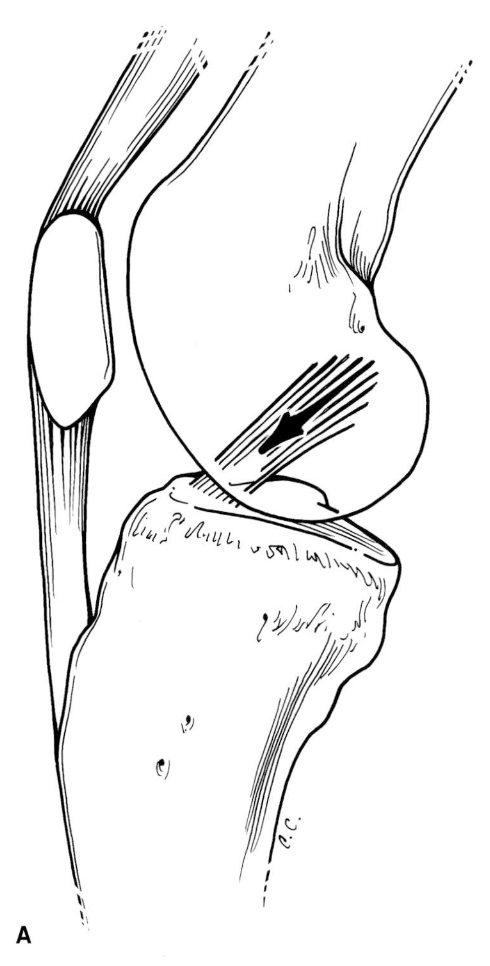

Fig. 72–1. *(A)* The quadriceps muscle functions as an antagonist to the intact anterior cruciate ligament. *(B)* The hamstrings not only function as antagonists to the intact posterior cruciate ligament, but *(C)* they increase joint load by tensioning the capsular ligaments through the capsular aponeurosis from the hamstring tendons.

tion, should be listed. Ongoing refinement of an existing classification or introduction of an additional category is possible only if supportive data are available.

Finally, if a classification is to be useful, it must be straightforward and intuitive. Schemes that require clinicians to refer constantly to complex tables or charts will never gain acceptance or be widely used. On the other hand, a system of classification based on anatomy is not easily understood without a solid foundation in anatomy. The sports medicine physician should be thoroughly familiar with the concepts of knee anatomy and how they relate to a classification system (see Chapter 63).

Historical Perspective

Hughston first presented his knee ligament classification to the American Academy of Orthopaedic Surgeons in January 1969. The publication of his work, the first comprehensive classification of ligament injuries, which appeared in 1976,[1,2] described patterns of ligament disruption in 157 patients. In a continuation of this series, Andrews and Axe reported on 968 knee ligament injuries.[3] Hughston has completed a 10-year prospective study of 826 patients.[4] In these three studies the methods were similar. Patients with severe acute or chronic injuries underwent a prescribed series of preoperative ligament tests, and the findings were carefully documented. Then patients underwent open operative procedures; thus, all injuries to capsular and intra-articular structures were explored and documented. The combinations of positive ligament test results were then correlated with the patterns of injury so that a predictive model was developed. In the first two studies, the findings were recorded in a protocol manner and the review was retrospective. In the third study, ligament tests were used to predict the anatomic injuries, and the accuracy of those predictions was verified by operative findings.

With the emphasis today on arthroscopic or minimal-incision surgery, it seems unlikely that classification validation of this magnitude will ever be repeated.

Conventions in this System

To standardize documentation of results, the Committee on the Medical Aspects of Sports of the American Medical Association advocated the following definitions, outlined in their 1968 handbook. A *sprain* is defined as an injury of ligamentous tissue, whereas a *strain* is a

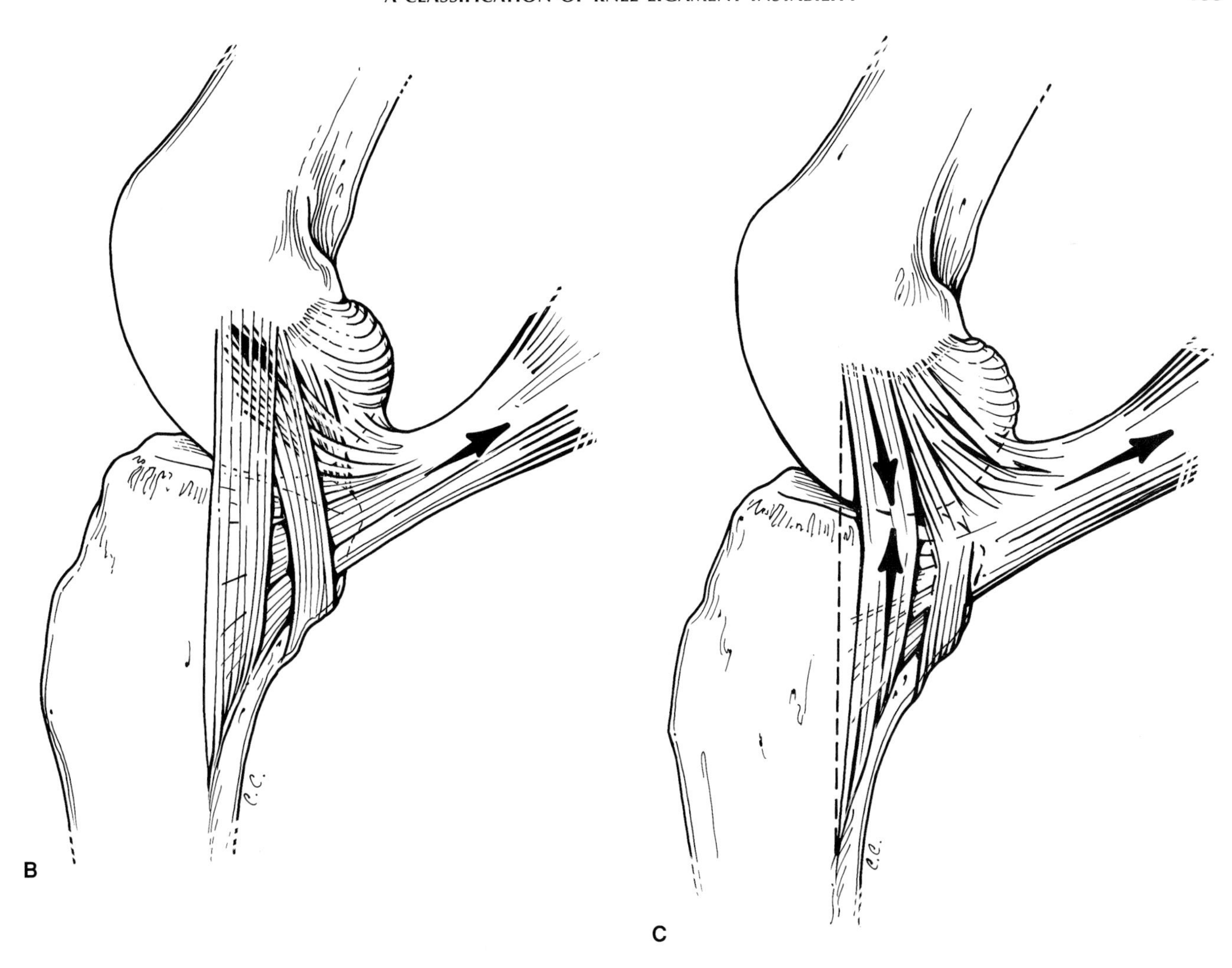

stretching injury to a muscle or its tendinous attachment to bone.

To standardize the severity of sprains, the gradations of mild, moderate, and severe are used. Both the degree of a sprain overall and the degree of a particular stability test used in characterizing that sprain are graded. A mild sprain (first degree) implies minimal tearing or stretching of fibers and is characterized by tenderness but no instability. A moderate sprain (second degree) is a disruption of more fibers (interstitial and partial tearing) and more tenderness, but only subtle abnormal motion. A severe sprain (third degree) is a complete disruption of the ligament with resulting instability. Severe sprains are further graded according to instability. Mild instability (1+) is translation of 5 to 9 mm (0 to 4 mm is considered physiologic) or rotation of 5° to 9° (0° to 4° is considered physiologic). Moderate instability (2+) is translation of 10 to 14 mm or rotation of 10° to 14°. Severe instability (3+) is greater than 15 mm of translation or 15° of rotation.

The knee motions are conceptualized as translations (linear displacement in one plane) or rotations (angular displacement about a given axis). The motions have six degrees of freedom: translations or rotations in the anterior-posterior (sagittal) plane, the medial-lateral (coronal) plane, and the compression-distraction (axial) plane (Fig. 72–2). In actuality, most motions, both normal and abnormal, involve some combination of rotation with translation. Furthermore, in the injured knee, the axis of the rotation can migrate during pathologic motion.

Most translations occur in the anterior-posterior plane, and it is common to characterize such motion as translation of the tibia relative to the femur. Translations in the medial-lateral plane can occur only with the most global disruptions, and the linear magnitude of compression-distraction translations is clinically negligible.

The most common rotation is the normal motion of flexion and extension in the sagittal plane. Likewise, some degree of axial rotation (tibial rotation coupled to knee flexion or to foot and ankle pronation and supination) is also normal, but an excessive rotatory subluxation of a tibial plateau is considered pathologic. Any significant rotation in the coronal plane (adduction or abduction rotation) is abnormal.

EXAMINATION OF THE TIBIOFEMORAL LIGAMENTS

A basic set of provocative examinations must be performed to elucidate injury to the tibiofemoral ligaments. Although other tests and variations of the ones discussed here have been described and may be helpful

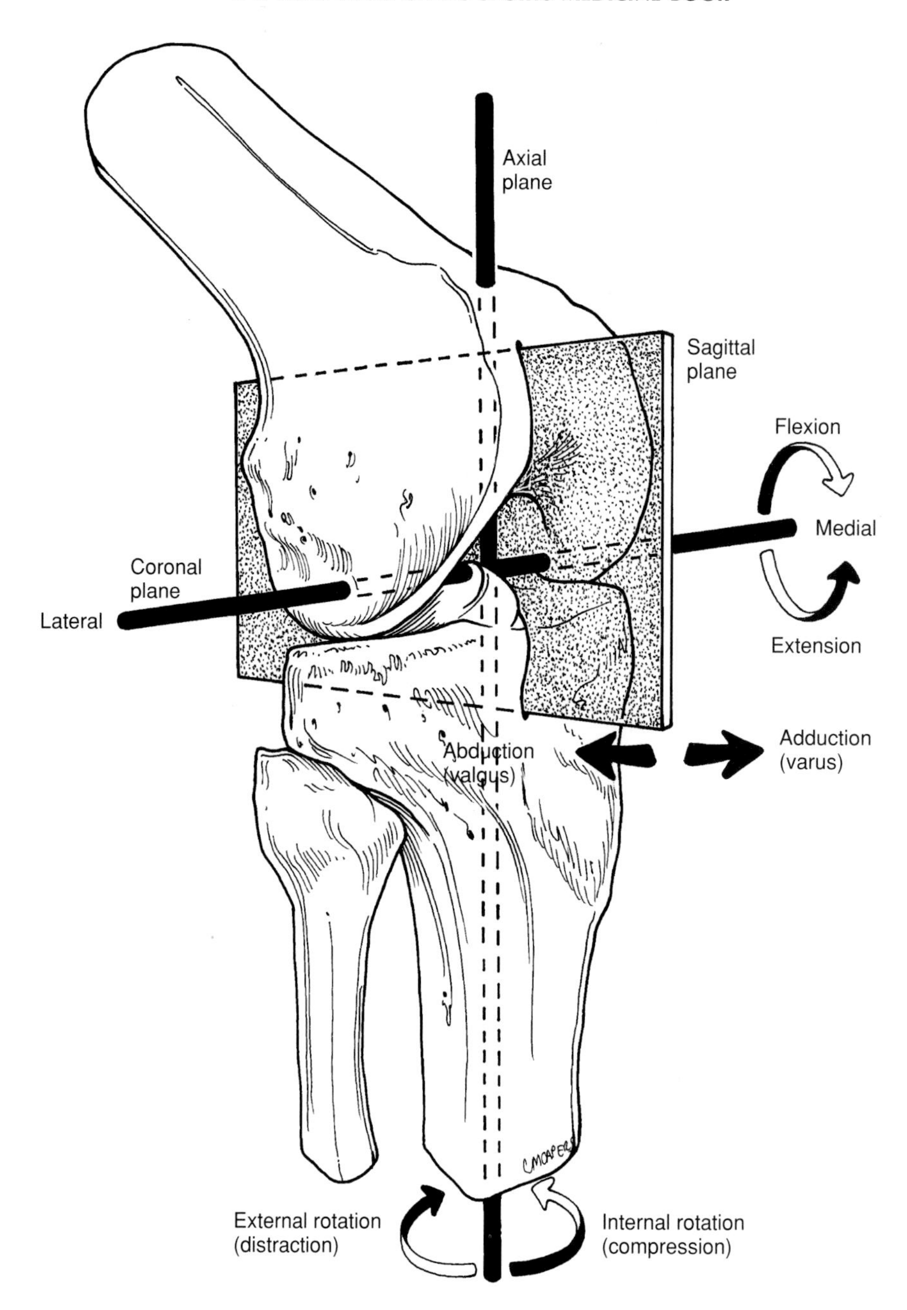

Fig. 72–2. A six-degrees-of-freedom model illustrates all possible rotations and translations about the knee.

in particular situations, these tests are considered the core of the examination. The tests are presented in the order in which they should be performed. Testing in this order necessitates a minimum of repositioning, which causes discomfort to and guarding by the patient, and tests progress from least noxious to more noxious ones.

The object of each test is to place the knee in such a position that a particular ligament, or set of ligaments can be isolated as the only ligament(s) resisting a particular pathologic motion. Tension is then placed on that ligament or set of ligaments, also by position of the knee, so they offer maximum resistance. If the ligament is intact, no pathologic motion should occur; if disrupted, no other ligament or group of ligaments can offer sufficient resistance to mask a positive reading.

For each test that follows, I describe why a position is chosen (Rationale) and what a positive finding means in the way of expected injury and classification (Interpretation). See Chapter 64, Physical Examination of the Knee, for a description of how the tests are performed. Some pairs of tests are performed simultaneously. Here, they are described in the order in which they should be performed (Table 72–1).

External Rotation Recurvatum Test

Rationale. As knee extension progresses to recurvatum, the arcuate complex alone prevents posterolateral subluxation, as distinguished from pure posterior translation.

Table 72–1. Examination of the Tibiofemoral Ligaments

Test	*Specific Instability*	*Injured Ligaments*
External rotation recurvatum	PLRI	Arcuate complex
Abduction 0°	SMI	PCL Medial middle third capsular ligament TCL POL ACL +/–
Adduction 0°	SLI	PCL Lateral middle third capsular ligament FCL Iliotibial tract fibers Arcuate complex* ACL +/–
Abduction 30°	Not specific	Medial middle third capsular ligament TCL POL ACL +/–
Adduction 30°	Not specific	Lateral middle third capsular ligament FCL Arcuate complex* ACL +/–
Lachman's test	Not specific	ACL
Anterior drawer 90° external rotation	AMRI	Medial middle third capsular ligament TCL POL ACL +/–
Posterior drawer 90° external rotation	PLRI	Lateral middle third capsule ligament FCL Arcuate complex*
Anterior drawer 90° neutral	ALRI	Lateral middle third capsular ligament FCL Iliotibial tract fibers ACL +/–
Posterior drawer 90° neutral	SPI	POL Arcuate ligament PCL ACL +/–
Anterior drawer 90° internal rotation	SAI	ACL PCL Lateral middle third capsular ligament FCL Arcuate complex* Medial middle third capsular ligament TCL POL
Posterior drawer 90° internal rotation	SPI	POL Arcuate ligament PCL ACL +/–
Pivot shift-jerk test	ALRI	Iliotibial tract fibers
Reverse pivot shift test	PLRI	Arcuate complex*

*Includes FCL.

Key: SMI, straight medial instability; PCL, posterior cruciate ligament; TCL, tibial collateral ligament; POL, posterior oblique ligament; ACL, anterior cruciate ligament; SLI, straight lateral instability; FCL, fibular collateral ligament; SPI, straight posterior instability; SAI, straight anterior instability; PLRI, posterolateral; AMRI, anteromedial: ALRI, anterolateral.

Interpretation. Posterolateral subluxation of the lateral tibial plateau indicates disruption of the arcuate complex and is specific for posterolateral rotatory instability.

Abduction Stress Test at 0°

The abduction stress 0° and adduction stress 0° tests are performed simultaneously.

Rationale. At 0° or hyperextension, the fibers of the posterior cruciate ligament become taut to the point of increasing joint contact forces (and thus stability). In this position, the posterior cruciate ligament is isolated as the ligament resisting abduction opening.

Interpretation. Abnormal opening at the mid-medial joint line, as described in the section on conventions, in either 0° or hyperextension, indicates damage to the posterior cruciate ligament and the medial capsular structures and signifies straight medial instability. The anterior cruciate ligament is likely to be damaged as well, though this test is not specific for anterior cruciate ligament disruption.

Adduction Stress Test at 0°

Rationale. At 0° or hyperextension, the fibers of the posterior cruciate ligament become taut to the point of increasing joint contact forces—and, thus, stability. In this position, the posterior cruciate ligament is isolated as the ligament that resists adduction opening.

Interpretation. Abnormal opening at the mid-lateral joint line in either 0° or hyperextension indicates damage to the posterior cruciate ligament and the lateral capsular structures and signifies straight lateral instability. The anterior cruciate ligament is likely to be damaged as well, although this test is not specific for anterior cruciate ligament disruption.

Abduction Stress Test at 30°

The abduction stress 30° and adduction stress 30° tests are performed simultaneously.

Rationale. At 30° of knee flexion, the fibers of the posterior cruciate ligament become relatively relaxed to resisting coronal plane rotation. The anterior cruciate ligament is in its most advantageous position to resist anterior translation. For resistance to coronal plane rotation, however, the capsular ligaments are most taut and must fail before the anterior cruciate ligament can experience a load from this form of stress. Thus, in this position, the middle third and posterior third medial capsular ligament complex is isolated as the structure that resists abduction opening.

Interpretation. Abnormal opening at the middle of the medial joint line indicates damage to the medial capsular structures and may signify rotatory instability. The anterior cruciate ligament is likely to be damaged as well, although this test is not specific for disruption of that structure.

Adduction Stress Test at 30°

Rationale. At 30° of knee flexion, the fibers of the posterior cruciate ligament have become relatively relaxed to resisting coronal plane rotation. The anterior cruciate ligament is in its most advantageous position to resist anterior translation. For resistance to coronal plane rotation, however, the capsular ligaments are tauter and must fail before the anterior cruciate ligament can experience a load from this form of stress. Thus, in this position, the middle third and posterior third lateral capsular ligament complex is isolated as the structure that resists adduction opening.

Interpretation. Abnormal opening at the middle of the lateral joint line indicates damage to the lateral capsular structures and can signify either anterolateral or posterolateral rotatory instability. The anterior cruciate ligament is likely to be damaged as well, although this test is not specific for anterior cruciate ligament disruption.

Lachman's Test, or Anterior Drawer Test in Extension

Rationale. The anterior cruciate ligament resists anterior translation, and in the first 20° of knee flexion the posterior cruciate ligament shares this function. Beyond 45° of flexion, the capsular ligaments are tauter than the anterior cruciate ligament and must fail before the anterior cruciate ligament is loaded. Therefore, to isolate and test the anterior cruciate ligament as the sole ligament resisting anterior translation, the knee should be flexed from 20° to 30°.

Interpretation. The amount of translation of the tibia on the femur signifies the amount of anterior cruciate ligament disruption. For greater accuracy, the examiner should grade the translation in millimeters, as precisely as possible. Although the three categories of severity (each representing a range of translation) are used clinically, the discipline of grading in millimeters makes one a better diagnostician. Lachman's test is specific for damage to the anterior cruciate ligament. It is not specific for any particular instability pattern; rather, it confirms whether anterior cruciate disruption is a component of that instability pattern.

Anterior Drawer Test at 90° in External Tibial Rotation

The anterior drawer and posterior drawer tests are performed simultaneously.

Rationale. As knee flexion increases to 90°, the posterior cruciate ligament is no longer positioned to resist anterior translation, nor does it increase joint contact forces. As noted previously, the anterior cruciate ligament is relaxed relative to the capsular ligaments. Therefore, if one assumes the contribution of the anterior third capsular ligaments is negligible, the middle third and posterior third capsular ligaments are isolated as the ones that resist anteromedial subluxation of the medial tibial plateau.

Confusion has arisen as a result of the study by Butler and coworkers that appeared to demonstrate that the anterior cruciate ligament was the primary restraint to anterior translation.[5] This conclusion should not have been reached, because their experimental model totally constrained tibial rotation; thus, loading of the capsular ligaments was delayed relative to loading of the anterior cruciate ligament. Furthermore, the appropriate question should not have been which ligamentous complex had the greatest tensile strength, but which ligament must fail first to allow the unconstrained tibia to translate anteriorly. If the appropriate experimental conditions are created, the capsular ligaments are the "primary" restraint to the anterior drawer test at 90°.

Interpretation. In a positive test, abnormal anteromedial subluxation of the medial tibial plateau can be sensed as the medial plateau translates forward in relation to the lateral plateau. With this motion, the examiner feels the medial anterior tibial rim become more prominent than the femoral condyle. Abnormal translation of the tibia on the femur signifies disruption of the medial capsular structures. This test is specific for anteromedial rotatory instability. It is not specific for anterior cruciate ligament disruption; however, with a pronounced positive result, there is likely to be damage to the anterior cruciate ligament as well.

Posterior Drawer Test at 90° in External Tibial Rotation

Rationale. In any position of knee flexion, the posterior cruciate ligament resists straight posterior translation. However, because the posterior cruciate ligament is located medially in the intercondylar notch, the lateral tibial plateau can drop back relative to the medial plateau with a coupled posterior translation–external axial rotation when the arcuate complex is damaged. This can occur even with an intact posterior cruciate ligament. At 90° of knee flexion, the arcuate complex is isolated to resist this motion, and placing the tibia in external rotation puts more tension on these ligaments.

Interpretation. In a positive test, abnormal posterolateral subluxation of the lateral tibial plateau can be sensed as the lateral plateau translates posteriorly with an axial rotatory component. With this motion, the examiner can feel the lateral anterior tibial rim drop out or become less prominent than the femoral condyle. Abnormal translation of the tibia on the femur signifies disruption of the lateral capsular structures. This test is specific for posterolateral rotatory instability. The anterior cruciate ligament may be damaged but it is usually intact in a knee with isolated posterolateral instability.

Anterior Drawer Test at 90° in Neutral Tibial Rotation

The anterior drawer and posterior drawer tests are performed simultaneously.

Rationale. The contribution of the capsular versus the cruciate ligaments to resisting anterior tibial translation was discussed earlier in the description of the anterior drawer test at 90° in external tibial rotation. Because external rotation of the tibia tensions the medial capsular ligaments to resist anterior tibial translation and tensions the posterior capsular ligaments to resist posterior tibial translation, internal rotation of the tibia would be expected to do the opposite. In fact, internal tibial rotation wraps the bundles of the posterior cruciate ligament to the point where, as with hyperextension of the knee, the posterior cruciate becomes the primary restraint to any abnormal motion. A compromise of sorts is to place the tibia in neutral rotation. In this position, the lateral capsular ligaments are relatively more tensioned than the medial capsular ligaments, but the bundles of the posterior cruciate ligament have not begun to wrap.

Interpretation. In a positive test, an abnormal anterolateral subluxation of the lateral tibial plateau can be sensed as the lateral plateau translates forward more than the medial plateau with axial rotation. With this motion, the examiner can feel the lateral anterior tibial rim become more prominent than the femoral condyle. Abnormal translation of the tibia on the femur signifies disruption of the lateral capsular structures. This test is specific for anterolateral rotatory instability. It is not specific for anterior cruciate ligament disruption, but, with a markedly positive test, the anterior cruciate ligament may be injured as well.

Posterior Drawer Test at 90° in Neutral Tibial Rotation

Rationale. In this test position, the posterior cruciate ligament becomes the primary resister of posterior translation. However, for translation of significant magnitude to occur, the posterior capsular ligaments must also fail. In our clinical experience, these ligaments fail simultaneously.

Interpretation. In a positive test, abnormal posterior translation of the tibial plateau can be sensed without any rotatory component. With this motion, the examiner can feel the anterior tibial rim drop back or become less prominent than the femoral condyle. The amount of translation of the tibia on the femur signifies disruption of the posterior capsular structures and of the posterior cruciate ligament if the translation is great enough. This test is specific for straight posterior instability. The anterior cruciate ligament may or may not be damaged. The test is not specific for anterior cruciate ligament disruption, but, with a pronounced positive result, there is likely to be damage to the anterior cruciate ligament as well.

Anterior Drawer Test at 90° in Internal Tibial Rotation

The anterior drawer and posterior drawer tests are performed simultaneously.

Rationale. Internal rotation of the tibia wraps and tensions the bundles of the posterior cruciate ligament. A positive test indicates posterior cruciate ligament disruption; however, for a translation of significant magnitude to occur, the anterior cruciate ligament and medial and lateral capsular ligaments must fail as well.

Interpretation. In a positive test, abnormal anterior translation of the tibial plateau can be sensed without any rotatory component. With this motion, the examiner can feel the anterior tibial rim become more prominent than the femoral condyles. The amount of translation of the tibia on the femur signifies disruption of medial and lateral capsular structures, the anterior cruciate ligament, and the posterior cruciate ligament if the translation is great enough (as described in the section on conventions). This test is specific for straight anterior instability.

Posterior Drawer Test at 90° in Internal Tibial Rotation

Rationale. While the neutral position of the tibia makes the posterior cruciate ligament the primary resister of posterior translation, internal rotation in a knee with a partially disrupted posterior cruciate ligament may diminish or extinguish the posterior drawer sign. This is due to the wrapping and tensioning of the elongated bundles. Should this occur (i.e., a positive posterior drawer test in neutral that diminishes with internal rotation), one may deduce that the posterior cruciate ligament remains partially intact.

Interpretation. Interpretation is essentially the same as that for the posterior drawer test in neutral.

Pivot Shift-Jerk Test

Rationale. Anterolateral subluxation of the lateral tibial plateau at or near extension can be resisted only by intact superficial and deep fibers of the iliotibial tract. Because of the medial position of the posterior cruciate ligament in the joint, the contribution of joint contact forces in the lateral compartment is negligible, particularly with adduction stress. The capsular ligaments are relatively relaxed as well. There is much confusion about the specificity of the pivot shift-jerk test for anterior cruciate ligament disruption. The confusion arises because the test detects anterolateral instability, and the incidence of associated anterior cruciate ligament disruption is very high in knees with anterolateral instability. Furthermore, if the anterior cruciate ligament is damaged, as with other tests described, the anterior translation component of the anterolateral subluxation is greater and the test result "feels" more positive to the examiner. Because it is possible to have a positive pivot shift-jerk test with an intact anterior cruciate ligament, this position should be thought of primarily as isolating the fibers of the iliotibial tract to resist anterolateral subluxation of the lateral tibial plateau.

Interpretation. The subluxation is usually occult. The reduction is dramatic and can best be perceived through the hand exerting the valgus stress. In more severe cases, it can be seen as well. A positive result indicates disruption of the iliotibial tract fibers and is specific for anterolateral rotatory instability.

Reverse Pivot Shift

Rationale. This test, along with the posterior drawer test at 90° in external tibial rotation, isolates the arcuate complex to resist posterolateral subluxation.

Interpretation. The perception, as with the jerk test, is of a sudden and dramatic joint dislocation. This finding indicates damage to the arcuate complex and is specific for posterolateral rotatory instability.

A CLASSIFICATION OF STRAIGHT AND ROTATORY KNEE LIGAMENT INSTABILITIES

Each instability is initially classified as acute or chronic, a distinction derived solely from the injury history. The distinction has important therapeutic considerations. Acute injuries are those that have occurred within 2 weeks. There is actually a subacute period lasting 2 to 4 weeks, and chronic injuries are at least 1 month old. For practical purposes, any injury older than 2 weeks is treated as a chronic one because it is at approximately that point that an acute repair of capsular ligaments can no longer be done and, if anything, a reconstructive procedure must be undertaken.

The classification has two broad categories: straight and rotatory instabilities (Fig. 72–3), depending on whether the posterior cruciate ligament is intact. If the posterior cruciate is disrupted to the point of being nonfunctional, the instability is straight (without a significant coupled rotation). If the posterior cruciate ligament is functional, the instability is rotatory, and instability classification is based on which capsular ligaments are disrupted (Fig. 72–4). While this is not exactly biomechanically accurate, for practical clinical purposes we accept the posterior cruciate ligament as the center of axial rotation for the proximal tibia.

By now, it should have become apparent that there are three pathologic axial rotations of the proximal tibia—anteromedial, anterolateral, and posterolateral subluxation of the lateral tibial plateau (Fig. 72–5). As noted before, posteromedial subluxation cannot occur because with an intact posterior cruciate ligament, the instability is prevented. When the posterior cruciate ligament is torn, rotation is uncoupled and the instability is straight.

Straight Instabilities

Straight instabilities occur when the posterior cruciate ligament is nonfunctional. Therefore, if tests that isolate the ligament are positive, the instability is straight. There are two uncoupled translations, anterior and posterior, and two uncoupled coronal plane rotations, abduction and adduction. Straight instabilities are usually due to severe injury because a powerful force is necessary to disrupt the posterior cruciate ligament. Massive associated trauma to the capsular ligaments should be anticipated.

STRAIGHT MEDIAL INSTABILITY AT 0° ABDUCTION

In straight medial instability, the abduction stress test at 0° of flexion is positive. The abduction stress test at 30° is also positive; however, at 0° a positive test signifies a straight instability. If Lachman's test is positive, the anterior cruciate ligament is torn as well.

With straight medial instability, there is uncoupled coronal plane rotation and the knee hinges open medially. The posterior cruciate ligament and all medial capsular ligaments are torn (Fig. 72–6). The anterior cruciate ligament is usually torn as well.

STRAIGHT LATERAL INSTABILITY AT 0° ADDUCTION

In straight lateral instability, the adduction stress test at 0° of flexion is positive. The adduction stress test at 30° is also positive; however, at 0° of flexion, a positive test signifies a straight instability. If Lachman's test is positive, the anterior cruciate ligament is torn as well.

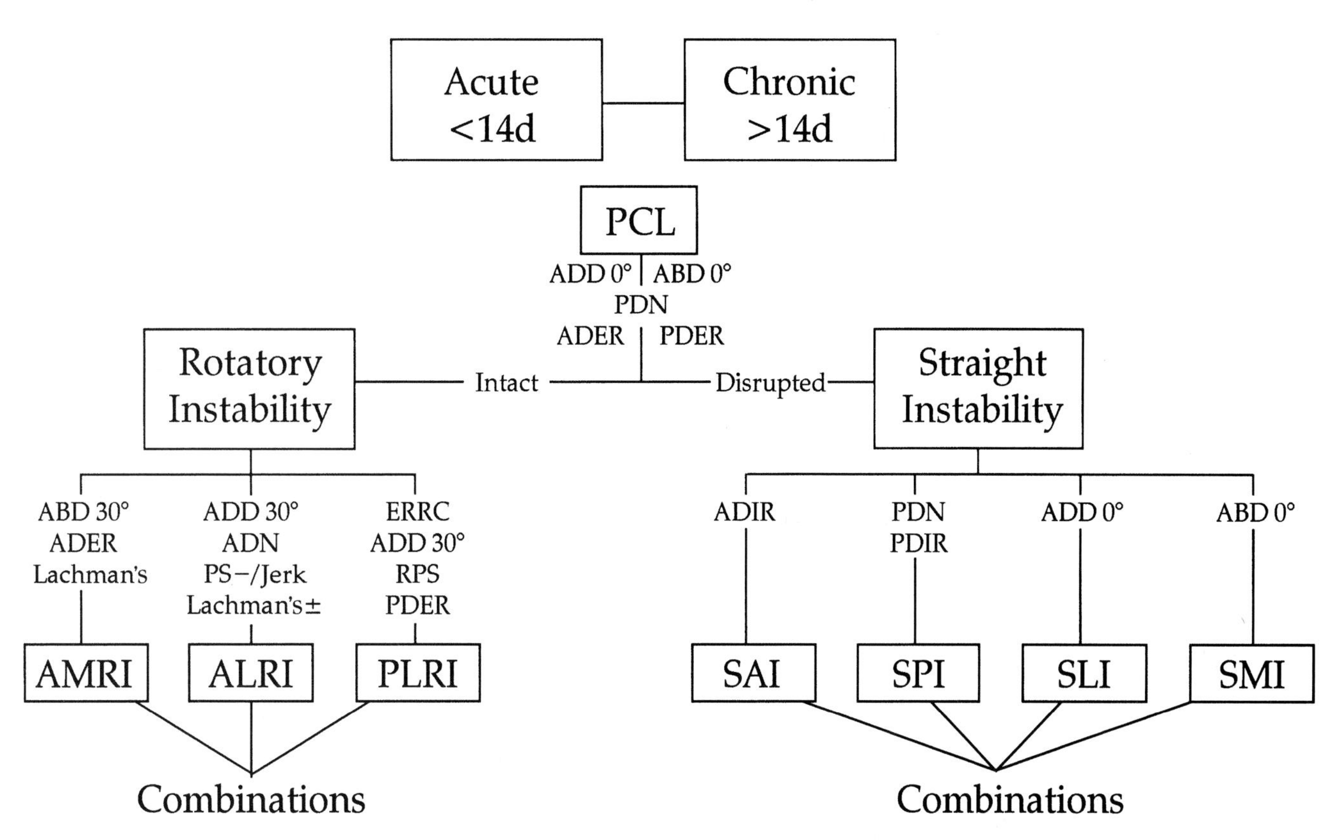

Fig. 72–3. Acute and chronic injuries are classified as straight or rotatory, according to the function of the posterior cruciate ligament.

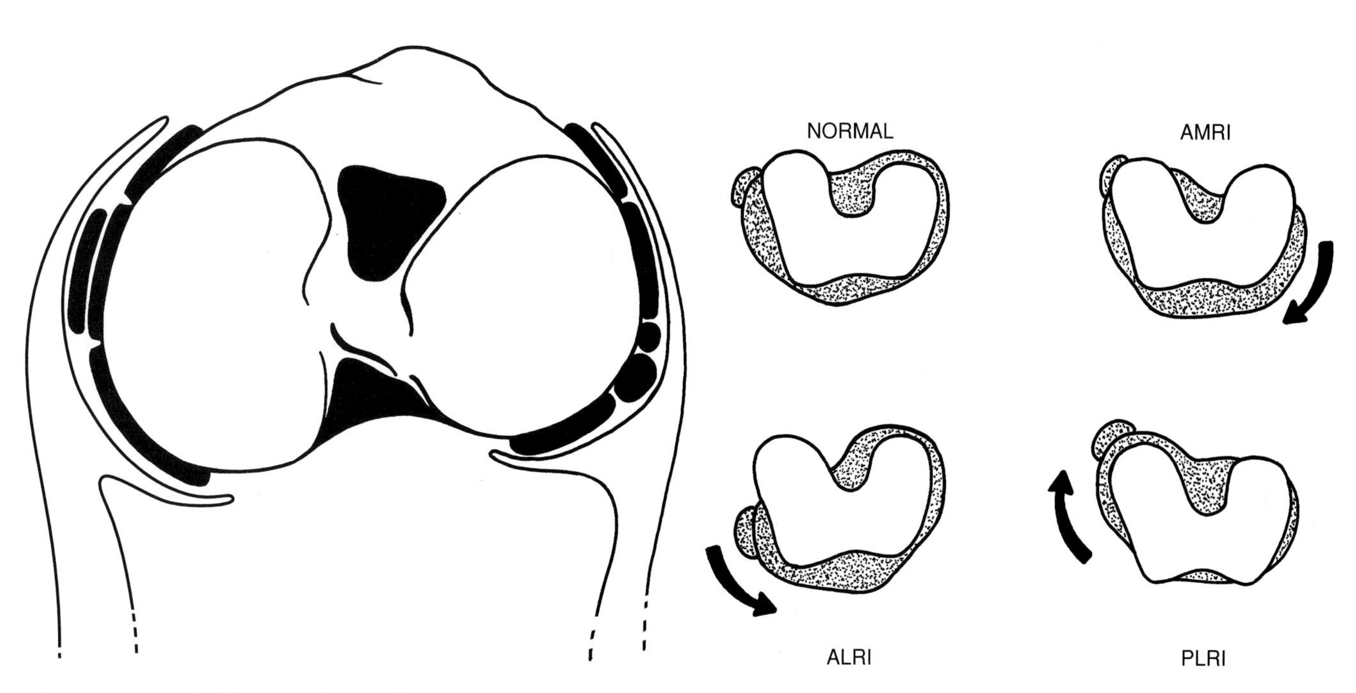

Fig. 72–4. Capsular ligaments that are the major determinants of rotatory instability.

Fig. 72–5. The three rotatory subluxations (tibia on femur) are anteromedial (AMRI), anterolateral (ALRI), and posterolateral (PLRI).

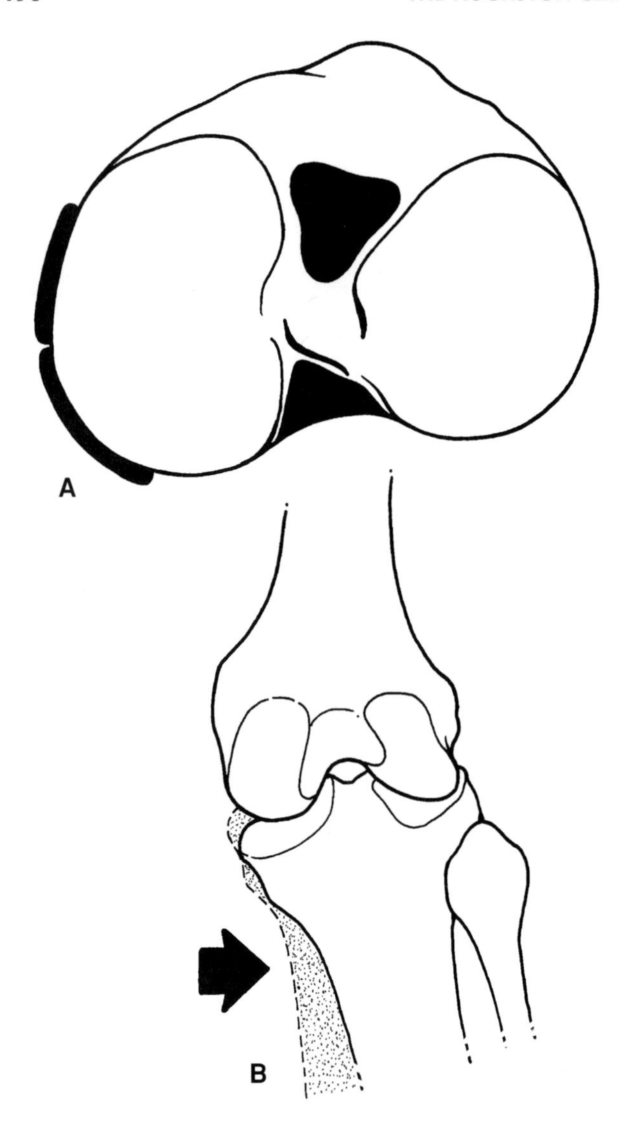

Fig. 72–6. *(A)* Straight medial instability is caused by damage to these ligaments. *(B)* Medial opening; arrow indicates the direction of stress application to perform the test.

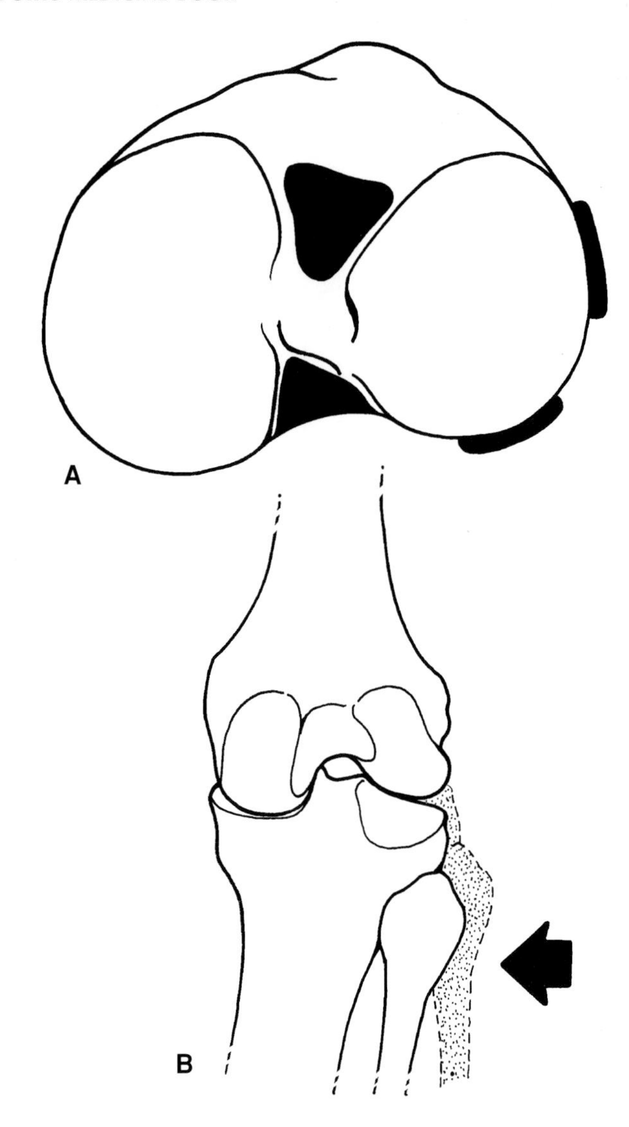

Fig. 72–7. *(A)* Straight lateral instability is caused by damage to these ligaments. *(B)* Lateral opening; arrow indicates the direction of stress application to perform the test.

With straight lateral instability, there is uncoupled coronal plane rotation and the knee hinges open laterally. The posterior cruciate ligament and all lateral capsular ligaments are torn (Fig. 72–7), and usually the anterior cruciate.

STRAIGHT ANTERIOR INSTABILITY: ANTERIOR DRAWER AT 90° FLEXION IN INTERNAL ROTATION

In straight anterior instability, the anterior drawer test at 90° of flexion in internal rotation is positive. In fact, all anterior drawer tests are positive; however, with the tibia in internal rotation, a positive test signifies straight instability.

With straight anterior instability there is uncoupled anterior translation of the tibia. No rotation occurs, indicating that the posterior cruciate ligament, anterior cruciate ligament, and all medial and lateral capsular ligaments are torn (Fig. 72–8).

It is appropriate at this point to discuss the four anterior drawer signs of tibiofemoral instability. Although the anterior drawer test at 90° is done in three rotational positions—external rotation, neutral, and internal rotation—there are four anterior drawer signs. Because combinations of rotatory instabilities are possible, anteromedial-anterolateral instability can exist. Curiously, although classified as rotatory, this instability exhibits little tibial axial rotation on the anterior drawer test. Thus, a positive anterior drawer test at 90° with the tibia in external rotation is consistent with anteromedial rotatory instability; in neutral rotation, it is consistent with anterolateral rotatory instability; and in external and neutral rotation, it is consistent with combined anteromedial and anterolateral rotatory instability. We then have two anterior drawer signs with no tibial axial rotatory component. The combined rotatory instability can be distinguished from the straight instability by a positive anterior drawer test in internal rotation as well.

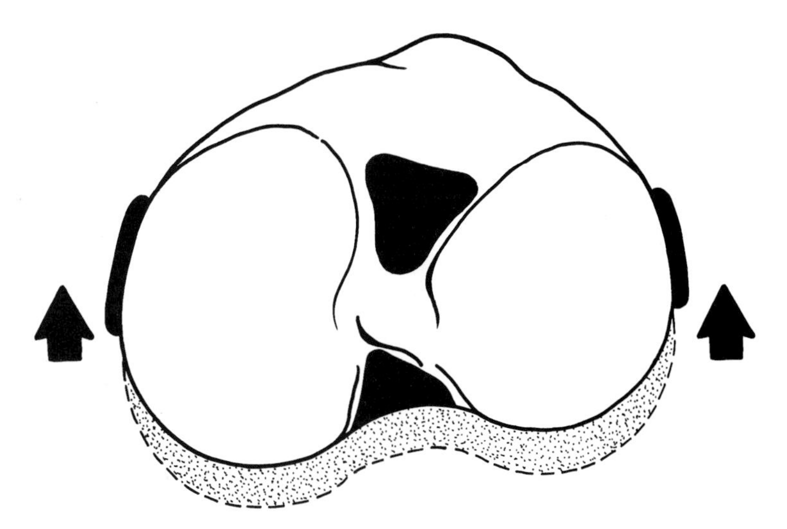

Fig. 72–8. Straight anterior instability is caused by damage to these ligaments.

STRAIGHT POSTERIOR INSTABILITY: POSTERIOR DRAWER AT 90° IN NEUTRAL POSITION

In straight posterior instability, the posterior drawer test at 90° with the tibia in neutral rotation or neutral and internal rotation is positive. In fact, all posterior drawer tests can be positive; however, a positive test in neutral or neutral and internal rotation of the tibia signifies straight instability.

With straight posterior instability there is uncoupled posterior translation of the tibia with no rotation. It is possible for the posterior cruciate ligament to have a relatively isolated tear since, during pure posterior translation with the knee in 90° of flexion, the posterior cruciate ligament fails before the posterior capsule is torn. More often, the posterior cruciate ligament, posterior oblique ligament, and arcuate complex are disrupted (Fig. 72–9). The anterior cruciate ligament must reverse orientation completely before it experiences the injury force and, therefore, it is torn in only the worst of injuries, such as dislocations.

Rotatory Instabilities

These instabilities occur when the tibia rotates about the axis of the intact posterior cruciate ligament in a direction governed by the injuries to the capsular ligaments. All tests for posterior cruciate ligament injury are negative. There are three basic classes of rotatory instability: anteromedial (AMRI), anterolateral (ALRI), and posterolateral (PLRI). In addition, any conceivable combination of these three can occur. Of the combinations, anteromedial-anterolateral rotatory instability is the most common, perhaps more common than ALRI. With regard to the three basic instabilities, the anterior cruciate ligament is rarely injured in cases of PLRI, is injured approximately 50% of the time in AMRI, and is injured 90 to 95% of the time in ALRI.

ANTEROMEDIAL ROTATORY INSTABILITY

AMRI is indicated by the combination of a positive abduction stress test at 30° (but negative at 0°) and a

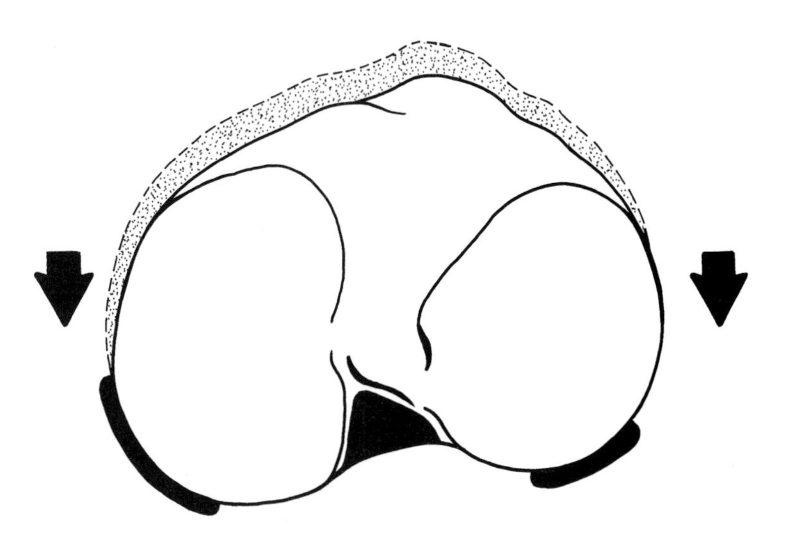

Fig. 72–9. Straight posterior instability is caused by damage to these ligaments.

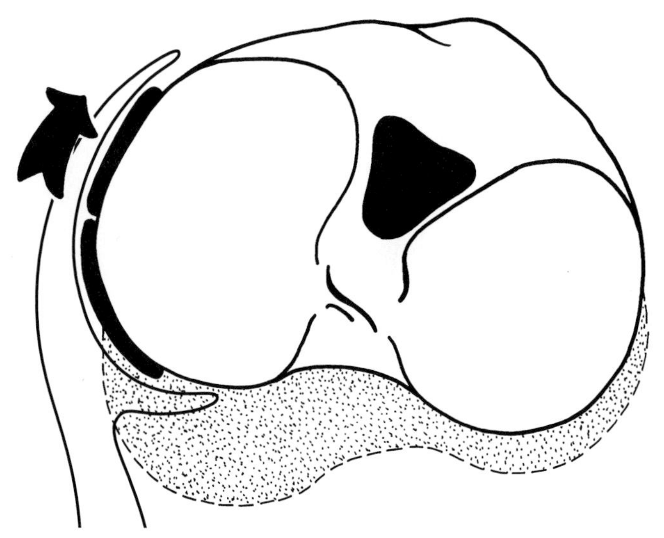

Fig. 72–10. Anteromedial rotatory instability. Arrow indicates the direction of tibial movement.

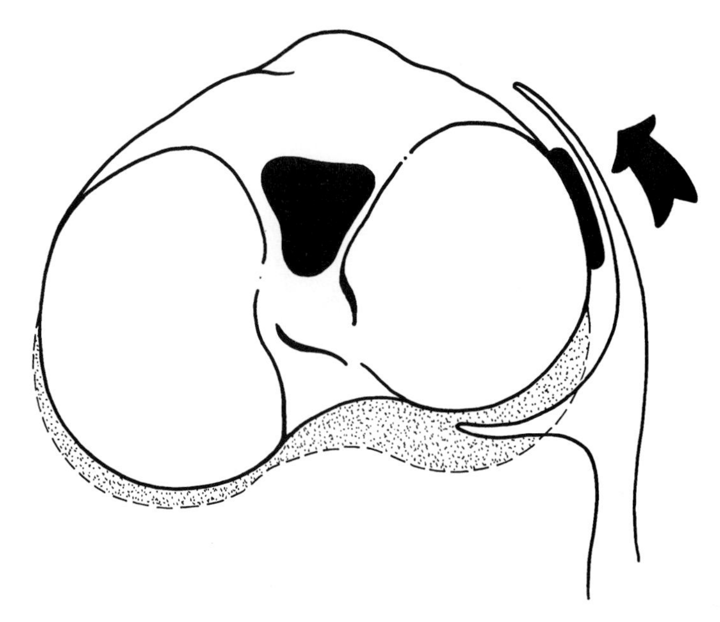

Fig. 72–11. Anterolateral rotatory instability. Arrow indicates the direction of tibial movement. Shaded area represents the iliotibial band.

positive adduction stress test at 90° in external rotation. Lachman's test is positive in about half the cases but is not a diagnostic criterion.

With AMRI, there is coupled axial rotation of the tibia with both abduction coronal plane rotation and anterior translation. The *sine qua non* of AMRI is anteromedial subluxation of the medial tibial plateau, which can occur only with disruption of the medial middle third capsular ligament, the tibial collateral ligament, and the posterior oblique ligament (Fig. 72–10). In addition, because of its attachment to these capsular structures, peripheral detachment of the medial meniscus can usually be found.

ANTEROLATERAL ROTATORY INSTABILITY

In ALRI, a positive jerk test is specific for the instability; however, the adduction stress test at 30° (but not at 0°) and anterior drawer at 90° in neutral rotation should also be positive. Lachman's test will be positive in most cases, but it is not a diagnostic prerequisite.

With ALRI, there is coupled rotation of the tibia on its axis with both adduction coronal plane rotation and anterior translation. The *sine qua non* of ALRI is anterolateral subluxation of the lateral tibial plateau, which can occur only with disruption of the lateral middle third capsular ligament, the fibular collateral ligament, and iliotibial tract fibers (Fig. 72–11). The presence of the popliteal hiatus and the morphology of the lateral meniscus and lateral compartment, as well as injury mechanisms, all contribute to the morphology of a meniscal tear. Thus, radial, flap, or complex body tears are more common than peripheral tears in the lateral meniscus.

POSTEROLATERAL ROTATORY INSTABILITY

In PLRI, the following combination of tests should be positive: the adduction stress at 30° (but negative at 0°), posterior drawer at 90° in external rotation, external rotation recurvatum, and reverse pivot shift. Lachman's test is usually negative. The adduction stress test at 30° is characteristically more accentuated in PLRI than in ALRI because of the roll-back of the tibia and the greater extent of damage to the arcuate ligament complex.

With PLRI, there is a coupled axial rotation of the tibia with both adduction coronal plane rotation and posterior translation. The *sine qua non* of PLRI is posterolateral subluxation of the lateral tibial plateau, which can occur only with disruption of the arcuate complex (Fig. 72–12).

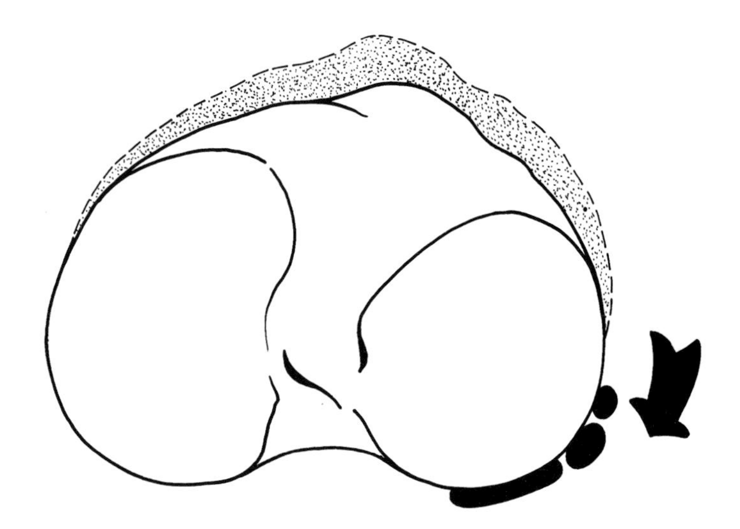

Fig. 72–12. Posterolateral rotatory instability. Arrow indicates the direction of tibial movement.

COMBINED ROTATORY INSTABILITIES

The most common combined patterns are AM-ALRI, AL-PLRI, and AM-AL-PLRI. Of these, AM-ALRI is the most common, and we suspect that it is more common than isolated ALRI. As expected, the positive tests required for the diagnosis and the injuries involved are simply combinations of those outlined for each of the isolated instabilities.

REFERENCES

1. Hughston, J. C., Andrews, J. R., Cross, M. J., and Moschi, A.: Classification of knee ligament instabilities. Part I. The medial compartment and cruciate ligaments. J. Bone Joint Surg. *58A*:159, 1976.
2. Hughston, J. C., Andrews, J. R., Cross, M. J., and Moschi, A.: Classification of knee ligament instabilities. Part II. The lateral compartment. J. Bone Joint Surg. *58A*:173, 1976.
3. Andrews, J. R., and Axe, M. J.: The classification of knee ligament instability. Orthop. Clin. North Am. *16*:69, 1985.
4. Hughston, J. C.: Knee Ligaments: Injury and Repair. St. Louis, Mosby Year-Book, 1993.
5. Butler, D. L., Noyes, F. R., and Grood, E. S.: Ligamentous restraints to anterior-posterior drawer in the human knee: A biomechanical study. J. Bone Joint Surg. *62A*:259, 1980.

SUGGESTED READINGS

Baker, C. L., Jr., Norwood, L. A., and Hughston, J. C.: Acute posterolateral rotatory instability of the knee. J. Bone Joint Surg. *65A*:614, 1983.

Brantigan, O. C., and Voshell, A. F.: The mechanics of the ligaments and menisci of the knee joint. J. Bone Joint Surg. *23*:44, 1941.

Fowler, P. J.: The classification and early diagnosis of knee joint instability. Clin. Orthop. *147*:15, 1980.

Hastings, D.: Sports related injuries of the knee and ankle. Ann. R. Col. Physicians Surgeons Can. *12*:205, 1979.

Hastings, D. E.: Knee ligament instability—a rational anatomical classification. Clin. Orthop. *208*:104, 1986.

Hsieh, H. H., and Walker, P. S.: Stabilizing mechanisms of the loaded and unloaded knee joint. J. Bone Joint Surg. *58A*:87, 1976.

Hughston, J. C., and Barrett, G. R.: Acute anteromedial rotatory instability. J. Bone Joint Surg. *65A*:145, 1983.

Hughston, J. C., and Jacobson, K. E.: Chronic posterolateral rotatory instability of the knee. J. Bone Joint Surg. *67A*:351, 1985.

Kennedy, J. C.: The Injured Adolescent Knee. Baltimore, Williams & Wilkins Co., 1979.

Kennedy, J. C., and Fowler, P. J.: Medial and anterior instability of the knee. J. Bone Joint Surg. *53A*:1257, 1971.

Marshall, J. L., and Rubin, R. M.: Knee ligament injuries—a diagnostic and therapeutic approach. Orthop. Clin. North Am. *8*:641, 1977.

Noyes, F. R., and Grood, E. S.: Classification of ligament injuries: Why an anterolateral laxity or anteromedial laxity is not a diagnostic entity. Instr. Course Lect. *36*:185, 1987.

Odensten, M., and Gillquist, J.: Functional anatomy of the anterior cruciate ligament and a rationale for reconstruction. J. Bone Joint Surg. *67A*:257, 1985.

Terry, G. C., and Hughston, J. C.: Associated joint pathology in the anterior cruciate ligament-deficient knee with emphasis on a classification system and injuries to the meniscocapsular ligament–musculotendinous unit complex. Orthop. Clin. North Am. *16*:29, 1985.

Wang, C. J., and Walker, P. S.: Rotatory laxity of the human knee joint. J. Bone Joint Surg. *56A*:161, 1974.

73

Lucien M. Rouse, Jr., Kenneth E. DeHaven, John Turba, and John M. Graham, Jr.

Anterior Cruciate Ligament Injuries

Acute Injuries

Lucien M. Rouse, Jr. and Kenneth E. DeHaven

Acute tears of the anterior cruciate ligament (ACL) are one of the most common injuries seen by sports medicine physicians. A typical scenario is this: An athlete involved in an agility sport decelerates and pivots on a planted foot. He feels a pop in the knee, falls, and is unable to continue play. Within an hour the knee swells. Radiographs taken in an emergency room that night are read as negative. After several weeks, the swelling resolves, the pain subsides, and the athlete returns to play, only to reinjure the knee when trying again to cut.

Most of those who treat athletic injuries, be they physicians, trainers, or therapists, would recognize this history as typical of an acute ACL tear, though, this injury frequently goes undiagnosed, and consequently is mismanaged. In a study by Noyes and coworkers looking at symptomatic chronic ACL tears,[1] the original treating physician made the correct diagnosis in only 6.8% of cases. It is thus incumbent upon those who treat athletic injuries on a regular basis to continue efforts to educate others in the health care professions, so that appropriate management of these patients is undertaken.

INITIAL EVALUATION

History

As in any other area of medicine, the diagnosis and management of an acute ACL injury depends on taking an accurate and complete history. The athlete can usually give a reasonably detailed account of the mechanism of injury. Most often, this involves deceleration on a planted foot, as in coming down from a rebound in basketball or cutting while running in sports such as soccer or football. Skiing is also a frequent cause of ACL tears, which can occur when the skier falls forward and catches the inside edge of the ski. This results in a combined external rotation and valgus force, with resultant combined injury to the medial collateral ligament and ACL (Fig. 73–1A). A second mechanism occurs when the skier coming down from a jump lands on one ski while leaning slightly backward. The tail of the ski hits first, causing the ski to snap down. This results in an anteriorly directed force to the tibia from the back of the rigid boot (Fig. 73–1B). A third mechanism occurs when the skier falls backward and catches the inside edge of the tail of the ski, which suddenly turns inward. This causes an internal rotation force with the knee flexed, resulting in disruption of the ACL (Fig. 73–1C).[2] Occasionally, the ACL can be torn in a hyperextension injury. This mechanism often causes injury to other ligamentous structures, including the posterior cruciate ligament and the collateral ligaments.

The majority of ACL injuries are not contact injuries; however, they can involve contact, such as a blow to the lateral aspect of the knee while the foot is planted. In evaluating a contact injury, one should be especially suspicious of associated ligament injuries, such as combined medial collateral ligament and ACL injuries.

Other factors considered in the history include whether the athlete heard or felt a "pop." Though not diagnostic, it is quite suggestive of an ACL tear. Was the athlete able to continue playing? It is unusual for an athlete to be able to participate after an acute ACL tear. A critical aspect of the history is swelling, both its extent and its timing. Although it is possible to have an acute ACL tear without developing a hemarthrosis, it is rare. This usually occurs within several hours after the injury. Conversely, traumatic hemarthrosis means the chances of at least a partial ACL tear are approximately 70%.[3,4] A history of being unable to straighten the knee

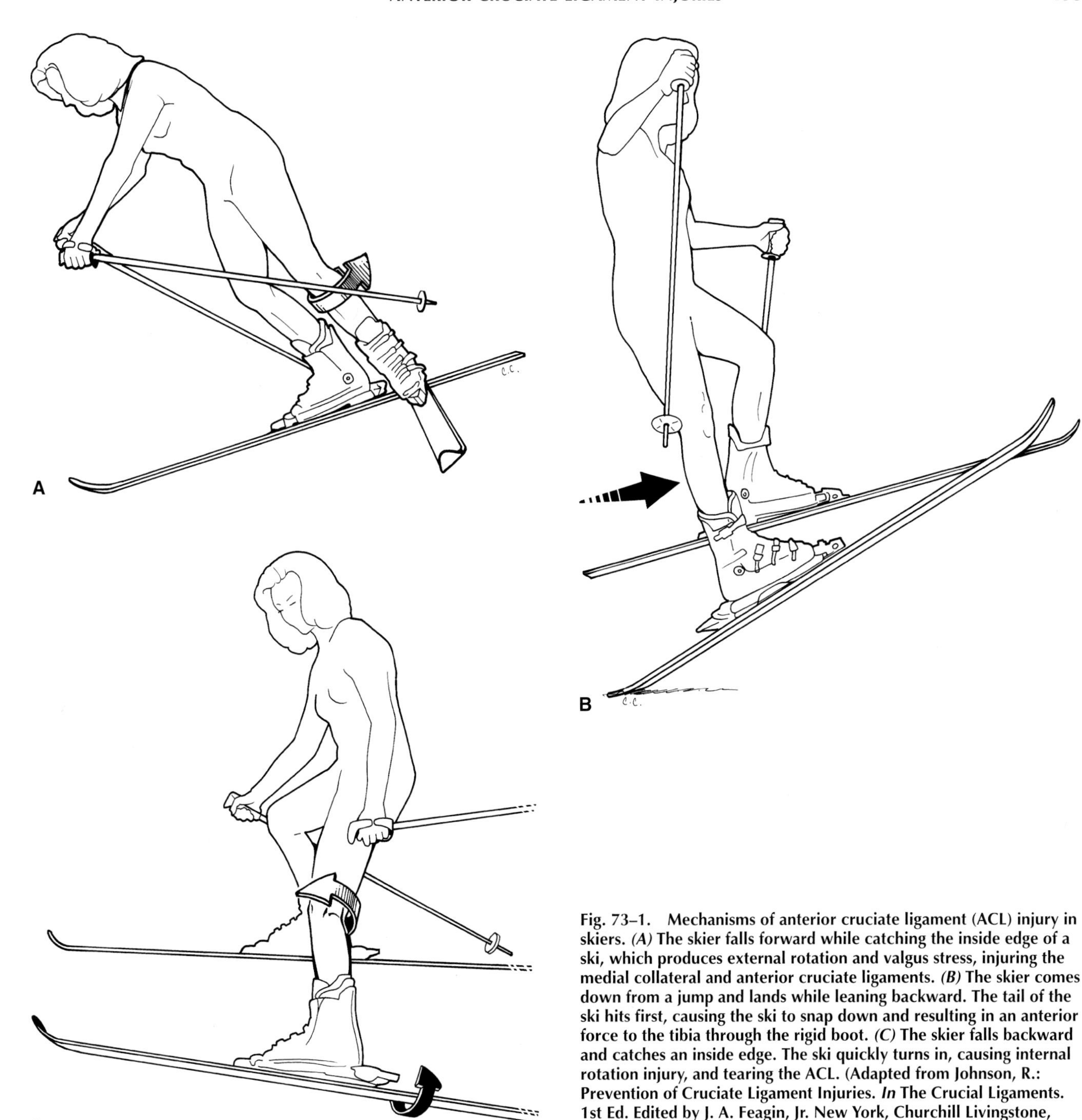

Fig. 73–1. Mechanisms of anterior cruciate ligament (ACL) injury in skiers. *(A)* The skier falls forward while catching the inside edge of a ski, which produces external rotation and valgus stress, injuring the medial collateral and anterior cruciate ligaments. *(B)* The skier comes down from a jump and lands while leaning backward. The tail of the ski hits first, causing the ski to snap down and resulting in an anterior force to the tibia through the rigid boot. *(C)* The skier falls backward and catches an inside edge. The ski quickly turns in, causing internal rotation injury, and tearing the ACL. (Adapted from Johnson, R.: Prevention of Cruciate Ligament Injuries. *In* The Crucial Ligaments. 1st Ed. Edited by J. A. Feagin, Jr. New York, Churchill Livingstone, 1988).

immediately after the injury may indicate a displaced meniscal tear.

The examiner should also inquire about previous knee injuries. Any treatment provided before presentation should be reviewed. Concomitant injuries should be assessed. Finally, many factors about the particular patient must be considered that would be important in decisions regarding treatment, such as age, activity level, goals, and socioeconomic considerations. These are reviewed in further detail later.

Physical Examination

A review of the physical examination of the knee is presented in Chapter 64. Specific aspects of the examination that relate to an ACL injury are reviewed. The examiner should first evaluate the opposite knee. There is significant individual variability in joint laxity; however, the difference in two legs of a given individual is usually minimal.[5] Examination of the contralateral knee allows for determination of what is normal for that patient. An assessment of that individual's normal range of motion is obtained. The examiner can also use this time to evaluate the patient's apprehension and ability to relax.

Examination of the injured knee begins with determination of an effusion. Again, a traumatic hemarthrosis should alert the examiner to the probability of an ACL tear. Range of motion is compared with that of the opposite leg. Limitations in flexion can be due to the effusion. Limits in extension, especially when present from the moment of injury, raise concern of possible locking due to a meniscal tear. Impingement of the remaining tibial stump of the ACL in extension can also cause an extension block.

The most important single test for assessing an ACL tear is Lachman's test (Fig. 73–2).[6] Both the amount of anterior tibial translation and the presence or absence of an end point are important parts of this examination. The patient's relaxation is critical to the accuracy of this test. The physician can assist in this by calmly reassuring the patient and by performing each part of the examination as gently as possible. Demonstrating a positive Lachman effect to the patient and family, as compared with the normal opposite side, can also help them understand the injury.

Other physical tests for an ACL tear should be performed, such as an anterior drawer test, tests for anteromedial rotatory instability (AMRI), and pivot shift examination. These are reviewed in Chapter 64, but they have been shown to be far less sensitive than Lachman's in detecting acute ACL tears.[6] A pivot shift test is often very difficult in the acute setting because of the patient's inability to relax adequately. If this is the case, multiple attempts to perform a pivot shift test should not be made.

The examiner should make a careful assessment of associated injuries. The incidence of significant meniscal tears is greater than 50% with an acute ACL tear.[3,4] Additional ligamentous and capsular injuries can occur and should be carefully evaluated in the examination. Associated injuries can significantly increase the risk of functional instability and future degeneration.

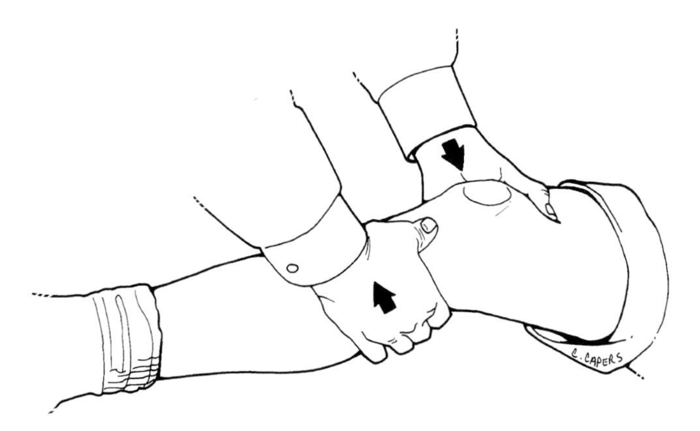

Fig. 73–2. Lachman's test, the most reliable one for an anterior cruciate ligament tear, should be performed with the patient as relaxed as possible, and findings should be compared with those from the opposite limb.

A proper clinical evaluation by an experienced examiner is usually all that is needed for the diagnosis of an ACL tear. Occasionally, the patient is unable to relax enough for an adequate examination. In this case, repeating the examination after several days to a week often allows a more thorough evaluation. Magnetic resonance imaging (MRI) should rarely be required to diagnose an ACL tear.

Diagnostic Studies

Plain radiographs of the knee should always be obtained, to rule out associated bone injuries. Standard views include anteroposterior, lateral, tunnel, and patellar profile views. Radiographic findings can occasionally include an osteochondral fracture. A small avulsion fragment from the proximal tibial insertion of the capsule may be seen in the anteroposterior view (Fig. 73–3). This lateral capsular sign, or Segond's fracture, should alert the examiner to the presence, not only of an ACL tear, but of associated lateral ligamentous and capsular injuries. Occasionally, the injury involves avulsion of the ACL insertion into the intercondylar tibial eminence. This is more prevalent in skeletally immature patients but it can occur in adults as well. In an adolescent, it is important to assess the status of the growth plates. Surgical reconstructions should be delayed or modified if the

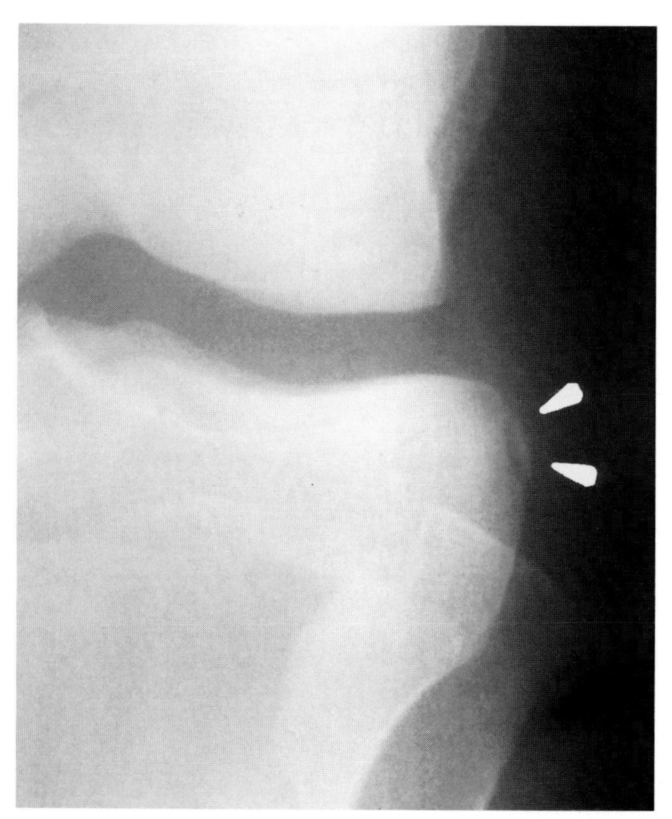

Fig. 73–3. Lateral capsular sign (Segond's fracture). Note the small bony fragment from the lateral tibia, just distal to the joint line. This represents tearing of the tibial insertion of the lateral capsule.

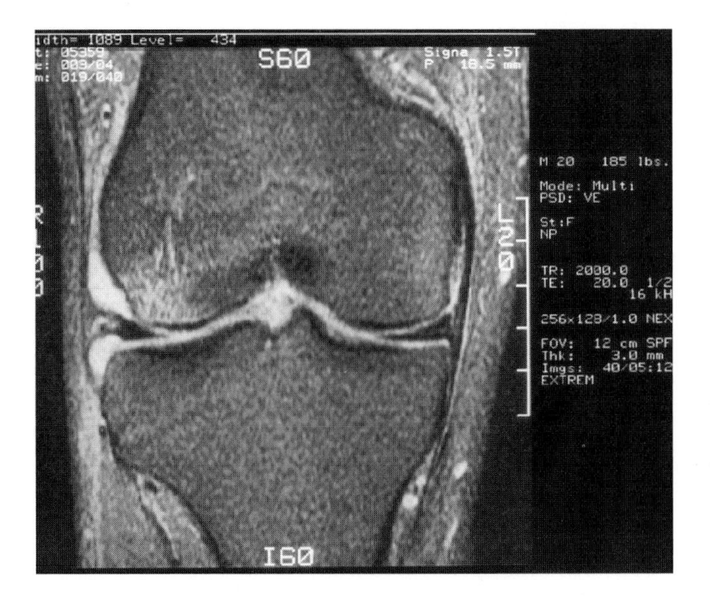

Fig. 73–4. MR image of an acute anterior cruciate ligament tear. Note increased signal intensity in the subchondral area of the lateral femoral condyle and the lateral tibial plateau. The significance of these "bone bruises" remains unclear.

patient has open growth plates. If a patellar tendon autograft is to be used for surgical reconstruction, changes in the tendon, as from Osgood-Schlatter disease or chronic patellar tendinitis, are important to recognize.

MRI is usually not necessary for the diagnosis of an ACL tear, but it can be useful for assessment of meniscal or articular cartilage injuries. A common MRI finding in acute ACL tears is the presence of increased subchondral signal in the femoral condyle or tibial plateau, especially laterally (Fig. 73–4).[7] The significance of these "bone bruises" is unclear; currently, they do not alter the treatment decisions.

If the patient opts for nonsurgical management of the ACL tear, MRI can be useful to determine the need for arthroscopic treatment of meniscus injury. For patients undergoing ACL reconstruction, the authors do not routinely perform MRI because concomitant intra-articular injury can be assessed at arthroscopy.

Instrumented ligament testing, such as a KT-1000, can be useful in the initial assessment.[5] This allows objective quantification of the amount of tibial translation. In the authors' practice, this is obtained for all acute ACL tears, though it is not necessary to make the clinical diagnosis of, or to treat, an ACL tear.

MANAGEMENT

Athletes who tear the ACL must understand that they have sustained a major injury to the knee. Multiple factors must be considered in deciding what treatment is best for each particular patient. This requires that the physician spend time not only to assess these factors but also to educate the patient about the nature of the injury and the different treatment options.

Associated injuries often influence the decision for operative or nonoperative treatment of the ACL tear. The presence of other ligament injuries often increases functional instability and often necessitates surgical treatment, not only of the ACL, but also of the associated injury. Since meniscal tears usually require surgical intervention, a peripheral tear that is amenable to repair may be the deciding factor in whether ACL reconstruction is done. There is clear evidence that the survival rate of a repaired meniscus is lower in an ACL-deficient knee.[8] Ultimately, the presence or absence of the associated injury, especially to the menisci and articular surfaces, may be the greatest influence on long-term prognosis for the patient's knee.[9]

The degree of generalized ligament laxity can also be a factor. Patients who have greater degrees of laxity on their normal side probably are at higher risk for functional instability with an ACL tear.

Age and activity level are important factors in treatment decisions. Although there continues to be controversy regarding exact treatment indications for acute ACL tears, especially isolated ones, there is general consensus regarding certain patients who represent a high-risk category for nonoperative management. Young, active patients involved in aggressive agility sports such as basketball, volleyball, football, or soccer are at high risk for reinjury if they stay in these activities.[1,10,11] "Physiologic" age and activity level are more important than chronologic age. The goals of the patient are important also.

Socioeconomic factors need to be considered. A worker involved in heavy physical labor may not be able to afford the many months of unemployment that a reconstruction may require. The patient's motivation and willingness to comply with a postoperative rehabilitation regimen are critical. Patients who are unwilling or unable to participate in their rehabilitation program should not be considered good candidates for surgical reconstruction.

The final decision about treatment should be the patient's rather than the physician's. This requires that much time be spent with the patient and family, to allow for adequate education about the nature of the injury and the advantages and disadvantages of each treatment option.

Nonoperative Management

In the management of patients with ACL tears, it is vital that the decision for nonoperative treatment does not result in no treatment. Nonoperative management must include treating associated lesions (such as meniscal tears), managing the acute phase of the injury, instituting a strengthening and functional rehabilitation program, establishing goals for return to activities, and counseling regarding sports and other activities that includes setting realistic goals.

About 50% of acute ACL tears are associated with significant meniscal injury. These meniscal tears need to be evaluated and managed appropriately. Frequently this involves diagnostic arthroscopy, with management of meniscal and other intra-articular injuries at that time.

With the advent of MRI, the necessity for diagnostic arthroscopy has been significantly decreased. If the MRI is negative for meniscal lesions, the ACL tear can usually be managed nonoperatively. Occasionally, arthroscopy will still be needed, as in the case of impingement of the residual stump of the ACL in extension. However, an examination under anesthesia and diagnostic arthroscopy should rarely be necessary to diagnose an ACL tear.

The acute phase of treatment consists of management of the effusion, regaining range of motion and muscle control, and restoring a normal gait pattern. Ideally, emergency treatment should commence on the field at the time of injury. This consists of icing the knee to minimize the initial bleeding and effusion. Also, an examination at this point is often more accurate because the patient is more relaxed. Once hemarthrosis and protective muscle guarding have developed, it is often much more difficult for the athlete to relax fully. Commonly, patients are seen several hours after the injury in an emergency room, or in the physician's office during the next couple of days. At that time there is usually significant hemarthrosis, and, again, the examination may be somewhat limited because of pain and limited motion. Usually, it is still possible to obtain enough relaxation to confirm a positive Lachman's test.

Use of a knee immobilizer is appropriate in this early phase, but it should not be worn full time and should not be used over the long term. Range of motion exercises should be instituted early. Ice should be used early and frequently, to help minimize and decrease the effusion.

It is important to re-establish a normal range of motion. Initial flexion gains are often easiest to obtain by having the patient sit with the thigh supported on a bench and the feet off the floor (Fig. 73–5A); the uninjured leg can then be used to provide active assisted motion. This allows for better relaxation, and usually the first 90° of flexion are rapidly regained in this position. Just as in an ACL reconstruction, it is also important to gain full extension early. Lying prone with the leg suspended over the edge of the table allows the patient to relax and more easily extend the knee (Fig. 73–5B). Failure to regain extension should cause the physician to suspect a possible displaced meniscal tear or impingement of the remaining tibial stump of the ACL. These concerns should be addressed and may require arthroscopic evaluation and treatment. As the initial pain of the injury resolves, patellar mobilization exercises are added. The usual course is for normal range of motion to be regained over several weeks. Although much less common than with surgical treatment, arthrofibrosis, with its excessive formation of intra-articular fibrotic tissue and resultant loss of motion, can occasionally occur. This must be addressed, just as with a surgically treated patient.

Initial strengthening exercises are begun, with the goals of re-establishing muscle control and establishing a hamstring-dominant gait. Athletes are taught isometric cocontractions with the knee at 45° of flexion. Hamstring-strengthening progressive resistance exercises are allowed throughout a full range of motion. Quadriceps-strengthening progressive resistance exercises are limited from 90° to 60°, to decrease anterior translation forces associated with full-arc extensions.

Closed–kinetic chain exercises, such as stationary bicycling, are allowed as soon as adequate range of motion is achieved. As pain and motor control improve, the athlete progresses to more vigorous closed-chain exercises, such as half squats, leg presses, and stair climbers. The closed-chain exercises cause less powerful anterior translation forces. These principles are discussed further in Chapter 79.

Crutches are used initially and a three-point gait pattern is taught, with progression of weight bearing allowed as tolerated. If the patient has a mechanical block to extension, this should be addressed before initi-

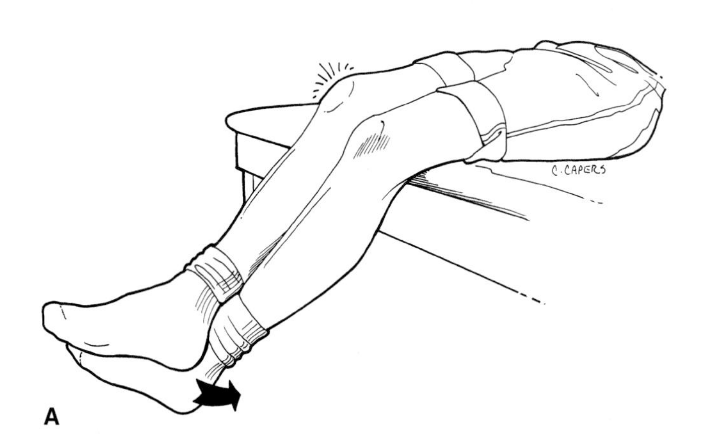

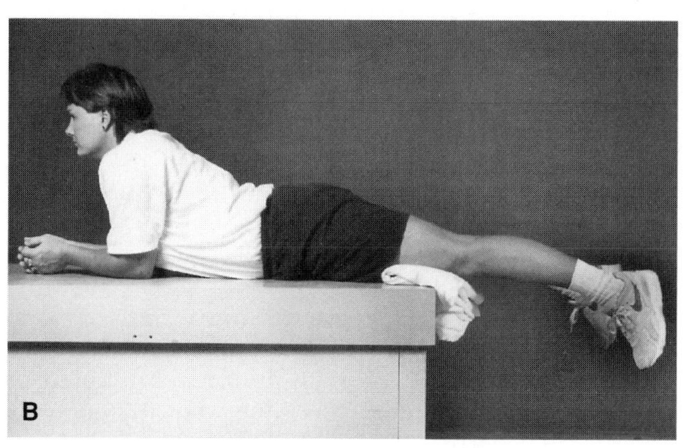

Fig. 73–5. *(A)* **Sitting position used to help regain initial flexion. The uninjured leg is used to provide active assisted support. Generally, the patient is able to relax in this position and to regain flexion more rapidly.** *(B)* **Prone position for regaining extension. This position again allows for more complete relaxation.**

ating full weight bearing. Biofeedback is used to reinforce use of hamstrings during initial gait training. When the patient is able to ambulate comfortably without a limp, the crutches are discontinued.

The functional phase of rehabilitation generally begins around 3 months, but the timing depends on meeting certain goals. Motion should have been regained with full extension and flexion approaching normal. The effusion should be resolved. Strength gains should be progressing, with hamstrings strength close (preferably 90% or better) to normal and quadriceps strength greater than 70% of normal. Next, the patient is fitted with a brace. An interval running program is initiated, beginning with straight-ahead jogging, progressing to increasing speeds, and finally to agility exercises. Balancing drills are emphasized to improve proprioception. Sport-specific drills are added. Strengthening exercises are continued.

The athlete is usually allowed to return to sport when the functional rehabilitation program has been successfully completed. Ideally, the athlete should have regained hamstrings strength equal to that in the uninjured knee, and quadriceps strength more than 80% of normal. We feel that return to sport guidelines should not be based solely on numbers obtained from an isokinetic machine but rather on an overall functional assessment of the patient's strength, endurance, and agility.

Throughout the rehabilitation process, continual counseling by all involved with the treatment of the athlete, including the physician, therapist, and trainer, should be emphasized. For athletes who elected nonoperative management of an ACL tear, we usually advise against returning to high-risk sports such as basketball, volleyball, soccer, and football. Although it is clearly possible to return to these types of sports with nonoperative management, the risk of reinjury with damage to the menisci or articular surfaces is significant.[1,10,11]

Operative Management

Patients who are athletically active, especially those involved with aggressive agility sports who want to try to maintain their active lifestyle, are usually managed with operative treatment of ACL tears. There are many factors to consider, including timing of surgery, evaluation and management of concomitant injuries, repair or reconstruction options, rehabilitation programs, and establishing realistic goals and expectations.

The timing of surgery has emerged as an important factor. In the past, surgery was often performed as soon as possible after the injury, often within the first week or two. Certainly, when primary repair of the ligament was attempted, this was necessary, but several recent studies have demonstrated a higher incidence of postoperative arthrofibrosis in patients treated within the first 3 weeks of injury.[12,13] Arthrofibrosis, one of the most difficult and prevalent complications of ACL surgery, is proliferation of intra-articular fibrous tissue, which can undergo cartilaginous, and even bony, metaplasia. This tissue limits range of motion, entraps the patella, and significantly compromises the results of the reconstruction. Treatment often involves surgical excision of this tissue and extensive postoperative rehabilitation. Even patients who are treated "successfully" and regain their motion still have more functional compromise than those who do not develop this difficult complication.[14] A delay in surgery of 3 weeks, or more, to allow range of motion to be regained and to allow the acute phase of the injury to resolve, appears to decrease the risk of arthrofibrosis.[12,13]

There are other factors, however, that influence the timing of surgery. The presence of multiple ligament injuries usually requires earlier surgical intervention, because repair of collateral and capsular ligaments is compromised by significant delays in surgery. Thus, patients who have combined ACL and collateral ligament injuries, especially those involving the posteromedial or posterolateral capsular ligaments, are usually treated with earlier surgical intervention. Preoperatively, every attempt is made to regain maximum range of motion, and the patient immediately begins postoperative range of motion exercises.

The presence of an extension block preoperatively also creates a difficult management decision. This problem is most often caused by a displaced meniscal tear, but the tibial stump of the ACL can also cause pain and impingement with extension. Though it is desirable to regain full extension before proceeding with ACL reconstruction, the patient should not be allowed to continue for prolonged periods with a significant extension block. The treatment options at that point consist of performing arthroscopy and addressing the cause of the mechanical block and then proceeding at that time with the reconstruction or performing a two-stage procedure. With the latter option, the mechanical block is treated arthroscopically. The patient continues with a rehabilitation program, and, when range of motion is regained, the reconstruction is performed. Although this involves two surgical procedures, a significant lack of extension preoperatively does increase the risk of postoperative arthrofibrosis with its associated difficulties.[12] The authors believe that each case should be evaluated individually considering all factors, including the degree of extension block, the overall pain level and the amount of swelling in the patient's knee, and individual patient preferences.

At the time of surgery a careful examination under anesthesia is performed and findings are compared with those from the opposite knee. This represents a unique opportunity to obtain a completely relaxed examination. Frequently with an acute injury, this is the first opportunity to demonstrate a pivot shift. Other ligament injuries should be carefully ruled out. Findings of this examination should be accurately documented. Diagnostic arthroscopy is then performed. Associated injuries, such as meniscal tears, articular surface injuries, and even osteochondral fractures, are frequently found. Treatment of these injuries is outlined in other chapters.

Surgical Options

Treatment options for the ACL tear include repair, repair with augmentation, extra-articular reconstruction, and intra-articular reconstruction. Primary repair of the ACL is seldom performed because of the high associated failure rate. A possible exception would be a patient with a tibial spine avulsion fracture, which can be repaired either open or arthroscopically (Fig. 73–6). The ACL should still be carefully evaluated since it can often be torn extensively in its substance in addition to the fracture, which could compromise the final stability.

Primary repair with augmentation remains a viable treatment option. Most often this involves use of the semitendinosus tendon to augment the repair. Though this procedure has met with good success, the authors think the approach has several disadvantages. Even with high-resolution MRI, it is difficult to assess the quality of the remaining ligament. Primary repair is most successful when the ligament has been torn from its femoral attachment without extensive intrasubstance tearing. This cannot be reliably determined without arthroscopic visualization, which can also be inconclusive. If the ligament is indeed found to be unsuitable for repair, primary reconstruction would then be elected. However, ideally, repair should be performed early after the injury, preferably within the first week or two. Thus, if a reconstruction is necessary, this would place the patient at some increased risk of arthrofibrosis or require a second anesthesia later. It is therefore our usual practice to delay the surgery, as outlined above, and proceed with primary reconstruction. One possible exception would be for pediatric or adolescent patients who have open growth plates and significant growth remaining and for whom surgical treatment is felt to be indicated.

Reconstruction options include autograft, allograft, and use of synthetic grafts. Synthetic grafts have resulted in unacceptably high failure rates with longterm followup. They are generally indicated only for salvage of a failed reconstruction, and the authors prefer other options even in that setting. They are definitely not indicated with a primary ACL reconstruction, except perhaps on an investigational basis.

The use of autograft versus allograft remains quite controversial. It is our preference to use autograft in a primary reconstruction. Though other graft sources have been used, currently the usual choices are the central third of the patellar tendon, the semitendinosus tendon or gracilis tendon, or both. The usual graft source in our practice is the central third of the patellar tendon.

There are many techniques of ACL reconstruction. The consistency and accuracy with which a surgeon performs reconstruction is more important than what tech-

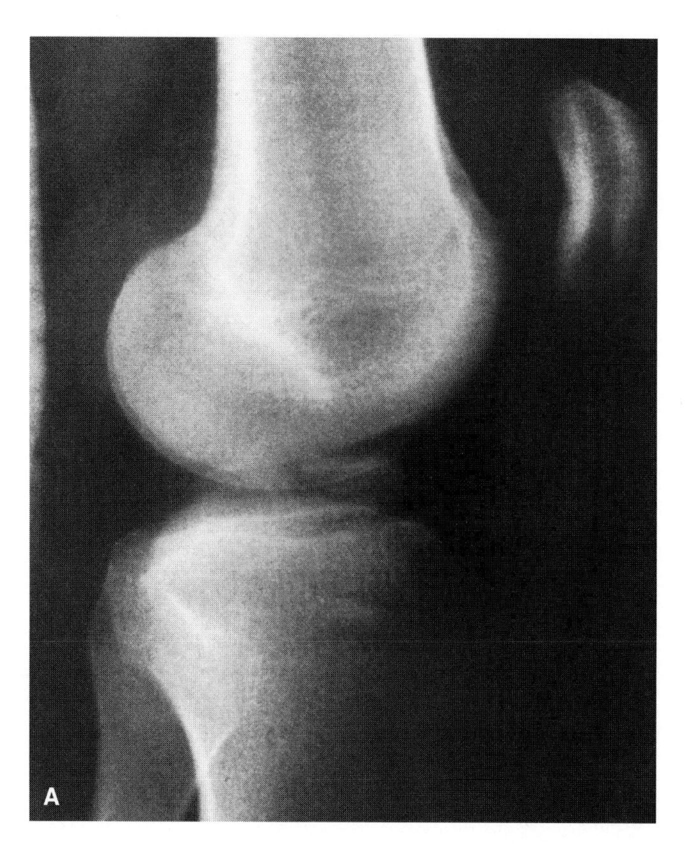

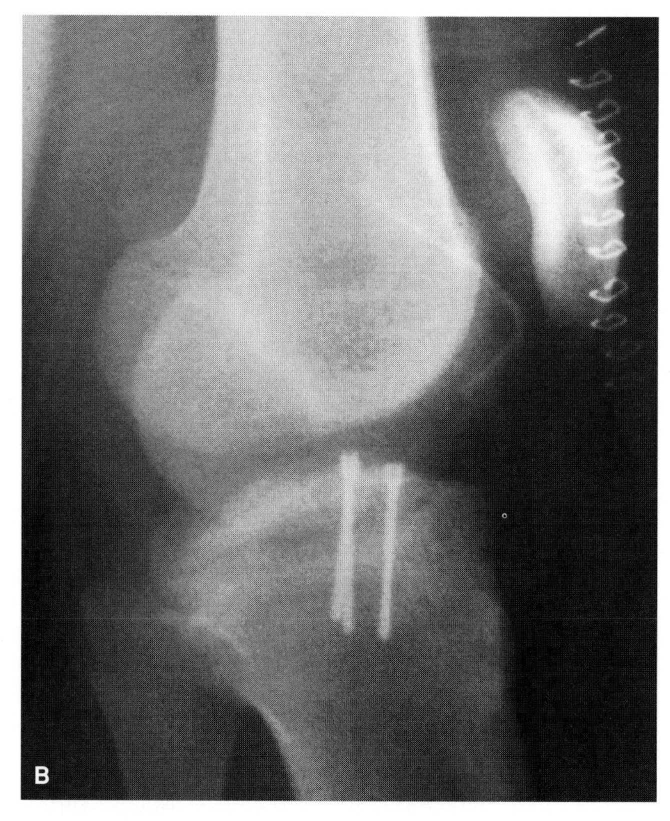

Fig. 73–6. Avulsion fracture of the tibial insertion of the anterior cruciate ligament. *(A)* Preoperative lateral radiographic view. *(B)* Postoperative radiograph after arthroscopically assisted reduction and fixation. In this case tearing of the ligament was not significant, but this is not always the case.

nique is used. The graft should be placed in an anatomic position. This requires adequate visualization, either arthroscopically or directly. Inaccurate placement of the graft results in abnormal strain, which either stretches out the graft or constrains the knee. Fixation of the graft should be adequate to allow early range of motion in the rehabilitation program.

Partial Anterior Cruciate Ligament Tears

Although they are less common than complete disruption, partial tears of the ACL can present difficult treatment decisions. Two important prognostic factors to consider in treating these injuries are what percentage of the ligament is torn and whether any instability is present.[15]

Tears involving less than 25% of the substance of the ligament have been shown rarely to progress to significant objective or functional instability, whereas tears involving more than 50% of the substance carry a high risk of progression. Even fairly mild increases in anterior laxity, as compared with the opposite side, indicate stretching (intrasubstance tearing) of the remaining ligament and are more likely to progress. Also, just like complete ACL tears, a significant percentage of partial ACL tears are associated with other significant intra-articular injuries that should be addressed.

The authors' management of a partial ACL tear involves, first, careful assessment of any increase in anterior tibial translation on Lachman's examination, as compared with the opposite side. This is sometimes best determined during an examination under anesthesia. The pivot shift examination is also compared with the opposite side. The amount of tearing of the ligament is then carefully assessed at arthroscopy. If the tear involves less than 50% of the ligament, the increased excursion on Lachman's test is less than 4 mm with a good end point, and the pivot shift examination is negative or trace, the patient is treated with the nonoperative protocol outlined earlier. If the tear involves more than 50% of the ligament, there is an increase in excursion on the Lachman test of more than 4 mm, or there is a positive pivot shift, the patient is treated for a complete tear.

POSTOPERATIVE REHABILITATION

The postoperative rehabilitation program is critical to the success of ACL reconstruction. Significant changes have been seen in postoperative management over the last decade,[12,16] evolving from immobilization in flexion to immediate range of motion with emphasis on obtaining full extension. Although the details of specific postoperative protocols vary, certain general principles apply.

Immediately after surgery, the patient is placed in a hinged brace, which is locked in full extension. The brace is intermittently unlocked, beginning on postoperative day 1, to allow flexion. Range of motion should be re-established as soon as possible. In our practice, we have found the use of an indwelling epidural catheter to be useful for the first postoperative day, to help patients initiate range of motion with less pain. Full terminal extension is emphasized, and the patient is encouraged to try to get to 90° of flexion within the first couple of days. The same techniques outlined in the section on nonoperative management are useful for surgical patients.

It is important to re-establish motor control of both the quadriceps and hamstrings in the initial postoperative period. We have found biofeedback techniques to be very useful for this. When adequate motor control has been demonstrated, weight bearing is initiated. With the brace locked in full extension, the patient is allowed to progress to full weight bearing. As motor control improves, walking is begun with the brace unlocked. This is initiated under a therapist's supervision, using biofeedback to establish a hamstrings-dominant gait pattern.

Strengthening exercises progress on a schedule similar to the nonoperative protocol. Stationary biking is instituted once adequate range of motion has been established. Other closed-chain exercises are added as strength and motor control improve. Progressive resistance exercises are begun within the first couple of weeks, using light weights. Hamstrings-resisted exercises are performed throughout a full range of motion, and quadriceps exercises are done in a limited arc from 90° to 60°.

Progression to functional rehabilitation depends on an adequate clinical picture, including restoration of range of motion, adequate muscle control and strength, and resolution of effusion. We think it is important for the patient to pursue a gradual progression of activities and for specific goals to be outlined for each patient. Although guidelines for progression can be given, the athlete needs to understand that there may be temporary setbacks and that progress has to be individualized. Return to sport is predicated, not only on adequate strength returns but also on successful completion of the functional rehabilitation program, including specific drills for the sport.

The time course for activity progression and return to sports is controversial. Return to full activity has been achieved as early as 4 months in some programs.[15] We remain concerned about the strength of the graft at that early time. Studies looking at strength to failure of the graft obviously cannot be done in humans, but biomechanical studies in animal models show considerable drop in graft strength over the first 6 weeks, with gradual improvement over a year. The average time for return to full sports for our patients is 9 months. Some return earlier if they have met their rehabilitation goals and have a specific reason for doing so.

The use of a functional ACL brace is also controversial. Certainly, if the reconstruction has been successful, a brace is not necessary to prevent anterior tibial translation, nor is it mechanically capable of substituting for an ACL at high functional loads. However, these braces are effective in resisting varus and valgus loads and hyperextension; this may provide protection from contact-induced reinjury, especially a blow to the lateral aspect of the knee. It is our practice to recommend these braces for sports for the first year after surgery; further use is based on patient preferences.

EXPECTATIONS AND LONGTERM OUTLOOK

Over the last two decades a tremendous amount of study and effort has been devoted to the ACL. As a result significant advances have been made in the diagnosis and management of this potentially disabling injury. Advancements in knowledge of the anatomy and biomechanics of the ACL have resulted in significant improvements in surgical techniques. Grafts of adequate strength, placed in an anatomic position and with adequate fixation, have allowed more aggressive rehabilitation, including full range of motion, while preserving the integrity of the reconstruction. The complication of arthrofibrosis is now more appreciated and has been significantly decreased with changes in the timing of surgery and in postoperative rehabilitation protocols.[12,13,16]

Emphasis on meniscal repairs, rather than meniscectomy, has resulted in the salvage of many menisci, which should decrease longterm arthritic changes.[8,9] Encouraging results concerning return to sports and restoration of stability have been reported,[16–18] with success rates better than 90% based on these criteria.

It is important not to define "success" just as return to sports or stable KT-1000 tests. Some athletes return to sports but at a less intensive level or at the same level but with some persistence of symptoms. Arthritic symptoms from loss of the menisci or articular surface injuries may not become apparent for years. The best reconstruction does not recreate a normal ACL or undo other associated injuries. It is still not known what the longterm results of these reconstructions, combined with current rehabilitation programs, will be, especially with regard to the eventual development of degenerative arthritis. The improved retention of the menisci and restoration of stability hold promise for better longterm results; though it remains to be seen whether the incidence of degenerative arthritis is, indeed, decreased 10 and 20 years after an injury, which will be the ultimate measure of success.

REFERENCES

1. Noyes, F. R., Mooar, P. A., Matthews, D. S., and Butler, D. L.: The symptomatic anterior cruciate-deficient knee. Part I: The longterm functional disability in athletically active individuals. J. Bone Joint Surg. *65A:*154, 1983.
2. Johnson, R. J.: Prevention of cruciate ligament injuries. *In* The Crucial Ligaments. 1st Ed. Edited by J. A. Feagin, Jr. New York, Churchill Livingstone, 1988.
3. DeHaven, K. E.: Diagnosis of acute knee injuries with hemarthrosis. Am. J. Sports. Med. *8:*9, 1980.
4. Noyes, F. R., Bassett, R. W., Grood, E. S., and Butler, D. L.: Arthroscopy in acute traumatic hemarthrosis of the knee. J. Bone Joint Surg. *62A:*687, 1980.
5. Daniel, D. M., et al.: Instrumented measurement of anterior laxity of the knee. J. Bone Joint Surg. *67A:*720, 1985.
6. DeHaven, K. E.: Evaluation of the acutely injured knee. *In* Arthroscopy: Diagnostic and Surgical Practice. Edited by S. Ward Casscells. Philadelphia, Lea & Febiger, 1984.
7. Rosen, M. A., Jackson, D. W., and Berger, P. E.: Occult osseous lesions documented by magnetic resonance imaging associated with anterior cruciate ligament ruptures. Arthroscopy, *7:*45, 1991.
8. DeHaven, K. E., Black, K. P., and Griffiths, H. J.: Open meniscus repair: Technique and two to nine year results. Am. J. Sports Med. *17:*788, 1989.
9. Lynch, M. A., Henning, C. E., and Glick, K. R., Jr.: Knee joint surface changes: Long-term follow-up meniscus tear treatment in stable anterior cruciate ligament reconstructions. Clin. Orthop. *172:*148, 1983.
10. Noyes, F. R., Matthews, D. S., Mooar, P. A., and Grood, E. S.: The symptomatic anterior cruciate–deficient knee: Part II: The results of rehabilitation, activity modification, and counseling on functional disability. J. Bone Joint Surg. *65A:*163, 1983.
11. Anderson, C., Odensten, M., Good, L., and Gillquist, J.: Surgical or nonsurgical treatment of acute rupture of the anterior cruciate ligament. J. Bone Joint Surg. *71A:*965, 1989.
12. Cosgarea, A. J., Sebastianelli, W. J., and DeHaven, K. E.: Prevention of arthrofibrosis following ACL reconstruction using one-third patellar tendon autograft. Am. J. Sports Med. (In press).
13. Harner, C. D., et al.: Loss of motion after anterior cruciate ligament reconstruction. Am. J. Sports Med. *20:*499, 1992.
14. Cosgarea, A. J., DeHaven, K. E., and Lovelock, J. E.: The surgical treatment of arthrofibrosis of the knee. Am. J. Sports Med. (In press).
15. Noyes, F. R., Mooar, L. A., Moorman, C. T. III, and McGinniss, G. H.: Partial tears of the anterior cruciate ligament. J. Bone Joint Surg. *71B:*825, 1989.
16. Shelbourne, K. D., and Nitz, P.: Accelerated rehabilitation after anterior cruciate ligament reconstruction. Am. J. Sports Med. *18:*292, 1990.
17. Clancy, W. G., Jr., Ray, J. M., and Zoltan, D. J.: Acute tears of the anterior cruciate ligament: Surgical versus conservative treatment. J. Bone Joint Surg. *70A:*1483, 1988.
18. Moran, D. J., and Andrews, J. R.: Arthroscopically assisted ACL reconstruction using patellar tendon autograft: Results after two years. Orthop. Trans. *15:*742, 1991.

Chronic Injuries

John Turba and John M. Graham, Jr.

Since ACL tears are often missed or dismissed by the patient as a knee sprain, orthopedists see more and more patients with chronic ACL injuries. A *chronic* lesion is defined as one that has been present 6 weeks or more, and by that time there is no chance for a primary repair. Because such patients are living with an unstable knee, specific problems may develop that lead them to seek medical attention.

Fred Allman made the statement, "The rupture of the anterior cruciate ligament is the beginning of the end in the athlete." We have to accept that athletic patients, as a rule, are highly motivated and will return to sporting activity no matter what we tell them. It is our job, therefore, to correct the instability and slow down the inevitable traumatic changes that will occur in these knees. It is also our job as physicians not to allow these types of knees to progress to a degenerative state, but to repair them before the loss of both menisci and the onset of the traumatic changes.

The term *anterior cruciate–deficient knee* is not synonymous with *chronic instability*. Opinions still vary about whether an isolated ACL tear (which is so rare as to be nonexistent) causes degenerative changes in the knee. The majority of ACL-tear patients have multiple injuries and usually exhibit rotatory instability patterns (see Chapter 72). Therefore, surgical treatment of these unstable knees often involves the repair or reconstruction of several structures.

HISTORY AND PHYSICAL EXAMINATION

Patients with a chronic ACL injury usually present complaining of giving way episodes and a general feeling of instability in the knee. They can typically recount an initial injury that was treated conservatively. The physical examination is outlined in previous chapters. The symptoms of instability should alert the examiner to the presence of ligament injury, and the injury should be classified as indicated by the outcome of specific physical tests.

The rotatory instabilities are defined as anteromedial, anterolateral, and posterolateral. Chronic instability has at least an anteromedial and an anterolateral component, and it may be combined with posterolateral rotatory instability. If one does not correct all components of rotatory instability according to the anatomic pathology, this approach will fail.

Anteromedial instability is defined by the anterior drawer test, done with the tibia in neutral and externally rotated positions. If the drawer tests in both external rotation and neutral position produce the same amount of excessive anterior translation of the tibia, the injury is basically confined to the posterior oblique ligament. If the drawer test in external rotation is increased 2 to 3 mm as compared with the anterior drawer in neutral, the anteromedial instability is moderately severe and other structures are injured as well.

With AMRI, the posterior oblique ligament is injured in both its tibial and its capsular arms, and the capsular arm of the semimembranosus tendon has been either attenuated or torn free. The vastus medialis obliquus (VMO) component can also be involved. The origin of the VMO at the medial femoral condyle can be ruptured free. This can lead to some very insidious patellofemoral problems.

Anterolateral rotatory instability is diagnosed by the presence of a pivot shift, or as we term it, *a positive jerk test*. With chronic instability, this is generally a 2+ or 3+ grade.

Posterolateral rotatory instability is diagnosed by having a positive posterolateral drawer, positive external rotation recurvatum test, and positive adduction stress at 30°. The patient with posterolateral instability can be diagnosed as having only one type of rotatory instability or combinations of any, even all three.

Meniscal tears and chondral lesions are often associated in athletes with a chronic ACL tear. Some of these injuries may have occurred at the time of the original trauma, whereas others may develop because of repeated episodes of giving way.

Delayed radiographic changes have been reported in unstable knees 2 to 10 years after injury[1,2]: osteophyte formation, flattening of the femoral condyles, medial joint narrowing, and osteoarthritis.

TREATMENT

Treatment of a patient with a chronic ACL injury must be individualized to best address the specific problem. Age, activity level, patient expectations, degree of initial injury, and accompanying factors such as degree of arthritis must be taken into account. Young people who place great demands on their knees and have repeated episodes of giving way despite bracing are best served with reconstruction. Older, more sedentary patients whose instability is less pronounced may need only nonoperative treatment.[3–5]

Essential to the issue of treatment of ACL injury is proper selection of surgical patients. Many patients respond well to nonoperative treatment. This includes restoration of full range of motion and strengthening of the involved extremity. Satisfactory muscle strength is more difficult to achieve in a patient with a chronic injury than in one with an acute injury because atrophy may have developed. In patients treated successfully (i.e., if functional instability is eliminated with rehabilitation), minimal operative intervention may be required. This may include arthroscopy for persistent mechanical symptoms such as locking or catching or persistent joint line pain or effusion. Partial meniscectomy, meniscal repair, synovectomy, or débridement of the ACL stump may assist the overall rehabilitation process and actually obviate operative stabilization.

Selecting patients for surgical stabilization is a complex, multifactorial process, especially those with chronic instability.[4,5] Many of the same criteria used to evaluate surgical candidates with acute injuries apply, but secondary instability, muscle atrophy, and arthritic changes figure in the decision-making process. Patients with symptomatic functional instability with repeated effusions and giving way despite bracing and an adequate trial of rehabilitation are candidates for stabilization. Injuries to the menisci and chondral surfaces associated with ACL tears, the age of the patient, and the degree of instability must be considered in evaluating the possibility of surgery. Activity level and the patient's expectations for return to sport warrant consideration as well and may be the single most important factor.[6]

Extra-Articular Reconstruction

For patients with anteromedial instability in which the external rotation drawer test result is equivalent to that of the neutral anterior drawer test, the injury is basically confined to the posterior oblique ligament. The ligament is attenuated at both its tibial and its capsular arms. This injury can be repaired by reconstructing both the tibial and the capsular arms, along with advancement of the tibial arm onto the tibial collateral ligament (Fig. 73–7). If the patient with AMRI has an

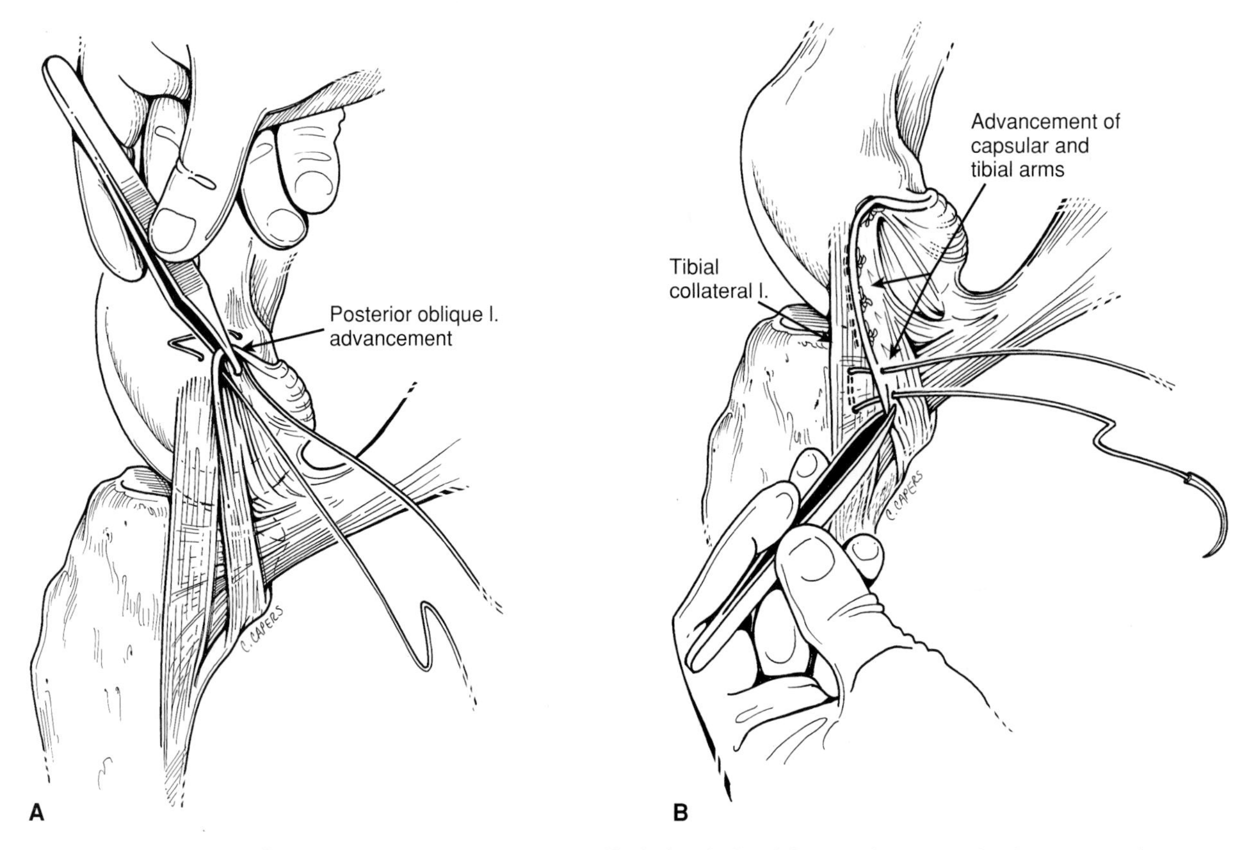

Fig. 73–7. Extra-articular repair for AMRI. Reconstruction of both the tibial and the capsular arms with advancement of the tibial arm onto the tibial collateral ligament.

external rotation drawer result 2 to 3 mm greater than that of the neutral anterior drawer test, the injury pattern generally falls into one of two categories. In both cases, the posterior oblique ligament is injured, both in its tibial and its capsular arms, but the capsular arm of the semimembranosus tendon may be involved and can be either attenuated or torn free. If the capsular arm of the semimembranosus is involved, the posterior oblique ligament will have to be reconstructed as described above, and then, having recognized the injury to the capsular arm of the semimembranosus tendon, that will have to be reconstructed as well. This reconstruction requires intimate knowledge of the anatomy of the semimembranosus tendon and dissecting it free so that it can be brought anterior and distal and sutured to the posterior oblique ligament to reconstruct this particular ligamentous component.

If both the tibial and the capsular arms of the posterior oblique ligament are avulsed from the tibial metaphysis, the status of the meniscus can make a difference in the treatment approach. If the patient previously had a complete meniscectomy, the posterior oblique ligament insertion into the tibial metaphysis anterior to the sheath of the direct arm of the semimembranosus tendon is visible. There is also a component of attenuation with the posterior oblique ligament. It is necessary to decorticate the tibial metaphysis to a base of bleeding bone and repair the ligament to the bone. After this step has been completed, one must reconstruct the posterior oblique ligament in the standard fashion. Any injury to the capsular arm of the semimembranosus tendon must be reconstructed as well. If the medial meniscus is intact, the situation is more difficult because the anatomy is not exposed. When one explores the tibial attachment of the posterior oblique ligament, there is a space of approximately 5 mm between the inferior border of the meniscus and the superior border of the attachment (Fig. 73–8A). One must probe this area carefully and, if amorphous tissue is encountered, this must be repaired. After the tibial metaphysis is repaired (Fig. 73–8B), the meniscal rim is reapproximated using No. 00 chromic sutures and the reconstruction of the posterior oblique ligament is carried out. The extent depends on the pathologic anatomy. If the patient with AMRI has a positive external rotation drawer and increased abduction with stress testing at 30°, the tibial collateral ligament should be reinforced with the sartorius muscle.

When the VMO component is present in the patient with AMRI—meaning that the origin of the VMO at the medial femoral condyle has ruptured free—the repair can be made by freshening the undersurface of the VMO along with the periosteum. The suture can be passed through the VMO and periosteum and then back to the VMO and sutured down. In the more severe cases, the angled drill hole technique should be used.

The extra-articular approach to the patient with anterolateral instability is directed at reconstruction of

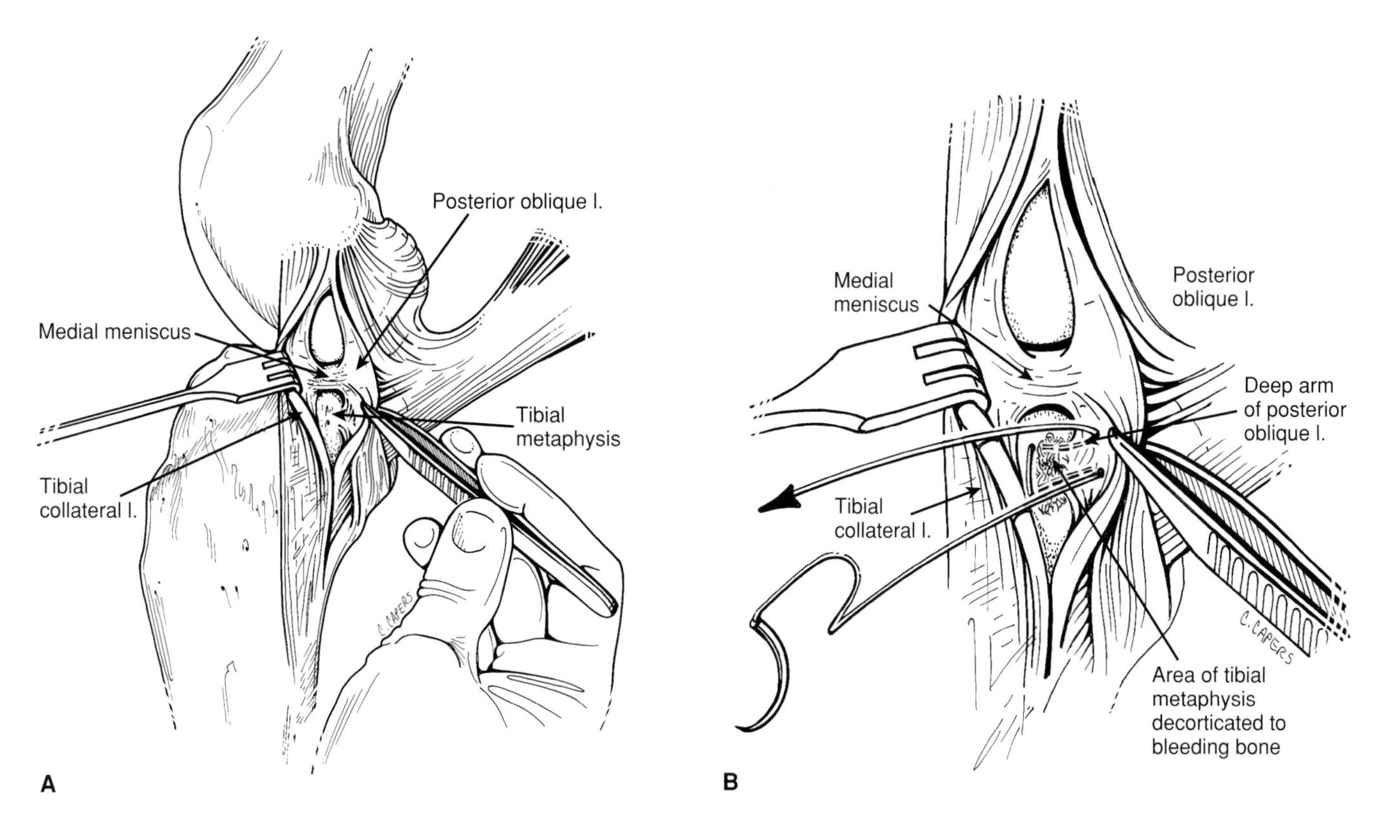

Fig. 73–8. Repair of the posterior oblique ligament to the tibial metaphysis.

the lateral middle third capsule, reconstruction of the iliotibial tract, and transfer of the long head of the biceps tendon into the reconstructed tract. Regarding dynamic transfer of the biceps, there are those who will assert that this has no function, but in athletes, the muscle becomes hypertrophic and in some can be extremely prominent, which indicates that it does have some function.

Posterolateral rotatory instability is extremely variable. If a posterolateral component is missed, anterolateral reconstruction only makes it worse. The physician must be careful and re-examine the contralateral knee, because in recurvatum there can be a posterolateral catch or jerk that can be misinterpreted as a positive anterolateral jerk. With experience, these two are easily distinguished. One should not reconstruct the posterolateral component unless there is a positive external rotation recurvatum or greater than a 1+ posterolateral drawer test. If the lateral meniscus is absent and there is a 2- to 3-mm opening with adduction stress, the posterolateral component should be reconstructed. The athlete without a meniscus will feel the 2- to 3-mm opening when cutting, whereas with the meniscus the opening is not felt.

Intra-Articular Reconstruction

For an active patient with chronic functional instability, especially with concomitant secondary instability, degenerative changes, or meniscal damage, intra-articular reconstruction warrants consideration. With technical advances, improved fixation techniques, and advanced rehabilitation, results are consistently good in the hands of experienced surgeons.

Autograft

Autogenous bone–patellar tendon–bone graft is likely the most popular technique. Popularized initially in the early 1980s by Clancy, this involves harvesting the central third of the patellar tendon with bone plugs from the inferior pole of the patella and the tibial tubercle.[7] This is usually accomplished through a single anterior longitudinal incision, preserving the peritenon (Fig. 73–9), harvesting the graft with bone plugs, and performing the reconstruction with arthroscopic assistance.[8,9] The single-incision technique involves interference screw fixation on the femur (Fig. 73–10) and interference screw or staple fixation to the tibia.[10] A double-incision technique may involve either interference fixation or use of a bicortical post on which to secure the sutures affixed to the graft. Advantages of this technique include the strength of the ligament, strong fixation with early consolidation of the bone plugs, and no concern about disease transmission. Disadvantages include donor site morbidity, including pain at the patellofemoral joint, and mechanical problems in addition to increased operative time because of the graft harvest.[11] Though repeat harvest of the central

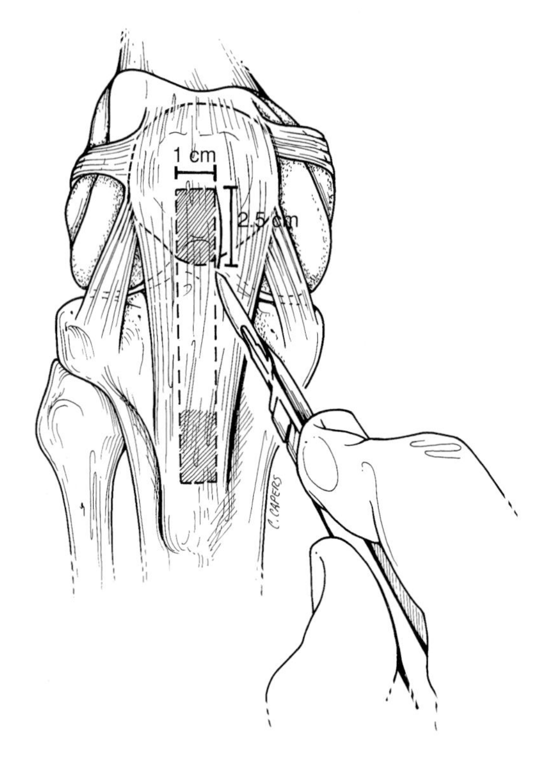

Fig. 73–9. Harvest of the central third patellar tendon graft through a single incision.

third of the patellar tendon has been reported for revision cases, graft strength and size are best in the primary reconstruction.

Hamstrings tendons (often semitendinosus and gracilis) have been used with success in chronic ACL reconstruction.[12] Harvesting the graft is somewhat easier and avoids potential problems with the patellofemoral joint. Several types of hamstrings substitution have been described. The one used most often involves transfer through a tibial tunnel that has a distally based stump. The tendons are routed through the knee and a femoral tunnel and then secured with either sutures or a bicortical post. Though this procedure is technically somewhat easier than a central-third patellar tendon graft, potential problems concern elongation and lack of firm fixation of the graft.

Allograft

Another alternative for intra-articular reconstruction is the cadaver allograft. Placement of the allograft and fixation of the bone plugs are identical to those for the autograft, often with a small single incision placed at the site of the tibial tunnel. Results have been promising; several successful series report minimal problems.[13,14] Anterior cruciate ligament allograft substitutes provide functional replacement for the ACL-deficient knee. Proponents cite less early morbidity as a significant advan-

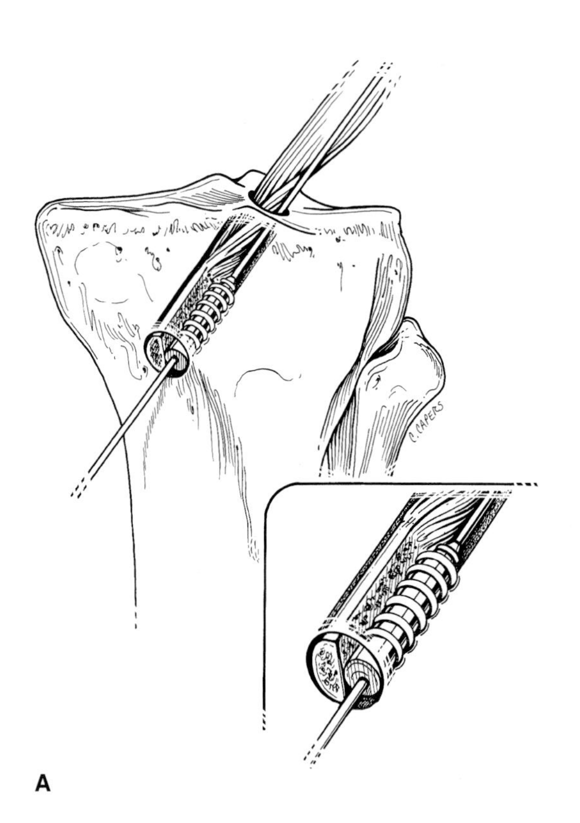

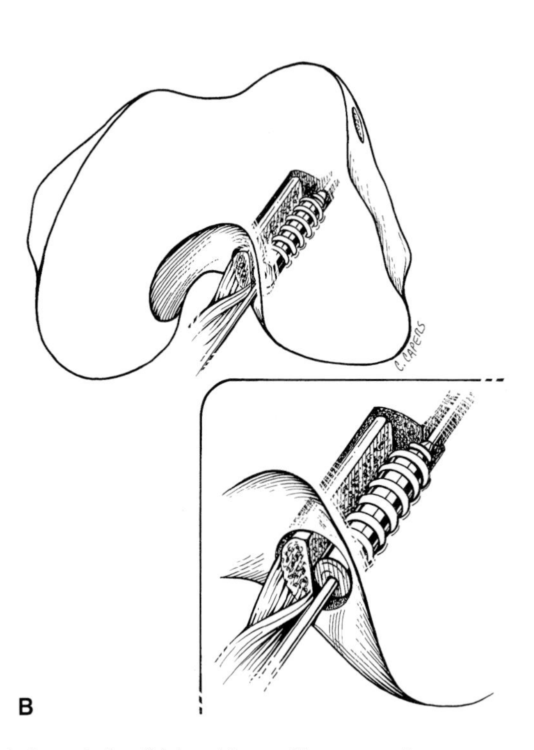

Fig. 73–10. Placement of the intra-articular graft through the tibial and femoral bone tunnels.

tage, with no trauma to the patellofemoral articulation. This decreases surgical time, minimizes surgical incisions, and may decrease time to functional return.

Longterm strength of allograft replacements may approach that of autografts, but no evidence suggests they are stronger.[15,16] Since revascularization takes longer with allograft than with autogenous bone–patellar tendon–bone graft, a longer period of protection may be warranted. Disease transmission continues to be a concern.

PROSTHETIC REPLACEMENT

Prosthetic replacement continues to be largely experimental because the ideal graft material and fixation method have yet to be developed. This approach has been accepted in varying degrees, but increased failure rates because of fatigue, synovitis, and early wear have continued to limit its general acceptance.[17]

EXTRA-ARTICULAR AUGMENTATION

The decision to proceed with extra-articular augmentation secondary to an intra-articular reconstruction depends on the surgeon's preference. The two-incision technique usually involves augmentation, though with a single anterior incision it is rarely undertaken. The degree of residual instability after intra-articular graft placement may be the principal reason for a secondary incision and additional augmentation.

REFERENCES

1. Jacobson, K.: Osteoarthritis following insufficiency of the cruciate ligaments in man. Acta Orthop. Scand. *48:*520, 1977.
2. McDaniel, W. J., and Dameron, T. B., Jr.: Untreated ruptures of the anterior cruciate ligament: A follow-up study. J. Bone Joint Surg. *62A:*696, 1980.
3. Amiel, D., Kleiner, J. B., and Akeson, W. H.: The natural history of the anterior cruciate ligament autograft of patellar tendon origin. Am. J. Sports Med. *14:*449, 1986.
4. Hughston, J. C.: Anterior cruciate deficient knee. Am. J. Sports Med. *11:*1, 1983.
5. Jackson, R. W.: The torn ACL: Natural history of untreated lesions and rationale for selective treatment. *In* The Crucial Ligaments. Edited by J. A. Feagin, Jr. New York, Churchill Livingstone, 1988.
6. Johnson, R. J., Beynnon, B. D., Nichols, C. E., and Renstrom, P. A. F. H.: Current concepts review—the treatment of injuries of the anterior cruciate ligament. J. Bone Joint Surg. *74A:*140, 1992.
7. Clancy, W. G. Jr., Nelson, D. A., Reider, B., and Narechania, R. G.: Anterior cruciate ligament reconstruction using one third of the patellar ligament augmented by extra-articular tendon transfers. J. Bone Joint Surg. *64A:*352, 1982.
8. Baker, C. L., and Graham, J.: Intraarticular ACL reconstruction using the patellar tendon: Arthroscopic technique. Orthopedics *16:*437, 1993.
9. Howe, J. G., Johnson, R. J., Kaplan, M. J., Fleming, B, and Jarvinen, M.: Anterior cruciate ligament reconstruction using quadriceps patellar tendon graft. Part I. Long-term followup. Am. J. Sports Med. *19:*447, 1991.
10. Kurosaka, M., Yoshiya, S., and Andrish, J. T.: A biomechanical comparison of different surgical techniques of graft fixation in anterior cruciate ligament reconstruction. Am. J. Sports Med. *15:*225, 1987.
11. Sachs, R. A., Daniel, D. M., Stone, M. L., and Garfein, R. F.: Patellofemoral problems after anterior cruciate ligament reconstruction. Am. J. Sports Med. *17:*760, 1989.
12. Zarins, B., and Rowe, C. R.: Combined anterior cruciate ligament reconstruction using semitendinosus tendon and iliotibial tract. J. Bone Joint Surg. *68A:*160, 1986.
13. Jackson, D. W., and Kurzweil, P. R.: Allografts in knee ligament surgery. *In* Ligament and Extensor Mechanism of the Knee: Diagnosis and Treatment. Edited by W. N. Scott. St. Louis, Mosby–Year Book, 1991.
14. Noyes, F. R., Barber, S. D., and Mangine, R. E.: Bone–patellar ligament–bone and fascia lata allografts for reconstruction of the anterior cruciate ligament. J. Bone Joint Surg. *72A:*1125, 1990.
15. Roberts, T. S., Drez, D., Jr., McCarthy, W., and Paine, R.: Anterior cruciate ligament reconstruction using freeze-dried ethylene oxide– sterilized, bone–patellar tendon–bone allografts. Two-year results in thirty-six patients. Am. J. Sports Med. *19:*35, 1991.
16. Shino, K., et al.: Reconstruction of the anterior cruciate ligament using allogeneic tendon: Long-term followup. Am. J. Sports Med., *18:*457, 1990.
17. Woods, G. A., Indelicato, P. A., and Prevot, T. J.: The Gore-Tex anterior cruciate ligament prosthesis. Two- versus three-year results. Am. J. Sports Med. *19:*48, 1991.

74 *Gene R. Barrett and Mervyn J. Cross*

Posterior Cruciate Ligament Injuries

Acute Injuries

Gene R. Barrett

The posterior cruciate ligament (PCL) is considered by many to be the principal stabilizer of the knee.[1,2] The knee is thought to rotate around this posterior and centrally located structure. Injury to the PCL is relatively uncommon as compared with the prevalence of anterior cruciate ligament (ACL) injuries, perhaps owing to the fact that it is twice as strong as the ACL. In several studies, PCL injury has been reported to account for 8 to 23% of all knee ligament injuries.[3–6] Approximately 50 to 90% of these injuries are sustained in motor vehicle accidents,[5,7] 40 to 50% occur during sports activities, and a small portion have other causes.[8–10] Injury to the PCL often occurs in people in their twenties.[9,11] This injury should always be considered in this younger age group, because of their more active lifestyle.

EXAMINATION

Mechanism of Injury

The most common cause of PCL injury is an anteroposterior blow to the tibia while the knee is flexed. This can happen several different ways. Hitting the tibia against the dashboard of an automobile when the knee is flexed is the "classic injury"; however, an "isolated" or interstitial tear of the PCL can occur when an athlete falls on a flexed knee when the foot is in plantar flexion (Fig. 74–1). This direct blow to the tibial tubercle transfers force through the PCL. The fact that the posterior capsule is lax and the PCL is tight during plantar flexion of the foot produces an isolated tear of the PCL. If the foot is dorsiflexed, the force is usually absorbed by the patella, unless the tibial tubercle strikes an elevated area such as another player's leg. An isolated PCL tear has also been observed with forced hyperflexion of the knee with the athlete's foot in dorsiflexion.[12]

A fourth mechanism of this injury is unexpected, sudden hyperextension of the knee. If the knee is forced into 30° of extension, the posterior capsule is torn, and next, the PCL; the ACL is usually torn also. Rotational forces with associated valgus or varus stress have also been described as mechanisms for PCL tears. In these

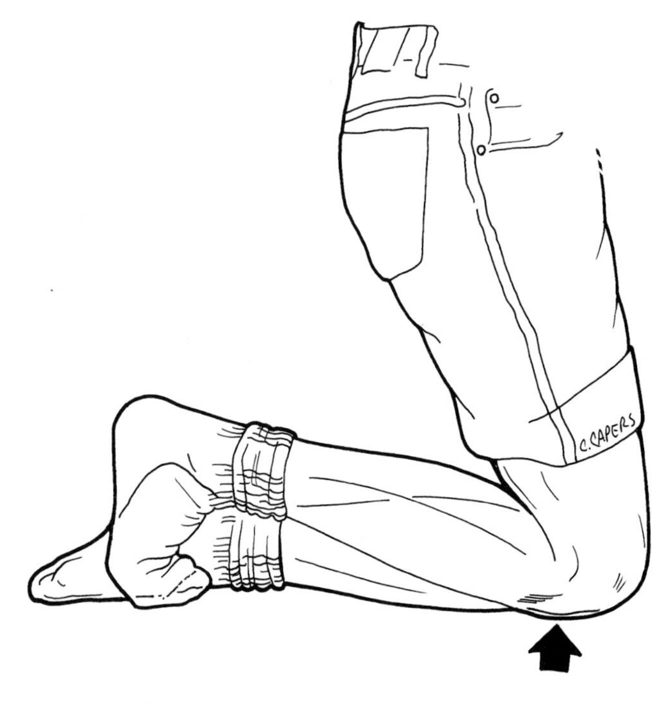

Fig. 74–1. **The mechanism of injury for an interstitial or isolated tear of the PCL can be a fall on the flexed knee with the foot in plantar flexion.**

cases, the medial or lateral collateral ligament is torn, and the ACL may or may not be torn. Valgus stress applied to the knee while it is in full extension causes medial compartment injury, and varus stress with the knee internally rotated and extended causes lateral compartment injury.

History

A careful description of the mechanism of injury can be critical in diagnosing PCL injuries. Physical examination often confirms injuries suspected from the history or the mechanism of injury. These are usually high-energy injuries, and they can be overlooked during the initial examination while the physician treats other more urgent injuries to the body.

Very minimal swelling with mild bloody effusion is typical of acute PCL injuries. The swelling generally occurs within the first 2 hours and is not the gross tense effusion that is more commonly seen with ACL injuries or patellar dislocation. Posterior knee tenderness, specifically in the popliteal fossa or posterolateral corner, can indicate a PCL tear. If there is an abrasion on the anterior aspect of the proximal tibia, a PCL tear must be ruled out. The patient often walks with the knee flexed, to avoid painful extension.

In a knee with multiple ligament disruptions, the examiner should suspect spontaneous reduction of a knee dislocation. Neurovascular assessment of the lower extremity is critical, and an arteriogram should be considered if there is any question of vascular injury. Peroneal nerve damage can occur from a varus force that injures the posterolateral ligaments. It has been reported that 10 to 30% of these injuries are associated with peroneal nerve injury.[13]

Physical Examination

On clinical examination of the knee, manifestations of PCL injury are often much more subtle than those of the typical ACL lesion. Quadriceps spasm can mask many of the test signs of PCL instability, and the patient should be totally relaxed when the examination is begun. Tests for PCL stability are based on posterior translation of the tibia in relation to the femur. Several tests are simple, and painless for the patient.

A positive *sag test* is one of the most characteristic findings. The tibial tubercle "disappears" or "drops back" on lateral inspection of the affected knee as compared with the normal side (Fig. 74–2). The test is performed with the knee and hip flexed to 90°. Gravity causes posterior displacement of the tibia in relation to the femur if the PCL is ruptured. Quadriceps spasm can prevent this tibial sag, or edema of the tibial tubercle can mask it.

The amount of posterior sag can be graded by measuring how far the anterior tibial plateau projects anterior to the femoral condylar surfaces. Normally, the anterior tibial margin should project about 1 cm in front of the femoral condyle when the knee is flexed

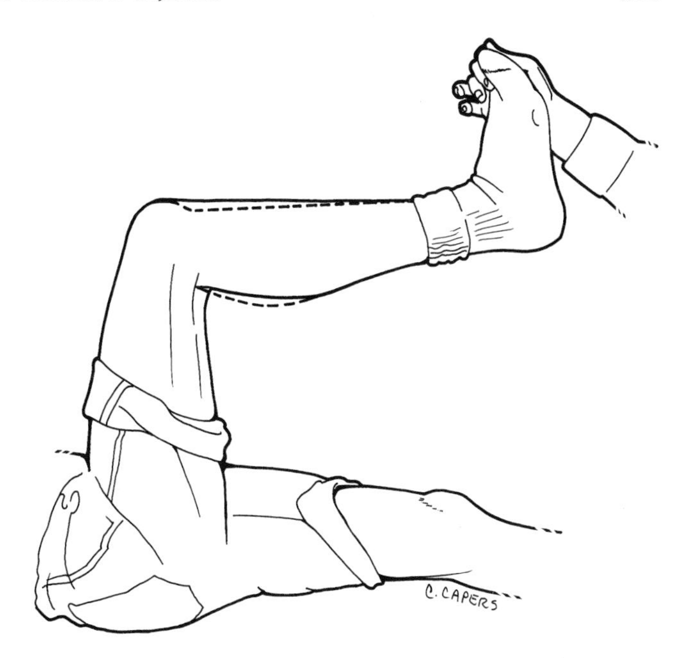

Fig. 74–2. A positive sag test result indicates a ruptured PCL.

90°. Posterior translation greater than that in the contralateral knee but with the tibial plateau prominence remaining anterior to the femoral condyles is noted to be a 1+ posterior drawer sign, which represents approximately 5 mm of posterior excursion. If the tibial plateau can be displaced posteriorly and is flush with the femoral condyles, a 2+ posterior drawer grade is assigned, which is approximately 10 mm of posterior displacement. If the tibial plateau is displaced posterior to the femoral condyles, it is graded as 3+ and represents more than 10 mm of abnormal posterior motion. An isolated PCL injury results in a 1+ or 2+ posterior sag, and usually no more. If a 3+ posterior drawer sign or sag is identified, additional ligament injury should be suspected.

The *posterior drawer test* is sensitive for PCL injury (Fig. 74–3). Frequently, the anterior drawer is misinterpreted in the presence of an ACL tear. With anterior movement, the examiner may be only reducing the posterior tibial displacement and not realize the tibia is actually resting posteriorly. Internal rotation of the tibia tightens up the PCL. If the posterior drawer test remains positive even with the tibia in internal rotation, the diagnosis of PCL injury is confirmed. This test is often used to distinguish between acute PCL and posterolateral injury. With a posterolateral injury findings of the external rotation recurvatum test are also positive.

The *quadriceps active test* is also done with the knee flexed 90°. When the patient tenses the quadriceps, the tibia is reduced into the normal position from its posterior position. *Godfrey's test* is done with both the hip and the knee flexed 90°. The examiner holds the patient's heel; the posteriorly displaced tibial tubercle is compared with the uninjured side and any difference is noted.[14]

Shelbourne's dynamic posterior shift test is done with the hip flexed 90° and the patient's heel supported in the

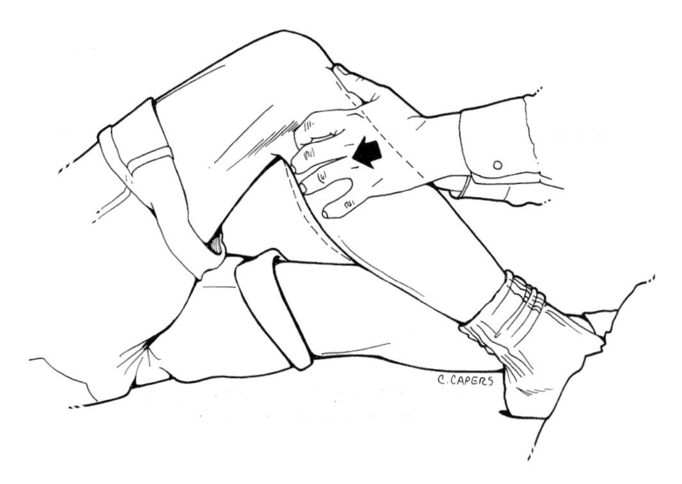

Fig. 74–3. The posterior drawer sign, in which a posterior force to the tibia creates posterior movement, is a sensitive test for PCL injury.

examiner's hand. The knee is extended slowly, allowing passive hamstrings tightness to accentuate the posterior position of the tibia. As the knee is fully extended, a clunk or jerk is felt as the knee reduces.[15] The *posterior Lachman's test* is done in the same flexed position (approximately 30°) as the anterior Lachman's test, but a posterior end point is felt.

Interpretation of the *reverse pivot shift test,* as described by Jakob, is controversial.[16] Some suggest that it indicates PCL injury, whereas most examiners think that it is best for detecting posterolateral rotatory instability. The reverse pivot shift is done by applying a valgus load to the flexed knee and then bringing the knee into extension. Reduction occurs when the knee is brought from the subluxated position (flexion) into extension. When the PCL and posterolateral structures are injured, this test is often markedly positive.

Differentiating PCL injury from posterolateral injury can at times be quite difficult. With posterolateral injury, the posterolateral drawer test and the external rotation recurvatum test are positive. With PCL injury these test results are negative. If with the knee in internal rotation the posterior drawer sign persists, PCL injury is verified.

Varus alignment of the leg usually increases the symptoms of posterolateral instability. A lateral shift in the stance phase of gait is noted. This helps the examiner differentiate PCL injury from posterolateral instability. The finding on pivot shift test is greater with combined PCL and lateral injuries.

Radiographic Evaluation

Posterior translation or sag of the tibia in the lateral view is the major finding of PCL injury on routine radiographs. Anteroposterior stress views of the knee are helpful, but they usually are not necessary to make the diagnosis. The displacement recorded on a stress radiograph may help the examiner grade the severity of the PCL injury. With an isolated tear, the tibia does not move posteriorly more than 5 mm on stress films. More than 10 mm of displacement indicates additional associated ligament injuries (i.e., posterolateral). Avulsion fractures of the posterior tibia, which can also be seen on routine radiographs, indicate PCL injury. Fracture of the fibular head, which is often seen in conjunction with PCL injury, indicates a lateral ligament complex injury.

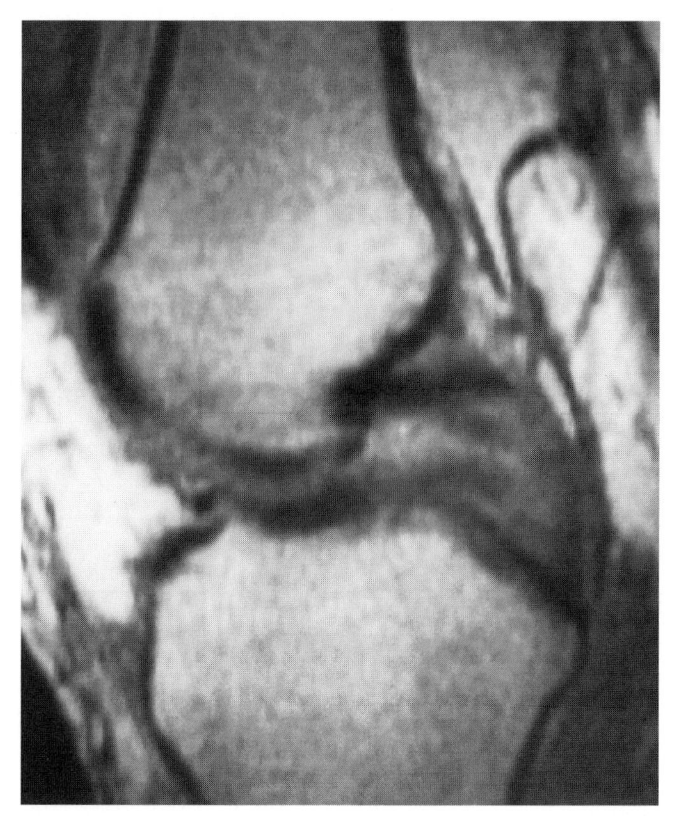

Fig. 74–4. MRI can show disruption of the PCL.

Magnetic resonance imaging (MRI) has become increasingly valuable for diagnosis of PCL injury. With acute injury, signal intensity is increased in the substance of the PCL (Fig. 74–4). Since this ligament is enclosed entirely in synovium, an interstitial tear can heal. MRI can be used to follow the process.

TREATMENT

Treatment for the acute PCL injury is controversial. There are several reports of excellent functional results without surgery.[12,17,18] It is generally thought that an isolated tear of the PCL is interstitial and should be treated nonoperatively. The diagnosis can be confirmed by MRI, routine radiography, and arthroscopy. Many of these tears heal, so that an end point is present on the posterior Lachman's test with 1+ excursion and an excellent functional result.

Bone avulsions are generally treated by surgical reattachment of the bone fragment with sutures or screws; though, if posterior translation is less than 10 mm, a case may be made for nonoperative treatment. Certainly, with associated ligament injury or excessive posterior excursion, reattachment of the bone fragment is recommended.[19–21]

Posterior cruciate ligament injury associated with other ligament injury is generally treated surgically. Any vascular injury should be repaired immediately and followed by ligament repair at the same operation. Examination under anesthesia is a very productive and integral part of this treatment. The diagnosis of PCL injury can be confirmed or expanded, depending on what other associated injuries are found. Arthroscopic examination is also indicated, to rule out associated pathologic conditions such as meniscus tears or osteochondral lesions.

Primary repair alone of PCL injuries has not been successful and is not recommended. Some form of augmentation is recommended with any repair. Associated ligament injuries should be repaired as "anatomically" as possible in the acute phase. The patellar tendon has been used, reportedly with success, for augmentation of PCL repair.[22] Other autograft tissues have been used, including gastrocnemius, semitendinosus, and gracilis, with limited success.[23,24] Allograft Achilles tendon has been used to augment repair as well. The addition of a synthetic splint when a weaker graft source such as semitendinosus or gracilis is used is recommended to maintain the tibia in the reduced position.[25]

REHABILITATION

Whether conservative or operative treatment is undertaken, rehabilitation of PCL injuries is very similar. Early motion is desirable, with strengthening of the quadriceps muscle group.

Emphasis is placed on quadriceps strengthening in the first 2 weeks after injury. During the next 4 weeks, hamstring strengthening is added to the quadriceps strengthening program. The player who has regained full range of motion, and strength, power, and endurance equal to that in the normal knee can return to normal activity. Functionally, these patients usually do well whether treated conservatively or with surgery.

REFERENCES

1. Hughston, J. C., Andrews, J. R., Cross, M. J., and Moschi, A.: Classification of knee ligamentous instabilities. Part I. The medial compartment and cruciate ligaments. J. Bone Joint Surg. *58A*:159, 1976.
2. Hughston, J. C., Andrews, J. R., Cross, M. J., and Moschi, A.: Classification of knee ligament instabilities. Part II. The lateral compartment. J. Bone Joint Surg. *58A*:173, 1976.
3. Clendenin, M. B., DeLee, J. C., and Heckman, J. D.: Interstitial tears of the posterior cruciate ligament of the knee. Orthopedics *3*:764, 1980.
4. Kennedy, J. C., and Grainger, R. W.: The posterior cruciate ligament. J. Trauma *7*:367, 1967.
5. Lysholm, J., and Gillquist, J.: Arthroscopic examination of the posterior cruciate ligament. J. Bone Joint Surg. *63A*:363, 1981.
6. O'Donoghue, D. H.: Surgical treatment of fresh injuries to the major ligaments of the knee. J. Bone Joint Surg. *32A*:721, 1950.
7. Trickey, E. L.: Rupture of the posterior cruciate ligament of the knee. J. Bone Joint Surg. *50B*:334, 1968.
8. Cross, M. J., and Powell, J. F.: Longterm followup of a posterior cruciate ligament rupture: A study of 116 cases. Am. J. Sports Med. *12*:292, 1984.
9. Hughston, J. C., Bowden, J. A., Andrews, J. R., et al.: Acute tears of the posterior cruciate ligament. J. Bone Joint Surg. *62A*:438, 1980.
10. Kennedy, J. C., Roth, J. H., and Walker, D. M.: Posterior cruciate ligament injuries. Orthop. Digest *7* (Aug./Sept.):19, 1979.
11. Moore, H. A., and Larson, R. L.: Posterior cruciate ligament injuries. Results of early surgical repair. Am. J. Sports Med. *8*:68, 1980.
12. Fowler, P. J., and Messieh, S. S.: Isolated posterior cruciate ligament injuries in athletes. Am. J. Sports Med. *15*:553, 1987.
13. Bergfeld, J. A., and DeMeo, P. J.: Posterior cruciate ligament injuries. Mediguide Orthop. *11*(3):1, 1992.
14. Godfrey, J. P.: Ligamentous injuries of the knee. Curr. Pract. Orthop. Surg. *5*:56, 1973.
15. Shelbourne, K. D., McCarroll, J. R., and Rettig, A. C., Benedict, F.: Dynamic posterior shift test. An adjuvant in evaluation of posterior tibial subluxation. Am. J. Sports Med. *17*:275, 1989.
16. Jakob, R. P.: Observation on rotatory instability of the lateral compartment of the knee. Acta Orthop. Scand. *52*:(Suppl):1, 1981.
17. Dandy, D. J., and Pusey, R. J.: The long-term results of unrepaired tears of the posterior cruciate ligament. J. Bone Joint Surg. *64B*:92, 1982.
18. Parolie, J. M., and Bergfeld, J. A.: Long-term results of nonoperative treatment of isolated posterior cruciate ligament injuries in the athlete. Am. J. Sports Med. *14*:35, 1986.
19. Ross, A. C., and Chesterman, P. J.: Isolated avulsion of the tibial attachment of the posterior cruciate ligament in childhood. J. Bone Joint Surg. *68B*:747, 1986.
20. Sanders, W. E., Wilkens, K. E., and Neidrie, A.: Acute insufficiency of the posterior cruciate ligament in children. J. Bone Joint Surg. *62A*:129, 1980.
21. Torisu, T.: Avulsion fracture of the tibial attachment of the posterior cruciate ligament. Clin. Orthop. *143*:107, 1979.
22. Clancy, W. G., Jr., Shelbourne, K. D., Zoellner, G. B., et al.: Treatment of knee joint instability secondary to rupture of the posterior cruciate ligament. J. Bone Joint Surg. *65A*:310, 1983.
23. Baker, C. L., Jr., Norwood, L. A., and Hughston, J. C.: Acute combined posterior cruciate and posterolateral instability of the knee. Am. J. Sports Med. *12*:204, 1984.
24. Lipscomb, A. B., et al.: Isolated posterior cruciate ligament reconstruction. Longterm results. Am. J. Sports Med. *21*:490, 1993.
25. Barrett, G. R., and Savoie, F. H.: Operative management of acute PCL injuries with associated pathology: Long-term results. Orthopedics *14*:687, 1991.

Chronic Injuries

Mervyn J. Cross

Patients with longstanding PCL rupture may present with symptoms related to instability or to laxity.[1] The patient complains of pain, catching, or swelling, which occur in the majority of patients (laxity related), or of recurrent episodes of instability. To understand the pathogenesis of these symptoms it is vitally important to understand the biomechanics of the knee and the contribution of the PCL to knee function.

Hughston and coworkers described the PCL as the centroid of the knee.[2] Their original classification of rotatory instability of the knee is based on the fact that the PCL is intact. They stated that patients complain of instability—the symptom of giving way—when they twist and turn. To understand the pathogenesis of these rotatory instabilities, it was necessary to classify them in the presence of an intact PCL. Disruption of the PCL deprives the knee of its centroid and of any possibility of *true* rotatory instability as defined by the original classification. This does not mean that the knee cannot twist and rotate, but it does not rotate above a central pivot point once the PCL is disrupted.

The PCL is dynamically supported by the quadriceps mechanism, one of the major muscle groups of the body. It is no coincidence that the major ligament of the body is supported by one of the major muscle groups. Proprioceptive control of the knee depends on an intact quadriceps mechanism.[3] If one can develop an efficient and strong quadriceps mechanism, it is possible proprioceptively to control posterior laxity of the knee, so that the patient will not complain of instability (Fig. 74–5). The static stability provided by the cruciate ligaments protects the patellofemoral mechanism and the menisci and stops the femur from being driven into the tibia in deceleration and descending movements.

When the PCL is ruptured, the increased laxity allows shearing forces to occur in the knee that give rise to the symptoms of swelling, catching, and pain. Increased incidence of meniscus tears, both medial and lateral, and of articular cartilage defects, and a markedly increased incidence of patellofemoral degeneration, articular defects, and arthrosis are observed. This knee joint instability can be controlled with adequate physical therapy and quadriceps rehabilitation. It is usually when this proprioceptive control[3] fails that the symptoms become manifest and progress.

The management of ruptures of the PCL can be divided into two main areas: isolated ruptures and intercurrent rupture of other ligaments. Isolated ruptures of the PCL are usually caused by a direct posterior force applied to the tibia, as in falling onto a bent knee. This is the most common mechanism of injury in sports for PCL rupture. Isolated rupture can also occur when the bent knee of a motorcyclist comes into contact with an object that strikes the anterior surface of the tibia in its upper area, driving the tibia posteriorly.

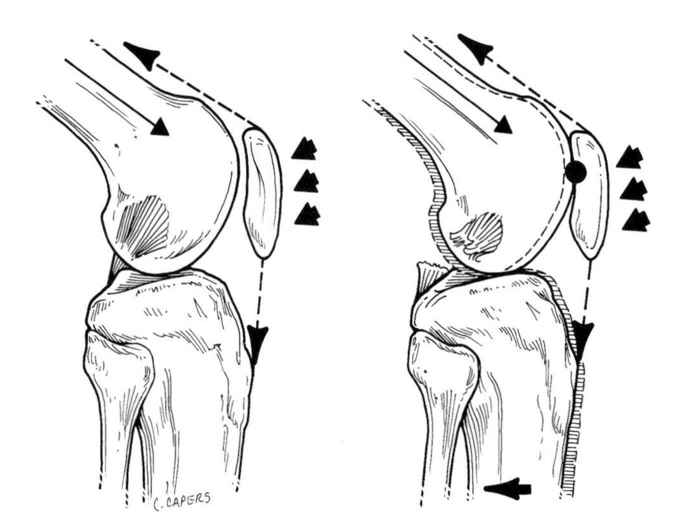

Fig. 74–5. A functioning quadriceps mechanism is necessary for proprioceptive control of the knee. The static stability provided by the cruciate ligament protects the patellofemoral mechanism and the menisci and stops the femur from being driven into the tibia in deceleration and descending movements.

Combined ruptures are usually associated with severe wrenching and twisting injuries, but they can occur in motor vehicle accidents or, more rarely, on the sporting field. Combined ruptures are usually associated with a fairly severe injury, possibly with a knee dislocation that reduces spontaneously.

HISTORY

The patient with an isolated rupture of the PCL presents with a swollen and painful knee. The diagnosis is commonly missed, particularly in the acute phase, and the patient's major complaint at the time of presentation may be anterior knee pain. It is uncommon for these patients to exhibit the instability reported in patients with ACL rupture and patellar subluxation. Patients with PCL rupture notice looseness or laxity in the knee, and their principal difficulties are in stopping after running and in descending stairs. Decelerating and running downhill present major problems.

Isolated ruptures of the PCL are commonly overlooked in patients who have been in a motor vehicle accident and fractured the femur. After the femur heals, the patient experiences persistent swelling, pain, and laxity in the knee. The injury often goes untreated in the acute phase because a knee ligament injury is a very low priority in a polytrauma patient.

Combined injuries of the PCL and other major ligaments are usually associated with posterolateral disruption, giving rise to severe subluxations and instability, particularly with hyperextension and varus force. Management of the combined injuries is different from that of an isolated injury. Patellofemoral changes, particularly in the trochlear groove and the articular surface of the patella, are associated with ligament laxity. The prevalence of lateral and medial meniscus tears, and damage to the femoral and tibial articular surfaces is also increased. All of these factors contribute to the increased incidence of osteoarthrosis.

TREATMENT

The treatment of these lesions is always based on a very careful history, a thorough clinical examination, and a complete assessment of the patient's current disability. The aim of therapy is to correct the disability and restore knee function. Conservative treatment consists of a very rigid and thorough exercise and rehabilitation program. Proprioceptive control mechanisms are taught, and the patient progresses under strict supervision until function is restored. Radiographs are important in the early stages because they may show a bone avulsion, which is easily corrected surgically. The majority of patients, however, have a rupture within the substance of the cruciate ligament.

SURGERY OF THE POSTERIOR CRUCIATE LIGAMENT

When surgery is indicated for PCL rupture, it is imperative that the tissue used be strong enough and that it be positioned isometrically in the tibia and the femur. This becomes an immediate problem because of the fan-shaped posterior cruciate ligament attaching to the femur (Fig. 74–6). I have attempted on numerous occasions to reproduce this fan shape by using multiple tendons; however, the difficulty in finding a tendon strong enough to be attached at different points often compromises the outcome.

Recent attempts at arthroscopic reconstruction of the PCL have been encouraged by the successes of arthroscopically assisted ACL-grafting techniques. Arthroscopic reconstruction of the PCL is plagued by a number of technical problems that need to be overcome before it becomes the standard treatment for longstanding PCL rupture. Briefly, the technical problems are those associated with placement of the tunnels and those associated with the anatomic aspects of the tunnels and the passage of the graft.

The anatomy of the posterior cruciate ligament is well-known. Because the tibial attachment lies so far posterior and inferior on the tibia, it is very difficult, arthroscopically, to see the exact point where it blends with the capsule. It is, therefore, a truly extra-articular attachment. This makes it very difficult to place arthroscopically. It is usually necessary to use a radiographically assisted technique to gain access for the placement of the tibial tunnel. The most commonly used method is to aim the guidewire centrally in the tibia at the junction of the sclerotic line that indicates the previous epiphyseal plate and the posterior tibial cortex (Fig. 74–7).[4] This anatomic site reproduces the tibial attachment of the PCL.

The femoral attachment is not difficult, from an arthroscopic point of view, because of its anterior placement in the notch on the lateral aspect of the medial femoral condyle. Also, a drill hole oriented toward the medial epicondyle of the femur affords a line of attachment quite suitable for endoscopic screw placement of the bone block in the femur.

In the technique currently in use the majority of the reconstruction is arthroscopically assisted; however, the posterior attachment and placement of the graft can be done via an open assisted technique through a posteromedial incision. It is recommended that the patellar tendon be taken from the opposite limb, to preserve the extensor mechanism on the injured side. This allows the normal side to regenerate a normal patellar tendon. It also makes it possible for one team to be taking the graft while the other team is preparing the knee and the intercondylar notch and performing the arthroscopy.

Technique

The injured knee is examined, and an adequate "notchplasty" is made, clearing out all the scar tissue from the ruptured PCL and being very careful to pre-

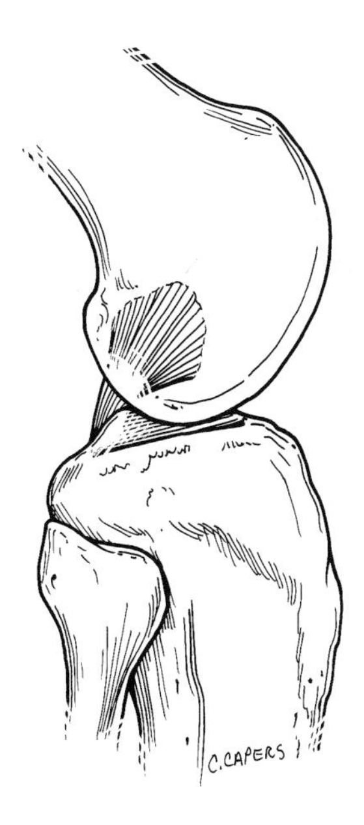

Fig. 74–6. The fan-shaped attachment of the PCL to the femur.

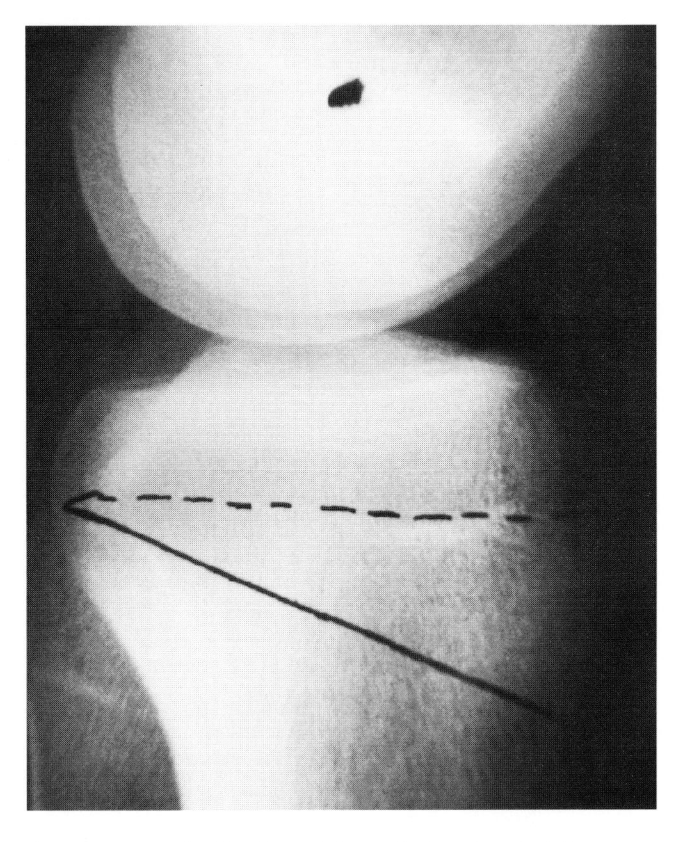

Fig. 74–7. A method for determining graft placement for PCL reconstruction using a radiographic technique and a guidewire.

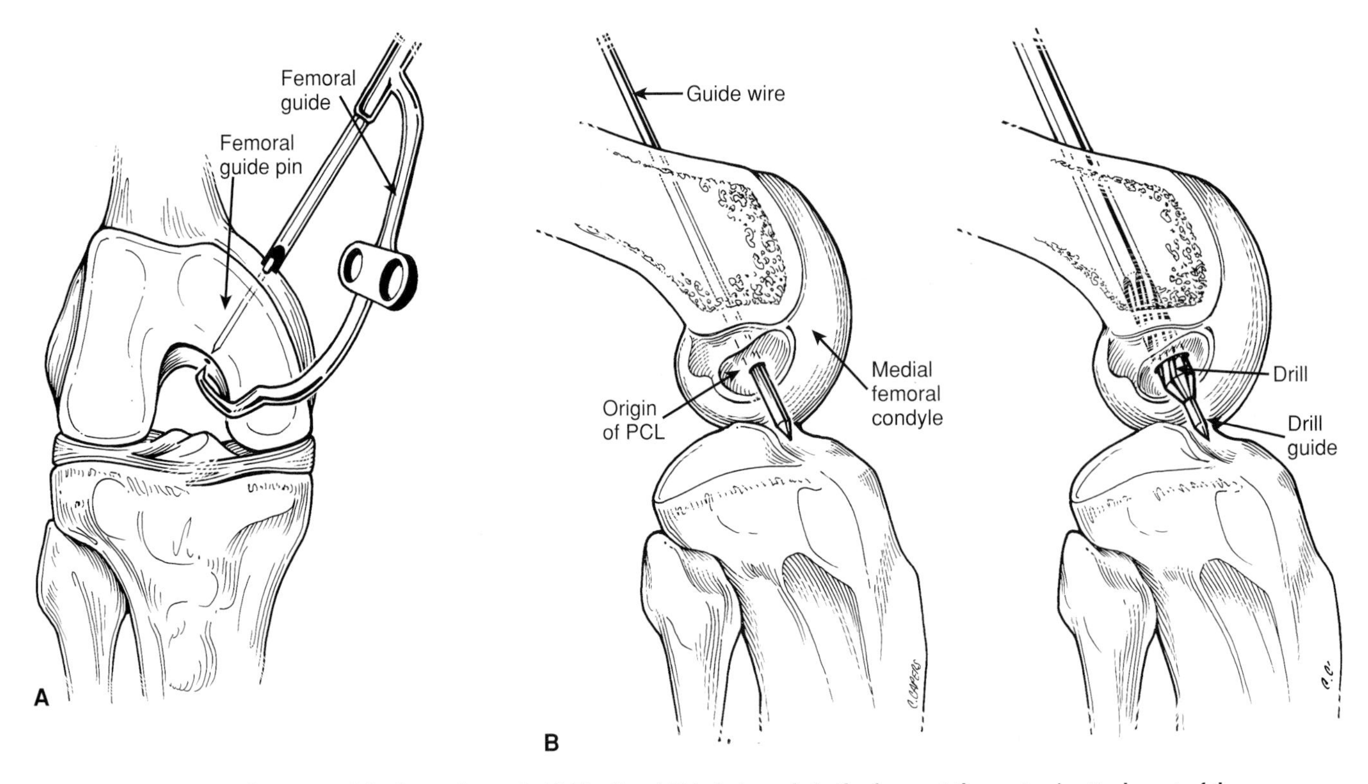

Fig. 74–8. Placement of the femoral tunnel. ***(A)*** **The first drill hole is made in the femur at the anatomic attachment of the PCL.** ***(B)*** **Once the attachment site of the PCL is located with the guidewire, it is possible to overdrill to the size of the graft.**

serve all the structures of the ACL. The menisci and all the articular surfaces are checked.

The first drill hole is made in the femur, and it is made at the anatomic attachment of the PCL, which is along the juxta-articular margin of the femur (Fig. 74–8A). Having made the drill hole, the area is plugged with a spigot and the posterior cruciate area is examined.

The arthroscope may be placed through the intercondylar notch to view the posterior aspect of the joint, but it is impossible to determine the exact attachment of the PCL by this technique because it blends with the capsule. The tibial tunnel is made using a guidewire and a radiographic technique, as described above, to locate the attachment site. Once this site is located with the guidewire, it is possible to overdrill to the size of the graft. I find that with the PCL, a 10-mm graft is usually necessary.

I think it is important to ensure that the lead bone block on the graft is no longer than 22 mm. It is difficult to pull a longer bone graft through the tibial tunnel and then pass it through the back of the joint around the sharp curve. The bone block can be sculptured in such a way that it passes easily through the tissues: slightly wedged anterior to posterior. A good block with suture leaders placed at right angles affords the surgeon more control over the block (Fig. 74–9).

Once the block is passed, it is possible to pass it through the joint and into the tunnel on the femoral condyle, where it is fixed with an endoscopic screw. This having been achieved, the leg is put through a range of motion to assess the isocentricity. If it is well and truly isocentric, the tibial block can then be fixed, usually with a post screw. This achieves adequate stability. After surgery, the knee is held in extension for 2 weeks in a brace, to allow the tissues to heal and settle.

Alternative surgical methods have been employed in the past, particularly using ligament augmentation devices: semitendinosus and gracilis tendons and, of

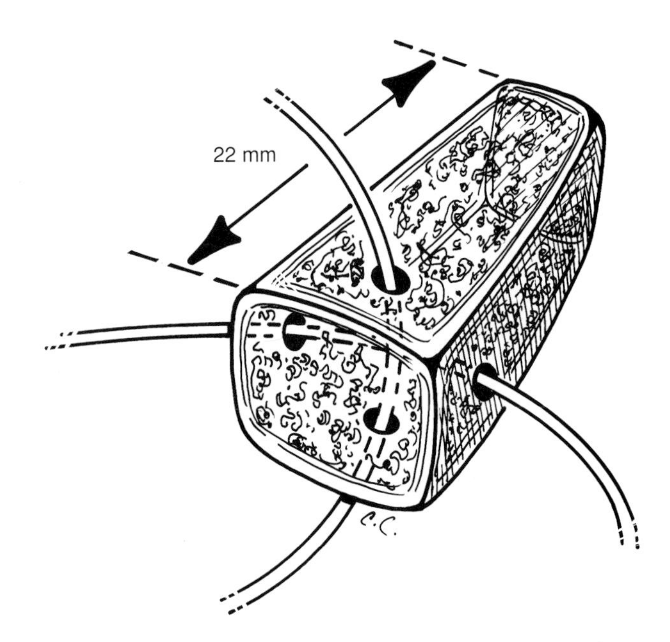

Fig. 74–9. Placing the suture leaders at right angles to each other affords the surgeon more control over the bone block.

course, allografts. I personally use only semitendinosus and gracilis for augmentation in repair of acute PCL ruptures. The semitendinosus and gracilis work extremely well for that purpose.

CONCLUSIONS

It has always been my intention to treat the patient's symptoms. I think that the patient who has combined ACL and PCL ruptures and a significant degree of instability related to the ACL rupture should be treated with ACL reconstruction. A PCL reconstruction should not be done at that time. If it is necessary later, the PCL can be reconstructed, but over many years and performing many cases I have never had to go back and do PCL reconstruction after having done the ACL reconstruction in such cases.

Other surgical techniques have been employed, and some surgeons have attempted to use double patellar tendons to make a stronger graft. I believe that this has now become obsolete, and that people are happy with the single patellar tendon graft if it is placed in good anatomic position. Other techniques have been described in which the operation was done in a two-stage technique. Results of these procedures have not been documented because of the scarcity of numbers and the absence of longterm followup.

It can be said that our understanding of PCL function is up to date with our understanding of the function of all other knee ligaments, but the solution to surgical PCL reconstruction is probably 10 years behind that of ACL reconstruction. This should provide an incentive to proceed with further investigation, with the aim of passing on our ideas, so that we may, in the near future, have an adequate surgical response for severe PCL instability.

REFERENCES

1. Cross, M. J., and Powell, J.: Long-term followup of posterior cruciate ligament rupture. A study of 116 cases. Am. J. Sports Med. *12*:398, 1984.
2. Hughston, J. C., Andrews, J. R., Cross, M. J., and Moschi, A.: Classification of knee ligament instabilities. Part I. The medial compartment. J. Bone Joint Surg. *58A*:173, 1976.
3. McCloskey, D. I., Cross, M. J., Honner, R., and Potter, E.: Sensory effects of pulling or vibrating exposed tendons in man. Brain *106*:21, 1983.
4. Claney, R.: Personal communication, 1991.

75

James R. Bocell, Jr.

Medial Collateral Ligament Injuries

Injuries to the knee are common in the world of sports, and a significant proportion are ligament disruptions. The number of knee injuries has risen in proportion to the increased number of participants in the many sporting opportunities that are available. As recreational sports have become increasingly popular and exercise equipment has improved, more people with little previous experience are embracing a more active lifestyle. Despite improvements in sports equipment and training philosophies and increased awareness of injury prevention, trauma to the knee ligaments continues to occur. It is imperative that sports physicians be knowledgeable in recognizing and treating these injuries. This requires a knowledge of anatomy, function, biomechanics, mechanisms of injury, physical findings, associated injury, and treatment options.

The medial ligament complex can be injured in isolation or in combination with other structures. If not properly treated, such injuries can delay return to sports, result in progressive deterioration of the joint, and possibly end a career.

ANATOMY

A thorough knowledge of local anatomy is essential for understanding the mechanics of the knee. Open repair of the damaged structures in the acute setting allows the physician to correlate the injured structures with the clinical instability. Recent trends in nonoperative management of some acute instabilities and the trend toward delayed reconstruction may deprive the surgeon of that opportunity. Every occasion available to inspect the anatomy in the acute phase provides the surgeon a valuable lesson in structure and function. A better understanding of the acute pathologic changes fosters understanding of the mechanics of proposed reconstructive procedures. There is also no substitute for dissection in the cadaver laboratory, as we strive to learn and understand.

A detailed description of the functional anatomy of the knee has been provided in Chapter 63. For the purposes of this chapter, however, it is important to review the anatomy and function of the medial ligament complex and to understand the complexity of the medial supporting structures. The expression *medial ligament complex* is more descriptive and encompasses the many discrete structures about the knee that work in concert.

The medial capsule, the deepest layer of the medial ligament complex, can be divided into three parts (Fig. 75–1): the anteromedial capsule or anterior third medial capsular ligament, the middle third medial capsular ligament, and the posteromedial capsule or posterior third medial capsular ligament. The anterior third (anteromedial capsule) is a thin structure that is reinforced by the medial extensor mechanism. Proximally, this becomes confluent with the distal quadriceps and medial patella. At the level of the meniscus, it is firmly attached to the periphery of that structure, and distally it is attached to the anteromedial tibia.

The middle third medial capsular ligament is a thicker structure and can be divided into meniscofemoral and meniscotibial portions (Fig. 75–2). The meniscofemoral portion originates at the medial femoral epicondyle and courses distally to the middle third of the medial meniscus, to which it is firmly attached. Distal to this structure it becomes the meniscotibial portion, which is attached to the medial aspect of the proximal tibia just below its articular surface. The middle third medial capsular ligament has been referred to as the *deep layer of the medial collateral ligament.* As will be shown, this structure is distinct from the overlying tibial collateral ligament, which has a different origin and insertion.

The posterior third medial capsular ligament comprises the posterior oblique ligament and oblique

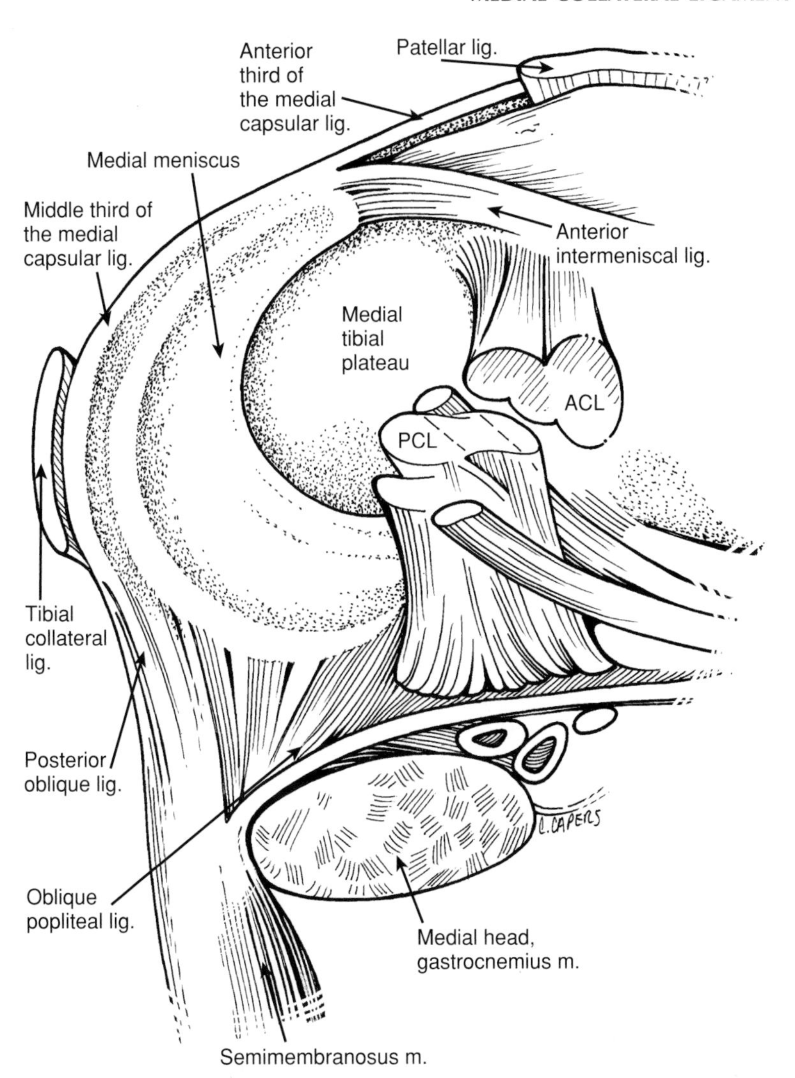

Fig. 75–1. The medial capsule is divided into three parts: the anteromedial capsule, the middle third medial capsular ligament, and the posteromedial capsule.

popliteal ligament. Both have their origins at the adductor tubercle, which is just posterior to the medial femoral epicondyle. These course distally and have strong attachments to the medial meniscus and the proximal tibia. Hughston and Eilers have described three divisions of the posterior oblique ligament:[1] the superficial, tibial, and capsular arms. The superficial arm courses distally over the anterior arm of the semimembranosus and attaches into the fascia of the pes anserinus. The tibial arm, the thickest portion of the posterior oblique ligament, courses distally and obliquely. There are strong attachments to the medial meniscus, and it is securely attached to the posteromedial tibia. The capsular arm of the posterior oblique ligament originates at the adductor tubercle and is confluent proximally with the oblique popliteal ligament. This passes posteriorly and continues as the attachment of the oblique popliteal ligament into the posterior aspect of the lateral femoral condyle.

Superficial to the medial capsular ligament is the tibial collateral ligament, which has been referred to as the superficial layer of the medial collateral ligament.[2] This structure is distinct from the underlying middle third medial capsular ligament. Proximally, it is attached to the medial femoral epicondyle, just superficial and slightly proximal to the attachment of the meniscofemoral portion of the middle third medial capsular ligament. It then courses distally along the medial aspect of the joint and attaches well below the joint line, onto the distal metaphyseal region medially. Because of its separation from the underlying medial capsular ligament and distal tibial metaphysis, the tibial collateral ligament glides anteriorly and posteriorly during flexion-to-extension motions.[3,4] Proximally, at the medial femoral epicondyle, the vastus medialis obliquus attaches to the tibial collateral ligament. The tibial collateral ligament does not attach to the medial meniscus.

The semimembranosus muscle-tendon unit provides dynamic support to the posteromedial corner. The tibial anterior arm attaches to the medial aspect of the proximal tibia, deep to the tibial collateral ligament. The inferior arm courses distally and obliquely to attach to the posteromedial aspect of the proximal tibia. The direct arm attaches posteriorly to the proximal tibia. The capsular arm inserts into and is continuous with the posterior oblique ligament and the oblique popliteal ligament.

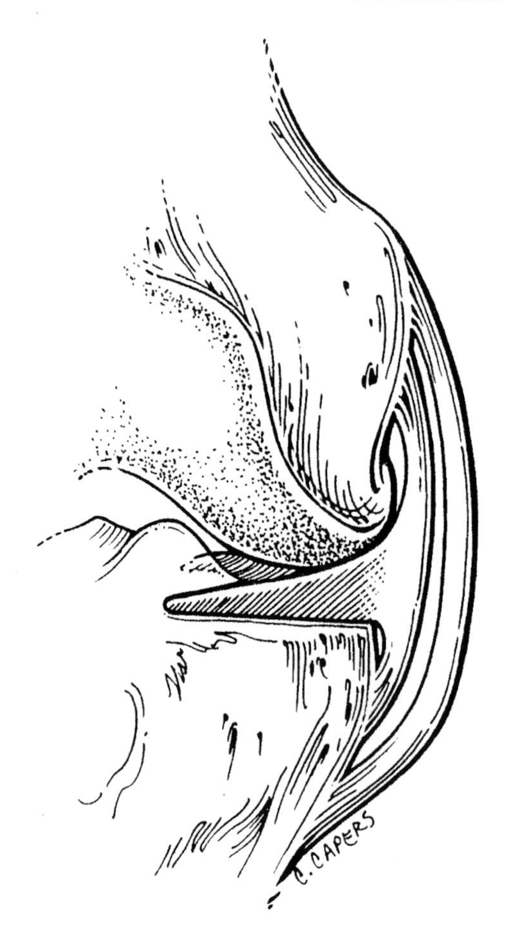

Fig. 75–2. The middle third capsular ligament is divided into meniscofemoral and meniscotibial portions.

The medial hamstrings—sartorius, gracilis, and semitendinosus muscles—insert via the pes anserinus tendon onto the anteromedial aspect of the proximal tibia, anterior to the attachment of the tibial collateral ligament. The pes anserinus tendon overlies the tibial collateral ligament, from which it is separated by the pes anserinus bursa.

FUNCTION AND BIOMECHANICS

The function of the medial ligament complex is to resist valgus and external rotation forces about the knee and, to a lesser degree, anterior tibial translation with the tibia in external rotation. A secondary function is protection of the medial meniscus by its strong medial capsular ligament attachments and the dynamic control exerted by the extensor mechanism on the anterior third of the medial capsular ligament and the semimembranosus on the posterior oblique ligament.[1,3] These dynamic actions move the anterior horn of the medial meniscus anteriorly in extension and the posterior horn posteriorly in flexion to retract those portions of the meniscus that would otherwise be pinched in the tibiofemoral articulation.

Although the function of the medial ligament complex is clear, there is considerable controversy about the contribution of specific anatomic structures to the stresses of valgus and external rotation. Although Hughston advocates anatomic repair of all damaged structures, he thinks that the posteromedial corner is essential to optimal function of the medial ligament complex and must be repaired to regain stability.[1,3] Although the posteromedial corner becomes more relaxed with increasing flexion, the dynamic force of the semimembranosus contracting through its capsular arm tightens the posterior oblique and oblique popliteal ligaments, increasing stability and resistance to valgus in external rotation forces.

Others think that the tibial collateral ligament is the most important structure, especially for resisting valgus stress, particularly in flexion.[5,6] In extension, the tibial collateral ligament and the posteromedial capsular structures are taut and contribute to stability in this position.

According to Müller,[4] the pes anserinus supplies dynamic input to the tibial collateral ligament, especially with the knee in extension. Because of the close anatomic relationship of the insertion of the tibial collateral ligament and the pes anserinus and their parallel orientation in this position, the pes anserinus theoretically functions as a dynamic tibial collateral ligament. The medial retinaculum is dynamized by the vastus medialis and its fibers that course from that muscle and the associated quadriceps tendon and insert about the proximal portion of the attachment of the tibial collateral ligament. They function as active medial stabilizers and thus enhance the function of the tibial collateral ligament. Finally, the semimembranosus muscle dynamically stabilizes the posteromedial corner by way of its capsular arm attachments into the oblique popliteal ligament and the posterior oblique ligament. In flexion, this dynamic contribution tenses the posteromedial capsular structures that normally become lax in flexion, creating a taut ligament complex. It is especially effective in resisting external rotation. In extension this muscle-tendon unit parallels the taut static stabilizers and enhances their strength.

EXAMINATION

Mechanism of Injury

Specific structures are more vulnerable when exposed to certain forces, and awareness of the injury mechanism increases the index of suspicion about what anatomic damage might be encountered. Many disruptions of the medial ligament complex occur as the result of "contact" stresses. Hughston and Barrett reported on 154 patients with acute anteromedial rotatory instability of the knee and found that 86% of them had sustained an injury as the result of a contact force applied to the lateral aspect of the knee or the proximal tibia when the foot was planted on the ground, resulting in a valgus and external rotation stress.[7] This can occur in any team sport, though it is more common in football, secondary to blocking. Football rules have been changed in recent years in an attempt to decrease the incidence of these injuries.

Stresses resulting in a pure valgus movement more typically result in disruption of the medial capsular ligament and overlying tibial collateral ligament. The combination of valgus movement and external rotation results in disruption of the posterior oblique ligament. As the valgus force increases, the tibial collateral ligament and middle third medial capsular ligament are also injured. This results in anteromedial rotatory instability. With increasing stress, the anterior cruciate ligament, which is a secondary stabilizer for the medial ligament complex, may be disrupted as well, increasing the severity of the anteromedial rotatory instability and potentially adding an element of anterolateral rotatory instability to the injury.[8]

Disruption of the medial ligament complex can also occur with "noncontact" injuries like a fall or sudden valgus stress, as when a snow skier "catches an edge" on an icy patch or a water ski suddenly caught in the water produces a sudden external rotation force. A cyclist who places a foot on the ground while moving, either to "brake" or to avoid a fall, may sustain the same type of injury. The medial ligament complex may also be injured in deceleration, cutting, twisting, and pivoting maneuvers. Frequently, however, this also results in disruption of the anterior cruciate ligament, producing combined instability with more serious consequences.

The forces that produce injury to the medial ligament complex can also cause other injuries. The anterior cruciate ligament may be involved, especially if stresses involve deceleration or twisting, pivoting, and cutting. The medial meniscus is firmly attached to the medial capsular ligament, and significant disruption and tearing of those structures may result in a peripheral tear of the medial meniscus. With extreme forces, the posterior cruciate ligament may be injured as well, either interstitially or with bone avulsion. With higher velocity and more violent injuries, a knee dislocation can occur; then the majority of the ligament structures about the knee may be damaged, in addition to the medial ligament complex. Finally, with increasing valgus stress, the bone may fail in the lateral compartment and a lateral tibial plateau fracture may result, in addition to the soft tissue injury on the medial side.

History

A careful and thorough history is essential. This includes documentation of the mechanism of injury, including the patient's perception as well as the observations of others (e.g., teammates, trainers, coaching staff). As the role of the sports medicine physician has become better defined, he or she is frequently on the sidelines and may have observed the incident firsthand. Game films may also provide a documentation of the mechanism of injury.

The report of an audible or palpable "pop" at the time of injury is helpful information. Though this is more common with disruption of the anterior cruciate ligament, it may be associated with avulsion of the tibial collateral ligament at its attachment.

The onset and severity of swelling must be ascertained. Swelling that occurs rapidly within the first 2 hours suggests an associated injury to the anterior cruciate ligament or a concomitant subluxation episode of the patella. With a pure medial complex ligament injury swelling is usually less pronounced. In a knee with major ligament injury, even with disruption of the anterior cruciate ligament, swelling may be relatively mild because of extravasation of the hemarthrosis into the soft tissues secondary to disruption of the synovial and capsular structures.

Functional instability may result from ligament instability, but it can be manifested in giving way secondary to reflex inhibition of the quadriceps because of pain and weakness from the injury. Because of muscle splinting and gait alteration, the patient may be able to walk without giving way. Therefore, it is not safe to rule out a major ligament injury because the patient has little swelling and can ambulate without giving way.

An injury associated with loss of motion, primarily limitation of extension, is usually thought to represent a meniscal tear with dislocation of the bucket-handle portion into the intercondylar notch. This is actually uncommon in medial ligament sprains, and limitation of extension usually occurs secondary to muscle spasm and pain as the medial ligament structures tighten with increasing extension. This "pseudolocking" usually occurs several hours after the injury.

Finally, it is important to inquire about previous injuries or symptoms in the knee, to determine what element of the patient's injury may be longstanding. The history of an injury to the uninvolved knee may also reveal a previous ligament injury that will alter the "baseline examination" findings of that leg as the examiner strives to determine what is "normal laxity" for that athlete.

Clinical Examination and Physical Findings

Although the physical examination has been covered in detail in Chapter 64, certain elements are worth emphasizing. All physical examinations start with inspection. This includes examination for antalgic gait and for external aids such as crutches or a splint. Swelling may be observed and its extent graded. A pure medial ligament injury may produce little or no intra-articular swelling, though localized swelling over the site of specific tissue damage usually begins within several hours. Skin changes may be evident as well, including abrasions secondary to the initial trauma, which may again help to substantiate the mechanism of injury. With late presentation, ecchymosis may be associated with the soft tissue injury. Erythema may be present in response to the acute inflammatory process or secondary to the direct trauma.

Palpation of the medial ligament complex frequently reveals a defect in the area of ligament disruption, and there is localized tenderness over the anatomic site of ligament damage. Range of motion frequently is limited: flexion can be decreased owing to pain from soft-tissue injury or to swelling. Pseudolocking, as mentioned above, is a limitation of extension that occurs some time after the injury and is secondary to muscle spasm and pain that occur with extension as the medial ligament complex tightens.

Clinical testing for ligament stability determines what combination of anatomic structures is injured as well as the severity of that injury. According to the *Standard Nomenclature of Athletic Injuries,*[9] damage to a ligament structure is defined as a *sprain.* There are three grades of sprain[10]: A Grade I, or first-degree, sprain represents microtearing of the ligament fibers with interstitial hemorrhage and localized tenderness but no demonstrable instability. A Grade II, or second-degree, sprain is defined as a result of moderate trauma with more ligament fiber involvement and alteration of ligament integrity. Minimal to mild clinical instability results. A Grade III, or third-degree, sprain is defined as a complete disruption of the ligament, usually resulting from severe trauma. This is associated with significant clinical instability. Evaluation of the knee for major clinical instability is, therefore, assessment for the presence or absence of a Grade III sprain.

Clinical tests for ligament stability define the type of instability as well as its severity. Instability is rated as mild (1+), moderate (2+), or severe (3+). A stability test that produces 0 to 5 mm of abnormal motion of the affected knee, as compared with the normal contralateral one, represents a 1+ instability. Abnormal motion or opening of the joint from 5 to 10 mm represents moderate instability. Greater than 10 mm of abnormal motion, again as compared with the normal side, is defined as severe instability. The severity of the instability depends on the degree of ligament sprain and the combination of affected ligaments.

The abduction stress test is the most important for evaluating the medial ligament complex. The patient is positioned supine with the thigh supported on the table. The patient can then relax without fear of the examiner dropping the leg or sudden movement that might produce pain. The leg is gently swung over to the side, and the examiner grasps the forefoot with one hand, applying pressure to the lateral aspect of the knee with the other hand (Fig. 75–3). The examiner then moves the foot back and forth repeatedly from the midline, applying counterpressure laterally at the knee. Abnormal motion can be evaluated and rated from 0 to 5 mm, 5 to 10 mm, or greater than 10 mm of pathologic "opening." Frequently there may be visible dimpling of the skin in soft tissues over the medial joint line with the more severe abduction instabilities. With increasing instability and greater involvement of more structures, including secondary restraints, the end point becomes softer and has been described as "mushy."

The abduction stress test is performed at both 30° of flexion and in full extension (Fig. 75–4). The posteromedial capsular structures are relaxed at 30° of flexion. The structures being evaluated are the tibial collateral ligament and the middle third medial capsular ligament. In extension, these ligaments are evaluated, but so are the posterior cruciate ligament and the posteromedial capsular structures.

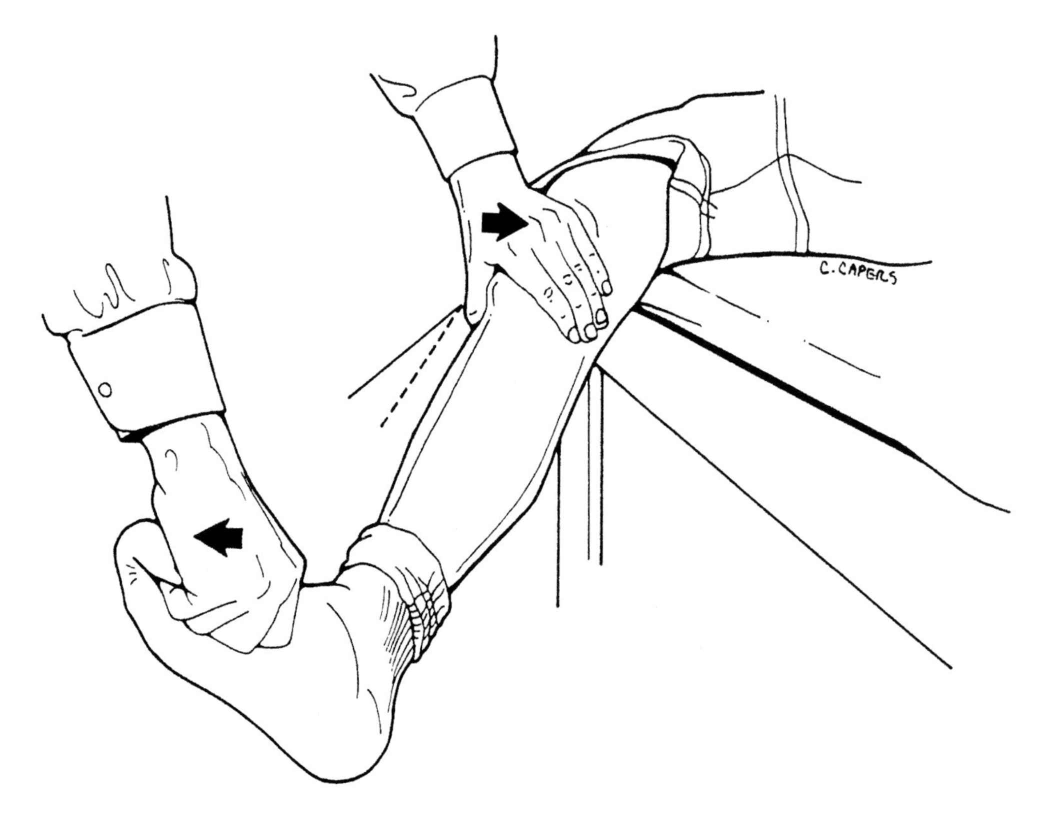

Fig. 75–3. The abduction stress test at 30° of knee flexion tests the integrity of the medial ligament complex.

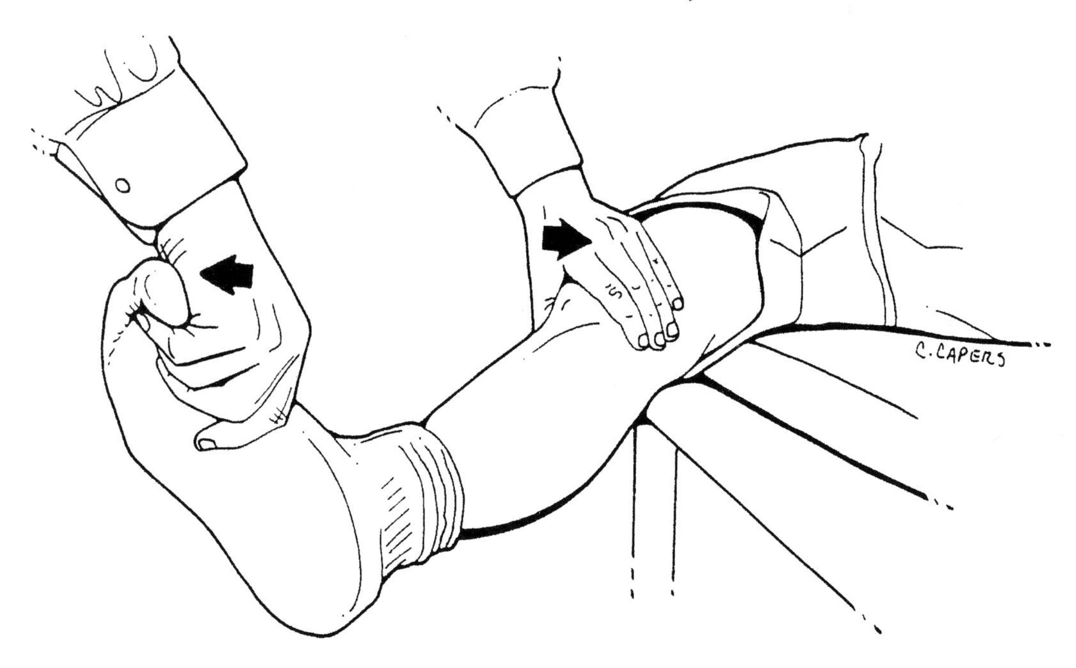

Fig. 75–4. The abduction stress test at full extension.

A thorough stability examination is always performed, testing the other secondary restraints, the cruciate ligaments, and the lateral ligament complex. There may be an increase in excursion on anterior drawer testing with the tibia in external rotation, with more involvement of the posteromedial capsular structures following an external rotation injury. A patient who experiences a great deal of discomfort from stability testing with hamstrings spasm and pseudolocking may benefit from a local anesthetic injected into the trigger point, to facilitate the return of extension. This may relieve discomfort and allow a more thorough examination.

Magnetic resonance imaging (MRI) has been helpful in confirming associated injury, principally the status of the anterior cruciate ligament, the lateral ligament complex, and the menisci. A ligament complex injury that might initially be treated nonoperatively might nonetheless require surgery if MRI suggests a concomitant meniscal injury that warrants surgical repair or an anterior cruciate ligament tear that might warrant reconstruction. In addition, we have detected several occult bone injuries, such as tibial plateau fractures, that were not evident even on retrospective review of plain radiographs. We have rarely performed arthrography since the advent of the MRI, and it is usually reserved for those who cannot tolerate the confinement of the MRI chamber. This has become less of a problem with advances in MRI technique.

The tibial collateral ligament and medial capsular ligaments usually fail in their substance(4); however, bone avulsions may occur as the strength threshold of the ligament complex is exceeded. Such an injury is usually a bone avulsion of the tibial collateral ligament from the medial femoral epicondyle. This is not to be confused with the Pellegrini-Steida calcification that is seen late on radiographic examination and is a result of calcification at the femoral attachment of the tibial collateral ligament in response to localized tearing of the ligament in this region.

Physeal injuries in a skeletally immature person may mimic a medial ligament disruption because of the opening that valgus testing produces in this situation. Other bone injuries may be associated (e.g., bone avulsion of the anterior cruciate ligament or intercondylar eminence fracture) and the lateral capsular sign,(11) which indicates avulsion of the middle third lateral capsular ligament from the tibia. Views should include anteroposterior, lateral, notch (tunnel), and infrapatellar views. Stress radiographs may be helpful to document the severity of the medial compartment instability and the presence of physeal injury.

TREATMENT

The goal of treatment is to restore stability to the knee, maximizing function and allowing the patient to return to previous activity levels. This involves protecting the injured structures from further damage, promoting healing, rehabilitating the lower extremity, and evaluating the knee for safe return to activity with minimal chance of reinjury.

For Grade III sprains of the medial ligament complex resulting in significant instability, the treatment has traditionally been open primary surgical repair in the acute setting. Many investigators, including O'Donoghue,(12,13) Hughston,(3,7) and Müller,(4) have documented their good results in the literature and have advocated early anatomic repair.

Numerous reports in the literature document excellent results following nonoperative treatment of Grade I and Grade II sprains of the medial ligament complex, and this approach has been widely accepted.[14–17] It should be stressed that nonoperative treatment of ligament injuries does not equal no treatment. Many surgeons now treat Grade III lesions nonoperatively as well if the anterior cruciate ligament is intact. Several orthopedists have reported excellent results treating Grade III tears of the medial collateral ligament nonoperatively with immobilization in a cast followed by a limited-motion cast brace.[18–20]

There is nevertheless a definite role for primary open repair of medial ligament injuries. Many continue to propose anatomic repair of medial ligament injuries, especially in the clinical situation with a 3+ or severe instability. The medial ligament injury, in combination with other ligament disruptions (e.g., severe posterior capsule disruption, torn posterior cruciate ligament, major posteromedial corner injury) warrants surgical repair. The combination of medial ligament injuries with other major ligament disruptions, especially the anterior cruciate ligament, when treated nonoperatively do not do as well as the "isolated" Grade III sprain of the medial ligament complex. Those with associated meniscal injuries, such as disruption of the capsular attachments to the medial meniscus, should be repaired primarily, because of the important function of that structure in joint stability and load transmission. Age and activity demands of the patient are always considerations when choosing between surgical and nonoperative treatment. It is assumed that athletes are active persons in good health who desire to return to their previous functional level.

When operative treatment is employed, the patient should undergo an examination under anesthesia combined with a precise determination of any associated damage. This requires inspection of the interior of the joint. Some have recommended this be performed through an accessory arthrotomy incision.[3] The current trend leans toward arthroscopic examination of the knee preceding primary ligament repair to carefully evaluate the articular surfaces for the presence of chondral fractures, the integrity of the anterior and posterior cruciate ligaments, and the status of the medial and the lateral meniscus. A medial hockey-stick incision is used to completely expose the medial ligament complex, to afford access to all structures. The disrupted ligaments are then repaired anatomically: avulsions are reattached to their anatomic attachments.

Special care must be taken to restore the normal relationship of the semimembranosus to the posterior medial corner, because this structure is important for dynamization of the posterior oblique and oblique popliteal ligaments. Injuries to the meniscal capsular attachments are obviously repaired at this time. Staples, if used, must be placed with caution. Reattaching the meniscofemoral portion of the middle third medial capsular ligament or the tibial collateral ligament distally to the cheek of the medial femoral condyle, as opposed to the medial femoral epicondyle, results in ankylosis because the altered attachment site of the medial ligament complex proximally changes the normal axis of motion, restricting extension and flexion.[3] This requires reoperation to restore normal motion. An example in point is illustrated by Figure 75–5. This patient was initially evaluated 2 years after open repair of the medial ligaments of her left knee following a skiing injury. Despite being placed into a limited motion brace postoperatively, she could not regain her motion. Closed manipulation was likewise unsuccessful. At the time of presentation, she lacked 17° of extension of the left knee, as compared with the right one. After removal of the staple with arthroscopic lysis of adhesions and débridement of the cheek of the medial femoral condyle, the patient was able to achieve full extension and flexion to 112°.

Nonoperative treatment of medial ligament disruptions requires a precise diagnosis. A thorough history, physical examination, and appropriate stability testing are required. If there is any question about the presence of associated injuries, especially to the anterior cruciate ligament or menisci, the situation warrants examination under anesthesia and operative arthroscopy. Treatment ranges from the use of crutches, to symptomatic splinting and bracing for a short time, to limited-motion bracing and protection for 4 to 6 weeks. Early protected

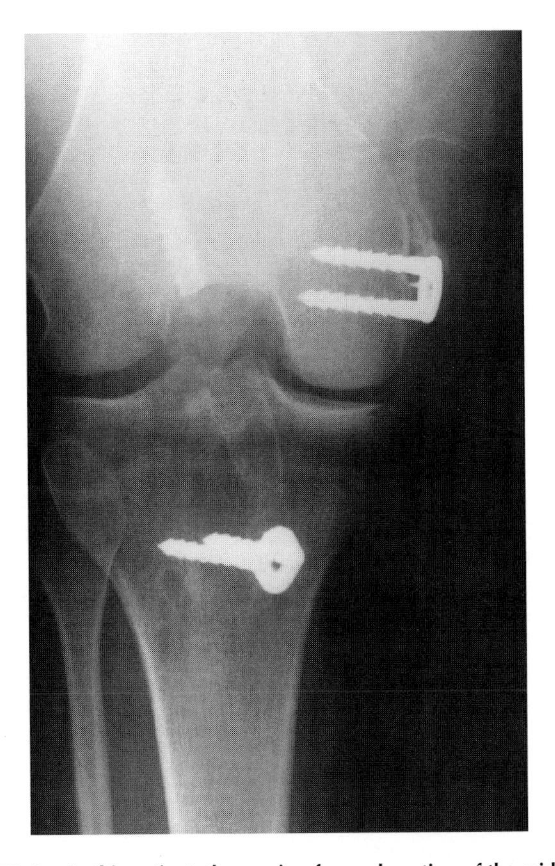

Fig. 75–5. In this patient, the meniscofemoral portion of the middle third capsular ligament was attached too far distally on the femur. This resulted in ankylosis, and the patient had to undergo staple removal and arthroscopic lysis of adhesions and débridement of the cheek of the medial femoral condyle.

weight bearing is usually allowed, depending on the severity of the instability and the patient's comfort. These specifics are covered in the next section.

Postoperative management and rehabilitation techniques have changed dramatically in the last several years. In the past, plaster immobilization for a 6-week course was recommended after primary repair or as definitive nonoperative treatment. In the literature, however, evidence of the deleterious effects of immobilization has accumulated.[21–24] Other experimental studies have reported delayed healing with immobilization and accelerated healing with motion.[25] Current trends, therefore, emphasize early motion to restore optimal ligament strength. While prolonged immobilization is to be avoided, the knee nevertheless needs to be protected during the mobilization process, to avoid disruption of the surgically repaired structures and to allow spontaneous healing of those managed nonoperatively. This can be provided by either a cast brace or one of the many rehabilitation braces currently available. These usually have adjustable devices (e.g., Velcro or adjustable straps) to allow changes in circumferential size to compensate for swelling and its resolution in the postoperative or postinjury period. This also facilitates dressing changes. The longitudinal medial and lateral struts protect against valgus stress and the adjustable hinges allow the physician to protect the knee against extremes of motion while allowing mobilization in the "safe range." After an acute repair, many surgeons restrict terminal extension to avoid stress to the posteromedial corner, especially after repair of those structures and the semimembranosus complex.

SPECIFIC CLINICAL SITUATIONS

Grade I Sprain of the Medial Ligament Complex

This athlete typically presents with a valgus stress resulting in an injury to the medial ligament complex. Pain is localized to the medial aspect of the joint. Although the patient is usually ambulatory, the gait may be antalgic and extension of the knee limited owing to spasm and pain. Physical examination usually reveals localized swelling and tenderness over the medial ligaments and no demonstrable instability. Treatment consists of crutch ambulation for protection and comfort, intermittent application of ice to the affected area to diminish pain and swelling, compression, elevation, and rest. Although this is an interstitial tear, there may be significant discomfort, and the patient may lack full extension. An injection of local anesthetic into the tender area may allow full extension and can enhance stability testing. Protected weight bearing with crutches is allowed. Isometric exercises are begun immediately and the patient rapidly advances to progressive resistive exercises. As discomfort decreases, crutches are discontinued and mobilization is begun. The rehabilitation program becomes more aggressive and is structured to restore strength, endurance, flexibility, and range of motion.

Grade II Sprain of the Medial Ligament Complex

A Grade II sprain is a more significant injury. Localized swelling over the injured structures and tenderness to direct palpation can be demonstrated. The patient may be ambulatory, again with limitation of extension secondary to pain and spasm, and may also benefit from a local anesthetic injection as a therapeutic measure. Mild instability may be detectable because of the increased severity of the ligament damage. Treatment is that outlined for Grade I sprains: crutches, rest, ice, elevation, and compression about the knee. Patients are usually more comfortable in a rehabilitation brace that allows full motion but offers protection against valgus stresses on the injured structures. Protected weight bearing with crutches is allowed. Again, isometric exercises are instituted immediately and the patient advances rapidly to progressive resistive exercises as comfort allows. Gentle stability testing is repeated on a weekly basis to evaluate progressive healing. Stability usually becomes maximal within several weeks. As discomfort diminishes and stability returns, the patient is allowed to discontinue crutches and the brace, and aggressive physical therapy is instituted. There may be more quadriceps atrophy since this is a more severe injury. It is important to document restoration of strength before the athlete resumes full activity.

Grade III Sprain of the Medial Ligament Complex

Although Grade III sprains represent complete disruption of the ligaments, this may not translate to a 3+ medial instability. It depends on what combination of ligament structures are involved and on the status of the secondary restraints. As previously noted, many surgeons have advocated nonoperative management of Grade I and II sprains, and more recently of Grade III sprains of the medial ligament complex.[14–20] Hughston,[3] however, cautions against confusing a Grade III sprain with a 3+ (severe) clinical instability and questions whether those reported Grade III sprains may, in fact, represent 2+ instability, which would be expected to do better with a nonoperative approach. He continues to recommend open primary repair in this situation.

A Grade III sprain is obviously a more severe injury. The patient has pain and localized swelling and the prevalence of limitation of motion secondary to spasm is greater. The patient may protect the knee, though initially in the immediate postinjury stage, there may actually be less discomfort with a Grade III sprain than with a Grade I or II lesion because the ligament is completely disrupted. Because this is a more severe injury, it is imperative to seek associated injuries, and the importance of a thorough history and physical examination cannot be overstated. If there is any question about which structures are damaged, the patient needs examination under anesthesia and direct inspection of the interior of the joint, which is usually performed arthroscopically. It is advantageous to place patients who present with a diffusely swollen knee, especially with hemarthrosis and marked limitation of motion, on crutches, combining that with a program of rest, ice, elevation, compression, bracing or splinting, and early exercises to reduce pain, swelling, and limitation of motion. This facilitates recovery and reduces the chance of postoperative fibrosis, should surgical repair be indicated.

As noted above, some authors propose nonoperative treatment even for severe instability of the medial ligament complex.[18–20] If this is undertaken, strict criteria must be observed, including the absence of any associated intra-articular damage, particularly meniscus or anterior cruciate ligament lesions. If at arthroscopy a medial meniscus capsular separation is identified, it must be surgically repaired by reattaching the capsular structures to the meniscus and restoring the capsular arm of the semimembranosus to the posteromedial corner. Associated disruption of the anterior cruciate ligament is a more severe injury that should be treated surgically, including reconstruction of the anterior cruciate ligament.

Postoperatively, the lower extremity is held in a limited-motion brace to protect against the extremes of motion. Traditional experience has dictated restriction of the last 30° of extension. Some surgeons are now treating Grade III sprains of the medial ligament with early protected motion from 0° to 90°, especially when combined with anterior cruciate ligament reconstruction. We recommend crutch ambulation and protection with a limited-motion brace for a full 6 weeks after open repair. Nonoperative treatment of a Grade III medial ligament injury does not change the physiology of ligament healing. We therefore recommend prolonged crutch ambulation and, again, protection with a limited-motion brace for 4 to 6 weeks. This is coupled with regular gentle stability evaluations of the knee to monitor progression of healing.

REHABILITATION

This regimen includes isometric exercises and leg raises and is rapidly advanced to progressive resistive exercises. Muscle atrophy is minimized by the initiation of this exercise program in the immediate postoperative period, avoiding immobilization, encouraging active motion, and using modalities such as a muscle stimulator if needed to help the athlete regain muscle control.

After postoperative protection is discontinued the full range of motion is restored with both active and passive modalities. Progressive weight bearing is allowed as stability, motion, and strength return. Muscle strength, flexibility, and endurance are all enhanced at this stage with specific aggressive exercises. Early closed–kinetic chain activities are instituted at this stage.

The goal of the final stage of rehabilitation is complete return of muscle strength, flexibility, and endurance. Neuromuscular coordination is regained with more advanced exercise techniques. A functional brace frequently allows the patient at this stage to engage in a more aggressive exercise routine, such as sports cord activities, to achieve this end. Functional strengthening and sport-specific exercise programs are employed, including agility drills. Return to sport is dictated by the return of motion, flexibility, strength, and endurance.

Isokinetic testing (Cybex, Biodex) is helpful in evaluating return of strength. Power and endurance can be evaluated, as can any patellofemoral problem or pain pattern by examining the torque curve produced during these tests. Side-to-side comparisons are helpful, and a 10% deficit compared with the normal side is thought to be significant, though this assumes a normal contralateral extremity for comparison purposes, which may not be available. Peak torque–body weight ratios for normal subjects have been determined by Wilke for the Biodex device.[26] A less than 10% deficit on side-to-side comparisons (assuming a normal contralateral extremity) and return of peak torque–body weight ratios to 90% of normal are desirable before the athlete can return to full athletic activity. It should be noted that the peak torque–body weight ratio varies with isokinetic testing speeds and the sex of the patient.

There is a great deal of controversy about the efficacy of prophylactic braces. They have not been shown consistently to be beneficial and are not recommended for the uninjured knee. Rehabilitation braces can be used to protect the knee after ligament repair or reconstruction and when a medial ligament injury is to be treated nonoperatively. There is also a significant amount of controversy over the use of functional braces as the athlete returns to the sports field. Because so much time is required for strengthening and remodeling healing ligament structures, we frequently use a functional brace initially when the athlete returns to competition. These are to be used for the short term, though their use may extend through the next season. The ultimate goal is to return the athlete to the arena with a stable knee and a strong lower extremity. In our experience, good muscle strength and neuromuscular coordination provide the best "bracing" to enhance performance and minimize the risk of further injury to the knee.

REFERENCES

1. Hughston, J. C., and Eilers, A. F.: The role of the posterior oblique ligament and repairs of acute medial (collateral) ligament tears of the knee. J. Bone Joint Surg. *55A*:923, 1973.
2. Warren. L. F., and Marshall, J. L.: The supporting structures and layers on the medial side of the knee: An anatomic analysis. J. Bone Joint Surg. *61A*:56, 1979.
3. Hughston, J. C.: Knee Ligaments: Injury and Repair. St. Louis, Mosby-Year Book, 1993.
4. Müller, W.: The Knee: Form, Function and Ligament Reconstruction. New York, Springer-Verlag, 1983.
5. Warren, L. A., Marshall, J. L., and Girgis, F.: The prime static stabilizer of the medial side of the knee. J. Bone Joint Surg. *56A*:665, 1974.
6. Grood, E. S., and Noyes, F. R., Butler, D. L., and Suntay, W. J.: Ligamentous and capsular restraints preventing straight medial and lateral laxity in intact human cadaver knees. J. Bone Joint Surg. *63A*:1257, 1981.
7. Hughston, J. C., and Barrett, G. R.: Acute anteromedial rotatory instability: Long-term results of surgical repair. J. Bone Joint Surg. *65A*:145, 1983.

8. Hughston, J. C., Andrews, J. R., Cross, M. J., and Moschi, A.: Classification of knee ligament instabilities, Part I. The medial compartment and cruciate ligaments. J. Bone Joint Surg. *58A*:159, 1976.
9. American Medical Association (AMA): Standard Nomenclature of Athletic Injuries. Chicago, AMA, 1966.
10. Bergfeld, J.: Symposium: Functional rehabilitation of isolated medial collateral ligament sprains. First-, second-, and third-degree sprains. Am. J. Sports Med. *7*:207, 1979.
11. Woods, G. W., Stanley, R. F., and Tullos, H. S.: Lateral capsular sign: X-ray clue to a significant knee instability. Am. J. Sports Med. *7*:27, 1979.
12. O'Donoghue, D. H.: Surgical treatment of fresh injuries to the major ligaments of the knee. J. Bone Joint Surg. *32A*:721, 1950.
13. O'Donoghue, D. H.: Treatment of acute ligamentous injuries of the knee. Orthop. Clin. North Am. *4*:617, 1973.
14. Derscheid, G. L., and Garrick, J. G.: Medial collateral ligament injuries in football: nonoperative management of Grade I and II sprains. Am. J. Sports Med. *9*:365, 1981.
15. Ellsasser, J. C., Reynolds, F. C., and Omohundro, J. R.: The nonoperative treatment of collateral ligament injuries of the knee in professional football players. J. Bone Joint Surg. *56A*:1185, 1974.
16. Fetto, J. F., and Marshall, J. L.: Medial collateral ligament injuries of the knee: A rationale for treatment. Clin. Orthop. *132*:206, 1978.
17. Hastings, D. E.: Non-operative management of collateral ligament injuries of the knee joint. Clin. Orthop. *147*:22, 1980.
18. Indelicato, P. A.: Non-operative treatment of complete tears of the medial collateral ligament of the knee. J. Bone Joint Surg. *65A*:323, 1983.
19. Indelicato, P. A., Hermansdorfer, J., and Huegel, M.: Nonoperative management of complete tears of the medial collateral ligament of the knee in intercollegiate football players. Clin. Orthop. *256*:174, 1990.
20. Jones, R. E., Henley, M. B., and Francis, P.: Nonoperative management of isolated Grade III collateral ligament injury in high school football players. Clin. Orthop. *213*:137, 1986.
21. Akeson, W. H., et al.: The connective tissue response to immobility: Biochemical changes in periarticular connective tissue of the immobilized rabbit knee. Clin. Orthop. *93*:356, 1973.
22. Evans, E. B., Eggers, G. W. N., and Butler, J. K.: Experimental immobilization and then remobilization of rat knee joints. J. Bone Joint Surg. *42A*:737, 1960.
23. Noyes, F. R.: Functional properties of knee ligaments and alterations induced by immobilization. Clin. Orthop. *123*:210, 1977.
24. Woo, S. L. Y., et al.: The biomechanical and morphological changes in the medial collateral ligament of the rabbit after immobilization and remobilization. J. Bone Joint Surg. *69A*:1200, 1987.
25. Binkley, J. M., and Peat, M.: The effects of immobilization on the ultrastructure and mechanical properties of the medial collateral ligament of rats. Clin. Orthop. *203*:301, 1986.
26. Wilke, K. E.: Dynamic muscle strength testing. *In* Muscle Strength Testing. Edited by L. Amundsen. New York, Churchill Livingstone, 1990.

76 *Todd A. Schmidt*

Posterolateral Rotatory Instability

Posterolateral rotatory instability (PLRI) is abnormal external rotation and posterior subluxation of the lateral tibial plateau in relation to the lateral femoral condyle. This abnormal rotation occurs only when the posterior cruciate ligament is intact. It can be an isolated instability or combined with anterolateral or anteromedial instability, or both. Posterolateral instability has more devastating functional consequences than other types of instability. The combination of a posterior cruciate tear with posterolateral instability causes straight lateral instability, which is differentiated from PLRI by an injury mechanism and an injury pattern that produce abnormal translation instead of rotatory subluxation.

Before 1976, the orthopedic literature had scattered reports and small series of injuries to the lateral ligaments of the knee.[1–6] In 1976, Hughston and coworkers described a classification of lateral knee ligament injuries based on "a correlation of functional anatomy and clinical and operative findings" in patients with both acute and chronic lateral instability.[7] They defined PLRI on the basis of findings during the physical examination and associated surgical findings. They described a single posterolateral functional unit, called the *arcuate complex*. The components of this complex are the fibular collateral ligament, the arcuate ligament, and the tendoaponeurotic unit formed by the popliteus muscle. In conjunction with these static structures are the reinforcements of the biceps femoris and the lateral head of the gastrocnemius.

Subsequent to the publication of the classification system of Hughston's group, there have been other clinical reports, anatomic studies, biomechanic evaluations, and descriptions of new clinical signs.[8–23] Careful study of this information helps the physician to make an accurate clinical diagnosis and to manage PLRI appropriately.

ANATOMY

The posterolateral anatomy of the knee is a complex interlinked musculotendoligamentous unit commonly referred to as *the arcuate complex* (Fig. 76–1). Seebacher paraphrases Kaplan to indicate that this complex structure is an evolutionary phenomenon of "adjustment of the sleeves of muscles that move the joint, providing balance and maximizing muscle efficiency."[11] Hughston states, "Functionally, each of the ligaments in the arcuate complex can be considered as an aponeurosis of the long and short head of the biceps and the central half of the popliteal muscle. Their complexity has resulted from the evolutionary digression of the proximal fibula distally from its previous femoral articulation. This distal migration allows for the rotation of the knee joint necessary to accommodate functional use of the knee in the erect posture."[24]

BIOMECHANICS

In the past 10 years, several studies of the biomechanics of the posterolateral portion of the knee have been published.[20–23] These scientific studies have helped clarify the restraints and limits of motion the posterolateral structures impose on movement of the knee when various forces are applied. Only the static effect of these structures can be studied in the cadaver model. In vivo, however, a dynamic influence supports these static structures. We have also found, at surgery, that the injury patterns typically are not the same as those that are created by selective cutting studies in cadavers.[25] Nonetheless, valuable information can be gained from these reports.

A deficit of the arcuate complex produces the greatest dysfunction and potential for impairment near the point of complete extension. Removal of these postero-

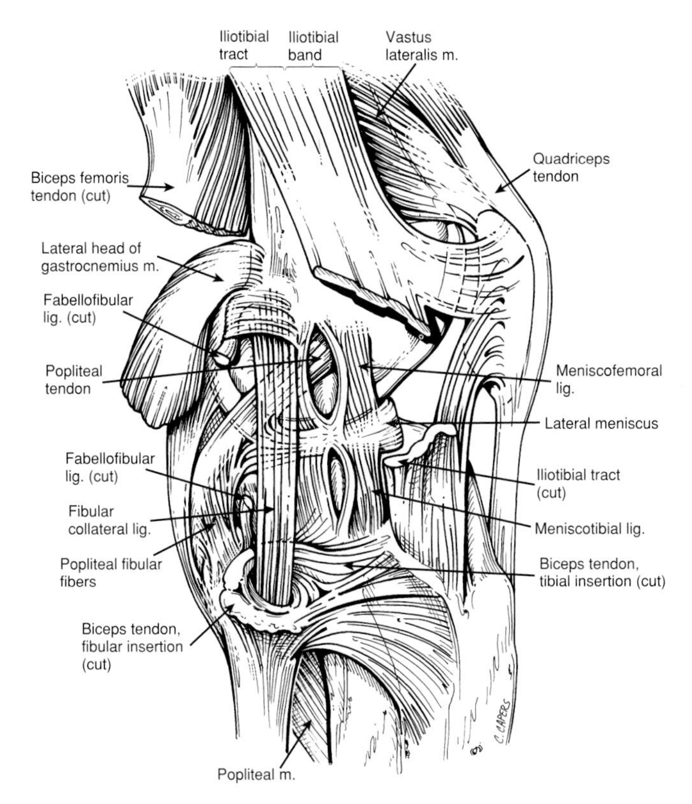

Fig. 76–1. Anatomy of the lateral aspect of the knee, including the arcuate ligament.

lateral restraints leads to increased external tibial rotation; the magnitude depends on the angle of knee flexion. When the arcuate complex alone is cut, external rotation is greater at 30° than at 90°.[25] When the posterior cruciate ligament is also sectioned, external rotation at 90° increases significantly, as does posterior translation of the tibia. In addition, the arcuate complex has been shown to act as the principal restraint to lateral opening. Posterolateral sectioning has also been shown to lead to an increase in internal rotation laxity and external rotation. When these structures fail, the anterior and the posterior cruciate ligaments are secondary restraints to adduction. When the posterolateral structures are cut, the anterior cruciate ligament also acts as the secondary restraint to internal rotation near extension and the posterior cruciate ligament is a secondary restraint to external rotation at 45° to 90° of flexion.

Isolated posterior cruciate ligament sectioning does not cause an increase in rotational laxity of the knee if the posterolateral capsule is intact. This indicates that, especially near extension, it is injury to the arcuate complex—not the posterior cruciate ligament—that causes PLRI.

MECHANISMS OF INJURY

For PLRI, the mechanism of injury is typically hyperextension and external rotation of the knee. We have found about half of all injuries to be contact injuries caused by a direct blow and half to be noncontact injuries caused by an indirect force applied to the knee.

A football tackle or block is the prototype of the contact injury. A direct blow to the extended knee, often from the anteromedial side, causes forceful hyperextension and simultaneous external tibial rotation (Fig. 76–2). About one fourth of our patients who sustain a contact injury present with an abrasion or ecchymosis over the anteromedial aspect of the knee. In approximately a fourth of our patients, PLRI is caused by a direct blow to the knee sustained while playing football.

Noncontact hyperextension injuries can occur in a number of ways. Usually, they are related to sudden or unexpected deceleration of the upper leg and body, which acts on the posterolateral structures of the knee as a lever on the fixed or planted foot. We have seen this frequently—in sports, falls, landing off balance, going over the handlebars of a motorcycle, or even stepping in a hole while walking.

With both contact and noncontact mechanisms, when the knee is extended the posterolateral capsule is the principal restraint. We rarely see concomitant posterior cruciate ligament tears with these injury mechanisms. Combined posterolateral and posterior cruciate ligament injuries typically occur from a direct anterior blow to the flexed knee;[26] though, with PLRI we do fre-

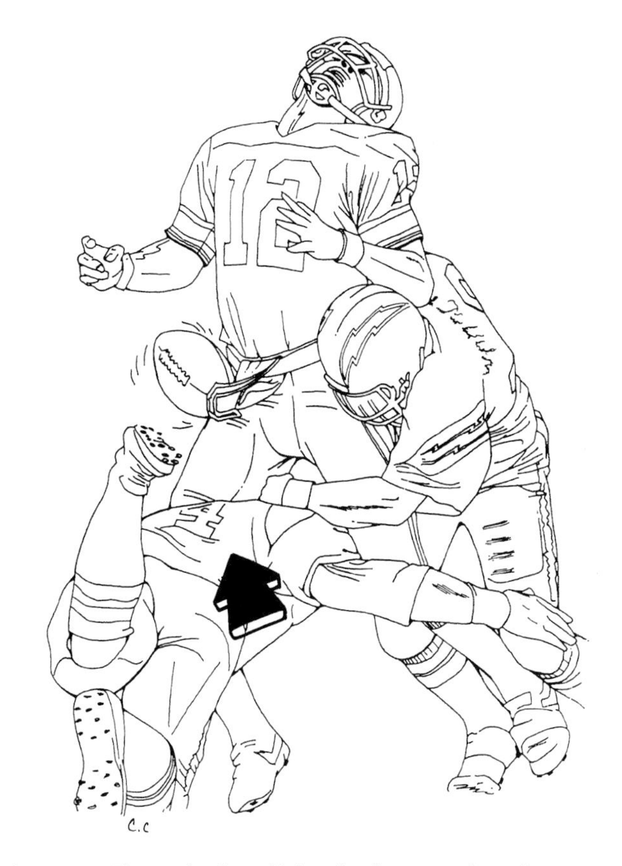

Fig. 76–2. The mechanism of injury for the posterolateral structures is often a direct blow to the extended knee from the anteromedial side, causing forceful hyperextension and simultaneous external tibial rotation.

quently see other instability patterns that are the result of injury to the posteromedial capsule or the anterior cruciate ligament and the iliotibial tract.

Iatrogenic damage to the arcuate ligament complex, though it is less common today than in the past, can occur if the surgeon does not fully understand knee anatomy and surgical techniques. Open meniscectomy or meniscal repair and anterior cruciate ligament and lateral extra-articular reconstructions have sometimes resulted in PLRI as a complication. Experience, education, and the emergence of arthroscopic techniques have led to a decline in iatrogenic PLRI.

CLINICAL PRESENTATION

When PLRI occurs in combination with other instabilities and ligament injuries, the patient usually seeks medical attention promptly. Typically, the patient cannot bear weight on the injured leg. With an injury that causes only PLRI, the patient may have little swelling and may be able to walk with only a limp. The injury may be thought to be "just a sprain." These patients may not seek medical attention until days or weeks after the injury.

With PLRI of long standing, the most frequent complaint is of "giving way backward" into hyperextension, which causes the patient unconsciously to assume a flexed-knee gait. Twisting, pivoting, and cutting are usually difficult. When pain accompanies this instability, it is usually localized along the medial joint line. After reviewing the patient's history, the physician confirms the diagnosis of PLRI by physical examination. Many clinical tests have been described, all variations of two unique tests: the posterolateral drawer test and the external rotation recurvatum test.

The posterolateral drawer test is performed with the knee in both 90° and 30° of flexion. The examiner holds the patient's knee and supports the leg by placing both hands on the proximal tibia with the thumbs on either side of the tibial tubercle. The leg and foot are rotated externally and repeated push and external rotation motion is applied (Fig. 76–3). The examiner looks and feels for posterior and external rotational translation of the tibia while pushing. The integrity of the posterior cruciate ligament is evaluated by testing the posterior drawer with the leg in neutral and internal rotation as well as by comparing the results of the posterolateral drawer test at 90° with that at 30°.

If a patient has PLRI and an intact posterior cruciate ligament, the posterior drawer sign is absent when the knee is rotated internally. The intact posterior cruciate ligament fibers are tightened with internal rotation and allow little anteroposterior motion. External rotation of the tibia relaxes the posterior cruciate ligament so that the arcuate complex is the principal stabilizing limit to motion. In addition, biomechanical studies have shown that the posterolateral drawer is most sensitive for assessing arcuate complex injury of the knees at 30° of flexion. Therefore, testing at both 30° and 90° assesses contributions to stability of both the arcuate complex and the posterior cruciate ligament.

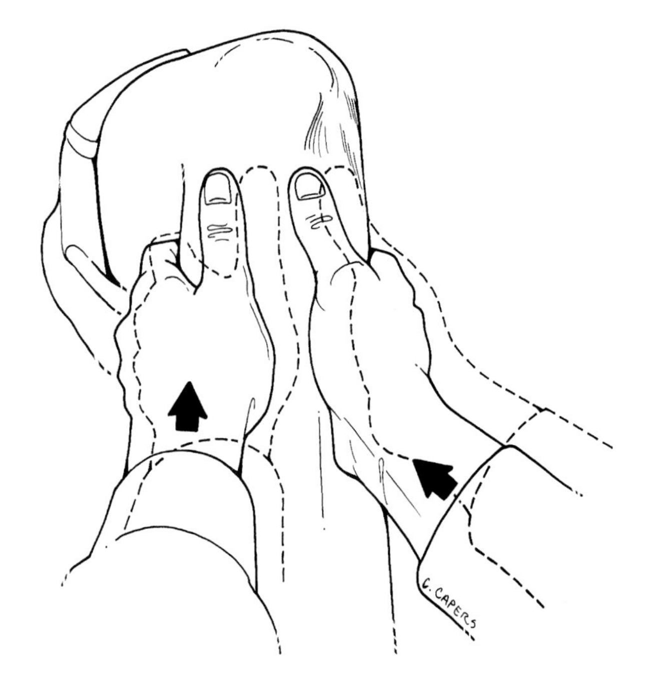

Fig. 76–3. The posterolateral drawer test is used to measure posterior and external rotational translation of the tibia.

The second test that is sensitive for PLRI, the external rotation recurvatum test, demonstrates abnormal motion of the femur in relation to the tibia when the knee is extended. The examination is performed on the supine patient with the legs extended. One of the examiner's hands is placed behind the knee to feel the relative motion of the tibia and femur. The opposite hand holds the medial forefoot and lifts the lower leg, placing the knee in maximum extension. Holding the foot in this manner allows the tibia to rotate externally and assume varus posture at the same time. In addition, recurvatum or relative hyperextension can occur. The anterior cruciate ligament comes into contact with the intercondylar shelf in extension. Thus, the degree of recurvatum is accentuated if the anterior cruciate ligament is torn. These motions can be both visualized and felt with the hand behind the knee. Visual side-to-side comparison is possible by holding the feet and extending both knees at the same time (Fig. 76–4). The external rotation recurvatum motion of the affected knee is compared with that in the unaffected knee.

Other tests are simply variations of the two described previously. Loomer described a modification of the posterolateral drawer test in which both hips and knees are flexed to 90° while the examiner grasps the foot.[16] While supporting and suspending the legs and looking up the axis of the tibia at the knee, the examiner externally rotates both feet maximally. The test is positive if, on side-to-side comparison, external rotation of the tibia is excessive, as indicated by viewing the direction in which the feet point. Cooper suggests doing the same test with the patient prone at both 30° and 90° of knee flexion.[18] The voluntary evoked posterolateral drawer sign was described by Shino and coworkers.[15] When seated, a patient with chronic posterolateral instability

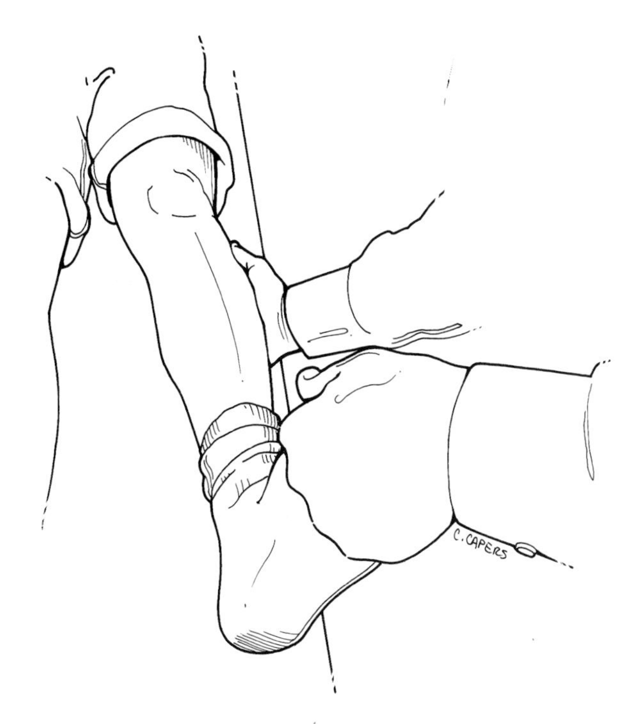

Fig. 76–4. Side-to-side comparison during the external rotation recurvatum test is done by lifting the patient's extremities by the big toe of each foot and watching for external rotation recurvatum in the injured extremity.

selectively contracts the biceps femoris, causing posterolateral subluxation, and then selectively contracts the popliteus to reduce it.

Two other tests use passive knee extension to assess tibial subluxation. In the reverse pivot shift test,[17] the examiner holds the patient's leg with the knee flexed and allows the tibia to slip into posterolateral subluxation. As the knee is straightened, valgus force is applied. As the knee approaches 20° less than full extension, one can see and feel a jerklike shift as the lateral tibial plateau is reduced under the femur. A variation of the reverse pivot shift is the dynamic posterior shift test.[14] In this test, the hip is flexed more to better control femoral rotation and to allow the hamstrings to tighten, thus applying an axial load to the joint. These tests are both variations of the posterolateral drawer test at 30°.

All tests for PLRI require careful comparison of the affected knee with the unaffected one.[18] There is a considerable range of normal laxity evident while performing the clinical tests for posterolateral rotatory instability.[25] The examination findings are clinically significant if they are present only in the injured knee.

Additional physical signs can be detected by assessing the skin and the peroneal nerve. Abrasions or ecchymosis on the medial side of the knee or upper shin are a clue that a direct blow was sustained in a site where it could injure the posterolateral ligaments. Because the peroneal nerve passes through the posterolateral aspect of the knee and is relatively fixed as it enters the leg, it is at risk for traction injury. Peroneal nerve function should be carefully assessed in patients with PLRI. Ten percent of our patients with acute PLRI have an injury to the peroneal nerve: half of the injuries are transient paresthesia, and the remainder complete palsy. Of patients with palsy, half recover and half have permanent loss of peroneal nerve function.

Radiographic examination is important when PLRI is suspected. As with any traumatic injury, subtle skeletal lesions may be seen. Shindell and coworkers described a radiographic finding ("the arcuate sign") that represents a fragment of bone avulsed from the fibular head.[12] Anatomically, it is a tear of the fibular arm of the arcuate ligament or the fibular collateral ligament insertion, or both. In an acutely injured knee the arcuate sign indicates posterolateral ligamentous injury.

Magnetic resonance imaging (MRI) is often useful in determining the presence or absence of ligamentous and osseous injuries of the posterolateral knee. However, it is often not helpful in assessing the specific pattern or exact location of arcuate complex injury. It is most helpful as an adjunct in the assessment of the integrity and anatomy of the cruciate ligaments and the menisci. It may be helpful if the clinical decision is whether to operate and what the operative procedure should be.

ACUTE POSTEROLATERAL ROTATORY INSTABILITY

We have found acute PLRI to be a relatively uncommon instability as compared with acute anterolateral or anteromedial rotatory instability. The diagnosis can usually be based on clinical examination findings, though sometimes the patient must be examined under anesthesia. Once the diagnosis of significant PLRI is made and related injuries are identified, a surgical plan is devised.

With PLRI, the arcuate ligament is always torn, most often near the tibia or fibula or transversely just proximal to the meniscus near the femoral origin. The fibular collateral ligament, popliteus, and short head of the biceps also tear frequently. The popliteus most often tears either near its femoral origin or at the musculotendinous junction, whereas the fibular collateral ligament usually tears near one end. When torn distally, the biceps tendon is often avulsed off the fibula as well. Surgical repair of these acute ligament or tendon injuries is accomplished with direct ligament-to-ligament and soft tissue–to–bone suture techniques.[8,27]

With isolated PLRI, the anterior cruciate ligament may be torn. A torn anterior cruciate ligament may also be part of the injury pattern of combined PLRI and ALRI. Meniscal tears are uncommon with isolated PLRI; however, with combined instabilities, lateral meniscal tears are common and frequently repairable.

We usually do not do intra-articular anterior cruciate ligament reconstruction at the same time as capsular and extra-articular repair of acute injuries that cause combined PLRI and ALRI. We find the posterolateral repair to be more secure when knee extension can be blocked for a period of 6 to 12 weeks. Because anterior cruciate ligament reconstruction should include full extension as part of early rehabilitation, we believe it best to achieve an early solid posterolateral repair and not risk potential complications caused by blocked extension after intra-articular surgery. Our results show it is rare for patients to have a residual instability that requires subsequent anterior cruciate ligament reconstruction.[26]

CHRONIC POSTEROLATERAL ROTATORY INSTABILITY

PLRI becomes chronic when initially it is missed, misdiagnosed, or mistreated. Careful attention to the patient's history and physical examination helps to make the diagnosis of this complex problem. Symptoms can be misleading if the condition has become chronic. The patient often experiences medial joint line pain because posterolateral subluxation increases the rotational and compressive forces on the medial compartment. Arthroscopic examinations to determine the cause of this medial pain are usually negative. Another common symptom in the chronic condition is the inability to "push off" with the affected leg. This occurs because the athlete does not have a solid end point that locks the knee in extension. The athlete often minimizes this functional disability by holding the knee in slight flexion.

With combined instability, PLRI can sometimes be overlooked because the examiner's attention is focused on the more obvious subluxations. This is often the case when ALRI is concomitant with an anterior cruciate ligament tear. When combined acute PLRI and ALRI is treated with reconstruction of the anterior cruciate ligament only, posterolateral instability can persist and cause the athlete functional problems. With chronic combined instability, if the surgeon's attention is focused solely on reconstruction of the anterior cruciate ligament, abnormal motions due to the combined laxity of the arcuate complex, lateral capsule, and iliotibial band injuries may persist.

In both of these situations, careful evaluation of the knee helps inform the decision about which surgical procedure to perform. For combined instability in which PLRI is severe, we have had good longterm results with extra-articular and capsular reconstruction. When the PLRI is the less severe subluxation, consideration can be given to combining intra-articular cruciate and extra-articular capsular surgery using modern surgical techniques. Three general methods of ligament reconstruction have been advocated for chronic PLRI: arcuate complex advancement and reefing; popliteal bypass; and fibular collateral ligament reconstruction.

With an arcuate complex advancement,[19,27] the common femoral osseous attachment of the fibular collateral ligament, popliteus, lateral head of the gastrocnemius, and arcuate ligament is osteotomized as a bone flap where these structures attach (Fig. 76–5A). When this flap is reflected, direct inspection and repair of the posterior half of the lateral meniscus and the popliteal hiatus is possible. The more distal portion of the arcuate ligament is then examined and stabilized to the tibia and fibula. This anchors the ligament so that, when the arcuate complex flap is advanced, pathologic looseness and excessive length are eliminated. The bone and arcuate complex flap is advanced anteriorly and fixed distally to a prepared bone bed (Fig. 76–5B). Just before the advancement and fixation, sutures are placed in the vertical posterior edge of the flap, along the medial

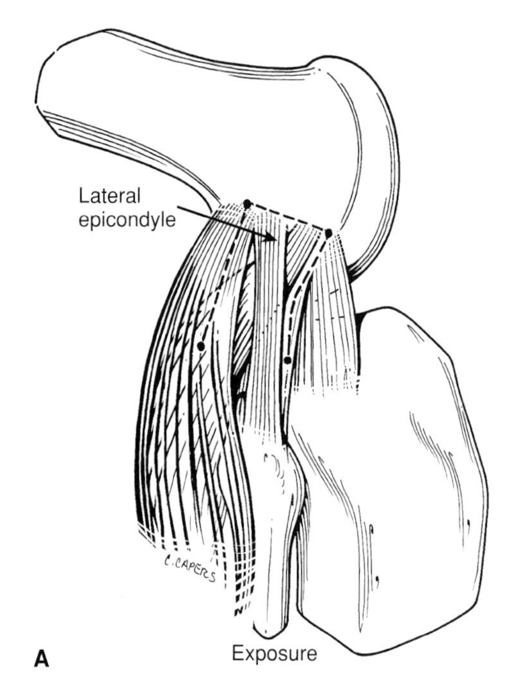

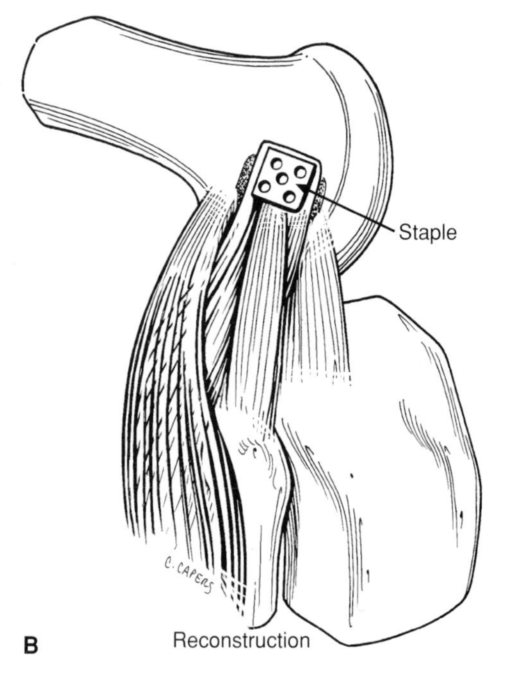

Fig. 76–5. *(A)* **Exposure for reconstruction of the arcuate complex. The femoral attachment of the fibular collateral ligament, popliteus, lateral head of the gastrocnemius, and arcuate ligament is osteotomized as a bone flap where these structures attach.** *(B)* **The bone and arcuate complex flap is advanced anteriorly and distally.**

edge of the gastrocnemius tendon–arcuate ligament. Once the complex is advanced and fixed to bone, the posterior sutures are tied, thus reefing and reconstructing the arcuate and fabellofibular ligaments and lateral head of the gastrocnemius. Proximally, the transferred and tightened tissue heals back to the original femoral bone bed, leaving the restored complex at its preinjury length and attachment sites. Repairs for associated instability may be done at the same time.

The popliteal bypass procedure has been described by several authors who believe that the popliteus tendon is the most important component of the arcuate complex.[28–30] They have suggested using a popliteal bypass procedure, passing a tissue substitute or augmentation such as a strip of iliotibial band, biceps tendon, free semitendinosus tendon, or an allograft through bone tunnels in the tibia and femur. The goal is to replicate the axis of the popliteal tendon, and thus its static function. No attempt is made to address the arcuate ligament or the dynamic aspect of the arcuate complex. The popliteal bypass functions, therefore, as a posterolateral tenodesis.

A third technique involves reconstruction of the fibular collateral ligament using the biceps tendon as a substitute.[31] The rationale is to cancel the action of the biceps femoris muscle, transferring its distally based tendon to create a new fibular collateral ligament and a lateral tenodesis. The tendon is left attached distally to the fibula and is transferred to the lateral femoral epicondyle, where it is fixed, ideally to the normal origin of the fibular collateral ligament. It is thought that the biceps transfer also "sweeps up the attached arcuate complex with it." Clancy, however, recommends against performing the procedure when the knee has sustained moderate or severe trauma and the biceps may have been ruptured from the fibula and the posterolateral capsule.

SUMMARY

Any physician who treats knee injuries should be familiar with and aware of PLRI when evaluating knee ligament injuries. Because chronic PLRI can be extremely disabling, the recommended treatment is early repair of all injured structures. When acute injuries to the posterolateral structures of the knee are overlooked, late reconstruction is possible and may be necessary.

REFERENCES

1. Platt, H.: On the peripheral nerve complications of certain fractures. J. Bone Joint Surg. *10*:403, 1928.
2. Watson Jones, R.: Styloid process of the fibula in the knee joint with peroneal palsy. J. Bone Joint Surg. *13*:258, 1931.
3. Highet, W. B., and Holmes, W.: Traction injuries to the lateral popliteal nerve and traction injuries to peripheral nerves after suture. Br. J. Surg. *30*:212, 1942.
4. Abbott, L. C., Saunders, J. B. D. M., Bost, F. C., and Anderson, C. E.: Injuries to the ligaments of the knee joint. J. Bone Joint Surg. *26*:503, 1944.
5. Novich, M. M.: Adduction injury of the knee with rupture of the common peroneal nerve. J. Bone Joint Surg. *42A*:1372, 1960.
6. Towne, L. C., Blazina, M. E., Marmor, L., and Lawrence, J. F.: Lateral compartment syndrome of the knee. Clin. Orthop. *76*:160, 1971.
7. Hughston, J. C., Andrews, J. R., Cross, M. J., and Moschi, A.: Classification of knee ligament instabilities. Parts I and II. J. Bone Joint Surg. *58A*:159, 1976.
8. Baker, C. L., Norwood, L. A., and Hughston, J. C.: Acute posterolateral rotatory instability of the knee. J. Bone Joint Surg. *65A*:614, 1983.
9. DeLee, J. C., Riley, M. B., and Rockwood, C. A., Jr.: Acute posterolateral rotatory instability of the knee. Am. J. Sports Med. *11*:199, 1983.
10. Grana, W. A., and Janssen, T.: Lateral ligament injury of the knee. Orthopedics *10*:1039, 1987.
11. Seebacher, J. R., et al.: The structure and function of the posterolateral aspect of the knee. J. Bone Joint Surg. *64A*:536, 1982.
12. Shindell, R., Walsh, W. M., and Connolly, J. F.: Avulsion fracture of the fibula: The "arcuate sign" of posterolateral knee instability. Nebraska Med. J. *69*:369, 1984.
13. Hughston, J. C., and Norwood, L. A., Jr.: The posterolateral drawer test and external rotational recurvatum test for posterolateral rotatory instability of the knee. Clin. Orthop. *147*:82, 1980.
14. Shelbourne, K. D., Benedict, F., McCarroll, J. R., and Rettig, A. C.: Dynamic posterior shift test. Am. J. Sports Med. *17*:275, 1989.
15. Shino, K., Horibe, S., and Ono, K.: The voluntarily evoked posterolateral drawer sign in the knee with posterolateral instability. Clin. Orthop. *215*:179, 1987.
16. Loomer, R. L.: A test for knee posterolateral rotatory instability. Clin. Orthop. *264*:235, 1991.
17. Jakob, R. P., Hassler, H., and Staeubli, H.-U.: Observations on rotatory instability of the lateral compartment of the knee. Acta Orthop. Scand. (Suppl. 191): 1, 1981.
18. Cooper, D. E.: Tests for posterolateral instability of the knee in normal subjects. J. Bone Joint Surg. *73A*:30, 1991.
19. Hughston, J. C., and Jacobson, K. E.: Chronic posterolateral rotatory instability of the knee. J. Bone Joint Surg. *67A*:351, 1985.
20. Nielsen, S., et al.: Rotatory instability of cadaver knees after transection of collateral ligaments and capsule. Arch. Orthop. Trauma Surg. *103*:165, 1984.
21. Grood, E. S., Stowers, S. F., and Noyes, F. R.: Limits of movement in the human knee. J. Bone Joint Surg. *70A*:88, 1988.
22. Gollehon, D. L., Torzilli, P. A., and Warren, R. F.: The role of the posterolateral and cruciate ligaments in the stability of the human knee. J. Bone Joint Surg. *69A*:233, 1987.
23. Markolf, K. L., et al.: Direct in vitro measurement of forces in the cruciate ligaments. Part II. J. Bone Joint Surg. *75A*:387, 1993.
24. Hughston, J. C.: Knee Ligaments: Injury and Repair. St. Louis, Mosby-Year Book, 1993.
25. Schmidt, T. A., Jacobson, K. E., and Hughston, J. C.: Acute posterolateral rotatory instability of the knee. Presentation at the 7th Annual Meeting of the Southern Orthopaedic Association, Maui, HI, 1990.
26. Baker, C. L., Jr., Norwood, L.A., and Hughston, J. C.: Acute combined posterior cruciate and posterolateral instability of the knee. Am. J. Sports Med. *12*:204, 1984.
27. Trillat, A.: Posterolateral instability. *In* Late Reconstructions of Injured Ligaments of the Knee. Edited by K. P. Schulitz, M. Krahl, and W. H. Stein. Berlin, Springer-Verlag, 1978.
28. Müller, W.: The Knee: Form, Function, and Ligament Reconstruction. Berlin, Springer-Verlag, 1983.
29. Bousquet, G., et al.: Stabilisation du condyle externe du genou dans les laxites anterieures chroniques: Importance du muscle poplite. Rev. Chir. Orthop. 72:427, 1986.
30. Jakob, R. P., and Warner, J. P.: Lateral and posterolateral rotatory instability of the knee. *In* The Knee and Cruciate Ligaments. Edited by R. P. Jakob and H.-U. Stäubli. Berlin, Springer-Verlag, 1992.
31. Clancy, W. G., Jr.: Repair and reconstruction of the posterior cruciate ligament. *In* Operative Orthopaedics. 2nd Ed. Edited by M. W. Chapman. Philadelphia, J. B., Lippincott, 1993.

77 *John Uribe*

Low-Velocity Dislocations of the Knee

Traumatic dislocation of the knee is a dramatic injury that results in extensive soft tissue damage, and frequently in neurologic or vascular compromise. It is described as an uncommon, even rare, injury. Meyers and Harvey reported seeing 53 cases over a 10-year period at Los Angeles County Hospital.[1] Hoover found 14 knee dislocations out of 2 million admissions to the Mayo Clinic,[2] whereas Shields and coworkers reported 26 cases over 28 years at the Massachusetts General Hospital.[3] The true incidence of this injury is likely much higher, and it appears to be increasing.[4] Many cases go unreported because the knee is frequently reduced at the scene of the injury or reduces spontaneously. Most published series are compilations of cases from large institutions seen over a number of years and treated by multiple physicians using a variety of different techniques. Consequently, proper management of this injury lacks consensus and remains controversial.

Dislocations of the knee can be a consequence of severe, or of very minimal, trauma. Those that result from high-energy trauma such as motor vehicle accidents, pedestrian-auto collisions, or falls farther than 5 feet are considered high-velocity dislocations. Low-velocity dislocations are most frequently caused by athletic trauma, usually from contact sports or falls from a height less than 5 feet. In published series of knee dislocations that report the individual mechanisms of injury, low-velocity dislocations account for approximately 25 to 30%.[3,5–7] Shelbourne and coworkers have the only published series of low-velocity dislocations, and it includes grossly unstable knees with complete tears of both cruciates and a collateral ligament.[8] Because the possible consequences of the injury and the management are similar, Shelbourne's group regards those injuries as dislocation followed by spontaneous reduction and likens them to frank dislocations. They report on 21 dislocations seen over a 7-year period, all due to sports-related trauma.

Kennedy classified knee dislocations into five types, according to the position of the tibia relative to the femur: straight (anterior, posterior, medial, lateral) or rotational.[9] Anterior dislocation appears to be the most common type,[10] though this classification is limiting, as it does not affect the treatment or the prognosis of the injury. A better approach is to classify the residual instability, as established by Hughston and colleagues.[11] This affords a better appreciation for the damaged structures, and, consequently, a more valid interpretation of results.

MECHANISM OF INJURY

Low-velocity knee dislocations can be the result of direct or indirect trauma. Kennedy demonstrated that hyperextension of the knee can result in anterior dislocation, with rupture of the posterior capsule at 30° of hyperextension (Fig. 77–1). Posterior dislocation usually results from direct trauma on the upper end of the tibia on a fixed femur or the lower end of the femur on a fixed tibia (Fig. 77–2). Varus forces produce medial dislocation with complete disruption of the lateral structures, and valgus forces may result in lateral dislocation with disruption of medial structures. Torsional stresses such as those produced by excessive rotation on a fixed tibia when changing direction rapidly or that produced by snow- or water skiing can cause rotatory dislocation (posteromedial, posterolateral, anteromedial, anterolateral).

Evaluation

A frank knee dislocation is usually quite obvious because there is marked deformity of the knee and a palpable step-off of the tibia in relation to the femur.

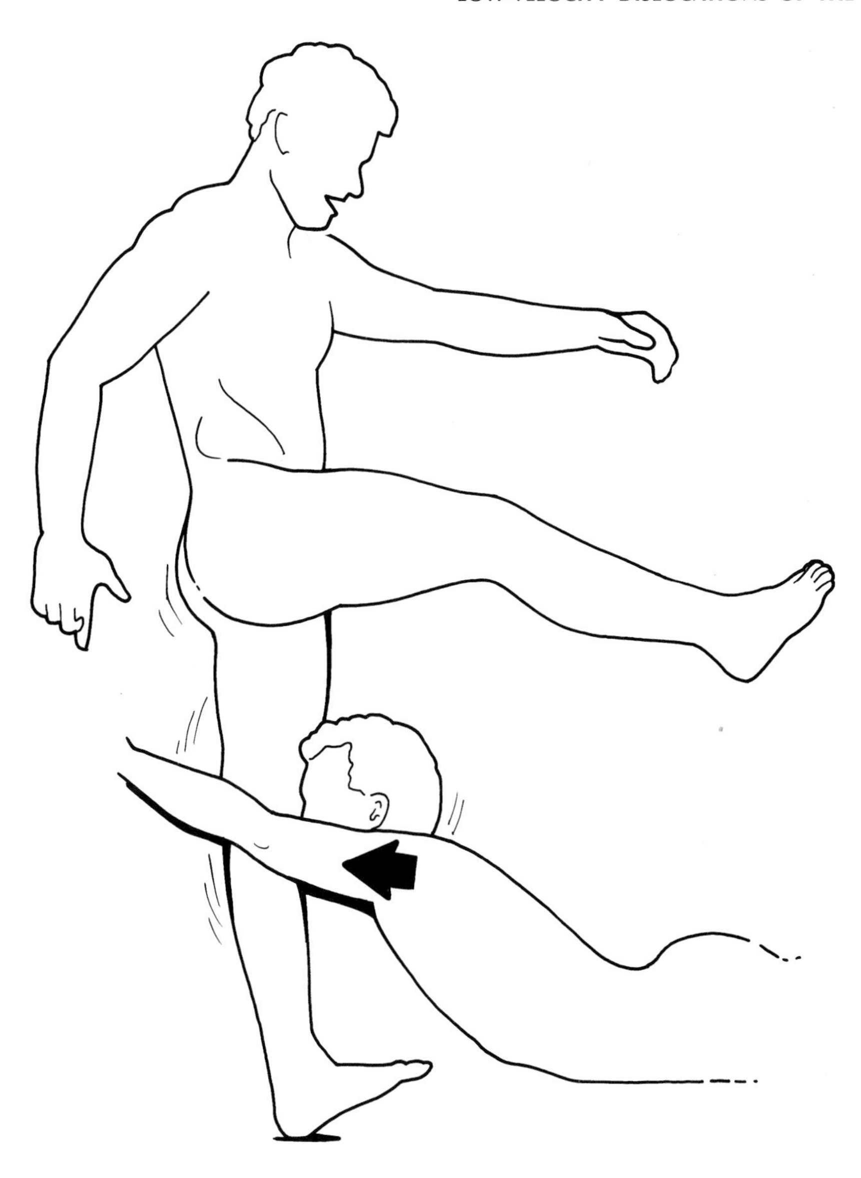

Fig. 77–1. Knee dislocation in sports can occur when a player such as a punter who planted a leg is struck across the knee, causing hyperextension dislocation.

Those knees with gross instability where Lachman's test is not only causing anterior subluxation of the tibia but reducing a posterior subluxation, and where the knee opens like a book with varus or valgus stress in full extension should be considered a dislocation that has spontaneously reduced. In the case of the clinically dislocated knee, a neurovascular examination should be carried out before reduction; though, often, this is not feasible because the athlete is in a great deal of pain, the hamstrings are in spasm, and removal of the shoes and tape may be too time consuming.

Reduction can usually be accomplished with relative ease. Heister described the technique in 1743 that today remains relevant: "The patient is placed on a bed or table. An assistant then holds the thigh firm above the knee while another extends the leg with the surgeon manipulating the knee into its natural place"[9] (Fig. 77–3). Open reduction may be necessary for posterior lateral dislocation if reduction is blocked by "buttonholing" of the medial femoral condyle and trapping of the medial hamstrings and collateral ligament. A "furrow" or "skin dimple" along the medial aspect of the knee may be evident; this is a clinical indication of the irreducibility.[12]

Dislocation of the knee is a true orthopedic emergency, and rapid realignment is essential. Reduction significantly relieves pain, which allows for more comprehensive examination. This sideline examination is the most informative until the patient is under anesthesia. On visual inspection, an already reduced knee may appear benign because the capsular disruption permits bleeding to spread into the calf rather than to collect as an effusion. The neurovascular status is assessed, with emphasis on comparison of the pedal pulses and the motor and sensory function of the peroneal nerve (Fig. 77–4).

After the neurovascular check, the emphasis of the physical examination is to determine the instability pattern of the knee and what residual ligaments are intact. Particular attention should be directed to the patellar

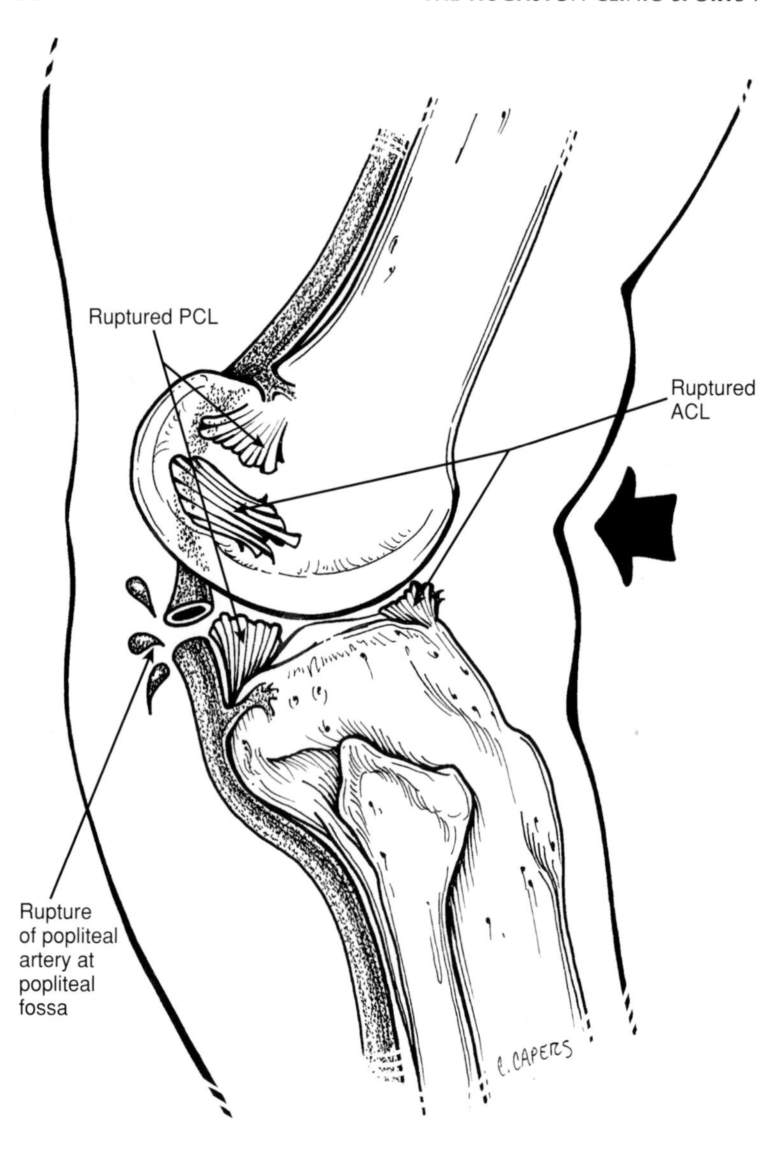

Fig. 77–2. Hyperextension of the knee can tear cruciates and cause traction injury of the popliteal artery.

tendon, which may also rupture with a knee dislocation and be overlooked. The examiner should determine the degree to which hyperextension is permitted as well as the degree of medial or lateral laxity with the knee in full extension (Fig. 77–5). It is not necessary to attempt a pivot shift or to stress the knee at 90° because this adds little to the diagnosis and is difficult to interpret. The knee is then immobilized at approximately 15° to 30° of flexion in either a posterior splint or a range of motion brace.

COMPLICATIONS

The popliteal artery originates in the tendinous hiatus of the adductor magnus muscle that holds it firmly against the femoral shaft. It then crosses the popliteal space and runs under the tendinous arch of the soleus, where, again, it is secured firmly to the tibia, making it susceptible to injury, particularly with hyperextension.[9]

The popliteal artery is injured in approximately 33% of knee dislocations (range, 16 to 64%).[6,10,13,14] Shelbourne thinks the risk is decreased in low-velocity dislocations, finding only 1 of 21 low-velocity dislocations with a popliteal artery injury.[8] McCoy and coworkers reported on four low-velocity dislocations, three of which had significant popliteal injury even though in two of those the pedal pulse was still palpable.[15] They emphasized that palpable pulses do not rule out an intimal tear that can later form a thrombus, a limb-threatening situation. Capillary refill is totally unreliable and it can be disastrous to mistake it as a sign of viability. If arterial repair is required, it should be performed within 6 to 8 hours, after which the need for amputation rises significantly.[16]

Siliski and Plancher recently reported on 3 of 40 knee dislocations resulting in above-knee amputations secondary to arterial injury, reinforcing the need for accurate assessment of the vascular status following a knee dislocation.[17] In our institution, all patients with frank knee dislocations and those with diminished pedal pulses undergo arteriography. All others are examined with duplex Doppler imaging and are closely monitored.

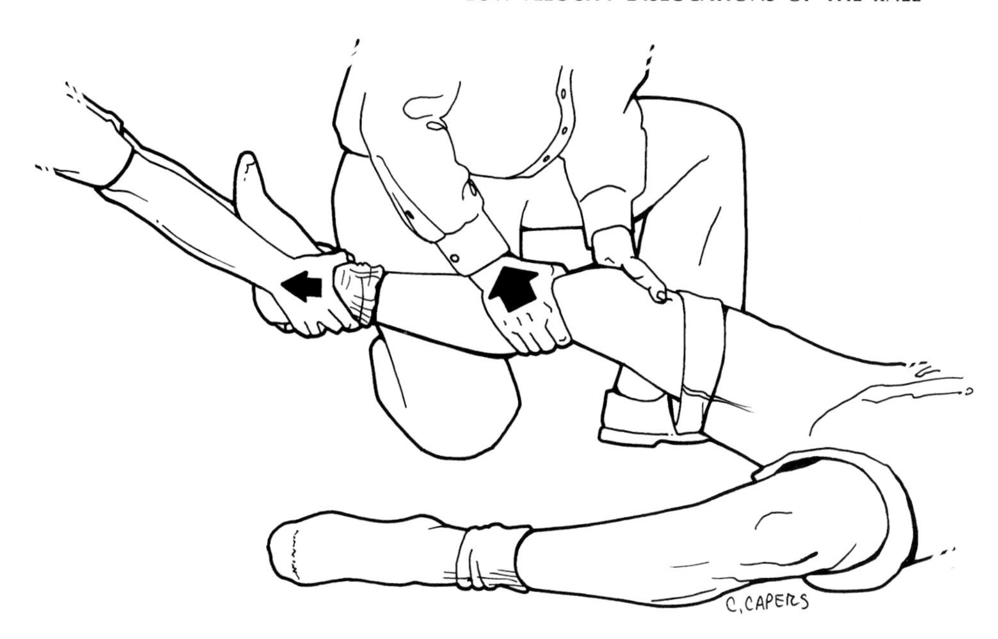

Fig. 77–3. During reduction of a dislocated knee, an assistant helps extend the knee while the surgeon manipulates it into correct position.

Nerve palsies are associated with 25 to 40% of knee dislocations.[18,19] The peroneal nerve, overwhelmingly the nerve most frequently injured, is particularly susceptible with medial dislocations. Approximately 50% of palsies remain permanent regardless of treatment, though those with partial involvement have a much better prognosis. The initial evaluation is therefore important in determining prognosis.

RADIOLOGY

Radiographs are valuable in determining the adequacy of reduction as well as the presence of bone fragments that may indicate soft tissue avulsions. We have found magnetic resonance imaging (MRI) to be extremely helpful, not only in determining the extent of ligamentous and subchondral injury but for preoperative planning. The surgical approach can be determined as well as the repairability of the cruciates, collateral ligaments, popliteal tendon, and menisci.

TREATMENT

There is considerable controversy regarding the ligamentous management of these injuries. There are essentially three basic approaches: (1) immobilization for 6 weeks[20]; (2) waiting 3 to 6 weeks, until range of motion is regained, before limited surgical intervention emphasizing reconstruction of the posterior cruciate and collateral ligaments[8]; and (3) early repair or reconstruction of all involved structures.[21] The problem lies in interpreting the results of the various forms of treatment because reported series lack a common method of evaluation and approaches to management of the injury vary much.

Overall, closed treatment provides a good functional result in approximately 68% of cases (i.e. better than 90° of flexion and stability). With a limited surgical approach, Shelbourne reports 19% return to the same level of athletic participation and 100% subjectively report good results overall.[8] Sisto and Warren, after repairing all damaged structures, reported 100% good overall results, and 77% of patients returned to some kind of athletic participation.[6] Our experience is very similar to that of Sisto and Warren. We found, as they noted, that ligament injuries in knee dislocations were often avulsions and thus amenable to anatomic repair, which today is much facilitated by the use of bone anchors. The overall common denominator for a good result appears to be early range of motion.

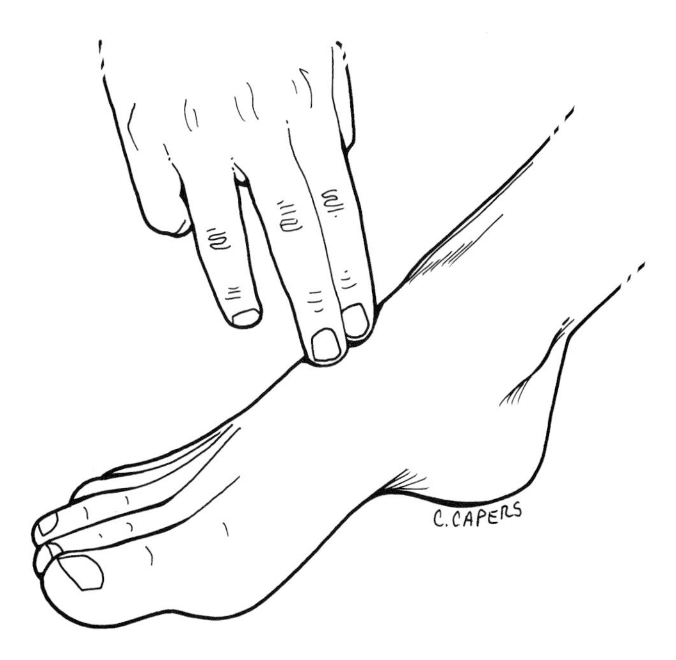

Fig. 77–4. Assessment of the neurovascular status in the reduced knee should include comparison with the opposite limb and checking of pedal pulses.

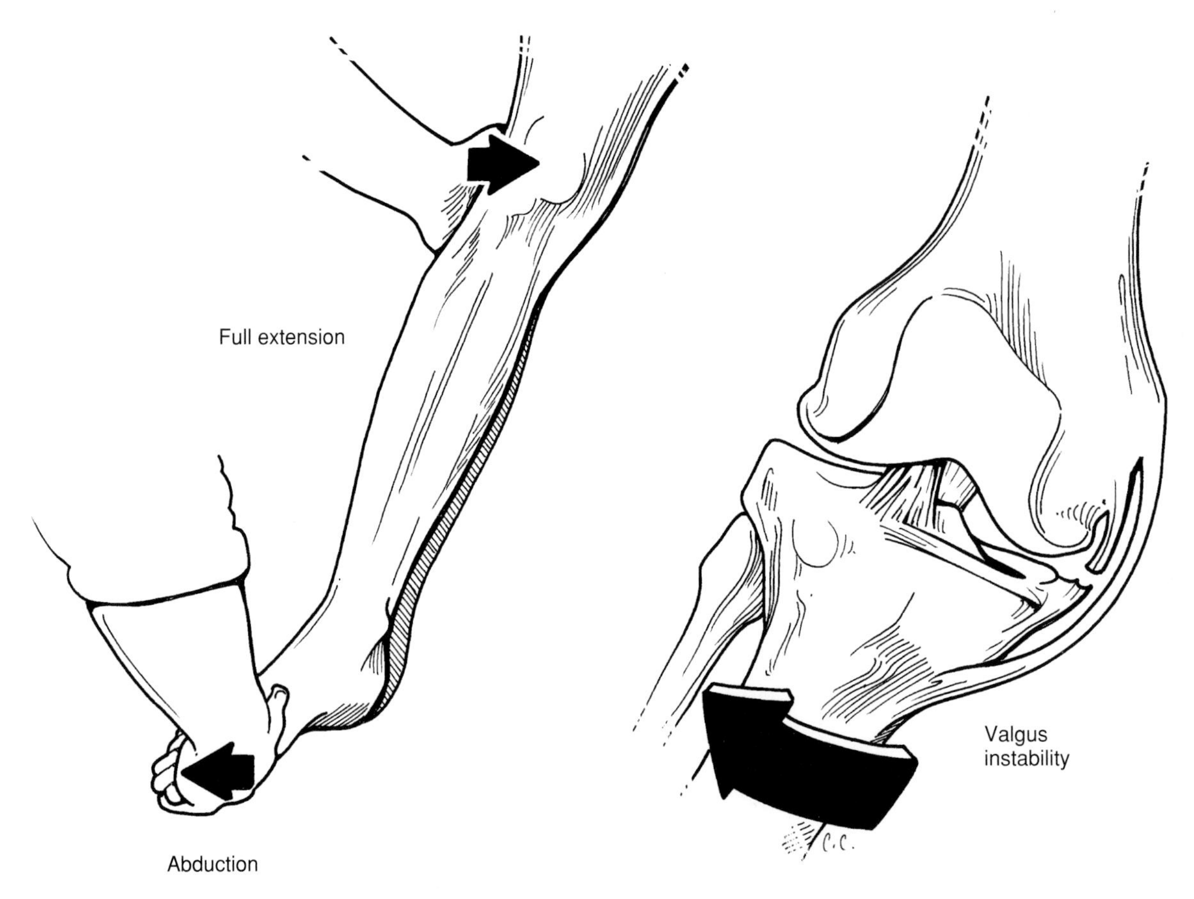

Fig. 77–5. Physical examination demonstrates valgus (or varus) instability with the knee in full extension.

Our current management protocol is to reduce the dislocation and assess neurovascular status, check stability of the knee in full extension and 30° of flexion, perform arteriography for all documented dislocations and for injuries with associated decreased pedal pulses or vascular symptoms, obtain MRI, and plan the surgical procedure. Precise knowledge of the anatomy is critical because this repair or reconstruction challenges the skills of the most experienced surgeon. The extremity is examined under anesthesia, and the knee is opened on the side of greatest instability, using a long parapatellar incision and carefully dissecting the layers. The interior of the joint is then examined before reattachment of the capsule, tendons, menisci, and collateral ligaments. Injury patterns vary, and complete dislocations can occur without disruption of both cruciates. If both the cruciates are disrupted, the central third of the patellar tendon is harvested, and, then, either through the defect or with arthroscopic assistance, the posterior cruciate or anterior cruciate ligament is repaired with reconstruction of the other.

Postoperatively, the patient is placed in an extension brace for the first week, followed by progressive weight bearing and range of motion exercises. Resistance exercises are started between the second and third month. Return to full activity is usually possible after 8 months to 1 year. Nonoperative management is reserved for older patients, those with low demands, and those whose injury is more than 21 days past.

SUMMARY

Low-velocity knee dislocation is a devastating injury and an orthopedic emergency. Rapid reduction with accurate assessment of the neurovascular status and appropriate workup is critical because neurovascular injury can complicate as many as 50% of these dislocations. A knee with gross instability, and tears of both cruciates, and a collateral ligament should be managed as a reduced knee dislocation. The sideline examination is the best opportunity to determine the degree and direction of instability. Early surgical intervention, with repair or reconstruction of all involved structures, followed by a rehabilitation program emphasizing progressive range of motion, can be expected to yield good to excellent results in the majority of cases.

REFERENCES

1. Meyers, M. H., Moore, T. M., and Harvey, J. P.: Traumatic dislocation of the knee joint. J. Bone Joint Surg. *57A*:430, 1975.
2. Hoover, M. W.: Injury of the popliteal artery associated with fracture and dislocation. Surg. Clin. North Am. *41*:1099, 1961.
3. Shields, L., Mital, M., and Cave, E.: Complete dislocation of the knee: Experience at the Massachusetts General Hospital. J. Trauma *9*:192, 1969.
4. Roman, P. D., Hopson, C. N., and Zenni, E. J., Jr.: Traumatic dislocation of the knee: A report of 30 cases and literature review. Orthop. Rev. *16*:917, 1987.

5. Frassica, F. J., Sim, F. H., Staeheli, J. W., and Pairolero, P. C.: Dislocation of the knee. Clin. Orthop. *263*:200, 1991.
6. Sisto, D. J., and Warren, R. F.: Complete knee dislocation: A follow-up study of operative treatment. Clin. Orthop. *198*:94, 1985.
7. Welling, R. E., Kakkasseril, J., and Cranley, J. J.: Complete dislocations of the knee with popliteal vascular injury. J. Trauma *21*:450, 1981.
8. Shelbourne, K. D., et al.: Low-velocity knee dislocation. Orthop. Rev. *20*:995, 1991.
9. Kennedy, J. C.: Complete dislocations of the knee joint. J. Bone Joint Surg. *57A*:430, 1975.
10. Green, N. E., and Allen, B. L.: Vascular injuries associated with dislocation of the knee. J. Bone Joint Surg. *59A*:236, 1977.
11. Hughston, J. C., Andrews, J. R., Cross, M. J., and Moschi, A.: Classification of knee ligament instabilities. Part I: The medial compartment and cruciate ligaments. J. Bone Joint Surg. *58A*:159, 1976.
12. Quinlan, A. G., and Sharrard, W. J. W.: Posterolateral dislocations of the knee. J. Bone Joint Surg. *40B*:660, 1958.
13. Jones, R. E., Smith, E. C., and Bone, G. E.: Vascular and orthopaedic complications of knee dislocations. Surg. Gynecol. Obstet. *149*:554, 1979.
14. O'Donnell, T. F., Jr., Brewster, D. C., Darling, B. C., Veen, H. and Waltman, A. A.: Arterial injuries associated with fractures and/or dislocations of the knee. J. Trauma *17*:775, 1977.
15. McCoy, G., Hannon, D., Barr, R., et al.: Vascular injury associated with low velocity dislocations of the knee. J. Bone Joint Surg. *69B*:285, 1987.
16. Miller, H. H., and Welch, C. S.: Quantitative studies of time factor in arterial injuries. Ann. Surg. *130*:428, 1949.
17 Siliski, J. M., and Plancher, K.: Dislocation of the knee. Presented at the Annual Meeting of the American Academy of Orthopaedic Surgeons, Las Vegas, 1989.
18. Almekinders, L. C., and Logan, T. C.: Results following treatment of traumatic dislocations of the knee joint. Clin. Orthop. *284*:203, 1992.
19. Thomsen, P. B., Rud, B., and Jensen, U. H.: Stability and motion after traumatic dislocation of the knee. Acta Orthop. Scand. *55*:278, 1984.
20. Taylor, A. R., Arden, G. P., and Rainey, H. A.: Traumatic dislocation of the knee joint. J. Bone Joint Surg. *54B*:96, 1972.
21. Reckling, F. W., and Peltier, L. F.: Acute knee dislocations and their complications. J. Trauma *9*:181, 1969.

78

Champ L. Baker, Jr.

Arthroscopy in the Treatment of Knee Disorders

HISTORICAL PERSPECTIVE

Over the past two decades, increased use of the arthroscope has revolutionized the ability of orthopedic surgeons to diagnose and concomitantly treat joint disorders. By providing new insights into the complexity of joint injuries, arthroscopy has also enabled orthopedic surgeons to better understand the intra-articular structures involved in various disorders. In particular, arthroscopy now plays an integral role in the management of athletic injuries of the knee joint.

During this period, significant progress has been made, in both equipment and technique. In the mid-1970s, one of the foremost arthroscopists in the United States asserted that hemarthrosis of the knee was a specific contraindication to the use of arthroscopy because visualization provided by the equipment at that time was inadequate. Subsequent development of fiberoptics, on-screen monitoring, and motorized equipment substantially enhanced visualization and improved the technical capabilities of arthroscopy. Thus, over time, we have better defined the diagnostic indications and greatly expanded the therapeutic horizon for knee arthroscopy. We now know that a hemarthrosis in the knee is one of the principal indications for using arthroscopy to detect intra-articular disorders.

The most important factor in the treatment of any athletic injury is the ability of the physician to make a quick, accurate diagnosis. The appropriate treatment plan, correct prognosis, and potential for return to activity by the patient all depend on the accuracy of the initial diagnosis. The availability of the arthroscope has much improved our diagnostic skills. Other sophisticated diagnostic modalities have also evolved, and magnetic resonance imaging (MRI), in particular, has in many instances proven better for diagnosing injuries because it is noninvasive and provides a complete picture of interstitial lesions as well as lesions of bone, cartilage, and ligament.

Although the arthroscope remains valuable as a diagnostic tool, its use as a therapeutic modality for joint disorders is the single most important factor in the advancement of care of athletic injuries. Its use has enabled athletes to overcome injuries and return to competition more quickly and safely than was thought possible a mere 15 to 20 years ago. For example, when a young football player twists his knee, suffers pain and swelling, is unable to play, and is missing out on practice, time becomes an extremely important factor in treating the injury. With the arthroscope, the orthopedic surgeon can accurately diagnose the intra-articular disorder and treat it at the same sitting. The minimally invasive nature of the procedure allows the athlete to return to practice and competition quickly, safely, and more efficiently than if the injury had been treated by open surgery. This extremely short postoperative recuperative period was not always possible before the advent of arthroscopic surgery.

When the arthroscope first came into common use, some orthopedic surgeons utilized it to perform diagnostic procedures using local anesthesia in the office setting. Arthroscopy quickly moved to the surgical suite, where it was employed as both a diagnostic and a therapeutic modality. More recently, interest has been renewed in using the arthroscope in the office to perform diagnostic and minimally invasive operative procedures. As health care reform alters the way medical care is provided, "office arthroscopy" may become more common. The future use of the arthroscope is uncertain, but at present it should be regarded as a surgical tool with which many procedures can be performed in the sterile environment of the surgical suite.

ANESTHESIA

Anesthesia for arthroscopy may be local infiltration at the portal sites and intra-articular injection, regional blocks, or general anesthesia for complete muscle relaxation. The choice is usually at the discretion of the operating surgeon, who may base the decision on what anatomic structures are involved and what operative procedure is planned. Currently, however, the majority of arthroscopic surgery in the United States is performed with either a spinal block or general anesthesia. This enables the surgeon to conduct a thorough ligament examination, which otherwise could be difficult in an acutely injured knee, and at the same time, to correlate ligament integrity with visualized intra-articular anatomy and disorders.

INSTRUMENTS

The following instruments are normally needed to perform arthroscopic procedures: (1) 4.0-mm diameter arthroscope with a 30° viewing lens, (2) 4.0-mm diameter arthroscope with a 70° viewing lens (optional), (3) video camera, (4) recorder, (5) pump (optional), (6) motorized shavers or bur, (7) probe, and (3) assorted hand instruments (e.g., grasper, clamps, curette).

USE OF TOURNIQUET

Some surgeons routinely use a tourniquet during the procedure, whereas others never use one. I normally do not use a tourniquet if I am performing the arthroscopy solely for diagnostic purposes or if I think a therapeutic procedure will be simple and brief. The advantage of using a tourniquet is that it aids visualization of the knee joint by providing a clearer field of view; though, with improved inflow-outflow techniques and the use of a pump, most visualization problems can be overcome without the use of a tourniquet.

ARTHROSCOPIC TECHNIQUE

The patient, under anesthesia, is positioned supine on the operating table. The leg is then prepared and draped. A leg holder is routinely used, so that the surgeon can apply pressure to open up the joint for better visualization when necessary (Fig. 78–1). The joint is distended with irrigating fluid through either the superomedial or superolateral portal, and the arthroscope, connected to a video camera, is introduced through an anterolateral portal. An anteromedial portal is established adjacent to the patellar tendon under the medial pole of the patella. A needle is used to localize this portal, to ensure that it is able to reach the posterior aspect of the medial joint. An alternative portal, the transpatellar tendon portal, has favor in Europe but is less common in the United States.

Systematic examination of the knee joint encompasses the patella, patellofemoral joint, medial compartment, medial meniscus, anterior and posterior horns of the menisci, anterior cruciate and posterior cruciate ligaments, lateral compartment, lateral meniscus, and intercondylar notch. The examination is augmented by inserting a probe through the medial portal to evaluate the consistency of the articular surface and to locate tears in the meniscus and determine if they are stable or unstable. For the examination to be complete, the arthroscope should be inserted adjacent to the anterior cruciate ligament, posterior to the notch, so that the surgeon can visualize the posterior aspect of the medial meniscus as well as the posterior aspect of the lateral meniscus, and look for loose bodies that may be present posteriorly. If necessary, a 70° arthroscope can be used for better visualization if a tear of the posterior horn of the medial meniscus is suspected, and in selected cases a posteromedial portal can be established and the arthroscope inserted posteromedially. It is the responsibility of the surgeon to carry out a thorough visual examination and palpation, to ensure a complete diagnostic evaluation.

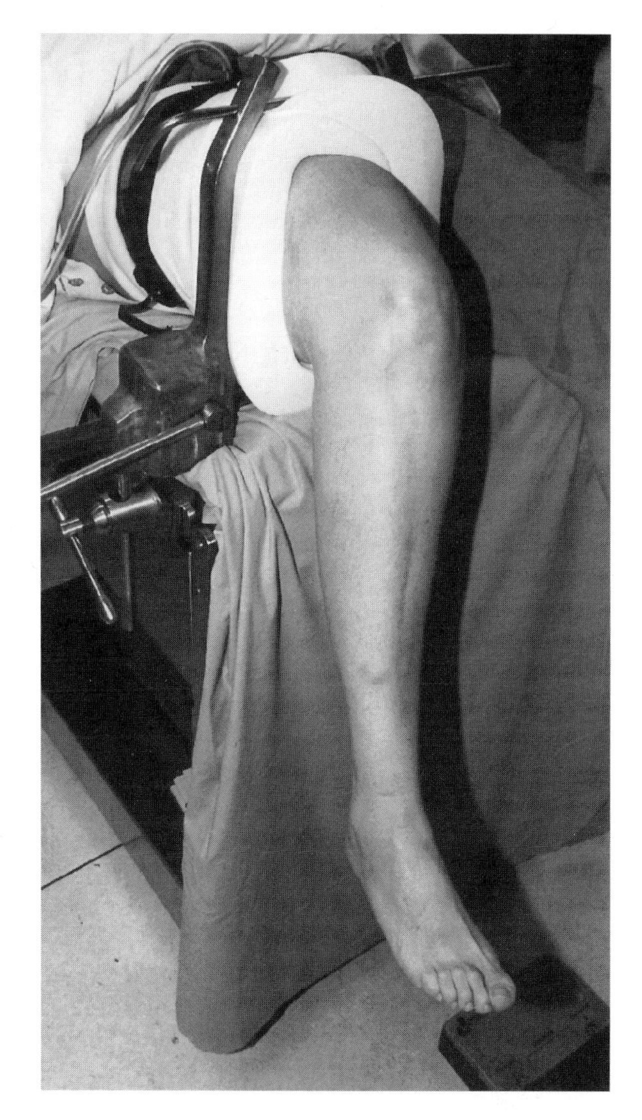

Fig. 78–1. Patient position for knee arthroscopy. The affected leg is in the leg holder.

After the procedure has been completed, excess fluid is expressed from the joint, and the portals are closed either with single stitches or with an adhesive bandage. A bulky wrap is then applied. A local anesthetic is often injected into the joint, to help minimize postoperative pain and swelling. An analgesic, such as ketorolac tromethamine (Toradol IM), may also be used, to help reduce postoperative discomfort. The patient is usually discharged the same day, prescribed partial weight bearing on crutches, and provided appropriate postoperative rehabilitation instructions.

SPECIFIC SURGICAL APPLICATIONS

Most common surgical procedures of the knee can be performed either by arthroscopy alone or by using the arthroscope as an adjunct to open surgery. In the case of athletic injuries, there are certain instances in which the arthroscope enables the patient to recover more quickly.

Hemarthrosis

Whenever an athlete suffers either a twisting noncontact or a contact injury to the knee and hears or feels a "pop," swelling of the joint may develop within an hour or two, maximizing within 12 to 24 hours. This effusion, referred to as a *hemarthrosis,* is a manifestation of blood in the joint secondary to intra-articular injury. The primary disorders associated with hemarthrosis are partial or complete rupture of the ACL, tears of the peripheral attachment of the medial or lateral meniscus, chondral fractures, and patellar subluxation or dislocation with possible loose bodies. The physician should consider all of these possibilities when conducting the initial examination of a patient with hemarthrosis.

Routine aspiration of the joint is not indicated, but it should be performed if the patient is markedly uncomfortable because of moderate or severe effusion or if a fracture or infection is suspected. Splinting the extremity and re-examining the patient a day or two after the injury often helps make the diagnosis. Most of the disorders that result in hemarthrosis are surgically correctable, and an athlete who presents with a hemarthrosis at the beginning of or during the playing season is a strong candidate for diagnostic and operative arthroscopy.

When the patient is examined under anesthesia, the surgeon can confirm the presence of ligamentous instability related either to the patellofemoral or the tibiofemoral joint. After the blood is evacuated, arthroscopic examination can confirm or rule out chondral fractures, intra-articular ligament injuries, and meniscal tears and separations. Often, once the diagnosis is made, the injury can be treated immediately and the patient can begin the appropriate rehabilitation program, which may allow him or her to return to play within the season. For example, an athlete who has patellar subluxation and an intra-articular loose body can be treated by removing the loose body, bracing the knee postoperatively, and beginning rehabilitation to allow early return to competition.

The most common injury causing hemarthrosis is rupture of the anterior cruciate ligament (Fig. 78–2); however, not all ligament tears need to be reconstructed

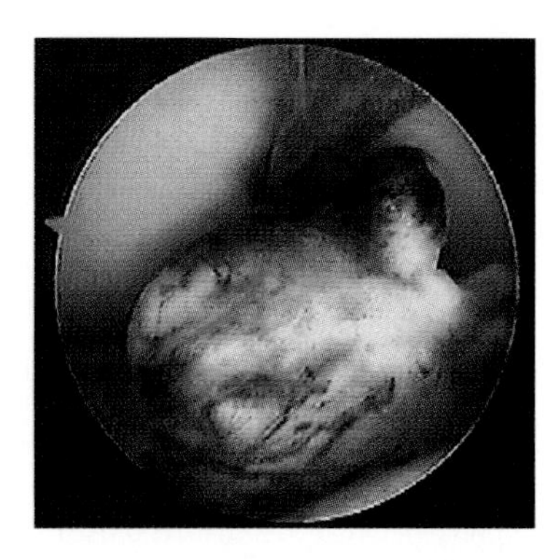

Fig. 78–2. Intra-articular view of an acute tear of the anterior cruciate ligament (ACL) with bleeding present.

initially, and the arthroscope can determine if the tear is partial or complete. Débridement of a complete tear that is blocking extension may be all that is needed to allow the patient to begin rehabilitation. This treatment approach may be appropriate, particularly if minimal instability is associated with the injury and the menisci are intact. In these cases, the athlete can often return to play during the season, particularly in football, and the surgeon can plan for reconstructive anterior cruciate ligament surgery at the end of the season.

If concurrent injuries (e.g., a peripherally detached meniscus) require immediate treatment, appropriate arthroscopic treatment of all injuries should be performed at that time and the joint should be stabilized.

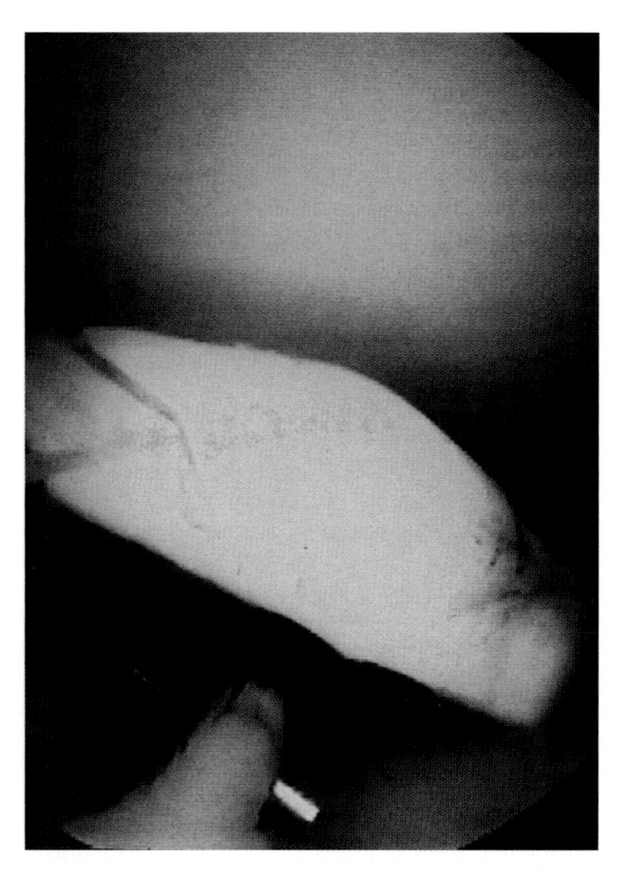

Fig. 78–3. Arthroscopic view of an intra-articular body from a patellar fracture.

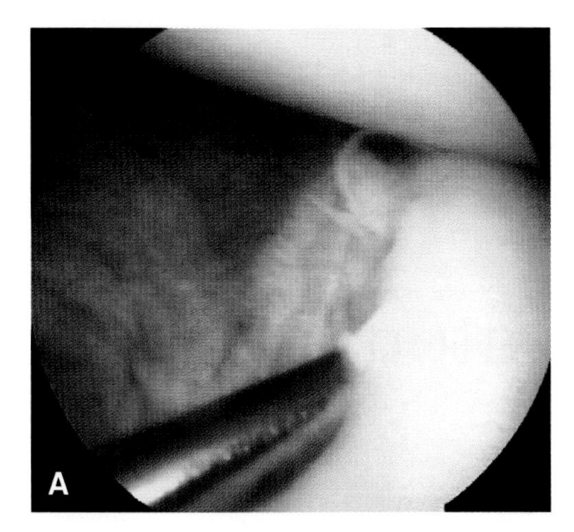

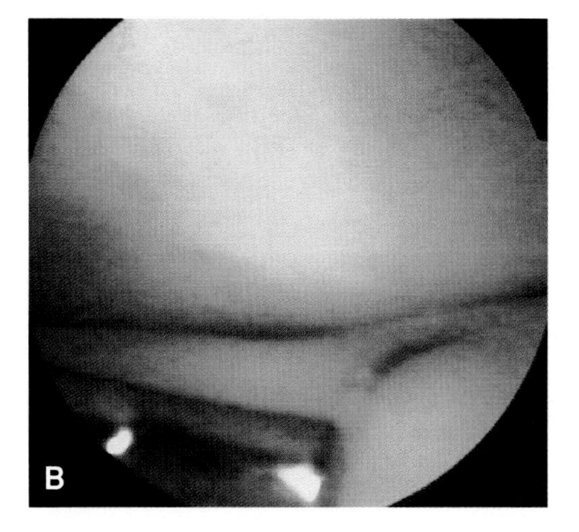

Fig. 78–4. ***(A)*** **Arthroscopic view of a meniscal rim tear through the peripheral vascular zone (the red-white zone).** ***(B)*** **Suture is placed in the inferior surface of the meniscus.**

In these cases, the athlete most likely will be forced to sit out the remainder of the season while undergoing rehabilitation.

Loose Bodies

Any mechanism of injury that causes subluxation of the knee joint, particularly of the patellofemoral joint, can result in a chondral or an osteochondral fracture. This may occur immediately, secondary to acute injury, or the fracture can develop over time, as the fragments gradually become larger until they produce symptoms of mechanical locking. When the patient complains of swelling, catching, and locking that prevents full extension or flexion of the knee, arthroscopic removal of these loose fragments (Fig. 78–3) is necessary. The minimal trauma associated with arthroscopic entry into the joint and removal of the fragments usually allows the athlete to return to competition very quickly.

Meniscal Disorders

Common tears of the meniscus include tears of the body, with mobile loose fragments, and peripheral separations. When the fragment is mobile or loose, arthroscopic removal of the fragment allows for quick and early return to athletic activity. If the meniscus itself is torn from its capsular attachment but is believed to be reparable, the repair can be accomplished either by arthroscopic technique alone or by open surgical technique after arthroscopic documentation. The arthroscope is helpful for localizing the tear (Fig. 78–4), and using an "inside-out" or "outside-in" technique for accurate placement of the sutures when reattaching the meniscus to the capsule.

Regardless of how the meniscus is repaired (i.e., arthroscopic or open technique), the patient will require a period of postoperative immobilization and recovery that will delay return to normal athletic activities. Thus, unlike repair of other knee joint injuries, for which arthroscopic treatment can be advantageous in minimizing recuperation, arthroscopic repair of a torn meniscus does not speed up recovery and subsequent return to competition. After meniscal repair, with or without concomitant ligament reconstruction, a recovery period of 3 to 4 months is usually necessary before the patient can return to unrestricted activity. Otherwise, there is increased risk of further damage to the cartilage before the repair has had adequate time to mature and heal.

SUMMARY

Over the past two decades, the care of knee injuries in athletes has been revolutionized by the availability of the arthroscope. The use of the arthroscope in the diagnosis of knee joint injuries offers orthopedic surgeons a quick, minimally invasive means of conducting a complete intra-articular examination and making an accurate diagnosis. Often, once the diagnosis is made, appropriate concomitant treatment to alleviate the patient's symptoms can be performed during the same arthroscopic procedure. In the hands of an experienced arthroscopist the risk of complications is minimal.

The arthroscope has eliminated the once common use of arthrotomy in the treatment of disorders such as meniscal tears, loose bodies, and patellar dislocations. In addition, the advent of arthroscopically assisted major procedures, such as ligament reconstruction, has resulted in less postoperative discomfort and quicker rehabilitation for the patient; however, use of the arthroscope does not expedite the maturation of scar tissue (e.g., torn anterior cruciate ligament) and there is still a prolonged period of recovery (as much as 6 to 9 months) before an athlete can return to sports.

Because of the minimally invasive nature of the arthroscope, significantly less trauma is associated with arthroscopic surgery as compared with an open procedure. Thus, the athlete-patient can often return to practice and sports activities within a very short time. The ability to treat a knee disorder arthroscopically is particularly advantageous when an athlete is injured during the playing season. In many cases, the joint disorder can be corrected and the athlete returned to competition within the season.

79 *Turner A. Blackburn, Jr.*

Rehabilitation of Ligamentous Knee Problems

HISTORICAL BACKGROUND

Rehabilitation of ligamentous knee injuries has changed drastically in the last decade. In the early 1980s, the surgery of choice was generally extra-articular repair or reconstruction. This extra-articular surgery required immobilization for 6 weeks, avoidance of weight bearing for some 8 to 12 weeks, and return to full activity after 6 to 9 months. Many surgeons were not pleased with the results of extra-articular surgery and searched for a way to substitute graft for the anterior cruciate ligament.

The early anterior cruciate ligament graft reconstructions were fraught with problems. Basic science research with animal models showed that it took as long as 18 months for the graft to gain normal strength.[1,2] (Today, we still do not know exactly when the graft reaches normal strength.) The initial strength of these grafts was not known at that time. Since rehabilitation programs for extra-articular reconstruction called for immobilization, this approach was tried for intra-articular reconstruction as well; however, many patients developed flexion contractures. Another problem was loss of good articular surface because of the lack of motion and of flexion contractures. Proprioception was lost because patients were forbidden to bear weight even longer than those who had extra-articular repairs.[3] New isokinetic devices were introduced at that time and, owing to poor understanding of the biomechanics and strength of the graft, improper use of the equipment led to many graft failures.

BIOMECHANICAL AND HEALING EFFECTS

Paulos and coworkers showed that quadriceps contraction with the knee in an open-chain position transmitted an anterior translation force to the tibia, especially with the knee between 0° and 45° of flexion.[4] This research definitely explained why high-intensity flexion-to-extension rehabilitation activities caused weak or poorly fixated grafts to rupture. Unfortunately, the effect of this research was to lessen the emphasis on quadriceps rehabilitation, even though quadriceps control is very important for knee function.

Henning and colleagues published a report of their findings using strain gauges in vivo in the anterior cruciate ligaments of two subjects.[5] This report supported the findings of Paulos' group, but they also found that the use of light-weight exercise (5 to 10 pounds) did not cause as much translation force. The most useful information was that, in closed-chain exercises, the forces of anterior translation were very moderate. So, though we once thought early weight bearing would damage the graft, it now appeared that there would not be enough force to harm it. In the weight-bearing position, the hamstrings moderate the pull of the quadriceps.

In 1983, Noyes and associates showed that the central one-third bone–patellar tendon–bone graft was anywhere from 40 to 50% stronger than a normal anterior cruciate ligament and the semitendinosus tendon had 75% the strength of a normal anterior cruciate ligament.[1] The combination of using the strongest graft, proper placement of the graft, a "notchplasty," and superior fixation has much accelerated the rehabilitation program for anterior cruciate ligament reconstruction.

With all the interest in the past decade on the intra-articular graft, many have forgotten that extra-articular surgery had been, and still is, a very effective way of controlling anterior instability in the knee.[6] In acute repairs of the medial compartment, the tissue healing response is quite good if repair occurs within 7 to 10 days of injury. At 6 weeks after repair, healing is far enough along to allow for gradual motion of the knee. On the lateral side, repair of the capsule is almost always augmented by an iliotibial band tenodesis, and sometimes by biceps advancement. By 3 to 6 weeks, healing has progressed enough to allow gradual range of motion to the knee.

The healing rate for the posterior cruciate ligament has not been studied in as much detail as that of the anterior cruciate ligament; therefore, clinical experience will have to demonstrate the healing rate for this structure. If the injury involves damage to other structures along with the posterior cruciate ligament, then, certainly, their repair is important to consider. If a central one-third bone–patellar tendon–bone graft is used to reconstruct the posterior cruciate ligament, the healing restraints and rehabilitation protocol would be similar to that described for the anterior cruciate ligament.

The posterolateral corner of the knee is generally reconstructed, even in the acute situation, with advancement of the arcuate complex. This requires the complex to heal into the femur. The reconstruction is stout enough at 6 weeks to allow gentle active motion, but one must remember that it is quite fragile during the 6- to 12-week postoperative period.

The anterior cruciate ligament is intracapsular but extrasynovial,[7] and though the anterior cruciate ligament has a good blood supply, injury to the ligament generally destroys the blood supply.[8] It is very difficult to know what program to follow when a diagnosis of a partial anterior cruciate ligament tear is made because of the different strengths and healing rates for partial tears of the anterior cruciate ligament.

It appears that the healing and inflammatory process in the knee after ligament injury is best allowed to calm down to allow for successful intra-articular surgery. This waiting period should be long enough to allow the knee to have full range of motion, reduced swelling, and good muscle tone. Once this is achieved, intra-articular surgery is appropriate. Problems with too early intra-articular intervention are flexion contractures, swelling, and pain.

The graft, whether it is autogenous or allogeneic, is thought to go through a standard collagen model repair, which shows that it is at its strongest initially, weaker at 9 to 12 weeks, after which it begins to gain strength again.[9] It is thought that revascularization occurs as early as 3 weeks in these grafts, but no one really knows how strong they are and how fast they heal.[10–12] If an allograft is done, it is important to know how it was sterilized and how it was stored, as these variables affect its strength and healing rate. Also, the capsular ligaments must not be forgotten in considering what rehabilitation program to use after anterior cruciate ligament injury associated with rotatory instability.

Unfortunately, we do not have enough scientific information at this point to base our programs on pure science. We have learned over the years at the Hughston Sports Medicine Center from athletes who have not followed the protocol, and the findings have been reiterated by others,[11] that patients with an intra-articular graft can be rehabilitated faster than basic science seems to indicate.

GUIDELINES FOR REHABILITATION

Performance Criteria

The goal of knee ligament rehabilitation is to return the patient to the highest level of functional activity. The rehabilitation program must be guided by the biomechanics of the knee joint and the healing constraints of the tissues involved. Once these are understood, a time-based rehabilitation program is clearly inadequate. Progress through the rehabilitation program should be based on performance criteria: the patient or athlete must reach certain critical levels of function before moving on to the next level. This is true regardless of how much time has gone by; the crucial factor is to await proper healing. The sooner motion can be introduced into the program, the healthier it is for the articular surfaces. The sooner weight bearing can begin, the sooner proprioceptive capability will improve. Knowing when to work passively for motion and when to work actively for motion is very important to the success of the outcome. As soon as the vastus medialis and the rest of the quadriceps muscles are functioning, the knee will be more stable and will function better.

Range of Motion

Methods to regain range of motion differ depending on the type of surgery. If the repair or reconstruction is extra-articular, the knee is usually immobilized in 45° to 60° of flexion, where the capsular structures are at their shortest possible length. The knee is immobilized in a limited motion brace for 4 to 6 weeks after surgery.

When rigid fixation is removed, range of motion exercises are started carefully. If extra-articular reconstruction or repair has been performed, range of motion into extension should only be done actively. The quadriceps is quite weak at this point, and the gradual increase in extension coming from active work ensures that the integrity of the surgery is preserved. Gaining 5° a week in extension is normal. As a final extension measurement after extra-articular surgery a 5° flexion contracture is acceptable. Only after 12 to 14 weeks should passive motion be used to gain extension. Flexion activities are begun passively and aggressively at the appropriate time. After extra-articular surgery, this is when the cast is removed, and full flexion might be hoped for by 12 weeks.

When extra-articular reconstruction is performed during the acute phase of injury, some patients are put in a limited range of motion cast-brace. Generally, the knee is held at 45° for 3 weeks. In the second 3 weeks, the cast-brace is opened up to an arc of 30° to 90°.

After intra-articular surgical procedures for anterior cruciate ligament and posterior cruciate ligament reconstruction, passive range of motion exercises are in

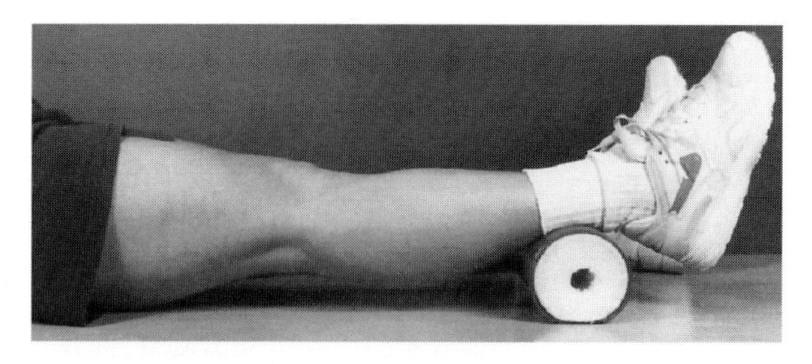

Fig. 79–1. Passive extension is gained by having the patient prop the ankle or heel on a pillow or bolster or lie prone extending the leg off the table with the knee supported.

order. The graft increases in size during the early healing period. Stress must be put on the graft initially so that full extension is maintained. This is a very important measure immediately after surgery. Passive extension is gained with the patient's ankle or heel propped on a pillow or bolster or with the patient lying prone with the leg extending off the bed and the knee supported (Fig. 79–1). Full extension is usually regained in 3 to 4 weeks. Flexion activities for intra-articular surgery begin on postoperative day 1. The patient should gain 90° of flexion within the first 4 to 5 days, and the complete range of flexion should be regained by 4 to 6 weeks.

Continuous Passive Motion

Salter has demonstrated that early motion encourages healing of damaged articular surfaces. He also showed that early motion reduced range of motion deficits. Thus, the concept of continuous passive motion (CPM) has been applied to knee ligament reconstruction. CPM is contraindicated for patients who had extra-articular surgery since passive motion is not appropriate for the integrity of the repaired or reconstructed tissues unless the individual case allows limited range of motion. After intra-articular surgery, both active and passive range of motion exercises begin immediately as does weight bearing. Therefore CPM, though not contraindicated, is not really necessary for the majority of patients treated with intra-articular surgery. Another thing to note about CPM is that the axis of the device is not able to follow the knee through a full range of motion. It may also apply inappropriate forces.[3]

Gait and Weight Bearing

Ambulation is an extremely important feature of the knee ligament rehabilitation protocol. It is necessary that weight bearing begin as soon as possible, but the important elements of range of motion and vastus medialis firing must be regained first so that normal gait results. The only time a patient is allowed to use an altered gait pattern is if the knee must be held in limited motion, as after an acute injury or an extra-articular repair. In these situations, rather than landing on the heel with the knee in extension (a position the knee is not capable of assuming) weight must be borne on the ball of the foot. The athlete will use crutches, place the ball of the foot down and contract the knee muscles to stabilize the knee and step through. Once range of motion and strength have improved and the protection phase for the ligament has ended, the athlete attempts normal heel-toe gait. Patients with an intra-articular reconstruction, whose motion is not restricted after surgery, should attempt the normal heel-toe gait as soon as possible.

Muscle Strengthening

Since slow-twitch muscle fibers are most affected by immobilization, high-repetition, low-weight exercises most efficiently restore function to those fibers. An injured body part cannot tolerate heavy weights or great stress during the healing phase. Initially the exercise regimen for the injured knee should be from five to ten sets of ten repetitions two to three times a day. Light weights may be used—probably no more than 10 pounds as the upper limit. This amount of weight should not put undue stress on any of the structures about the knee during healing.[5] The hip musculature and the hamstrings seem to respond well to five sets of ten repetitions once or twice a day. The quadriceps muscles need much more stimulation and should be worked two to three times a day with more repetitions. It is important that, during quadriceps exercises, the knee be taken to the fullest possible degree of extension with the leg lifts. Allowing the knee to sag or flex increases stress on the extensor mechanism. Once closed-chain activities are begun, it is important to start slowly, since the knee muscles must control the entire body's weight. Depending on the activity, 10 to 50 repetitions are most appropriate.

Proprioception

Proprioception is an extremely important part of the rehabilitation program. Certainly, early weight bearing prevents the loss of many of the components of proprioception, but specific activities to improve balance and kinesthetic awareness are very important. Simple things can be used, such as standing and balancing on one leg, rising up on the ball of the foot and balancing, and even closing the eyes. Equipment is available to test proprioception and balance and to help train for this important facet of rehabilitation. As the athlete progresses into functional activities, these proprioceptive activities will contribute much. Most of the important proprioception about the knee comes from its muscular support, so the muscles are the focus of much of the rehabilitation program.

Bracing

Postoperative braces should be selected for their ability to be accurate in their range of motion adjustments and to allow flexion and extension stops as necessary. Some surgeons only use straight immobilizers after patellar tendon grafting because they remove them quite soon. It must be remembered that functional braces usually come with a 10° extension stop. This stop should be eliminated in the immediate postoperative situation because it only encourages flexion contractures in the knee. Once the athlete is ready to engage in vigorous activities, this stop may be reactivated. To try to control a nonreconstructed knee, the 10° stop would be beneficial.

Rehabilitation After Multiple Knee Operations

It is often difficult to determine what rehabilitation protocols to follow when multiple surgeries—extra- and intra-articular—have been performed about the knee. Meniscal repair also complicates matters. If the surgery is purely extra-articular, following the protection guidelines mentioned earlier would be very important. If extra-articular and intra-articular surgery are combined, the intra-articular surgery protocol takes precedence in informing the rehabilitation process. This is also true if there is a meniscal repair.

Total Fitness

It is extremely important, during the rehabilitation program for the knee injury, that the athlete's total body fitness not be ignored. The bicycle is an excellent machine for maintaining cardiovascular fitness. It helps strengthen the legs and is a good "heart" exercise. Certainly, upper body ergometers, and even swimming, may help to keep the athlete conditioned. Just because the lower extremity is injured does not mean that the upper body cannot be exercised appropriately for the athlete's sport.

REHABILITATION OF ACUTE AND CHRONIC INJURIES TO KNEE LIGAMENTS

Nonoperatively Treated Medial Compartment Injuries

Our experiences with medial compartment injuries at the Hughston Sports Medicine Center have led us to devise a protocol that allows for nonoperative treatment of these injuries. The criteria of eligibility for this nonoperative treatment are (1) that there has been no meniscal or anterior cruciate ligament injury, and (2) that instability is in the mild to moderate range. Controlled range of motion appears to be the best way to allow these injuries to heal. A hinged immobilizer that prevents the athlete from extending the knee the last

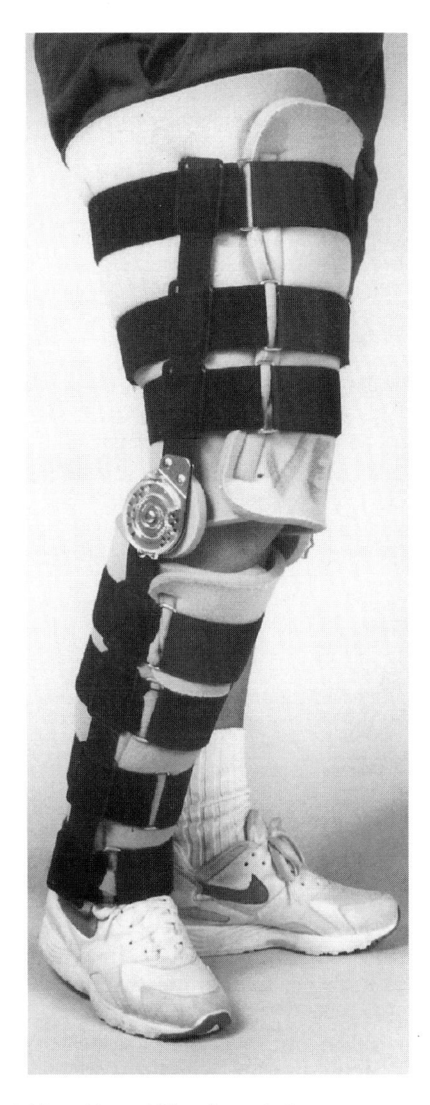

Fig. 79–2. A hinged immobilizer is used after surgery to prevent unwanted extension and flexion while allowing motion within the permissible range.

20° allows for protected weight bearing and spares the knee the stress put on the capsule when the knee is fully extended (Fig. 79–2). Full flexion is allowed. Weight bearing is protected with crutches for at least 3 weeks.

Knee exercises can be started immediately. It is recommended that the athlete work on quadriceps sets, terminal knee extensions, straight leg raises, and hamstring curls, along with exercises for the hip flexors, hip abductors, and hip extensors. All of these are done in a many-repetitions, little-weight mode. Bicycling can begin as soon as the athlete is comfortable.

Ligaments can be tested weekly to monitor their healing. Once joint openings have decreased, the athlete may advance from partial weight bearing to full weight bearing and progress out of the immobilizer. This may take 4 to 6 weeks. Once the athlete is bearing full weight, closed-chain exercises are started (Table 79–1). Isotonic and isokinetic work may also begin once the lig-

Table 79–1. Functional Exercise Continuum

Closed-chain continuum
- Leg press with rubber tubing and progress to machines
- Wall slides or mini-squat, mini-trampoline
- One-leg sissy squat
- Tubing squats, two legs progressing to one
- Step-ups and side step-ups
- Hops against tubing side to side, two legs, one leg, one leg agility, plyometrics

Ambulation continuum
- No weight bearing
- Partial weight bearing
- Walk 2 miles
- Stride/jog 2 miles
- Sprint 40 yards
- Cutting
- Deceleration
- Sport specific

Functional testing
- General hop test: one jump, three jumps, timed, and side to side
- Figure-of-eight run
- Sprint speed
- Endurance run
- Agility run: T test
- Proprioceptive testing
- Carioca
- Isokinetic testing

aments are healing. The athlete progresses through the functional exercise continuum until able to pass functional testing and return to full activity.

Acute Anterior Cruciate Ligament Injury with Anterolateral Rotatory Instability

When the acute injury is diagnosed as anterolateral rotatory instability, there is usually a full or partial tear of the anterior cruciate ligament and a middle-third lateral compartment tear of the capsule, with possible iliotibial tract injury. A capsular injury needs protection just as the anterior cruciate ligament injury does. It is difficult to know how strong the partially torn anterior cruciate ligament may be, and, thus, to outline a specific progressive protocol. Obviously, if the anterior cruciate ligament is torn completely the protocol does not have to include protection for it, but the capsular component does need protection.

If the protocol demands protection of a partially torn anterior cruciate ligament, only very light resistance should be used for quadriceps work. Heavier quadriceps work can be done in the 90° to 45° range, where anterior translation force is less. A hinged immobilizer at 20° protects the capsular ligaments. Weight bearing should be controlled with crutches.

Exercises consist of quadriceps sets, terminal knee extensions, straight leg raises, hamstrings curls, and strengthening of the hip abductors, hip extensors, and hip adductors. Once the athlete is functioning well in the immobilizer and with crutches, he or she may begin general closed-chain activities such as minimal squats, cycling, rubber tubing squats, and light leg press activities. The athlete may progress into more functional activities in 4 to 6 weeks (Tables 79–1, 79–2), depending on healing as judged by time and ligament testing.

Once the athlete begins more aggressive activities, it is advisable to use a functional brace. This should build confidence and may help the athlete return to full activity as soon as possible. Many times the program outlined above is what the athlete will work through while waiting for the appropriate time for surgery.

Operatively Treated Anteromedial Rotatory Instability

The patient who undergoes—in the acute phase or later—a surgical procedure for anteromedial rotatory instability has the knee kept locked at anywhere from 45° to 60° in a hinged immobilizer. During this time, quadriceps and hamstrings sets are encouraged, along with straight leg raises and strengthening of the hip abductors, hip adductors, and hip extensors. The patient is allowed toe-touch weight bearing with crutches.

In the acute phase, the immobilizer hinge is opened for motion from 30° to 70°. For a chronic injury the brace stays at the set range of motion for 6 weeks.

Use of the immobilizer is discontinued at 6 weeks and the athlete begins a general active range of motion and muscle-strengthening program. As described earlier, extension is gained through active motion and flexion through active and passive motion. Quadriceps sets, terminal knee extensions, straight leg raises, and exercises for the hip flexors, adductors, abductors, and extensors are all done in an open-chain fashion with no more than 5 pounds of resistance, as tolerated. The patient with acute anteromedial rotatory instability may progress a bit faster with range of motion exercises.

Table 79–2. Rehabilitation Protocol for Patients with Acute Nonoperatively Treated Rotatory Instability (AMRI, ALRI)*

Phase	*Activities*
Immobilization	Hinged brace allowing 20° to full extension for 3 to 6 weeks, depending on ligament laxity tests
Ambulation	Two-crutch touch-down weight bearing One-crutch as quadriceps improves Full weight bearing once brace use is ended Begin running in brace as tolerated Full range of motion when out of brace
Exercise	Strength exercises at 5 to 10 sets a day using no more than 10-pound weights Quadriceps sets Terminal knee extensions Straight leg raises with terminal knee extensions Hip flexion Hip extension Hip adduction Hip abduction Hamstrings curls
Functional progression	Weight room and aggressive closed-chain activities (see Table 79–1)

*Key: AMRI, anteromedial rotatory instability; ALRI, anterolateral rotatory instability.

Weight bearing is partial at 6 weeks and progresses to full weight bearing as knee extension and quadriceps control improve. Generally, the patient is bearing full weight at 10 to 12 weeks. The functional exercise continuum is followed, and more strenuous isotonic and isokinetic exercises are done as tolerated.

Once the athlete can meet the functional guidelines, he or she may return to full activity. A functional brace is not always necessary and is used on a p.r.n. basis.

Operatively Treated Anterolateral-Anteromedial Rotatory Instability

The patient who undergoes extra-articular surgery for anterolateral or anterolateral-anteromedial rotatory instability usually has the knee locked in a hinged immobilizer at 45° after surgery (Table 79–3). The acutely injured athlete may have limited range of motion from 30° to 70° after 3 weeks. The patient with a chronic injury should be immobilized for 6 weeks. Only touch-down weight bearing is allowed for the first 6 weeks; then weight bearing gradually increases. At 6 weeks, the immobilizer is removed, though it may be used during sleeping hours, to prevent passive extension of the knee. Range of motion is increased using active exercises for extension and passive motion for flexion. The athlete works with quadriceps setting, terminal knee extensions, straight leg raises, and strengthening of the hip adductors, abductors, and extensors during the immobilization stage and the stage between removal of the immobilizer and full weight bearing.

Once weight bearing with crutches is comfortable, the closed-chain continuum can be started. As the athlete progresses through the functional exercise continuum, he or she works toward returning to sport-specific activities. Generally, this takes 6 to 8 months.

The rehabilitation protocol after intra-articular surgical reconstruction follows a different route because it is not a capsular repair or reconstruction (Table 79–4). The biggest difference is that full extension is required from postoperative day 1. The patient's knee should be held in a full-extension immobilizer, and full extension of the knee must be ensured (The physician should not rely on the immobilizer or the hinge markings for this.) Patients are allowed touch-down weight bearing to tolerance. The immobilizer is taken off for exercises the first day after surgery, where, again, passive extension is

Table 79–3. Suggested Aggressive Protocol After Anterolateral or Anteromedial Extra-Articular Procedures

Postoperative day	
1–4	Hinged postoperative brace (45°)
	Gait: initially non–weight bearing
	Transcutaneous electronic nerve stimulation and ice
	Quadriceps sets
	Hamstrings sets
	Ankle pumps
	Straight leg raises and flexion-to-extension 70° to 40° in the hinged postoperative brace
4–5	Dressing change
	Immobilizer set 90° to 40°
	Gait: touch-down weight bearing
	Exercises performed in the brace, as above with addition of terminal knee extension, hamstrings curls, hip flexion, and hip extension
10–12	Stitches out
	Patient allowed to shower
	Immobilizer set 90° to 40°
	Gait: touch-down weight bearing
	Exercises as for days 1 through 5
Postoperative status	
3 wk	Hinged postoperative brace set 90° to 20°
	Gait: partial weight bearing
	Exercises out of brace
	Exercises as for days 1 through 5, plus straight leg raises with terminal knee extensions, flexion to extension 90° to 0°, flexion activities
6 wk	Hinged postoperative brace set 90° to 10°
	Gait: partial weight bearing to full weight bearing (2 to 4 wk)
	Maintain 10° flexion contracture
	Exercise as at 3 wk
	Biking when range of motion is sufficient
	Well leg and upper body program
12 wk	Gait: full weight bearing with no brace
	Exercises as at 6 wk
	Side step-ups, swimming program, walking program, weights to 10 pounds as tolerated
4 mo	Exercises as for 12 wk, plus weight room activities
	More aggressive closed-chain activities
5–7 mo	Functional activities
	Continued weight bearing
	Weight training
	Progressive running and agility skills
	Return to sport when testing and functional activities are within normal limits

Table 79–4. Rehabilitation After Intra-Articular Patellar Tendon Graft

- Immediately postoperative
  - Compression dressing, ice
  - Locked hinged brace 0° (treat extra-articular or meniscal repair combined with intra-articular reconstruction as intra-articular reconstruction)
  - Proper elevation
  - Ankle pumps encouraged, muscle stimulation and biofeedback and quadriceps sets
  - CPM
- Postoperative day 1
  - Patient out of bed
  - Gait: weight bearing to tolerance
  - Ankle pumps
  - Quadriceps sets, terminal knee extensions or heel lifts
  - Obtain full passive extension out of brace
- Postoperative day 2
  - Dressing change
  - Begin working to 90° of flexion out of brace
  - Unlock brace as patient becomes more comfortable
  - Gait: weight bearing to tolerance with crutches
  - Stimulation to train quadriceps
  - Exercises (out of brace): quadriceps sets, heel lifts, flexion activities, straight leg raises with heel lift, hamstrings stretches, passive extension, and full flexion, as tolerated
- Postoperative day 3
  - Gait: weight bearing to tolerance with crutches
  - Exercises out of brace: quadriceps sets, heel lifts, flexion activities, straight leg raises with heel lift, hamstrings stretching, passive extension to 0°, hip flexion, flexion to extension 90° to 45°, active range of motion 90°+ as tolerated, and hamstrings curls
  - Functional exercises such as mini-squats and rubber tubing leg presses started and progressed
- Status postoperatively 2–3 wks to 6 wks
  - Brace 0° to full flexion, decrease use as comfortable, replace with knee sleeve as comfortable
  - Gait: weight bearing to tolerance with crutches, progress to full weight bearing as quadriceps develop
  - Exercises: biking as tolerated, 30 to 60 minutes
  - Gradually increase progressive resistance exercises to 5 pounds on exercises for day 3 above
  - 90° to 45° flexion to extension for quadriceps training
  - Squats as tolerated, step-up standing, knee flexion progressed, hip extension
  - Hip abduction, hip adduction
  - Rubber tubing, squats (single and double), leg press
  - Walking program
  - Safe isokinetics
  - Proprioception exercises
  - Continue exercises from the first 6 wks using weights up to 10 pounds
  - Steps
  - Closed-chain activities
  - Progress proper quadriceps-strengthening activities
  - Isokinetic testing
- Status postoperatively 12 wks
  - Isokinetic testing
  - Begin running program as strength and knee conditions permit
- Status postoperatively 4–6 mos
  - Functional brace for support (p.r.n.)
  - Agility programs
  - Sport-specific activities
  - Return to sport when testing and functional activities are within normal limits

emphasized and active assisted flexion is begun. The patient begins quadriceps setting and terminal knee extension and is assisted with electrical stimulation and biofeedback to get a good quadriceps contraction. Straight leg raises are begun when the patient is comfortable. Flexion to 90° is encouraged by 5 to 7 days. This motion progresses, as tolerated, over the next week to 10 days.

Quadriceps sets, terminal knee extensions, straight leg raises, hip flexion, hamstrings curls, aggressive knee flexion, and minimum standing knee bends are continued when the patient leaves the hospital. Other hip exercises are begun as soon as they do not cause discomfort. The straight-knee immobilizer is discontinued once gait activities become normal. Crutches are used until quadriceps strength is appropriate and gait is steady. Cycling can be started as soon as wounds have healed and there is enough range of motion. Light resistance is used with the exercises, with a goal of 10 pounds within 6 to 10 weeks. High-resistance, isokinetic, and isotonic open-chain extension exercises are avoided until 4 to 6 months. It is hoped that the athlete can return to full activity, on average, after 6 to 7 months.

Nonoperatively Treated Posterior Cruciate Ligament Injuries with Posterolateral Rotatory Instability

The acute or chronic nonoperatively treated posterior cruciate ligament injury is treated quite simply with low-stress, open-chain exercises, beginning with quadriceps sets, terminal knee extensions, straight leg raises, and exercises for hip flexors, adductors, abductors, and extensors. Hamstring exercises may be avoided at first and added once the ligament has had some time to heal. Quadriceps work should be done from 60° to 0° in the flexion-to-extension mode and in the straight leg raise mode.

Weight bearing is controlled initially with crutches, and the athlete is allowed to progress as quadriceps control increases. Generally, a brace is not used unless the athlete is uncomfortable. The athlete may progress to functional activities through the continuum, as comfort allows.

The acute posterolateral rotatory instability is a capsular injury, and full extension is detrimental to the healing of this structure. An immobilizer with an extension lock at 20° is necessary for acute knee injuries for up to 6 weeks. The exercises described above are used, but the athlete does not place the knee in full extension.

Operatively Treated Posterior Cruciate Ligament Injuries with Posterolateral Rotatory Instability

In a direct repair of the posterior cruciate ligament it is important to take the weight of the tibia off the repair. Therefore a long-leg brace with heel cup is important. Also, it is extremely important when elevating the leg, that the patient supports the leg behind the tibia and not at the heel, so that no force is being levered back onto the posterior cruciate ligament. The postoperative cast is worn 4 to 6 weeks with the knee flexed at 60° to 70°. The foot is included in the cast. Once the cast is removed, the patient wears a long-leg brace, but no weight is borne until quadriceps control is regained, 8 to 10 weeks after surgery. All quadriceps exercises are encouraged, but hamstrings strengthening is delayed until the 3-month mark. Cycling and closed-chain exercises are used once range of motion is comfortable and weight bearing status permits.

If a graft is used, such as patellar tendon or semitendinosus, or an allograft, the protection described before is important, but, as with the intra-articular graft for the anterior cruciate ligament, the patient begins immediate motion. In fact, the protocol for the intra-articular posterior cruciate ligament graft is the same as that for the anterior cruciate ligament, except that we try to protect from posterior shear.

The postoperative routine for an arcuate complex advancement for posterolateral rotatory instability must also be handled extremely carefully. Postoperatively, the joint is placed in a cast at 60° to 70° flexion with the foot incorporated and a pelvic band to keep the leg from rotating externally and putting stress across the posterolateral corner. There must be adequate support beneath the tibia, and the heel must not rest on the bed when the patient is supine. The patient can perform quadriceps sets and straight leg raising with the cast in place.

At 6 weeks, the cast is removed and a long-leg brace with a dial-lock hinge and heel cup is worn. It is very important that extension comes gradually and slowly with active quadriceps contraction. Flexion can be gained with active assisted motion. The brace is locked at 60°, and, as the patient is able to extend further, it is locked into further extension. The brace should not put any stress on the reconstructed structures, so the position should always be less than the amount of active knee extension. It is important to protect the knee from shear forces when exercising, with support at the proximal tibia posteriorly.

Terminal knee extensions, straight leg raises, and limited flexion-to-extension exercises all are done, along with strengthening of the hip flexors, adductors, abductors, and extensors. Hamstrings strengthening is begun at 12 weeks. The patient is allowed partial weight bearing once 20° of active extension is reached, progressing from a toe-heel gait to a heel-toe gait as extension improves. Increasing extension gradually is extremely important. Once the athlete has obtained good range of motion and stability is good on ligament testing, the functional continuum can be used.

RETURN TO SPORT

The return to full activity is very important to the athlete. Obviously, a person returning to a sedentary life does not have to reach for high functional goals. Being able to lift one's body weight on a step, walk, and get up out of a squat or up from a chair is all that is necessary. For those going on to more athletic endeavors, a carefully planned program must be used to allow the person to return safely to fullest capacity.

This progression is accelerated by the use of closed-chain exercises. It is very important to set reasonable goals to ensure that athletes practice functional activities so they can build on them and progress. Table 79–1 gives a simple outline of a continuum of functional exercise, but the specifics of a particular sport require planning of activities that simulate the sport's moves.

The return to activity depends on a number of variables. Certainly, enough healing time must pass so that the ligament is sturdy. Strength is very important and can be measured isokinetically, but it must also be measured functionally; tests such as the hop test, figure-of-eight runs, and agility runs all should be evaluated.

Postoperatively, knees have a tendency to swell and become irritated by vigorous practice in running sports, so athletes must be helped through these early return to sport activities, to allow the knee to calm down. Even though athletes may be returning to sport as early as 6 or 7 months, it is likely to be a full year or more before they can forget about the knee and concentrate on the sport.

REFERENCES

1. Noyes, F. R., Butler, D. L., Paulos, L. E., and Grood, E. S.: Intra-articular cruciate reconstruction. I. Perspectives on graft strength, vascularization and immediate motion after replacement. Clin. Orthop. *172*:71, 1983.
2. Noyes, F. R., DeLucas, J. L., and Torvik, P. J.: Biomechanics of anterior cruciate ligament failure. An analysis of strain rate sensitivity and mechanisms of failure in primates. J. Bone Joint Surg. *56A*:236, 1974.

3. Noyes, F. R., Barber, S. D., and Mangine, R. E.: Abnormal lower limb symmetry determined by function hop tests after anterior cruciate ligament ruptures. Am J. Sports Med. *19*:513, 1991.
4. Paulos, L. E., Noyes F. R., Grood, E., and Butler, D. L.: Knee rehabilitation after anterior cruciate ligament reconstruction and repair. Am J. Sports Med. *9*:140, 1981.
5. Henning, C. E., Lynch, M. A., and Glick, K. R., Jr.: An in-vivo strain gauge study of elongation of the anterior cruciate ligament. Am J. Sports Med. *13*:22, 1985.
6. Andrews, J. R., and Sanders, R.: "mini-reconstruction" technique in treating anterolateral rotatory instability (ALRI). Clin. Orthop. *172*:93, 1983.
7. Ameil, D., Kuper, S., and Akeson, W. H.: Cruciate ligaments. Response to injury. *In* Knee Ligaments—Structure, Function, Injury, and Repair. Edited by D. D. Akeson and W. O'Connor. New York, Raven, 1990.
8. Arnoczky, S. P.: Blood supply to the anterior cruciate ligament and supporting structures. Orthop. Clin. North Am. *16*:15, 1985.
9. Paulos, L. E., Butler, D. L., Noyes, F. R., and Grood, E. S.: Intra-articular cruciate reconstruction. Replacements with vascularized patellar tendon. Clin. Orthop. *172*:78, 1983.
10. Arnoczky, S. P.: The vascularity of the anterior cruciate ligament and associated structures: Its role in repair and reconstruction. *In* The Anterior Cruciate Deficient Knee: New Concepts in Ligament Repair. Edited by D. W. Jackson and D. Drez. St. Louis, C.V. Mosby, 1987.
11. Shelbourne, K. D.: Team Concept Meeting, Sports Physical Therapy Section, American Physical Therapy Association, December, 1991.
12. Paulos, L. E.: Knee rehabilitation after anterior cruciate ligament reconstruction and repair. J. Orthop. Sports Phys. Ther. *13*:2, 1991.

80 *Robert R. Burger*

Knee Braces

With the increased media exposure enjoyed by high-profile sports and athletes over the past 25 years, knee braces have gained widespread acceptance among competitive athletes. Early knee braces evolved from the methods of cast-bracing but were cumbersome and precluded athletic activity. Historically, supportive taping for the unstable knee was the standard of care for injured athletes, and, until the 1960s, very few braces were available. Knee braces were widely noticed after the national exposure of Joe Namath and the Lenox Hill brace in the late 1960s. This fueled the perception among athletes and coaches that knee braces are not only an option but frequently standard equipment for competitors or athletes at high risk for knee ligament injuries.

Because of the ever increasing number of knee braces currently available, team physicians have an essential role: distinguishing the *science* of knee bracing from the *business,* so as to make educated and informed recommendations on their use and appropriateness.

CLASSIFICATION OF KNEE BRACES

In response to the increasing popularity and demand for knee braces, in 1984 the Sports Medicine Committee of the American Academy of Orthopaedic Surgeons (AAOS) held its first symposium to evaluate the status of knee bracing.[1] The committee recognized that, despite the large number of commercially available braces at the time, scientific data needed to justify widespread use of knee braces were limited. This committee classified knee braces in three basic categories: prophylactic, rehabilitative, and functional. Prophylactic braces include those designed to protect the knee from injury or reduce the severity of injury. Rehabilitative braces include those used to allow the injured knee, whether treated operatively or nonoperatively, protected motion during the healing phase. Functional braces are designed to provide protection and stability to the unstable knee. It should be noted that such designations are to some degree arbitrary, since many braces could be classified in more than one category. For the sake of completeness, a fourth category, patellar braces, should also be recognized. Each class of knee braces will be evaluated separately, to review the functional goals, design variations, and indications for use.

PROPHYLACTIC KNEE BRACES

Prophylactic knee braces were designed with the goal of protecting from injury. Common designs, including the McDavid (McDavid Knee Guard, Inc., Clarendon Hills, IL) and Anderson (Omni Scientific, Inc., LaFayette, IN) braces, consisted of laterally based, hinged supports developed to protect the medial collateral ligament (MCL) from injury sustained in a direct contact valgus blow. Alternative designs have expanded in complexity, and manufacturers often imply (whether it is scientifically proven or not) that they afford protection to other ligaments, including the anterior cruciate ligament (ACL), in both contact and noncontact injuries.

The ideal prophylactic knee brace would be one that could be proven to decrease the severity and frequency of disabling knee injuries while allowing the athlete to maintain normal speed and agility. Such a brace would need to be lightweight and form fitting, to minimize additional energy expenditure, since muscle fatigue could also predispose the athlete to injury. The brace would have to protect the knee and demonstrate no increased risk for ankle or leg injuries. Additional criteria for an ideal brace include comfort, durability, accessibility, and cost effectiveness. Unfortunately, the ideal brace does not exist, and the variability in brace design and effectiveness, as well as the lack of well-controlled clinical trials, makes it difficult to evaluate whether any brace successfully meets all these goals.

Brace Design

The rationale behind most knee brace designs is to absorb the direct or indirect stress placed on the knee during an athletic maneuver, thus lessening the chance of injury. Initial brace designs were intended to redirect the force of lateral impact away from the knee joint to points above and below. Theoretically, more recent designs decrease the absolute strain on the knee ligaments, not only by dissipating the impact force above and below the joint but also by increasing the duration of impact loading on the knee.

For simplicity's sake, prophylactic knee braces can be subgrouped into two types: (1) lateral bar-based hinged designs fitted with a hyperextension stop and (2) medial and lateral-based designs incorporating straps or plastic cuffs with a polycentric hinge.

Early protective braces consisting of lateral hinge designs were used to minimize the force of direct contact lateral blows to knees, thus protecting the MCL. Variations in such braces include single-axis, dual-axis, or polycentric-axis designs, which may alter or restrict the normal axis of knee motion in one or more planes. Braces of this type are intended to statically restrain abnormal knee motion, especially in response to a valgus stress. Common examples of these types include the McDavid, Anderson, and Protective Knee Guard (Donjoy, Carlsbad, CA; (Fig. 80–1).

The second type of preventive knee brace uses a plastic cuff or strap suspension system incorporating medial and lateral supports held together with a polycentric hinge. Many of these braces cannot be classified simply as prophylactic braces, since they can also be used as functional, or even rehabilitative, braces. Examples include the Losse Knee Defender (Donjoy, Carlsbad, CA) and the Am-Pro Knee Guard (American Prosthetics, Davenport, IA), as well as other braces marketed primarily as functional braces and designed to protect the ACL-injured knee.

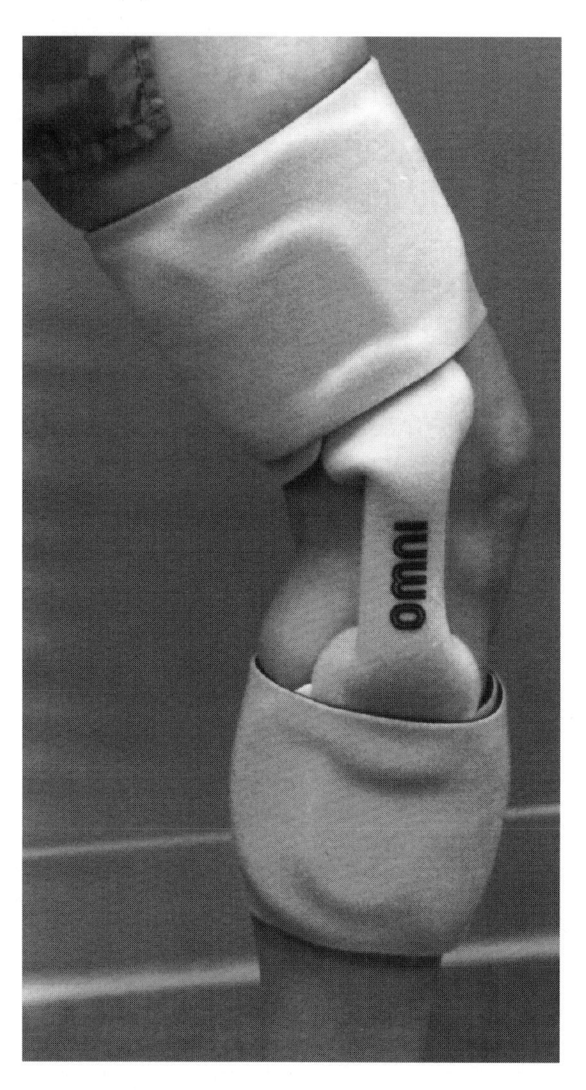

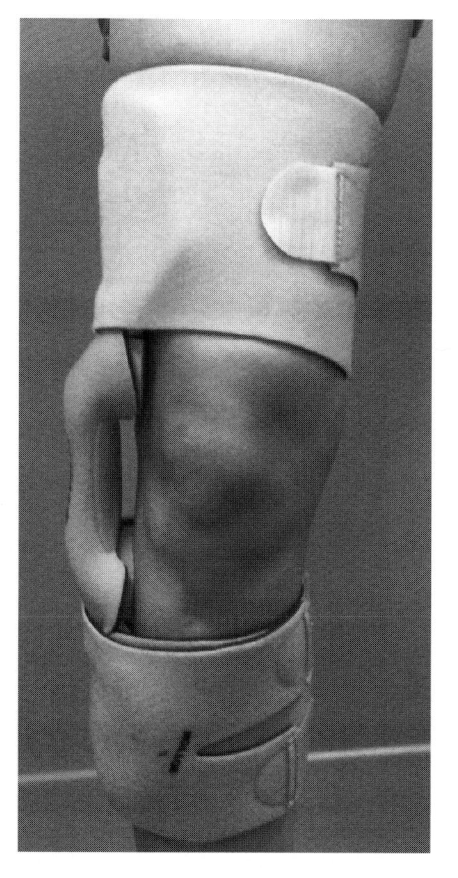

Fig. 80–1. The Anderson knee stabler (Omni Scientific Inc., Concord, CA).

Laboratory Studies

Numerous studies have been performed on cadaver knees and artificial knee models to evaluate the effectiveness of various knee braces. These studies, while not directly applicable to the clinical setting of the on-field injury, provide helpful insights. Laboratory studies clearly demonstrate that all braces do not provide equal protection.[2,3] Therefore, extrapolating results and drawing conclusions from controlled trials with a specific type of brace to apply to all types of prophylactic braces is misleading. Paulos and France and their respective coworkers concluded from basic science testing of several brace designs that force distribution and energy absorption determine the effectiveness of a given brace, and they determined that longer, stiffer braces protect better from injury.[4,5] Additionally, they suggested that knee braces are most effective for larger-mass, low-velocity impacts with the limb fixed and the knee in extension.

Such studies are limited by the inability to duplicate the complex force vectors of high-energy stresses on the knee. Additionally, studies in vitro do not adequately reflect the effects of loading, position of foot and knee at injury, and dynamic muscle response to the forces imposed on the knee at injury. Furthermore, no relationship has been proven between the performance of a brace under laboratory conditions and its performance on the athletic field.

Clinical Trials of Bracing

Several clinical trials of prophylactic knee braces in football have shown contradictory results. Quillian, Schriner, and Hansen and coworkers observed lower rates of MCL injuries when prophylactic braces were worn.[6–8] Hewson's group found no difference in the incidence of knee injuries, whereas Rovere's noted an increased rate of knee injuries with prophylactic braces.[9,10] Taft and colleagues found lateral bracing to be ineffective for decreasing the number of meniscal or ligamentous injuries, and, in a multi-institutional National Collegiate Athletic Association study, Teitz and associates found that prophylactic knee braces do not prevent knee injuries and may in fact be harmful.[11,12] Grace's group likewise found knee bracing to be ineffective in preventing injury and noted a higher rate of foot and ankle injuries when braces were worn.[13] In a controlled, prospective clinical trial of prophylactic braces performed by Sitler and colleagues at West Point in seven-man intramural football leagues, bracing seemed to be effective in decreasing the rate of knee injuries (both total and MCL) in defensive players only.[14] There was no difference in the overall severity of knee injuries, with or without braces. Sitler's group concluded that prophylactic knee braces are most effective at protecting the MCL during direct contact lateral blows to the knee with the foot in a fixed, loaded position.

Given the fact that, at best, these studies provide inconclusive evidence that prophylactic knee bracing in any way decreases the rate or severity of knee injuries and could possibly even increase the risk of injury, the AAOS and the American Academy of Pediatrics have published position statements that do not recommend the use of prophylactic knee braces at this time.[1,15] Clearly, more research is necessary to better identify which athletes are at high risk for serious knee injury and to determine what role, if any, prophylactic knee braces may have in lowering the risk of injury.

REHABILITATIVE BRACES

Rehabilitative knee braces were developed as an extension of the principle of protecting the injured ligaments with splinting or casting to allow adequate healing. Salter and coworkers and Noyes and colleagues demonstrated the beneficial effects of maintaining knee motion on the articular cartilage, and Gerber and associates noted improved ligamentous healing of knee injuries when motion over a controlled arc was maintained.[16–18] Rehabilitative braces were designed to allow protected motion of injured knees, whether treated operatively or nonoperatively, while preventing abnormal varus or valgus stress on the healing knee.

The basic design most often includes medial and lateral support arms, a hinge system to allow knee motion, and thigh and calf enclosures that incorporate straps for support and suspension. Often, flexion and extension stops are added to limit the arc of motion (Fig. 80–2).

The advantages of rehabilitative braces include easy application and removal, comfort, lightweight protection, static stability, and off-the-shelf accessibility. Additional benefits include ease in obtaining postoperative knee motion, lower rates of ankylosis, and less frequent need for subsequent knee manipulation.[19] Potential problems with rehabilitative braces include the possibility of dependent edema below the brace straps, fitting difficulties for patients with severe angular deformities or extremes of leg size, improper fitting or placement of the hinges, and limited means of ensuring compliance with brace wear. Despite these drawbacks, rehabilitative braces have been well accepted by injured athletes, and they facilitate early aggressive rehabilitation.

FUNCTIONAL BRACES

Functional braces were designed to allow athletes with an unstable knee to continue participating at the highest possible level by minimizing pain, swelling, and instability. Originally designed for ACL injuries, these braces were envisioned to allow the athlete to cut, decelerate, and change directions by controlling the pivot shift.[20] Ideally, such braces would also protect the knee from further injury.

Functional braces work by minimizing the absolute displacement or rotation of the tibia on the femur. Mechanisms by which these braces act include prevention of knee hyperextension and increased resistance to displacement. Other theoretical, but as yet unproven,

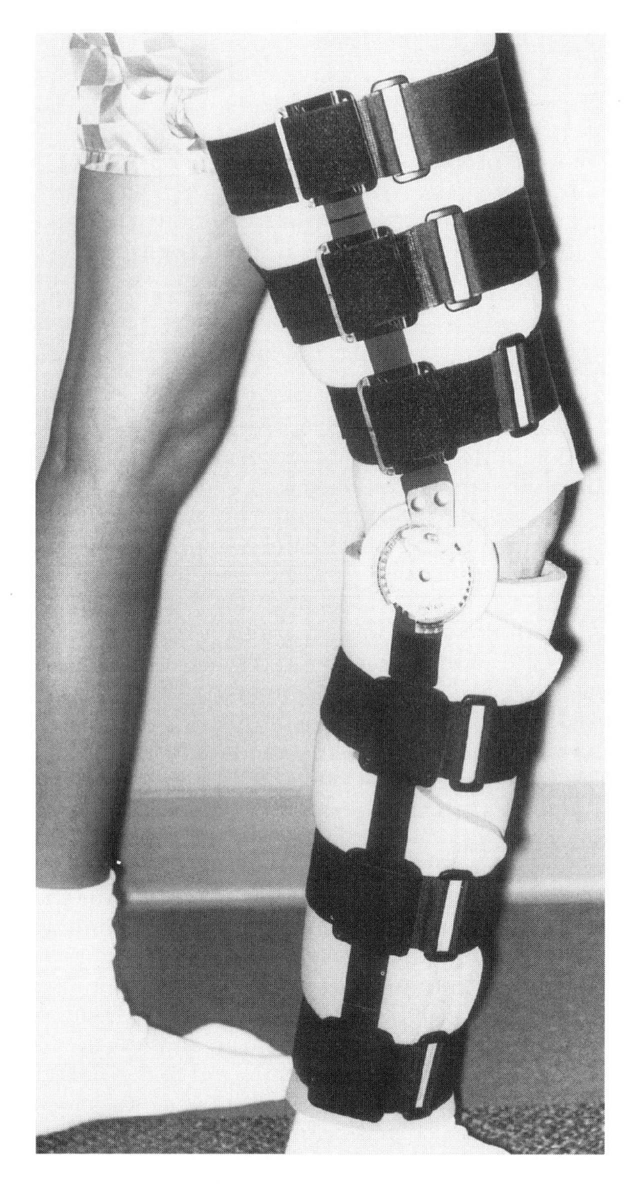

Fig. 80–2. Vantage long-leg brace (Vantage Orthopaedics, Cincinnati, OH).

mechanisms of brace protection include augmentation of limb proprioception and alteration of limb position during cutting. By these means, functional braces ideally should prevent or minimize episodes of giving way associated with the pivot shift. How well any brace functions depends not only on its protective ability but also on its ability to duplicate the normal combination of rolling and gliding motions of the knee while controlling abnormal motion.

Design Types

Two major designs have been used for functional braces: (1) hinge-post-strap and (2) hinge-post-shell. The Lenox Hill brace (Lenox Hill Brace Shop, New York, NY), originally designed to control anteromedial rotatory instability in Joe Namath's knee, is the prototype strap-design brace (Fig. 80–3). Other braces of this type include the Feanny (Medical Design, Grand Prairie, TX) and the Donjoy 4-Point Brace (Donjoy, Carlsbad, CA). Hinge-post-shell designs, consisting of a semirigid plastic shell that encompasses both thigh and calf, were developed to improve on the soft tissue contact area and brace suspension. Other theoretical benefits include increased brace stiffness and rigidity. Common examples of shell-design braces include the CTi (Innovation Sports, Carlsbad, CA), Generation II Polyaxial Brace (Generation II Orthotics, Vancouver, B.C.), the Townsend Brace (Townsend Industries, Bakersfield, CA), and the Donjoy RKS (Donjoy, Carlsbad, CA). Although off-the-shelf functional braces are available, most braces used today are custom designed. Figure 80–4 depicts several commonly used functional braces.

Brace Effectiveness

Functional braces are designed for the closed kinetic chain of knee gait, and laboratory studies on the effectiveness of braces at controlling instability often cannot replicate the loaded state of the knee during sports or the dynamic impact of muscle control. Studies in vitro suggest that functional braces are effective at controlling anteroposterior translation when very low loads are applied to the braced knee, but functional braces may be limited in their ability to control knee laxity when subjected to the powerful forces imposed during athletic participation.[21–26] Most athletes with unstable knees believe the brace improves performance in running and cutting, and in one study 91% of patients thought the knee brace was beneficial.[20, 27–29] The use of a brace does not, however, return the athlete to “normal,” so functional bracing should not be considered an adequate substitute for reconstructive knee surgery in a competitive athlete who desires to maintain the highest level of function. Nonetheless, athletes report a high level of satisfaction with functional braces, subjectively noting a decrease in symptoms of instability, relief of pain, and a sense of protection from brace wear. It has also been speculated that functional braces may be effective after ACL reconstruction by reducing the repetitive loads on the ACL substitute, thus decreasing creep of the graft.

Indications for Functional Braces

No clear-cut indications for functional bracing have been set forth, and most recommendations for use are empirical, citing anecdotal successes in selected athletes. Functional braces have typically been used in one of three ways: (1) postoperatively, (2) instead of operation, and (3) prophylactically. Prophylactic knee braces were discussed earlier. Use of functional knee braces in nonoperatively treated patients with unstable knees seems to decrease the frequency of instability episodes, although no scientific studies document proven effectiveness.

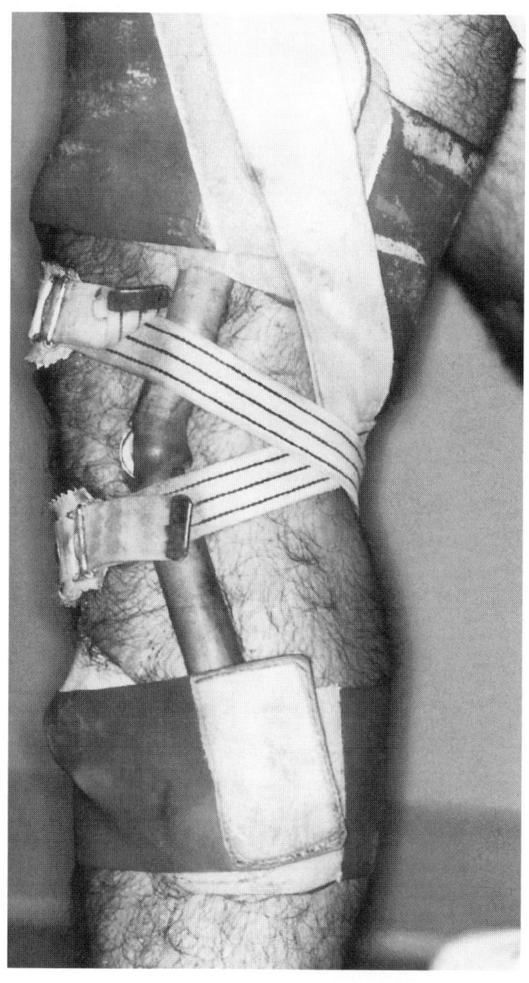

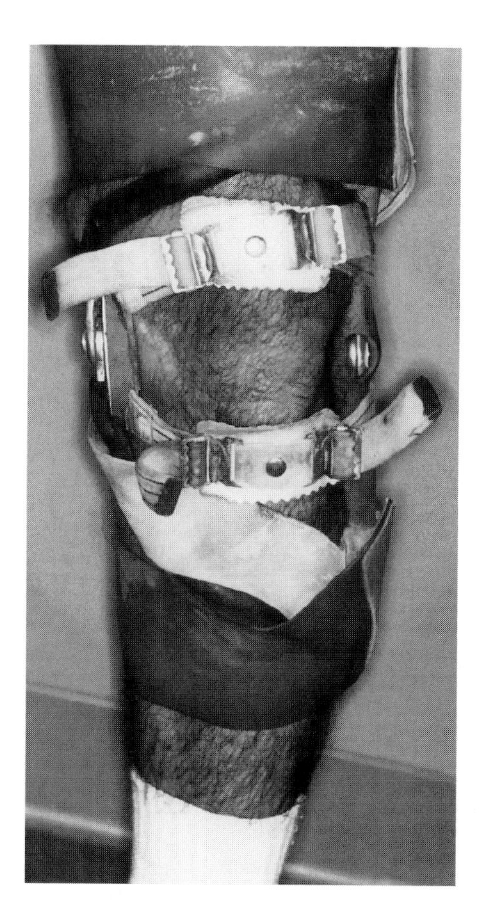

Fig. 80–3. The Lenox-Hill derotation brace (Lenox Hill Brace Shop, New York, NY).

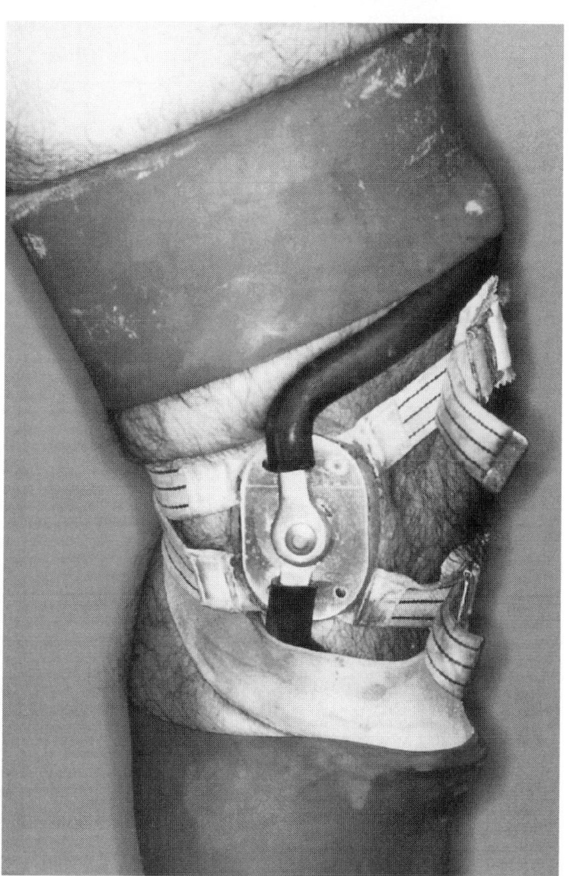

These braces have also been useful for patients whose knee instability is secondary to a neuromuscular disease that precludes surgical stabilization.

Use of functional braces following knee ligament reconstruction remains controversial, and variations in treatment range from wearing the brace for any further sporting activity, wearing it only during the first year after surgery to allow maturation of the grafted ligament, and using functional braces only for athletes when surgery produces suboptimal results and residual instability. It is evident that no strict criteria for use of functional knee braces currently exist.

Limitations

Current limitations on the use of functional braces include lack of controlled clinical studies that demonstrate proven effectiveness. No studies as yet have shown that braces clearly protect injured or reconstructed knees from further injury or minimize the development of post-traumatic arthritis. Current braces adversely affect speed and agility and have been proven to increase energy consumption, which may itself make the knee more vulnerable to further injury.[30–32] Athletes frequently complain of problems with brace migration and slipping during sporting activity.[27] Other problems include improper fitting and loss of suspension. Brace

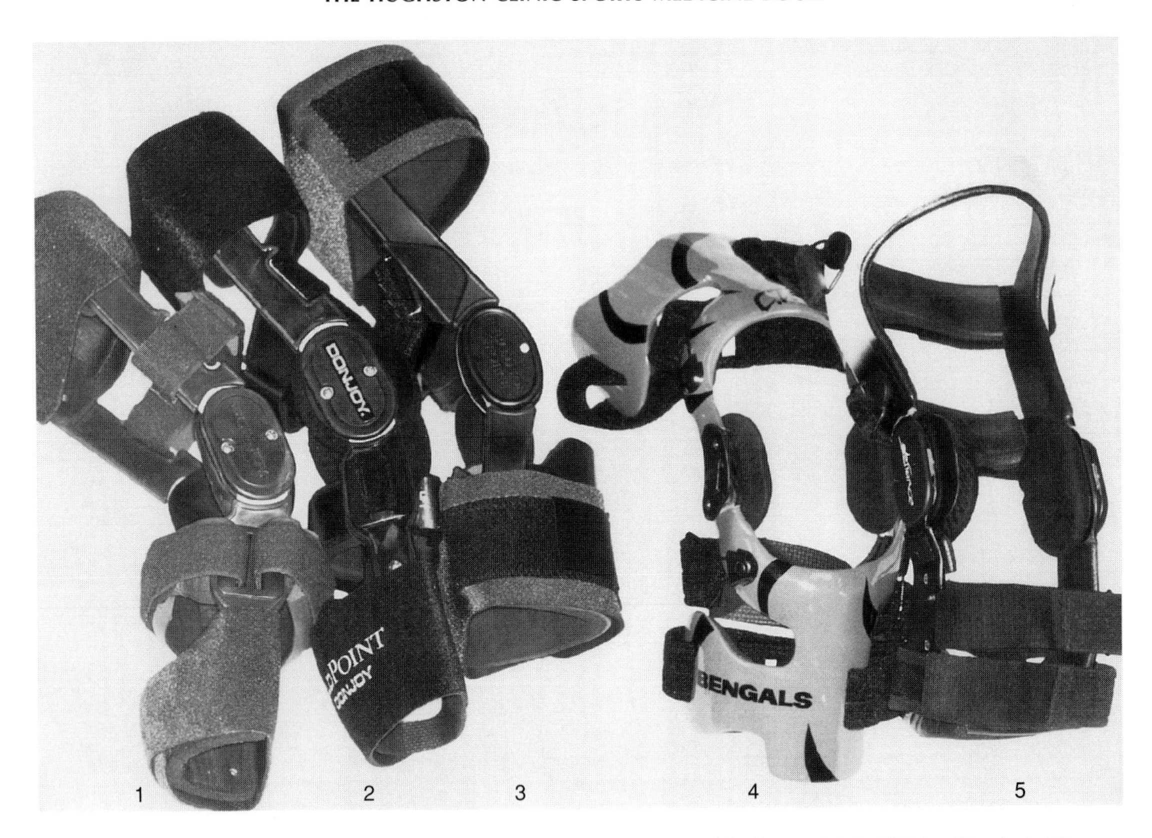

Fig. 80–4. Common functional knee braces: (1) 4-Point brace (DonJoy, Carlsbad, CA); (2) Gold Point (DonJoy); (3) Bledsoe Force Brace (Medical Technology, Inc., Grand Prairie, TX); (4) CTi 2 (Innovation Sports, Irvine, CA); (5) Defiance (DonJoy).

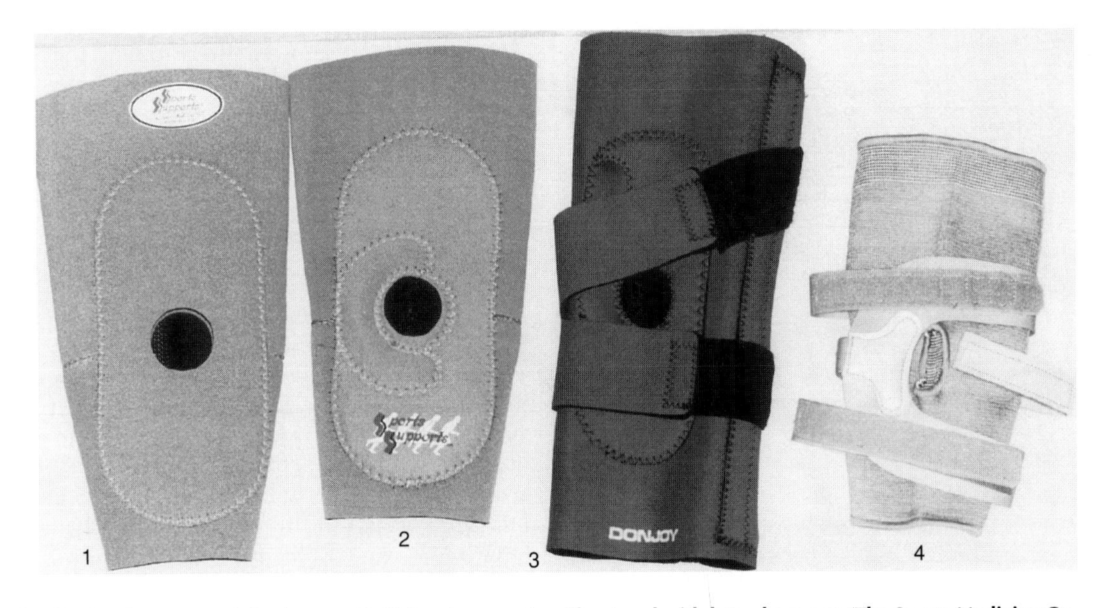

Fig. 80–5. Common patellar braces: (1, 2) Sports supports without and with lateral support (The Sports Medicine Co., Irvine, TX); (3) lateral patellar knee support (DonJoy); (4) Palumbo patellar stabilizing brace (Dynorthotics, Vienna, VA).

wear from repeated use is a potential problem, as is the cost, including insurance reimbursement and brace modifications.

Future Directions

Future advances in the science of knee bracing depend on the development of lighter, more cost-effective braces that better control abnormal knee motion while imposing no restriction on athletic performance. Furthermore, longterm clinical studies are needed to determine if functional braces prevent the development of arthritic changes or subsequent injuries in unstable knees. Research is necessary to determine if the protective effect of knee braces is purely mechanical, or if they provide any significant proprioceptive, or even psychological, benefit for competitive athletes.

PATELLAR BRACES

Patellar braces were developed with the primary goal of diminishing symptomatic lateral patellar subluxation. Most braces are constructed of a neoprene or elastic sleeve, frequently combined with either a buttress pad or a strapping system for additional support. Although patellar braces have been purported to dynamically stabilize the patella and improve sensory feedback, they most likely act as a static restraint by mechanically decreasing lateral displacement of the patella on the femur. Other potential benefits include a warming effect on the knee and reduction of knee swelling. Numerous patellar braces are available, and most can be fitted off the shelf (Fig. 80–5).

Patellar braces are often used on the athletic field and during activities of daily living, in part because of the frequency of anterior knee pain, but also because of the relatively low cost and easy accessibility of such braces.

Few studies are available that address the benefits of patellar braces, and they should be considered only as an adjunct to a rehabilitation program including strengthening and flexibility exercises.

Lysholm and coworkers did note an increase in peak quadriceps force generated in 88% of patients wearing these braces, but scientific testing and clinical trials have not as yet demonstrated the proven efficacy of patellar braces.[33]

SUMMARY

The use of knee braces has increased significantly over the past 25 years, and competitive athletes have readily accepted them as necessary equipment that allows for continued sports participation. Critical analysis of knee braces reveals that most recommendations for brace wear are empirical, and there is a clear need for controlled clinical trials to determine the most appropriate uses for knee braces in sports. Knee braces should be viewed, not as a panacea, but as a helpful adjunct to patient education and comprehensive rehabilitation. With continuing modifications in brace design and increased emphasis on duplicating the biomechanics of the normal knee, team physicians need to closely monitor the evolving science of knee braces, so as to make informed decisions about their efficacy and usefulness.

REFERENCES

1. Drez, D. J. Jr. (Ed.): American Academy of Orthopaedic Surgeons: Knee Braces—Seminar Report. Chicago, IL, American Academy of Orthopaedic Surgeons, 1984.
2. Baker, B. E., et al.: A biomechanical study of the static stabilizing effect of knee braces on medial stability. Am. J. Sports Med. *15*:566, 1987.
3. Baker, B. E., et al.: The effect of knee braces on lateral impact loading of the knee. Am. J. Sports Med. *17*:182, 1989.
4. Paulos, L. E., et al.: Biomechanics of lateral knee bracing. Part I. Response of the valgus restraints to loading. Am. J. Sports Med. *15*:419, 1987.
5. France, E. P., et al.: The biomechanics of lateral knee bracing. Part II. Impact response of the braced knee. Am. J. Sports Med. *15*:430, 1987.
6. Quillian, W. W., Simms, R. T., Cooper, J. S., et al.: Knee bracing in preventing injuries in high school football. Int. Pediatr. *2*:255, 1987.
7. Schriner, J. L.: A two-year study of the effectiveness of knee braces in high school football players. J. Osteopathic Sports Med. *1*:21, 1987.
8. Hansen, B. L., Ward, J. C., and Diehl, R. C.: The preventive use of the Anderson knee stabler in football. Physician Sportsmed. *13(9)*:75, 1985.
9. Hewson, G. F., Jr., Mendini, R. A., and Wang, J. B.: Prophylactic knee bracing in college football. Am. J. Sports Med. *14*:262, 1986.
10. Rovere, G. D., Haupt, H. A., and Yates, C. S.: Prophylactic knee bracing in college football. Am. J. Sports Med. *15*:111, 1987.
11. Taft, T. N., Hunter, S. L., and Funderburk, C. H.: Preventive lateral knee bracing in football. Presented at the 11th Annual Meeting of the American Orthopaedic Society for Sports Medicine. Nashville, Tennessee, July, 1985.
12. Teitz, C. C., et al.: Evaluation of the use of braces to prevent injury to the knee in collegiate football players. J. Bone Joint Surg. *69A*:2, 1987.
13. Grace, T. G., et al.: Prophylactic knee braces and injury to the lower extremity. J. Bone Joint Surg. *70A*:422, 1988.
14. Sitler, M., et al.: The efficacy of a prophylactic knee brace to reduce knee injuries in football: A prospective, randomized study at West Point. Am. J. Sports Med. *18*:310, 1990.
15. American Academy of Pediatrics: Knee brace use by athletes. Pediatrics *85*:228, 1990.
16. Salter, R. B., et al.: The biological effect of continuous passive motion on healing of full-thickness defects in articular cartilage: An experimental investigation in the rabbit. J. Bone Joint Surg. *62A*:1232, 1980.
17. Noyes, F. R., Mangine, R. E., and Barber, S.: Early knee motion after open and arthroscopic anterior cruciate ligament reconstruction. Am. J. Sports Med. *15*:149, 1987.
18. Gerber, G., Jakob, R. P., and Ganz, R.: Observations concerning a limited mobilisation cast after anterior cruciate ligament surgery. Arch. Orthop. Trauma. Surg. *101*:291, 1983.
19. Buss, D. D., et al.: Arthroscopically assisted reconstruction of the anterior cruciate ligament with use of autogenous patellar-ligament grafts. Results after twenty-four to forty-two months. J. Bone Joint Surg. *75A*:1346, 1993.
20. Nicholas, J. A.: Bracing the anterior cruciate ligament deficient knee using the Lenox Hill derotation brace. Clin. Orthop. *172*:137, 1982.
21. Wojtys, E. M., et al.: A biomechanical evaluation of the Lenox Hill knee brace. Clin. Orthop. *220*:179, 1987.

22. Wojtys, E. M., Loubert, P. V., Samson, S. Y., and Viviano, D. M.: Use of a knee brace for control of tibial translation and rotation. J. Bone Joint Surg. *72A*:1323, 1990.
23. Hofmann, A. A., Wyatt, R. W. B., Bourne, M. H., and Daniels, A. V.: Knee stability in orthotic knee braces. Am. J. Sports Med. *12*:371, 1984.
24. Branch, T., Hunter, R., and Reynolds, P.: Controlling anterior tibial displacement under static load: A comparison of two braces. Orthopedics *11*:1249, 1988.
25. Beck, C., Drez, D., Jr., et al.: Instrumented testing of functional knee braces. Am. J. Sports Med. *14*:253, 1986.
26. Cook, F. F., Tibone, J. E., and Redfern, F. C.: A dynamic analysis of a functional brace for anterior cruciate ligament insufficiency. Am. J. Sports Med. *17*:519, 1989.
27. Mishra, D. K., Daniel, D. M., and Stone, M. L.: The use of functional knee braces in the control of pathologic anterior knee laxity. Clin. Orthop. *241*:213, 1989.
28. Bassett, G. S., and Fleming, B. W.: The Lenox Hill brace in anterolateral rotatory instability. Am. J. Sports Med. *11*:345, 1983.
29. Colville, M. R., Lee, C. L., and Ciullo, J. V.: The Lenox Hill brace. Am. J. Sports Med. *14*:257, 1986.
30. Houston, M. E., and Goemans, P. H.: Leg muscle performance of athletes with and without knee support braces. Arch. Phys. Med. Rehabil. *63*:431, 1982.
31. Zetterlund, A. E., Serfass, R. C., and Hunter R. E.: The effect of wearing the complete Lenox Hill Derotation Brace on energy expenditure during horizontal treadmill running at 161 m/min. Am. J. Sports Med. *14*:73, 1986.
32. Highgenboten, C. L., Jackson, A., Meske, N., and Smith, J.: The effects of knee brace wear on perceptual and metabolic variables during horizontal treadmill running. Am. J. Sports Med. *19*:639, 1991.
33. Lysholm, J., Nordin, M., Ekstrand, J., and Gillquist, J.: The effect of a patella brace on performance in a knee extension strength test in patients with patellar pain. Am. J. Sports Med. *2*:110, 1977.

81

Leland C. McCluskey

Functional Anatomy of the Ankle and Foot

Injuries to the ankle and foot are quite common during sports activities. Because the joints of the ankle and foot are closely linked to those of the knee and hip, disorders in one area affect the biomechanics of the entire extremity. A clear understanding of the functional anatomy and related biomechanics of the ankle and foot enables clinicians better to diagnose and treat most injuries to this part of the lower extremity.

THE ANKLE

Bone Anatomy

The distal tibia consists of the concave plafond and the medial malleolus. The plafond is the weight-bearing portion of the tibia and has an anterior concavity to resist talar translation. The medial malleolus has two small eminences (colliculi) separated by a groove. The deep deltoid ligament is attached in the intercollicular groove and to the posterior colliculus. The superficial deltoid ligament is attached farther anterior, which is important in recognizing the origin of avulsion fractures.

The lateral malleolus, located at the distal end of the fibula, is positioned approximately 1 cm distal and posterior to the medial malleolus. It has a medial facet for articulation with the talus, a fossa at the articulation with the tibia, and a posterior sulcus for passage of the peroneal tendons.

Motion resulting in upward and downward movement of the foot occurs about a single axis that is oriented obliquely to the long axis of the leg, that passes between the medial and lateral malleoli, and that is directed laterad, posteriorly, and 20° to 25° distally.[1,2]

The malleoli also provide a medial and a lateral buttress to the talus, which serves as an important link between ankle and foot. Movements of the talus with respect to the tibia and tarsal bones are realized by passive transmission of forces by the ligaments. No tendons attach to the talus, a bone composed of a head (which articulates with the navicular bone of the foot), a neck, and a body. The body has a lateral process, a posterior process, and an articular dome. The lateral process of the talus forms both the lateral third of the talar articulation with the posterior calcaneal facet and the superolateral articulation with the distal fibula. The posterior process of the talus is formed by the medial and lateral tubercles, between which lies a groove containing the flexor hallucis longus tendon (Fig. 81–1). Testing the tendon can help localize disorders in this area.

The lateral tubercle of the posterior process is larger and lies farther posterior than the medial one. The os trigonum, located just posterior to the lateral tubercle, is a separate ossification center that persists as an unfused accessory bone in about 6.5% of adults.[3] It fuses into an elongated lateral tubercle (called Stieda's process) in approximately 50% of adults. A fracture of the lateral tubercle (Shepherd's fracture) can cause posterior impingement symptoms similar to those seen with a symptomatic os trigonum.

Ankle Ligaments

The lateral and medial tibiofibular ligaments (syndesmosis) help stabilize the ankle joint (Fig. 81–2). The biomechanical properties of these ligaments and their orientation allow a normal amount of rotation and motion while maintaining stability.

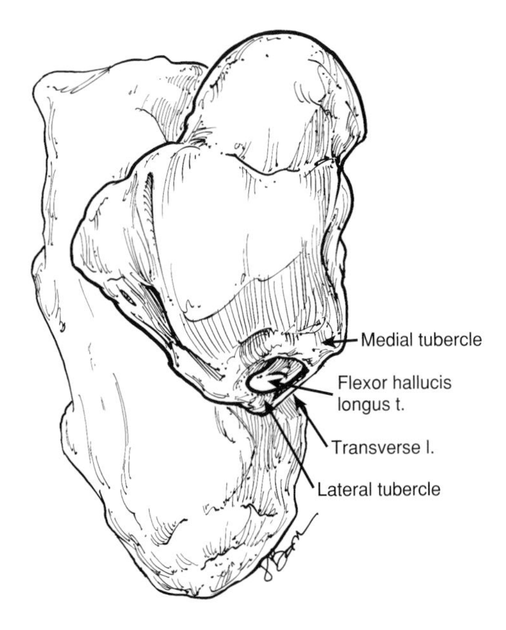

Fig. 81–1. Superior view of the talar dome demonstrates the flexor hallucis longus between the medial and lateral tubercles of the talus.

The lateral ligaments are the anterior talofibular, the calcaneofibular, and the posterior talofibular. The anterior talofibular ligament is an intra-articular thickening of the anterolateral capsule that extends from the anterior border of the distal fibula to the distal anterolateral neck of the talus. It measures approximately 2 cm long and 1 cm wide.

The calcaneofibular ligament is a cordlike extracapsular structure that arises from the anterior part of the fibula and that runs from the inferior aspect of the lateral malleolus distally and posteriorly to a small tubercle on the lateral aspect of the calcaneus. It forms the posteromedial wall of the peroneal tendon sheath and spans both the ankle and the talocalcaneal joints. This anatomic relationship explains the high incidence of injury to the peroneal tendon associated with severe ankle sprains. The ligament is relaxed in the normal standing position and with plantar flexion. Placing the foot in dorsiflexion and inversion tenses the ligament.

The posterior talofibular ligament, the strongest of the lateral ligaments, runs horizontally from the distal fossa of the fibula to the lateral tubercle on the posterior process of the talus. The ligament is relaxed in neutral position and in plantar flexion and tensed in dorsiflexion.[4] Though the lateral talocalcaneal ligament is not a true structure of the ankle joint, it blends with the fibers of the anterior talofibular ligament proximally and attaches to the calcaneus adjacent to the calcaneofibular ligament.

The deltoid, the major medial ligament, is a strong triangle-shaped ligament composed of a broad superficial portion and a more important short deep portion. The fibers of the superficial deltoid are directed more in the sagittal plane, whereas the deep deltoid fibers are nearly horizontal. The superficial fibers run in a continuous sheath from the medial malleolus. The deep deltoid originates on the undersurface of the medial malleolus, near its tip, and runs a horizontal course within the joint to the medial surface of the talus. The tendons of the tibialis posterior and flexor digitorum longus cross superficially over the deltoid ligament.

The distal tibiofibular articulation is supported by the four strong syndesmosis ligaments (i.e., the anterior inferior, posterior inferior and transverse tibiofibular and the interosseous ligament). The anterior inferior and posterior inferior tibiofibular ligaments run from superior to inferior in corresponding sites on the anterior and posterior aspects of the syndesmosis. The strong transverse tibiofibular ligament runs from the posterior articular tip of the distal tibia to the fibula and

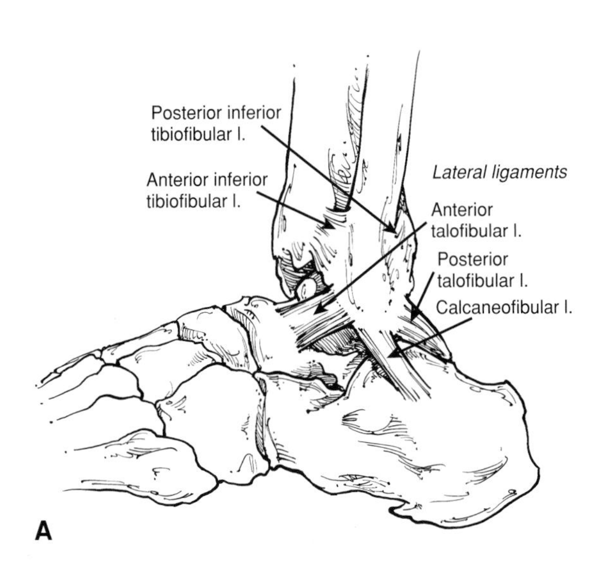

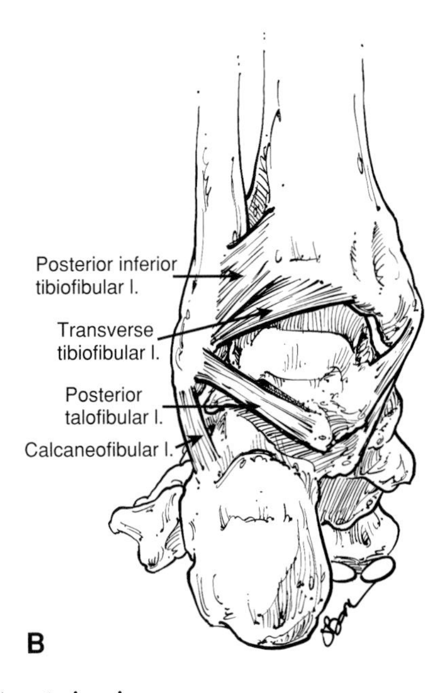

Fig. 81–2. Ankle ligaments, *(A)* lateral and *(B)* posterior views.

is almost continuous with the inferior margin of the posterior inferior tibiofibular ligament. The name given to the distal portion of the interosseous membrane, is the *interosseous ligament,* is the strongest of the tibiofibular ligaments.

ACHILLES TENDON

The Achilles tendon, the largest, thickest, strongest tendon in the body, can sustain forces of four to seven times body weight.[5] It is formed by the gastrocnemius and soleus muscles, whose primary function is plantar flexion of the ankle, and it links this muscle complex with the calcaneus.

The gastrocnemius muscle arises from two heads on the posterior surface of the femur, just proximal to the condyles. The muscle bellies converge into a median raphe and an aponeurosis, which forms a third to half of the Achilles tendon. The soleus muscle extends from the posterior aspect of the tibia, the interosseous membrane, and the fibula. Because the soleus is 75% Type I (slow-twitch) fibers and only crosses the ankle joint, it is more likely than the gastrocnemius to exhibit atrophy as a result of immobilization. The two muscles join to form the Achilles tendon in the middle of the calf. From there, the tendon twists almost 90° posterolaterally, to its insertion into the posterior tubercle of the calcaneus.

Although no true synovial sheath surrounds the tendon, an outer covering, the paratenon, is formed by the enveloping superficial crural fascia. The retrocalcaneal bursa lies between the distal tendon and the superior tip of the posterior calcaneus (bursal projection). This bursa does have a synovial lining and can become inflamed, especially in persons with a "hatchet-shaped" calcaneus or Haglund's deformity. The superficial Achilles tendon bursa lies between the tendon and the skin and can also become inflamed. A careful examination must be performed to distinguish between these lesions (Fig. 81–3).

THE FOOT

To achieve bipedal gait, the human foot has the unique ability to be both flexible and rigid. After heel strike, the foot becomes flexible to adjust to uneven surfaces and to be able to absorb several times the body's weight during running. Before pushing off, the foot converts to a rigid lever with heel inversion. Most patients with foot injuries have limitations of one of these two dual functions or difficulty converting from one to the other.

The skeleton of the foot contains 26 bones: the hindfoot is made up of the talus, calcaneus, navicular, and cuboid; the midfoot contains three cuneiforms and five metatarsals; and the forefoot contains the distal metatarsals and 14 phalanges (Fig. 81–4). The bones of the foot are bound together by ligaments, muscles, and tendons into two arches, one longitudinal and one transverse. The longitudinal arch has a medial and a lateral portion. The medial longitudinal arch is formed by

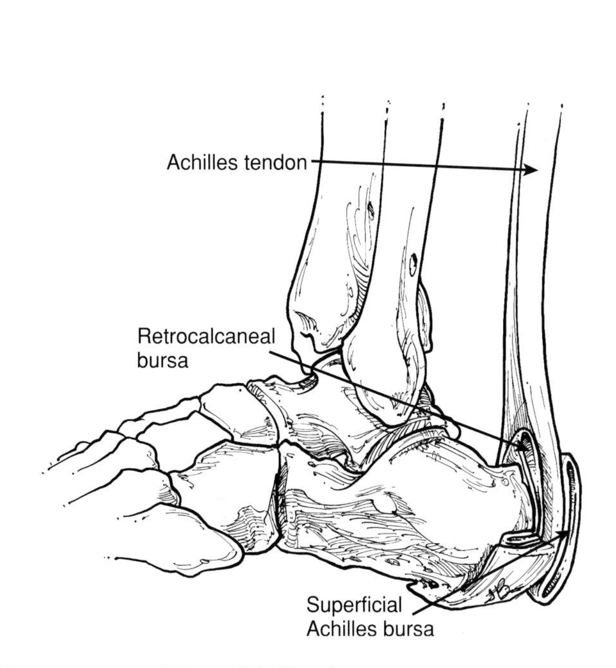

Fig. 81–3. Lateral view of hindfoot bursas.

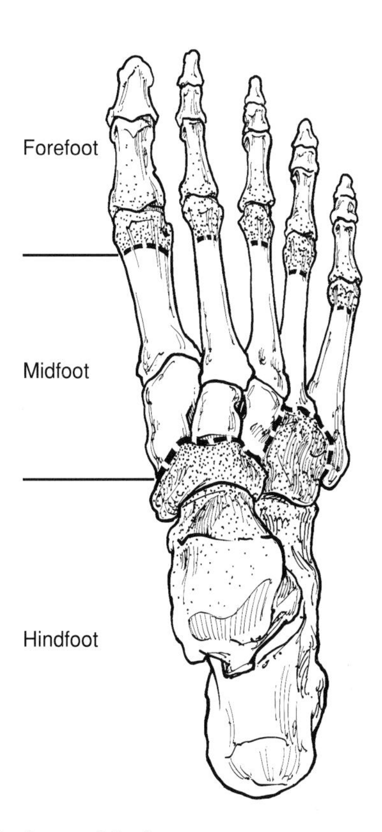

Fig. 81–4. The bones of the foot.

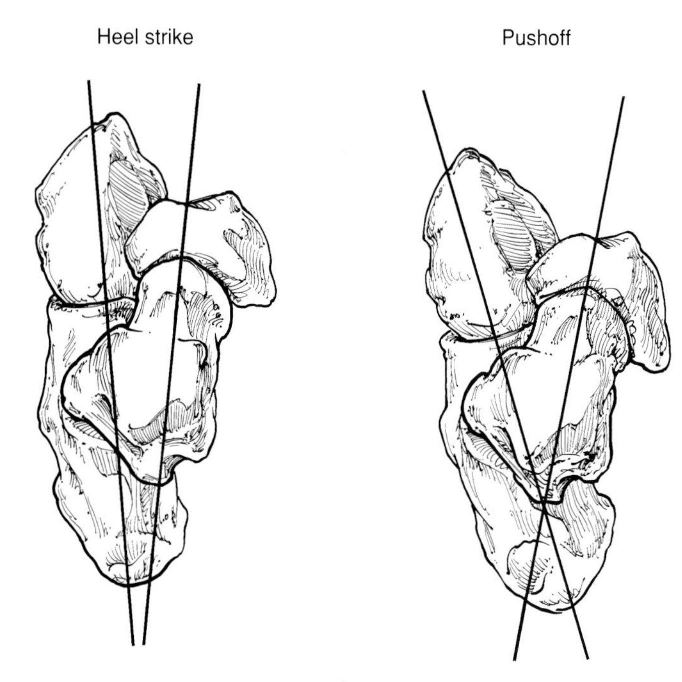

Fig. 81–5. Talonavicular and calcaneocuboid axes, which unlock the hindfoot (parallel) and lock the hindfoot (divergent).

the talus, calcaneus, navicular, cuneiform tarsals, and the first, second, and third metatarsals. The lateral longitudinal arch is formed by the calcaneus and the cuboid tarsals, plus the fourth and fifth metatarsals. The transverse arch results from the placement of the distal row of tarsals and the five metatarsals. The plantar ligaments, particularly the spring ligament, support the arches and are supplemented in this function by the posterior tibial tendon and the plantar aponeurosis.

The soft tissues, including the plantar fascia (through the windlass mechanism) and the intrinsic and extrinsic muscles, affect the skeletal orientation and function of the foot. The plantar fascia originates from the medial tubercle of the calcaneus and inserts principally into the proximal phalanx, the flexor tendon sheaths, the plantar ligaments, and the skin. The intrinsic muscles originate and insert in the foot itself and are divided into four layers on the plantar side and one major muscle on the extensor side. The extrinsic muscles to the foot arise in the calf and cross the ankle joint to insert into the foot.

Hindfoot

The hindfoot is the link between the ankle and foot, enabling the foot to convert from being flexible after heel strike to a rigid lever at push-off. At heel strike, the hindfoot is in valgus, which "unlocks" the foot by allowing the calcaneocuboid and talonavicular axes to be parallel. At push-off, the hindfoot inverts to a varus position, which locks the foot by forcing the calcaneocuboid and talonavicular axes to diverge farther (Fig. 81–5).

The talocalcaneal (subtalar) joint consists of the posterior, anterior, and middle facets. The sinus tarsi is the opening just anterolateral to the posterior facet and is the insertion for the extensor digitorum brevis muscle, the lateral talocalcaneal ligament, and the extensor retinaculum. The tarsal canal is a smaller area between the posterior and middle facets, where the interosseous ligament is located, as well as the artery of the tarsal canal to the talus.

The tarsal tunnel is on the medial side of the hindfoot (Fig. 81–6). The posterior tibial tendon, located immediately distal and posterior to the medial malleolus, has a broad insertion into the navicular, the spring ligament complex, the metatarsal bases, and, to a lesser degree, into the other tarsal bones. This broad insertion produces varying degrees of torque on the different segments of the tendon, which may permit segmental lengthening, and subsequent dysfunction, of the tendon. Blood supply to the tendon is lacking near the tip of the medial malleolus, where the tendon can rupture. Posterior to the posterior tibial tendon, in sequence, are the flexor digitorum longus tendon; the posterior tibial artery, vein, and nerve; and the flexor hallucis longus tendon. The flexor retinaculum forms the roof of the tarsal tunnel; then, distally, it divides to encompass the abductor hallucis muscle. Finally, the deep fascia of the abductor is confluent with the plantar fascia.

The first branch of the lateral plantar nerve is the nerve to the abductor digiti quinti muscle (Baxter's nerve), which is often involved in heel pain syndrome. This nerve courses beneath the deep fascia of the abductor hallucis muscle, then makes nearly a 90° turn to traverse the heel between the quadratus plantae and the flexor digitorum brevis muscles (Fig. 81–7). The flexor digitorum brevis insertion into the calcaneus forms the heel spur noted in many patients with heel pain syndrome. The plantar fascia, which originates from the medial tubercle of the calcaneus slightly superficial to the flexor digitorum brevis insertion, has medial, central, and lateral segments. These segments insert principally into the proximal phalanx, the flexor tendon sheaths, the plantar ligaments, and the skin.

The anterior tibial tendon is the major dorsiflexor of the ankle and foot, and secondarily inverts the hindfoot and midfoot. It counteracts the tendency of the per-

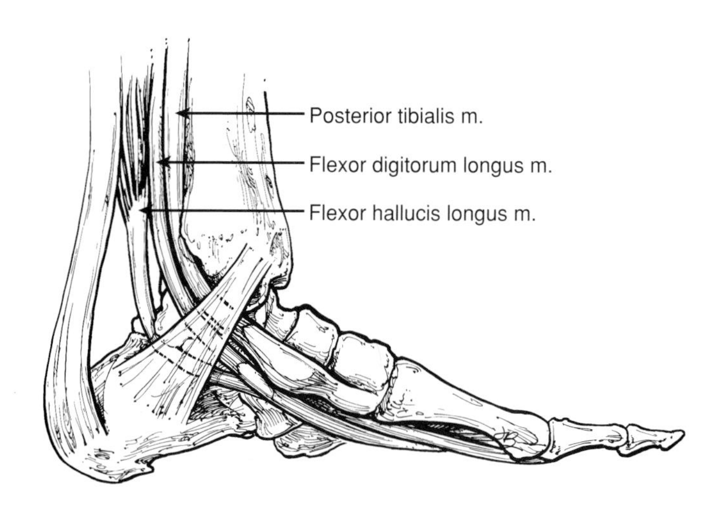

Fig. 81–6. Medial view of the tarsal tunnel.

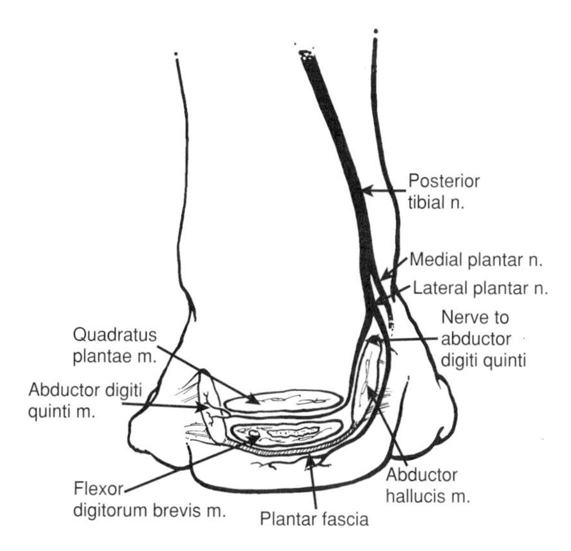

Fig. 81–7. Coronal section of the heel demonstrates the course of the lateral plantar nerve to the abductor digiti quinti, which is associated with heel pain syndromes.

oneus longus tendon to achieve plantar flexion of the first metatarsal. The anterior tibial tendon also works as a decelerator of the foot during heel strike.

On the lateral side of the heel, the peroneal tendons are located just posterolateral to the fibula. The peroneus brevis inserts into the base of the fifth metatarsal, and the peroneus longus enters the plantar side of the foot through a groove in the cuboid and inserts across the foot into the base of the first metatarsal. The peroneal tendons are major dynamic ankle stabilizers, helping to deter the common inversion ankle sprain. The peroneus brevis principally everts the ankle and subtalar joint, whereas the peroneus longus is a main plantar flexor of the first metatarsal–medial forefoot column. Secondarily, it assists in eversion of the ankle. Loss of peroneus longus function may result in eversion weakness and produce a dorsal bunion.

The sural nerve, which travels 1 cm posterior and parallel to the peroneal sheath, provides sensation to the lateral border of the foot. The deep peroneal nerve, located adjacent to the dorsalis pedis artery, runs deep to the extensor retinaculum to the first web space. The superficial peroneal nerve, located adjacent to the peroneus tertius tendon, provides sensation to the dorsum of the foot. These nerves, along with the tibial nerve, are commonly involved in ankle injuries.

Midfoot

The navicular, cuboid, three cuneiforms, and metatarsal bases make up the midfoot. Lisfranc's fracture-dislocation involves the tarsometatarsal (TMT) joints. Of particular interest is Lisfranc's ligament itself, which is located between the medial cuneiform and the second metatarsal base and stabilizes the second metatarsal.

The plantar muscles in the foot are divided into four layers. The first layer is composed of the flexor digitorum brevis, the abductor hallucis, and the abductor digiti quinti muscles. The second layer is composed of the flexor digitorum longus, the quadratus plantae, the flexor hallucis longus, and the lumbricals. Of note, the flexor digitorum longus attaches to each muscle or tendon in this layer. The flexor hallucis longus and flexor digitorum longus are attached at the knot of Henry. The quadratus plantae inserts into the flexor digitorum longus, and the lumbricals arise from the medial aspect of the flexor digitorum longus tendons. The third layer is composed of the flexor hallucis brevis, the flexor digiti minimi, and the two heads of the adductor hallucis muscle. Within the fourth layer are the three plantar and the four dorsal interossei (the central ray in the foot is the second ray; in the hand it is the third ray). These four layers are covered superficially by the plantar fascia aponeurosis.

Forefoot

The forefoot consists of the five metatarsals and three phalanges of each toe, except for the great toe, which has only two phalanges. The second metatarsal is usually the longest and has the least TMT joint motion, which predisposes it to stress fractures. The second metatarsophalangeal (MTP) joint is also at risk for synovitis and instability. The plantar plate is the major stabilizer of the MTP joint and, together with the intrinsic muscles, prevents the dorsal subluxation so often associated with hammertoe and chronic synovitis.

The first MTP joint is unique and is often involved in sports injuries when the tendinous and ligamentous balance is disturbed. The sesamoid bones develop in the flexor digitorum brevis tendons and the fibrous plantar pad. The sesamoids are normally separated by the cristae of the metatarsal head. The sesamoid complex includes multiple tendon and ligament insertions, including the lateral sesamoid ligament, the deep transverse metatarsal ligament, and the adductor hallucis tendon into the lateral sesamoid and the abductor hallucis tendon and medial sesamoid ligament into the medial sesamoid (Fig. 81–8).

The main function of the extensor digitorum longus tendon is dorsiflexion of the proximal phalanx through

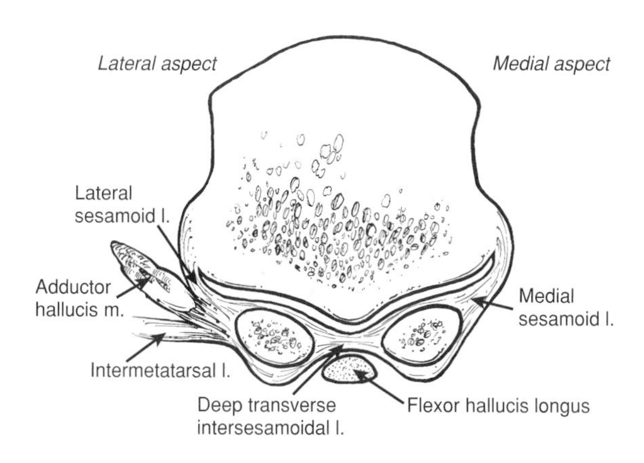

Fig. 81–8. The sesamoid complex.

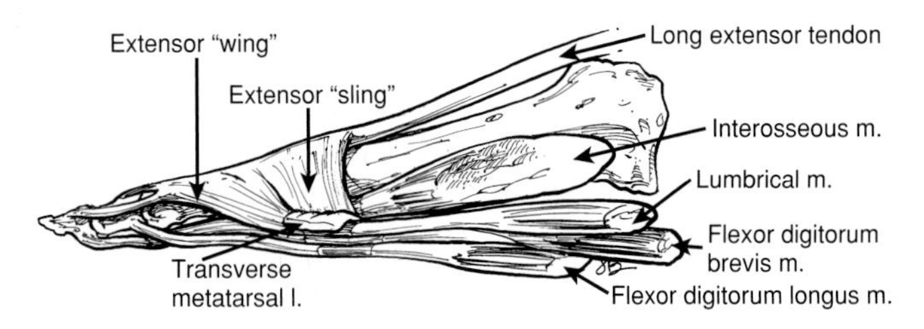

Fig. 81–9. Lateral view of the toe.

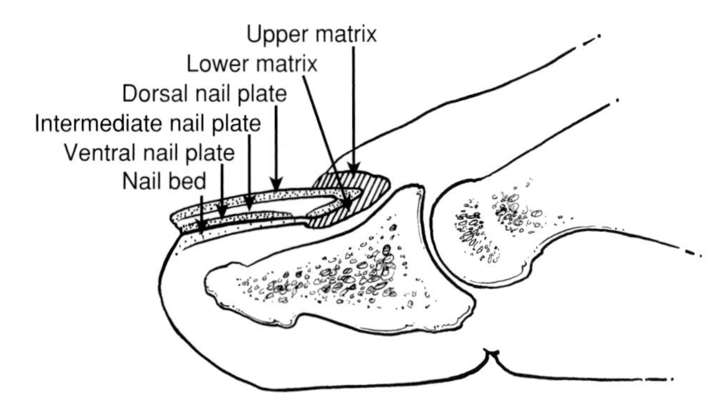

Fig. 81–10. The human nail and its matrix.

the extensor "sling" (Fig. 81–9). It also inserts into the middle phalanx as the central slip and into the distal phalanx as the lateral band. The effect on the interphalangeal joints is weak, particularly with dorsiflexion of the toe.

The extensor "wing," or "hood," is more distal and allows the intrinsic muscles (the lumbricals and interossei) to dorsiflex the proximal interphalangeal (PIP) and distal interphalangeal (DIP) joints. The interosseous muscles insert mainly into the proximal phalanx itself, which make them the chief plantar flexor of the MTP joints, but they contribute to the extensor wing as well. The interosseous tendons pass dorsal and the lumbricals pass plantar to the deep transverse metatarsal ligament. Both tendons pass plantar to the central axis of the MTP joint and dorsal to the PIP and DIP axes. Each toe except the fifth has a tendon from the extensor digitorum brevis muscle. The flexor digitorum brevis and –longus course plantar to the toe, the flexor digitorum brevis splitting and inserting into the middle phalanx, while the flexor digitorum longus inserts into the base of the distal phalanx. Pathologic claw toe or hammertoe is best understood by noting the antagonistic muscles that act on the MTP and interphalangeal joints.

The interdigital nerve passes plantar to the deep transverse metatarsal ligament, along with the lumbrical tendons. At this level, the nerve can undergo perineural fibrosis (Morton's neuroma), most commonly at the third web space and occasionally at the second space.

Finally, the anatomy of the nail should be mentioned. The nail plate rests on the nail bed and arises from the nail matrix, or root. The matrix begins at the level of the lunula and extends proximally close to the DIP joint and deep to the periosteum of the distal phalanx. This anatomy must be well understood for partial or complete matricectomy to be successful (Fig. 81–10).

REFERENCES

1. Inman, V. T.: The Joints of the Ankle. Baltimore, Williams & Wilkins, 1976.
2. Close, J. R.: Some applications of the functional anatomy of the ankle joint. J. Bone Joint Surg. *38A*:761, 1956.
3. Burman, M. S., and Lapidus, P. W.: The functional disturbances caused by the inconstant bones and sesamoids of the foot. Arch. Surg. *22*:936, 1931.
4. Storemont, D. M., Morrey, B. F., An, K. N., and Cases, J. R.: Stability of the loaded ankle: Relation between articular restraint and primary and secondary static restraints. Am. J. Sports Med. *13*:295, 1985.
5. Scheller, A. D., Kasser, J. R., and Quigley, T. B.: Tendon injuries about the ankle. Orthop. Clin. North Am. *11*:801, 1980.

82

David Tremaine

Physical Examination and Ancillary Tests of the Ankle and Foot

The clinical history and physical examination are dictated by whether the problem is acute or chronic and by the mobility of the patient. In addition, the examiner must be aware that many acute injuries are superimposed on pre-existing chronic problems, such as recurrent ankle sprains or shin splints. In most cases, pain or discomfort in the ankle and foot are caused by local afflictions, the point of pain corresponding to the site of the disorder. Using a standardized form can help you conduct a thorough and appropriate history and examination (Fig. 82–1). Findings from the history and examination help determine if radiographs and ancillary tests, such as diagnostic aspirations and injections, bone scintigraphy, computed tomography (CT), magnetic resonance imaging (MRI), and ankle arthroscopy are needed to help make the correct diagnosis.

CLINICAL HISTORY

The nature of the injury or main complaint should first be documented. Is it acute, acute-recurrent, chronic, secondary to induced or overuse trauma, or related to other joint or functional limitations? In addition to any exacerbating and mitigating factors, coexisting medical conditions (e.g., diabetes, gout, neurologic disorders) or physical problems (e.g., hip deformity, myelodysplasia, cerebral palsy), and other relevant personal or family history should be noted. Any treatment provided before the current examination should also be noted.

Mechanism of Injury

If there was trauma to the ankle or foot, the physician should note what type of sporting activity was involved and try to determine the mechanics of the injury and its effect on the extremity. Too often, the mechanism of injury is misinterpreted and its magnitude not properly appreciated. The clinical appearance of the ankle or foot right after the injury, or even several days later, may be misleading and may not accurately represent the degree of trauma. During this period, even radiographs may not sufficiently demonstrate the true nature of the injury. Asking the patient to act out the injury can provide a better medical description and understanding. Specifically, determining the position of the foot at the time of injury, the direction of any impacting force, and the amount of angulation of the injured part can clarify the severity of the injury.

Proper Descriptive Terms

By convention, we describe the position of the distal injured part in relation to the proximal part. For example, a *plantar flexion, inversion ankle injury* implies that the foot-talus complex was plantar flexed and inverted relative to the tibia. It is important to understand that the functional motions of the foot are multiplanar. Descriptions of single-plane and three-plane motions, for examination purposes, are provided in Table 82–1. Using these terms clarifies communication with orthopedists, neurologists, radiologists, and other specialists who might have to be consulted.

Pain and Swelling

After trauma, pain and swelling are important features of the history. Pain is recorded for severity (mild to severe), quality (burning versus aching), onset (acute versus delayed), and localization, and swelling, for dif-

HUGHSTON ORTHOPAEDIC CLINIC, P.C.
COLUMBUS, GEORGIA

FOOT AND ANKLE SHEET

Patient Name ________________________ Date ______________

Chart No. ______________ Age ______________ Sex ______________

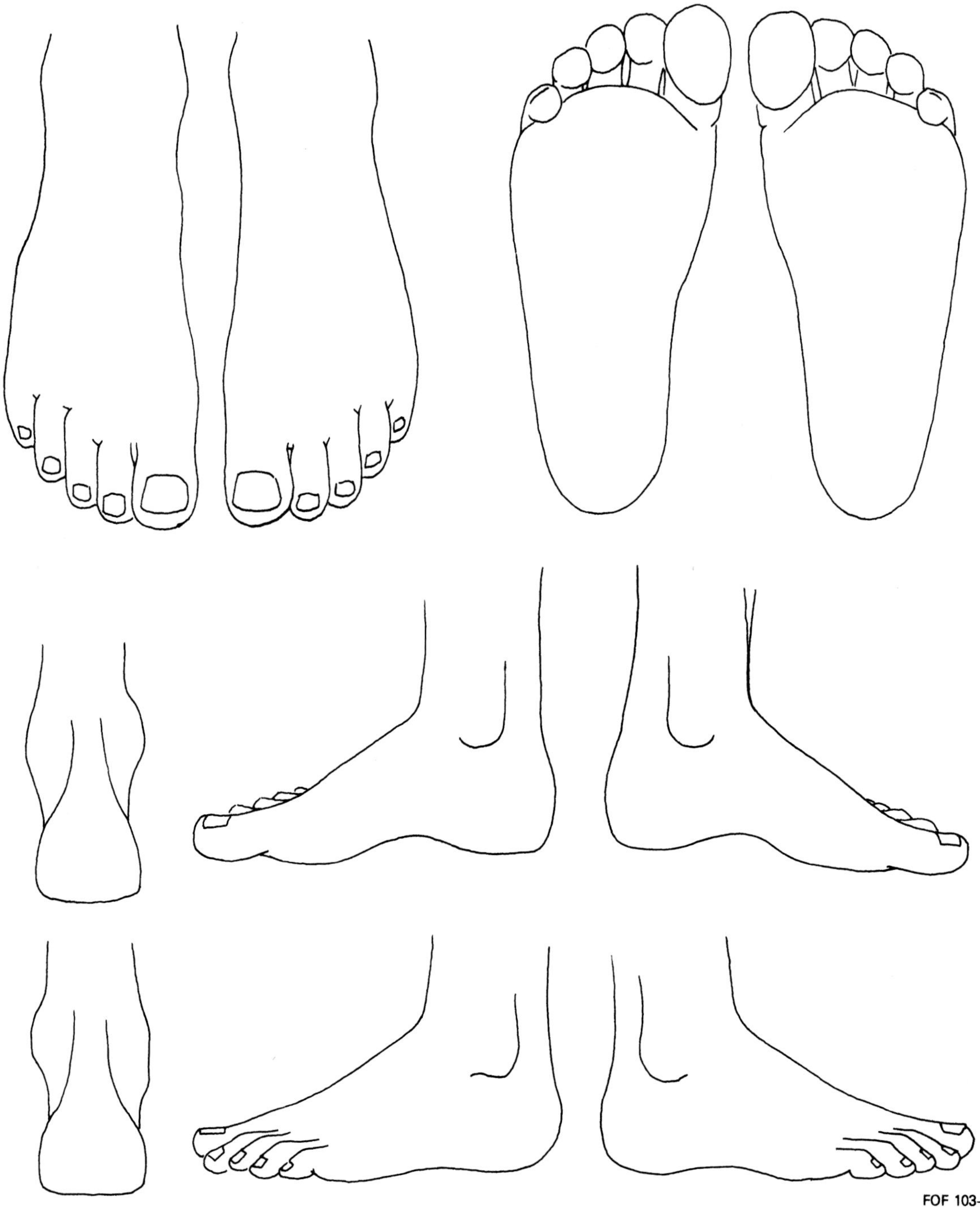

FOF 103-484

RIGHT LEFT

HISTORY:

WHAT:

HOW:

WHEN:

WHERE:

____

____

PHYSICAL EXAM: ANKLE

	ECCHYMOSIS	TENDERNESS	SWELLING
Medial	______	______	______
Lateral	______	______	______
Anterior	______	______	______
Posterior	______	______	______

Heelcord______ INSTABILITY:

Ant. Tib______ Drawer______

Post. Tib______ Inversion______

Peroneals______

FOOT

Planus______ Tenderness______

Cavus______ Deformity______

Rigidus______

NEUROVASCULAR X-RAY

Dorsalis Pedis______ Fracture______

Posterior Tib.______ Deformity______

Sensation______ Degenerative______

DIAGNOSIS

____

Fig. 82–1. Standardized form for recording findings of the history and physical examination of the ankle and foot.

fused or localized quality and for how soon after the injury it developed.

Chronic, Overstress, or Recurrent Injuries

When an athlete suffers chronic, overstress, or recurrent injury, the history should include the patient's sports activity and the specific sport movement that causes or aggravates the problem. Factors such as changes in training technique, improperly fitting or worn equipment, and environmental conditions need to be considered. Assistance from the coach or trainer is frequently needed to obtain an accurate history in this regard.

Table 82–1. Descriptive Terms for Documenting Examination of the Ankle and Foot

Single-Plane Motions
Abduction: Lateral movement of the forefoot on the midfoot
Adduction: Medial movement of the forefoot in relation to the midfoot
Varus (inversion): Inward tilt of the foot
Valgus (eversion): Outward tilt of the foot
Dorsiflexion of the foot: Backward bending of the foot at the ankle
Dorsiflexion of the toes: Bending of the toes toward the sole of the foot
Plantar flexion of the foot: extension of the foot so that the forefoot is depressed with respect to the position of the ankle
(N.B.: Dorsiflexion and plantar flexion of the ankle joint or foot are described in relation to more proximal joints.)
Equinus: Plantar flexion of the foot in relation to the tibia
Cavus: Plantar flexion of the forefoot in relation to the hindfoot
Internal (or *external*) *rotation:* Rotation of the distal segment relative to the proximal segment of the joint being described
Three-Plane Motions
Pronation of the foot: The combination of dorsiflexion, eversion, and abduction
Supination of the foot: The combination of plantar flexion, inversion, and adduction

PHYSICAL EXAMINATION

Physical examination of the ankle and foot proceeds systematically, to optimize diagnosis and minimize additional trauma to the extremity. During the examination, both of the patient's lower extremities should be completely exposed, so that the affected ankle and foot can be compared with the contralateral limb. The examiner begins by carefully observing the patient's gait, noting if and how it is affected. (In a busy practice, this part of the examination is frequently omitted.) After gait analysis, the ankle and foot should be carefully inspected with the patient in the standing position. After inspection, each structure of the ankle and foot should be palpated for tenderness. Next, the neurovascular status of the ankle and foot should be assessed. Only after all of these have been accomplished are range of motion and stability tests conducted. Otherwise, further damage can be inflicted on an already injured ankle or foot. Stress testing is often delayed until appropriate radiographs are obtained to rule out fractures or dislocations, so that further disruption or displacement does not occur.

Gait Analysis

Many ankle and foot problems become noticeable or are accentuated by faulty, interrupted body mechanics during ambulation. Walking is a complex, largely automatic function controlled by the neuromuscular system, which maintains balance and produces the motor signals that sequence muscle firing and limb positioning in space. Both functions can be affected by injuries. As the patient walks, the examiner should watch from the side and from the front, paying close attention to hip motion, knee motion, and ankle and foot motion in each phase of gait (heel strike, midstance, toe-off, and swing). The movement from one right-heel contact with the floor to the next right-heel contact constitutes a complete gait cycle. Factors in gait analysis are balance, step length, and cadence, and the examiner should look in particular for patellar squinting, abnormal thrust or timing, proper heel eversion shortly after heel strike, and heel and midfoot inversion from midstance through push-off.

Inspection

From the side, a normal foot forms a right angle with the leg. Talipes equinus, a fixed flexion deformity, causes the patient to stand with the heel raised off the ground. Talipes calcaneus, on the other hand, is a fixed dorsiflexion deformity that prevents the patient from placing the forefoot on the ground, resulting in most of the body's weight being placed on the heel. It is important also to note any abnormalities of the foot's longitudinal arch. In pes planus, the arch is flattened and frequently heel valgus is associated. In contrast, cavus foot has a high arch. Viewing the foot from behind, the examiner notes deformity or malposition of the heel. In talipes valgus the foot is abducted, or everted. In talipes varus, the foot is adducted, or inverted.

Deformities of the lesser toes may be congenital or acquired. Causes of acquired disorders include improperly fitted shoes, trauma, and neuromuscular diseases. The most common disorders of the lesser toes are hammer toes and claw toes. In hammer toe, the metatarsophalangeal (MTP) joint is extended, the proximal interphalangeal (PIP) joint is flexed, and the distal interphalangeal (DIP) joint is extended. In claw toe, the PIP and DIP joints are flexed, causing excessive extension of the MP joint and giving the toe its characteristic clawed appearance. Often, all the lessor toes are involved.

The presence of calluses and their anatomic sites should also be noted. Calluses can indicate areas of excessive weight-bearing pressure, such as the bottom of the forefoot in talipes equinus or the heel in talipes calcaneus. The abnormal toe posture in hammer toe causes increased pressure in the shoe on both the top and base of the toe, resulting in painful calluses. The patient with claw toe can experience painful calluses at the pressure points of each affected toe. The location of calluses can also provide valuable information about the mechanics of the patient's foot. Lateral midfoot and significant lateral heel calluses indicate excessive supination, whereas medial forefoot calluses indicate excessive pronation. Calluses localized on specific metatarsals, such as a second or third metatarsal head, suggest insufficiency of the great toe with forefoot supination problems. A first ray callus denotes plantar flexion of the first ray. Diffuse metatarsal calluses indicate global cavus foot problems or equinus of the ankle-hindfoot complex.

An exostosis, a bony prominence of the foot, can occur as a bunion in the area of the first metatarsal head. An exostosis may also be found at the joint of the first metatarsal and cuneiform or at the posterolateral aspect of the calcaneus. Likewise, a bunionette can occur on the lateral aspect of the fifth metatarsal. All of these conditions can result in pain due to pressure from the patient's shoe.

After trauma, the ankle and foot should be inspected for ecchymosis and swelling, which if present should be carefully localized (i.e., medial or lateral ankle, hindfoot, midfoot, or forefoot) to aid in the diagnosis. For example, ecchymosis on the medial side of the heel after an ankle sprain indicates a greater degree of injury, such as disruption of additional subtalar joint ligaments or osteochondral fractures. The progression of swelling and the degree of associated skin tenseness can be warnings of compartment syndrome. This problem has been emphasized in leg injuries, but it can be equally serious in the foot.

Palpation

After inspection, the examiner should systematically palpate each structure of the ankle and foot (i.e., ankle ligaments, subtalar joints, Achilles tendon, plantar fascia, base of the metatarsal joints) for tenderness, beginning away from the suspected site of injury or abnormality and leaving the most painful area for last. It is important to palpate both proximal and distal to the suspected site of injury. Point tenderness helps to localize the injury and assess its extent. Crepitation with palpation suggests tendinitis or fracture.

Single fingertip pressure should be applied to each area with the fingertip placed directly on the localized anatomic point, without irritating adjacent tissues. Before the examiner removes the pressure, the patient should have adequate time to respond at each point. Inadequate response time will produce inaccurate examination findings. Strain or rupture of the plantar fascia can be assessed by palpating the fascia's insertion into the medial tuberosity of the os calcis while the toes are passively dorsiflexed. In patients with plantar fasciitis, the Achilles tendon is usually tight, and tenderness can often be elicited on the inner portion of the foot and just in front of the heel.

Neurovascular Testing

To evaluate the vascular status, the dorsalis pedis and posterior tibial pulses are palpated and capillary circulation is assessed. With impending compartment syndrome, the pulses are frequently bounding, secondary to the shunting of the blood through the major vessels, away from the microcirculation.

Nerve testing should include the sensory, motor, and autonomic systems. It is important to conduct a technically correct sensory examination, since gross pressure will be felt even when there is complete laceration of that nerve. Usually, careful light touch or safety pin–point identification applied to relevant dermatomes is adequate. Both extremities should be assessed sequentially, and the patient should be able to feel the appropriate sensation (i.e., a safety pin prick should feel like a pin prick). The patient is also asked if the sensation is the same or different in the two extremities.

Tinel's sign is a cutaneous tingling produced by pressing on or tapping the nerve trunk that has been damaged or is healing following trauma. Testing is best performed by applying percussion over the appropriate sensory nerves. Tinel's sign may be the only positive diagnostic test of a neuroma or tunnel syndrome, which can occur after even minor soft tissue injuries. Tarsal or anterior tibial tunnel syndrome is frequently associated with biomechanical excesses in the foot—forefoot varus with compensatory hindfoot pronation or hindfoot varus with compensatory midfoot or forefoot pronation, among others. Both put abnormal tension on the posterior tibial nerve or its branches. Though nerve conduction studies and electromyographic findings are helpful, they are often nonspecific or negative.

The autonomic nervous system should also be examined. Reflex sympathetic dystrophy syndrome or lesser causalgia symptoms can occur after ankle and foot injuries and are not always related to significant trauma. They can occur after fracture-dislocations or mild ankle sprains. They also are not age related; the problems have been noted in teenaged, middle-aged, and elderly athletes. Signs such as mottling of the ankle or foot, diffuse swelling, anhidrosis, nondermatomal sensory changes, stiffness of multiple joints, and pain symptoms out of proportion to the diagnosed injury should alert the examiner to the possibility of these complications.

Range of Motion Testing

The active range of motion of the ankle and foot should be compared with that of the opposite extremity. The ankle joint is capable of dorsiflexion and plantar flexion. The normal range of dorsiflexion is 10° to 20° past a right angle with the leg; that of plantar flexion is 30° to 40° past neutral.

With the foot held in the subtalar neutral position, the amount of tibial varus of the leg, the amount of subtalar varus in relation to the leg, and the forefoot axis in relation to the hindfoot axis are noted. Single-plane motion of the foot is demonstrated by inversion and eversion of the subtalar joint, dorsiflexion and plantar flexion of the ankle, abduction and adduction of the forefoot, and internal and external rotation of the foot.

Movement at the subtalar joint is evaluated passively by holding the patient's lower leg with one hand and rotating the heel and foot into inversion and eversion with the other hand (Fig. 82–2). Subtalar joint motion characteristically has two thirds more inversion than eversion. Motion at the midtarsal joint is also demonstrated passively by steadying the patient's heel with one hand and rotating the forefoot with the other. A decrease in the range of motion may be due to a disorder such as tarsal coalition. Flexibility of the first metatarsal is tested.

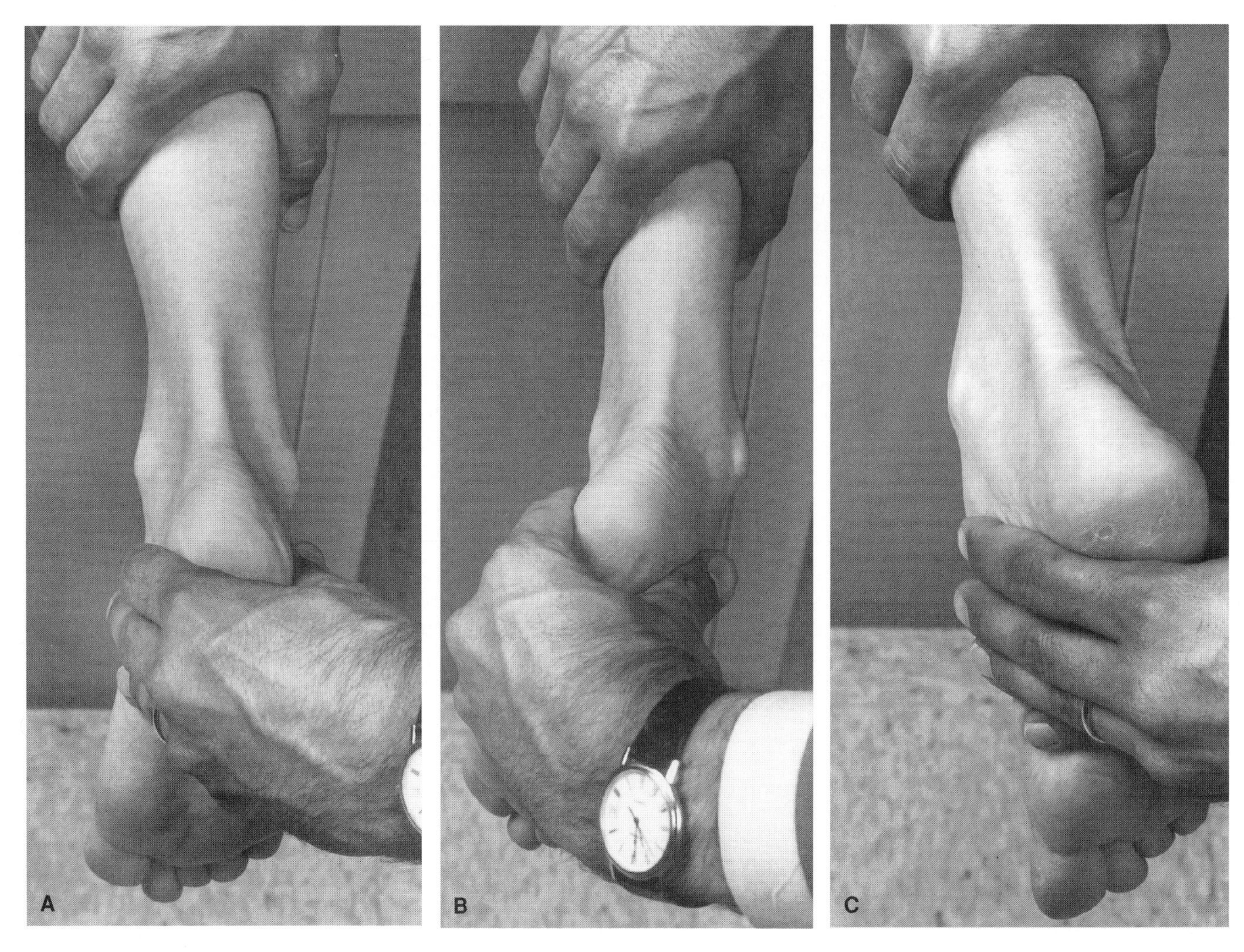

Fig. 82–2. **Subtalar joint movement is evaluated by passively holding the patient's lower leg with one hand. Beginning in the neutral position *(A)*, the examiner rotates the heel and foot into inversion *(B)* and eversion *(C)* with the other hand.**

Testing Ankle Ligament Stability

The anterior ankle drawer stress test is performed to evaluate the integrity of the anterior talofibular ligament. With the patient's ankle in slight plantar flexion, the examiner grasps the posterior aspect of the calcaneus with one hand and applies pressure superiorly against the calcaneus to decrease the tension on the ankle joint. Then, placing the other hand around the lower tibia to stabilize it, the examiner attempts to bring the calcaneus and talus forward on the tibia (Fig. 82–3). If excursion is excessive compared with that of the unaffected ankle, the anterior talofibular ligament may be injured.

The inversion stress test (or talar tilt test) assesses the integrity of the calcaneofibular and anterior talofibular ligamentous portions of the lateral ligaments. It is performed with the ankle in neutral position or only slight plantar flexion. In plantar flexion, the anterior talofibular ligament is taut and the calcaneofibular ligament is more relaxed. This helps to distinguish injuries to the two ligaments. By stabilizing the tibia with one hand and applying varus stress at the level of the calcaneocuboid joint with the other hand, the examiner tilts the talus into inversion (Fig. 82–4). The movement produces a "soft" end point often associated with pain when the patient has sustained a severe lateral ligament injury. The eversion stress test evaluates the deltoid ligament by moving the calcaneus and talus into eversion (Fig. 82–5).

Next, side-to-side motion of the talus and calcaneus is examined as a unit, to assess the integrity of the tibiofibular ligament. If the mortise of the ankle joint is widened, as in syndesmosis injuries, the talus can be moved sideways, producing a "thud" as it hits the fibula (thus the name, *clunk test*).

Testing Tendons

To test the peroneus longus tendon, the examiner attempts to dorsiflex the first metatarsal while the patient everts the foot. Resistance indicates an intact or functioning tendon. The recently described *painful os peroneum*

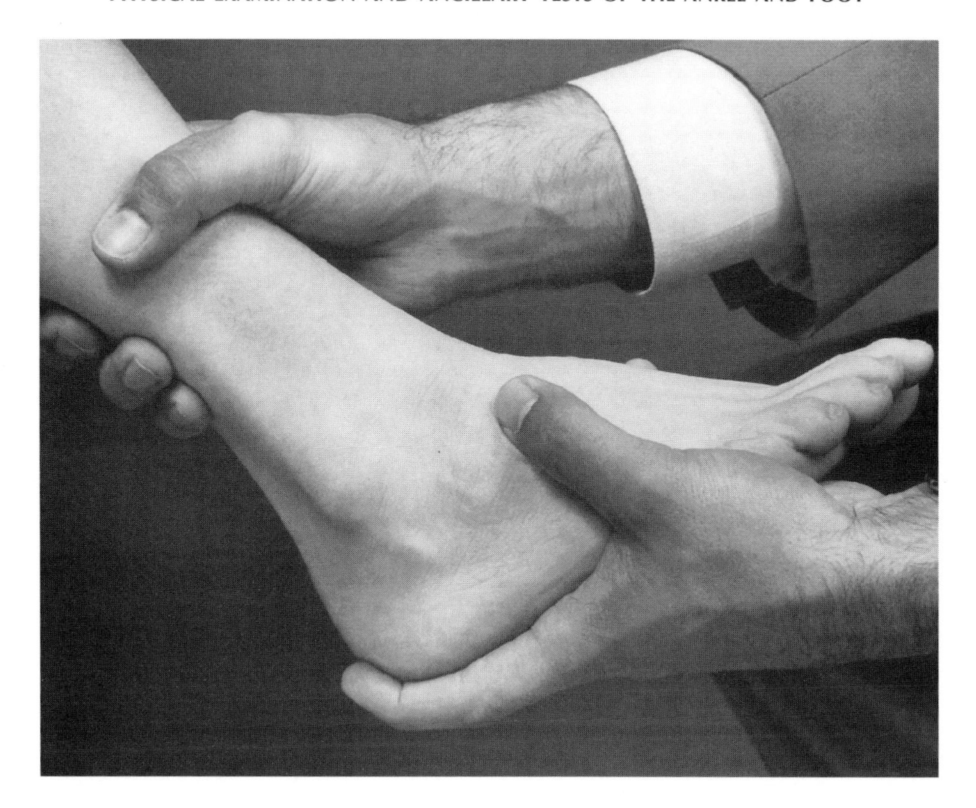

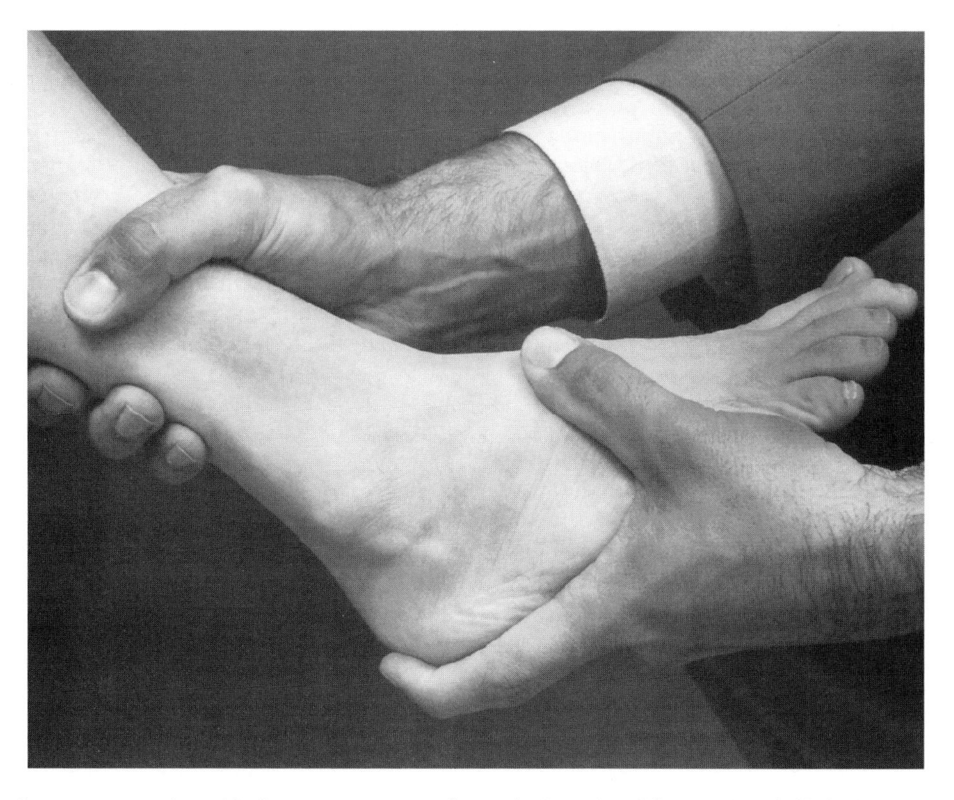

Fig. 82–3. Anterior ankle drawer stress test evaluates the integrity of the anterior talofibular ligament.

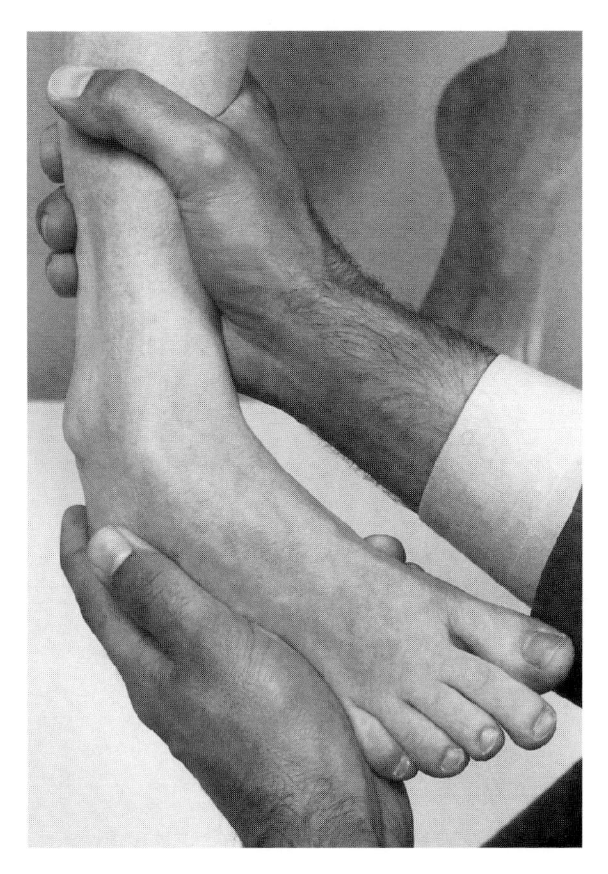

Fig. 82–4. Inversion stress test (or talar tilt test) assesses the integrity of the calcaneofibular and anterior talofibular ligaments.

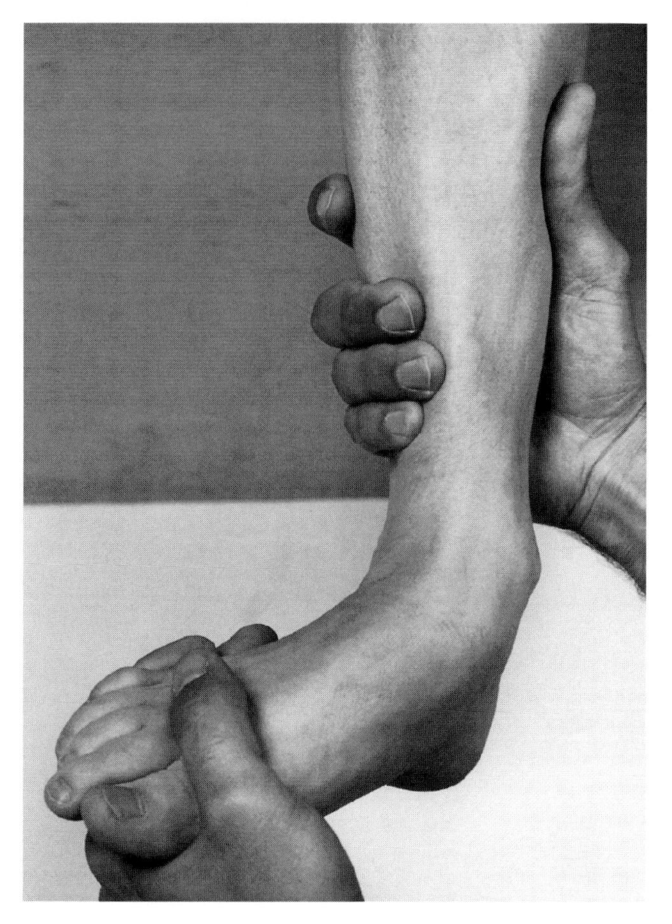

Fig. 82–5. Eversion stress test evaluates the deltoid ligament.

syndrome (POPS) is associated with degenerative changes or rupture of the peroneus longus tendon, or with fracture or degenerative changes of the os peroneum. This injury or condition is identified by pain on palpation of the tendon at the calcaneocuboid tunnel and the area just proximal to it. Subluxating peroneal tendons, associated with some ankle sprains, are believed to be secondary to a deficient, lax, or ruptured superior peroneal retinacular ligament. This problem can be identified by palpating the peroneal tendons at the fibular groove with the patient's foot in dorsiflexion and eversion.

Resisted inversion of the foot, starting with the foot in the everted position, tests the strength of the posterior tibial muscle-tendon unit. The long flexors lie directly behind the posterior tibial tendon. To distinguish joint injuries from tendon injuries, the joint should be tested with the tendon in the maximum relaxed position. For the long flexors, this is done with the toes and midfoot in maximal plantar flexion. If pain occurs with ankle motion and is not significantly increased by positioning the tendons on stretch (i.e., by dorsiflexion of the great toe or lessor toes), then the joint, and not the tendon, is affected.

Testing the Achilles Tendon

Flexibility of the Achilles tendon is determined by dorsiflexing the patient's foot with the midtarsal joints locked in inversion. This is done with the knee extended to evaluate the gastrocnemius muscle and with the knee flexed to evaluate the soleus muscle (Fig. 82–6). One-legged toe rises help detect subtle weakness in the posterior calf muscles. Having the patient attempt 10 toe rises lends more objectivity to this test. In Thompson's test, commonly used to evaluate Achilles tendon rupture, the patient is placed prone and the calf is squeezed from the medial to the lateral aspect while the examiner looks for plantar flexion. If there is no flexion or only a trace, tendon rupture must be suspected. It is very important not to misdiagnose Achilles tendon rupture as an ankle sprain.

RADIOGRAPHIC EVALUATION

Ankle and foot radiographs are a necessary part of most postinjury evaluations and can further aid in the diagnosis. The localizing symptoms and clinical findings determine which views to order. Similar views of the unaffected ankle or foot may be taken for comparison.

Routine Radiographs of the Ankle

If the patient has sustained an ankle injury, routine anteroposterior (AP), lateral, and mortise views may be needed to rule out coexisting fractures. Many of the

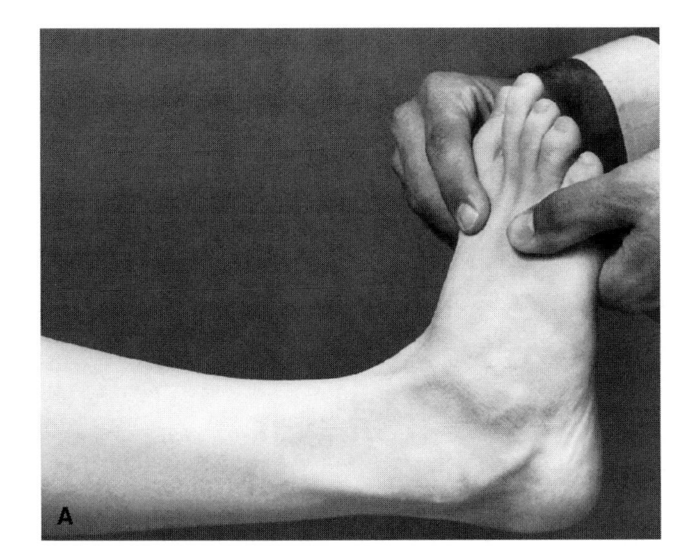

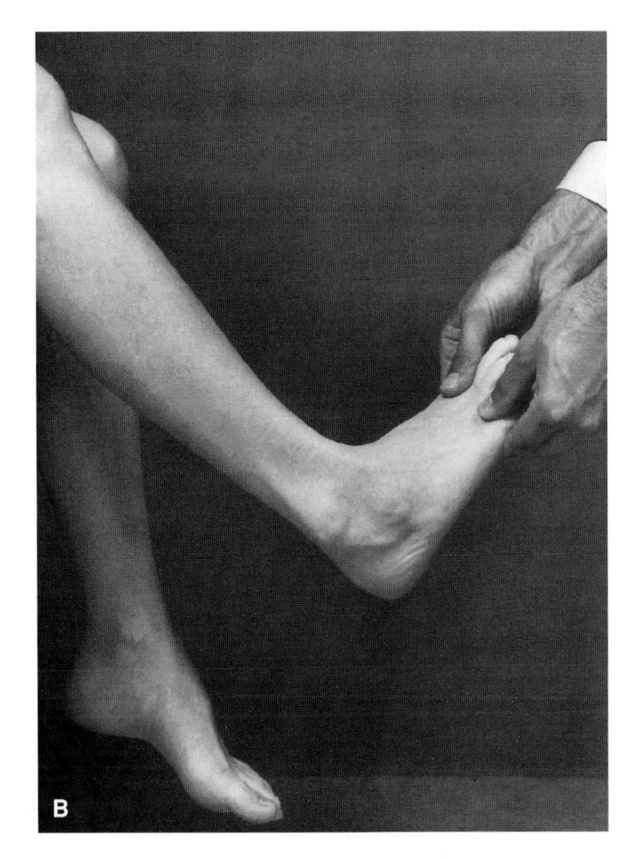

Fig. 82–6. The Achilles tendon is tested by *(A)* dorsiflexing the foot with the midtarsal joints locked in inversion. The gastrocnemius muscle is tested with the knee extended. *(B)* The soleus muscle is tested with the knee flexed.

residual problems associated with ankle sprains are secondary to fractures of the osteochondral talus, the anterior process of the calcaneus, or the lateral process of the talus, and, on occasion, to foot fractures.

Stress Radiographs of the Ankle

Stress radiographs can be helpful in further assessing ankle stability. Both AP and varus stress radiographs should be obtained. The inversion stress test (talar tilt) or the anterior drawer test is performed while the radiograph is being taken. Particular attention should be paid to the subtalar joint, which is often seen on the AP stress view and the lateral view. Brodén's views are particularly helpful for evaluating the posterior subtalar joint.

Routine Radiographs of the Foot

Standard views of the foot are the AP, lateral, and medial oblique views. Occasionally, an ankle and foot series may be needed to properly assess the injured structures. The reverse-foot oblique view is helpful for detecting medial column and medial foot injuries and first metatarsal–medial sesamoid problems. To properly evaluate the MTP joint of the great toe, a sesamoid view should be taken to rule out fracture, dislocation, and osteonecrosis.

Stress Radiographs of the Foot

Stress radiographs of the foot—primarily abduction and pronation—help detect Lisfranc's dislocation that has spontaneously reduced, whereas routine foot radiographs may be normal. When the forefoot is stressed, the foot dislocates completely. Subtle findings that may be observed include mild compression of the cuboid, a small avulsion off the medial base of the first metatarsal, or a fracture at the base of the second metatarsal or medial cuneiform by Lisfranc's ligament. Small disruptions in the lines between the second metatarsal and the medial cortex of the middle cuneiform on the AP view and interruption of the line of the fourth metatarsal in line with the medial cuboid on the oblique view also suggest a significant Lisfranc's injury.

DIAGNOSTIC ASPIRATION AND INJECTION

If following injury an osteochondral fracture is suspected that cannot be demonstrated on radiographs, aspiration of effusion from the injured site may be necessary. Fat globules in the aspirated fluid or blood indicate communication with the intramedullary canal, usually owing to an osteochondral fracture. Aspiration of a tense effusion can also significantly relieve pain symptoms and enhance rehabilitation.

Local injections of xylocaine into the subtalar joint, second MTP joint, or between the third and fourth metatarsals to relieve symptoms of Morton's neuroma are also helpful diagnostically. The examiner should carefully evaluate the degree of pain relief immediately after the injection and record these findings.

ANCILLARY IMAGING TESTS

In most cases, an accurate history, thorough physical examination, and appropriate radiographs are sufficient to correctly diagnose ankle and foot problems; however, when the diagnosis is difficult or the injury extremely severe, more sophisticated ancillary imaging modalities may be needed. These tests are costly and time consuming, and before ordering them the physician should ask an important question: "Will the information I obtain alter my planned course of treatment?" Ankle arthroscopy is now being performed more often. Other joints in the foot are also being examined by arthroscope, but experience is limited to date.

Bone Scan

A bone scan is particularly helpful for nondescript ankle or foot pain. Any disorder or condition that results in active bone turnover will be demonstrated. Stress fractures, osteochondral fractures, osteomyelitis, active arthritis, and bone tumors can be localized, but specificity is poor. In addition, in many athletes, several areas of increased bone uptake are noted. These patients have often experienced a number of previous episodes of stress reactions that were never documented, and they can confound the diagnosis. An extremely valuable use of bone scans is evaluating for reflex sympathetic dystrophy. This difficult diagnosis can be made when the appropriate clinical symptoms are coupled with diffuse bone uptake.

Computed Tomography

For acute trauma, CT may augment plain radiography and further delineate small or minimally displaced fractures, entrapped tendons, or subtle subluxations. CT is also helpful in grading osteochondral fractures and congenital tarsal coalitions, which are frequently associated with recurrent ankle sprains. CT also demonstrates in greater detail the extent of arthritis and Lisfranc's injuries and talocalcaneal disorders when plain radiographs are not adequate. Single-photon emission CT (SPECT) allows even more accurate localization of subtle disorders.

Magnetic Resonance Imaging

MRI is very sensitive for detecting stress fractures, bone contusions, and hyperemic degeneration. It is the most sensitive imaging modality for assessing osteonecrosis, osteochondritis dissecans, and subchondral fractures. MRI is a valuable tool for evaluating ligaments, tendons, and soft tissue injuries of the ankle and foot. The deltoid, spring, and fibular ligaments are well visualized, and ankle tendon evaluation is more accurate with MRI than with CT.

With MRI it is possible to distinguish tendinitis from tenosynovitis, peritendinitis, or synovial proliferation and scarring (i.e., stenosing tenosynovitis), though mild forms of these lesions can be totally missed by MRI. In addition, it is difficult to differentiate tendinitis from early frank tendon rupture. However, the extent of chronic tendinitis, particularly in the Achilles tendon, can be evaluated by MRI. Similarly, it is useful in diagnosing sesamoid fractures or distinguishing osteonecrosis from flexor hallucis longus tendinitis. Diagnosis of a tarsal coalition is facilitated when the coalition is fibrous. Foreign bodies (e.g., thorns, wood chips) that are not identifiable on routine radiographs can be seen with MRI. At present, MRI has not been useful for evaluating plantar fasciitis.

83

Peter M. Cimino and James L. Beskin

Soft Tissue and Overuse Injuries in the Lower Leg

Muscle Strains, Shin Splints, Chronic Exertional Compartment Syndromes, and Nerve Entrapment Syndromes

Peter M. Cimino

MUSCLE STRAINS

Muscle strains are partial disruptions of the muscle-tendon unit that result from powerful eccentric contractions. Eccentric muscle contractions are those in which the muscle lengthens as it creates tension. For example, eccentric action takes place during a biceps curl exercise, when the lifter lowers the weight as the arm extends. These actions occur when an athlete attempts to decelerate a limb, as in the example, or the total body. Disruption, which usually occurs at the musculotendinous junction, is followed by an intense inflammatory reaction and subsequent fibrosis.[1]

Classifications

First Degree. Tear of only a few muscle or tendon fibers results in mild swelling, pain, and disability. The patient is still able to produce a strong but painful muscle contraction.

Second Degree. A moderate number of muscle or tendon fibers are disrupted, but the muscle-tendon unit remains intact. The patient experiences a moderate amount of pain, swelling, and disability and is able to produce only a weak and painful attempt at muscle contraction.

Third Degree. Complete rupture of the muscle-tendon unit is characterized by the patient's extremely weak attempt at muscle contraction.

Treatment

Treatment of muscle strains consists of early application of ice, along with elevation of the affected extremity. Gradual range of motion exercises are initiated shortly after icing down the injured extremity. Oral nonsteroidal anti-inflammatory medications may relieve pain. Physical therapy modalities, including ultrasound, anaphoresis, and electrical muscle stimulation, are commonly employed. The patient may return to athletic activity after pain and swelling have subsided and muscle strength and function are sufficient to tolerate the planned athletic endeavors.

SHIN SPLINTS

Exercise-induced pain in the lower leg is common in sports. The several names for pain in the medial part of the tibia include *medial tibial syndrome, medial tibial stress syndrome, tibial periostitis,* and *shin splints.* Athletes often experience pain in this area, especially if they have been running for some time and make a change in running surface, running technique, or shoe type, among other factors.

The cause of the pain is still unknown. It may be the result of an inflamed periosteum or an avulsion of the periosteum of the posteromedial distal tibia. Pain and tenderness are localized to the area immediately posterior to the tibial ridge, extending 6 to 10 cm (Fig. 83–1). An anatomic variation, such as pes cavus or overpronation, is commonly associated with shin splints.

Radiographs should be obtained to rule out a stress fracture. In chronic cases of shin splints, there may be mild thickening or undulation of the posterior distal tibia. A bone scan is usually normal or shows mild, diffuse uptake along the painful area.

Initial treatment for shin splints consists of a period of rest whose duration depends on the individual's degree of pain. Anti-inflammatory medications are of questionable benefit. Stretching and careful warm-up before athletic activity should be stressed. Any anatomic variation should be corrected with a semirigid foot orthosis. Running athletes should wear a proper running shoe that provides both shock absorption and a firm heel contour.

CHRONIC EXERTIONAL COMPARTMENT SYNDROMES

Compartment syndrome is a condition in which increased tissue pressure within a limited space compromises circulation and function of the contents of that space. Traditionally, we think of the leg as having four compartments (i.e., anterior, lateral, superficial posterior, and posterior), which are bounded by bone and thick fascial covering. During strenuous exercise, there is an increase in muscle volume and pressure inside these fascial compartments because of their limited ability to expand.[2] In some cases, the rise in pressure may compromise local blood flow to the muscle belly, resulting in ischemic pain.

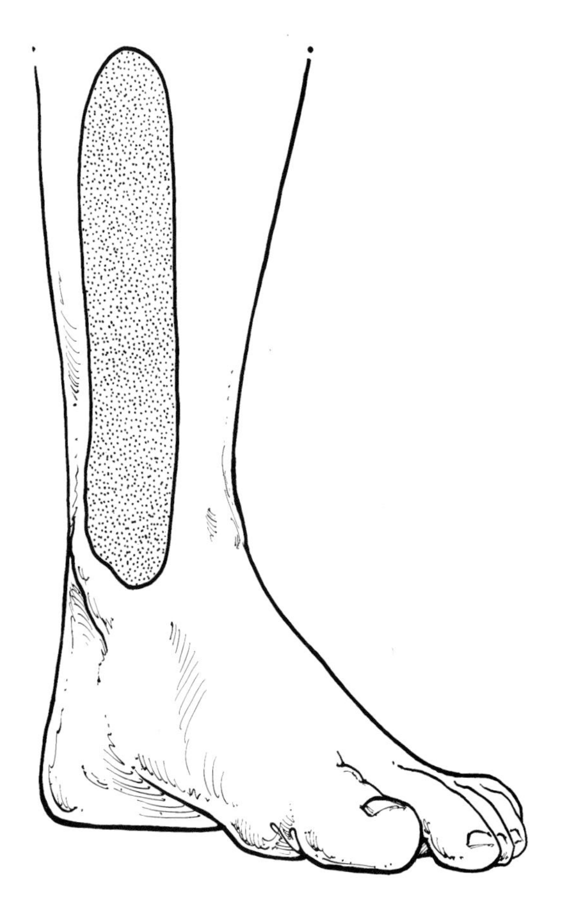

Fig. 83–1. Area of involvement in shin splints.

Chronic exertional compartment syndrome is a subtle, reversible condition seen in athletes and has a different clinical presentation than acute compartment syndrome. The latter, which generally occurs after a traumatic accident or a surgical procedure when a dressing or splint is too tight, is an emergency that requires immediate surgical intervention.

History

Chronic compartment syndrome usually involves the anterior or posterior compartment, or both. Lateral compartment syndrome is extremely rare. Leg pain occurs after the athlete has been exercising (usually running) for some time, and the onset is often predictable because it starts about the same time during the exercise. The pain is described as a dull ache that increases during exercise to the point where activity has to be stopped.

The pain is localized to the involved muscles of the entire compartment. Athletes with anterior compartment syndrome complain of diffuse pain centered over the anterior compartment, and may, at the onset of the pain, experience dysesthesia on the dorsum of the foot. Athletes with posterior compartment syndrome complain of pain along the posteromedial border of the distal two thirds of the tibia, radiating toward the ankle and medial arch of the foot, with possible concomitant dysesthesia along the medial border of the foot.

Between 75 and 90% of patients have bilateral symptoms, although, oftentimes, symptoms are worse in one leg.[2] Some patients complain of numbness, tingling, or weakness in the leg or foot. Rest always alleviates the pain, but it takes some time for relief to occur, especially as the syndrome becomes more severe. A prolonged period of rest does not relieve the problem; the symptoms usually recur after the athlete returns to the sport activity.

Physical Examination

Physical examination usually does not reveal any abnormalities. Tenderness and increased tension in the involved compartment may be palpated if the patient has been exercising prior to the examination. Passive stretching of the involved muscle after exercise may increase the pain. When only one leg is affected, comparing the two leg circumferences may reveal muscle atrophy. Although each of these compartments contains a major nerve, symptoms or signs of nerve dysfunction are rare.

Diagnosis

The differential diagnosis includes stress fracture, periostitis or shin splints, muscle strain and tendinitis, and deep venous thrombosis. Radiographs should be obtained to rule out bone abnormalities. Patients with paresthesia or numbness should be evaluated with electromyography (EMG) and nerve conduction velocity studies for evidence of nerve dysfunction.

The diagnosis of chronic compartment syndrome is based on the typical history of exercise pain, supplemented with intracompartmental pressure measurements taken at rest and just after exercise. Increased pressure after exercise with prolonged time for normalization of the pressure are the parameters most commonly used for determining chronic compartment syndrome.[3,4] Increased pressure alone, without the characteristic clinical history, is not considered sufficient to make the diagnosis.

Treatment

There is general consensus that conservative, nonsurgical treatment of chronic exertional compartment syndrome is successful only if the patient gives up the activity that precipitates the symptoms. Nonsurgical treatments, such as physiotherapy, ultrasound, orthotics, and anti-inflammatory drugs, have not proven effective in relieving symptoms.

Because most athletes who seek medical care want to continue their exercise activities, surgery is usually recommended; fasciotomy is the treatment of choice.[5] Surgical release of the involved compartment usually relieves symptoms and enables the athlete to resume previous activities (Fig. 83–2). Immediately after surgery, range of motion exercises of the knee, ankle, and foot are started. Weight bearing is permitted as tolerated. Normal activities can be resumed rapidly once the wound has healed.

NERVE ENTRAPMENT SYNDROMES

Nerve entrapment syndromes frequently are a secondary phenomenon to problems such as lower extremity edema, compression syndrome, bone impingement, and joint instability. Nerves that may be affected include the superficial and deep peroneal nerves, the sural nerve, the posterior tibial nerve and its branches, and the interdigital nerve (Fig. 83–3). Often, these nerve problems are functional; that is, the nerve is entrapped only during athletic activity.

Thus, it is important to obtain an accurate history and perform both a static and a functional physical examination. Because standard tests do not always demonstrate the symptoms, exertional activity is often necessary before testing. For example, nerve conduction delays may occur only during treadmill exercise. Correction of the underlying condition may resolve symptoms. If conservative measures fail, surgical decompression at the site of entrapment becomes necessary.

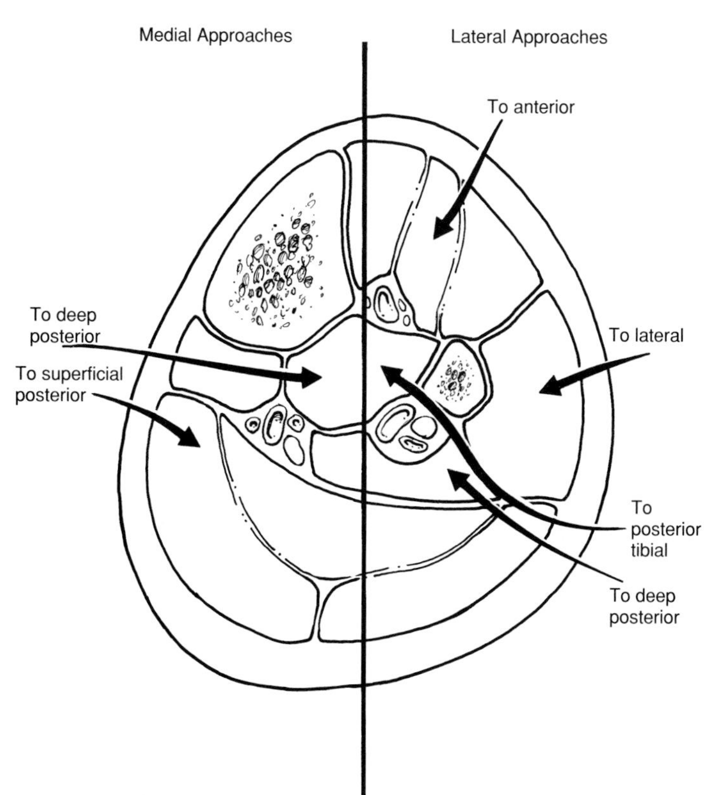

Fig. 83–2. Lateral and medial approaches for release of compartments in compartment syndromes.

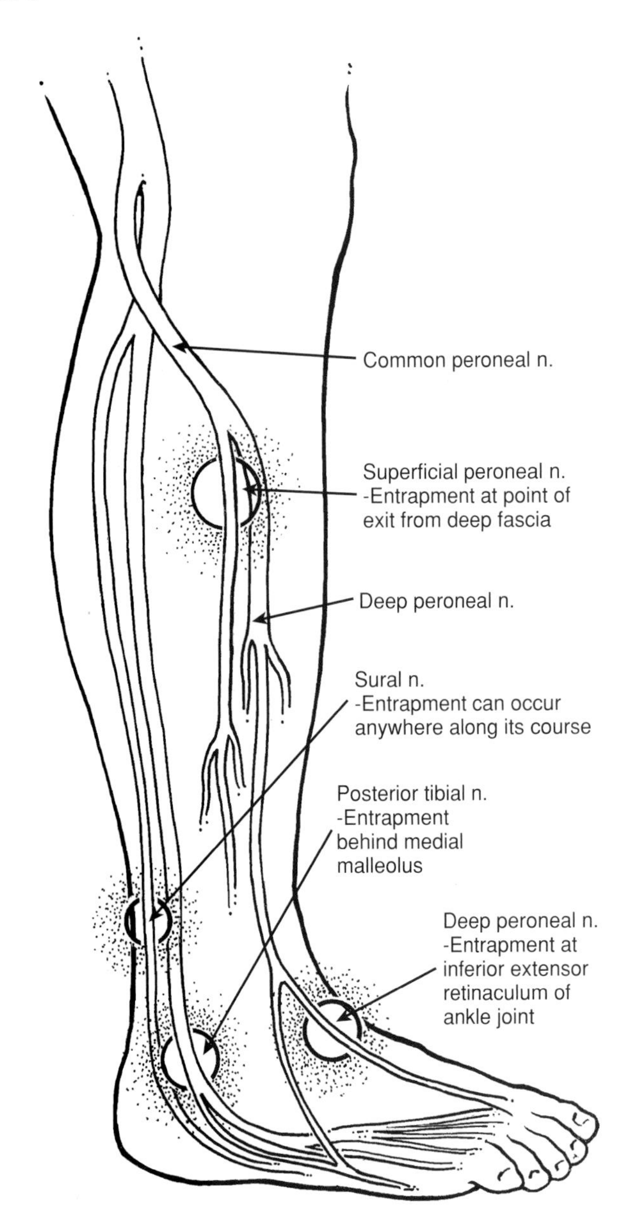

Fig. 83–3. Nerves that may be affected by nerve entrapment syndromes.

Superficial Peroneal Nerve Entrapment (Anterolateral Compartment Syndrome)

Entrapment of the superficial peroneal nerve usually occurs at its exit point from the deep fascia. Many patients have fascial defects at the intermuscular septum between the anterior and lateral compartments, and the nerve may be impinged as it courses around the edge of the fascia.[6] A muscle bulging through the defect can compress the nerve, and chronic ankle sprains may subject the nerve to recurrent stretching.

Entrapment causes pain over the outer border of the distal calf and the dorsum of the ankle and foot. Numbness and paresthesia may occur along the nerve distribution. The pain is typically worse with physical activities such as walking, jogging, running, and squatting. Nocturnal pain is rare.

The physical examination should include the lower back and the region where the common peroneal nerve sweeps around the neck of the fibula. Point tenderness is present at the site where the nerve emerges from the deep fascia. Pain may also be elicited by palpating the impingement site while passively plantar flexing and everting the patient's foot.

Deep Peroneal Nerve Entrapment (Anterior Tarsal Tunnel Syndrome)

The most common site of entrapment of the deep peroneal nerve is under the inferior extensor retinaculum at the level of the ankle joint. The nerve is placed under maximum stretch as the foot is positioned in plantar flexion and supination. Trauma (e.g., repeated ankle sprains) often plays a role. Tight-fitting shoes or ski boots have also been implicated as a causative factor.[7] Patients complain of pain in the dorsum of the foot with occasional radiation into the first web space. The pain usually occurs during athletic activity and subsides with removal of the shoe and with rest.

Again, examination includes the lower back, the region where the common peroneal nerve sweeps around the neck of the fibula, the entire course of the nerve throughout the anterior compartment of the leg, and the dorsum of the foot. Depending on the area of entrapment, pain may be elicited by either dorsiflexion or plantar flexion of the foot. Decreased sensation may be noted in the first web space.

Sural Nerve Entrapment

The sural nerve travels along the lateral border of the Achilles tendon and continues inferior to the peroneal sheath in a subcutaneous position. It provides sensation to the lateral heel and the lateral aspect of the fifth toe and fourth web space. Entrapment can occur anywhere along its course, resulting in shooting pain and paresthesia. On physical examination, the nerve should be palpated from the popliteal fossa to the toes. Local tenderness and Tinel's sign are characteristic. Occasionally, numbness is noted.

Entrapment of the Posterior Tibial Nerve and Its Branches

The posterior tibial nerve may be entrapped at several locations in its course as it exits the deep posterior compartment of the lower leg and runs distally behind the medial malleolus before branching into the lateral and medial plantar nerves. Traditional tarsal tunnel syndrome occurs behind the medial malleolus, under the retinacular ligament. Common symptoms include pain and numbness in the plantar aspect of the heel and foot. Pain is exacerbated by pressure to the compressed nerve adjacent to the medial malleolus.

The first branch of the lateral plantar nerve can be entrapped at the superior edge of the abductor hallucis longus muscle or just inferior to the muscle where it joins the plantar fascia. Athletes with hypermobile, pronated feet may be particularly susceptible to chronic stretching of this nerve. Nerve stretching or compression can be caused by ankle joint instability or chronic ankle edema. The most common complaint is chronic heel pain that radiates from the medial inferior aspect of the heel proximally into the medial ankle region. The pain may even radiate across the plantar aspect of the heel to the lateral aspect of the foot. Frequently, the pain is worse in the morning, when engorgement of the venous plexus adds to the compression. The pain is often exacerbated by running, and it can even occur when the athlete runs on the ball of the foot. A characteristic finding is tenderness over the first branch of the lateral plantar nerve, deep to the abductor hallucis longus muscle. Pressure at the site of compression reproduces the symptoms and causes pain to radiate both proximally and distally. Instability and swelling problems should be corrected before surgical intervention and may very well provide relief of symptoms and obviate surgical decompression.

Entrapment of the medial plantar nerve occurs in the region of the master knot of Henry at the inferior aspect of the talonavicular joint. This condition (also called *jogger's foot*) classically affects joggers, particularly those who run with excess heel valgus or hyperpronation of the foot. As with patients who have entrapment of the lateral plantar nerve, there often is a history of ankle injury in the presence of a chronically unstable lateral ankle. The pain often radiates distally into the medial toes and may radiate proximally into the ankle. The pain is worse when running on level ground, especially around curves, but it can also be induced by workouts on stairs. Characteristically, there is tenderness on the medial plantar aspect of the arch of the foot and in the region of the navicular tuberosity. The pain may be reproduced by everting the heel or by having the patient stand on the ball of the foot. Tinel's sign may be noted. Decreased sensation usually is present only after the patient has been running.

In rare cases, the medial hallucis nerve is entrapped as it exits the distal abductor hallucis muscle. This syndrome, which produces pain in the medial aspect of the first metatarsophalangeal joint in the area of the tibial sesamoid, is often mistaken for tibial sesamoiditis.

Interdigital Nerve Entrapment (Morton's Neuroma)

As, during push-off, the foot is in plantar flexion and the toes in dorsiflexion, the interdigital nerves between the second and third and the third and fourth metatarsals may be compressed by the intermetatarsal ligament. This causes neuritic radiation of pain into the affected web spaces and toes. Often, the pain also radiates proximally. The differential diagnosis includes herniated lumbar disc, metatarsalgia of the metatarsal heads, metatarsal stress fracture, and subluxation or capsulitis of the metatarsophalangeal joint. Initial treatment involves the use of a wider shoe and a metatarsal pad, to change the relative position of the metatarsals. If the pain persists in spite of conservative treatment, the nerve is excised.

REFERENCES

1. Garrett, W. E., Jr., et al.: The effect of muscle architecture on the biomechanical failure properties of skeletal muscle under passive extension. Am. J. Sport Med. *16*:7, 1988.
2. Rorabeck, C. H., and Macnab, I.: The pathophysiology of the anterior tibial compartmental syndrome. Clin. Orthop. *113*:52, 1975.
3. Rorabeck, C. H., et al.: The role of tissue pressure measurement in diagnosing chronic anterior compartment syndrome. Am. J. Sports Med. *16*:143, 1988.
4. Mannarino, F., and Sexson, S.: The significance of intracompartmental pressures in the diagnosis of chronic exertional compartment syndrome. Orthopedics *12*:1415, 1989.
5. Rorabeck, C. H., Fowler, P. J., and Nott, L.: The results of fasciotomy in the management of chronic exertional compartment syndrome. Am. J. Sports Med. *16*:224, 1988.
6. Styf, J.: Entrapment of the superficial peroneal nerve: Diagnosis and results of decompression. J. Bone Joint Surg. *71B*:131, 1989.
7. Lindenbaum, B. L.: Ski boot compression syndrome. Clin. Orthop. 140:109, 1979.

Achilles Tendon Injuries

James L. Beskin

The Achilles tendon, the largest and strongest tendon in the body, endures forces of four to seven times body weight and is one the most common sites of injury to athletes.[1] The causes of injuries to the Achilles tendon are multifactorial and are not related simply to events that occur during exercise. Recognizable patterns of tendon disease permit correct diagnosis and selection of proper treatment.

RISK FACTORS

Anatomic variations of the lower extremity that affect limb alignment and joint mobility contribute to Achilles tendon injuries. These include decreased passive ankle dorsiflexion and subtalar range of motion, forefoot varus,[2] hyperpronation, limb angular or torsional malalignments,[3] variation in the shape of the calcaneus (e.g., Haglund's bump) that may cause direct mechanical pressure on the tendon during exercise, and limited vascular perfusion typically found in the central portion of the tendon.[4]

Exogenous conditions that are present during exercise can be critical in evaluating Achilles tendon problems. Training errors, type of activity, and strenuousness of exercise are all variables that warrant consideration. Clearly, some sports are associated with a higher incidence of Achilles tendon problems than others. In almost all cases, rupture is due to strenuous activity that results in forceful eccentric or concentric contraction of the gastrocnemius-soleus muscle group.[2,5] In contrast, Achilles tendinitis is most commonly associated with less strenuous activities, such as jogging or running, which rarely result in acute, complete rupture. Instead, these athletes usually develop chronic, degenerative changes that lead to inflammation, partial rupture, and tendinosis.

Aging factors are also important. Age-related changes are often manifested by loss of flexibility. Achilles tendon injury is associated with diminished flexibility, and the rate of rupture is highest in athletes in their 30s and 40s.[2]

Genetic factors may also play a role; current data suggest that some persons with Type O blood are congenitally at greater risk for developing Achilles tendon problems. In addition, men have a significantly higher incidence of Achilles tendon ruptures that cannot be fully explained on the basis of activity and sports participation alone.

Certain systemic diseases are known to predispose to Achilles tendon symptoms. Many of the arthritides can cause enthesopathy or tenosynovitis that present as Achilles tendinitis. Other systemic conditions such as gout, hyperlipidemia, and diabetes have also been associated with Achilles tendon problems. On rare occasions, the adverse effects of pharmacologic agents, such as fluoroquinolone antibiotics (e.g., ciprofloxacin), systemic corticosteroids, and local corticosteroid injections may result in Achilles tendinitis or rupture.[6–8]

PATHOPHYSIOLOGY

Figure 83–4 shows the different tissues within the Achilles musculotendinous unit. The tendon is composed of densely packed collagen fibers and is not, in itself, very vascular. These tendon fibers are grouped into bundles by a fibrous connective tissue (the endotenon). The surrounding layer (the paratenon) consists of loose connective tissue that enhances tendon gliding.[3] The Achilles tendon lacks a true synovial sheath but is surrounded by a pseudosheath (i.e., the epitenon or peritenon).

The blood supply to the tendon is provided by vessels entering from the muscular origin and bony insertion of the Achilles tendon. The mesotenon, or vinculum, on the anterior surface of the tendon provides an important pathway for blood vessels to the tendon between its origin and insertion. There is a critical zone of limited perfusion in the area 2 to 6 cm above the tendon insertion, which corresponds to the area of most frequent rupture.[4]

Two areas of protective bursal tissue lie near the insertion of the Achilles tendon. Both the retrocalcaneal and the precalcaneal bursas have synovial cell linings that may manifest systemic inflammatory disorders as well as local inflammatory responses to mechanical irritation.

Not all forms of "tendinitis" affect the Achilles tendon equally.[9–11] Some patients experience an inflammatory process limited to the paratenon tissues, a condition

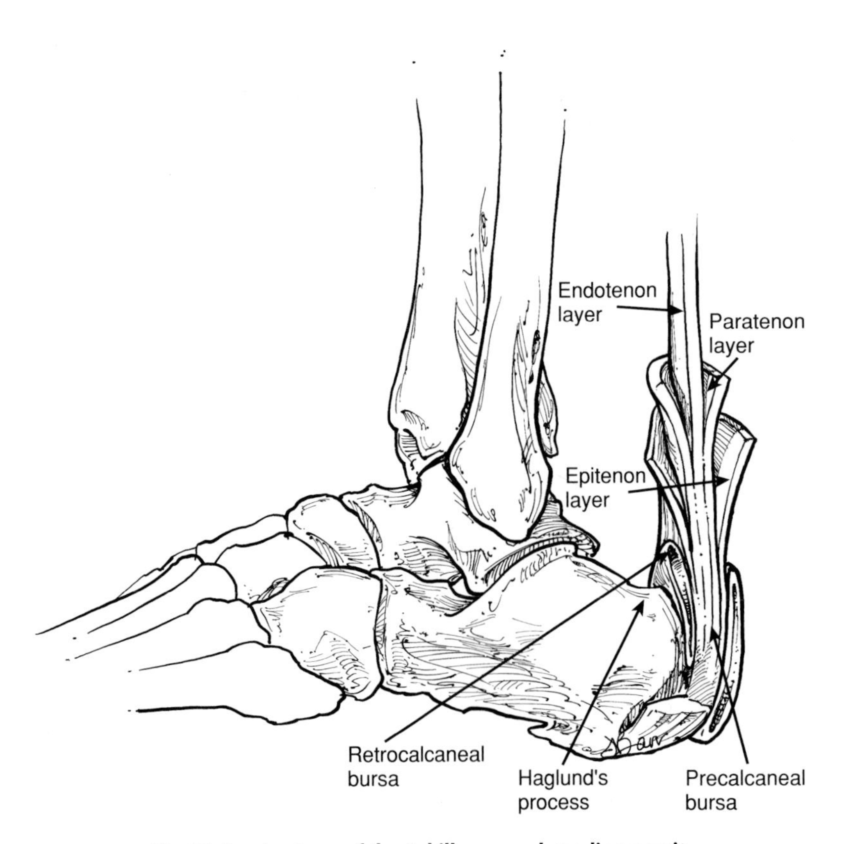

Fig. 83–4. Anatomy of the Achilles musculotendinous unit.

now referred to as *paratenonitis*. In other patients, the tendon itself is damaged and degenerates, resulting in "tendinosis." In many instances, paratenonitis progresses to tendinosis. Tendon degeneration can occur and progress without clinical evidence of inflammation. Marked vascular and metabolic changes may occur in paratenonitis.[10] These changes may impede the mechanical gliding of the Achilles tendon, which in turn increases mechanical irritation. Hypoxia from diminished blood flow may result in pain and limit the capacity of the tendon tissue to regenerate.

The architecture of the Achilles tendon can also be an important factor in tendon failure. The spiral design of the tendon fibers may contribute to a "wringing" effect that could compromise blood flow to the central third of the tendon.[11]

ACHILLES TENDINITIS

The anatomic distinction of noninsertional and insertional tendinitis can be used to divide patients with Achilles tendinitis into groups with similar attributes.[12]

Noninsertional Tendinitis

Patients with noninsertional tendinitis typically present with pain 2 to 6 cm above the Achilles tendon insertion. Pain usually occurs after exercise and is often present early in the morning. As the condition worsens, symptoms may occur during exercise or become constant.

Physical examination reveals local thickening and tenderness along the course of the tendon. Crepitus may be present during the early acute phase of injury. Many patients have lost flexibility of the gastrocnemius-soleus muscles, evidenced by diminished ankle dorsiflexion when the knee is held in extension. Other predisposing anatomic factors, such as foot or extremity malalignments, should be sought.

In some cases, paratenonitis occurs independently, and often it antedates the pathologic changes in the Achilles tendon itself. In other cases, the tendon is damaged and degenerated, resulting in tendinosis. Tendinosis typically is associated with chronic paratenonitis, but it can occur in otherwise asymptomatic persons. The clinical significance of these two subsets of noninsertional tendinitis, paratenonitis and tendinosis, lies in their treatment and results.[9,10]

Distinguishing isolated paratenonitis from tendinosis can be difficult on clinical grounds alone. Pain associated with acceleration or exertion has been found to correlate with surgical findings of tendinosis. Chronic symptoms (longer than 16 weeks), as well as failure to respond to rest and conservative care, should also raise the suspicion of tendinosis.

Routine radiographs are not diagnostic but may reveal calcification in the tendon that is compatible with chronic degenerative changes. Ultrasound is the most readily available and cost-effective means to evaluate the tendon for qualitative changes or partial tears. Magnetic resonance imaging (MRI) is conceivably the most accurate means of determining if the symptoms are due to tendon involvement; however, limited availability and high cost presently limit its use as a screening tool for all patients with "tendinitis." MRI should be reserved for patients whose tendinitis is resistant to conservative treatment and for preoperative planning when surgery is contemplated.

For patients with isolated paratenonitis, cessation of the aggravating activity and control of the inflammatory process often allow healing to occur. Treatment consists of rest, stretching, cold therapy, and orthotics to elevate the heel or control pronation. Nonsteroidal anti-inflammatory drugs (NSAIDs) can provide some analgesic effects, and they may be used on a trial basis during the acute phase of injury. However, their efficacy remains controversial, and they can have serious side effects.

Equally controversial is the use of corticosteroids. Clearly, enough data exist to condemn intratendinous injections, which are likely to further weaken the tendon.[7,8] In addition, the reduced symptoms after injection may permit a higher level of activity, which in turn increases the risk of failure of an Achilles tendon compromised by tendinosis. Because of these findings and the technical difficulty of proper placement of the medication, I strongly caution against the use of injectable corticosteroids. If they are used, structured rehabilitation and protection from high-demand exercises for at least 4 to 6 weeks are prudent.

There have been encouraging reports of using other agents, including glycosaminoglycan polysulfate (GAGPS) and heparin, to control the reactive tissue adhesions associated with paratenonitis. The ability of GAGPS to inhibit the formation of thrombin and fibrin is thought to reduce the establishment of immature scar tissue and resultant adhesions.[13]

For cases of paratenonitis unresponsive to conservative treatment, a limited surgical approach to decompress the tendon and cause lysis of adhesions within the paratenon is worthwhile. In the presence of tendinosis, ability to heal is limited and, likewise, prognosis for recovery with conservative care is less promising. Therefore, if 4 to 6 months' conservative treatment fails to relieve the patient's pain, surgical intervention is recommended.[9,14–16] In severe cases of tendinosis, recovery is usually slow; many patients require 6 to 8 months or longer to return to intensive activity.

Insertional Tendinitis

Insertional tendinitis is distinguished by localization of the patient's symptoms to the distal aspect of the tendon. The symptoms and signs of this entity may overlap with those of other conditions of the heel, particularly retrocalcaneal or precalcaneal bursitis and Haglund's bump (Fig. 83–5). Insertional tendinitis is not readily subdivided into pathologic subgroups involving the paratendinous and tendinous tissues.

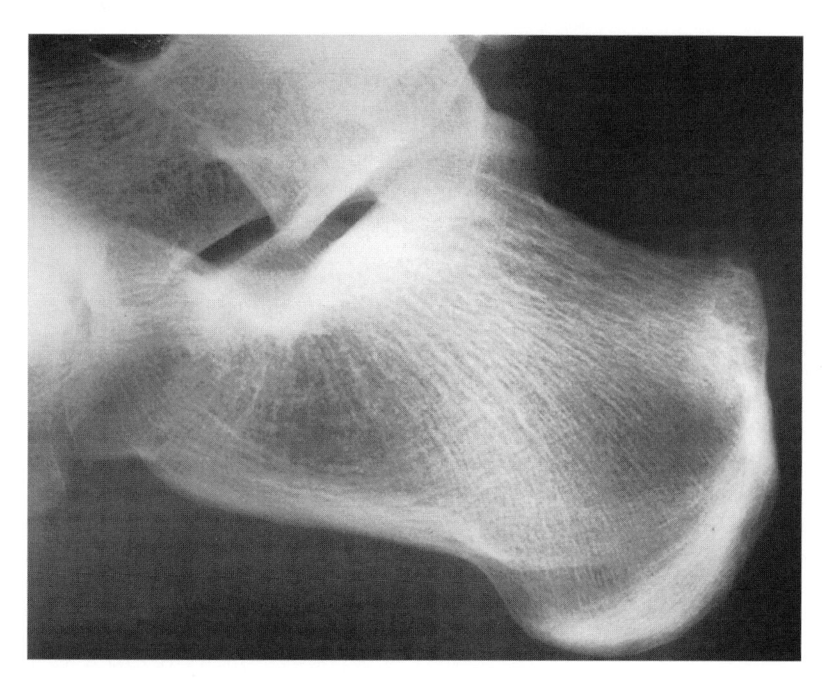

Fig. 83–5. Radiograph demonstrates chronic insertional tendinitis and reactive bone over Haglund's process.

Symptoms may, however, be similar to those of noninsertional tendinitis, with pain during or after exercise. Often, focal redness and warmth are associated with tenderness at the Achilles insertion. Most often, the symptoms are on the posterolateral side, where thickening of the tissues is usually evident. The proximal aspect of the tendon remains relatively normal. Physical examination may also reveal tightness of the gastrocnemius-soleus muscles or other foot or limb malalignments.

Radiographic findings are inconsistent but may include spurs at the site of the Achilles insertion on the calcaneus and, occasionally, calcification in the distal portion of the tendon. Many patients also demonstrate an abnormally prominent Haglund's process. In some cases, MRI may be helpful in determining if the primary disorder lies in the tendon substance or in the adjacent tissues.

Treatment is directed at reducing tensile forces and contact pressure on the distal Achilles tendon. Limiting the patient's activity while working on stretching and controlled strengthening exercises is usually helpful. Cushioning the heel counter of the shoe and adding a temporary heel lift also help reduce symptoms. When appropriate, orthotics should be used to limit pronation or to accommodate other foot malalignments. NSAIDs, cold therapy, and ultrasound may be helpful during the acute phase.

Chronic cases need further scrutiny for other underlying disorders. Enthesopathy of the Achilles tendon is commonly associated with a number of rheumatic disorders that may make the usual treatments less effective. Similarly, rheumatic diseases, as well as the mechanical factors mentioned above, may affect the adjacent bursal tissues, and this can mimic insertional tendinitis. When the retrocalcaneal or precalcaneal bursas are contributing sources of pain, careful injection of corticosteroids into the bursal tissue is justified. There is minimal increased risk of Achilles tendon rupture when the injection material is limited to the bursal area. Injections into the tendon fibers should be avoided.

Unfortunately, the surgical results for salvage of refractory cases of insertional tendinitis are not as predictable as for the noninsertional tendinitis group.(11,15) Nevertheless, patients should be considered for surgical débridement of the distal tendon if conservative management fails to relieve symptoms. It is usually advisable to remove the prominent calcaneal process at the time of surgery as well.

ACHILLES TENDON RUPTURE

Acute, complete rupture of the Achilles tendon is a relatively infrequent diagnosis as compared with other Achilles tendon problems, but it is a potentially disabling injury. The overall incidence of rupture is reported to be increasing, possibly because of changes in recreational activity as well as increased clinical awareness of the problem.(5,17,18)

Achilles rupture typically occurs in men in their 30s or 40s, usually without warning. Most often, they are recreational athletes participating in basketball, soccer, racquet sports, or other activities that impose forceful eccentric or concentric contracture of the gastrocnemius-soleus muscles.

Although the exact cause of Achilles tendon rupture remains obscure, multiple risk factors appear to be involved. Most notable are the findings of limited vascular perfusion at the usual site of rupture.(4) Factors affecting anatomic limb alignment and genetic makeup are evidently important as well.(2,5) Excessive or uncoordinated muscle contracture is also a potential cause of rupture. The tendon is more likely to rupture after a period of inactivity or when the muscle is fatigued. It is likely that some of the causative factors are not mutually exclusive but instead contribute, to a greater or lesser degree, toward failure of the Achilles tendon.

Diagnosis

Diagnosis is based principally on clinical findings. The presenting history is remarkably consistent: most athletes recount no prodromal symptoms and are completely surprised by the abrupt pain of the rupture. Many report feeling certain that someone else kicked or struck their leg. Although most patients are unable to continue their sports participation, the severe pain usually is temporary, leading some to postpone medical care by assuming the injury is just a "sprain." A prolonged limp with plantar flexion weakness eventually prompts them to seek medical attention.

In a few patients, the correct diagnosis may be missed initially. This usually happens because the remaining muscle function of the ankle is capable of providing some resistive plantar flexion force to the casual examiner. However, the combined forces of the toe flexors and the posterior tibial tendon provide less than 15 to 30% of the potential plantar flexion force available from an intact Achilles tendon.[1] For this reason, patients with Achilles tendon rupture present with a shortened stride from weakened push-off and an inability to perform a single-limb toe rise.

The most reliable way to diagnose an acute Achilles tendon rupture is with Thompson's test, which is easily performed by having the patient lie prone with the feet suspended in the air (Fig. 83–6A).[19] By firmly squeezing each calf, it will become apparent that there is no passive movement of the ankle in which a complete rupture has occurred. Failure to move the ankle with this maneuver constitutes a positive test that is nearly 100% reliable. The additional finding of a palpable defect in the area of the tendon is also confirmatory of a suspected rupture (Fig. 83–6B).

Radiographs are not helpful in making the diagnosis but are justified for evaluating other potential associated disorders and in identifying the rare avulsion fracture off the posterior calcaneal tuberosity. The clinical symptoms and signs usually obviate sophisticated imaging modalities (e.g., MRI, ultrasound). Such studies, however, may be useful for assessing tendon apposition when nonsurgical techniques are chosen or for evaluating late or chronic ruptures.

Treatment

Acceptable results can be obtained from both nonsurgical and surgical treatment options. The choice must be based on the individual patient's situation, and, to some extent, on the skills and preferences of the physician.

Nonsurgical treatment, while generally successful, clearly leaves the patient at higher risk of re-rupture.[20,21] This complication often occurs early in the recovery phase, usually less than 6 months after the injury. Complications related to immobilization, such as cast sores and deep venous thrombosis, occur with equal frequency in both nonsurgical and surgical treatment and are generally minimal. However, the prolonged immobilization in equinus position required by nonsurgical treatment does increase the rehabilitation time.

Nonsurgical treatment is most successful when initiated within 48 hours of injury; functional results and risk of re-rupture are comparable to those of surgical repair.[21] The patient's foot should be placed in "forced plantar flexion" in a short-leg cast for 4 weeks, followed by 4 weeks of "semiequinus" casting. A heel raise is used for another 4 weeks after cast removal, followed by the initiation of progressive rehabilitative exercises.

Most agree that surgical apposition of the ruptured tendon ends is the most consistent means of regaining gastrocnemius-soleus power.[18,22,23] This re-establishes the proper musculotendinous length and creates tension on the retracted muscle during healing, which may help to reduce atrophy. Some of the current repair techniques are strong enough to allow casting in a neutral ankle position, or even to permit some limited early range of motion of the ankle.[24,25] Consequently, surgically treated patients generally achieve earlier return to functional activity and do not have to undergo the prolonged process of regaining ankle dorsiflexion associated with equinus casting. In addition, the risk of re-rupture is considerably lower in surgically repaired tendons.[18,22,23,25]

Though early repair is desirable, skin conditions should be optimized and swelling should be controlled before proceeding with surgery. Postoperative results are usually the same, as long as the surgery is performed within 2 to 3 weeks after injury.[22,23,25] The primary concern with surgical repair is the potential morbidity associated with wound complications, chief among them skin slough and infection. However, modern surgical techniques and proper soft tissue handling have much reduced the high rates seen in earlier surgeries. Possible anesthetic complications are another consideration in selecting patients for open repair.

In deciding which patients would benefit from surgery, the physician must first determine if there are any underlying conditions that could increase the risk of peri- or postoperative complications. Age itself is not a contraindication, but other coexisting conditions, such as peripheral vascular disease, diabetes, and heart disease, may make nonsurgical treatment the prudent choice. Generally, surgical repair of the Achilles tendon should be reserved for healthy, active persons who desire to return to a high level of activity.

Postoperative care is dictated by the needs and motivation of the patient. In cooperative, reliable patients, the three-bundle repair tolerates early range of motion.[25] A dorsiflexion block splint or removable protective brace is advisable. In many cases, protection with a cast for 4 to 6 weeks is best. In all circumstances, touch-down weight bearing is necessary during the first 3 to 4 weeks after repair. Afterward, a gradual increase

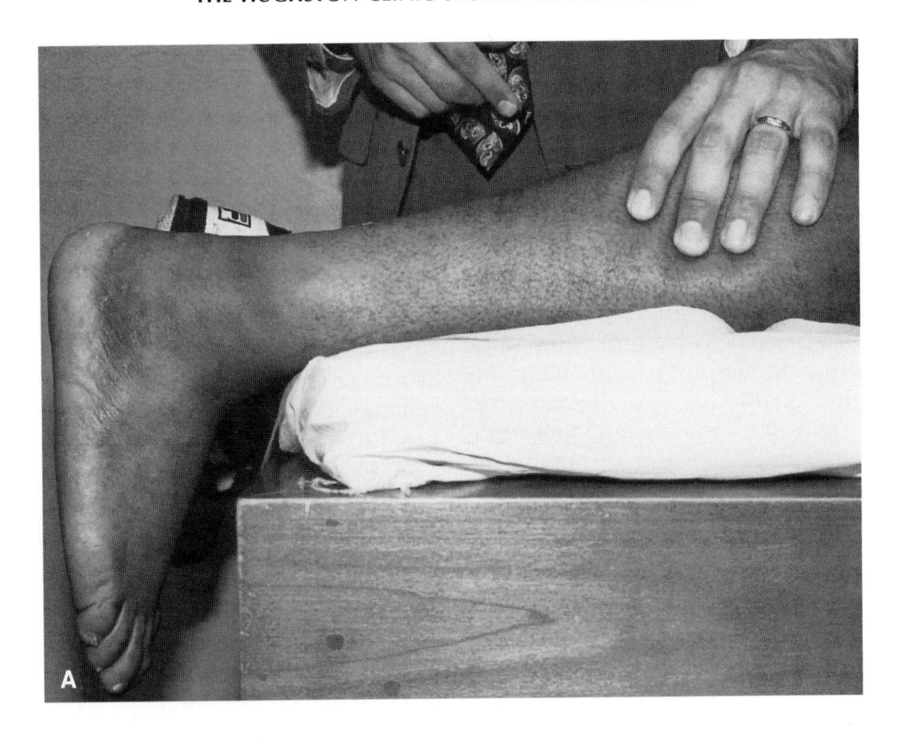

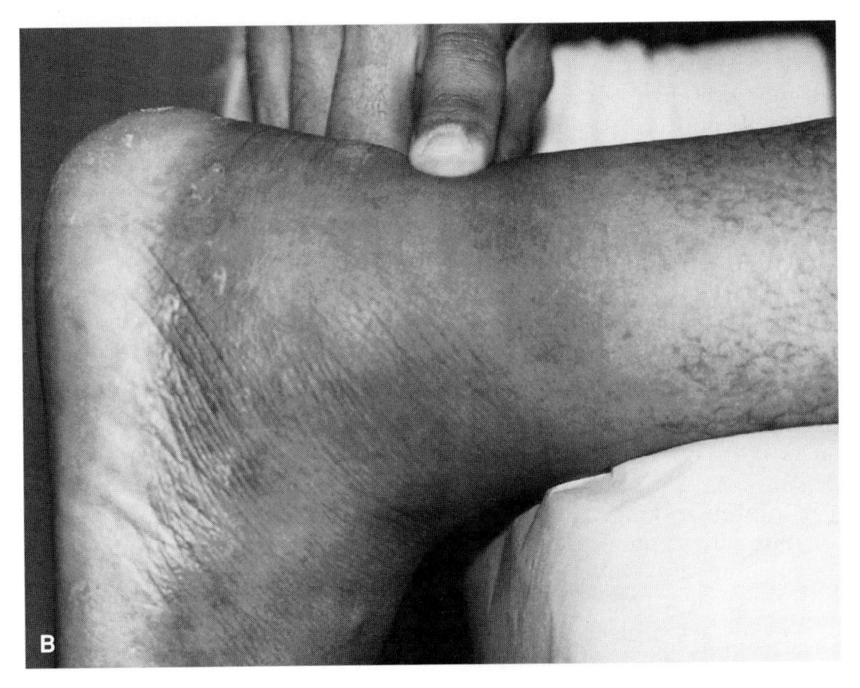

Fig. 83–6. *(A)* A positive Thompson's test associated with a ruptured Achilles tendon: the foot cannot be plantar flexed with this maneuver. *(B)* Identification of a palpable defect in the typical location of Achilles rupture.

to full weight bearing in a cast or protective brace is allowed. All surgical repairs need cast or brace protection for at least 6 to 8 weeks after surgery.

Progressive resistive exercises are started, along with continued work on regaining flexibility of the ankle. Most patients are allowed to resume sports activity 4 to 6 months after surgery. Patients who perform range of motion exercises early in their rehabilitation program may experience less muscle atrophy and be able to return earlier to activity.[24,25] Longterm results, however, do not indicate that any one rehabilitation technique has a distinct advantage over others.[25]

REFERENCES

1. Scheller, A. D., Kasser, J. R., and Quigley, T. B.: Tendon injuries about the ankle. Orthop. Clin. North Am. *11*:801, 1980.
2. Kvist, M.: Achilles tendon injuries in athletes. Ann. Chir. Gynaecol. *80*:188, 1991.
3. Galloway, M. T., Jokl, P., and Dayton, O. W.: Achilles tendon overuse injuries. Clin. Sports Med. *11*:771, 1992.
4. Carr, A. J., and Norris, S. H.: The blood supply of the calcaneal tendon. J. Bone Joint Surg. *71B*:100, 1989.
5. Jozsa, L., et al.: The role of recreational sport activity in Achilles tendon rupture. Am. J. Sports Med. *17*:338, 1989.
6. Ribard, P., et al.: Seven Achilles tendinitis including 3 complicated by rupture during fluoroquinolone therapy. J. Rheumatol. *19*:1479, 1992.
7. Kleinman, M., and Gross, A. E.: Achilles tendon rupture following steroid injection. J. Bone Joint Surg. *65A*:1345, 1983.
8. Mahler, F., and Fritschy, D.: Partial and complete ruptures of the Achilles tendon and local corticosteroid injections. Br. J. Sports Med. 26:7, 1992.
9. Puddu, G., Ippolito, E., and Postacchini, F.: A classification of Achilles tendon disease. Am. J. Sports Med. *4*:145, 1976.
10. Kvist, M. H., et al.: Chronic Achilles paratenonitis: An immunohistologic study of fibronectin and fibrinogen. Am. J. Sports Med. *16*:616, 1988.
11. Schepsis, A. A., and Leach, R. E.: Surgical management of Achilles tendinitis. Am. J. Sports Med. *15*:308, 1987.
12. Clain, M. R., and Baxter, D. E.: Achilles tendinitis. Foot Ankle *13*:482, 1992.
13. Sundqvist H., Forsskahl, B., and Kvist, M.: A promising novel therapy for Achilles peritendinitis. Int. J. Sports Med. *8*:298, 1987.
14. Nelen, G., Martens, M., and Burssens, A.: Surgical treatment of chronic Achilles tendinitis. Am. J. Sports Med. *17*:754, 1989.
15. Leach, R. E., Schepsis, A. A., and Takai, H.: Long-term results of surgical management of Achilles tendinitis in runners. Clin. Orthop. *282*:208, 1992.
16. Allenmark, C.: Partial Achilles tendon tears. Clin. Sports Med. *11*:759, 1992.
17. Hattrup, S. J., and Johnson, K. A.: A review of ruptures of the Achilles tendon. Foot Ankle *6*:34, 1985.
18. Wills, C. A., Washburn, S., Caiozzo, V., and Prietto, C. A.: Achilles tendon rupture. Clin. Orthop. *207*:156, 1986.
19. Thompson, T. C., and Doherty, J. H.: Spontaneous rupture of tendon of Achilles: A new clinical diagnostic test. J. Trauma *2*:126, 1962.
20. Inglis, A. E., Scott, W. N., Sculco, T. P., and Patterson, A. H.: Ruptures of the tendo Achillis: An objective assessment of surgical and nonsurgical treatment. J. Bone Joint Surg. *58A*:990, 1976.
21. Carden, D. G., et al.: Rupture of the calcaneal tendon. J. Bone Joint Surg. *69B*:416, 1987.
22. Inglis, A. E., and Sculco, T. P.: Surgical repair of ruptures of the tendo Achillis. Clin. Orthop. *156* :160, 1981.
23. Jacobs, D., et al.: Comparison of conservative and operative treatment of Achilles tendon rupture. Am. J. Sports Med. *6*:107, 1978.
24. Carter, T. R., Fowler, P. J., and Blokker, C.: Functional postoperative treatment of Achilles tendon repair. Am. J. Sports Med. *20*:459, 1992.
25. Beskin, J. L., Sanders, R. A., Hunter, S. C., and Hughston, J. C.: Surgical repair of Achilles tendon ruptures. Am. J. Sports Med. *15*:1, 1987.

84

Rene K. Marti and Niek van Dijk

Ankle Sprains

Ankle sprains, the most common of all ankle injuries, are especially likely to be sustained in sports and recreational activities.[1] The lateral ligaments are the most frequently sprained joint structures; however, the tibiofibular syndesmosis and the medial ligament (the deltoid ligament) can also be injured. Despite the fact that ligamentous injuries of the ankle occur so frequently, all too often, the typical ankle sprain is either disregarded or undertreated.

It is generally agreed that untreated or inadequately treated trauma to the ankle ligaments may have serious sequelae, such as persistent pain, swelling, unsteady gait on uneven ground, and chronic instability.[2] Watson Jones' historic statement, "It is worse to sprain an ankle than to break it" is still valid.[3] It is believed that permanent instability of the talus after a sprain is due to failure to distinguish between a simple sprain and a rupture of the lateral ligaments at the time of injury. Thus, accurate diagnosis is important for correct treatment and optimal outcome. Fortunately, most ankle sprains respond well to appropriate conservative treatment, and surgery is necessary only when nonsurgical approaches do not work.

In the 1960s, diagnostic and treatment protocols almost uniformly consisted of stress radiographs and plantar immobilization of the injured ankle. In the 1970s, even more aggressive protocols were started, including arthrograms and anatomic reconstruction of the ligaments during surgery.[4–8] At present, functional treatment is the rule and less importance is attached to differentiating between single and multiple ligament injuries. Consequently, stress radiographs and arthrographic examination are regarded as excessive. The physician relies more on the history and physical examination, though in the case of ankle injuries, many orthopedists consider the acute-phase physical examination unreliable.

PREDISPOSING FACTORS FOR ANKLE SPRAINS

The extent of tissue damage associated with trauma depends not only on the mechanism and magnitude of the forces acting on the ankle but also on the position of the foot and ankle during the trauma. Predisposing factors that contribute to supination trauma to the ankle include (1) pes cavovarus (hollow foot), (2) crus varum, and (3) a previous supination injury.

This is easy to understand because in a cavovarus foot, the talus is already situated more or less above the calcaneus, in a partially supinated position. With crus varum, the subtalar joint is not able to compensate for the valgus malposition. Finally, a previous supination injury, resulting in an elongated anterior talofibular ligament (ATFL), impedes appropriate reaction by the active stabilizers.

LATERAL LIGAMENT SPRAINS

Lateral stability of the ankle joint is provided by the ATFL during plantar flexion and the calcaneofibular ligament (CFL) during dorsiflexion. The ATFL plays a key role in transmitting rotatory forces from the fibula to the talus and is considered the most important stabilizing ligament of the joint. However, the ATFL is the weakest of the three lateral ligaments, having the least elastic transformation property. Insufficiency of the ATFL leads to instability that is similar to anterolateral rotatory instability in the knee.

Mechanism of Injury

The lateral ligaments are injured secondary to "inversion" or varus tilt only when the ankle is incompletely loaded (e.g., during initial foot contact with the ground) and may occur because of internal rotation (Fig. 84–1).[9] During walking, the foot is in plantar flexion when it is placed on the ground; thus, the ATFL is the first ligament to be tensed. As the ATFL approaches vertical orientation to the ground with full plantar flexion, the CFL approaches vertical orientation with slight dorsiflexion.

If the lateral edge of the foot is not supported and the peroneal musculature does not temporarily prevent further inversion, part of the capsular ligament complex may rupture. The ATFL is the first to rupture with such forced inversion of the ankle. Rupture of the ATFL is always associated with rupture of the joint capsule because the ligament is incorporated into the capsule.

Rupture of the ATFL because of forced inversion allows anterior subluxation of the talus out of the ankle mortise. In the horizontal plane, the talus rotates on the medial malleolus and the intact deltoid ligament, using this ligament as a kind of axis. On the lateral side, because of the subluxation, the convex edge of the talus can abut the sharp anterior edge of the distal tibia and produce an osteochondral lesion. Longterm degenerative changes can be expected when recurrent subluxations overtax the joint.

Forced plantar flexion, in combination with adduction, causes rupture of the ATFL, followed by partial rupture of the CFL. If continued force is applied, the CFL ruptures completely, followed by rupture of the posterior talofibular ligament (PTFL). Isolated rupture of the capsule, partial rupture of the ATFL, and isolated rupture of the CFL are all rare injuries.

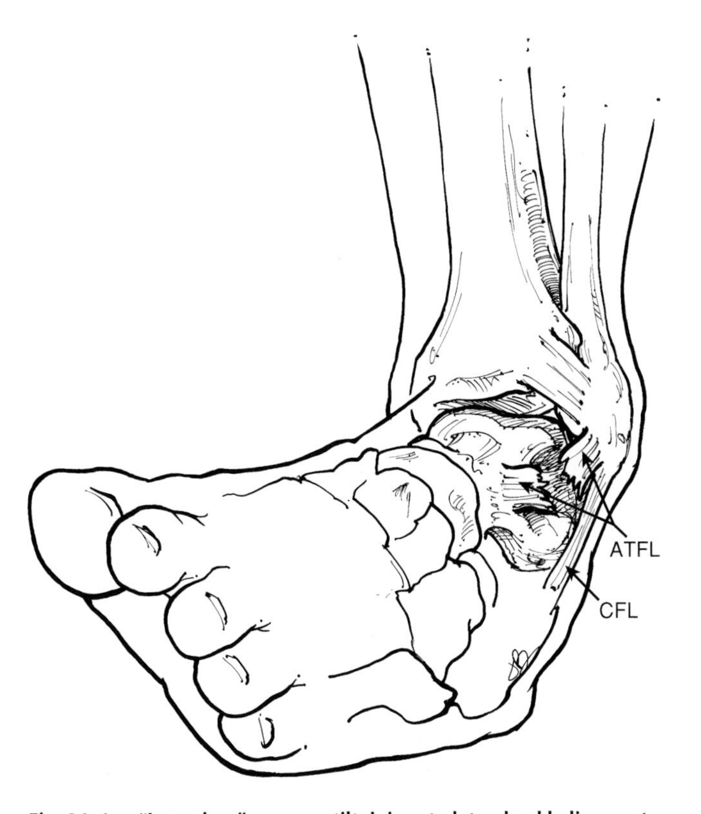

Fig. 84–1. "Inversion," or varus tilt, injury to lateral ankle ligaments.

Classification of Injuries

There is some variation in different schemes for grading of ligament injuries. O'Donoghues's Grades I, II, and III are anatomically based and require stress tests or invasive arthrography and tenography to accurately grade the injury. Some orthopedists consider Grade III sprains to be the rare case in which all three lateral ligaments are completely torn, as in a dislocated ankle. Most, however, associate Grade III injuries with complete disruption of the ATFL and CFL.[10] We prefer to classify acute ankle sprains as mild, moderate, or severe, an approach that, basically, corresponds to Grades I, II, and III, respectively (routine stress radiographs views and invasive tests are not performed).

With mild sprains, 48 hours after the injury, swelling is minimal, range of motion good, and the patient is able comfortably to bear weight without needing crutches. With moderate sprains, swelling is more pronounced, range of motion limited to about 0° to 30° of flexion, and the patient usually needs to use crutches or a cane to bear weight on the involved extremity. Most sprains fall into this category. Severe sprains cause marked swelling, ecchymosis laterally, and minimal pain-free range of motion, and the patient is unable to bear weight on the affected limb.

Clinical Diagnosis

Athletes who sustain ankle sprains should be evaluated with a complete history, physical examination, and radiographs to ensure an accurate diagnosis and appropriate treatment.

History

The history often is helpful in determining the mechanism of injury. The patient can usually reproduce the mechanism by demonstrating the precipitating events with the uninjured ankle. When taking the history, it is also important to differentiate between low-velocity and high-velocity trauma. In addition, any history of chronic joint instability or of previously treated or untreated ligament injury is relevant. Reconstruction of the mechanism of injury and signs and symptoms such as swelling, the "snap," and other subjective symptoms do not necessarily reflect the severity of the injury.

Physical Examination

The initial examination normally reveals a diffusely swollen, plantar flexed, ecchymotic, tender ankle. Tenderness usually is found anterolaterally at the ankle, and often along the CFL as well. The medial side of the ankle and the syndesmosis frequently are tender and swollen in association with lateral injuries; however, clinical examination of the ankle within the first couple of days of injury is often unreliable.

There are several advantages to performing the physical examination when pain and swelling have subsided (usually within 4 to 7 days after the injury). Pressure pain is more localized at the site of actual tissue or ligament damage. The presence of a hematoma is an important indication of ankle ligament injury and, if one exists, the discoloration is more evident. Finally, because of diminished pain and swelling, there is less reactive muscle tension present and stability testing is tolerated better.

Generalized joint laxity should be noted. The examiner should also look for pes cavus (or, conversely, pes planus) since pes cavus, associated with rigid varus hindfoot position, predisposes athletes to recurrent ankle sprains. Tarsal coalition should be suspected, particularly in adolescents with recurrent sprains. The patient often has a rigid pes planus deformity with peroneal muscle spasm. A complete neurovascular checkup should also be performed since concomitant superficial and deep peroneal nerve and sural nerve injuries that may be present often are overlooked initially.[11] The peroneal tendons can be subluxated, dislocated, or ruptured, particularly with dorsiflexion injuries.

The keystone of the delayed physical examination is the stability test, which can be repeated without harming the patient. The extent of lateral ligament damage and instability is evaluated primarily by the anterior drawer test and the inversion stress test (talar tilt test). The degree of demonstrable mechanical instability during the examination depends on the position of the ankle joint. In dorsiflexion, the joint is very resistant to anterior subluxation forces, whereas in plantar flexion this resistance is quite low. The anterior drawer test principally assesses the ATFL; however, the CFL and PTFL also produce some stability during the examination, particularly when the ankle is dorsiflexed. The inversion stress test evaluates mainly the integrity of the CFL, in addition to the ATFL.

The anterior drawer test is performed with the patient's ankle in neutral and plantar flexion (Fig. 84–2). The tibia is stabilized with one hand, while the other hand directs an anterior force to the heel. When the ATFL is ruptured and force is applied to the talus in an anterior direction, the anterolateral edge of the talus shifts approximately 1 cm forward, out of the ankle mor-

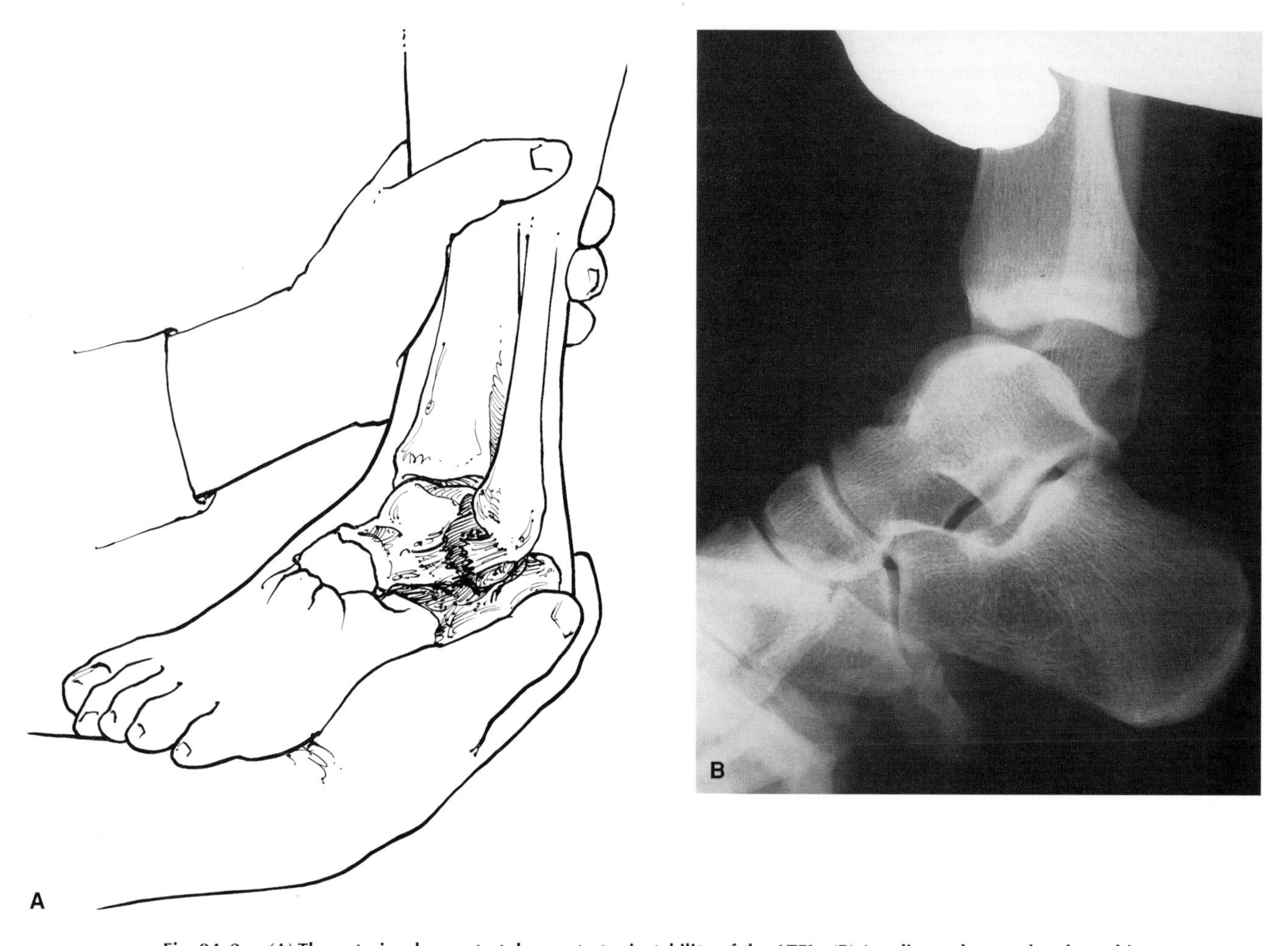

Fig. 84–2. *(A)* The anterior drawer test demonstrates instability of the ATFL. *(B)* A radiograph may also show this instability pattern.

tise. The center of rotation is the intact deltoid ligament.

In practice, the anterior drawer phenomenon can be demonstrated in every patient with an ankle ligament rupture. However, without anesthesia, this clinical diagnosis can only be made immediately after the injury, before swelling and reactive muscle rigidity have developed, or a few days after the injury, when the swelling and pain have resolved.

The inversion stress test is performed with the ankle in a neutral position or slight plantar flexion, to place more tension on the CFL (Fig. 84–3). The examiner stabilizes the tibia with one hand while with the other hand applying varus stress at the level of the calcaneocuboid joint. Although the inversion stress test provides the best noninvasive means of evaluating the integrity of the CFL, it does not distinguish between single- and double-ligament tears. The test is best used to assess chronic symptoms of instability.

The delayed physical examination provides information that is not surpassed in value by any other diagnostic modality, even the "gold standard," arthrography. Absence of palpation pain at the site of the ATFL excludes ankle ligament rupture. The combination of a negative anterior drawer test and the absence of hematoma discoloration is consistent with an intact capsular ligament. A combination of palpation pain at the site of the ATFL, lateral hematoma discoloration, and a positive anterior drawer test almost always indicates an ankle ligament injury. Finally, almost half of all ankle ligament injuries are associated with palpation pain at the level of the syndesmosis without the presence of a syndesmosis rupture, or at the area of the medial malleolus.

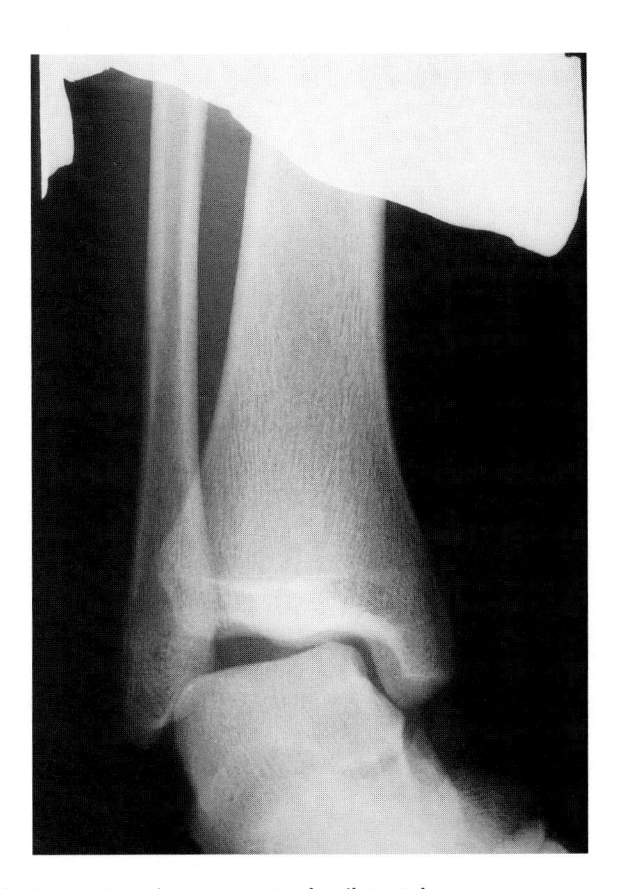

Fig. 84–3. **Inversion stress test (talar tilt test) demonstrates instability of the CFL.**

Radiographic Evaluation

Plain anteroposterior (AP) and lateral radiographs enable the clinician to detect ligament-avulsion fractures and to rule out other bone lesions. Stress radiographs allow the talar shift to be documented and compared with the stress test results obtained during the physical examination. The uninjured ankle should be compared in exactly the same position.

Most orthopedists accept a difference in talar tilt equal to or greater than 6° as corresponding to a difference of more than 3 mm in the anterior drawer test and regard it as evidence of an ankle ligament injury. With the inversion stress test, a talar tilt greater than 10°, as compared with the opposite ankle, represents significant chronic instability.

Because the reliability and reproducibility of stress radiographs depend on the amount of pain and degree of muscle tension and the position of the ankle during imaging, the best results are obtained if the patient is under general anesthesia. Routine use of stress radiographs is not recommended, however, because they do not much improve the diagnostic accuracy over that obtained by stress testing during the physical examination.[12]

Ancillary Diagnostic Studies

Arthrography, especially if performed within 48 hours of the injury, is regarded as the gold standard for evaluating a severe, multiple lateral ankle ligament injury.[13–15] Differentiating between an isolated ATFL injury and multiple ligament injuries is possible by observing if there is leakage into the peroneal tendon sheath. It is not possible to distinguish between an anterolateral capsule tear, a partial rupture of the ATFL, and complete rupture of the ATFL.

Tenography is considered by some to be the best modality for detecting multiple ligament rupture,[16] but an isolated ATFL injury cannot be detected by tenography, and differentiating between an isolated ATFL injury and multiple ligament injuries has no therapeutic consequences. These invasive studies are not necessary for the evaluation of most ankle sprains. They should be performed only if treatment decisions depend on the results. For example, if single- or double-ligament tears are treated in exactly the same way, arthrography or tenography is not indicated. Because we manage acute lateral ligament sprains nonsurgically, we do not try to document severity of ligament damage with arthrography (or stress radiography).

The role of ultrasonography in the evaluation of ankle ligament injuries is still unclear and has found only limited application. In our studies, however, it has shown much sensitivity and moderate specificity, and it might be a good noninvasive supplementary diagnostic technique. The value of computed tomography (CT) and of magnetic resonance imaging (MRI) are still being debated, and their use depends much on the individual clinician.

Differential Diagnosis

Because these injuries can accompany an ankle sprain, the differential diagnosis should include peroneal tendon disorders (subluxation, dislocation, rupture); superficial peroneal or sural nerve injury; injury to the syndesmosis; subtalar joint spasms; fractures of the lateral malleolus, fifth metatarsal base, os trigonum, or lateral process of the talus; and several intra-articular lesions (e.g., osteochondral fractures and impingement lesions).

Treatment

The paramount goal when treating an ankle ligament injury is complete recovery without residual symptoms. Possible treatments include immobilization (either by elastic bandage or plaster casting), surgical treatment, or functional management. We believe all first-time acute sprains (mild, moderate, severe) should be treated nonsurgically with early functional mobilization implemented by an immediate rehabilitation program.

A recent survey of treatments of acute tears of the lateral ligament complex of the ankle concluded that functional treatment with a short period of protection followed by early range of motion exercises and neuromuscular training is the method of choice, even initially in competitive athletes. This provides patients the quickest recovery of full range of motion and return to work and physical activity without producing any more mechanical or functional instability than casting alone or surgery.[17] No significant difference was observed in the treatment results of isolated ATFL rupture and of multiple ligament injuries.

These conclusions are substantiated by our own study consisting of a randomized series of 122 patients who had one or more ruptured ankle ligaments. Four treatment approaches—taping alone, elastic bandaging alone, surgery and taping, and surgery and elastic bandaging—are being evaluated. At the time of this writing, no statistically significant differences have been noted in the clinical results (as measured by symptoms of giving way, clinical anterior drawer test, and stress radiographs) of the four groups. Functional treatment alone or following surgery has resulted in similar good outcomes in approximately 85% of cases.

The goal of initial treatment is to minimize pain, swelling, and stiffness. Some orthopedists prefer casting, initially, for varying periods of time, depending on the severity of the injury, citing patient comfort, compliance, and ability to bear weight. No data show that immobilization in any position promotes ankle ligament healing. We prefer to avoid casting, if at all possible, because of the potentially deleterious effects of immobilization, such as muscle atrophy and joint stiffness. Casting is reserved for persons with severe pain and swelling and so much guarding that they will not move the ankle through any range of motion. The cast is removed after approximately 1 week, and an elastic bandage or pneumatic compression splint is applied.

Most patients with acute ankle sprains can be kept comfortable enough with an elastic bandage or a pneumatic splint (Fig. 84–4). This permits them to start at least partial weight bearing immediately and, at the same time, to begin dorsiflexion and plantar flexion range of motion exercises as tolerated. The ankle is rested with elevation and ice. As soon as the patient is able, strengthening begins with isometric exercises and advances to progressive isotonic and isokinetic resistance exercises. When the patient's strength permits, proprioceptive exercises are started. The tilt board and balance disc are helpful for restoring proprioception. After normal strength has returned, running and agility activities are allowed. Heel cord stretching should be emphasized throughout rehabilitation, to prevent recurrent ankle sprains.

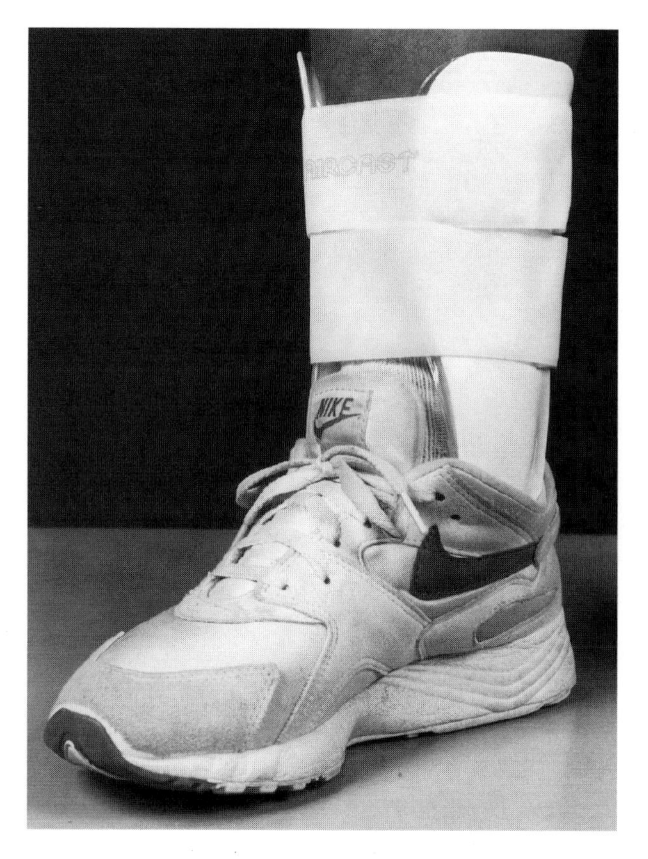

Fig. 84–4. Use of pneumatic compression splint to protect a sprained ankle.

How long an elastic bandage or pneumatic splint should be used depends on the severity of the injury, the activity involved, and the level of the athlete. If the swelling is minimal, several days is usually sufficient. If there is an obvious hematoma or more severe pain owing to the swelling, a 6-week taping protocol is recommended after the swelling has subsided. Persons who participate in recreational activities normally do not have the luxury of being taped and usually do quite well with any of the commercially available protective splints upon returning to activity. The splint is discontinued when the person feels comfortable and confident. The exception is those who have had several previous sprains; in this case, we recommend continued protection whenever the person is participating in agility sports.

Indications for Surgery

Our indication for surgery is no longer based on the traditional grading (i.e., severity) of ligament injury. Differentiation between high- and low-velocity trauma and the degree of damage to the articular cartilage are more important criteria. Surgical intervention is reserved for patients who have chronic functional instability (giving way) and documented mechanical instability and who have not benefited from nonsurgical treatment and for selected other cases, mainly young athletes involved in ball sports who are predisposed to lateral ligament injuries.

ATFL insufficiency plays a key role in disrupting the normal biomechanics of the ankle joint. There is no doubt that chronic instability leads to secondary reactions such as osteochondritis, fatigue fractures of the anterior aspect of the medial and lateral malleoli, osteophytes, and, finally, arthrosis. In ball sports, especially with soccer players, anterolateral rotatory instability, very often including the subtalar joint, is the major factor that leads to those changes. Significant damage to both ankles as a consequence of recurrent dislocations is frequently seen.

This is why we still prefer surgical treatment of injuries secondary to high-velocity trauma in young, active athletes, especially when they have predispositions for recurrent dislocations such as crus varum, pes cavus, hindfoot varus with limited eversion, and tight Achilles tendon. Surgery in the acute setting also permits treatment for those rare cases in which a coexisting ankle injury requires surgical intervention (e.g., displaced fracture, displaced osteochondral lesion of the talus, peroneal tendon rupture or dislocation), though such infrequently are associated with ankle sprains.

Functional treatment after surgery is mandatory. Immediately postoperatively, a dorsal splint is applied and maintained for 3 to 5 days. After the splint is removed, a prescribed exercise schedule is initiated. Seven days after surgery, the sutures are removed, the joint is protected with either an elastic bandage or pneumatic splint for 5 weeks, and rehabilitation is continued, as previously described. Full weight bearing is permitted, as tolerated. The entire postoperative regimen is conducted on an ambulatory basis.

SYNDESMOSIS SPRAINS

Injuries to the ligaments of the tibiofibular syndesmosis usually, but not always, are associated with ankle fractures. The "frank" ankle diastasis without fracture can be either a straight, lateral fibular subluxation (Type I); straight, lateral fibular subluxation with plastic deformation of the fibula (Type II); posterior, rotatory subluxation of the fibula (Type III); or superior dislocation of the talus (Type IV).[18]

Diagnosis

If the patient's history and the mechanism of injury are not the usual inversion injury that results in a lateral ligament sprain, a syndesmosis sprain should be suspected. An example would be an athlete who is stopped and then pushed back on a planted foot, resulting in an eversion–external rotation injury (Fig. 84–5). On physical examination, tenderness over the distal tibiofibular and deltoid ligaments and the squeeze test at the midcalf level help confirm the diagnosis.

AP, lateral, and mortise radiographs of the ankle should be obtained whenever syndesmosis injury is suspected. If routine radiographs are normal, stress views with external rotation may confirm the diagnosis. Arthrography and scintigraphy also have been reported to help demonstrate syndesmosis disruptions.[19–21]

Treatment

Treatment depends on the severity of the injury and the degree of instability. If no instability is demonstrated on stress tests, the patient is permitted to bear weight as tolerated, using an elastic bandage or pneumatic splint for protection while progressing through a rehabilitation program similar to that for an inversion sprain. A longer recovery period can be expected than that for a typical inversion sprain.

If a patient has normal radiographs but demonstrates laxity on stress testing, the ankle is immobilized with a long-leg cast for approximately 6 weeks, and frequent followup radiographs are obtained during the first 3 weeks. If radiographs show acute disruption of the syndesmosis or if the patient develops diastasis during conservative treatment, surgical intervention with screw fixation is necessary for stabilization.

After the wounds are healed, a postoperative splint is applied, range of motion exercises are started immediately, and protective weight bearing is permitted as tolerated. The screw is removed 8 to 12 weeks after surgery, and rehabilitation is accelerated. The athlete usually is able to return to activity 3 to 4 months following surgery.

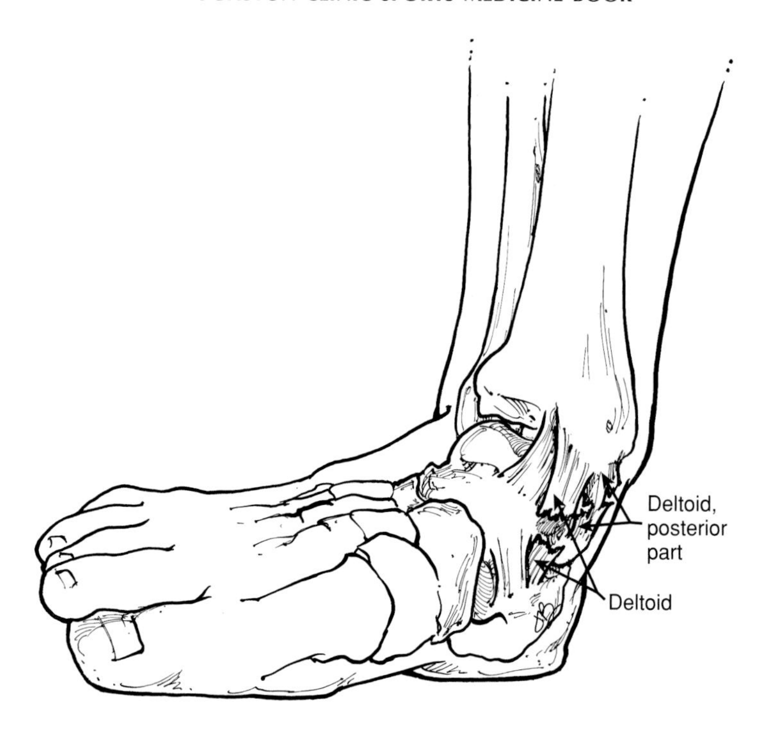

Fig. 84–5. Eversion and external rotation injury resulted in a syndesmosis sprain.

MEDIAL LIGAMENT SPRAINS

Forced external rotation and abduction (whether combined with forced plantar flexion or neutral position of the ankle or neither) causes partial rupture of the medial deltoid ligament (Fig. 84–6). Isolated tears of the deltoid ligament are extremely rare and normally have no clinical consequences. Tears of the deltoid ligament typically are associated with a syndesmosis injury or fibular fracture. Because the deltoid ligament offers significant restraint to internal rotation during axial loading, it can also be injured during sprains to the lateral ligaments.

Diagnosis

On physical examination, tenderness can be elicited over the deltoid ligament and over the anterior syndesmosis, lateral malleolus, or proximal fibula, depending on the presence of other injuries. Ankle joint stability and posterior tibial tendon function should be evaluated. Routine and stress radiographs can help assess stability and determine treatment.

Treatment

The rare isolated deltoid ligament tear or a deltoid ligament injury associated with a stable syndesmosis sprain is managed nonsurgically with protected mobilization or cast immobilization. Surgery for an unstable syndesmosis rupture is described above. The deep deltoid ligament is approached surgically only when it is necessary to extricate it to reduce the ankle joint.

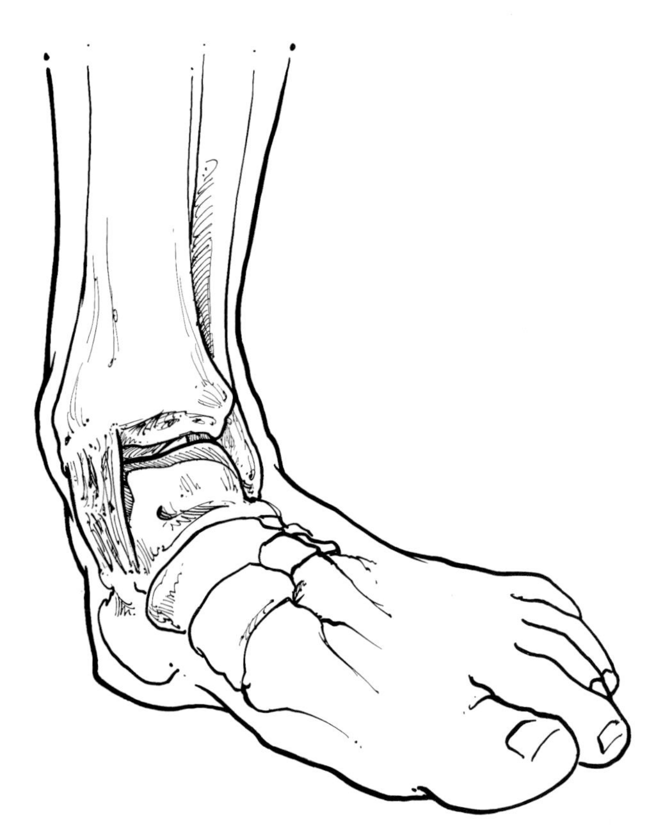

Fig. 84–6. Forced external rotation and abduction injury resulted in partial rupture of the deltoid ligament.

RESIDUAL SYMPTOMS

The large percentage of residual complaints seemingly unrelated to the form of primary treatment is difficult to explain. Residual symptoms, which occur frequently, include recurrent dislocation, functional instability, and pain, stiffness, and swelling during or after activity. In many cases, these residual findings are manifested on the medial side of the ankle joint. The most important causes of these symptoms are impaired proprioception, decreased muscle coordination and strength, weakness of the peroneal muscle, synovitis (including adhesions and synovial impingement), and chondral and osteochondral lesions.

In general, a larger percentage of residual symptoms is observed after a short followup period. With longer followups, the symptoms depend not only on the severity of the initial trauma but also on additional trauma associated with recurrent dislocations. A higher level of activity puts greater demands on the involved ankle joint. In patients without functional instability, it is particularly difficult to interpret and treat ongoing pain.

In patients who rupture one or more of the lateral ankle ligaments following inversion trauma, impingement can occur between the medial malleolus and the medial facet of the talus. This can lead to microscopic cartilage damage, especially in athletes who sustain high-velocity trauma. In these cases, surgical repair and functional postoperative treatment are indicated to restore normal biomechanics and prevent arthritic changes in younger, very active athletes.

RECURRENT INSTABILITY

Recurrent instability of the ankle joint is a clinical diagnosis. The patient's history is more important than objective findings such as talar tilt, but there is no good correlation between functional instability and demonstrable mechanical instability. Thus, before surgery is considered, an aggressive rehabilitation program should be implemented, even for patients with true mechanical instability and recurrent sprains. Many patients with chronic functional instability have improved dramatically as a result of appropriate rehabilitation.

Recurrent dislocations, unsteadiness in walking, and inability to participate in sports activities are reasons for surgical intervention. Before surgery, the patient should be prepared with conservative treatment, including coordination and muscle training and the use of adequate shoes. After surgery, the ankle is immobilized in a plaster splint for as long as 5 days. The patient is then allowed to perform dorsal and plantar flexion exercises. After the wound has healed and joint function is restored, a below-knee walking cast is worn for approximately 6 weeks.

REFERENCES

1. Brooks, S. C., Potter, B. T., and Rainey, J. B.: Treatment for partial tears of the lateral ligament of the ankle: A prospective trial. Br. Med. J. *282*:606, 1981.
2. Rijke, A. M., Jones, B., and Vierhout, P. A. M.: Stress examination of traumatized lateral ligaments of the ankle. Clin. Orthop. *210*:143, 1986.
3. Watson-Jones, R.: Fractures and Joint Injuries. 4th Ed. London, E & S Livingstone, 1955.
4. Niethard, F. U.: Die Stabilitat des Sprunggelenkes nach Ruptur des lateralen Bandapparates. Arch. Orthop. Unfallchir. *80*:53, 1974.
5. Reichen, A., and Marti, R. K.: Die frische fibulare Bandruptur. Helv. Chir. Acta *42*:23, 1975.
6. Prins, J. G.: Diagnosis and treatment of injury to the lateral ligaments of the ankle. Acta Chir. Scand. (Suppl.):*486*:3, 1978.
7. Raaymakers, E. L. F. B., van Bergen Henegouwen, D. P., van Os, J. H., and Marti, R. K.: Operatieve behandeling van de laterale enkelbandruptuur. Geneesk Sport *12*:25, 1979.
8. Gronmark, T., Johnsen, O., and Kogstad, O.: Rupture of the lateral ligaments of the ankle: A controlled clinical trial. Injury *11*:215, 1980.
9. Storemont, D. M., Morrey, B. F., An, K. N., and Cass, J. R.: Stability of the loaded ankle: Relation between articular restraint and primary and secondary static restraints. Am. J. Sports Med. *13*:295, 1985.
10. Cass, J. R., and Morrey, B. F.: Ankle instability: Current concepts, diagnosis, and treatment. Mayo Clin. Proc. *59*:165, 1984.
11. Meals, R. A.: Peroneal-nerve palsy complicating ankle sprain: Report of two cases and review of the literature. J. Bone Joint Surg. *59A*:966, 1977.
12. van Dijk, C. N.: On diagnostic strategies in patients with severe ankle sprain. Thesis, University of Amsterdam, 1994.
13. Spiegel, P. K., and Staples, O. S.: Arthrography of the ankle joint: Problems in diagnosis of acute lateral ligament injuries. Radiology *114*:587, 1975.
14. van den Hoogenband, C. R., and van Moppes, F. I.: Die Behandlung der lateralen Ligamentrupturen des oberen Sprunggelenkes mit der Coumans-Bandage und direkter Mobilisation. Eine prospective Vergleichs-studie. Hefte Unfallheilkunde *189*:1030, 1987.
15. Mayer, F., Herberger, U., Reuber, H., and Meyer, U.: Vergleich der Wertigkeit gehaltener Aufnahmen und der Arthrographie des oberen Sprunggelenks bei Verletzungen des lateralen Bandkapselapparates. Unfallchirurg. *90*:86, 1987.
16. Bleichrodt, R. P., Kingma, L. M., Binnendijk, B., and Klein, J. P.: Injuries of the lateral ankle ligaments: Classification with tenography and arthrography. Radiology *173*:347, 1989.
17. Kannus, P., and Renstrom, P.: Treatment for acute tears of the lateral ligaments of the ankle joint. J. Bone Joint Surg. *73A*:305, 1991.
18. Edwards, G. S., Jr., and DeLee J. C.: Ankle diastasis without fracture. Foot Ankle *4*:305, 1984.
19. Brostrom, L., Liljedahl, S. O., and Lindvall, N.: Sprained ankles II: Arthrographic diagnosis of recent ligament ruptures. Acta Chir. Scand. *129*:485, 1965.
20. Katznelson, A., Lin, E., and Militiano, J.: Ruptures of the ligaments about the tibiofibular syndesmosis. Injury *15*:170, 1983.
21. Marymont, J. V., Lynch, M. A., and Henning, C. E.: Acute ligamentous diastasis of the ankle without fracture: Evaluation by radionuclide imaging. Am. J. Sports Med. *14*:407, 1986.

85

J. William Van Manen

Traumatic Ankle and Foot Injuries

The foot and ankle are commonly injured areas of the body, and the distribution of injuries in sports as a whole seems to parallel non–sports-related injuries. Whereas approximately 15% of football injuries and 18% of baseball injuries affect the ankle and foot, in basketball and tennis this figure increases to more than 40%. In terms of numbers of injuries, the foot and ankle are major sites of athletic disability. It is apparent that a good understanding of the anatomy—and of the injury—is very important for those who manage injuries in this area.

EMERGENT CARE OF FOOT AND ANKLE TRAUMA

In the absence of life-threatening injuries, the key to emergency care is to prevent further injury. Further injury may occur in several ways: tissue ischemia, infection, or further mechanical trauma. Knowledge of these can allow one to recognize and take action to minimize the consequences.

Tissue Ischemia

Loss of arterial blood supply owing to disruption of the artery is rare in the foot and ankle, but a severely displaced ankle or foot injury is a common cause of loss of arterial blood flow. Loss of circulation for more than 2 to 4 hours may result in irreversible ischemic changes. Immediate assessment of pulses, followed by prompt reduction of the dislocation, should prevent this complication by restoring circulation early.

A second cause of ischemic injury is a condition called *compartment syndrome*. This is a common sequela of tibial fractures, but it is less frequently recognized in the foot. Crushing injuries, calcaneus fractures, and tarsometatarsal joint injuries commonly result in compartment syndrome.

Swelling and severe pain (out of proportion to apparent injury) are the hallmarks of presentation. Good pulses and normal skin color are *not* findings that rule out compartment syndrome. If a patient is still experiencing severe pain despite immobilization, compartment syndrome must be considered. Compartment syndrome may evolve over several hours, so followup for 12 to 24 hours of the patient with "at risk" injuries is necessary. Swelling and bleeding into a compartment may elevate pressure so that capillary blood flow ceases. Left untreated, the structures in the compartment suffer ischemic tissue injury. Surgically opening the compartment allows interstitial pressures to return to normal and prevents permanent ischemic injury.

Infection

Infection of open wounds is another mechanism by which further tissue injury can occur. One of the goals of emergency management of open wounds is to minimize the risk of infection. Clinical judgment is used to decide how aggressive the treatment needs to be for prevention. At minimum, wound cleaning and sterile bandaging are required. If the wound is large, soft tissue injury is extensive, and gross contamination is present, or if an open fracture exists, tetanus prophylaxis, early use of systemic antibiotics, and surgical débridement are required.

One open injury in the foot deserves particular attention. Puncture wounds to the foot that occur when the object passes through an athletic shoe can result in *Pseudomonas* infection. These injuries look innocuous and are often followed by several days of minimal discomfort. Increased pain and local signs of infection should be aggressively evaluated and treated. Broad-spectrum antibiotic prophylaxis has been recommended for such wounds, and aggressive surgical care and appropriate antibiotic coverage are needed if infection occurs.

Mechanical Trauma

Finally, and equally important in the prevention of further injury, is the time-honored practice of splinting the injured extremity. Splinting can prevent a closed fracture from becoming open. Hemorrhage is minimized by immobilization because clot-disrupting motion is avoided. Pain control is also optimized and splinting allows the patient to be moved about safely.

INJURIES TO THE ANKLE AND HINDFOOT

Ankle Fractures

Ankle fractures are among the most common major joint injuries. Though many injuries around the ankle are technically "ankle fractures," only those that involve disruption of the ankle mortise are normally considered ankle fractures. The ankle mortise is the osseous and ligamentous structures within which the talus is cradled. Injuries to the ankle mortise are usually due to indirect forces (adduction, abduction, or rotation between the lower leg and foot) and can occur in virtually any sports activity.

Initial evaluation of an ankle injury involves asking the athlete how the injury occurred: Was there an audible "pop"? Could the athlete bear weight on the injured extremity? Was any deformity observed? The physical examination should first document the neurovascular status of the affected extremity and then localize sites of tenderness. (Tenderness may be elicited all the way up to the knee in certain ankle fractures.) Any deformity should be noted. The injury should be splinted to prevent further injury.

Radiographs of the ankle in a routine trauma series include anteroposterior (AP), lateral, and mortise (20° internal rotation oblique) views. If pain or tenderness is present proximal to the ankle, two views of the lower leg are also required. The radiographs should be evaluated for (1) the presence or absence of a medial malleolar fracture or widening of the space between the medial malleolus and the talus; (2) the presence or absence of a fibular fracture, its relationship to the tibial plafond (i.e., at, above, or below), and the orientation of the fracture (e.g., transverse, oblique, comminuted); (3) displacement of the distal tibiofibular joint (to assess competence of the syndesmosis); and (4) displacement of the talus from its normal anatomic position beneath the tibia.

Using a system for classification of ankle fractures allows better communication when discussing treatment options. The Lauge-Hansen system is based on the mechanism of injury and foot position, and direction of force at the time of injury (Table 85–1). This information can be inferred from the fracture pattern.

Ankle fractures may be treated with or without internal fixation. The final results appear to be most closely correlated with how accurately the reduction is obtained and maintained. An isolated, nondisplaced fracture of the distal medial malleolus or lateral malleolus may be managed by immobilization in a weight-bearing short-leg cast or even a brace. A nondisplaced bimalleolar fracture may require a long-leg cast with the knee in flexion to ensure control. In either case, weekly assessment with radiographs for 3 to 4 weeks is necessary to ensure that this position is not lost.

Table 85–1. Lauge-Hansen Classification System for Ankle Fractures

Supination-Adduction
- Stage I: Transverse fracture of the fibula distal to the plafond or rupture of the lateral ligament complex
- Stage II: Includes vertical fracture of the medial malleolus

Supination-Eversion
- Stage I: Injury to the anterior tibiofibular ligament
- Stage II: Spiral-oblique fracture of the fibula at the level of the plafond
- Stage III: Fracture of the posterior lip of the tibia
- Stage IV: Transverse fracture of the medial malleolus or rupture of the deltoid ligament

Pronation-Adduction
- Stage I: Transverse fracture of the medial malleolus or rupture of the deltoid ligament
- Stage II: Rupture of the anterior and the posterior tibiofibular ligaments
- Stage III: Includes short oblique fracture of the lateral malleolus

Pronation-Eversion
- Stage I: Transverse fracture of the medial malleolus or rupture of the deltoid ligament
- Stage II: Includes rupture of the syndesmosis
- Stage III: Spiral-oblique fracture of the fibula proximal to the plafond
- Stage IV: Avulsion fracture of the posterior lip of the tibia

Displaced fractures may be reduced and held with closed management; however, the more unstable the injury, the less likely it is that such a treatment approach will be able to obtain and maintain acceptable reduction. Unstable or unreducible fractures are usually best managed by open reduction and internal fixation.

Stable internal fixation allows for early motion, which can minimize muscle atrophy and osteoporosis. After the fracture has healed, the athlete can return to sports activities when he or she regains 80 to 90% of normal muscle strength. In uncomplicated cases, time lost from practice is usually 3 to 6 months. Return to preinjury status depends on the sport, but it may take 6 to 12 months.

Distal Tibial Physeal Fractures in the Adolescent

The external rotatory forces that cause supination–external rotation and pronation–external rotation fracture patterns in adults can cause a peculiar intra-articular fracture in adolescents. During adolescence, the distal tibial physis closes medially first. Then, over a number of months, the "fused" portion of the physeal plate expands more and more laterad, until the physis is completely closed.

Ankle injuries that occur during the transition period of open physeal growth to fusion of the epiphysis are called *transitional fractures.* Juvenile Tillaux and triplanar fractures are intra-articular fractures in which that portion of the epiphysis that is not yet fused to the metaphysis is displaced. These fractures are complex, and plain radiographs are not adequate for proper evaluation. Accurate assessment of fracture configuration and displacement requires computed tomography (CT; Fig. 85–1).

Growth anomalies are not common after these injuries because so little growth potential remains in the physis. These fractures usually reduce easily but are often difficult to hold to less than 2 mm of residual displacement. Because arthritic changes can be expected over the long term if residual displacement is 2 mm or greater, internal fixation may be required to stabilize the fracture sufficiently. Healing and full return of normal function can be expected within 3 to 6 months after injury.

Osteochondral Fractures of the Ankle

Osteochondral fractures of the ankle most often occur as part of an ankle sprain, when the talus, tilting out of the mortise, strikes the lateral or medial malleolus. The articular surface of the joint is affected, and the fracture is usually located in the most lateral or medial margins of the talar dome. The medial lesion is more posterior than the lateral one. The articular portion of the fibula or medial malleolus can also sustain an osteochondral injury. Nondisplaced fractures should be immobilized in a cast for 6 to 8 weeks. If, after this, a symptomatic nonunion occurs, fragment excision can relieve symptoms. Small displaced fractures require removal. Osteochondritis dissecans of the talus may be a chronic consequence of an osteochondral fracture.

The classification system most often used for osteochondral fractures is that of Berndt and Harty. This system is based on the radiographic appearance of the lesion. Stage I is a compression fracture; Stage II is partial separation of the osteochondral fragment; Stage III is complete separation of the fragment with displacement; and Stage IV is a displaced osteochondral fracture. Variations of this classification system have been made using CT, magnetic resonance imaging (MRI), or arthroscopic appearance of the lesion.

These injuries are not rare, but since they are often subtle or not visible on initial radiographs because they

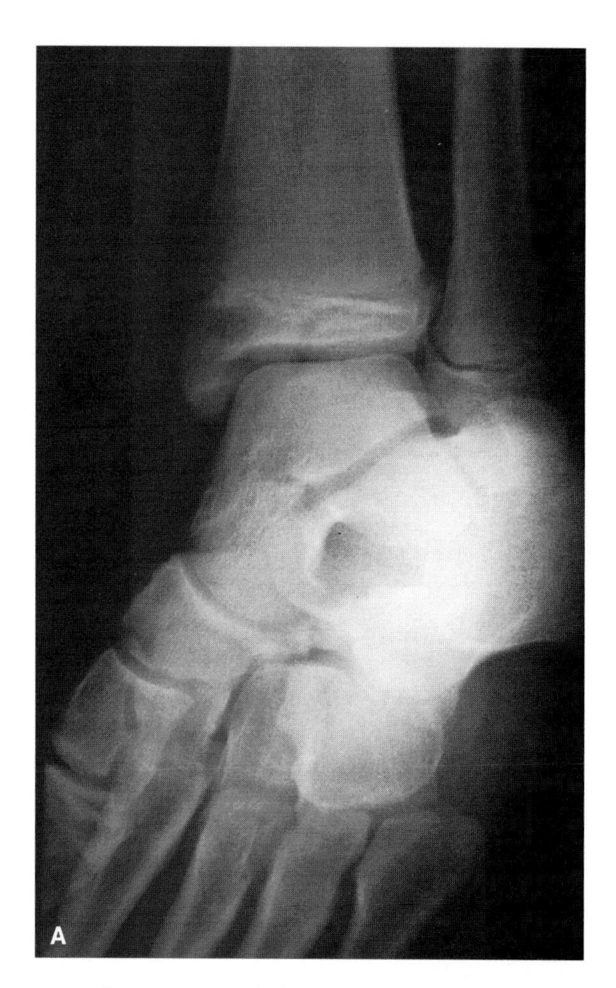

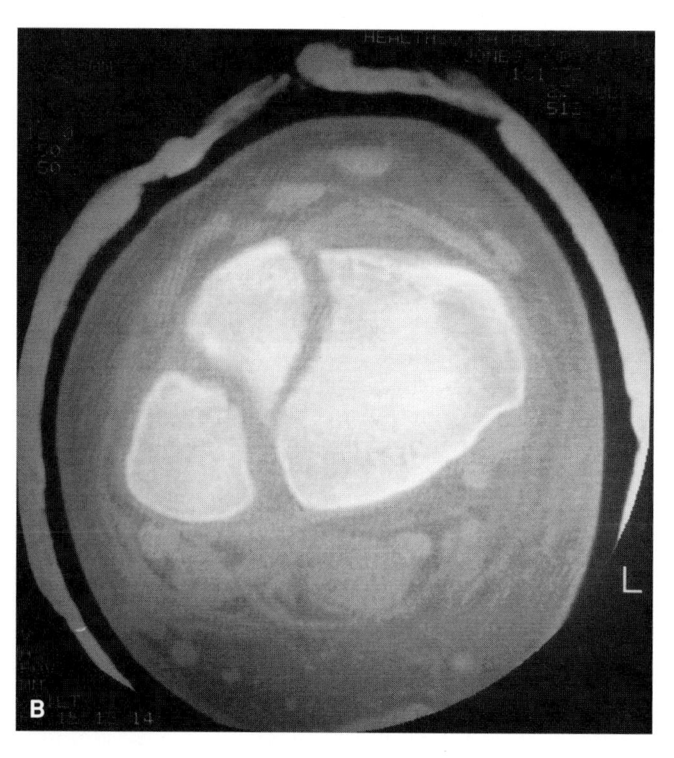

Fig. 85–1. *(A)* A fairly benign-looking fracture of the epiphysis of the distal tibia. *(B)* CT of the same individual shows 4 to 5 mm displacement. This degree of displacement is associated with significant risk of post-traumatic arthrosis.

are either undisplaced or the x-ray projection does not allow visualization, delayed diagnosis is common.

Osteochondral fractures are a common cause of unexplained chronic ankle pain after a sprain. Activity-related pain, swelling, joint catching, weakness, or joint instability may continue for months or years before the diagnosis of an osteochondral lesion is made.

Even if radiographs are normal at the time of initial injury, repeating the radiographic examination is justified if pain is still present 3 to 4 months later. Bone resorption and repair at the injury site may make the fracture visible on followup examination. When the index of suspicion is high but radiographs are negative, bone scan or MRI can identify the presence of an osteochondral fracture (Fig. 85–2).

Treatment of osteochondral fractures depends on the stage of the lesion and the extent of the patient's symptoms. Asymptomatic, nondisplaced lesions do not require treatment. Symptomatic Stage I and II lesions often respond well to 6 weeks in a short-leg cast. Medial Stage III lesions also may become asymptomatic after a period of immobilization. Medial Stage IV lesions and lateral Stage III and IV lesions do not respond well to conservative management and require excision. Other lesions that continue to be symptomatic despite immobilization should also respond well to surgical excision.

Surgery can be performed by open arthrotomy or by arthroscopic techniques with good to excellent results expected in 80 to 90% of patients. Longterm results (more than 5 to 10 years followup) have shown progressive symptomatic and radiographic changes consistent with arthrosis in 30 to 60% of patients.

Fractures of the Posterior Process of the Talus

Fractures of the posterior process of the talus are not common injuries; however, they should be considered when a patient has chronic posterior ankle pain. The posterior process varies in size and may have an accessory ossicle associated with it, the os trigonum. The lateral tubercle of the posterior process is the common site of injury and is best seen on lateral radiographs of the

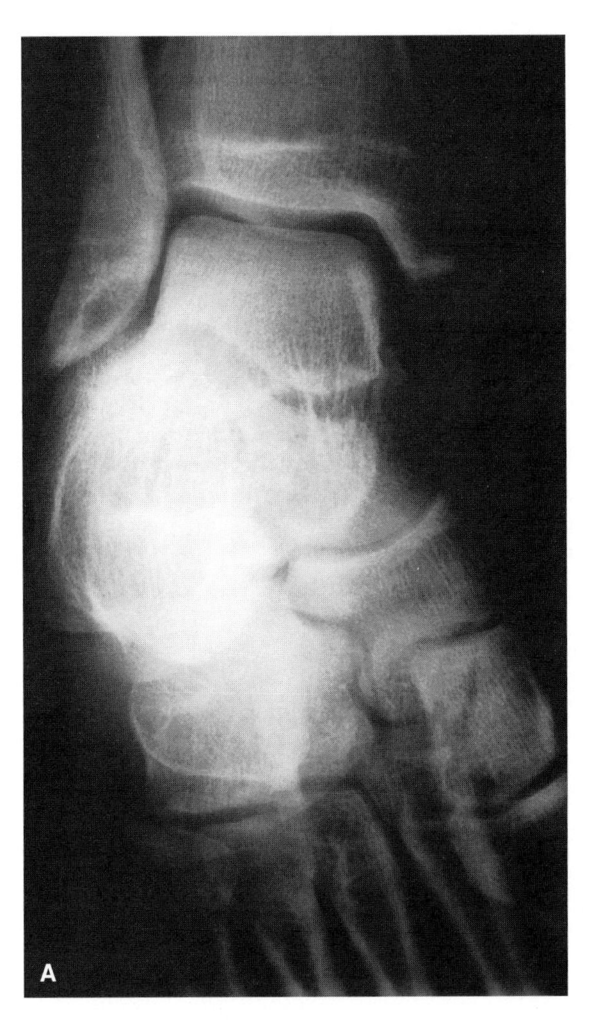

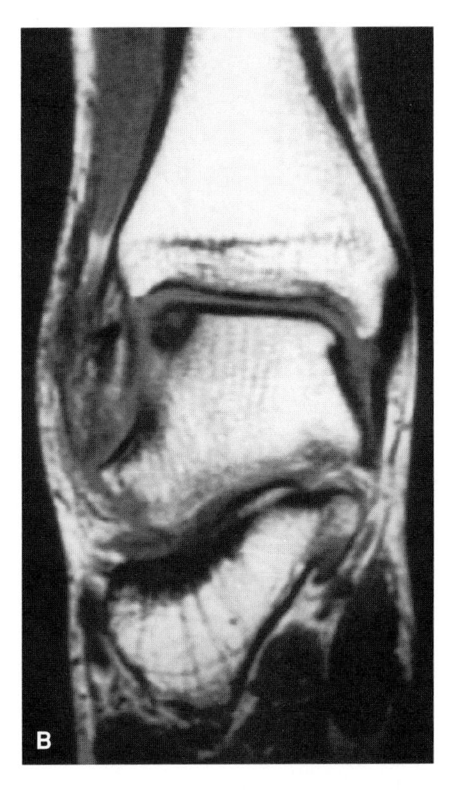

Fig. 85–2. A normal mortise view showed no abnormalities in the talus *(A)*, but this patient had chronic pain and underwent MRI, which revealed a lateral talar osteochondral injury *(B)*.

foot. A fracture can occur as an avulsion of the posterior talofibular ligament during an inversion injury, but an injury caused by direct compression of the posterior process between the calcaneus and tibia during forced plantar flexion is more commonly described (Fig. 85–3). This can occur acutely or as a result of repeated trauma, leading to, in essence, a stress fracture.

The diagnosis is made on clinical grounds. The patient complains of deep posterolateral ankle pain aggravated by activities that force plantar flexion of the foot (e.g., downhill walking or running or the *demi pointe* and *en pointe* position in dance). Tenderness can be elicited with pressure over the posterior talus. Pain may also be noted when flexor hallucis longus function is resisted or when the ankle is forced into plantar flexion.

The injury is best noted on lateral radiographs of the foot. An acute fracture is recognized by irregularity of the fracture margins, whereas os trigonum is characterized by smooth, rounded margins. Radiographs support the clinical findings, but if the clinical impression is uncertain, the presence of an ossicle does not confirm the diagnosis. In these cases, a bone scan may be performed. A positive scan strongly supports a causal relationship between the os trigonum and posterior ankle pain.

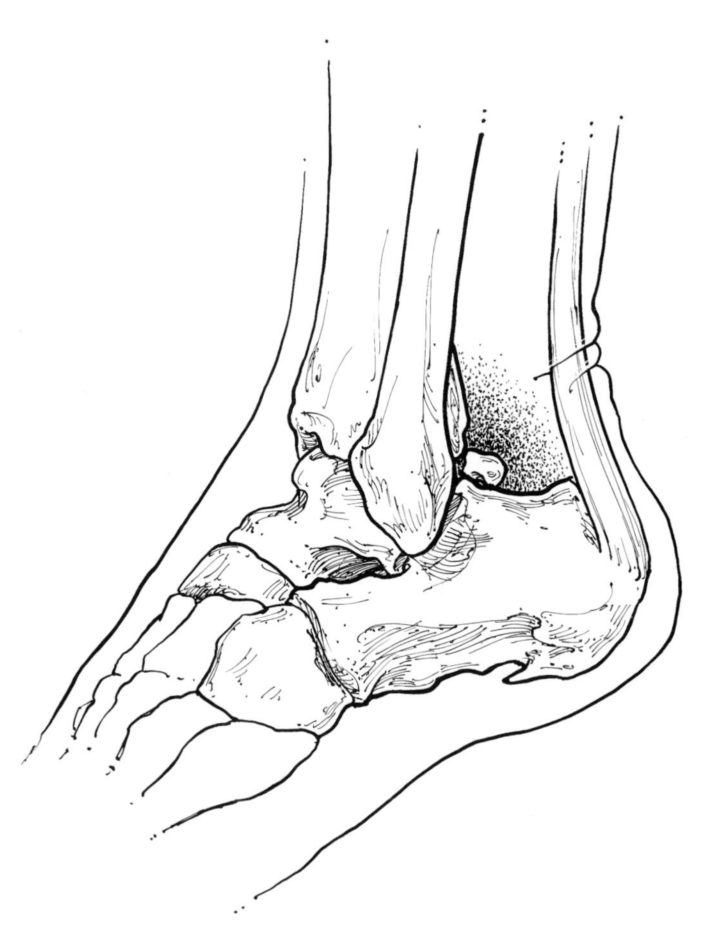

Fig. 85–3. A rendition of a posterior os trigonum–type fracture shows how, on forced plantar flexion, the posterior process can be squeezed between the posterior margin of the tibia and the posterior edge of the subtalar joint on the calcaneus.

Initial treatment is conservative. Immobilization for 4 to 6 weeks has been recommended, and, for an acute fracture, avoidance of weight bearing is also advised. When conservative measures fail to satisfactorily relieve the symptoms, surgical excision is warranted. Although pain relief can be expected, some orthopedists have reported that a significant percentage of patients continued to experience chronic, persistent pain. After surgery, the athlete can usually return to practice within 1 to 3 months.

Talar Neck Fractures

Talar neck fractures are uncommon injuries that are generally due to high-energy trauma. Two very important points must be made about this injury. First, any fracture displacement causes distortion of the subtalar mechanism. For this reason, anatomic reduction is necessary. Second, since the majority of this bone is covered by articular cartilage, the vascular supply is limited. Thus the risk of avascular necrosis is significant after injury.

Subtalar Dislocations

Subtalar dislocations can occur medially or laterally. Medial dislocation is the result of an inversion injury and has been referred to as the *basketball foot.* The dislocated foot is obviously deformed, often with severe tenting of the skin across the talar head. The tension in the skin can result in necrosis, so prompt reduction under anesthesia is recommended.

Reduction is accomplished in a closed fashion in the majority of cases and is usually stable. Only a short period of immobilization (2 to 3 weeks) is recommended because the most common complication is subtalar joint stiffness. Return to normal function is permitted at 6 to 8 weeks if the patient's strength and comfort level are adequate. Strapping of the foot for practice and competition is recommended for 6 to 9 months.

Plantar Fascia Ruptures

Plantar fascia rupture should be suspected when sudden, severe pain occurs in the arch of the foot. Most patients so affected have been athletes who previously had symptoms of or were treated for plantar fasciitis. Many patients have received cortisone injections for plantar fasciitis.

The acute episode is characterized by swelling, and often ecchymosis, located in the arch. Treatment is symptomatic, and return to activity is usually possible within 3 to 6 weeks. Symptoms of pre-existing, chronic plantar fasciitis appear to resolve after resolution of the acute injury.

INJURIES THAT MIMIC ANKLE SPRAINS

Sprains involving the lateral ligaments of the ankle joint have been discussed in another chapter; however, a number of structures on the lateral side of the ankle and foot are vulnerable to the same mechanism of injury. All too often, these injuries are lumped together under the rubric of "ankle sprains." Knowledge of the anatomy and proper examination allow more specific diagnosis. Specific diagnosis has more than academic interest. Treatment and prognosis vary with the type of injury, so the tendency to consider each injury as "just another sprain" must be resisted.

Syndesmosis Sprains (High Ankle Sprains)

Injuries to the ligaments of the distal tibiofibular joint are common. They cause a significant amount of pain and rarely allow the athlete to continue competition the day of injury. They are commonly misdiagnosed as "ankle sprains." The area of tenderness lies over the distal tibiofibular joint, higher on the ankle than a "true" ankle sprain. External rotation of the foot within the mortise as well as tibiofibular compression at midcalf level causes pain at the ankle.

Initial treatment is symptomatic and is geared toward returning the athlete to activity. Strapping may be helpful in controlling symptoms. These injuries, however, have been shown to require two to three times longer recovery before return to competition. Fortunately, chronic pain and instability generally are not seen with these injuries.

Avulsion Fractures of the Tuberosity of the Fifth Metatarsal (Dancer's Fractures)

The peroneus brevis muscle forcefully contracts during inversion injuries, often avulsing its insertion site at the tuberosity (base) of the fifth metatarsal. This injury should not be confused with the more troublesome Jones' fracture, which is discussed later.

Treatment is directed toward the symptoms and toward prevention of severe displacement of the fracture. Therefore, athletic activity should be restricted for at least 6 weeks, and permitted only after good (80%) eversion strength and full muscle control are obtained. Nonunion of these injuries is common, but fibrous healing usually is not symptomatic and does not need treatment.

Dislocations of the Peroneal Tendons

The peroneal retinaculum may be injured by a forceful contraction of the peroneal tendons on a dorsiflexed foot. Within a few hours of injury, swelling on the lateral aspect of the ankle is indistinguishable from that associated with an ankle sprain. Once the swelling is severe, it may be difficult to recognize the tendency of the tendons to move in and out of their normal position. Ankle motion is painful with these injuries, as it is with ankle sprains, so the major differentiating feature on physical examination is the site of maximal tenderness. In an ankle sprain pain is worst anterior to the fibula, whereas with dislocation of the peroneal tendons, tenderness is maximal on the posterior aspect. Radiographs normally show no bone injury, though occasionally an avulsion fracture of the posterior lip of the fibula is seen.

Treatment of this acute injury in an athlete should be surgical repair because the results are excellent in most cases. The prevalence of instability of the tendons after nonoperative management has been reported at 30 to 75%.

Recurrent peroneal tendon subluxation is a cause of recurrent ankle pain or instability in athletes. The patient often complains of painful popping. Because these injuries are commonly misdiagnosed as ankle sprains in the acute setting, the correct diagnosis is usually made weeks or months after the initial injury.

With a chronic lesion, the diagnosis is easily made. The examiner may both observe and palpate the tendons being dislocated from their anatomic position by having the patient evert the foot against resistance in plantar flexion and dorsiflexion. The treatment for symptomatic, chronic peroneal tendon dislocation is surgery. Numerous surgical procedures have been described, but simple surgical repair appears to work as well as any of the reconstructive procedures.

"Ankle Sprains" in Skeletally Immature Athletes

Inversion trauma to the ankle of a skeletally immature athlete frequently causes separation of the distal fibular physis, or growth plate, and spares the lateral ankle ligaments (Fig. 85–4). Physeal fractures are commonly misdiagnosed as ankle sprains because spontaneous reduction usually occurs and radiographs reveal no bone abnormality. The correct diagnosis is made by localizing the site of maximum tenderness and swelling over the distal fibular physis.

Differentiating these injuries is important because, unlike ankle sprains, for which immobilization is controversial, physeal fractures require immobilization to minimize the risk of displacement. Protection with a short-leg walking cast for 4 weeks is recommended. Displaced fractures require reduction, and open reduction and internal fixation may occasionally be necessary.

Injuries to the distal fibular physis due to inversion injuries rarely result in growth abnormalities. While potential for a growth disturbance is small, the athlete's parents should be made aware of the possibility at the initial evaluation. Growth arrest, if it were to occur, can cause severe valgus deformity of the ankle. Return to athletic activity is allowed when full, pain-free range of motion and strength have been restored, usually 6 to 8 weeks after the injury.

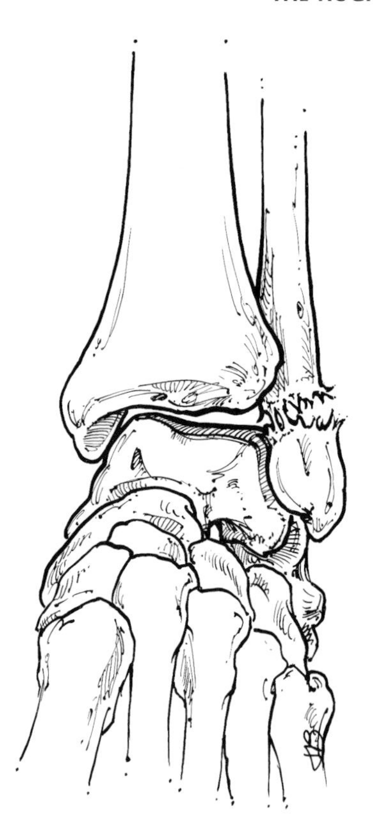

Fig. 85–4. **An inversion injury to the ankle in an immature athlete can avulse the distal physis of the fibula.**

INJURIES TO THE MIDFOOT

The midfoot is a site that is frequently injured in sports, and the area of it most frequently injured is the tarsometatarsal joint (Lisfranc's fracture). Overuse injuries such as stress fractures of the navicular or cuboid bones are sometimes seen in gymnasts and distance runners. Vague, activity-related pain in a runner's midfoot can be shown to be a stress fracture by bone scintigraphy. Rest is required for healing. An accessory navicular may be the cause of medial arch pain, and if immobilization does not relieve the symptoms, surgical excision may be necessary.

Lisfranc's Fractures

Injuries to the tarsometatarsal joints are not uncommon in sports and dance. In football, the injury can result from a blow to the back of the heel when the toes are firmly planted to the ground and the foot in plantar flexion. In baseball, the injury may occur during a slide. In dancers, the injuries occur in a fall from *en pointe* or *demi pointe* position.

As the dorsal ligaments of the joint rupture, the foot collapses into plantar flexion at the tarsometatarsal joint. Fractures of the bases of the metatarsals and of the cuneiforms are frequently associated with the ligamentous injury. Spontaneous reduction often occurs and it is typically so complete that radiographic changes are very subtle. These apparently "slight" changes seen on radiographs are very important to recognize, because only anatomic reduction achieves consistently satisfactory results.

Significant trauma to the tarsometatarsal joint does not allow continued sports participation. Swelling is often severe, but only localized swelling is possible, even in significant injuries. Tenderness can be elicited along the dorsal aspect of the midfoot. Indirect stressing of the joints also results in pain.

Good radiographs are required to assess these injuries. On the lateral view, alignment of the dorsal margin of the first metatarsal with the lateral cuneiform should be anatomic. Anteroposterior views should reveal perfect alignment of the medial edges of the second metatarsal and intermediate cuneiform. The oblique view should reveal the same relationship for the third metatarsal and the lateral cuneiform. The oblique view also allows assessment of the articulation of the cuboid and the fourth and the fifth metatarsal. Fractures of the bases of the metatarsals, a transverse fracture of the base of the second metatarsal, or cuboid fracture should all suggest the possibility of severe ligament injury.

Treatment of these injuries requires anatomic reduction. Subtle displacements are sometimes difficult to discern, even for the trained eye, so physical examination (sometimes under anesthesia) is required to assess stability and, thus, the need for internal fixation. Clinical results are directly correlated with the degree of reduction obtained, but recovery may take several months.

Jones Fractures

Fractures of the metatarsals are usually treated symptomatically and rarely cause longterm problems. The exception is Jones fracture, a transverse fracture at the proximal metaphyseal-diaphyseal junction of the fifth metatarsal. Whether in the acute or the chronic phase, its natural history includes significant risk of delayed union or nonunion. The Jones fracture can present acutely, with sudden onset of pain at the time of injury, no prodromal symptoms, and radiographic signs consistent with acute injury. With a subacute fracture a period of mild discomfort precedes the acute injury and radiographs show a periosteal reaction. The chronic form is nonunion characterized by intramedullary sclerosis.

An acute fracture can be treated by immobilization in either a weight-bearing or non–weight-bearing short-leg cast. Clinical and radiographic union usually are evident in 8 to 12 weeks. Today, most orthopedists recommend non–weight-bearing immobilization. Subacute fractures are treated likewise and appear to have similar results; however, the athlete should be made aware that healing may be protracted and that surgery may be needed in some cases to obtain union. The delayed healing associated with many Jones fractures can result in longterm disability, especially in athletes.

Treatment of chronic nonunion of the fifth metatarsal in an athlete is surgical. Either bone grafting or intramedullary screw fixation works satisfactorily (Fig. 85–5).

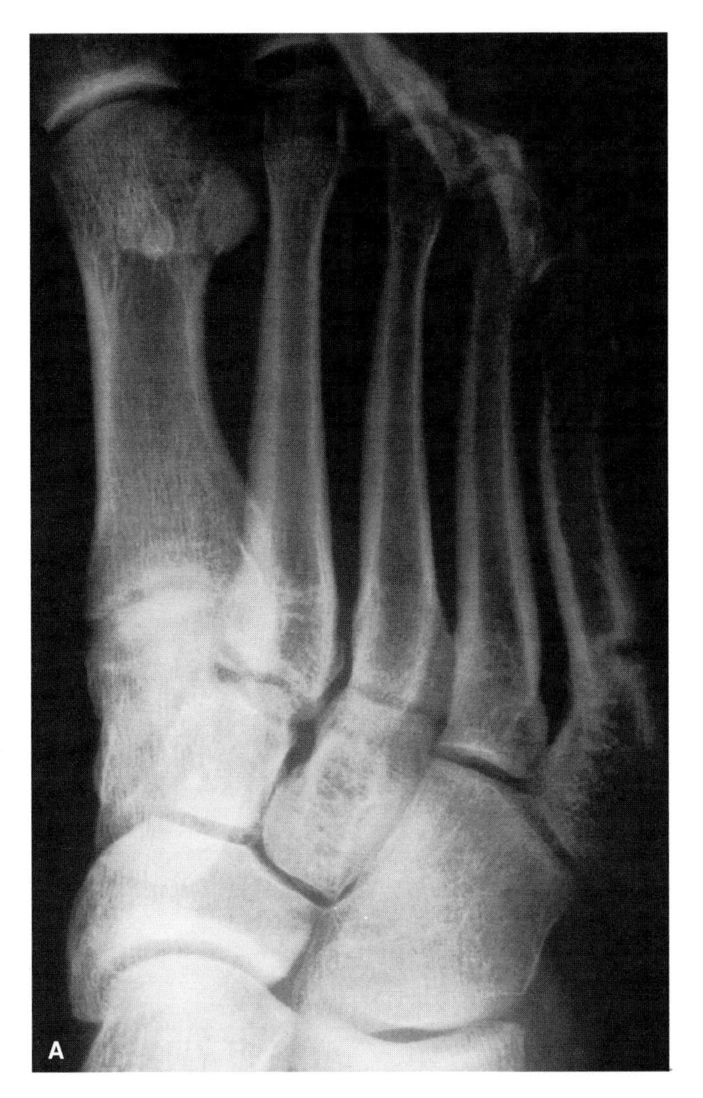

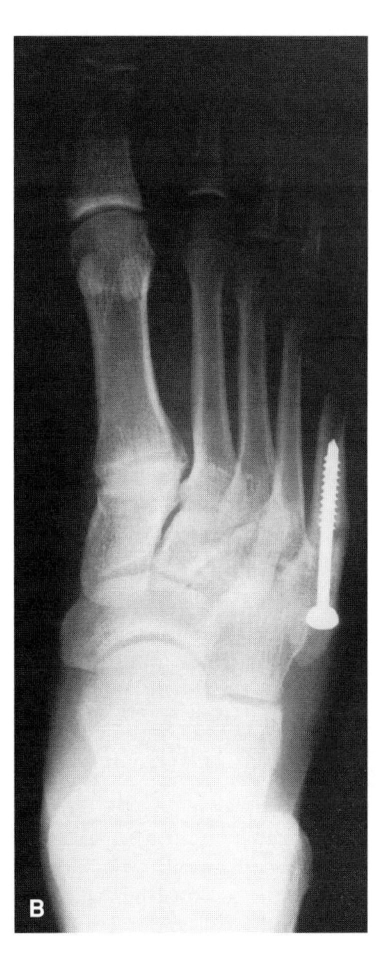

Fig. 85–5. *(A)* **Typical appearance of a chronic nonunion of a Jones fracture. Note the early intramedullary sclerosis, the gaping of the fracture site laterally and the deviation of the metatarsal distal to the fracture.** *(B)* **Six weeks after intramedullary fixation with a screw without bone grafting, the lesion was not tender and bone formation is noted across the lateral fracture site.**

INJURIES TO THE FOREFOOT

Most significant injuries to the forefoot involve the first metatarsophalangeal joint. Injuries (usually fractures) of the lesser toes are often best treated with "buddy taping" until pain subsides. Activities can be continued, as tolerated. Injuries to the great toe can lead to much more disability, as would be expected considering its importance in normal gait mechanics.

Turf Toe

Sprains of the first metatarsophalangeal joint were given the name *turf toe* by Bowers and Martin in 1976, when the injury was attributed to hard artificial turf playing surfaces. Coker and coworkers found that sprains of the first metatarsophalangeal joint in college football players resulted in twice as many missed practices as ankle sprains. In most cases, the injury occurs as a result of hyperextension of the joint. Use of lighter, more flexible shoes appears to have increased the risk of these injuries.

Athletes with these injuries present with pain and swelling. Tenderness and painful motion in the joint can be elicited during physical examination. Swelling and discomfort tend to worsen during the 24 hours after an acute injury. Radiographs may show a capsular avulsion fracture involving the first metatarsal head or the base of the proximal phalanx. Fractures to the sesamoid bones can also be seen with this injury.

Treatment for this injury is rest. A compression dressing, elevation, and ice are useful adjuncts to counteract swelling and pain in the acute phase. Resting the foot can be difficult to enforce, however, because neither the athlete nor the coach can understand why a "simple toe sprain" should restrict activity. Cortisone injections are contraindicated for management of this injury.

Severe injuries can take 3 to 6 weeks to heal, and a too early return to practice can result in a longer period of disability. Taping the toe to resist dorsiflexion forces can both provide pain relief and control swelling. Shoes with stiff soles or a shoe insert can also resist toe dorsiflexion and provide some protection. With proper care, the prognosis for recovery is excellent. Even patients with the more severe injuries return to preinjury activities; however, symptoms of some degree persist in a significant number of athletes.

Injury to the Great Toe Sesamoids

Injury to the sesamoid bones of the great toe may occur as a result of a single acute episode, as seen in turf toe, but more often no specific causative event can be recalled. Pain can be due to fracture, osteochondritis dissecans, sesamoiditis, bursitis, or even from a callus located beneath a sesamoid. The athlete complains of pain in the ball of the foot with weight bearing, but the exact location may be vague. Physical findings usually are normal, except for exquisite tenderness over the affected sesamoid.

Radiographs can confirm the presence of a fracture, but differentiating between an undisplaced fracture and a bipartite sesamoid can be difficult. Other changes that may be seen include a "mottled" appearance, cystic changes, or collapse of the sesamoid that may indicate osteochondritis dissecans (avascular necrosis) of the sesamoid. Pain referable to a sesamoid, but with normal radiographs, is termed sesamoiditis.

Most sesamoid pain is treated with rest and padding of the area to relieve pressure. When symptoms persist, excision of the sesamoid is warranted for pain relief. Gradual return to sports activities is allowed approximately 6 weeks after surgery.

BIBLIOGRAPHY

Acker, J. H., and Drez, D., Jr.: Non-operative treatment of stress fractures of the proximal shaft of the fifth metatarsal (Jones fracture). Foot Ankle *7*:152, 1986.

Berndt, A. L., and Harty, M.: Transchondral fractures (osteochondritis dissecans) of the talus. J. Bone Joint Surg. *41A*:988, 1959.

Bowers, K. D., Jr., Martin, R. B.: Turf-toe: a shoe-surface related football injury. Med. Sci. Sports. *8*:81, 1976.

Clanton, T. O., Butler, J. E., and Eggert, A.: Injuries to the metatarsophalangeal joints in athletes. Foot Ankle *7*:162, 1986.

Coker, T. P., Arnold, J. A., Weber, D. L.: Traumatic lesions of the metatarsophlangeal joint of the great toe in athletes. Am. J. Sports Med. *6*:326, 1978.

Das De, S., and Balasubramaniam, P.: A repair operation for recurrent dislocation of peroneal tendons. J. Bone Joint Surg. *67B*:585, 1985.

DeLee, J. C.: Fractures and dislocations of the foot. *In* Surgery of the Foot and Ankle. 6th Ed. Edited by R. A. Mann and M. J. Coughlin. St. Louis, C. V. Mosby, 1993.

Green, N. E., and Bruno, J., 3rd.: *Pseudomonas* infections of the foot after puncture wounds. South. Med. J. *73*:146, 1980.

Hopkinson, W. J., et al.: Syndesmosis sprains of the ankle. Foot Ankle. *10*:325, 1990.

Mann, R. A.: Biomechanics of the foot and ankle. *In* Surgery of the Foot and Ankle. 6th Ed. Edited by R. A. Mann and M. J. Coughlin. St. Louis, C. V. Mosby, 1993.

Mubarak, S. J., and Hargens, A. R.: Compartment Syndromes and Volkmann's Contracture. Philadelphia, W. B. Saunders, 1981.

Richardson, E. G.: Injuries to the hallucal sesamoids in the athlete. Foot Ankle *7*:229, 1987.

Rockwood, C. A., Green, D. P., and Bucholz, R. W.: Fractures in Adults. 3rd Ed. Philadelphia, J. B. Lippincott, 1991.

Torg, J. S., et al.: Fractures of the base of the fifth metatarsal distal to the tuberosity. J. Bone Joint Surg. *66A*:209, 1984.

Zelko, R. R., Torg, J. S., and Rachun, A.: Proximal diaphyseal fractures of the fifth metatarsal—treatment of the fractures and their complications in athletes. Am. J. Sports Med. *7*:95, 1979.

86 *Peter D. Candelora and Stephen C. Hunter*

Overuse Foot Injuries

Heel Pain

Peter D. Candelora

Although heel pain is a common foot complaint of athletes, the actual origin of the painful heel syndrome is unknown. Some possible causes to be considered include a heel bruise, heel pad trauma, calcaneal stress fracture, plantar fasciitis, tarsal tunnel syndrome, and rupture of the plantar fascia. The precipitating factor can be a sudden increase in activity level, start up of vigorous exercise, or an overuse syndrome due to repetitive trauma.[1] The painful heel can be caused by training errors, abnormal anatomic or biomechanical factors, loose-fitting heel counters in shoes, inflexible soles, inadequate shock absorption at the heel, or inappropriate training surface.

HEEL BRUISE

A heel bruise is often observed in a foot that has a very mobile fat pad.[2] Palpation of the medial tubercle of the calcaneus elicits tenderness. Treatment consists of physical therapy with pulsed ultrasound, to reduce inflammation, and point stimulation, to decrease pain while massaging the fat pad to manually produce lysis of adhesions. A heel cup can be used to help with shock absorption. Cortisone injection may be considered if conservative treatment is unsuccessful; however, fat necrosis can occur as a result of the injections.

HEEL PAD TRAUMA

Repetitive heel pad trauma causes the fat and septa to flatten and spread, resulting in a decreased ability to absorb shock.[2] The heel tends to be painful in the morning and improves shortly after activity begins. The symptoms may be due to transudate, which settles in the heel pad overnight and forms a gluelike fibrin that causes adhesions. After the athlete takes a few steps, the adhesions break up and the symptoms diminish.

CALCANEAL STRESS FRACTURE

Calcaneal stress fracture is usually seen in persons who are inactive and suddenly begin a vigorous sport activity. It is also seen in athletes who perform repetitive activity such as jogging. For athletes, the fracture can be caused by a sudden increase in the intensity or duration of training. Hindfoot varus, causing excessive pronation and internal tibial torque, seems to predispose to stress fractures.[3]

The patient complains of either a sharp, persistent, and sometimes progressive pain, or a deep, dull ache over the calcaneus. A complaint of pain on impact can suggest this problem. Sometimes, pain is elicited by squeezing the medial and lateral borders of the calcaneus. Point tenderness is present on the plantar aspect of the calcaneus.

Early plain lateral radiographs can demonstrate as many as 50% of stress fractures; later, radiographs reveal a higher percentage, when callus formation can be better appreciated. Special lateral views at 45° to the horizontal may also help detect a stress fracture.[4] Bone scans are more specific for early detection of fractures.

Treatment includes complete cessation of the sporting activity and rest until the fracture has healed. For comfort and protection, a short-leg cast may be used for immobilization. Weight bearing and resumption of activity start only when the pain has resolved.

PLANTAR FASCIITIS

The term *plantar fasciitis* refers to a number of disorders associated with the insertion of the plantar fascia at the calcaneal medial tubercle on the plantar surface of the os calcis. It can represent a periosteal avulsion, microtear, or inflammation of the fascia (Fig. 86–1). It is the most common diagnosis for pain at the inferior aspect of the heel.[5] This entity may truly be an overuse syndrome, if repetitive trauma causes microscopic fascial tears and subsequent inflammation.

The patient, often a walker or runner, complains of sharp heel pain, usually, but not always, at the medial process of the calcaneal tuberosity. Sometimes the pain lessens with activity, though it may also be described as a burning sensation or a dull ache felt during activity. Weight bearing exacerbates the pain; rarely is there any swelling. Only 20 to 30% of cases are bilateral.[5]

On physical examination, tautness of the fascia may be noted. Decreased flexibility (i.e., tight Achilles tendon) is an important contributing factor.[6,7] The pain may be elicited by passively stretching the fascia and Achilles tendon, dorsiflexing the foot, or having the patient stand on the toes. Although radiographs show spur formation in 50% of cases, the spurs are not the cause of the pain.[5] Bone scintigraphy or magnetic resonance imaging (MRI) can help elucidate the diagnosis.[8] Electromyographic and nerve conduction studies are normal.

Treatment is usually conservative. Rest and nonsteroidal anti-inflammatory drugs (NSAIDs) can be used for pain relief. Limited dorsiflexion indicates decreased flexibility of the ankle and foot. Heel cord stretching exercises to stretch the Achilles tendon and fascia should be employed. Training techniques and shoe wear should be reviewed.

Training on soft surfaces such as grass can be beneficial. Icing for 20 to 30 minutes following athletic activity may be helpful.

A soft orthotic with a Tuli heel cup should be used. If the athlete has a varus or pronation biomechanical anomaly of the foot, corrective orthotics should be considered. For refractory cases, the use of ankle-foot orthotic night splints with 5° of dorsiflexion has shown good results.[9]

Improvement is usually slow and very gradual. Monthly evaluations should be conducted to provide

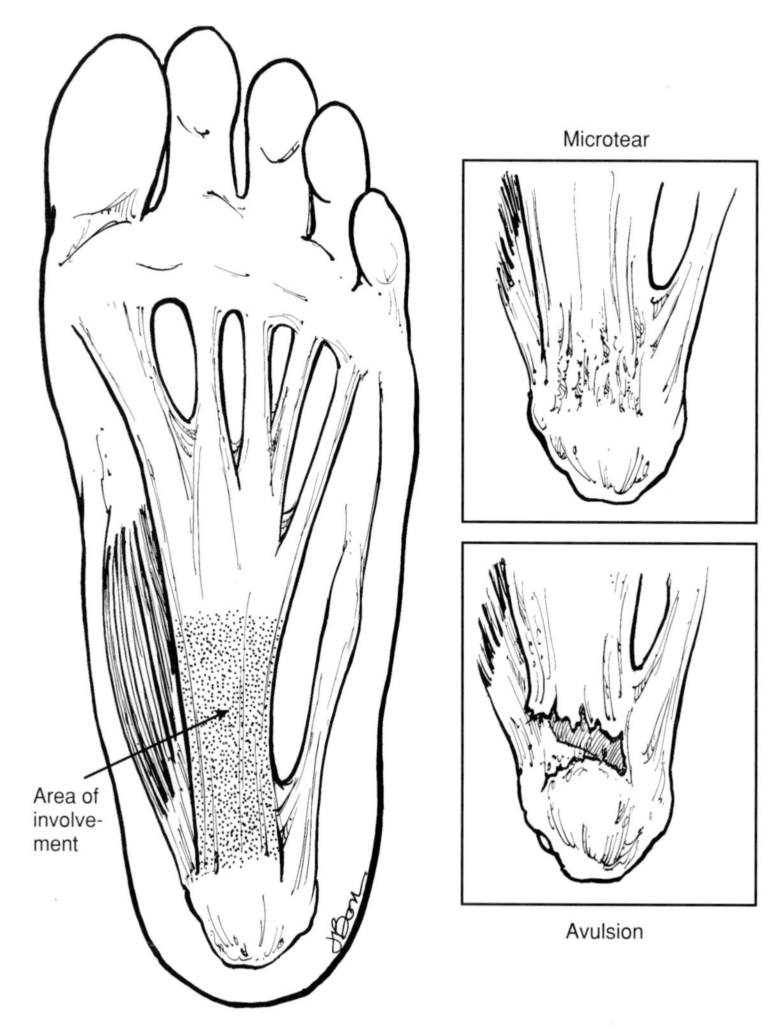

Fig. 86–1. Disorders at the insertion of the plantar fascia at the calcaneal medial tubercle on the plantar surface of the os calcis that can cause plantar fasciitis include periosteal avulsion, microtear, and inflammation of the fascia.

the patient continued support and to document progress (e.g., check degree of dorsiflexion, heel stretching, amount of tenderness, compliance with treatment program). Treatment can go on for over a year. The general rule is that how ever long the problem existed is at least how long it will take to resolve it.

If conservative treatment is unsuccessful, cortisone injection into the medial tubercle may be justified; however, repeated injections can cause plantar fascia rupture or atrophy of the heel pad because of fat necrosis. If all else fails, surgical release of the plantar fascia can be considered, but results vary significantly and current expectations of postoperative success are not as great as they were in the past.

TARSAL TUNNEL SYNDROME

Tarsal tunnel syndrome is entrapment of the posterior tibial nerve in the flexor retinaculum or either or both of the nerve's branches (i.e., the medial and lateral plantar nerves) as they traverse the abductor hallucis muscle (Fig. 86–2). In athletes, the most commonly implicated causes of this problem are heel varus or valgus, fractures, dislocations, and direct pressure (os trigonum).[10–13]

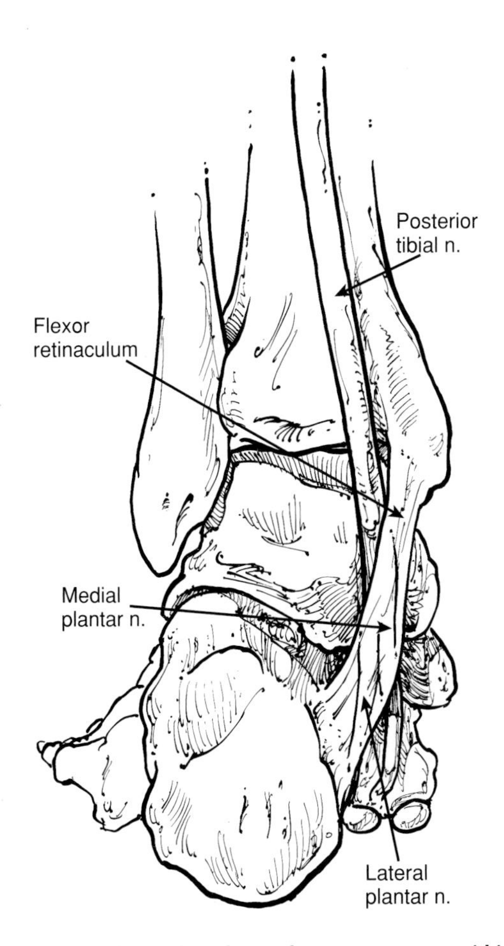

Fig. 86–2. Tarsal tunnel syndrome due to entrapment within the flexor retinaculum of the posterior tibial nerve, or either or both of its branches (i.e., medial and lateral plantar nerves).

Athletes who participate in activities that can result in recurrent or repetitive trauma, such as long distance runners, are most susceptible, especially if while running they exhibit excessive pronation or valgus or external rotation of the foot. Tarsal tunnel syndrome has occasionally been seen in athletes who compete in sports that require a squatting position that results in extreme dorsiflexion of the ankle (e.g., jockeys),[14] and in skiers secondary to compression from ski boots.[10]

Symptoms can include pain in the medial malleolus radiating to the sole of the foot, heel, and occasionally up the calf and leg; paresthesia, dysesthesia, and hyperesthesia; and burning or numbness on the plantar aspect of the foot or toes. Sensory loss may be in the distribution of the medial or lateral plantar nerves, but in most cases, the paresthesia is difficult to delineate clearly.

Pain is poorly localized. Runners may complain of gradual onset of burning heel pain or aching in the arch. Activity usually exacerbates the pain, and cramping in the longitudinal arch is not uncommon. The athlete may also report night pain or pain during rest. Pain may be relieved when the shoes are removed or the feet are elevated.

During the physical examination, abnormal biomechanical alignment of the foot should be assessed by looking for excessive varus or valgus heels, excessive external rotation of the foot, or a high arch. Examining the athlete's shoes may reveal areas of increased wear on the heels or potential impingement in the arch of the foot (causing compression of the medial plantar nerve).

The diagnosis of tarsal tunnel syndrome can be made by eliciting Tinel's sign over the posterior tibial nerve or abductor hallucis. Sometimes, dorsiflexion, inversion, or eversion reproduces the symptoms. Tenderness may be present over the abductor hallucis or proximal or distal to the posterior tibial nerve (Valleix's phenomenon). Pain is usually not found at the insertion of the plantar fascia (as it is in plantar fasciitis). There may be swelling over the course of the posterior tibial nerve from a space-occupying lesion.

Anteroposterior (AP), lateral, and oblique radiographic views should be taken to delineate any soft tissue masses, bony anomalies, or traumatic disorders that might create a space-occupying lesion. MRI may be performed if a mass is believed to be the cause of the syndrome.[15,16] Although the results of electromyographic and nerve conduction studies may be abnormal, they are not always dependable.[14] Sensory action potentials are the most sensitive electrophysiologic test.[17] Pain relief following injection of cortisone and xylocaine directly into the tarsal tunnel can help clinch the diagnosis.

Conservative treatment consists of rest and icing, NSAIDs, change of shoe wear, correction of shoe tightness, additional arch support (though some feel that arch support should be avoided so as not to cause compression over the abductor hallucis[13]), and the use of orthotics to correct abnormal foot biomechanics.[10] Injection of cortisone and xylocaine may also be considered. Several weeks to several months of conservative management should be attempted before trying more aggressive treatment. If conservative measures are not successful, surgical decompression of the tarsal tunnel may be necessary.

RUPTURE OF THE PLANTAR FASCIA

Rupture of the plantar fascia is rare but should be considered when an athlete engaged in a sport that involves a great deal of running or jumping complains of acute heel pain after intense activity. There is localized tenderness and swelling.[18] As swelling decreases, a defect may be palpable at the site of the lesion.

Conservative treatment consists initially of avoidance of weight bearing, use of crutches, and icing for 15 minutes three times a day until the symptoms subside (usually within 2 weeks). Once the pain has resolved, weight bearing can gradually be started. Support to the ruptured area can be provided by a pad or soft orthotic in the shoe and by taping. Crutches should be used until full weight bearing and normal walking are possible. Full training can be resumed when the athlete is able to stand on tiptoe without pain. If conservative measures are not successful, surgical transection of the plantar fascia may be necessary.

HEEL PAIN IN PEDIATRIC AND ADOLESCENT ATHLETES

Heel pain in pediatric and adolescent athletes can be due to the causes already discussed or to others. In some cases, the pain may not have a demonstrable cause. Sever's syndrome, osteochondritis of the apophysis of the calcaneus, can develop in children between ages 5 and 12 years.[19] Point tenderness at the apophysis along with a history of repetitive trauma to the heel or excessive push-off activity (creating traction stress injury) can suggest this syndrome. Treatment consists of rest, decreased activity, heel cord stretching exercises, and the use of a soft heel cup and a quarter-inch heel lift until symptoms resolve.

Tarsal coalition (usually between the calcaneus and the navicular or the calcaneus and the talus) can cause heel pain and is usually seen in athletes in the second decade of life. Physical findings include limited subtalar motion or peroneal muscle spasm on attempted motion.[20] Oblique radiographs and computed tomography can help in the diagnosis. Treatment consists of immobilization with a short-leg cast for 6 to 8 weeks. Weight bearing is allowed during this period. If this does not alleviate the problem, either resection of the coalition or triple arthrodesis is a surgical option; however, most patients can be managed conservatively.

If an obvious cause for heel pain cannot be determined, rest, icing, NSAIDs, and heel cups can be tried on an empirical basis. Continued participation in the sporting activity should be discouraged, and repeated examinations should be conducted to ensure completeness of evaluation. General advice on proper training, warm-up techniques, and the appropriate level of activity should be provided to both the athlete and the athlete's parents.

REFERENCES

1. Harvey, J. S., Jr.: Overuse syndrome in young athletes. Clin. Sports Med. *2*:595, 1983.
2. Kulund, D.: Pain under the heel in runners. Virginia Med. *115*:340, 1988.
3. Lehman, W.: Overuse syndrome in runners. Am. Fam. Physician *29*:157, 1984.
4. Amis, J., Jennings, L., Graham, D., and Graham, C. E.: Painful heel syndrome: Radiographic and treatment assessment. Foot Ankle *9*:91, 1988.
5. Schepsis, A., Leach, R. E., and Gorzyca, J.: Plantar fasciitis. Etiology, treatment, surgical results, and review of the literature. Clin. Orthop. *266*:185, 1991.
6. Kibler, W. B., Goldberg, C., and Chandler, T. J.: Functional biomechanical deficits in running athletes with plantar fasciitis. Am. J. Sports Med. *19*:66, 1991.
7. Warren, B. L.: Plantar fasciitis in runners: Treatment and prevention. Sports Med. *10*:338, 1990.
8. Berkowitz, J., Kier, R., and Rudicel, S.: Plantar fasciitis: MR imaging. Radiology *179*:665, 1991.
9. Wapner, K. L., and Sharkey, P. F.: The use of night splints for treatment of recalcitrant plantar fasciitis. Foot Ankle *12*:135, 1991.
10. Jackson, D. L., and Haglund, B.: Tarsal tunnel syndrome in athletes. Am. J. Sports Med. *19*:61, 1991.
11. Jackson, D. L., and Haglund, B. L.: Tarsal tunnel syndrome in runners. Sports Med. *13*:146, 1992.
12. Murphy, P. C., and Baxter, D. E.: Nerve entrapment of the foot and ankle in runners. Clin. Sports Med. *4*:753, 1985.
13. Rask, M. R.: Medial plantar neurapraxia (Jogger's foot). Clin. Orthop. *134*:193, 1978.
14. Cimino, W. R.: Tarsal tunnel syndrome: Review of the literature. Foot Ankle *11*:47, 1990.
15. Zeiss, J., Ebraheim, N., and Rusin, J.: Magnetic resonance imaging in the diagnosis of tarsal tunnel syndrome. Clin. Imaging *14*:123, 1990.
16. Kerr, R., and Frey, C.: MR imaging in tarsal tunnel syndrome. J. Comput. Asst. Tomogr. *15*:280, 1991.
17. Oh, S. J., Sarala, P. K., Kuba, T., and Elmore, R. S.: Tarsal tunnel syndrome: Electrophysiologic study. Ann. Neurol. *5*:327, 1979.
18. Leach, R., Jones, R., and Silva, T.: Rupture of the plantar fascia in athletes. J. Bone Joint Surg. *60A*:537, 1978.
19. Crosby, L., and McMullen, S.: Heel pain in an active adolescent? Consider calcaneal apophysitis. Physician Sportsmed. *21*(4):89, 1993.
20. Sullivan, J. A.: Recurring pain in the pediatric athlete. Pediatr. Clin. North Am. *31*:1097, 1984.

Forefoot Problems

Stephen C. Hunter

Overuse of the foot can be defined as performing an activity to the point at which the osseous and soft tissue structures are stressed or fatigued beyond their tolerance. This can occur in an athlete with a completely "normal" foot, but it is more likely to happen in a foot that has pre-existing problems. Abnormalities, such as ligament laxity, musculotendinous weakness, or ankylosis of a forefoot joint may set the stage for overuse injuries of the forefoot. Obviously, structural deformities that affect the mechanical function of the foot can increase the risk of overuse injuries.

STRESS FRACTURES

Metatarsal Stress Fracture

A stress fracture of a metatarsal is a disruption of the bony architecture of the shaft of the metatarsal bone. It usually occurs after repetitive loading causes bone failure and fracture. Activities such as marching, long distance running, and dancing can produce stress fractures.

The patient feels pain and may limp because of pain on weight bearing. Some swelling may be present. The diagnosis is often made on a clinical basis, as radiographs may not show evidence of a fracture until weeks after the injury, when new bone forms.

The treatment of choice for metatarsal stress fractures is rest and limited weight bearing. Often, the use of crutches is sufficient, but immobilization by casting may be indicated if the patient has significant pain. Although painful symptoms may persist for 2 to 3 weeks and healing may require 6 to 8 weeks, the overall prognosis is excellent for most patients.

An athlete with a metatarsal stress fracture can be allowed to return gradually to his or her sports activities when all symptoms have abated and radiographs demonstrate good healing of the fracture. Rigid protective footwear can help during the initial period of return to sports activities.

Sesamoid Stress Fracture

Stress fractures of the sesamoids are also caused by excessive functional overload, though they are not a common phenomenon. Localized pain over the sesamoid that is exacerbated by weight bearing or palpation is diagnostic. The fracture is discernible on radiographs and may persist as fibrous union.

Sesamoid stress fractures are treated with rest and splinting. A donut orthotic can be used to protect the pressure point. Casting is rarely necessary. With continued activity, symptoms may persist for months, and nonunion is a possibility. Chronic cases may require surgery to debride or repair nonhealing sesamoid fractures.

An athlete who responds to conservative treatment can return to sports activities gradually. A shoe insert is often helpful to provide splinting of the great toe.

REACTIVE SYNOVITIS

Turf Toe

The term *turf toe* evolved because it affects players who injure the great toe while playing on artificial turf.[1–3] Turf toe is caused by forced dorsiflexion of the metatarsophalangeal joint of the great toe, which jams the proximal phalanx against the metatarsal head because the plantar capsule restricts dorsiflexion. Resultant injuries include sprains of the collateral ligaments, dorsal joint compression, plantar ligament avulsion, and dislocation and fracture of the sesamoids.

Initial treatment of turf toe consists of rest, ice, compression, and elevation. NSAIDs can be useful. After acute symptoms have abated, heat modalities (e.g., whirlpools), active and passive toe motion exercises, and foot-strengthening exercises are beneficial. Protection with a stiff orthotic shoe insert that limits dorsiflexion of the great toe is necessary during rehabilitation.

The athlete should not return to sports activities until all symptoms have resolved; however, the prognosis for turf toe is good, especially a first episode treated early.

Metatarsalgia

Pain beneath the metatarsal heads that is exacerbated by functional activities is often caused by inflammation of the metatarsal bursas or increased pressure points over isolated metatarsal heads.[4,5] The most common cause of metatarsalgia is increased weight-bearing pressure over one metatarsal head. This can irritate the soft tissues about the metatarsal head and cause buildup of callus (transfer lesion). Secondary calluses over the metatarsal heads can compound the pain. Differential diagnoses include stress fractures, neuromas, and avascular necrosis of the metatarsal head.

Focal pressure problems are managed by redistributing the pressure load of the foot. This can be achieved with special shoe inserts designed to lift a prominent metatarsal head. Cutouts of an orthotic insert that accommodate a callus prominence also relieve pressure. In addition, calluses should be trimmed and the athlete's footwear should be examined for deformities that may cause focal pressure points.

Metatarsalgia inflammation can be relieved by foot soaks and NSAIDs. Once the symptoms have resolved, the athlete's prognosis is good and he or she should be able to return to sports activities. The use of orthotics that provide cushioning beneath the metatarsal heads helps prevent recurrence.

Neuritis

Neuritis in the forefoot is due to irritation and resultant inflammation of the intermetatarsal nerves as they branch to become digital sensory nerves. These nerves pass along the plantar surface of the foot beneath the intermetatarsal ligament before coursing up to the toes. The risk of compression and irritation of the nerves in these areas is significant, especially between the third and fourth toes because this nerve is less mobile.

Irritation of the nerves causes inflammation and fibrosis, and subsequently vasculitis, which can stimulate

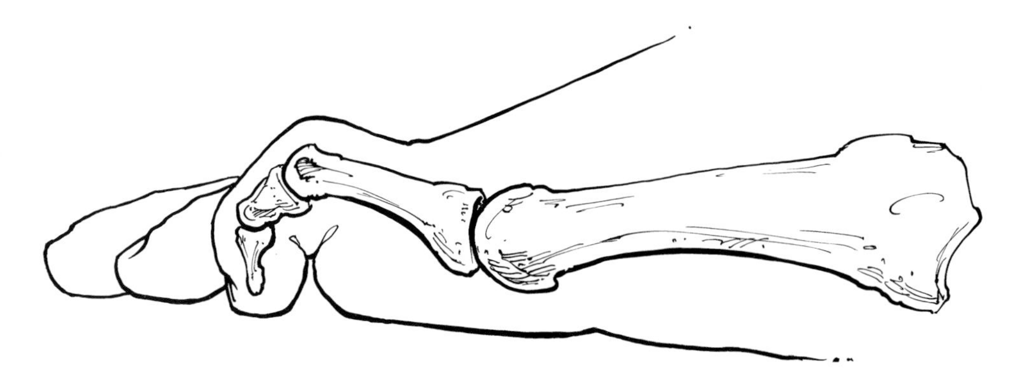

Fig. 86–3. In hammertoe, the metatarsophalangeal joint is extended, the proximal interphalangeal joint is flexed, and the distal interphalangeal joint is extended.

formation of scar tissue about the nerve. A fibrotic pseudotumor, called *Morton's neuroma,* creates an enlarging mass that increases pressure on the nerve and compounds the problem.[6,7]

In its early stages, the condition may respond to conservative treatment, including rest, soaking, protective padding, and NSAIDs. Corticosteroid injections may resolve the inflammation. Chronic neuromas, however, respond poorly to conservative measures and cause significant pain and functional disability. Surgical removal of the neuroma may be necessary to treat these conditions. Although the patient loses some feeling in the toes, it does not cause any disability. Neuromas are not a common athletic problem, but when they are diagnosed and treated appropriately, affected athletes should be able to return to sports activities without problems.

AGGRAVATED DEFORMITIES

Bunions and Bunionettes

Bunions are bony prominences on the medial aspect of the first metatarsal head. A bunionette is a bony prominence on the lateral aspect of the fifth metatarsal head. They are usually asymptomatic unless secondary pressures cause bursal inflammation and pain. These bony prominences are usually caused by congenital metatarsal splaying. They can be accentuated by constricting footwear that forces the toes away from the medial and lateral metatarsal heads. Irritating pressure over the prominences can also be due to constrictive footwear.

The simplest treatment is footwear that has an ample toe box. Braces are not helpful, and donut pads large enough to relieve the pressure over the prominence may not fit in shoes. Severe deformities that cause significant symptoms may require surgical correction. If surgery is necessary, the athlete may be restricted from sports activities for a prolonged period as the bone and ligament repairs heal.

Small Toe Deformities

There are two common small toe deformities (i.e., hammertoe and claw toe) that can cause pain and functional disability in the forefoot.[5,8] These deformities may be congenital or acquired. The acquired type are usually caused by ill-fitting footwear that cramps the toes into abnormal postures. The deformities can occur in one or more toes. The second toe is frequently affected since in some people it is longer even than the great toe.

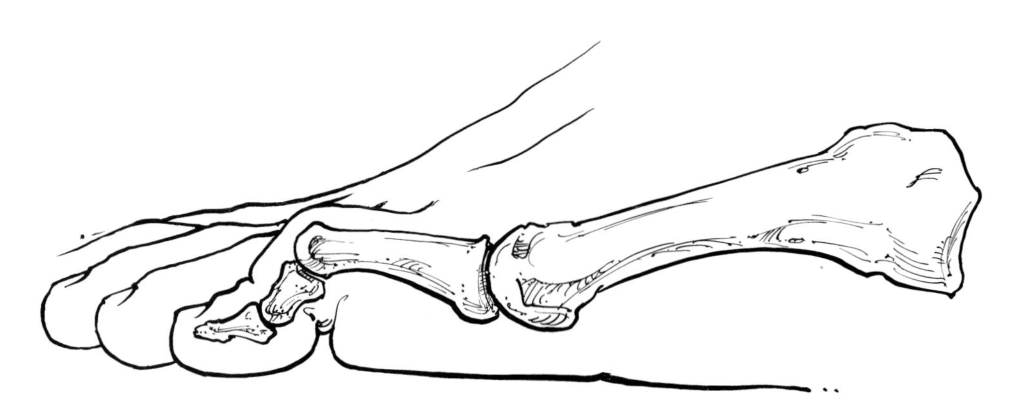

Fig. 86–4. In claw toe, the proximal and the distal interphalangeal joint are flexed, causing excessive extension of the metatarsophalangeal joint.

In hammertoe, the metatarsophalangeal joint is extended, the proximal interphalangeal joint is flexed, and the distal interphalangeal joint is extended (Fig. 86–3). This abnormal posture causes increased pressure in the shoe on both the top and base of the toe, resulting in painful calluses.

In claw toe, both interphalangeal joints are flexed, causing excessive extension of the metatarsophalangeal joint and giving the toe its characteristic clawed appearance (Fig. 86–4).[9] The patient develops painful corns and calluses at the pressure point of each affected toe.

Conservative treatment consists of using shoes with toe boxes large enough to accommodate the toe deformities. Splinting and taping may help if the deformities are not contracted. Pressure calluses that form on the tips and prominences of the toes need to be padded. Surgery may be required to correct severe rigid deformities.[10] Fortunately, hammertoes and claw toes are not common problems in athletes.

REFERENCES

1. Coker, T. P., Arnold, J. A., and Weber, D. L.: Traumatic lesions of the metatarsophalangeal joint of the great toe in athletes. Am. J. Sports Med. *6*:326, 1978.
2. Sammarco, G. J.: Turf toe. Instr. Course Lect. *42*:207, 1993.
3. Rodeo, S. A., et al.: Turf-toe: An analysis of metatarsophalangeal joint sprains in professional football players. Am. J. Sports Med. *18*:280, 1990.
4. Gould, J. S.: Metatarsalgia. Orthop. Clin. North Am. *20*:553, 1989.
5. Bordelon, R. L.: Management of disorders of the forefoot and toenails associated with running. Clin. Sports Med. *4*:717, 1985.
6. Shichikawa, K.: Morton's metatarsalgia. Rheumatism *22*:30, 1966.
7. Alexander, I. J., Johnson, K. A., and Parr, J. W.: Morton's neuroma: A review of recent concepts. Orthopedics *10*:103, 1987.
8. Coughlin, M. J.: Mallet toes, hammertoes, claw toes, and corns. Postgrad. Med. *75*:191, 1984.
9. Garth, W. P., Jr., and Miller, S. T.: Evaluation of claw toe deformity, weakness of the foot intrinsics, and posteromedial shin pain. Am. J. Sports Med. *17*:821, 1989.
10. Turan, I.: Deformities of the smaller toes and surgical treatment. J. Foot Surg. *29*:176, 1990.

87 *David F. Martin and Walton W. Curl*

Arthroscopy in the Treatment of Ankle Disorders

In recent years, ankle arthroscopy has gained general acceptance, both as a diagnostic tool and as a means for surgically treating a variety of ankle conditions.[1–7] As a result, it has become a valuable procedure for sports medicine physicians. Because of the irregular shapes of the bones around the ankle joint, accurate imaging of the area can be difficult.[8] Ankle joint arthroscopy is an excellent tool for identifying intra-articular disorders, and it can be applied when, though extra-articular causes have been ruled out, the athlete continues to experience symptoms in the joint despite conservative treatment.[9]

The procedure can also help physicians treat ankle problems in season. Arthroscopic surgery has a relatively low morbidity and a reasonably rapid recovery time that allows the athlete to return to sports activity quickly and safely. In many cases, recovery time is shorter than after an open surgical procedure.[10] Even though arthroscopic instruments have improved much, and despite the small incisions, aggressive surgery can be performed. This makes appropriate pre- and postoperative rehabilitation extremely important. The results of arthroscopic procedures in athletes' ankles are enhanced when range of motion, strengthening, and agility conditioning are emphasized.

Arthroscopy of the ankle joint should not be taken lightly or considered to be a benign technique. Complications can occur that permanently damage the ankle.[6,11] Thus, the procedure must be used advisedly. When an athlete has no mechanical symptoms and examination reveals minimal physical findings, arthroscopy may have no significant benefit. In this case, conservative management, with emphasis on conditioning exercises, should be the first line of treatment. If, despite conservative treatment, an athlete has a demonstrable intra-articular disorder, mechanical symptoms, or continued swelling, ankle arthroscopy can be extremely valuable in making the correct diagnosis and rendering appropriate treatment.

INDICATIONS

As the techniques of ankle joint arthroscopy have been refined, indications for its use have increased.[6,12] Caution remains key, since many uses of arthroscopy have not been evaluated for longterm results.[1,3–5,13–15] It is helpful to classify the indications for ankle arthroscopy into four general categories that cover injuries to athletes of all ages.

The first category is soft tissue disorders—synovitis, impingement, adhesions, and instability. Next are osteochondral disorders, which include chondromalacia, transchondral talar dome fractures, loose bodies, and osteophytes. Third is arthritic conditions, which can be due to post-traumatic degeneration, degenerative disease, rheumatoid arthritis, or infection. The final category is persistent ankle pain, the cause of which may be unclear. In these cases, it is important to be aware of the possibility of reflex sympathetic dystrophy (RSD).

Previously, evaluation and treatment for many of these disorders required arthrotomy, which resulted in significant morbidity. It is difficult to properly assess intra-articular conditions of the entire ankle joint through a single arthrotomy. Arthroscopy, on the other hand, is less invasive and permits good visualization anteriorly, posteriorly, medially, and laterally. Thus, this important weight-bearing joint can be fully and safely evaluated without arthrotomy, and valuable information can be obtained for determining necessary treatment, planning postoperative rehabilitation, and developing recommendations for longterm activity. For example, a recreational athlete with mild degenerative changes accompanying a meniscoid lesion can be cautioned to avoid impact-loading activities and to modify sports participation accordingly.

Arthroscopy is also less invasive than arthrotomy, and intra-articular disorders can be treated with significantly less morbidity, allowing for quicker return to sports activities.[10] Operative procedures that can be performed arthroscopically include synovectomy, lysis of adhesions, lateral ligamentous reconstruction, débridement of transchondral talar dome fractures, removal of loose bodies, and meniscoid or osteophyte excision.[6,14,16–19]

There are a number of contraindications to ankle arthroscopy. Though most are rare in athletes, they must nonetheless be considered. It is generally accepted that extravasation is not a problem around the ankle; however, significant edema or soft tissue swelling impedes arthroscopy. The presence of edema limits the mobility of the arthroscope within the joint and obscures portal anatomy. Severe degenerative joint disease and ankle joint ankylosis can narrow the joint space and cause technical difficulty with getting the arthroscope and other instruments into the joint itself. Patients with compromised skin conditions or skin breakdown around the ankle joint should not undergo arthroscopy until the problem is treated. A good example of this is an ankle that has been taped for support and develops a rash. Such rashes can be superinfected with *Staphylococcus* organisms. Other potential contraindications include generalized infection, neuromuscular abnormalities, and anesthesia risks.

INSTRUMENTATION

Instrumentation has improved substantially since the early 1980s, which has made possible significant advances in ankle arthroscopic surgery.[12] A video system is now considered essential. Whereas, early on, the most commonly used arthroscope was 2.7 mm in diameter, today a 4.5-mm arthroscope is most often used. The 2.7 mm scope can still be extremely useful for small patients with tight joints. In most cases, the 30° arthroscope is used and a 70° arthroscope is available to more closely examine the medial and lateral gutters and the posterior aspect of the joint.

The arthroscope and cannulas have been modified to make ankle joint arthroscopy easier.[19] Arthroscopes have been made shorter to enhance maneuverability. Cannulas are interchangeable among scopes and shavers. Cannulas should not have sideholes at their tip so they can be left in a portal once it is established and avoid repetitive trauma and extravasation of fluid into subcutaneous tissues that contain the sensory nerves. Other important equipment includes an inflow system for fluid (with or without a pump), special hand instruments, a tourniquet system, syringe–spinal needle–intravenous tubing to permit initial joint distension, and, perhaps, a distraction device.

TECHNIQUE

Procedural Cautions

Surgical technique for arthroscopy of the ankle joint must be meticulous, to avoid damaging articular surfaces. The ankle joint is stabilized by a strong medial and lateral ligament complex that makes the joint extremely tight.[12] Because of the small size of the joint, the ligaments are located much closer to the axis of distraction, thus restricting access. In addition, the ankle joint transmits extraordinary forces from the foot to the leg.[20] The talar dome has a small surface area, as does the tibial plafond. Owing to the constrained nature of the tibiotalar articulation, the cartilage must withstand great forces per unit of area during athletic activity. This makes damage to even a small portion of the articular cartilage a serious incident.[19]

The peripheral nerves course very close to the capsule of the ankle joint; so, a sound anatomic basis for portal placement is critical. Nerve damage is a serious complication since it can leave portions of the weight-bearing areas of the foot without sensation.[6] An insensitive foot is unacceptable for an athlete. Nerve damage can also occur from an "inside-out" problem. The ankle capsule is not as thick as that of other joints, and a powerful or aggressive shaving instrument can easily shave out through the capsule and injure the adjacent neurovascular bundles.[19] Thus, power instruments should never be operated in the ankle except under direct visualization.

Patient Positioning

The positioning of the patient for ankle joint arthroscopy varies, depending on the preference of the surgeon and the traction method used, if any.[12] The first method described involves placing the patient in the supine position and stabilizing the lower extremity with a knee holder. The foot of the table is lowered, and the foot and ankle hang free (Fig. 87–1).[1,5] This allows use of gravity or manual manipulation for distraction. In addition, a loop of Kling or Kerlex material can be used to distract the ankle.[21] We have used a commercially available mechanical traction device and ankle stirrup, which permits accurate control of the amount of distraction and access to both the anterior and the posterior aspects of the joint.

Other positions include the semilateral decubitus position (used without traction) and the supine position with flexed hip and knee and foot holder (with invasive distraction).[12,22] Each position allows ease of access to a different area of the ankle joint, and the decision about which to use depends on the particular ankle disorder and the individual patient.

Anesthesia

Appropriate anesthesia is also extremely important. The tightness of the ankle joint makes arthroscopy

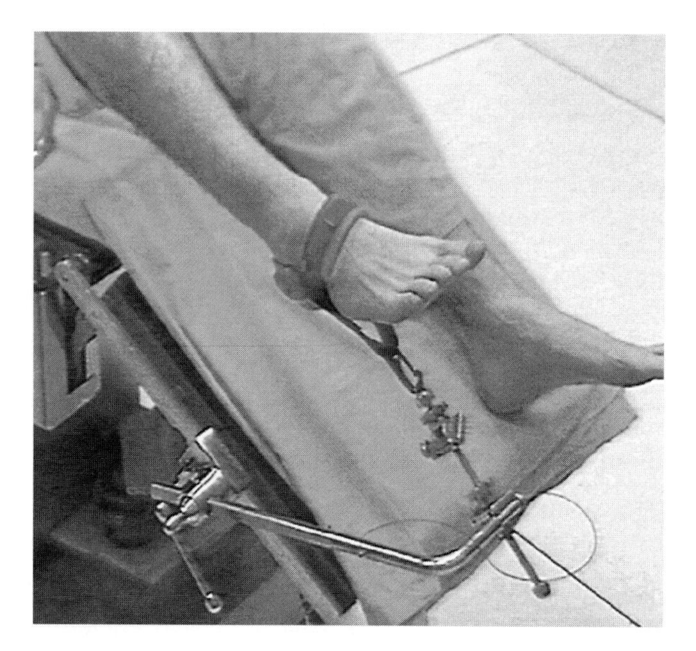

Fig. 87–1. Patient in the supine position for ankle arthroscopy.

difficult, and without proper muscle relaxation the joint surfaces are at greater risk of iatrogenic injury. Thus, in most cases, a general anesthetic or a spinal epidural anesthetic is required for complete muscle relaxation. Local anesthesia is appropriate only in limited cases of specific, isolated disorders.[7]

Establishing Portals

Before beginning the arthroscopic procedure, it is important to outline the surface anatomy with a marking pen, since extravasation of fluid can quickly distort the anatomy. To exsanguinate the area the leg is elevated and a tourniquet is applied. As the joint is distended with saline injection, the ankle dorsiflexes slightly; this confirms intra-articular needle placement.

In establishing portals, the scalpel should be used on the skin only, then the subcutaneous tissue should be carefully spread down to the joint capsule with a hemostat. Following this, we prefer to use a sharp trocar under control, as it cuts its way through the capsule rather than tearing through, as would a blunt trocar. Also, less pressure is needed to pass the sharp trocar, and establishment of the portal is better controlled.

The most common portals used are anterolateral, anteromedial, and posterolateral. The anterolateral portal is established just lateral to the peroneus tertius tendon at the level of the joint line. The structure at greatest risk here is the subcutaneous intermediate dorsal cutaneous branch of the superficial peroneal nerve. This nerve can usually be palpated or visualized just under the skin with gentle inversion and plantar flexion.[6] The anteromedial portal is established just medial to the tibialis anterior tendon. The saphenous vein, which is located in this area, can be avoided by direct visualization with the aid of transillumination. The posterolateral portal, used to view posterior disorders, is established close to the Achilles tendon, to avoid the sural nerve. The anterocentral, posteromedial, and trans-Achilles tendon portals are not recommended.[1,6,11,23]

Examination and Treatment

After the necessary portals have been established, based on what disorders are believed to be present, the arthroscopic examination can be conducted. The majority of space available for the arthroscope and instrumentation lies anterior to the tibial plafond, so the surgeon should "aim anterior" when entering the joint. This helps to protect the articular cartilage from scuffing. Because the portals over the anterior aspect of the ankle joint are quite close together, triangulation is difficult.

After the arthroscopic procedure (examination or treatment) has been completed, the joint is injected with Marcaine and epinephrine to help control postoperative pain and bleeding. Good portal closure is accomplished with either sutures or Steristrips. This is important in the ankle, because the capsule is located so close to the skin. When placing sutures, care has to be taken to avoid subcutaneous veins and nerves.[10]

SPECIFIC PATHOLOGIC CONDITIONS AND TREATMENT

The most common conditions encountered in athletes are soft tissue and osteochondral disorders. The ankle sprain is believed by some to be a precursor to synovitis or impingement syndromes.[11,18,24–30] Soft tissue problems in the ankle joint may also be due to overuse injuries in athletes. Osteochondral disorders include chondromalacia lesions of the talus or tibial plafond and transchondral talar dome fractures. In athletes, they may be a result of either acute or overuse injury.

These entities are amenable to arthroscopic evaluation and treatment when they do not respond to conservative therapy. The workup may include a repeat physical examination, radiography, computed tomography (CT), bone scan, or magnetic resonance imaging (MRI). If one of the above conditions is recognized and the athlete desires to return to competition, arthroscopy should be considered.

Anterolateral Impingement

Soft tissue impingement of the ankle was first recognized as hyalinized tissue in the anterolateral aspect of the ankle joint and was termed a *meniscoid lesion* (Fig. 87–2).[30] More recently, a similar lesion that caused impingement in the ankles of soccer players was reported.[25] Other reports have described anterior fibrous bands and redundant ligamentous tissue impinging in the anterior aspect of the ankle joint and impinge-

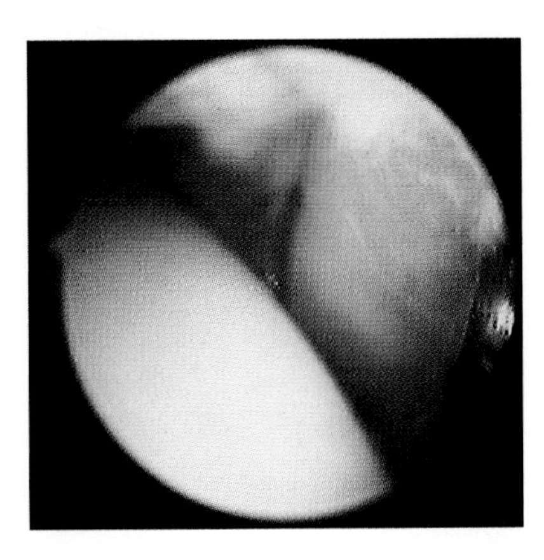

Fig. 87–2. Meniscoid lesion.

ment of the inferior border of the tibiofibular ligament in the anterolateral aspect of the ankle.[18,31] In this patient population, excellent longterm results (relief of symptoms) have been achieved with arthroscopic resection of the inflamed, impinging tissue.[11,14–31]

Managing athletes with chronic pain after a lateral ankle injury can be problematic. Very often, there are no signs of ligamentous laxity, but patients continue to show signs of intra-articular disorders such as swelling, clicking, popping, and "giving way" of the joint. These athletes may have anterior or anterolateral synovitis and impingement. While the origin of this tissue in unclear, it has been proposed that it may be the result of partial ligament injury with hemarthrosis and subsequent inflammation leading to excess synovitis and scar tissue, which then impinges in the joint space during ankle motion.[11,18,26,28]

When an athlete has this syndrome, conservative treatment—rest, splinting, nonsteroidal anti-inflammatory medications, physical therapy, and possibly cortisone injection—is the first line of therapy. If the symptoms persist, arthroscopic synovectomy with removal of all anterior and lateral impinging tissue should be considered. A power shaver is used under direct visualization, and care is taken to debride all the way to the lateral border of the talus and then over its edge into the lateral gutter. All anterior impinging synovium is also excised. Range of motion is observed intra-articularly, to ensure that all impinging tissue has been removed. Excellent results with return to activity and only minimal residual symptoms can be expected in the majority of these patients.[11,24,26,28,29]

Transchondral Talar Dome Fractures

There has been controversy as to whether transchondral talar dome fractures of the ankle joint represent spontaneous avascular necrosis of underlying bone (as in osteochondritis dissecans) or the result of a traumatic event.[32] The traumatic origin theory has gained acceptance, and any athlete with a history of ankle injury and continued pain, swelling, "giving way," clicking, and crepitus should be evaluated for a transchondral talar dome fracture. This includes radiographs, and possibly CT, to better delineate the bony margins of the lesion, and MRI to help determine if the overlying cartilage is intact.

Transchondral talar dome fractures, which occur either anterolaterally or posteromedially, have been classified into four stages.[33] Stage I is a small area of compression of subchondral bone (with intact cartilage), Stage II is a partially detached but nondisplaced osteochondral fragment, Stage III is a completely detached but nondisplaced osteochondral fragment, and Stage IV is a completely detached and significantly displaced osteochondral fragment (Fig. 87–3).

Stage I and II lesions are often asymptomatic, and, initially, conservative treatment is recommended.[34] Although patients with Stage III lesions are usually symptomatic, they can also be managed conservatively.[32] Stage IV lesions should be treated surgically, since the loose fragment in the joint could cause further damage. In general, arthroscopic management of these lesions includes débridement of any loose or partially detached fragments of cartilage and bone along with curettage and possible drilling of the bony bed.

Because medial lesions are generally deep and involve larger fragments of bone, initially they should be treated less aggressively, with just drilling as a first procedure and a longer period of immobilization to encourage healing.[32] If this treatment approach fails, arthroscopic débridement and curettage usually produce an excellent outcome.[2,6,15,32,35,36] Athletes who continue to have problems most often complain of pain and swelling associated with activity.[6] Medial lesions with significant posterior extension need to be approached carefully. It is difficult to treat these lesions completely from an arthroscopic approach, and very often transmalleolar portals or open malleolar osteotomy is required for thorough débridement of the bony bed.[32] Invasive distraction may also be necessary for medial lesions. Lateral transchondral talar dome fractures are not as technically demanding as medial lesions, and they respond very well to arthroscopic treatment. Athletes are usually able to return to sports activities within 2 months after arthroscopic débridement.[2]

Anterior Osteophytes of the Ankle

Anterior osteophytes in the ankle can produce impingement and significant symptoms in athletes who repeatedly dorsiflex their ankles.[10,32] This condition has been reported in dancers and football players.[37,38] These osteophytes can occur on the tibia or the talus and can severely limit dorsiflexion.[32]

The lesions are classified as Grade I if there is synovial impingement with cartilaginous extrusions and osseous spurring up to 3 mm, Grade II if there is osteochondral reaction exostosis with an osteophytic reaction greater than 3 mm, Grade III if there is significant exostosis with fragmentation and concurrent spurring on the talus (Fig. 87–4), and Grade IV if there is a degenerative process involving the anterior aspect of the ankle.[10,19]

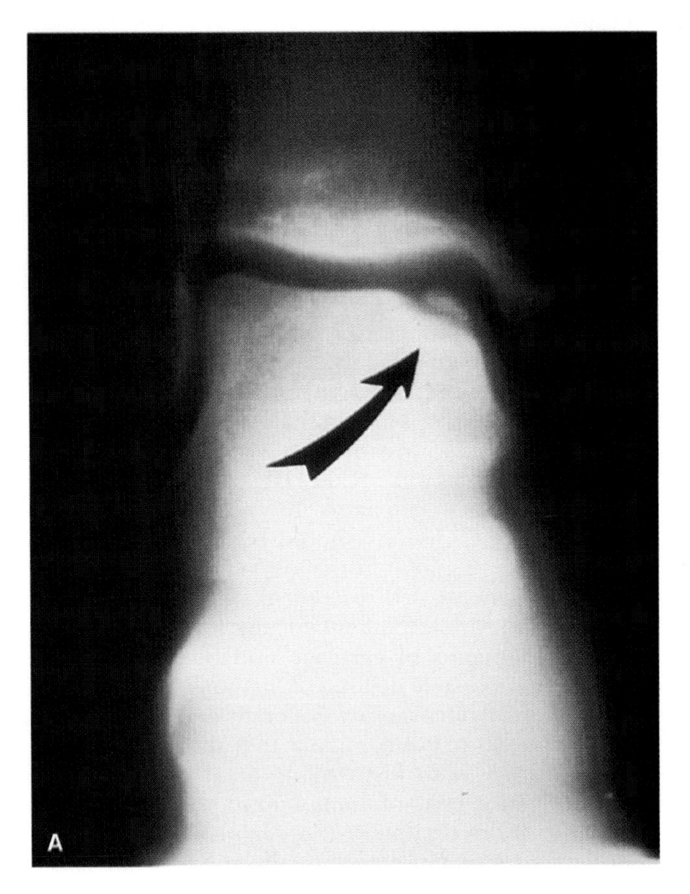

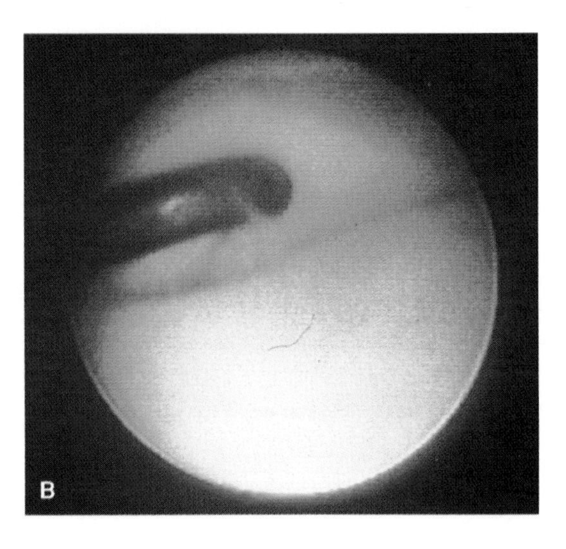

Fig. 87–3. (A) CT shows Stage III transchondral talar dome fracture. (B) Arthroscopic view of same lesion.

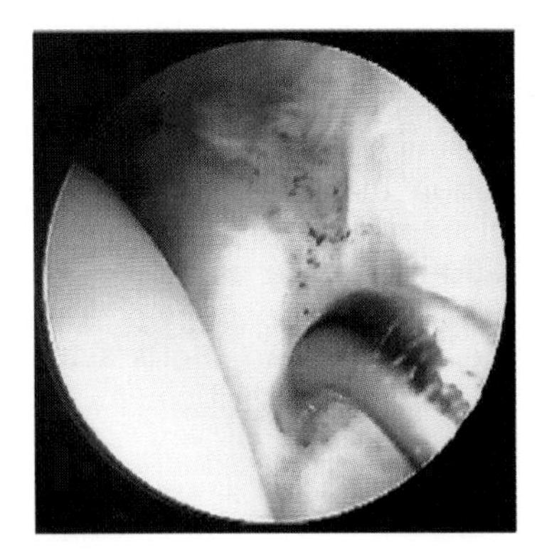

Fig. 87–4. Grade III osteophyte of the anterior ankle.

Grade IV lesions are not amenable to arthroscopic treatment.[19]

If conservative therapy is not successful in treating anterior osteophytes, arthroscopy and débridement should be considered. Usually, a large amount of anterior synovitis is present, which should be debrided first. Following this, spurs may be removed with an arthroscopic bur or a small osteotome.[32] When this procedure is accomplished arthroscopically, good results can be expected and the recovery time is shorter than with open treatment.[10,32] The type of lesion has a significant impact on the rate of recovery and return to athletic competition, with a Grade IV lesion taking longer to heal.[10]

POSTOPERATIVE REGIMEN

The regimen following ankle arthroscopy is similar for all of the procedures discussed. A compression dressing is applied and ice and elevation are encouraged for 24 to 48 hours. Active range of motion exercises and toe-touch weight bearing are started as soon as the patient can tolerate. Weight bearing is advanced quickly, and patients begin physical therapy 1 to 2 days after surgery.

This therapy should first concentrate on decreasing inflammation and swelling and improving range of motion. After that, the focus should be on increasing strength and agility. Agility training is extremely important for athletes who have undergone ankle arthroscopy. The rehabilitation program should involve the entire lower extremity, to ensure adequate return of strength in the thigh as well.

Return to sports activity should be expected within 6 to 8 weeks. Criteria for return to sport should stress function, and, more important, sport-specific function. Range of motion and strength should approach approximately 80% of normal before the athlete can return to athletic activity. Single-leg hopping and agility should also approach normal levels.

COMPLICATIONS

Complications do occur with operative ankle arthroscopy. Those encountered most commonly include paresthesia, nerve transection, hemarthrosis, infection, sinus tract formation, osteomyelitis, articular scuffing, fluid extravasation, instrument breakage, deep vein thrombosis, pin tract infection, and fracture. There is a learning curve with arthroscopy that can be accelerated with cadaver study.[1,5,6,12]

Close attention to technique, along with sound anatomic knowledge and sensitive handling of the instruments, is very important. When placing portals, great care must be taken to protect cutaneous nerves. Hemarthrosis and infection can be significant postoperative problems, and the surgeon must pay strict attention to hemostasis and consider prophylactic antibiotics for patients who may require them.[6,11] With appropriate patient selection, careful technique, and close follow up, excellent results can be achieved with minimal morbidity.

REFERENCES

1. Andrews, J. R., Previte, W. J., and Carson, W. G.: Arthroscopy of the ankle: Technique and normal anatomy. Foot Ankle *6*:29, 1985.
2. Baker, C. L., Andrews, J. R., and Ryan, J. B.: Arthroscopic treatment of transchondral talar dome fractures. Arthroscopy *2*:82, 1986.
3. Drez, D., Jr., Guhl, J. F., and Gollehon, D. L.: Ankle arthroscopy: Technique and indications. Clin. Sports Med. *1*:35, 1982.
4. Drez, D., Jr., Guhl, J. F., and Gollehon, D. L.: Ankle arthroscopy: Technique and indications. Foot Ankle *2*:138, 1981.
5. Carson, W. G., Jr., and Andrews, J. R.: Arthroscopy of the ankle. Clin. Sports Med. *6*:503, 1987.
6. Martin, D. F., et al.: Operative ankle arthroscopy: Long-term followup. Am. J. Sports Med. *17*:16, 1989.
7. Ferkel, R. D., and Fischer, S. P.: Progress in ankle arthroscopy. Clin. Orthop. *240*:210, 1989.
8. Kingston, S.: Magnetic resonance imaging of the ankle and foot. Clin. Sports Med. *7*:15, 1988.
9. Fallat, L. M.: Accuracy of diagnostic arthroscopy of the ankle joint. J. Foot Surg. *26*:26, 1987.
10. Scranton, P. E., and McDermott, J. E.: Anterior tibiotalar spurs: A comparison of open versus arthroscopic débridement. Foot Ankle *13*:125, 1992.
11. Martin, D. F., Curl, W. W., and Baker, C. L.: Arthroscopic treatment of chronic synovitis of the ankle. Arthroscopy *5*:110, 1989.
12. Guhl, J. F.: Ankle arthroscopy: Special equipment, operating room set-up, and technique. *In* Operative Arthroscopy. Edited by J. B. McGinty, et al. New York, Raven Press, 1991.
13. Heller, A. J., and Vogler, H. W.: Ankle joint arthroscopy. J. Foot Surg. *21*:23, 1982.
14. Parisien, J. S.: Diagnostic and operative arthroscopy of the ankle: Technique and indications. Bull. Hosp. Joint Dis. Orthop. Inst. *45*:38, 1985.
15. Parisien, J. S., and Shereff, M. J.: The role of arthroscopy in the diagnosis and treatment of disorders of the ankle. Foot Ankle *2*:144, 1981.
16. Barber, F. A., et al.: The anatomy of ankle arthroscopic surgery. Surg. Rounds Orthop. *1*:22, 1987.
17. Hawkins, R. B.: Ankle instability from an arthroscopist's perspective. *In* Operative Arthroscopy. Edited by J. B. McGinty, et al. New York, Raven Press, 1991.
18. Bassett, F. H., et al.: Talar impingement by the anterioinferior tibiofibular ligament: A cause of chronic pain in the ankle after inversion sprain. J. Bone Joint Surg. *72A*:55, 1990.
19. Scranton, P. E., et al.: Symposium: arthroscopy of the ankle and foot. Contemp. Orthop. *26*:67, 1993.
20. Nuber, G. W.: Biomechanics of the foot and ankle during gait. Clin. Sports Med. *7*:1, 1988.
21. Yates, C. K., and Grana, W. A.: A simple distraction technique for ankle arthroscopy. Arthroscopy *4*:103, 1988.
22. Parisien, J. S.: Instrumentation in arthroscopic surgery of the ankle. *In* Ankle Arthroscopy: Pathology and Surgical Technique. Edited by J. F. Guhl. Thorofare, NJ, Slack, 1988.
23. Voto, S. J., et al.: Ankle arthroscopy: Neurovascular and arthroscopic anatomy of standard and trans-Achilles tendon portal placement. Arthroscopy *5*:41, 1989.
24. Meislin, R. J., et al.: Arthroscopic treatment of synovial impingement of the ankle. Am. J. Sports Med. *21*:186, 1993.
25. McCarroll, J. R., et al.: Meniscoid lesions of the ankle in soccer players. Am. J. Sports Med. *15*:255, 1987.
26. Ferkel, R. D.: Soft tissue pathology of the ankle. *In* Operative Arthroscopy. Edited by J. B. McGinty, et al. New York, Raven Press, 1991.
27. Zimmer, T. J.: Chronic and recurrent ankle sprains. Clin. Sports Med. *10*:653, 1991.
28. Ferkel, R. D., et al.: Arthroscopic treatment of anterolateral impingement of the ankle. Am. J. Sports Med. *19*:449, 1991.
29. Stone, J. W., and Guhl, J. F.: Meniscoid lesions of the ankle. Clin. Sports Med. *10*:661, 1991.
30. Wolin, I., et al.: Internal derangement of the talofibular component of the ankle. Surg. Gynecol. Obstet. *91*:193, 1950.
31. McGinty, J. B., et al.: Symposium: Arthroscopy of joints other than the knee. Contemp. Orthop. *9*:71, 1989.
32. Ewing, J. W.: Arthroscopic management of transchondral talar dome fractures (osteochondritis dissecans) and anterior impingement lesions of the ankle joint. Clin. Sports Med. *10*:677, 1991.
33. Berndt, A. L., and Harty, M.: Transchondral fractures (osteochondritis dissecans) of the talus. J. Bone Joint Surg. *41A*:988, 1959.
34. Canale, S. T., and Belding, R. H.: Osteochondral lesions of the talus. J. Bone Joint Surg. *62A*:97, 1980.
35. Lundeen, R. O.: Medial impingement lesions of the tibial plafond. J. Foot Surg. *26*:37, 1987.
36. Parisien, J. S., and Vangsness, T.: Operative arthroscopy of the ankle: Three years' experience. Clin. Orthop. *199*:46, 1985.
37. Kleiger, B.: Anterior tibiotalar impingement syndromes in dancers. Foot Ankle *3*:69, 1982.
38. O'Donoghue, D. H.: Impingement exostoses of the talus and tibia. J. Bone Joint Surg. *39A*:835, 1957.

IV

REHABILITATION

88 *Joe Gieck*

Rehabilitation of the Lower Leg, Ankle, and Foot

When rehabilitating the lower leg, ankle, or foot after overuse injury or other trauma, the best advice for the athlete is, *Let the leg be the doctor.* Rehabilitation should be guided by how the extremity responds to exercise, at whatever level is appropriate. If the rehabilitation program causes pain and swelling during or after exercise, especially the morning after, the level of activity should be reduced. This applies to the number of different exercises, their sets and repetitions, and the amount of weight being used. When the athlete can perform the exercises without developing symptoms, the level of activity can be increased accordingly.

Athletes who have difficulty adjusting to this principle usually are compulsive about their workouts (and, so, abuse themselves) and have poor coping skills in injury management. Injury and its necessary rehabilitation can be a frustrating process for athletes, but unless they comply with the underlying principle of adjusting their level of activity to the level of pain, athletes usually begin training too soon, which prolongs the injury process, impedes healing, and further delays return to pain-free competition.

The point in the playing season is also important when dealing with lower extremity injuries. At the beginning of a competitive season, the principles of pain-free exercise are rigorously observed; whereas, toward the end of the season, an athlete may safely continue to compete even with some pain and inflammation. Athletes who are experiencing pain at the beginning of the season should be counseled to back off until they can perform pain free. Toward the end of the season, rest and rehabilitation can be delayed until the season is over, at which time the pain-free exercise principles again apply.

OBJECTIVES OF REHABILITATION

Rehabilitation of the lower extremity is based on progressing through a sequence of specific and incremental objectives: (1) pain relief; (2) ambulation without limping; (3) regaining range of motion and strength; (4) training for proprioception; (5) training for endurance, power, speed, and agility; and (6) return to competition. Athletes who comply with the regimen return safely to activity sooner. Mistakes in rehabilitation are either progressing too rapidly and having to cut back on activity or demonstrating no progress after completing a sequence and thus retarding progress.

Pain Relief

During the early stages of injury, the principal goal of rehabilitation is pain relief. The acronym is RICE, for *r*est, *i*ce, *c*ompression, and *e*levation. Initially after the injury, the affected extremity should be wrapped with a snug elastic bandage. The athlete should elevate and rest the extremity and then apply ice for approximately 20 minutes out of each hour until retiring for the night. Nonsteroidal anti-inflammatory drugs (NSAIDs) may be used to control pain.

The following day, cold and electrical stimulation help reduce inflammation. The cryokinetic principle, ISE, is then applied[1]: *i*ce, *s*tretching, and *e*xercise. Ice is applied for 20 minutes to the injured area while active stretching is performed by the patient. At the end of this session, passive range of motion exercise is continued, followed by resistance exercise (usually for three sets of ten repetitions).

Hydrotherapy is an appropriate modality because active exercise can be implemented during the treatment. The criteria for switching from cold to heat include no active swelling, full pain-free range of motion, no inflammatory heat in the limb, and maximal response to cold treatment.[1] Contrast baths may be used before switching to heat entirely; they enhance circulation without producing some of the edematous effects of heat.

The athlete usually begins treatment in a 102°F whirlpool for 3 minutes, then switches to cold water (55 to 65°F) for 2 minutes. As the athlete tolerates this, the ratio of hot to cold time is changed to 4:1. Ending the session with cold treatment helps control swelling that may develop during heat therapy. Temperatures below 55°F are of no physiologic benefit and may cause frostbite. Intermittent compression and massage are also effective means of decreasing edema. Reducing edema more effectively relieves pain by removing the noxious mechanical stimulus over the injured soft tissue.

Ambulation

High-voltage electrical stimulation in conjunction with a cold whirlpool is an especially effective modality for relieving pain and swelling and helping the athlete regain normal ambulation without limping. Stimulation treatment is provided for 15 minutes, followed by walking for 5 minutes, and the two are then repeated. This treatment is performed two to four times a day. A crutch or cane may be used to help the athlete ambulate.

Pain-free ambulation without limping is an especially important goal because limping exacerbates the inflammatory process by maintaining pressure on injured tissue. The athlete starts with slow, straight walking on flat, and then on undulating, surfaces. Next come slow S-pattern walks on undulating, and then—undulating, hilly, surfaces. As the athlete progresses, the pace of walking is accelerated.

Range of Motion and Strength

Pursuit of the dual objectives of regaining range of motion and strength starts when the athlete can perform the necessary movements and exercises without pain. These movements and exercises are performed in a slow and gentle manner, to prevent further inflammation. As a general rule, exercises are first performed for about 5 minutes and gradually extended to 30 minutes. Exercise modalities include pool walking, backward walking, bicycling, Stairmaster, Nordic track, and Versaclimber.

Proprioception

As the athlete is able to tolerate these challenges, proprioception exercises are added, to restore what has been lost because of the injury. Proprioception receptors in ligaments and tendons are especially vulnerable to disruption. Proprioceptive exercises (e.g., balance; leaning forward and backward; bending down, touching the floor and returning to an upright position; heel raises; and ball catching and throwing) begin on a flat hard surface, progress to a soft surface, and then to a proprioception device (Fig. 88–1). The exercises are performed with the eyes first open and then closed. Three sets are performed hourly for 30 seconds. The athlete begins with weight distributed bilaterally and progresses to unilateral weight bearing.

Endurance, Power, Speed, and Agility

Endurance, power, speed, and agility exercises are added as the athlete progresses through the rehabilitation program. Progress may be rapid after a minor injury or may take several months after more serious

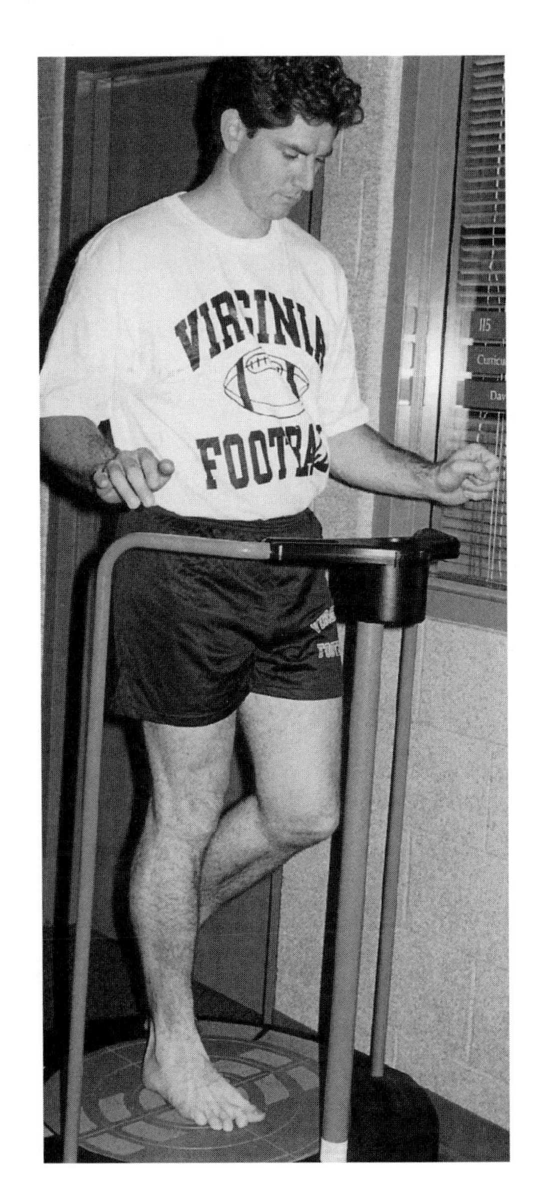

Fig. 88–1. Proprioception exercise device.

trauma. After the athlete is able to walk fast, he or she starts a walking-jogging regimen of 50 steps of each, then progresses to full jogging. During this sequence, proprioception exercises are continued. Next, the athlete starts a jog-run regimen of 50 steps each and begins limited sports activities. From there, the athlete progresses to full running and plyometric exercises. Athletes can return to their sport after regaining the agility necessary for that activity.

Criteria for Return to Activity

Before returning to activity, athletes should have full pain-free range of motion and normal strength, endurance, and power in the affected extremity. They should be able to complete functional activities appropriate to their sport without pain. This includes regaining full running speed, ability to cut 90° to the left and right at full speed, ability to run a figure-of-eight pattern at full speed (accelerate and decelerate around pylons), ability to hop equally on both extremities for distance and time, and dynamic control of any instability. The athlete should also show a strong desire to return to the sport.

If an athlete insists on continuing to practice or compete while a lower extremity injury is still in the inflammatory stage, it is important that ice be applied to the affected area immediately after the activity for approximately 20 minutes, to reduce additional inflammation secondary to the exertion. Although the athlete is not ideally progressing past the stage of inflammation before return to sports participation, this often occurs because he or she does not properly follow the rehabilitation program or is not aware of the correct sequence.

SHIN SPLINTS

Shin splints, an inflammatory condition that causes pain in the lower leg, is normally due to overuse injury. Often, the condition is constantly being exacerbated as the athlete trains and thus it can become chronic. Muscle weakness and decreased flexibility can contribute to shin splints or be a result of the condition.

Shin splints can happen early in the season in an unconditioned athlete who participates in a high-intensity running program within a short period of time or in a conditioned athlete who is putting more stress on the lower legs than they can tolerate, as when an athlete used to running 20 miles a week suddenly increases to 40 miles. Ideally, mileage should not be increased by more than 10% a week. An athlete who trains on a crowned surface, a soft or sandy surface, or an excessively hard surface, or who suddenly changes surfaces while involved in an intensive training program, is also at risk of developing shin splints.

Shin splints can occur in either the anterior or posterior compartments of the lower leg, though the latter site is more common. The inflammatory condition is usually situated posterior to the medial tibial ridge and confined to the lower third of the tibia.[2] Posterior compartment shin splints are frequently caused in part by improper lower leg biomechanics. For example, a foot that overpronates adds extra stress to the posterior tibialis tendon with each stride as it tries to eccentrically control the mechanics of the foot during running. Poor shoe support and a tight Achilles tendon compound the problem.

Anterior shin splints are caused by repetitive dorsiflexion during running. They are often associated with a tight Achilles tendon, which may be the result of an ankle that did not regain full dorsiflexion in rehabilitation following a previous ankle sprain. When dorsiflexion is limited, the anterior tibialis tendon has to overcome increased dorsiflexion resistance and the added stress of the tight Achilles tendon. This burden, added to the eccentric activity of the anterior tibialis as it decelerates the foot at heel strike, is often more than enough to produce the inflammatory response of anterior shin splints. A weak anterior tibialis is overstressed during running because the foot is uncontrolled at heel strike and a resultant foot slap occurs. Running downhill accentuates this stress. Fatigue and the addition of incline running are classic mechanisms of anterior shin splints.

Treatment for shin splints usually consists of applying heat before activity and cold after activity for approximately 20 minutes. If an athlete participating in competition has acute pain before activity, cold is applied both before and after. Aspirin taken immediately before exercise can also be beneficial. NSAIDs may be used for chronic shin splints.

Rehabilitation for athletes with shin splints consists of stretching exercises and exercises to regain range of motion (Fig. 88–2) and strength (Fig. 88–3). If biomechanical abnormalities are present, they must be corrected if treatment is to be successful.[3] Overpronation plus heel valgus, the most common abnormality, is often easily corrected with the appropriate orthotic appliance. Taping may help support the longitudinal arch of the foot.

Rest is a critical factor if shin splints are to be successfully treated. Many athletes want pain relief but also want to be able to continue to participate in their sport, yet one cannot continue to abuse tissue and at the same time expect relief. This is where alternative methods of cross-training, whenever possible, are important. For example, cross-country runners can maintain a good level of fitness through intensive pool training and bicycle riding. In addition to alternative workouts, superficial hot and cold therapy and NSAIDs can also help athletes who, though injured, have to prepare for an important meet.

COMPARTMENT SYNDROME

Compartment syndromes can be a result of chronic shin splints or of trauma.[3] Acute compartment syndromes require aggressive intervention to prevent muscle necrosis and neuropathy. Athletes with chronic com-

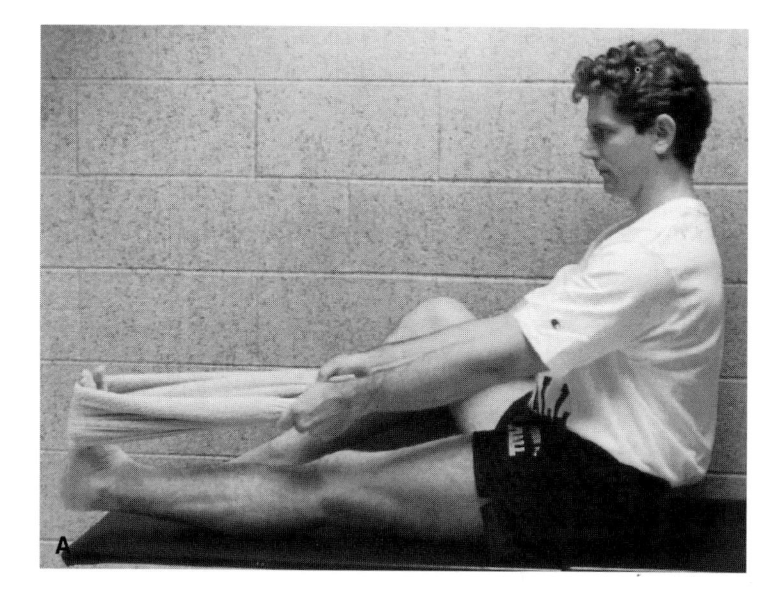

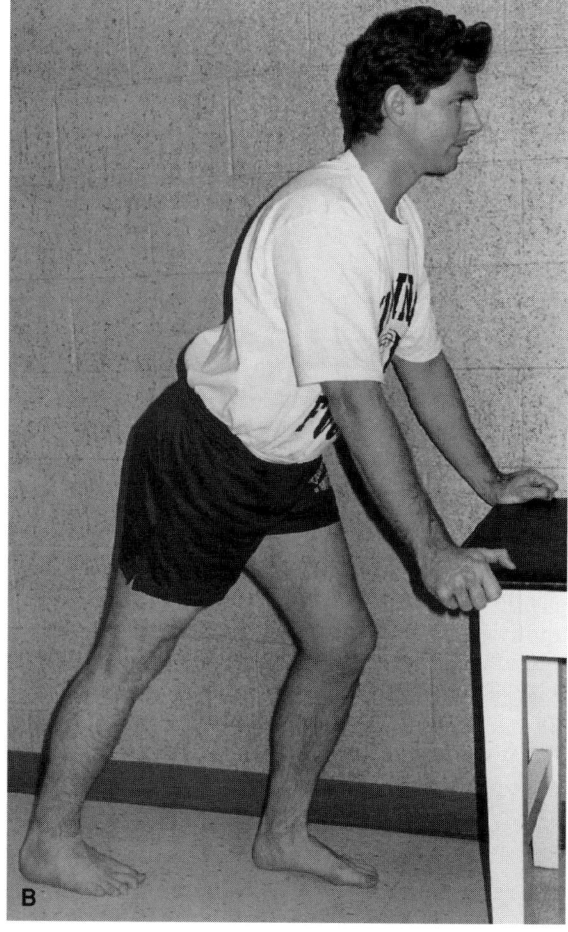

Fig. 88–2. (A–B) Range of motion exercises for dorsiflexion.

partment syndrome complain of gradual continual deep pain, often of an aching nature, that begins at a certain level of athletic activity. A common example is the cross-country runner who experiences this type of pain 15 minutes into the workout and the pain increases in intensity as running continues. Another example is the field hockey player who can practice and play short sprints but is unable to complete endurance requirements.

In these cases, only rest provides relief, and the usual rehabilitation procedures have no lasting positive effects. Fasciotomy is usually indicated for athletes who wish to continue in competition. After surgery, rehabilitation is begun as tolerated by the athlete, following the previously mentioned guidelines of regaining range of motion, strength, proprioception, endurance, power, speed, and agility. If an athlete suffers neuropathy secondary to compartment syndrome, it may take 6 months or longer to recover complete function, provided the nerves remain intact.

GASTROCNEMIUS-SOLEUS COMPLEX INJURY

The classic mechanism of injury to the gastrocnemius-soleus complex is sudden strain—as a result of improper warm-up or fatigue at the end of an exercise period or when the athlete attempts to extend a workout beyond normal limits.[4] Occasionally, overuse causes a problem, but that is usually limited to the Achilles tendon.

For the athlete who limps while walking, treatment should be immediate partial weight bearing or none. The RICE principle, described previously, is applied. A wrap is then reapplied to the calf, and the athlete is provided crutches or a cane with instructions to bear weight only to the point of discomfort but not to limp. It is important to maintain a pain-free gait. With minor injury, often the use of a wrap and a heel lift to reduce passive dorsiflexion during ambulation suffice.

The next day, the athlete should continue with the ISE routine. Active dorsiflexion to gently stretch the calf, followed by passive range of motion exercises, can be accomplished with a towel (see Fig. 88–2A). The towel is also used to perform resistive plantar flexion exercises. As these exercises cease to be challenging, the standing stretch and flat heel raises are begun. The routine progresses to passive stretching and resistive exercise off a step, then to the use of a calf machine (see Fig. 88–3). As improvement is noted, the heel lift is removed and the athlete is acclimated to a flat court or field shoe. Pool exercises and backward walking may be started at

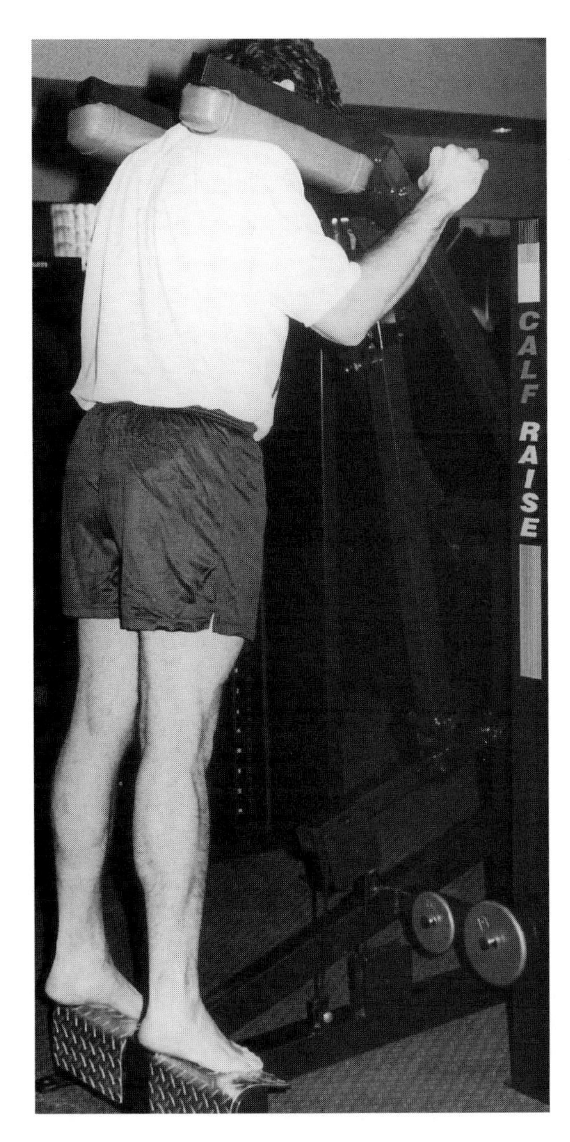

Fig. 88–3. Calf machine exercise for gastrocnemius-soleus strength.

an early stage as less pressure is exerted during pool walking and less dorsiflexion is needed during backward walking. Return to activity should follow the rehabilitation sequence described previously.

ACHILLES TENDON INJURY

Injury to the Achilles tendon is most often due to overuse, resulting in tendinitis. The athlete usually has compromised dorsiflexion and decreased plantar flexion strength. This loss is either a result of the insult to the tendon or was previously present and led to the tendinitis. A common problem is the athlete who jogs on his or her toes, adding additional eccentric stress to the Achilles tendon. There may also be a history of increasing training mileage more than the recommended 10% a week or suddenly starting training on hills.

The foot should be examined for abnormal pronation, which may lead to undue stress on the Achilles tendon. In addition, the runner's footwear should be evaluated for proper fit, and if necessary, adjustments should be made or the shoe should be discarded if it is worn out. The athlete's running technique should also be observed for proper mechanics.

The athlete needs to be advised to manage the injury by first eliminating or limiting whatever is abusing the tendon. Tendinitis is, in a way, a self-protective mechanism to prevent rupture and, in the athlete who heeds the warning it is usually self-limiting. Without cooperation, rehabilitation is doomed to failure. The rehabilitation program for athletes with Achilles tendinitis is similar to that for gastrocnemius-soleus injury. The calf machine provides appropriate exercises for those with Achilles tendinitis (see Fig. 88–3).[5] The 7-day regimen consists of three sets of ten repetitions at slow speed with no pain on days 1 and 2; moderate speed with no pain on days 3, 4, and 5; and fast speed with slight discomfort allowed on days 6 and 7.

Rupture of the Achilles tendon usually occurs in the middle-aged athlete secondary to a sudden, stressful eccentric contraction, but it is being seen more often now in younger athletes who continue to abuse the tendon. The athlete's history is tendinitis that takes longer and longer to become pain free during a run. The athlete may feel a "pop" followed by loss of plantar flexion and present clinically with either a slap gait or a gait that is externally rotated because he or she cannot actively achieve plantar flexion.

Treatment may be surgical or nonsurgical, followed by immobilization for 6 to 8 weeks. There is some evidence that early, limited weight bearing aids early alignment of collagen fibers, strengthening the repair. After the cast is removed, the athlete begins gentle passive and active range of motion exercises and progresses as tolerated. In addition to the previously mentioned routine for gastrocnemius-soleus injury, early pool walking is a good exercise that is usually tolerated well. Heavy resistance is added as the athlete regains pain-free ambulation without limping (see Fig. 88–3).

ANKLE INJURIES

With lateral ankle sprains, dorsiflexion is lost immediately, and the athlete assumes a flat-footed gait because of painful dorsiflexion during normal walking. Functional evaluation can be accomplished with the heel raise. An athlete who cannot bear weight fully on the toes usually takes longer than a week to return to competition. An athlete who can bear weight but cannot hop on the involved extremity normally takes at least a week to return. High sprains involving the tibiofibular ligaments are the slowest to heal.

Early running on an injured ankle accelerates degenerative changes in the joint. For this reason, it is especially important that the athlete's ankle be fully rehabilitated and all of the criteria for return be met (e.g., pain-free running without any sign of a limp) before the ankle is taped and the athlete is allowed to participate in sports.

For minor to moderate sprains, active range of motion is begun the day after the injury with adjunctive cryotherapy. This is easily accomplished in a cold whirlpool. Only dorsiflexion and plantar flexion are performed. Inversion-eversion range of motion is not performed as that only exacerbates the inflammatory process caused by the sprain. Stretching is indicated, unless there is an abnormal loss of inversion-eversion. In most cases of minor and moderate sprains, this does not occur.

Progression of stretching into dorsiflexion begins with towel stretches and then wall stretches, first as double-leg and finally as single-leg stretches. Stretches should be done both with the knee bent (Achilles) and straight (upper gastrocnemius), to obtain maximum range of motion. In the wall stretches, if the athlete does not feel the Achilles being stretched, the foot of the flexed knee should be moved backward until the tendon can be felt to stretch. Stretching should be done before the ankle is taped, to maintain as much dorsiflexion as possible, since the most common mechanism of a sprain is inversion and plantar flexion, and, for the ankle, plantar flexion is a compromised position. Bicycling and walking down stairs (emphasizing keeping the heel of the trailing leg on the step as long as possible) are also excellent means of regaining normal dorsiflexion.

An ankle that has not been fully rehabilitated will exhibit loss of dorsiflexion. Preseason screening should be done to determine if athletes have adequate dorsiflexion (approximately 20°). A functional squat test can easily and quickly determine this; the athlete should be able to fully squat while holding the heels flat on the floor (Fig. 88–4). Those without adequate dorsiflexion must lift the heels from the floor to maintain their balance. The degree of deficit is determined by the number of inches the heels come off the floor when the full squat position is assumed.

Plantar flexion usually is not lost except when the ankle has been immobilized for an extended period. In these situations, range of motion exercises are best accomplished after the ankle has been in a warm whirlpool. Manual stretching is then applied to the affected ankle. Prolonged immobilization can also result in capsular restrictions of the talocrural, subtalar, midtarsal, and tibiofibular joints. Mobilization exercises are used to loosen these restrictions.

Regaining strength usually is not a problem, because the small tendons around the ankle do not press on swollen soft tissue and cause reflex inhibition in the involved muscle. Isometric exercises are begun early and performed in multiple positions for six seconds in each position, repeated daily. Three motions of the ankle joint (i.e., dorsiflexion, inversion, and eversion) can easily be strengthened with the use of elastic tubing (Fig. 88–5). Isokinetic and isotonic exercises may be added as tolerated.

Manual dynamic resistance is a very effective and inexpensive mode of exercise. Plantar flexion is the one motion that requires more extensive exercise to fully regain strength. The use of heavy weights with few repetitions (e.g., three sets of ten repetitions with the knee flexed and extended) is necessary to restore normal strength to the gastrocnemius-soleus (see Fig. 88–3). Isokinetic and isotonic testing should be performed to determine if plantar flexion strength has been regained.

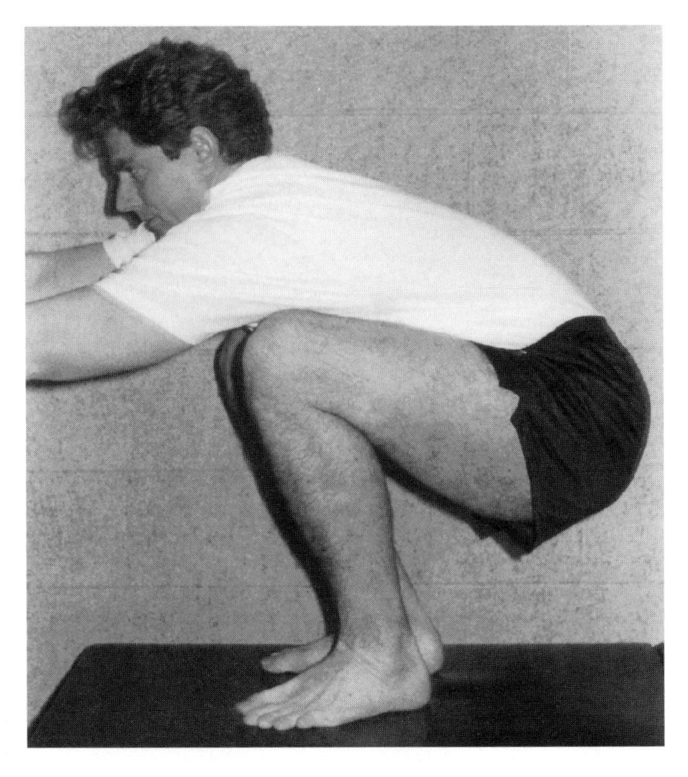

Fig. 88–4. Functional squat test.

Of major concern following ankle injury is loss of proprioception. Balance testing of athletes with poorly rehabilitated ankles showed that proprioceptive loss is often significant.[6] This lack of proprioception may explain why so many athletes subsequently experience ankle sprains even though they have regained normal range of motion, strength, and endurance levels. Thus, it is critical that the athlete perform appropriate proprioception exercises (see Fig. 88–1). Many taping studies also indicate that tape acts basically as a proprioceptive device.

Exercises to increase endurance, power, speed, and agility are then performed in the progression previously described. Again, the athlete is taped and returned to competition when he or she can ideally meet the criteria for return to activity.

LONGITUDINAL AND METATARSAL ARCH STRAINS

Constant pounding, either at the beginning of a training period or from trying to increase mileage too quickly, can injure the soft tissue of the longitudinal arch of the foot. Excessive foot pronation and valgus heel posture exacerbate the problem. Rehabilitation consists of increasing strength in the toe flexors and posterior tibialis (as it also supports the arch) with towel curls and inversion exercises. Heel cord stretching is also important because a tight heel cord accentuates

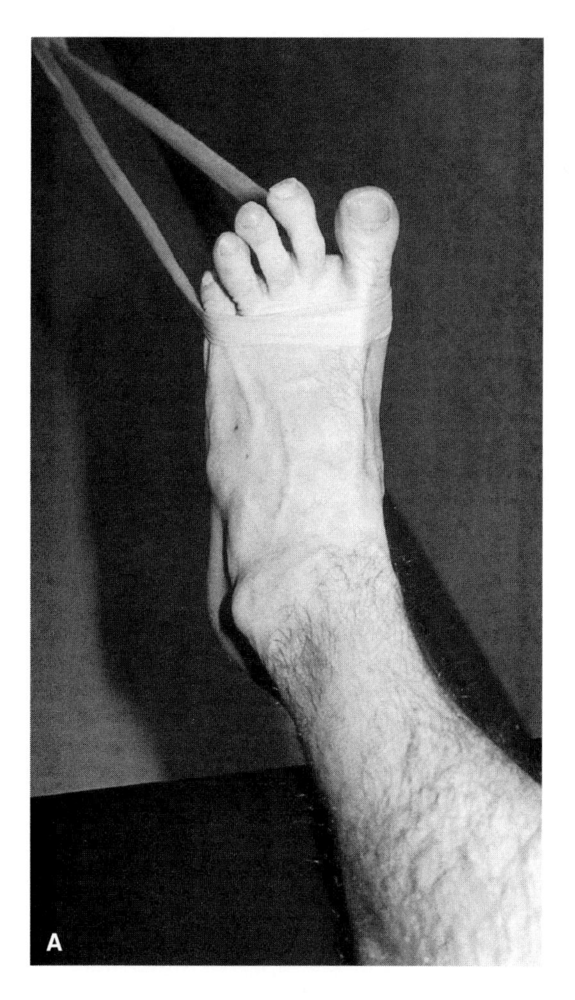

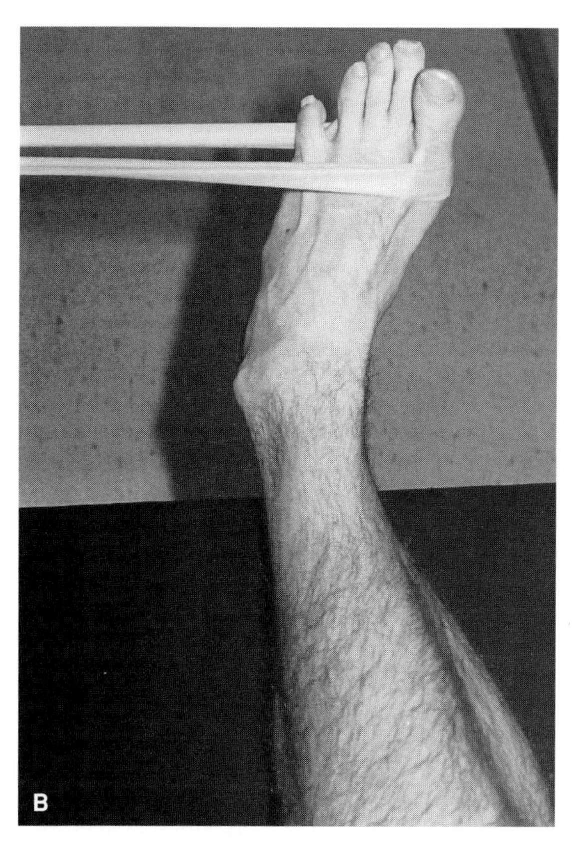

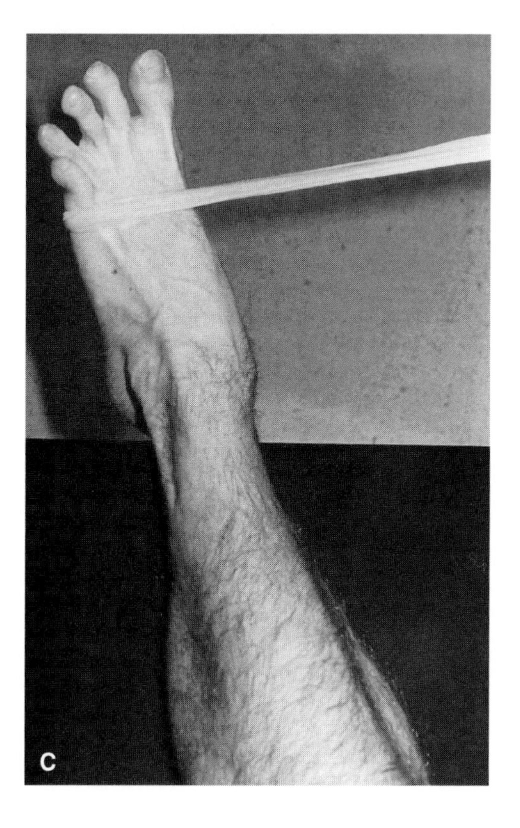

Fig. 88–5. Strengthening exercises for ankle sprains: *(A)* Dorsiflexion strengthening. *(B)* Inversion strengthening. *(C)* Eversion strengthening.

pronation during running. External support may be provided by taping the longitudinal arch. When taping, the ankle should be dorsiflexed and the toes flexed to elevate the arch and shorten the toe flexors.

When exercise and taping are not sufficient, an orthotic device may be necessary, especially with pes planus. A semirigid device is easily tolerated by the athlete and helps dissipate the high levels of force at the foot, while it functions as a mobile adaptor. Orthotics can be made easily and inexpensively for the competitive athlete and can effectively control biomechanical problems of the foot.

Metatarsal arch strain may occur in conjunction with longitudinal arch strain, as a result of added pronation or independently as a result of a pounding exercise routine on a hard surface. Toe flexor exercises, along with the use of a metatarsal pad, usually alleviate symptoms. The pad should be fitted so that the metatarsal heads (usually two and three) are supported proximally and the pad is not pressing directly on the area of soreness (Fig. 88–6). The pad may be glued into the shoe or incorporated into the orthotic for the athlete with longitudinal arch problems.

PLANTAR FASCIITIS

Plantar fasciitis, most common in older athletes and those who are putting in excess mileage, is an injury of

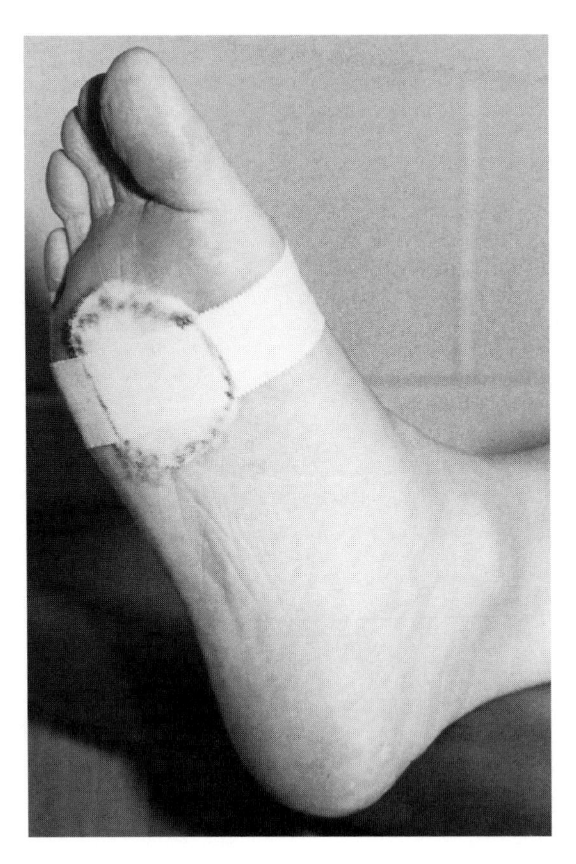

Fig. 88–6. Metatarsal pad.

overuse. Running up inclines and on asphalt surfaces also adds stress to the fascia. Pain may be associated with passive range of motion of the toes, which stretches the plantar fascia, especially when the ankle is dorsiflexed. The single most important means of managing this problem is to eliminate the abuse factor; however, it is not unusual for the condition to take 2 to 3 months or longer to improve, even when the abuse is curbed. Athletes often get frustrated and "push through the pain," exacerbating the already inflamed condition.

Contrast treatments and ultrasound may help relieve pain. Transverse friction massage for 6 to 8 minutes every other day can help increase blood flow to the area and aid healing. Taping of the arch may help relieve discomfort, especially when a tight medial pull of the tape over the posteromedial aspect of the plantar surface is emphasized. Orthotics with a deep heel cup and a medial heel wedge (and medial arch support for the pes planus foot) usually decrease stress and enable the athlete to attain a pain-free gait.

TURF TOE

Turf toe results in pain and limited range of motion of the first metatarsophalangeal joint. Initial treatment is aimed at relief of pain. A rigid steel or plastic innersole may help. Taping the metatarsophalangeal joint in either slight hyperflexion or slight hyperextension (depending on the mechanism of injury) and anchoring it to the second toe eliminate some of the stress to the joint and permit the athlete earlier return to activity.

Because the joint capsule is often involved, loss of joint motion may result. Athletes need at least 70° of hyperextension to run, and loss of joint motion seriously lessens their ability to do so by changing running mechanics, which can lead to overuse injuries elsewhere. The athlete can be taught early mobilization and stretching exercises that should be performed a number of times daily. If further motion loss is noted, a rigid surface may be added to the athlete's orthotic to take pressure off the first metatarsophalangeal joint.

REFERENCES

1. Kulund, D. N.: The Injured Athlete. 2nd Ed. Philadelphia, J. B. Lippincott, 1988.
2. Schuech, P.: Tibialis posterior shin splints: Diagnosis and treatment. Athl. Train. *19*:271, 1984.
3. Andrews, J. R., and Harrelson, G. L.: Physical Rehabilitation of the Injured Athlete. Philadelphia, W. B. Saunders, 1991.
4. Prentice, W. E.: Rehabilitation Techniques in Sports Medicine. St. Louis, Mosby College, 1990.
5. Curwin, S., and Stanish, W. D.: Tendinitis: Its Etiology and Treatment. Lexington, MA, Collamore, 1984.
6. Glencross, D., and Thornton, E.: Position sense following joint injury. J. Sports Med. Phys. Fitness *21*:23, 1981.

89 *Herbert L. Silver and Robert M. Poole*

Therapeutic Modalities in Sports Rehabilitation

Sports physical therapy has served to shift the focus of orthopedic rehabilitation away from the treatment of symptoms toward emphasis on functional outcomes. In sports medicine, the desired functional outcome is rapid return of the athlete to competition. This goal is achieved with the aid of physical therapists and their unique knowledge of the pathophysiology of musculoskeletal injury and thorough understanding of how healing can be safely and rapidly achieved. The appropriate use of therapeutic modalities is part of this knowledge.

Therapeutic modalities are often used to control pain, but in sports medicine, though the difference may at times be subtle, the goal of using these modalities is to increase function. For example, one reason for using cold to treat an acute ankle sprain is its analgesic effect. In sports medicine, the principal goal of using cold is early control of swelling, which limits the loss of range of motion and makes possible earlier use of muscle through this greater range. This combination results in less swelling and earlier return to functional activity. Rather than using this modality to treat pain, which is an end in itself, in sports medicine this modality is used to achieve greater function.

It is safe to assume that injury to vascularized tissue initiates the process of inflammation and repair.[1] Inflammation is a nonspecific response; regardless of how the injury occurred, the basic response is the same; however, the body must be able to respond to any contingency, so this response may be more than is necessary for some situations.[2] The degree of inflammation depends on the severity of the injury. Mismanagement of, or failure to manage, the initial inflammatory stage is a principal cause of complications seen in a sports medicine practice. Controlling the inflammatory response with therapeutic modalities has been shown to be beneficial.[3] Understanding inflammation, and how therapeutic modalities may be beneficial or detrimental to this process, allows the practitioner to skillfully manage the acute phase of injury and provide appropriate and timely treatment.

Once the inflammatory process is under control, the practitioner must work with the body so that soft tissue repair follows an appropriate course. Applying therapeutic heat too early in the process or too intensely not only prolongs inflammation but may cause reinjury—a nontherapeutic outcome. Heat, cold, sound, and light are not themselves therapeutic: only when they are applied at the appropriate time in the appropriate doses do they become useful to the injured athlete. Understanding the physiology of injury and tissue repair helps the clinician make appropriate decisions about therapeutic modalities during this phase of healing.

Controlling Early Inflammation

After an acute injury, edema interferes with normal circulation and nutrition of the tissues; it also limits range of motion and prolongs the presence of chemical irritants that contribute to pain. This leads to loss of function, increased pain, and prolonged rehabilitation. Clinicians have noted the benefits of early applications of *i*ce, *c*ompression, and *e*levation (ICE) to control this process. This protocol modulates the inflammatory response and improves the outcome.[3] Any modality or combination of modalities that can control this nonspecific response certainly aids early return to function.

The application of cold has several immediate effects in the early stages of inflammation:

1. It reduces swelling and extravasation of blood into the skin and surrounding tissues.[4, 5]
2. It slows metabolism, reducing oxygen demand and preventing some of the necrosis that results from oxygen deprivation.
3. It reduces the release of vasodilators such as histamine, which would otherwise increase the swelling.[6]
4. It reduces muscle spasms.[3, 5]
5. It decreases pain, which allows for increased passive and active motion.

A review of animal studies by Michlovitz does not support the notion that cryotherapy by itself prevents or reduces edema.[6] In the animal studies cited, researchers applied cold, either continuously over a 24-hour period or several times within 24 hours, at temperatures from 5 to 30°C. Compared with controls, animals treated within 2 hours after injury using ice bags or water baths at temperatures at or below 20°C exhibited more swelling. Michlovitz points out that the researchers in these studies did not use compression or elevation during or after treatment, as is common practice. These studies point out the need for caution when using cryotherapy immediately after trauma (within the first 2 hours) or using cold water baths below 20°C. Also, cryotherapy should always be combined with compression, elevation, and exercise, as discussed below. In support of the ICE protocol, Michlovitz cites human studies in which cold plus compression significantly decreased the duration of disability.[6]

Compression increases pressure outside the microvessels. Since escape of fluids and cells is partially dependent on pressure gradients,[1] increasing the pressure outside the microvessels stems this process. The lymph system consists of open-ended vessels in tissue spaces throughout the body. These vessels have one-way valves that allow lymph to flow only toward the heart. The lymphatic system works by pressure gradients as well. By increasing pressure around the "open ends," edema is forced into the lymph vessels.[7] When the vessels become engorged with fluid, the valves can become incompetent and the system fails. This results in swelling that cannot resolve on its own and requires interven-

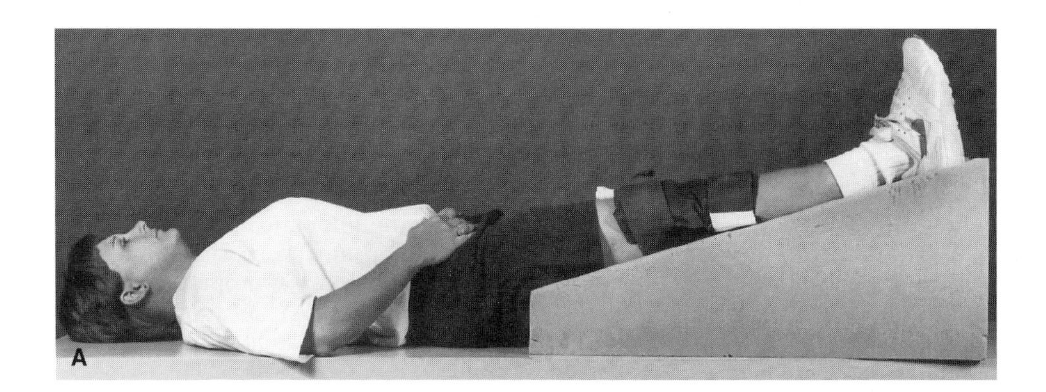

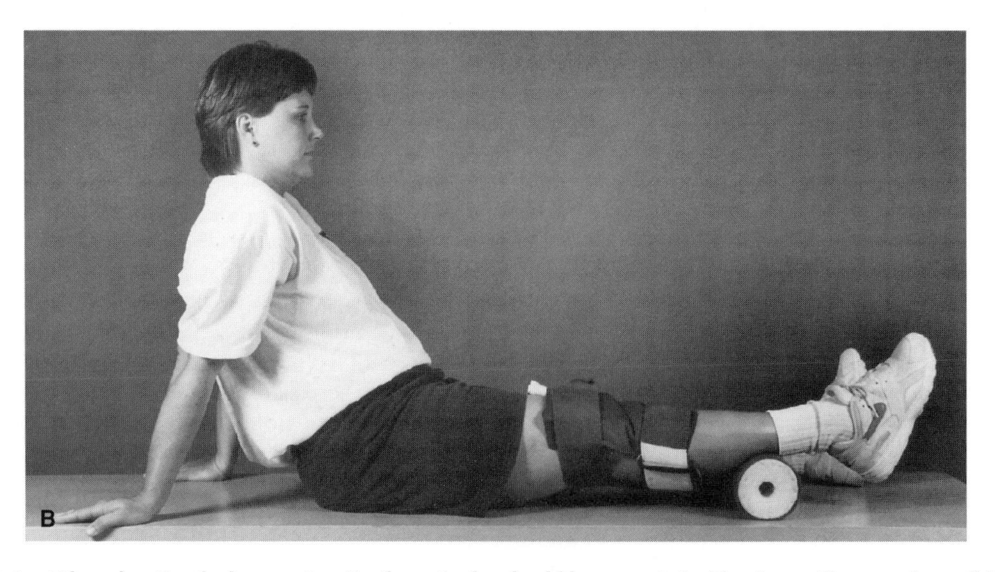

Fig. 89–1. When elevating the lower extremity, the entire leg should be supported with a foam pillow or other solid support *(A)*. The leg should not be supported at a single concentrated point *(B)* because this may interfere with the vascular or lymphatic system.

tion. It is also possible that, after some time, the lymph vessels become distended, which may lead to long-term failure and chronic swelling. To prevent these complications, compression may be applied both proximal and distal to the area of injury, if possible, to limit swelling and to maintain the patency of the lymphatic system.

Elevation of the injured area creates a gravity pressure gradient to facilitate lymph drainage. Elevation also decreases blood pressure in the injured area, reducing the volume of fluid that leaks from the damaged blood vessels (Fig. 89–1).

Exercise is prescribed to maintain motion and prevent contractures from forming. Gentle active motion creates a "muscle pump" that aids movement of fluids through the lymphatic system toward the heart. The contraction of the surrounding muscle compresses the lymph vessels. The orientation of the valves forces lymph toward the heart.[7] A further benefit of early motion is to prevent reflex inhibition, which commonly occurs in muscle surrounding an injured joint. Muscle inhibition prevents active contractions in these muscles. Use of electrical muscle stimulation in these situations is discussed later.

To control acute swelling, cold, compression, elevation, and exercise are combined. How well this "combination technique" can be applied depends on what area is involved and what resources are available. The combination technique is much easier to apply over peripheral joints of the arms and legs (ankle, knee, wrist, elbow) than in the shoulders, neck, or back.

Contraction of the musculature surrounding a joint is important. For example, once a good quadriceps contraction can be consistently developed, swelling in the knee diminishes. Likewise, for ankle sprains, once weight bearing is sufficient, the muscles of the leg help pump out the edema.

However, in an acute injury of the knee, swelling inhibits the quadriceps muscles. In this situation, prolonged elevation of the joint above the heart plus a compressive wrap or stocking is used. Although cryotherapy is usually emphasized, when considering the mechanics of swelling and edema control, the importance of prolonged elevation and compression after surgery or an acute injury cannot be overemphasized. When elevation and compression can be used appropriately, ice should be considered an adjunctive, rather than a primary, treatment.

CRYOTHERAPY

Therapeutic cooling (cryotherapy) occurs through either conduction or evaporation. Conduction, the most common method, causes loss of heat from the tissues through direct contact with the cooling agent. The degree of tissue temperature change depends on these variables: type of cooling agent; temperature of the cooling agent; duration of treatment; mode of application; and conductivity of the area being cooled.

Ice massage produces a greater degree of cooling than a gel pack. More internal heat is transferred from the tissues to melt the ice than to raise the temperature of the gel pack. Also, with ice massage, evaporation adds to the overall change in tissue temperature.

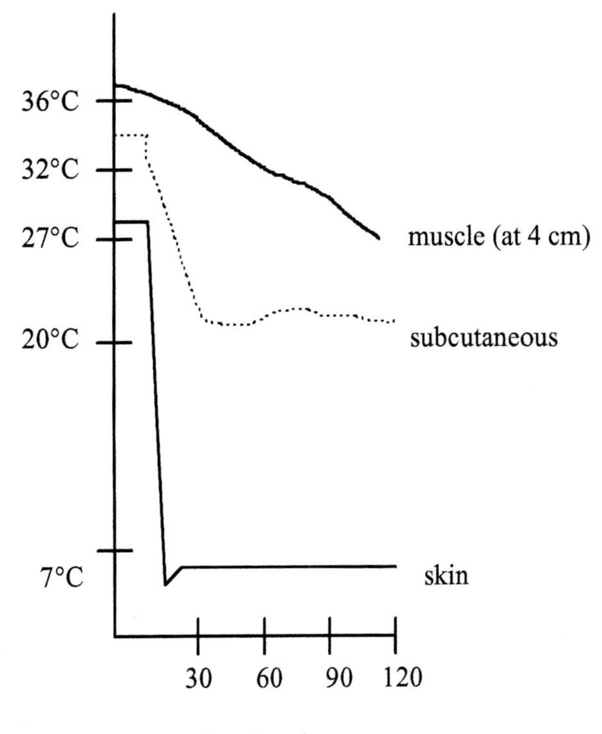

Fig. 89–2. Temperature changes of various types of tissue during ice pack application to the calf. (Adapted from Bierman, W. and Friedlander, M.: The penetrative effects of cold. Archives of Physical Therapy. *21*:585, 1940.)

The greater the temperature difference between the skin and the cooling source, the greater is the resulting change in temperature.[6] Duration of treatment also plays an important role. Though the skin reaches its maximum cooling point in approximately 15 minutes, subcutaneous fat can continue to cool for approximately 50 minutes. Muscle at a depth of 4 cm is still decreasing in temperature after 2 hours (Fig. 89–2).[8] In a study on dog knees, after continuous application of an ice pack for 1 hour, it took more than 60 minutes for the tissue temperature to return to resting values.[9]

Indications and Application Techniques

Therapeutic applications of cold are indicated for the following acute and chronic sports lesions: sprains, strains, contusions, fractures, minor burns and abrasions, heat illness, acute phase of inflammatory bursitis, tendinitis, tenosynovitis, and muscle spasm (acute or chronic). Ice packs are the most inexpensive method of applying therapeutic cold. A plastic bag or towel filled with chipped, flaked, cubed, or crushed ice may be applied directly to the skin. Commercial cold packs contain a gel and are usually cooled to between 0°C and −10°C. Treatment time varies, but 15 to 30 minutes is sufficient to lower muscle temperatures at 4 cm depth by 2 to 3°C. Because of the risk of frostbite, applications of ice packs and gel packs that are colder than 0°C should be monitored closely by checking the skin every 20 minutes.

A terry cloth towel may be used for cryotherapy by placing it in a bucket of crushed ice and water. The towel is very cold when applied because ice particles stick to it. Since the towel warms rapidly, it must be changed every 4 to 5 minutes.[10]

Massage with an ice cube is an excellent, and usually convenient, method of icing a relatively small superficial area of inflammation. An ice cube from an ice tray may be used, but a more convenient chunk results from freezing water in a styrofoam cup. The styrofoam is peeled away, and the ice is used to massage the inflamed area in a circular motion for 5 to 10 minutes, until the area is numb. This treatment works very well over the epicondyles of the elbow, the patellar tendon, and collateral ligaments of the knee and the ligaments of the ankle.

Ice massage may also be used over muscle, both for contusions and for decreasing muscle spasms (e.g., in the back and hamstrings). These applications can be longer—up to 15 minutes.

Immersion in a bucket of cold water and ice may be used for larger areas. Depending on the ratio of ice to water, the temperature will be cool (19 to 26°C), cold (12.5 to 19°C), or very cold (0 to 12.5°C).[11] Because immersion is one of the more uncomfortable methods of applying cold, the temperature must be adjusted to make the treatment tolerable. Very good results may be achieved when using the cool to cold ranges mentioned above; it is not necessary to always use the coldest range. To control swelling, treatment is applied for 10 to 20 minutes. For pain relief, treatment continues until anesthesia is produced. In a very cold ice bath, this takes less than 5 minutes.

In studies cited earlier by Michlovitz, subjects treated within the first 2 hours after injury using temperatures below 20°C had more swelling than untreated controls. Therefore, precaution should be taken to avoid (1) applying cold *too soon* after injury, (2) using temperatures considered *too cold*, and (3) applying cold for *too long*. More research is needed to establish better guidelines.

Vapocoolant sprays (fluoromethane and ether chloride) may be used to rapidly cool an area for analgesic effect. Because this type of cold is only superficial and does not cool tissue beneath the surface, its effect is only analgesic and not anti-inflammatory. As an analgesic the method is quite useful. It allows rapid local pain reduction, which facilitates active and passive exercise. It may be inadvisable, after using this, to allow the athlete to return to uncontrolled activity, since the potential for reinjury is greater when pain is effectively blocked. This treatment could be used for a mild contusion (e.g., a baseball hit into the shin) so the athlete can continue to play. The potential for serious injury in this situation is small. For analgesia, the area is sprayed. Caution should be taken, since repeated applications can lower skin temperature to 4°C, causing skin damage.[10]

Vapocoolant sprays are also convenient for acute muscle spasms. The muscle is stretched as far as comfort allows and is then sprayed unidirectionally, from the muscle attachment farthest from the contracted joint toward the joint. The spray is held approximately 2 feet from the muscle and moved at about 4 inches per second, covering the muscle at least twice. After the muscle is sprayed, additional force is applied and the muscle is gently stretched. The therapist then uses the hands to warm the skin, and the treatment is repeated as many as three times.

Contraindications and Precautions for the Use of Cryotherapy

Contraindications for cryotherapy include (1) cardiac dysfunction, including angina pectoris, (2) open wounds older than 48 to 72 hours (vasoconstriction may delay healing), (3) arterial insufficiency, (4) hypersensitivity to cold (cold urticaria, Raynaud's phenomenon), and (5) peripheral neuropathies, including diabetes, which compromises sensation.[11] Several precautions should be considered as well: temperature range, duration of treatment, and timing of treatment in relation to the onset of injury. It is suggested that the duration of cryotherapy not exceed 30 minutes. Care should be taken to avoid applying cold directly over a superficial nerve, particularly the peroneal nerve at the fibular head. Injuries have been reported when cold is applied to this area for longer than an hour.[6] Frostbite does not result from short-term application of cold directly to the skin; however, several cases of cold skin "burn" have been reported when gel packs cooled below 0°C were applied directly to the skin.[10]

COMPRESSION

A compressive wrap, such as an Ace bandage or Tubigrip, may be combined with the ice pack to provide compression. The Tubigrip is more "user friendly" for home application over the ankle, knee, wrist, or elbow because the material is inherently compressive and its compression does not depend on wrapping skill (Fig. 89–3). It is easy to apply Tubigrip, and the only major complication may be a tourniquet effect if the ends of the tube roll.

The athlete is instructed to keep the compressive wrap on at all times during the first several days after an injury, to help control swelling. After the first several days, the wrap is used only during the day. The importance of controlling inflammation in the early stages cannot be overemphasized, and continuous application of compression is imperative.

Mechanical Application of Cryotherapy and Compression

An ideal combination of cryotherapy and compression may be found in such devices as the Cryocuff (Aircast,

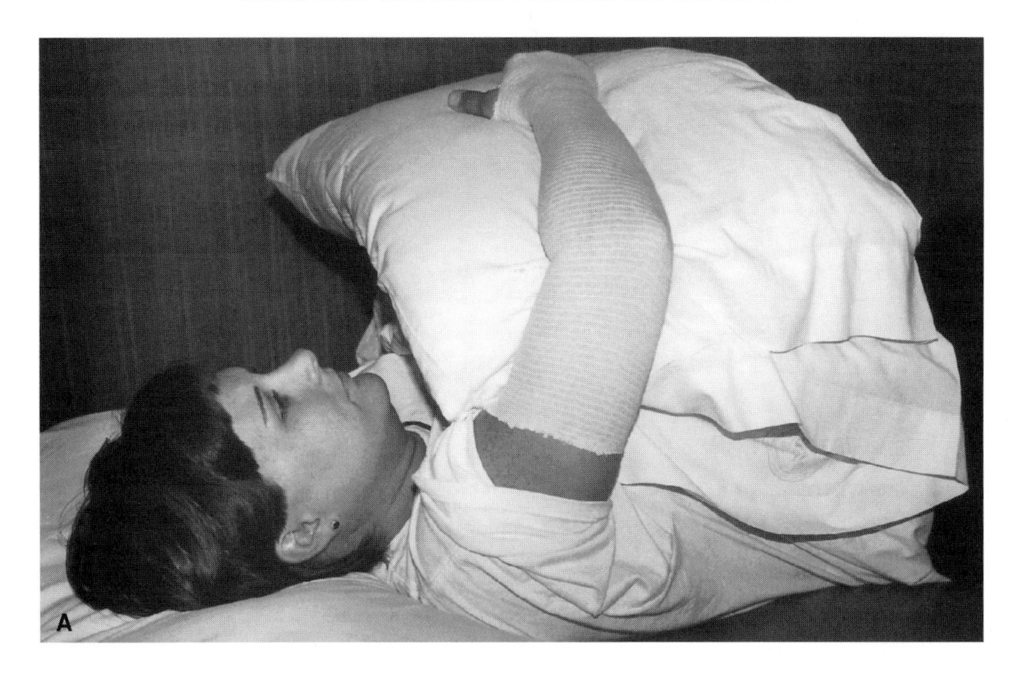

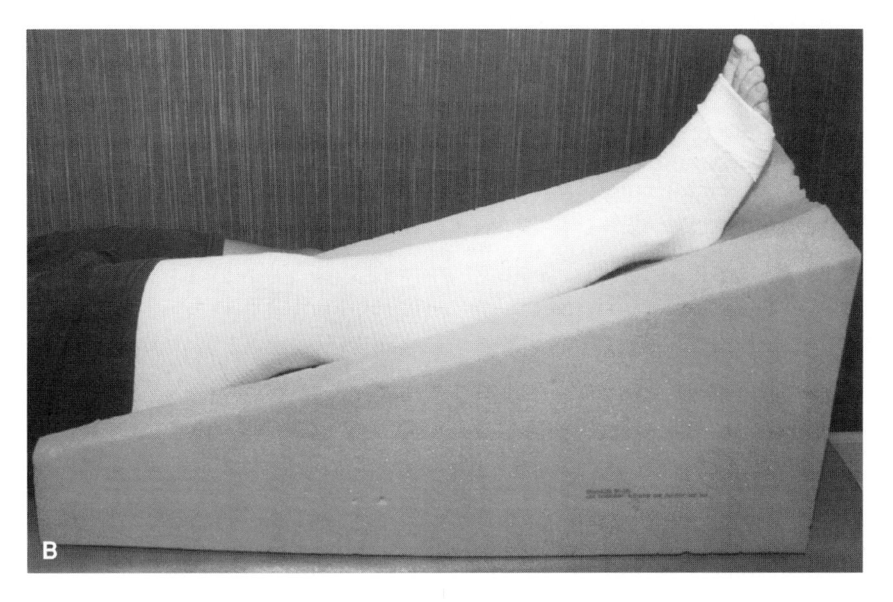

Fig. 89–3. The Tubigrip is easy for the patient to use at home and comes in various sizes to fit (A) the arm or (B) the leg.

Summit, NJ) or Cryotemp (Jobst Institute, Toledo, OH). The Cryocuff is a simpler device that uses a vacuum bottle of ice and water as the cooling agent (Fig. 89–4). Pressure depends on how high above the treated area the bottle is raised. For safety, the maximum pressure gradient is limited by the length of the connecting hose, so it is very difficult to apply too much pressure. Both units use specific cuffs designed for individual joints.

The Cryotemp relies on a mechanical pump to apply pressure and to circulate cold water (10 to 25°C). A sleeve is applied to the elevated extremity through which the water circulates. The amount of pressure, duration of pressure, and temperature of the cooling agent may be set. Intermittent pressure provides a pumping action to reduce edema. A new model of the Cryocuff that uses an air pump to cycle pressure mechanically is ideal for continuous application to an acute injury to an extremity joint or for postsurgical application.

ULTRASOUND

Pulsed Ultrasound

Pulsed ultrasound (US) has been suggested for use on acute inflammation.[12] The commonly cited rationale

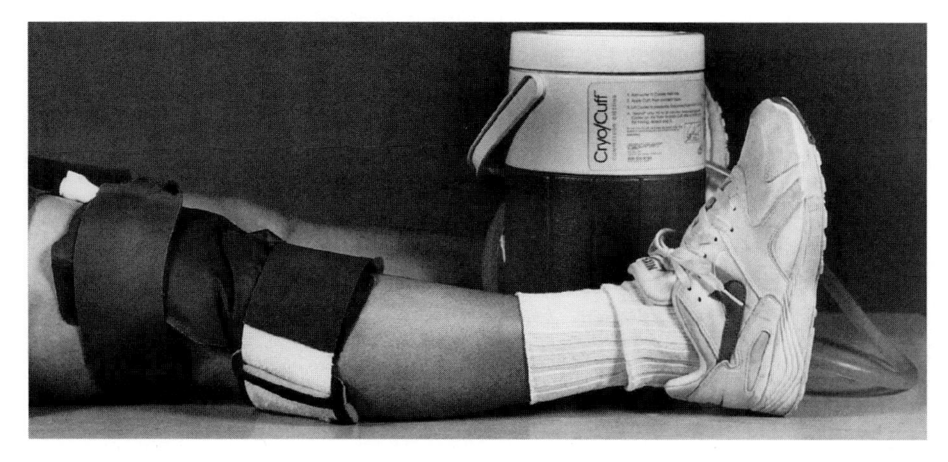

Fig. 89–4. The Cryocuff uses a thermos of ice and water, which can be raised to different heights to control the amount of pressure in the cuff.

for the use of US is that it increases circulation and tissue heating. In contrast, US at low intensity (less than 0.5 mV/cm^2) and pulsed at a 20% duty cycle has been suggested, to allow the injury to pass through the inflammatory stage more quickly.[13] Used in this way, low intensity and cycled, the nonthermal therapeutic effects of US, cavitation and acoustic streaming, are believed to modify cell membrane permeability. This allows for diffusion of metabolites and facilitates transport of ions, and possibly of some molecules, across cell membranes.[12] Unlike the early use of ice, one of the goals of which is to limit release of inflammatory agents such as histamine, a single treatment of pulsed ultrasound applied during the early inflammatory stage stimulates the release of histamine and other chemotactic agents that attract neutrophils and monocytes to the wound site. By facilitating this process, rather than limiting the inflammatory process, as with cryotherapy, the goals of the early stage of inflammation (e.g., débridement) are achieved earlier. This should result in earlier resolution of the injury and allow an earlier return to activity. It must be emphasized that, with low-intensity pulsed US, tissue heating is avoided. In the early stages of inflammation, continuous duty cycles of US at intensities greater than 0.5 W/cm^2 are contraindicated.

Pulsed Ultrasound Treatment

When using US for therapy, the physician should keep in mind the following variables: duration of treatment; effective radiating area of the soundhead (ERA); duty cycle; size of area to be treated; depth of tissue to be treated; and thermal versus nonthermal treatments.

Treatment time must take into account the effective radiating area (ERA) of the particular soundhead. This information is supplied in the instruction manual with the individual unit. The area to be treated is divided into treatment zones measuring 1½ times the ERA. For an acute injury, each of these zones is treated for 1 to 2 minutes. With an ERA of 5 cm^2 and a treatment area of 7.5 cm^2 (the area of an inflamed lateral epicondyle), treatment would take between 1 and 2 minutes to achieve the nonthermal benefits desired for an acute injury.

Ultrasound frequency depends on what soundhead is supplied. The US frequency is selected based on the depth of the tissue: 3 MHz for superficial tissues and 1 MHz for deeper tissue. Nonthermal effects suggested for use in acute injuries are achieved with the pulsed US at a 20% duty cycle and an intensity of no more than 0.5 mV. The sound head is slowly moved over this area in an overlapping circular motion. Each treatment zone, as defined above, is treated for 1 to 2 minutes.[12]

The use of pulsed US to increase the tensile strength of tendon has also been studied.[12,13] Some researchers suggest that low-intensity pulsed US increases the tensile strength of tendon. Such increases are noted only during the first several weeks of healing; after 8 weeks, treated and untreated controls develop similar levels of strength. This treatment may be beneficial in allowing earlier return of function with less risk.

Continuous Ultrasound

Continuous US is indicated when tissue heating is desired. US selectively heats tissues with high collagen content: tendon, cartilage, ligament, and bone. The heating effect is particularly concentrated at the interfaces of these tissues. Selective heating is used to facilitate stretching of contracted deep connective tissue. Precise temperature levels are needed to achieve an appropriate stretch without causing injury. Since it is impossible to measure tissue temperatures in the clinic, the potential for injury may in fact increase when deep connective tissue is stretched in this manner.[14]

When highly vascularized tissue such as muscle is treated with continuous US, the tissue does not heat; rather, circulation increases to dissipate the heat. Very little heating (1 to 2°C) actually takes place in the muscle, but blood flow increases significantly and remains elevated as long as 60 minutes after treatment ends.[13,15] Local increases in blood flow may be beneficial in the treatment of muscle spasms and to aid tissue healing in various conditions.

PHONOPHORESIS

Topical application of anti-inflammatory medications assisted by US, called phonophoresis, has also been used to control inflammation. Molecules are driven and dispersed by US waves.. The medication must be appropriate for use with US, in that it must not block the transmission of sound waves. If the medication is first thoroughly rubbed into the skin, the problem of transmission block can be avoided.

The most commonly used anti-inflammatory medications are hydrocortisone cream, in 0.5%, 1%, 5%, or 10% concentration, and salicylate. Hydrocortisone in concentrations over 1.0% is controlled and requires a physician's prescription, but according to Kahn it adds no benefit as only so much medication can be absorbed, no matter what the concentration.[16] Salicylate (Myoflex cream) is an over-the-counter nonsteroidal preparation. The mechanism of action of these medications is similar to that when they are taken orally, though with phonophoresis systemic responses are avoided.

IONTOPHORESIS

The mechanism of iontophoresis is different from that of phonophoresis, in that the medications are in appropriate solutions that allow ions to be repelled by a like-charged direct current. Many practitioners have avoided iontophoresis in the past because of chemical burns, which occur as hydroxide ions build up under the cathode (negative electrode) as a result of the dissociation of water molecules. Recent advances have been made in buffering the medications or adding a buffering agent to the electrode. Also, advances in the materials used in the electrodes reportedly allows better release of the medications and greater safety as well (Fig. 89–5).

Dexamethasone sodium phosphate is the only medication approved by the U.S. Food and Drug Administration for iontophoretic introduction, and it is the one most commonly used. It is possible to use this medication in the acute stage of inflammation; however, it is more commonly used for persistent inflammation. Other medications have been suggested for introduction by iontophoresis as well (Table 89–1).

ELECTRICAL STIMULATION

Electrical stimulation using a monophasic pulsed current device as delivered by high-voltage stimulators has been shown to reduce edema formation in frogs,[17] hamsters,[18] and rats[19]; however, positive results were seen only if the stimulation was used in the first hours after injury and if the cathode was used as the stimulating electrode. These studies suggest that some of the regimens currently practiced may be used too late in the course of the injury or may use an incorrect waveform (other than cathodal high voltage) or pulse parameters. Based on these studies, high-voltage pulsed current (HVPC) at 120 pulses per second (pps), at an intensity of 90% of that required to produce a muscle contraction, is applied to the injured area with the cathode for 30 minute treatments up to 4 times within the first 8 hours of injury.[20]

Some researchers have reported the effects of electrical muscle stimulation on local blood supply.[21]

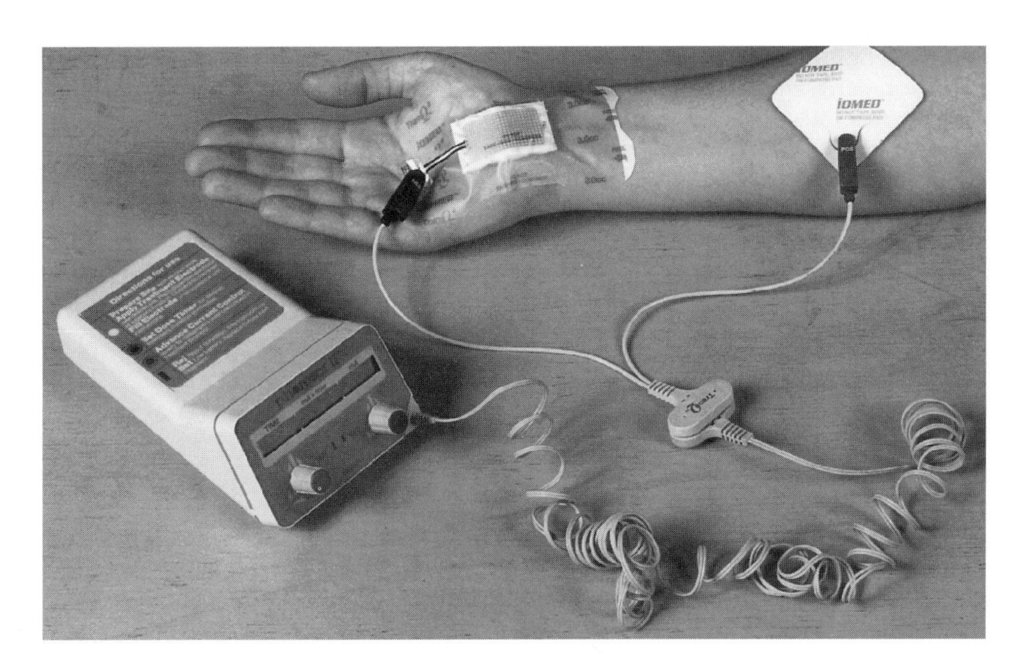

Fig. 89–5. The Transcue II electrode by Empi allows better release of the medications and improved safety than older types of electrodes.

Table 89–1. Currently Used Ions: Properties and Sources

Hydrocortisone: 1% ointment, various local sources, positive pole; anti-inflammatory; avoid ointments with "paraben" preservatives; used for arthritis, tendinitis, myositis, bursitis
Mecholyl: mecholyl ointment, (Gordon Labs, Upper Darby, PA); positive pole; vasodilator, analgesic; used for neuritis, neurovascular deficits, sprains, edema
Lidocaine: from xylocaine 5% (Astra Pharmaceutical Co., Westboro, MA); positive pole; anesthetic analgesic; used for neuritis, bursitis, painful range of motion
Acetic acid: 10% stock solution, cut to 2%; negative pole; used for calcific deposits, myositis ossificans, frozen joints
Iodine: from Iodex (with methyl salicylate); negative pole; sclerolytic, antiseptic, analgesic; used for scar tissue, adhesions, fibrositis
Salicylate: from Myoflex (Adria Labs, Columbus, OH) ointment, 10% salicylate preparation, or Iodex *with* methyl salicylate (Medtech Labs Inc., Cody, WY); negative pole; decongestant, analgesic; used for myalgias, rheumatoid arthritis
Magnesium: from 2% solution of magnesium sulfate (Epsom salts); positive pole; antispasmodic, analgesic, vasodilator; used for osteoarthritis, myositis, neuritis
Copper: 2% solution, copper sulfate; positive pole; caustic, antiseptic, antifungal; used for allergic rhinitis, dermatophytosis (athlete's foot)
Zinc: from zinc oxide ointment 20%; positive pole; caustic, antiseptic; enhances healing; used for otitis, ulcerations, dermatitis, other open lesions
Calcium: from calcium chloride, 2% solution; positive pole; stabilizer or irritability threshold; used for myospasm, frozen joints, trigger finger, mild tremors (non-Parkinsonian)
Chlorine: from table salt (NaCl), 2% solution; negative pole; sclerolytic; used for scar tissue, adhesions
Lithium: from lithium chloride or lithium carbonate, 2% solution; positive pole; specifically for gouty tophi
Hyaluronidase: from Wydase (Wyeth, Philadelphia, PA); solution to be mixed as directed on vials; positive pole; absorption agent for edema, sprains

(Kahn, J.: Principles and Practice of Electrotherapy. 3rd Ed. New York, Churchill Livingstone, 1994. p. 138.)

Though no research has demonstrated that electrical stimulation decreases edema after the first day of injury, such stimulation is beneficial in cases where muscle function is inhibited (e.g., after knee injury, particularly patellar dislocations, or in postsurgical knees). Currier and coworkers reported a significant increase in blood flow when stimulating the gastrocnemius muscle with a 2500-Hz sine wave at 50 pps (similar to what "Russian stimulators" and "medium-frequency" generators produce) at 10 to 30% of maximum voluntary contraction (MVC).[22] In a similar study using HVPC at 30 pps at up to 30% MVC to stimulate the gastrocnemius, the treated subjects did not experience increased blood flow at the popliteal artery, whereas a group exercising at 30% MVC did exhibit increased blood flow.[23]

We suggest that common "muscle-stimulating" devices that (1) use a frequency around 2500 Hz and (2) can be adjusted to 50 pps be used at intensities that produce a comfortable but visible contraction of the quadriceps muscles. *On* times of 8 seconds and *off* times of around 20 seconds, with a total treatment time of 5 to 15 minutes, are used. This treatment is used only if there is no active muscle contraction and usually is discontinued when active muscle contractures are restored, usually in fewer than five sessions.

CONTRAST BATHS

Contrast baths are commonly used after the acute phase of inflammation. Theoretically, the contrast of heat and cold creates vasodilation and contraction of blood and lymph vessels, producing a "pumping" action to remove edema from the region. This treatment may serve to "unclog" lymph vessels by heating and to control the detrimental effects of heat by cooling the area immediately after. Various protocols are followed, usually beginning with heat and ending with cold. The cycle may be repeated several times. The physician using contrast baths should consider the level of inflammation in deciding how warm or hot the bath should be and the duration of this phase of the treatment. Also, the duration of the cooling phase can be adjusted. For example, early in the subacute phase, the initial bath would be warm rather than hot and of shorter duration; this is followed by a relatively long cold treatment. Later in the subacute phase, the initial bath may be hot and last longer and the length of the cooling phase is a matter of less concern.

SUMMARY

Therapeutic modalities are most effective when combined with therapeutic exercise and integrated into an overall rehabilitation program. There are many unanswered questions about which modalities work best and which parameters are most effective. With an understanding of the physiology of injury and the mechanism through which therapeutic modalities intervene in this process, effective outcomes may be achieved.

REFERENCES

1. Reed, B., and Zarro, V.: Inflammation and repair and the use of thermal agents. *In* Thermal Agents in Rehabilitation. 2nd Ed. Edited by S. L. Michlovitz. Philadelphia, F. A. Davis, 1990.
2. Peacock, E. E.: Wound Repair. 3rd Ed. Philadelphia, W. B. Saunders, 1984.
3. Gieck, J. H., and Saliba, E. N.: Application of modalities in overuse syndromes. Clin. Sports Med. *6*:427, 1987.
4. Wadsworth, H., and Chanmugan, A. P.: Electrophysical Agents in Physiotherapy. Australia, Science Press, 1983.
5. Loane, S. R.: Cryotherapy-using cold to treat injuries. *In* Sports Medicine: Fitness, Training, Injuries. Edited by O. Appenzeller. Baltimore, Urban & Schwarzenberg, 1988.
6. Michlovitz, S. L.: Cryotherapy: The use of cold as a therapeutic agent. *In* Thermal Agents in Rehabilitation. 2nd Ed. Edited by S. L. Michlovitz. Philadelphia, F. A. Davis, 1990.
7. Williams, P. L., and Warwick, R. (eds.): Gray's Anatomy. 36th Ed. Philadelphia, W. B. Saunders, 1980.
8. Bierman, W. and Friedlander, M.: The penetrative effect of cold. Arch. Phys. Ther. *21*:585, 1940.
9. Wakim, K. G., Porter, A. N., and Krusen, K. H.: Influence of physical agents and of certain drugs on intra-articular temperature. Arch. Phys. Med. *32*:714, 1951.
10. Poole, R. P., Lee, B. C., and Blackburn, T. A. *In* Physical Modalities in Rehabilitation: Sports Medicine for the School Age Athlete. Edited by Reider, B. Philadelphia, W. B. Saunders, 1990.
11. Hayes, K. W.: Manual for Physical Agents. 4th Ed. Norwalk, CT, Appleton & Lange, 1993.
12. Dyson, M.: Role of ultrasound in wound healing. *In* Wound Healing: Alternatives in Management. Edited by L. Kloth, J. M. McCulloch, and J. A. Feedar. Philadelphia, F. A. Davis, 1990.

13. Enwemeka, C. S.: Enweba, Lecture notes, Update of Modalities, Fall Meeting, Physical Therapy Association of Georgia, 1993.
14. Cummings, G.: Personal communication. Georgia State University, Department of Physical Therapy, 1993.
15. Griffin, J., and Karselis, T. C.: Physical Agents for Physical Therapists. 2nd Ed. Springfield Ill, Charles C Thomas, 1982.
16. Kahn, J.: Principles and Practice of Electrotherapy. 2nd Ed. New York, Churchill Livingstone, 1991.
17. Taylor, K., Fish, D. R., Mendel, F. C., and Burton, H. W.: Effect of a single 30-minute treatment of high voltage pulsed current on edema formation in frog hind limbs. J. Am. Phys. Ther. Assoc. *72*:63, 1992.
18. Reed, B. V.: Effect of high voltage pulsed electrical stimulation on microvascular permeability to plasma proteins. J. Am. Phys. Ther. Assoc. *68*:491, 1988.
19. Mendel, F. C., Wylegala, J. A., and Fish, D. R.: Influence of high voltage pulsed current on edema formation following impact injury in rats. J. Am. Phys. Ther. Assoc. *72*:668, 1992.
20. Bettany, J. A., Fish, D. R., and Mendel, F. C.: Influence of high voltage pulsed direct current on edema formation following impact injury. J. Am. Phys. Ther. Assoc. *70*:219, 1990.
21. Currier, D. P.: Neuromuscular stimulation for improving muscular strength and blood flow, and influencing changes. *In* Clinical Electrotherapy. 2nd Ed. Edited by R. Nelson and D. P. Currier. Norwalk, CT, Appleton & Lange, 1991.
22. Currier, D. P., Petrilli, C. R., and Threlkeld, A. J.: Effect of graded electrical stimulation on blood flow to healthy muscle. J. Am. Phys. Ther. Assoc. *66*:937, 1986.
23. Walker, D. C., Currier, D. P., and Threlkeld, A. J.: Effects of high-voltage pulsed electrical stimulation on blood flow. J. Am. Phys. Ther. Assoc. *68*:481, 1988.

Appendix. Sample Program: Physical Modalities in the Treatment of an Acute Patellar Dislocation

Acute phase: days 1–3

Goal: Control swelling and pain

Treatment options:

1. Pulsed US at <0.5 mV/cm^2 at 20% duty cycle along insertion of medial gastrocnemius for between 2 and 3 minutes for days 1 and 2.

or

Cryotherapy with ice pack or compression cryotherapy units (Cryocuff or Cryotemp) for 20–30 minutes several times a day.

2. Compression: When using either US or cryotherapy, these are combined with compression using Tubigrip or other compressive dressings. Dressing is left on continuously for the first 3 days; then it may be used only during the day if swelling has subsided at night.

3. Elevation: Elevate the knee above the heart, making sure the ankle is above the knee. This may be combined with ankle pumps and quadriceps sets if tolerated.

Goal: Protect the injured joint

Treatment:

1. Straight-leg immobilizer.
2. Crutches and weight bearing as tolerated.

Goal: Facilitate quadriceps activity and maintain hamstrings flexibility

Treatment:

1. Exercise of quadriceps sets, terminal knee extensions, sitting hip flexion, and hamstrings stretching. These exercises are performed only if tolerated at this early stage.

Subacute phase: days 3–7

Goal: Control swelling

Treatment options:

1. Continue cryotherapy several times a day, as needed.
2. Continue compression dressing during the day and include nighttime compression if needed.
3. Elevate leg above heart as much as possible.
4. Begin electric stimulation with either high-voltage, medium-frequency, or Russian stimulator to facilitate active quadriceps contraction, 35–50 pulses per second, intensity set as high as tolerable, or, where visible muscle contraction is noted, 8 seconds on with 12- to 20-second rest period. The knee is positioned to perform terminal knee extension (TKE), and the patient attempts contractions during the *on* time. If the patient is unable to lift the foot, the therapist may assist by lifting the foot and gently reducing assistance until the patient achieves an active contraction. Many times active TKEs are performed after one treatment session on previously inhibited quadriceps. Emphasize active quadriceps sets and TKEs once the patient can perform independently and discontinue electric stimulation.
5. Lymphatic massage, massaging the quadriceps toward the heart, facilitating lymphatic drainage.
6. Iontophoresis with dexamethasone to vastus medialis obliquus insertion where tender. (Option: May use US, low-intensity 20%, over area before using iontophoresis. This reduces skin resistance, allowing quicker permeability.)
7. Phonophoresis with Myoflex at 1.0 W/cm^2 continuous for 4 to 7 minutes over VMO insertion.

Goal: Strengthening and flexibility

Treatment:

1. Exercise: Quadriceps sets, TKEs, sitting hip flexion, hamstrings stretching, passive flexion to point of pain, biking when passive range of motion is >115°. Closed-chain activities as tolerated.
2. *Gait:* Discontinue immobilizer when closed-chain activities are tolerated. May use knee sleeve. Begin single crutch and emphasize normal gait pattern.

Return to Activity: 1 week after injury and beyond

Criteria:

1. Full active extension and passive knee flexion.
2. Swelling only after exercise that can be controlled by ice, compression, and elevation.
3. Similar bilateral hamstrings flexibility.

Treatment:

1. Exercise: Emphasize closed-chain activities, plyometrics when tolerated, and sport-specific activities. May continue ice, compression, and elevation if needed while progressing exercise program.

90 *William D. Jones*

Resistance Training and Flexibility Maintenance

The use of strength and conditioning can be traced back to the early civilizations, to the medical *gymnastai* whose major duties were to condition athletes and maintain high performance levels.[1] Several authors have suggested that proper resistance training can increase speed of movement and flexibility.[2–4] Resistance training includes "free" weights, machines with weight stacks, machines using hydraulics, isokinetic machines, elastic bands, and body weight—anything that offers resistance to the muscles involved. Training with resistance, regardless of the apparatus, should be done with the specific sport or activity in mind. For example, any individual seeking "general fitness" as a goal can use a resistance program tailored to the appropriate level and the final goals of that individual. Another specific goal would be rehabilitation after surgery or an injury. Resistance training has historically been the foundation for such rehabilitation because the forces used to strengthen the muscles can be controlled to avoid injury to a repaired structure.[5,6] The type of surgery or injury dictates the methods to be used.

Some sports, like Olympic weight lifting, are based on resistance exercise. In competition, weight lifters must perform two lifts: the clean and jerk and the snatch. While it sounds simple, this sport actually requires a great deal of strength, power, and flexibility to compete. The highest human power outputs ever recorded have been produced by high-level weight lifters.[7] Likewise, the sport of body building requires extreme levels of muscle hypertrophy and low levels of body fat. The object is the "body ideal," and judging criteria include symmetry, muscularity, size, and presentation. Weight training is the primary "tool" of the sport; however, many competitors have incorporated aerobic activity into their training to control the level of body fat.

The sport of power lifting requires the athlete to lift maximum weights in the deadlift, squat, and bench press. It requires a tremendous amount of strength. The name is misleading, as power is not actually tested, since speed is not a major component of the sport. Skill is also required, but not as much as for Olympic weight lifting.

Other sports have primary objectives other than aesthetics or pounds lifted. Resistance training should be applied as a secondary component to overall conditioning in these sports and should complement the particular sport.

Although weight training has been used for specific and general conditioning for years, misconceptions still abound:

Fat turns into muscle, or muscle turns to fat when you stop training. Muscle and fat cells have two different structures. As training progresses it may seem that fat turns to muscle; however, this change in appearance is probably from the addition of lean body weight. It may also seem that muscle turns to fat during a hiatus in training, but the phenomenon is actually muscle atrophy. The appearance of fat usually results if the athlete does not adjust calorie intake.

High repetitions with low weight achieves definition of muscle. Muscle definition comes from lack of fat, not a particular weight training schedule. Aerobics, along with a restricted diet, reduces the proportion of body fat.

I don't want to look like Mr. or Ms. America . . . that's too big. This is the last thing anyone should ever worry about. An increase in size takes months and years; body changes are gradual. No one ever wakes up in the morning to discover they did one too many sets the day before.

I don't want to become muscle bound. "Muscle bound" describes a lack of elasticity in the muscles. The size of a muscle does not determine a person's flexibility. A study found that Olympic weight lifters are second only to gymnasts in flexibility.[8]

RESISTANCE TRAINING

Modes of Resistance

Although any type of resistance can cause an increase in strength and power, theory and research strongly indicate that free weights produce superior results.[9–11] Individual choices and preferences, practicalities, and safety must also be addressed.[12]

For safety, and perhaps for legal reasons, spotters may be essential during some free weight exercises (e.g., squat, bench). Machines may be safer in this respect, since the weight cannot fall on the lifter. No studies have compared the numbers or types of injuries that occur with free weights and machines; however, injuries can occur with both systems.

Free weight training takes more skill than using machines, and some of that skill so acquired may carry over into the performance of the sport. More of the body is used during free weight training for stabilization. Most machines and pulley system resistance can isolate muscles better than free weights. At times this is good for rehabilitation, and sometimes for body building. Muscles rarely work in isolation during sports participation.

With free weights it takes more time to adjust the weights, whereas in most machines it is a simple matter of moving a "pin." Most machines afford minimum increases of 10 to 15 pounds (depending on the manufacturer), whereas free weights can be adjusted by as little as 2½ pounds. Free weights are also generally cheaper than machines.

Physiologic Results

The reduction of resting heart rates via exercise has been commonly cited as evidence of increased cardiovascular fitness.[12,13] Studies have shown that highly weight-trained athletes have lower than average resting heart rates.[14–17]

Blood pressure changes resulting from resistance exercise have been the subject of controversy, depending on the reporting source. Blood pressure increases with isometric exercise,[18] as well as immediately after weight training.[19] However, these increases are similar to responses to other high-intensity exercise.[20] Significant decreases in resting systolic pressures have also been noted with resistance training.[21,22] Though there may be high peaks of blood pressure during resistance exercise, overall, there are also some benefits. Though the body adapts to changes that occur during exercise, persons with a history of cardiovascular disease should proceed under a physician's care and with proper instruction.

Maximum aerobic power ($\dot{V}O_2max$) is defined as the point at which oxygen consumption "plateaus" and shows no further increase with additional workload.[13] Resistance training is not regarded as a superior form of exercising to increase $\dot{V}O_2max$; however, some circuit training studies and some noncircuit studies show a 4 to 9% increase in $\dot{V}O_2max$.[21,23–25]

Body composition studies have shown significant increases in lean body mass and loss of body fat in men and women of all ages who perform resistance training.[21,26–28]

BASIC CONCEPTS AND PRINCIPLES

To understand why it is important that training be sport specific, one must understand energy production and how the body uses energy for different tasks. Training programs can be changed and adapted to help the athlete become more efficient, both in performance and in the amount of time spent training, based on the type and level of exercise needed for the individual's sport.

Energy Systems

Adenosine triphosphate (ATP) is a highly specialized chemical substance that provides "useful" energy and is important in muscle contraction, which equates with strength and power.[29] Adenosine triphosphate can be replenished (on a basic level) by three energy systems.

The ATP-CP (stored phosphagen) system is anaerobic. As ATP is used, energy can be immediately replenished by creatine phosphate, which donates a phosphate molecule to reform ATP. This system is used to provide energy immediately, but it cannot be sustained. Thus, it is used mainly for initiation of action and short-term events (0 to 45 seconds)[30] with short rests between. To train the ATP-CP system, exercise should be performed at maximum intensity for up to 30 to 45 seconds with 45 to 90 seconds of absolute rest between sets.[31]

The lactic acid (anaerobic glycolysis) system is taxed during relatively continuous all-out exertion lasting 45 seconds to 3 minutes. It also provides energy at the beginning of a period of exercise, before the aerobic system takes over. To train the lactic acid system, work should be performed at high intensity for 2 to 3 minutes and light activity during rest intervals of 4 to 6 minutes between sets.[31]

The aerobic system provides energy during continuous submaximal activity lasting longer than 3 to 4 minutes. To improve aerobic capacity, work should consist of 15 to 180 minutes at 60 to 80% of maximum heart rate.[31] The body never works exclusively aerobically or anaerobically. Thus, adequate training is needed in all systems, to enhance tolerance of heavy anaerobic work and improve recovery.

Elements of Training

The basic principles of training apply not only to resistance training but to other areas of training as well.

Volume is equal to duration (time) and frequency (sessions per day or week). The volume of training can be estimated by the total repetitions in a given period.[12] *Intensity* (load) is equal to the power output (rate of work) and can be estimated by the average weight lifted.[12] *Variation* is included because the body tends to adapt to stresses. Periodic changes in exercises, methods, volume, and intensity are necessary. Done in a correct manner (i.e., periodization), variation can help reduce the possibility of overtraining and injury and take the athlete to peak performance levels.[12] *Specificity* is important because training adaptations are specific to the cells and their structural and functional elements.[32,33] With this in mind, volume and intensity can be varied within the specificity guidelines. *Overload* refers to the practice of taxing muscles beyond their present capacity. This is necessary to increase the size or functional ability of the muscle fiber.[34] Without overload there would be little or no increase in performance. *Reversibility* refers to the fact that training effects are transient. To sustain the effects of training, an athlete must continue to apply all of the training principles.[35]

Understanding the types of contractions involved in training help one appreciate the goals of certain training techniques. There are three basic types of voluntary muscle contraction.

Isometric. The muscle contracts but its length does not change.[34]

Concentric. The muscle contracts and as it does, it gets shorter.[34] This is also sometimes referred to as a *positive motion,* or *positive work.*

Eccentric. The muscle lengthens as it contracts.[34] The movement begins at the end range of a concentric contraction (maximum "shortened" position). The resistance is then slowly released to the end range ("lengthened") position. Eccentric contractions are sometimes referred to as *negatives,* or *negative work.* Although eccentric contractions have been shown to develop the greatest amount of tension in a muscle, negative work alone has not been shown to be superior to concentric work alone.[36]

Since the body works constantly in combinations of isometric, concentric, and eccentric contractions, no single area should be emphasized over others during training.

There are four basic methods of producing an increase in strength and power. A general understanding of these will bridge the communication gap between physician, therapist, coach, and athlete.

Isometrics. With isometric exercise the muscle contracts against resistance without changing its length or the angle of the joint the muscle crosses (no movement). An example is pushing against an immovable object without changing limb position. These types of exercises are more useful during rehabilitation, but generally they are not useful for enhancing athletic performance because strength develops only at the angle at which the exercise is performed.[37]

Isotonics. Isotonic exercises, the kind most commonly performed, use resistance through an available range of motion—with free weights, body weight, or machines, among others.

Isokinetics. Isokinetic exercises are done on a machine that regulates speed of movement. The resistance is considered varied, or accommodating, since, regardless of the force applied, speed is constant. These machines are most commonly used in a rehabilitation setting. Though they may be used as an adjunct to strength training, they violate the specificity principle in that few human movements contain phases of constant limb angular velocity.[34]

Plyometrics. The majority of training activities involve contractions in which a muscle acts, first eccentrically, then concentrically.[34] Plyometrics is a training technique that involves eccentric-to-concentric sequences of muscle activity.[34] During the eccentric phase the muscle is preloaded and able to store elastic energy. It immediately contracts concentrically, using the stored energy.[34] The goal of plyometric training is to reduce the amount of time between the eccentric phase and initiation of the concentric phase, in hope of increasing power.[38] Plyometrics should be introduced gradually into the overall program, since they increase the intensity of training; they should also be sport specific.

TRAINING THEORY AND APPLICATION

Periodization of training is a concept in which the basic principles of training are used and manipulated in such a way as to reduce the chance of overtraining while bringing about peak performance.[12,39] Usually, there are five stages of training[12,40]: hypertrophy, basic strength, strength and power, peaking, and active rest.

The hypertrophy stage prepares the body for the increasing intensity of training to follow. Generally it consists of 3 to 4 weeks of low-intensity, high-volume workloads. Training can be one to three times per day for 3 to 4 days per week. After warm-up sets, the athlete performs three to ten work sets of eight to twelve repetitions.

The goal during the basic strength stage is to increase strength and build a foundation for power work. This stage may last 4 to 5 weeks and uses high intensity and moderate to high volume. Training sessions are done one to three times per day 3 to 5 days per week. The athlete should perform three to five work sets of four to six repetitions.

The strength and power phase concentrates on power development and generally lasts 3 weeks. Work is done at high intensity and low volume 3 to 5 days per week and training one or two times a day. Three to five work-sets at two to three times is typical.

The peaking stage lasts about 3 weeks. During this period optimal peak training is reached. Strength and power can also be maintained, to a certain degree, at this stage. The intensity of a workout can range from very high to low; however, the volume is always low. Training may be from 1 to 5 days per week, once a day. After a proper warm-up, one to three work sets are performed at one to three repetitions. As the volume of work decreases, more time is spent on technique.

The active rest period allows the athlete to take a break from regular training for a few days to a few weeks and engage in other active exercise. This periodization program can be repeated continually to enhance the athlete's capabilities. The periodization of resistance training should complement the periodization of the particular sport involved.

FACTORS OF STRENGTH DEVELOPMENT

Hypertrophy of muscle fiber has long been touted as the reason for strength gain, and, indeed, it may be the most important factor during sustained training periods.[41] However, strength is determined not only by size but by the ability of the nervous system to appropriately activate the muscle.[42] It has been shown that weight training can recruit higher-threshold motor units more effectively than less intensive training, and it appears to enhance synchronization and summation of motor unit firing.[43–46] The neural factors may help explain early training gains in strength in the absence of hypertrophy.[47]

Hyperplasia continues to be a controversial subject. Although some evidence supports the theory of gaining new muscle fibers via exercise,[48] it is generally thought that new fibers forming in humans via satellite cells appear to replace only necrotic ones, so that there is no net increase in fibers.[49]

Strength training can be applied to both young and old athletes with positive results. In general, muscle mass increases in parallel with body mass during the prepubertal phase of growth. Moderate strength training can take place, but maximum lifts should not be done by adolescents because of potential problems at the epiphyses of the bones.[50]

During prepuberty there is no difference between boys and girls with respect to strength trainability (top young female gymnasts may perform 40 pull-ups).[50] After puberty, men become stronger than women in general. However, woman can train using the same principles as men and substantially increase their overall strength. All motor properties (strength, endurance, skill) are adaptable throughout life and can be improved by training.[50] Older persons may require longer recovery periods between exercise sessions.

Muscle soreness is a common problem during training. This usually happens 12 to 48 hours after exercise and is referred to as delayed-onset muscle soreness. Empirical evidence suggests the delay is 12 to 24 hours for young athletes and 24 to 48 hours for older ones.[12] There are several theories as to why this occurs: lactic acid,[51] tonic muscle spasms,[52] connective tissue or torn tissue,[53,54] and tissue fluid.[55]

Lactic acid is not a metabolic waste product because a major portion of it is apparently used for energy.[13] It is also completely removed in about 1 hour and 40 minutes (50% in 25 minutes; 75% in 50 minutes).[56] "Active recovery" (light to moderate exercise) facilitates the recovery process as compared with passive procedures and also provides a means for faster lactic acid removal.[13] Obviously, this is not the cause of delayed-onset soreness. Electromyographic studies have not supported the tonic muscle spasm theory.[57] The remainder of the theories have to do with some type of cell damage.

It has been shown that eccentric exercises frequently produce delayed soreness.[12] This does not mean one should avoid the eccentric phase of exercise. The body functions normally under synchronized concentric, eccentric, and co-contractions. The athlete should train to minimize the amount of postexercise soreness by practicing periodization. It should also be noted that athletes adapt to some eccentric exercise.

FLEXIBILITY

Flexibility is the term commonly used to refer to range of motion about a particular joint.[34] While flexibility is a necessary component of training in regard to possibly decreasing injury, it has probably been over-rated and overdone in most training programs. The goal of flexibility is to induce a plastic, rather than elastic, change in connective tissue, since such changes are more lasting over time.[34] When plastic changes are induced tissue is weakened, but, since flexibility training occurs in conjunction with other training, no long-term "weakness" should result.[34]

The absolutely necessary amount of flexibility depends on the sport. It is as much or a little more than the joint and muscle must move during a particular sport. Obviously, some sports require more flexibility than others, and athletes should be trained according to the specificity principle (e.g., football lineman do not need the flexibility of gymnasts).

Flexibility is easily maintained during resistance training by incorporating flexibility exercises into the overall program. This can take 5 to 10 minutes during warm-up or cool-down. It has been shown that more permanent changes in flexibility occur during the cool-down phase.[34] Resistance training does not hinder flexibility as long as full range of motion is used. Some studies even indicate that weight training generally enhances flexibility.[8,58,59]

Ways To Enhance Flexibility

While maintenance of flexibility is relatively easy, enhancement can take time, just as gaining strength and power does.

Static stretching. Static stretching involves holding a muscle in the stretched position for a time (generally 15 seconds to 1 minute). Static stretching is done slowly and is considered the stretching method least likely to cause injury or soreness.[60] There is a question, however, about how static flexibility can relate to dynamic capabilities.

Ballistic stretching. Ballistic stretching uses momentum to provide stretch; it is also known as *bouncing*. There may be a risk of injury from this type of work; however, it may be appropriate for higher-level athletes, because sport activities are usually ballistic.[60]

Proprioceptive neuromuscular facilitation (PNF). Various methods (contract relax-agonist contract, hold relax, contract relax) involve active contractions followed by passive motion into the "new" range. These are designed to take advantage of neural effects of inhibition.[34,61] Many of the stretches must be done with assistance. They have been touted as the best way to achieve flexibility; though reviews do not verify this.[34]

All three examples of flexibility training work. There does not appear to be any clear and simple evidence indicating which one is most effective.[34] All features of the sport and the athlete must be taken into account to determine which may be more appropriate.

CONCLUSION

The sport an athlete competes in must be totally analyzed from the standpoint of strength and flexibility and for its metabolic, environmental, and societal aspects as well. Resistance and flexibility training are only parts of an athlete's overall program.

REFERENCES

1. Harris, H. A.: Greek Athletes and Athletics. London, Hutchinson & Co., 1964.
2. Chui, E. F.: Effects of isometric and dynamic weight-training exercises upon strength and speed of movement. Res. Q. *35*:246, 1964.
3. Clark, D. H., and Henry, F. M.: Neuromotor specificity and increased speed from strength development. Res. Q. *32*:315, 1961.
4. Whitley, J. D., and Smith, L. B.: Influence of three different training programs on strength and speed of a limb movement. Res. Q. *37*:132, 1966.
5. DeLorme, T. L.: Restoration of muscle power by heavy resistance exercise. J. Bone Joint Surg. *27*:645, 1945.
6. DeLorme, T. L., and Watkins, A. L.: Techniques of progressive resistance exercise. Arch. Phys. Med. *29*:263, 1948.
7. Garhammer, J.: Power production by Olympic weightlifters. Med. Sci. Sports Exerc. *12*:54, 1980.
8. Jensen, C. R., and Fisher, A. G.: Scientific Basis of Athletic Conditioning. Philadelphia, Lea & Febiger, 1979.
9. Stone, M. H.: Considerations in gaining a strength–power training effect. Nat. Strength Cond. Assoc. J. *4*(1):22, 1982.
10. Sylvester, L. F., Stiggins, C., McGown, C., and Bryan, G.: The effect of variable resistance and free-weight training programs on strength and vertical jump. Nat. Strength Cond. Assoc. J. *3*(6):30, 1981.
11. Wathen, D.: A comparison of the effects of selected isotonic and isokinetic exercises, modalities, and programs on the vertical jump in college football players. Nat. Strength Coaches Assoc. J. *2*:47, 1980.
12. Stone, M. H., and O'Bryant, H. S.: Weight Training: A Scientific Approach. Edina, MN, Burgess International, 1987.
13. McArdle, W. D., Katch, F. I., and Katch, V. L.: Exercise Physiology: Energy, Nutrition, and Human Performance. Philadelphia, Lea & Febiger, 1991.
14. Saltin, B., and Astrand, P. O.: Maximal oxygen uptakes in athletes. J. Appl. Physiol. *23*:353, 1967.
15. Morganroth, J., Maron, B. J., Henry, W. L., and Epstein, S. E.: Comparative left ventricular dimensions in trained athletes. Ann. Intern. Med. *82*:521, 1975.
16. Stone, M. H., Nelson, J. K., Nader, S., et al.: Short-term weight training effects on resting and recovery rates. Athl. Training *18*:69, 1983.
17. Kusinitz, I., and Keeny, C. W.: Effects of progressive weight training on health and physical fitness of adolescent boys. Res. Q. *29*:294, 1958.
18. Bartels, R. L., Fox, E. L., Bowers, R. W., and Hiatt, E. P.: Effects of isometric work on heart rate, blood pressure, and net oxygen cost. Res. Q. *39*:437, 1968.
19. Wescott, W., and Howeff, B.: Blood pressure responses during weight training exercise. Nat. Strength Cond. Assoc. J. *5*(1):67, 1983.
20. Astrand, P. O., Ekblom, B., Messin, R., and Rozenek, R.: Intra-arterial blood pressure during exercise with different muscle groups. J. Appl. Physiol. *20*:253, 1965.
21. Stone, M. H., Wilson, G. D., Blessing, D., and Rozenek, R.: Cardiovascular responses to short term Olympic style weight training in young men. Can. J. Appl. Sports Sci. *8*:134, 1983.
22. Hagberg, J. M., Ehsani, A. A., Goldring, D., et al.: Effect of weight training on blood pressure and hemodynamics in hypertensive adolescents. J. Pediatrics *104*:147, 1984.
23. Gettman, L. R., and Pollock, M. L.: Circuit weight training: A critical review of its physiological benefits. Physician Sportsmed. *9*(1):45, 1981.
24. Wright, J. E., Patton, J. F., Vogel, J. A., et al.: Anaerobic power and body composition after 10 weeks of circuit weight training using various work:rest ratios (abstract). Med. Sci. Sports Exerc. *14*:170, 1983.
25. Hickson, R. C., Rosenkoetter, M. A., and Brown, M. M.: Strength training effects on aerobic power and short-term endurance. Med. Sci. Sports Exerc. *12*:336, 1980.
26. Johnson, C. C., Stone, M. H., Lopez, S. A., et al.: Diet and exercise in middle-aged men. J. Am. Dietary Assoc. *81*:695, 1982.
27. Brown, C. H., and Wilmore, J. H.: The effects of maximal resistance training on the strength and body composition of women athletes. Med. Sci. Sports *6*:174, 1974.
28. Moritani, T., and deVries, H. A.: Potential for gross muscle hypertrophy in older men. J. Gerontol. *35*:672, 1980.
29. Billeter, R., and Hoppeler, H.: Muscular basis of strength. *In* Strength and Power in Sport. Edited by P. V. Komi. London, Blackwell Scientific, 1991.
30. Kraemer, W. J., and Fleck, S. J.: Anaerobic metabolism and its evaluation. Nat. Strength Conditioning Assoc. J. April-May, 1982.
31. Knortz, K. A.: Muscle physiology applied to geriatric rehabilitation. *In* Topics in Geriatric Rehabilitation. Edited by C. B. Lewis. Frederick, MD, Aspen, 1987.
32. McCafferty, W. B., and Horvath, S. M.: Specificity of exercise and specificity of training: A subcellular review. Res. Q. *48*:358, 1977.
33. Sale, D. G., and MacDougall, J. D.: Specificity in strength training: A review for the coach and athlete. Can. J. Appl. Sport Sci. *6*:87, 1981.
34. Enoka, R. M.: Neuromechanical Basis of Kinesiology. Champaign, IL, Human Kinetics, 1988.
35. Thorstensson, A.: Observations on strength training and detraining. Acta Physiol. Scand. *100*:491, 1977.
36. Johnson, B. L., and Adamczyk, J. W.: A program of eccentric-concentric strength training. Am. Corrective Ther. J. *29*:13, 1975.
37. Fleck, S. J., and Schutt, R. C., Jr.: Types of strength training. Orthop. Clin. North Am. *14*:449, 1983.
38. Albert, M.: Eccentric Muscle Training in Sports and Orthopaedics. New York, Churchill Livingstone, 1991.
39. Schmidtbleicher, D.: Training for power events. *In* Strength and Power in Sport. Edited by P. V. Komi. London, Blackwell, 1992.
40. Stone, M. H., et al.: A theoretical model of strength training. Nat. Strength Cond. Assoc. J. *4*(4):36, 1982.
41. Komi, P. V., and Karlsson, J.: Skeletal muscle fibre types, enzyme activities and physical performance in young males and females. Acta Physiol. Scand. *103*:210, 1978.
42. Sale, D. G.: Neural adaption to strength training. *In* Strength and Power in Sport. Edited by P. V. Komi. London, Blackwell Scientific Publications, 1992.
43. Guyton, A. C.: Textbook of Medical Physiology. Philadelphia, W. B. Saunders, 1981.
44. Hayes, K. C.: A theory of the mechanism of muscular strength development based upon EMG evidence of motor unit synchronization. *In* Biomechanics of Sports and Kinanthropometry. Miami, FL, Symposia Specialists, 1978.

45. Komi, P. V.: Neuromuscular performance: Factors influencing force and speed production. Scand. J. Sports Sci. *1*:2, 1979.
46. Sale, D. G., MacDougall, J. D., Upton, A. R., and McComas, A. J.: Effect of strength training upon motoneuron excitability in man. Med. Sci. Sport Exerc. *15*:57, 1983.
47. Moritani, T., and deVries, H. A,.: Neural factors versus hypertrophy in the time course of muscle strength gain. Am. J. Phys. Med. *58*:115, 1979.
48. Gonyea, W. J., Sale, D., Gonyea, F., and Mikesky, A.: Exercise induced increases in muscle fiber number. Eur. J. Appl. Physiol. *55*:137, 1986.
49. MacDougall, J. D.: Hypertrophy or hyperplasia. *In* Strength and Power in Sport. Edited by P. V. Komi. London, Blackwell Scientific, 1991.
50. Israel, S.: Age related changes in strength and special groups. *In* Strength and Power in Sport. Edited by P. V. Komi. London, Blackwell Scientific, 1991.
51. Assmussen, E.: Observations on experimental muscle soreness. Acta Rheumatol. Scand. *1*:109, 1956.
52. deVries, H. A.: Prevention of muscular distress after exercise. Res. Q. *32*:177, 1961.
53. Hough, T.: Ergographic studies in muscular soreness. Am. J. Physiol. *7*:76, 1902.
54. Friden, J., Segar, J., Sjostrom, M., and Ekblom, B.: Adaptive response in human skeletal muscle subjected to prolonged eccentric training. Int. J. Sports Med. *4*:177, 1983.
55. Stauber, W. T.: Eccentric action of muscles: Physiology, injury and adaptation. Exerc. Sports Sci. Rev. *19*:157, 1989.
56. Hermausen, Machlum, L. S., Pruett, R., et al.: Lactate removal at rest and during exercise. *In* Metabolic Adaption to Prolonged Physical Exercise. Edited by H. Howald and J. R. Poortmans. Basel, Birkhauser, 1975.
57. Abraham, W. M.: Factors in delayed muscle soreness. Med. Sci. Sports *9*:11, 1977.
58. Fox, E. L.: Sports Physiology. Philadelphia, W. b. Saunders, 1984.
59. O'Shea, J. P.: Scientific Principles and Methods of Strength Fitness. Reading, MA, Addison-Wesley, 1976.
60. Corbin, C. B., and Lindsey, R.: Concepts of Physical Fitness with Laboratories. Dubuque, IA, Wm. C. Brown, 1985.
61. Knott, M., and Voss, D. E.: Proprioceptive Neuromuscular Facilitation: Patterns and Technique. New York, Hoeber-Harper & Row, 1968.

91 *Laura Stokes*

Aerobic Conditioning

Though our society is enthralled with sports and the athletes who participate, on a whole, people have a very poor understanding of what it means to be physically fit. Most exercise physiologists assert that physical fitness encompasses body composition, flexibility, muscle strength and endurance, and cardiovascular strength and endurance. An athlete, or a regular exerciser, is not wholly fit unless the training program includes all of these components. The term *aerobic exercise* has been coined to describe activities that induce metabolism of fats or carbohydrates while the body uses oxygen. They are sustained, prolonged activities. On the other side of the coin are activities that require quick bursts of intensive activity, usually of less than 2 minutes' duration; these are termed *anaerobic,* exercises that do not use oxygen.

ANAEROBIC AND AEROBIC METABOLIC PATHWAYS

To maintain existing cells, to grow new tissues, and to perform work with cells, the body needs a steady supply of chemical energy. Most of that energy comes from catabolic breakdown of the nutrients the body absorbs. The energy extracted from the nutrients by oxidation (removal of electrons) is transferred to energy-carrying molecules within the cells, such as adenosine triphosphate (ATP). Two common pathways that cells use to extract energy from nutrients are anaerobic and aerobic metabolism.

Under aerobic (oxygen-using) conditions the cells are operating at an efficiency as high as 41%, about 20 times more efficient than under anaerobic conditions. In addition, the by-products of aerobic reactions are water and carbon dioxide, compounds the body is well equipped to handle and that do not lead to muscle fatigue.

When muscles are working, the cells are constantly selecting the most appropriate and most "cost-effective" (i.e., energy-preserving) system to perform the required activity. If the cells are forced to work long at a level of intensity that consumes oxygen faster than it can be supplied, the cells become oxygen deficient. Under these circumstances they can no longer maintain aerobic metabolism and shift to anaerobic energy production. In this mode the cells continue to produce energy for work though much less efficiently, and concomitantly lactic acid builds up in muscles. Sustaining this level of intensity soon leads to muscle fatigue and loss of contraction strength. Though no oxygen is required during the anaerobic activity, oxygen is needed when that activity ceases, to remove the acidic metabolites. The longer anaerobic activity is sustained, the greater is the "oxygen debt" for the tissues. This, in part, explains the hyperventilation that most often follows anaerobic activity, even when the muscle tissues are no longer being used.

Anaerobic Threshold

The level of exercise below which the cells maintain aerobic metabolism and above which they must switch to anaerobic metabolism is referred to as the *anaerobic threshold* (AT). In the 1920s and 1930s, researchers demonstrated that blood lactate increases exponentially with exercise intensity. As exercise intensity increases, blood lactate remains constant or even declines during light work (less than 50% Vo_2max). At work loads demanding 50 to 70% Vo_2max, blood lactate begins to increase with exercise intensity. During exercise, the blood lactate concentration increases linearly over time, with a slight increase around 2 mmol/L and then a sharp exponential increase at about 4 mmol/L. This last increase is termed the lactate threshold, blood lactate breaking point, early lactate, or anaerobic threshold. Recently, researchers have come to the conclusion that more lactate is being released into the bloodstream than is simultaneously being cleared. Thus, the only "threshold" aspect of blood lactate response is that it is the first measurable evidence that lactate release and clearance are unbalanced; it does not reflect a sudden "turning on" of a different energy system.

It is important to exercise at the anaerobic threshold. This allows for slower reduction of muscle glycogen stores than if the athlete were pushing beyond the threshold. Maffulli and coworkers observed a strong correlation between the natural racing speed of 112 endurance athletes and the running speed of the same athletes at their anaerobic threshold, as determined in field and laboratory studies.[1] This indicates that, during competition, the trained athlete's body naturally paces itself to run at its optimal, most efficient speed. This also supports the principle of training at the anaerobic threshold, which can be modified and raised until it reaches the individual's genetic ceiling.

Aerobic Power

The ability of the body to supply oxygen to the working muscles, and therefore perform the requisite sustained activity, has been termed *aerobic capacity*, or *power*. Aerobic power is the maximal amount of oxygen that can be consumed per minute during maximal exercise. Maximal oxygen consumption (Vo_2max) is calculated in terms of volume of oxygen consumed (in liters) per unit of time (in minutes). It is used to express the absolute power of the cardiorespiratory system to deliver and allow the body to perform aerobic work. It is often best, for purposes of comparison, to normalize this value in terms of the amount of tissue that is being supplied with that oxygen. To correct for this, body weight is brought into the calculations:

$$Vo_2max = ml/kg \times min^{-1}.$$

Maximal aerobic power can be affected by a number of controllable and uncontrollable factors. Among the controllable ones are the athlete's percentage of body fat, training regimen, and psychological attitude. Manipulating the controllable factors is the basis of any good conditioning program. The most significant uncontrollable factors affecting aerobic power are genetics, gender, and age.

Prepubescent girls and boys show no significant difference in Vo_2max values; however, after puberty the peak aerobic power of women is, on average, 70 to 75% that of men. The values reach their peak at 18 to 20 years of age for both sexes and decline gradually thereafter. Aging decreases Vo_2max approximately 9% for each decade of life after age 25 years.[2] It is not known if this is due to the aging process or to a reduction in physical activity. One longitudinal study showed that, after 18 years, nonexercisers lost 41% of Vo_2max whereas exercisers lost only 13%.[3] Interestingly, a 65-year-old man's average maximum aerobic power is about equal to that of a 25-year-old woman.[4] This gender discrepancy may be explained by two major factors. Since women have a higher percentage of body fat and Vo_2max is often expressed in terms of gross body weight (not just lean body mass), women's values may be unfairly skewed. Women also have a naturally lower hemoglobin concentration, which reduces their oxygen-carrying capacity and therefore their Vo_2max.

Tests for Maximal Aerobic Power

The testing and determination of maximal aerobic power can be as costly as opened circuit or gas analysis or as simple as monitoring recovery heart rate after a step test or as easy to administer to groups as a 12-minute walk-run. Unless the sports medicine practitioner is already equipped, he or she will probably want to select the most reliable field test with his or her capabilities to determine an athlete's maximal aerobic power.

Numerous studies show how to use a bench to determine maximal aerobic power via a submaximal test. This procedure is inexpensive and uses no special equipment other than a bench, a stopwatch, and a metronome. The original test had a subject step up and down at a constant rate of 30 step-ups per minute on a bench 20 inches high for a period of 5 minutes.[5] The subject's pulse was measured for 30 seconds at 1 minute into the recovery stage. A number of researchers have tried to modify the test, keeping the concept of repeated stepping up and down on a bench but allowing for variation in participant's leg length and individual height by modifying the height of the step,[6,7] changing the time of the test to 3 minutes, measuring heart rate during exercise, and using a graded step test in which the height of the bench increases 2 cm every minute or 4.5 cm every 2 minutes.

Using a bicycle ergometer to test aerobic power has inherent advantages and disadvantages. The stationary upright position makes data collection easy (e.g., blood pressure, Electrocardiographic (ECG) monitoring, drawing blood for lactate analysis), it provides a modicum of safety for the subject, and the equipment is relatively inexpensive. There are two major drawbacks to this method. Bicycling is a non–weight-bearing activity, which eliminates the factor of the subject's body mass if determining oxygen consumption in terms of body mass ($ml/kg \times min^{-1}$). The other drawback ties into the specificity of training certain muscle groups. Most sports participants have a component of running rather than cycling in their sport; therefore, an exercise test performed walking or running would better match the skills they have already developed.

Tests have been developed that use walking or running as the activity. Some have been designed for the field and some can be done only on a treadmill in the laboratory. Two common field tests are the 1-mile run (for school-aged children) and the 12-minute run-walk. In the 1-mile run, the children are asked to run-walk 1 mile in the shortest time possible. For the 12-minute run-walk, established by Cooper, the subject walks or runs for 12 minutes, and the goal is to cover as much distance as possible. When comparing the distance covered with a graded exercise test, the VO_2max values for 115 military personnel correlated fairly well.[8] Both of these tests can be administered en masse on a track or a flat, measured surface; though, if a subject is not motivated or misjudges pacing, values may be skewed.

Exercise tests performed on a treadmill allow the exercise technician to study a number of different parameters, such as blood pressure, ECG, and oxygen consumption. Many of these tests are designed so that the intensity of exercise increases progressively, typically at 3-minute intervals, to attain a steady state at that intensity. The test continues until the subject is exhausted or the physician stops the test. Since the exercise is progressive or graded, the tests have been termed *graded exercise tests* or GXTs (Table 91–1).

It is important to discourage the use of the treadmill handrails as much as possible during testing, because using them can falsely reduce estimation of VO_2max. The common protocols—the Bruce, the Balke, and the Ellestad—were designed for different purposes. The Balke protocol is designed to measure physical fitness, whereas the Bruce and Ellestad protocols are used to examine cardiovascular function.

A number of newly developed submaximal tests are described in the literature, and most can be administered if a treadmill is available.[9–11] The best options for testing aerobic power are probably a well-developed graded exercise test that works the athlete to maximum capacity (requiring the practitioner to own expensive equipment), a bench step test administered with the mentioned modifications, or a field test of a 12-minute walk-run, as outlined by Cooper.[12]

Also, the practitioner looking at exercise tests needs to know the sample demographics of the normative data and make sure that they reflect the test population of concern. Some studies do indicate that the test used for adults is applicable to children also.[13,14]

Table 91–1. Commonly Used Treadmill Protocols Showing Format of Speed, Grade and Minutes of Testing.*

BRUCE PROTOCOL

Stage	Speed (m.p.h.)	Grade %	Min.	MET[1] Requirement* Men	Women	Cardiac
I	1.7	10	1	3.2	3.1	3.6
			2	4.0	3.9	4.3
			3	4.9	4.7	4.9
II	2.5	12	4	5.7	5.4	5.6
			5	6.6	6.2	6.2
			6	7.4	7.0	7.0
III	3.4	14	7	8.3	8.0	7.6
			8	9.1	8.6	8.3
			9	10.0	9.4	9.0
IV	4.2	16	10	10.7	10.1	9.7
			11	11.6	10.9	10.4
			12	12.5	11.7	11.0
V	5.0	18	13	13.3	12.5	11.7
			14	14.1	13.2	12.3
			15	15.0	14.1	13.0

[1]MET=energy requirement of resting metabolism (3.5 ml O_2 consumed per kg of body weight per min).
*MET values are for each minute *completed*. Note that women and cardiac patients achieve *lower* $\dot{V}O_2$ for equivalent work load. Holding on to front rail *increases* the apparent MET capacity.

NAUGHTON-BALKE PROTOCOL

Speed (m.p.h.)	Grade (%)	Min.	METS
3.0 (Constant)	2.5	2	4.3
	5.0	2	5.4
	7.5	2	6.4
	10.0	2	7.4
	12.5	2	8.4
	15.0	2	9.5
	17.5	2	10.5
	20.0	2	11.6
	22.5	2	12.6

MODIFIED BALKE PROTOCOL

Speed (m.p.h.)	Grade (%)	Min.	METS
2.0	0	3	2.5
2.0	3.5	3	3.5
2.0	7.0	3	4.5
2.0	10.5	3	5.4
2.0	14.0	3	6.4
2.0	17.5	3	7.4
3.0	12.5	3	8.5
3.0	15.0	3	9.5
3.0	17.5	3	10.5
3.0	20.0	3	11.6
3.0	22.5	3	12.6

(American College of Sports Medicine: Guidelines for Exercise Testing and Prescription. 4th Ed. Philadelphia, Lea & Febiger, 1991.)

EXERCISE PRESCRIPTION

The goal of the aerobic fitness program is to increase VO_2max. Increased VO_2max allows more oxygen to be supplied to the working muscles, which increases the amount of energy produced. This increased ability to deliver oxygen to the muscles occurs because of various physiologic changes associated with training: greater cardiac stroke volume, increased capillarization to the muscles, increased numbers of red blood cells (and, therefore, hemoglobin content), increased myoglobin, and increased number of mitochondria, among others.

Before sports participation the athlete should receive a medical clearance. Information related to clearance can be gathered in a questionnaire, physical tests, or physician-supervised tests such as graded exercise tests. The American College of Surgeons recommends that individuals with a history of cardiovascular problems and previously inactive people older than 35 years should have a graded exercise test before beginning a fitness program.

The American College of Sports Medicine has issued guidelines on the development of individual exercise prescriptions[2]:

Mode of activity: Any activity that uses large muscle groups, that can be sustained for a prolonged period, and that is rhythmic and aerobic, e.g., running-jogging, walking-hiking, swimming, skating, bicycling, rowing, cross-country skiing, rope skipping, and various endurance game activities.
Intensity of exercise: Physical activity corresponding to 40 to 85% Vo_2max or 55 to 90% of maximal heart rate. It should be noted that exercise of lower intensity may provide important health benefits and may increase fitness for persons who were previously sedentary and "low fit."
Duration of exercise: Continuous or discontinuous aerobic activity for 15 to 60 minutes.
Frequency of exercise: Three to five days per week.
Rate of progression: In most cases, the conditioning effect allows individuals to increase the total work done at each session. With continuous exercise, this is achieved by increasing intensity, duration, or some combination of the two. The most significant conditioning effects are observed during the first 6 to 8 weeks of the exercise program. The exercise prescription may be adjusted as these conditioning effects occur; the adjustment depends on participant characteristics, new exercise test results, and/or exercise performance during exercise sessions.

These guidelines fit both beginning exercisers and seasoned athletes who, during a season of competition, may be exercising as often as 6 or 7 days a week. (For guidelines on muscle strengthening, see Chapter 90.)

It is important to make sure that the exercise program is individualized, setting work loads or intensities within safe limits. The program should progress very slowly for 2 to 3 weeks, particularly for new or rehabilitating athletes. A good general guideline is that the subject should be able to talk while performing the aerobic exercise. If this is not possible, the intensity of the program should be reduced.

Intensity is the one factor that varies for each person, and it is the one area that can most be manipulated. Limitations may be imposed by the equipment, the athlete's economy of movement, or physical status, or simply the boredom associated with performing a repetitive task. The concept of increasing the load using weights is supported in the literature.[15] Load carriage to the torso, hands, and ankles is applicable only if the activity is a weight-bearing one; however, because of possible problems—elevated blood pressure, biomechanical changes in stride patterns,[16] possible problems to joint capsules—it is recommended that the athlete increase the speed of work rather than the load, if possible. The major benefit to increasing load carriage may be a psychological one, in that if exercisers feel they are "doing more" they are more likely to stay motivated and to stick with the program.

The guidelines of the American College of Sports Medicine use the athlete's heart rate to measure intensity of exercise. Target heart rate is determined by the following formula:

220 – (Age in years) = Maximum heart rate

Maximum heart rate – Resting heart rate = Heart rate reserve

(Heart rate reserve × 0.70) + Resting heart rate = Lower target heart rate

(Heart rate reserve × 0.85) + Resting heart rate = Upper target heart rate

For example, a 36-year-old with a resting heart rate of 68 beats per minute (bpm) would have a maximum heart rate of 184 (220 – 36) and a heart rate reserve of 116 (184 – 68). The lower target heart rate would be 149 ([116 × 0.70] + 68) and the upper target heart rate would be 166 ([116 × 0.85] + 68).

Ratings of perceived exertion (RPE) can be another useful device for setting exercise prescriptions. They can allow self-regulation of intensity as best suits the athlete's needs. The athlete is asked to quantify the amount of strain or difficulty experienced while performing an activity. One of the most widely used scales of RPE is Borg 15, a 15-point RPE scale, from 6 to 20 (Table 91–2).[17] Often, the selected value matches the exercise participant's heart rate by a multiple of 10 (e.g., someone who was exercising and had attained a heart rate of approximately 140 bpm would select an RPE of 14). With this scale, a value of 12 or 13 represents approximately 60% of maximum heart rate. A rating of 16 matches 85% of maximum heart rate. Following the American College of Sports Medicine guidelines above, most athletes want to exercise in the 12- to 16-RPE range. If the 10-point scale is used, the values are between 4 and 6 RPEs. Approximately 10% of exercisers inappropriately select abnormal or unrealistic RPE scores for their activity. This obviously precludes their using RPEs to establish an exercise prescription.

It is best to use the RPE during a graded exercise test and then to extrapolate that sensation of intensity to the training session. The athlete selects the RPE during the test and is then asked to remember the values and how they related to his or her feelings during that stage of the graded exercise test. How well an athlete can accurately implement the production technique is poorly documented; however, using RPE values, researchers have successfully taught athletes to replicate treadmill

Table 91–2 RPE scales. Original scale (6 to 20) on left and revised scale (1 to 10) on right.

Category RPE Scale		*Category-Ratio RPE Scale*	
6		0	Nothing at all
7	Very, very light	0.5	Very, very weak
8		1	Very weak
9	Very light	2	Weak
10		3	Moderate
11	Fairly light	4	Somewhat strong
12		5	Strong
13	Somewhat hard	6	
14		7	Very strong
15	Hard	8	
16		9	
17	Very hard	10	Very, very strong
18		•	Maximal
19	Very, very hard		
20			

(Borg, G. A.: Med. Sci. Sports. Exerc. *14*:377–387, 1982.)

running intensities while running in the field and to extrapolate exercise training intensity from results of a graded exercise test.[18] RPE can be a complementary tool, along with target heart rate, to provide appropriate feedback to the athlete attempting to achieve his or her desired exercise intensity.

The energy requirement of resting metabolism has been determined to be 3.5 ml of oxygen consumed per kilogram of body weight per minute. This has been arbitrarily assigned the value of 1 MET. METs are another measure of the specific intensity of an athlete's exercise prescription. After a graded exercise test, a $\dot{V}O_2max$ value will have been determined for the athlete. By dividing this value by 3.5 the practitioner can determine the athlete's maximum MET value. Using the available charts, such as that presented in Table 91–3, various activities can be selected for the athlete that provide exercise at the appropriate intensity. This is done by taking 40 to 85% of the maximum MET value (or, for fit persons, 70 to 85%) and matching those values to the specific activity (see Table 91–3).[2]

It is impossible to overstate the importance of selecting an activity that the participant enjoys. People quickly lose interest in a program that is boring. This leads to noncompliance, and participants never attain the greatest possible benefits from exercise. Research has shown that it is also necessary to select activities that mimic the athlete's sport or use the same large muscle groups. A basketball player should not just swim or ride a bike for aerobic activity; running is necessary to get the full benefit of training. Rathnow and Mangum support the need to keep the athlete's training single mode (SM) (e.g., walk or jog only) versus multimode (MM) (e.g., walking-jogging, cycling, and using an arm crank).[19] Although the lack of variability in the training activities may lead to boredom, the practitioner's responsibility is to keep the conditioning program as singularly modal as possible, so that expected increases of aerobic power can be produced. It is still possible to keep the workout challenging by interspersing various intervals of work and rest.

One of the most important parts of a training regimen is pure repetition of the activity, to train neural pathways to perform in proper sequence or to become coordinated. This conserves the economy of the movement. Increasing coordination (i.e., economy) allows an

Table 91–3 Leisure Activities in METs: Sports, Exercise Classes, Games, Dancing

	Mean	*Range*		*Mean*	*Range*
Archery	3.9	3–4	Horseshoe pitching	—	2–3
Backpacking	—	5–11	Hunting (bow or gun)		
Badminton	5.8	4–9 +	Small game (walking, carrying light load)	—	3–7
Basketball			Big game (dragging carcass, walking)	—	3–14
Game play	8.3	7–12 +	Judo	13.5	—
Nongame play	—	3–9	Mountain climbing	—	5–10 +
Billiards	2.5	—	Music playing	—	2–3
Bowling	—	2–4	Paddleball, racquetball	9	8–12
Boxing			Rope skipping	11	—
In-ring	13.3	—	60–80 skips/min	9	—
Sparring	8.3	—	120–140 skips/min	—	11–12
Canoeing, rowing, kayaking	—	3–8	Running		
Conditioning exercise	—	3–8 +	12 min per mile	8.7	—
Climbing hills	7.2	5–10 +	11 min per mile	9.4	—
Cricket	5.2	4.6–7.4	10 min per mile	10.2	—
Croquet	3.5	—	9 min per mile	11.2	—
Cycling			8 min per mile	12.5	—
Pleasure or to work	—	3–8 +	7 min per mile	14.1	—
10 mph	7.0	—	6 min per mile	16.3	—
Dancing (social, square, tap)	—	3.7–7.4	Sailing	—	2–5
Dancing (aerobic)	—	6–9	Scuba diving	—	5–10
Fencing	—	6–10 +	Shuffleboard	—	2–3
Field hockey	8.0	—	Skating, ice or roller	—	5–8
Fishing			Skiing, snow		
From bank	3.7	2–4	Downhill	—	5–8
Wading in stream	—	5–6	Cross-country	—	6–12 +
Football (touch)	7.9	6–10	Skiing, water	—	5–7
Golf			Sledding, tobogganing	—	4–8
Power cart	—	2–3	Snowshoeing	9.9	7–14
Walking (carrying bag or pulling cart)	5.1	4–7	Squash	—	8–12 +
Handball	—	8–12 +	Soccer	—	5–12 +
Hiking (cross-country)	—	3–7	Stair climbing	—	4–8
Horseback riding			Swimming	—	4–8 +
galloping	8.2	—	Table tennis	4.1	3–5
trotting	6.6	—	Tennis	6.5	4–9 +
walking	2.4	—	Volleyball	—	3–6

(American College of Sports Medicine: Guidelines for Exercise Testing and Prescription. 4th Ed. Philadelphia, Lea & Febiger, 1991.)

athlete to expend less energy for a given task than a less coordinated one does.

Since most activities involve some degree of running, the practitioner should be acquainted with general guidelines for running style. Minor exceptions should be made for each individual's distinct anatomy and physiology. When running, the foot should land under the knee, not ahead of it, with the heel striking before the rest of the foot, but not emphatically. The toes should stay in line with the heel. All motion of the arms and legs should be directed forward in an easy circular action, as in pedaling a bicycle. The arms should be held loose with the hands relaxed. It is very important to avoid any side-to-side swinging of the arms, which is a common problem for women. The stride should be several inches longer than the walking stride. The body should stay low but erect, and the head should bob up and down as little as possible.

"Two-a-day" training sessions are a favorite of coaches in many sports. However, this extra emphasis and work demand, if not properly administered, can either provide no benefits or actually be deleterious to the athlete's performance. Costill and coworkers found no benefit in requiring swimmers to perform two-a-day training sessions of 1½ hours each as compared with a matched group of swimmers performing one daily session of 1½ hours.[20] They also did not find much in the literature to support the notion of two-a-day.

Training Techniques

Before selecting the training technique, the exercise prescriptionist should understand all of the necessary components of a single exercise session. Each aerobic session should include a warm-up phase, endurance training, and a cool-down portion. The warm-up phase is designed to increase muscle temperature and increase function. Warming up is done by performing light aerobic work such as walking or slow jogging and mild stretching exercises and calisthenics for 5 to 10 minutes. This allows for dilatation of peripheral vessels, increasing oxygen supply to the working muscles before the demand for that oxygen becomes great. This reduces the chance of early muscle fatigue. At the end of the warm-up, the body should be close to the lower range of the target zone, whether that be determined by heart rate, RPE, or MET. The endurance or aerobic portion should last 15 to 60 minutes. It should include activities that involve large muscle groups and elicit values within the established target zone. The cool-down period should include activities of decreasing intensity that slowly return the body to near resting state. The importance of the cool-down period cannot be overlooked. It is thought that many cardiovascular accidents occur because of improper cool-down. These three components need to be included, regardless of what training technique the athlete uses.

The best way to approach the development of an appropriate training program is first to analyze the physiologic components of the participatory sport. Noble has developed a physiologic training theory.[21] He recommends looking at a sport, in terms, not of the skills or strategies involved, but of what metabolic systems are at work. The first step is to determine the type, frequency, duration, and intensity of the movements performed during the activity. This knowledge is then coupled with selection of the metabolic systems that need to be trained. Each activity can be broken down into relative percentages for each specific metabolic pathway (Fig. 91–1). With this knowledge the training of the various pathways can be made proportional to what the activity demands.

To gain improvement in a system the demand on that system must be increased significantly above the normal demands of daily activities. This is the *overload principle*. The manipulation of the frequency, intensity, or duration of the activity creates the necessary overload. It is best when the body is overloaded in a progressive manner, over time. This can be defined as progressive resistance. The body adapts to loads placed on it, to once again achieve homeostasis.

Various training techniques have been developed that manipulate frequency, intensity, and duration to create overload. These techniques can be divided into two major categories, continuous and interval training. Continuous training methods are those that provide no rest periods and are best applied to athletes whose sport is predominantly aerobic. Continuous training can be long, slow distance (LSD); moderate-duration, high-intensity; or Fartlek. It is important that the intensity is set so that the workload remains submaximal.

In LSD training, the athlete typically works at 60 to 70% of Vo_2max, which places the pace of the activity well below that of racing or competition. These sessions should last 30 minutes to more than 2 hours on some days.[22]

Moderate-duration, high-intensity training pushes the intensity of the training exercise to the limits of the anaerobic threshold (AT). Keeping the intensity just below the AT allows the athlete to perform near race pace, and the session may be referred to as *pace,* or *tempo, training.* The benefit of using this training method is to acclimate the body to working at the AT, thus increasing the amount of time that the athlete can perform at that intensity during competition.[22]

Fartlek, or Swedish speed play, intersperses periods of activity of varying intensity, such as jogging, with sprints. This method places greater emphasis on the anaerobic metabolic system than LSD; however, it is important to remember that it is still continuous, with no rest periods. Some athletes feel that this technique helps alleviate boredom during training.

In interval training, periods of rest are interspersed with work bouts. Duration of the rest period can be determined by time, distance, or measured heart rate. It has been indicated that interval training helps athletes train neural pathways to respond to competition pace and to exercise longer at the outer limits of aerobic metabolism. This also allows for more high-intensity exercise to be performed in a single training session. Lower ratios of work bout to rest period (e.g., 1:2 or 1:3), with work

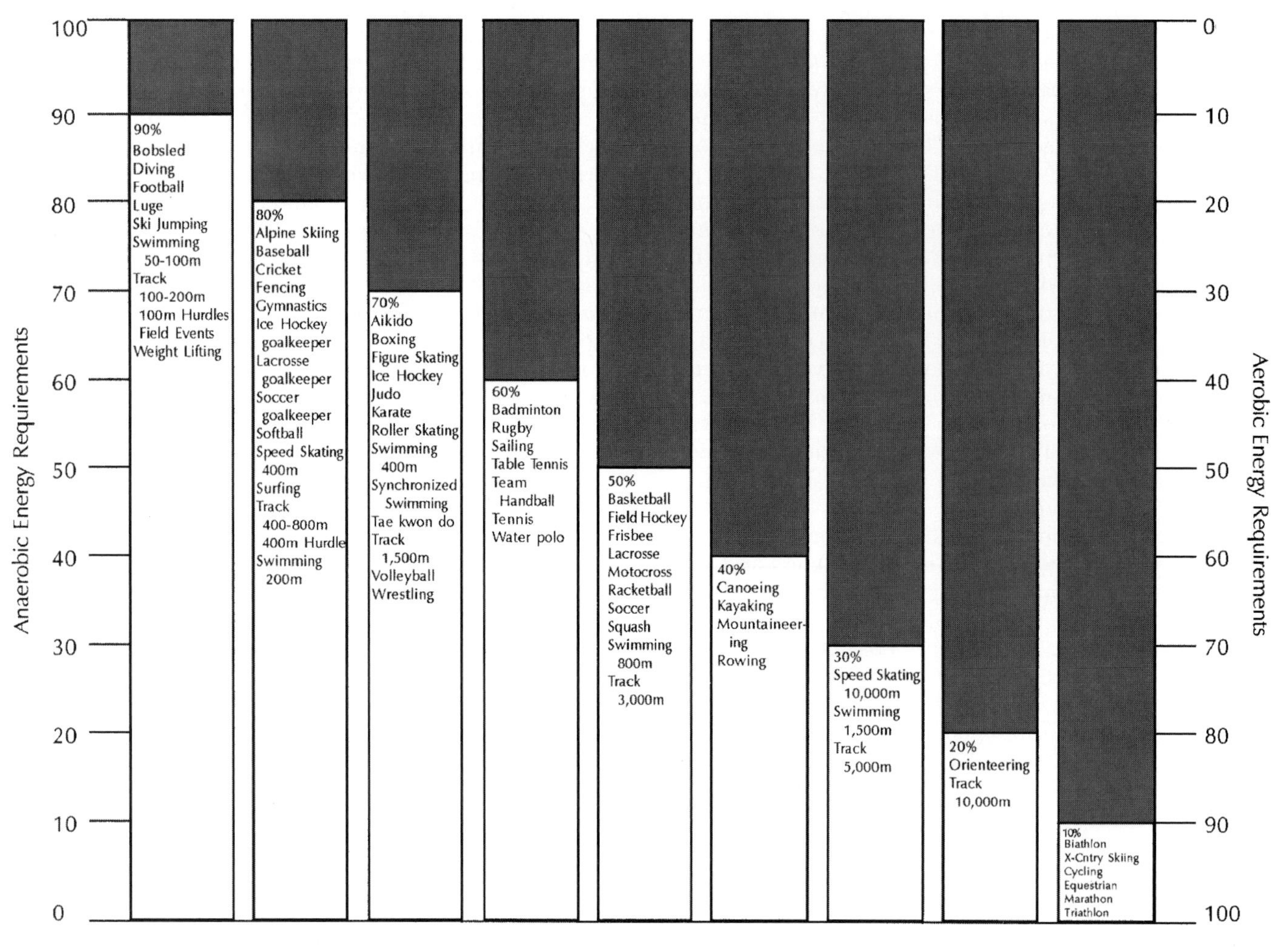

Fig. 91–1. Anaerobic and aerobic energy requirements for different sports. (Sharkey, B. J.: Coaches' Guide to Sport Physiology, Champaign, IL, Human Kinetics Publishers, 1986.)

bouts that are shorter (1 to 2 minutes) and much more intensive (90 to 100% of maximum) are better for training anaerobic capacity. Researchers disagree about the length of the work bouts and rest periods. It is thought that both short (10 to 40 seconds) and long (3 to 5 minutes) intervals should be incorporated in the training regimen. If the interval workout is performed at maximum speed, the work interval should be short and the rest interval from 10 seconds to 2 minutes. The longer intervals should be performed at 80 to 90% of maximum speed, with rest intervals of 3 to 15 minutes. During rest it is best to continue mild exercise, because it has been shown that exercise at an intensity of 30 to 40% of maximum is the best way to remove accumulated lactic acid. Both continuous and interval training can result in similar improvements in aerobic power, as long as the total energy expenditure of the two is equal.[23]

REHABILITATING THE RUNNER

The physician or coach must make intelligent decisions when establishing an individual athlete's rehabilitation exercise prescription. Ways to continue training the athlete without placing further stress on the injury need to be explored. For athletes whose sport has a running component, a possible injury may be a stress fracture in the tibia or the fibula, shin splints, plantar fasciitis, or tendinitis of the heel cord. These types of injuries require the athlete to stop running for awhile, which raises concern about loss of aerobic power.

A common solution to this problem is to select other aerobic activities. Because of the specificity of the training effect mentioned earlier, it is best not to substitute cycling or lap swimming to augment the program but rather to run in water. Water running is believed to supply the necessary aerobic benefits without the impact trauma of running on land. A number of commercially available vests mildly increase an athlete's buoyancy; though, because of cost limitations, some coaches have successfully trained their athletes to perform both deep water running (DWR) and shallow water running (SWR) unsupported.[24] Although research has shown that treadmill running elicits a higher Vo_2max and maximum heart rate than either DWR (2.5 to 4 m depth) or SWR (1.3 m depth), the injured athlete derives benefit.

Water running may be the next best thing to land running; however, some athletes state that they feel a major biomechanical difference between water and land running.[25] This might cancel out some of the specificity of the training effect. More research needs to be directed to this question.

If weight bearing is allowed, injured runners may use the following guidelines: Initially, athletes should be able to walk 2 miles at a pace of 14 to 15 mph without pain, limp, or swelling. The next stage is to jog 10 to 20 minutes on a soft, flat, level surface. Runners should increase running time 5 minutes per week up to 45 minutes or the preinjury time. They should then sustain this duration for 2 weeks on the same soft, level surface. If after 2 weeks they are pain free, not limping or swelling, they may gradually increase work intensity at their own pace. Speed and interval work can be resumed at a moderate level. Intervals should be increased 3 to 5% per week until 100% of original workout speed and distance are regained. Runners need to be sensitive to their body and not have preconceived notions about a timetable for return to full activity. This rough outline may need to be followed more slowly, or faster, depending on the individual case. The eventual goal for any runner should be set at 90% of maximum heart rate or 80% of maximum performance speed for a given training distance.

REFERENCES

1. Maffulli, N., Capasso, G., and Lancia, A.: Anaerobic threshold and performance in middle and long distance running. J. Sports Med. Phys. Fitness *31*:332, 1991.
2. Pate, R. R., et al. (eds.): Guidelines for Exercise Testing and Prescription. 4th Ed. Philadelphia, Lea & Febiger, 1991.
3. Kasch, F. W., et al.: The effect of physical activity and inactivity on aerobic power in older men (a longitudinal study). Physician Sportsmed. *18*(4):73, 1990.
4. Astrand, P. O., and Rodahl, K.: Textbook of Work Physiology: Physiological Bases of Exercise. 2nd Ed. New York, McGraw-Hill, 1977.
5. Brouha, L.: The step test : a simple method of measuring physical fitness for muscular work in young men. Res. Q. Exer. Sport *14*:31, 1943.
6. Francis, K., and Brasher, J.: A height-adjusted step test for predicting maximal oxygen consumption in males. J. Sports Med. Phys. Fitness *32*:282, 1992.
7. Francis, K., and Culpepper, M.: Validation of a three minute height-adjusted step test. J. Sports Med. Phys. Fitness *28*:229, 1988.
8. Cooper, K. H.: A means of assessing maximal oxygen intake. J.A.M.A. *203*:201, 1968.
9. George, J. D., et al.: Development of a submaximal treadmill jogging test for fit college-aged individuals. Med. Sci. Sports Exerc. *25*:643, 1993.
10. Latin, R. W., and Elias, B. A.: Predictions of maximum oxygen uptake from treadmill walking and running. J. Sports Med. Phys. Fitness *33*:34, 1993.
11. Ebbeling, C. B., et al.: Development of a single-stage submaximal treadmill walking test. Med. Sci. Sports Exerc. *23*:966, 1991.
12. Cooper, K. H.: Aerobics. New York, Bantam Books, 1968.
13. Rowland, T. W.: Does peak Vo_2 reflect Vo_2max in children?: Evidence from supramaximal testing. Med. Sci. Sports Exerc. *25*:689, 1993.
14. Drabik, J.: The general endurance of children aged 8-12 years in the 12-min run test. J. Sports Med. Phys. Fitness *29*:379, 1989.
15. Shoenfeld, Y., et al.: Walking: A method for rapid improvement of physical fitness. J.A.M.A. *243*:2062, 1980.
16. Maud, P., Stokes, G., and Stokes, L.: Stride frequency, perceived exertion, and oxygen cost response to walking with variations in arm swing and hand held weights. J. Cardiopul Rehabil *10*:294, 1990.
17. Borg, G., Hassmen, P., and Lagerstrom, M.: Perceived exertion related to heart rate and blood lactate during arm and leg exercise. Eur. J. Appl. Physiol. *56*:679, 1987.
18. Glass, S. C., Knowlton, R. G., and Becque, M. D.: Accuracy of RPE from graded exercise to establish exercise training intensity. Med. Sci. Sports Exerc. *24*:1303, 1992.
19. Rathnow, K. M., and Mangum, M.: A comparison of single- versus multi-modal exercise programs: Effects on aerobic power. J. Sports Med. Phys. Fitness *30*:382, 1990.
20. Costill, D. L., et al.: Adaptations to swimming training: Influence of training volume. Med. Sci. Sports Exerc. *23*:371, 1991.
21. Noble, B. J.: Physiology of Exercise and Sport. St. Louis, Mosby College, 1986.
22. Pate, R. R., and Branch, J. D.: Training for endurance sport. Med. Sci. Sports Exerc. *24*:S340, 1992.
23. Adeniran, S. A., and Toriola, A. L.: Effects of continuous and interval running programmes on aerobic and anaerobic capacities in schoolgirls aged 13 to 17 years. J. Sports Med. Phys. Fitness *28*:260, 1988.
24. Town, G. P., and Bradley, S. S.: Maximal metabolic responses of deep and shallow water running in trained runners. Med. Sci. Sports Exerc. *23*:238, 1991.
25. Bishop, P. A., Frazier, S., Smith, J., and Jacobs, D.: Physiologic responses to treadmill and water running. Physician Sportsmed. *17*(2):87, 1989.

92 *Jon M. Hay*

Taping, Splinting, and Fitting of Athletic Equipment

Protective equipment is important to the athlete, much as an offensive line is important to the football quarterback. If any part of that line breaks down, the quarterback can be reached by the opposing team and may be injured. Likewise, if any part of the protective equipment breaks down or fits improperly, injurious forces can reach the athlete. Protective equipment is designed to disperse energy received by the opposing force, absorb and deflect blows, limit undesired motion, and protect from sharp objects.[1]

Even though different equipment is made for different types of sports, the materials must be of the finest quality, to ensure protection. Regulation of protective equipment has been made possible through such organizations as The American Society for Testing and Materials (ASTM), The Canadian Standards Association (CSA), and The National Operating Committee on Standards for Athletic Equipment (NOCSAE).[1–6] These organizations have helped set the criteria that equipment-producing companies must meet. The state high school associations have also contributed to making the athletic environment safer by formulating rules and regulations for equipment use. In collegiate sports, the National Collegiate Athletic Association has a policy on all equipment used in sports it governs.[7]

Protective equipment is also a huge legal concern. To protect everyone involved from any type of litigation, the following steps should be taken:[3]

Purchase the equipment from reputable manufacturers.
Buy the safest equipment that resources allow.
Make sure that every piece of equipment is assembled correctly.
Maintain the equipment properly.
Use the equipment for the purpose for which it was designed.
Warn athletes about possible hazards when using this equipment.
Use great caution when constructing or customizing any piece of equipment.
Do not allow an athlete to use defective equipment.

All equipment should be routinely inspected. Often athletes will try to customize equipment that has already been purchased. Many manufacturers have a disclaimer that indicates they are not responsible if equipment is modified after purchase. Athletes must be told that if they modify their piece of equipment, they are putting themselves at risk. If the athlete is injured while wearing modified equipment, the manufacturer is not liable.

HEAD

When it comes to contact or collision sports, protection of the head is one of the most important areas. Great care has been taken to protect the head from fast projectiles, such as hockey pucks and baseballs, and from hard blows taken in sports such as football.

Football Helmets

The coach, trainer, or equipment manager fitting a football helmet must make sure that the helmet has a NOCSAE stamp on its back portion.[1–3,5–8] This seal of approval indicates that the helmet has been tested to withstand the minimum tolerated forces for which it is rated.

Helmets fall into two categories: (1) padded and (2) air and fluid filled. When fitting a football helmet, the following criteria should be checked, and rechecked periodically throughout the season:

- The helmet should fit snugly around all parts of the head and the base of the skull.
- The gap between the eyebrow and the front edge of the helmet should be 3/4 inch (two fingerwidths). (Fig. 92–1A).
- The ear holes should be centered over the ear openings (Fig. 92–1B).
- The cheek pads should be snug (Fig. 92–1C).
- The chin strap should be centered.
- The face guard should be attached securely to the helmet, allowing unobstructed vision.[1–4, 6,9]

To verify the fit the fitter should (1) pull down on the face mask, (2) try turning the helmet, (3) push down on the helmet, and (4) pull back and forth on the face mask. None of these maneuvers should produce movement.[1–4,6,9] The fit of the helmet should be rechecked after the first 3 to 4 days of practice, and periodically throughout the season.

Batting Helmets

Unlike football helmets, baseball batting helmets are designed to withstand the high-velocity impact of a small projectile.[1,5] Unfortunately, few data on batting helmets are yet available. These helmets usually consist of a very hard shell with a foam liner. They typically have ear flaps that cover both sides of the head with foam padding on the inside to protect against blows.[1,5] Some observers have suggested putting external padding onto the helmet or redesigning it completely for better protection of ball players.[5]

Ice Hockey

The ice hockey helmet has the same general purpose as the baseball batting helmet: to protect the athlete from very small, high-velocity missiles. The difference is that hockey players sustain multiple hits from hockey sticks and pucks *and* blows similar to those football players take, as in being blocked or falling onto the ice. Ice hockey helmets have a hard shell with a liner that is designed to absorb and disperse the force of blows to the head.[1,5]

Lacrosse

Lacrosse helmets are made of a very hard protective shell with a four-point chin strap that is padded for protection.[1,5]

FACE GUARDS

Football

The face guards in football are made of very heavy steel with a plastic coating.[2,5] The helmet should have at least two bars, and the upper part of the face guard should be mounted 3 inches above the face opening. The distance from the face guard to the nose should be 1.5 inches, or roughly three fingerwidths (Fig. 92–2).[1,3,4,9]

Ice Hockey

Face guards used by ice hockey players are made of either a hard clear plastic or steel wire, or a combination of the two.[2,5] They must be able to withstand high-velocity point impacts from hockey pucks and sticks as well as blunt impacts with opponents, the ice, or a wall. Face guards must meet the ASTM and CSA standards.[5] The chin straps, like those for lacrosse and football, should be padded.

Lacrosse

Face guards in lacrosse are made of a steel wire but are not quite as strong as those used in football and hockey. They are worn a specified distance from the face. Currently, there is no requirement for women lacrosse players to use a face shield or a face guard.[5,7]

Baseball

Face shields or guards are worn mainly by catchers. They are usually made of heavy steel wire. The catcher's face guard includes a throat protector, which is attached to the face mask and is usually left dangling over the player's throat.[7] Many youth leagues mandate that players wear a face protector when at bat and in the field.[5]

MOUTH

According to the American Dental Association (ADA), mouth guards prevent more than 200,000 injuries per year.[10] If the mouth guard is fitted and worn correctly, it can help prevent tooth loss and temporomandibular problems. It can also help cushion the chin bone against blows that can cause cerebral concussions.[1,2,7,8,10–12] Mouth guards come preformed off the shelf, but they can also be form fitted or custom fitted.[2,3,7,8,11] Many high school associations and the NCAA mandate that mouth guards be worn in both practices and games.[1–3,5,7,8,11,12] It is also mandatory that all mouth pieces be yellow.[5,7]

EYES

Each sport has different requirements for eye protection. For some sports, like football, a face shield might be satisfactory to protect the eyes, whereas in racquetball, because of the small projectile, it is best for the ath-

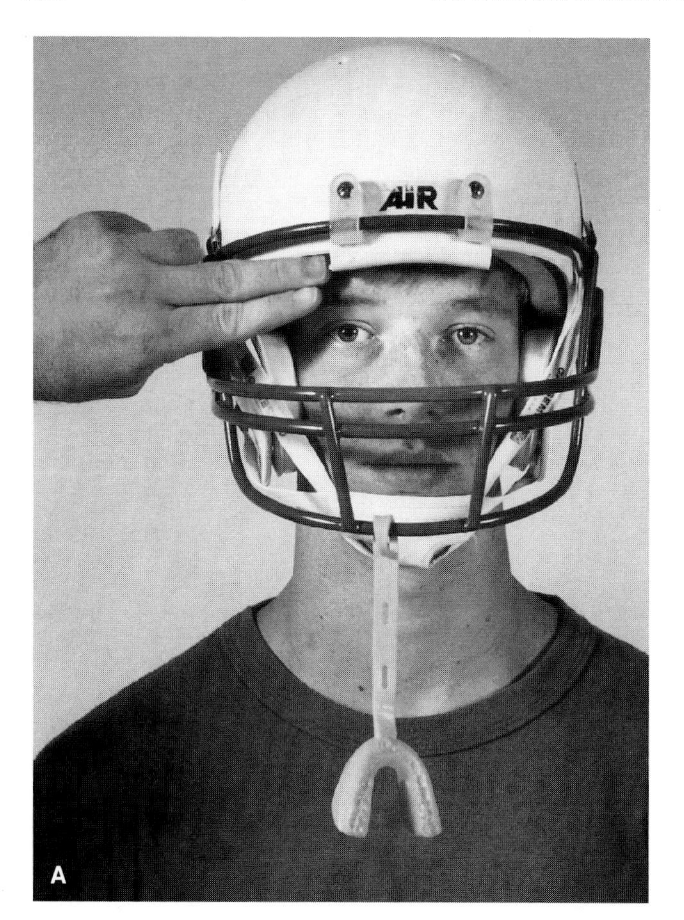

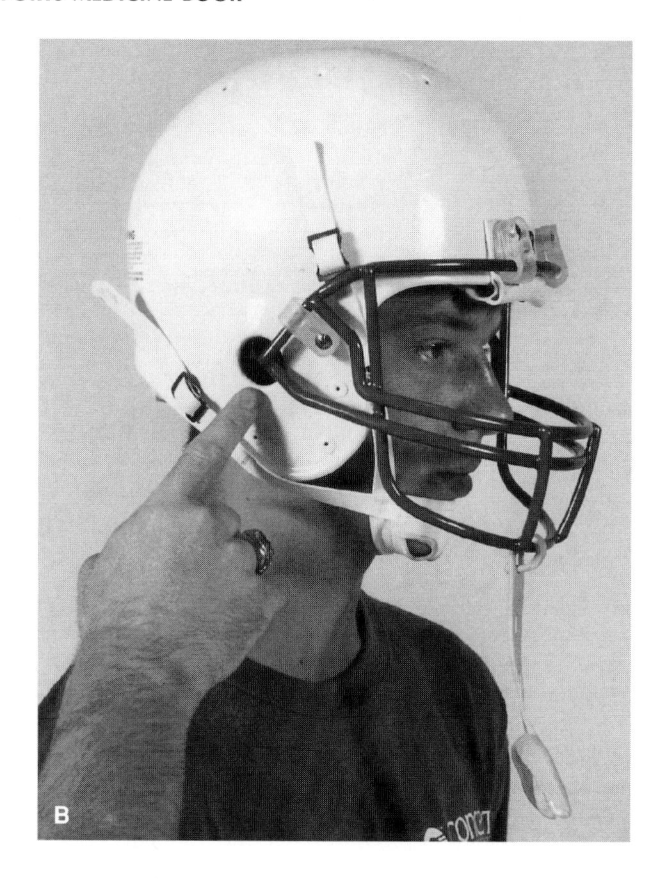

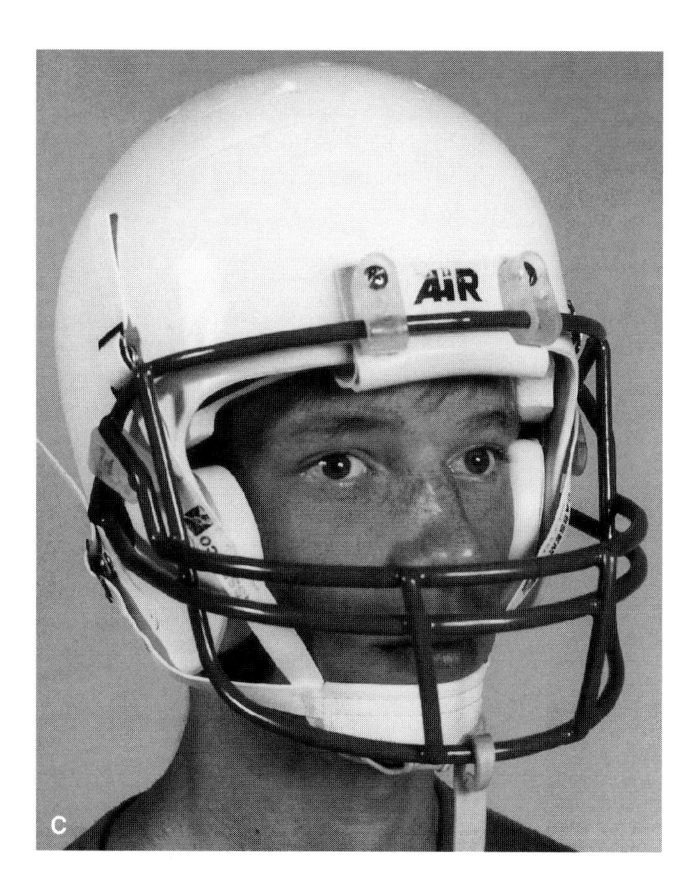

Fig. 92–1. In fitting a helmet there must be a ¾ inch space between the eyebrow and the front edge of the helmet *(A)*, the ear holes must be centered over the ears *(B)*, and the cheek pads must be snug *(C)*.

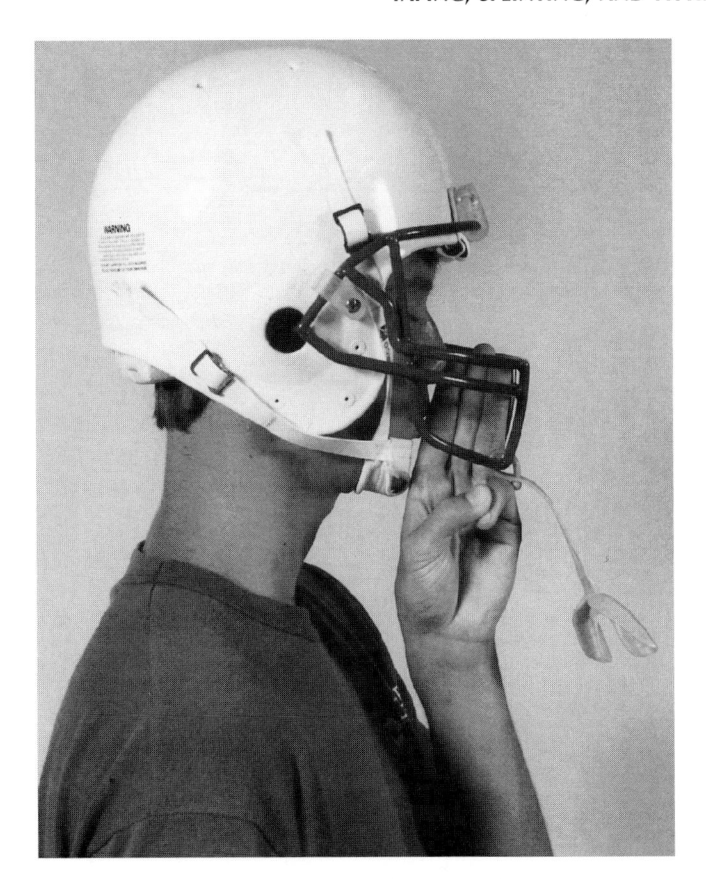

Fig. 92–2. The face guard should be three fingerwidths from the face.

lete to wear a more rigid eye protector. The best material used for eye protectors today is a polycarbonate plastic, a substance 7.6 times better able than cast resin to withstand the impact of high-velocity projectiles.[13] It is also the only material currently approved for eye protection by the ASTM.[1]

Contact lenses are not recommended for eye protection simply because, once they are set on the eye, they act like part of it. They can also roam around the surface of the eye. Likewise, glasses are not suitable eye protection, because they can shatter on impact, leaving the athlete at risk. Eye guards that cover the entire eye area are more highly recommended than eye guards that have a frame and an open space, particularly for sports such as racquetball, squash, and tennis. Open eye guards can still leave the eye unprotected.[13,14] Racquetballs traveling at high speeds can squeeze through the open area and forcefully strike the eye.

EARS

Ear guards are used predominantly in boxing and wrestling. They are designed to prevent ear injuries, the most common being "cauliflower ear." Most other contact sports, such as football, use full-head protection in the form of a helmet that includes protection of the ear.[1,3,6,7,9]

NOSE

Nasal protection usually comes in the form of premolded devices that can be purchased off the shelf or custom fitted. They can be made of hard plastic or a material such as Orthoplast. Unfortunately, very little data are available to indicate the level of protection these devices offer.

UPPER BODY

Shoulder

When we think of protecting the shoulder in a collision sport we usually think of football. Shoulder pads for football depend on the player's position. Quarterbacks and receivers use smaller, flatter pads; linemen use bulkier ones.[1,3,4] When fitting shoulder pads, the following criteria should be observed:

The inside pad should cover the tip of the shoulder (Fig. 92–3A).
The outside pad should cover the deltoid (Fig. 92–3B).
Neck motion should be unrestricted (Fig. 92–3C).
The pads should fit snugly against the body, not too tightly or too loosely.
The pad should not restrict the motion of the arms necessary to play the position.[1–4,9] A special pad can be used to protect an injured shoulder (e.g., with an acromioclavicular sprain).[9,15] These pads can be custom made or off the shelf, such as spider pads or "shoulder savers."[9] They can be placed beneath the regular shoulder pads.

Neck

Football is the sport commonly thought of in association with neck protection. Neck collars can usually be attached to the shoulder pads.[2] They come in many different types and generally come off the shelf rather than being customized.[4] Unfortunately, when budgets are strict, sometimes athletes, coaches, or trainers make neck rolls themselves. Such action can leave a coach or trainer open to liability.[3,4]

Chest and Ribs

Chest protectors are used mainly by catchers in baseball and softball and the umpires in these sports. In football and ice hockey, chest protection is often built into the shoulder pads.

For fencing, the NCAA has made it mandatory for women to wear chest protectors. Breast support is another area of concern for women athletes. In sports that involve running and jumping, such as basketball, track and field, and lacrosse, a sports bra is quite useful, to prevent excessive stretching of the Cooper's ligaments. Unfortunately, conventional bras do not provide enough support in this area.

Rib protection is also quite important, especially in collision or contact sports. Many rib protectors can be

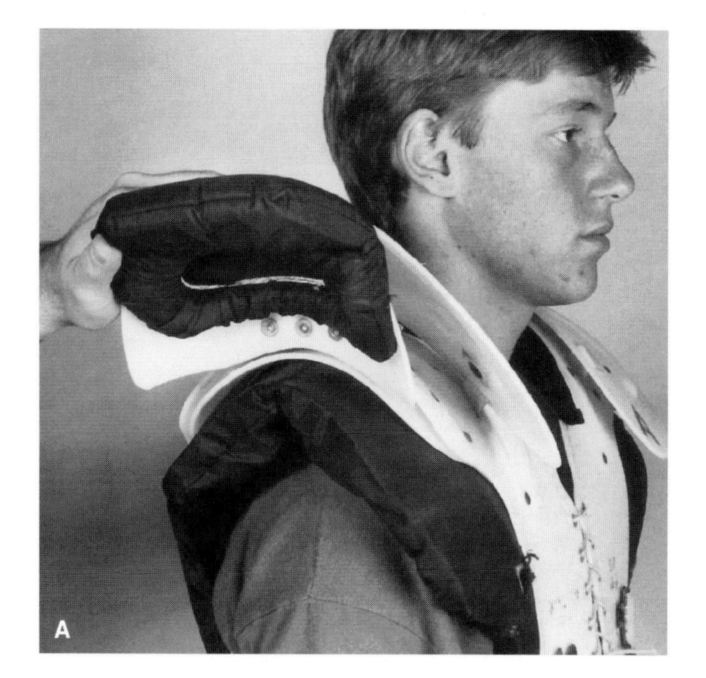

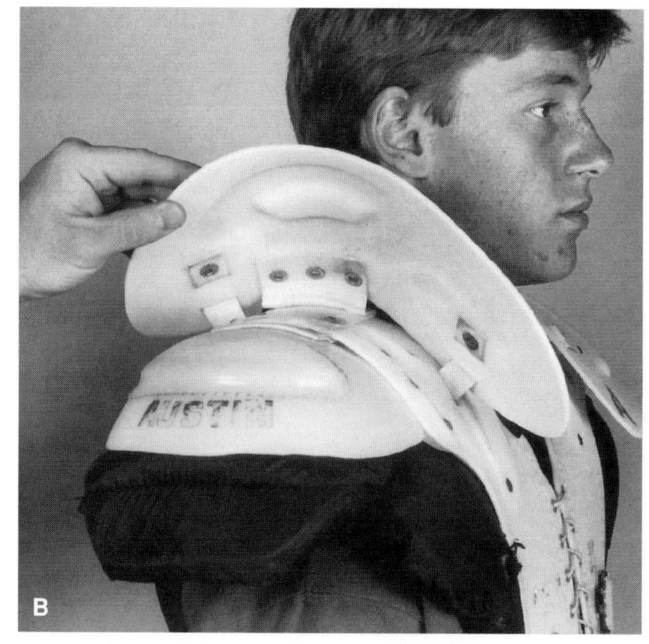

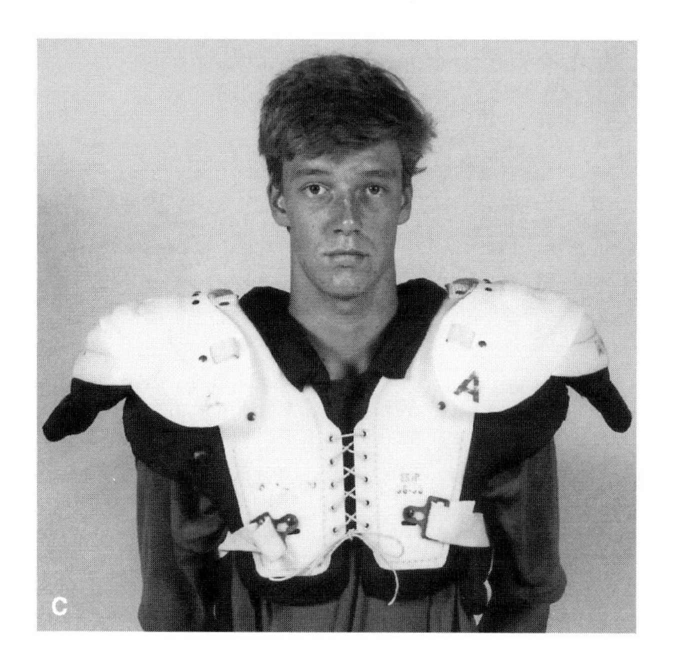

Fig. 92–3. **In fitting shoulder pads the inside pad must cover the tip of the shoulder *(A)*, the outside pad must cover the deltoid *(B)*, and neck motion must not be restricted *(C)*.**

purchased off the shelf.[4] They consist of pads to protect the ribs suspended from a harness worn over the shoulders (Fig. 92–4). Most of them are used by quarterbacks, fullbacks, and halfbacks.[2,5]

Elbow and Forearm

Elbow and forearm protection is used mainly in collision sports. Like other protectors, they can range from off-the-shelf types to custom-made products. They are usually made of a hard plastic shell with a foam liner. These kinds of elbow and forearm protectors are designed to protect the elbow from injury or to prevent a pre-existing injury from becoming worse. Tennis elbow straps can also be considered protective equipment because they are used to allow the athlete to perform while preventing an elbow injury from becoming worse.[2]

Hand

Hand protection is extremely important, in contact and noncontact sports. In contact sports, hand protection usually involves protecting the dorsal surface, to disperse direct blows. In noncontact sports (baseball, golf),

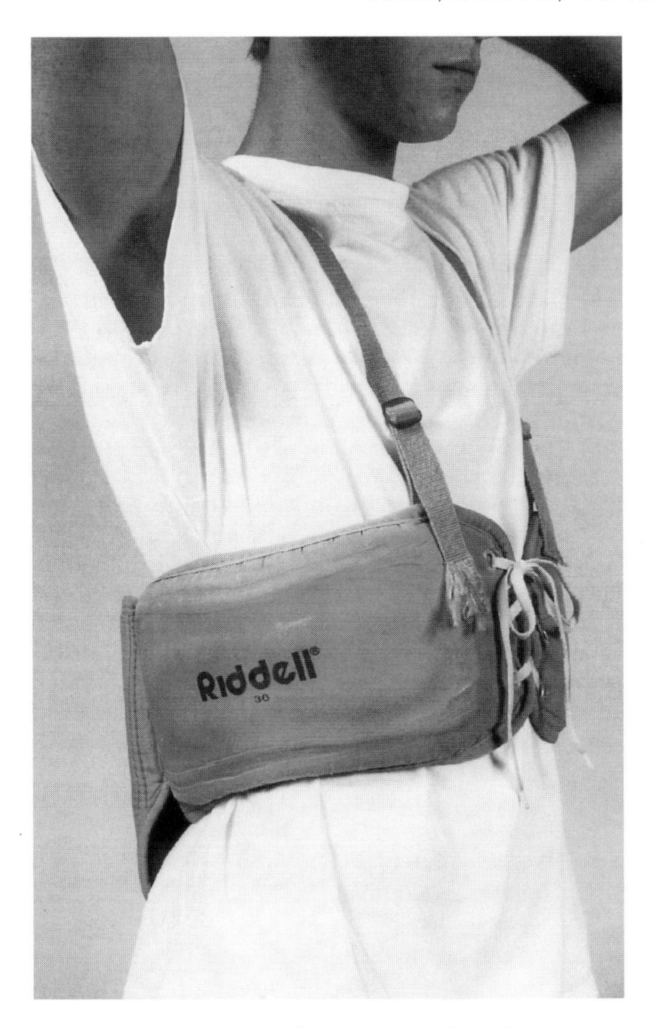

Fig. 92–4. A rib protector can be worn attached to a harness.

gloves are sufficient protection. They prevent friction when using a bat or club. In gymnastics, hand protection comes in the form of straps to support the hand and wrist and from chalk to help prevent friction that creates blisters.

LOWER BODY

Hip and Thigh

Hip and thigh protection is very common and important in contact sports like football, lacrosse, and ice hockey. Football players are required to wear hip, buttock, and thigh pads, which cannot be less than ½ inch thick. If a player has an injury such as a hip pointer, the hip pads may be modified; a bubble pad or modified thigh pad may be used.[2,11]

Knee

Like thigh pads, knee pads should be no less than ½ inch thick.[6] They are used mainly in football and wrestling, and occasionally in men and women's basketball. Knee protection can come in the form of straps such as the Chopat or Levine. These straps are used for rehabilitation of patellar tendinitis, and they allow athletes to play with little or no pain. If the athlete is using a functional knee brace, many high school associations and the NCAA mandate that there be at least ½ inch of padding over exposed metal areas, particularly for contact sports.[7] Knee pads can also come in the form of neoprene sleeves with built-in patellar stabilizers, to prevent patellar subluxation or dislocation.[2,9]

Lower Leg, Ankle, and Foot

Shin guards can be purchased ready made or custom fitted. They are designed for high- or low-velocity impacts—being hit by a ball or hockey puck or being kicked by an opponent. Sometimes padding supplied on ready-made guards is too thin; an athlete may need additional padding, particularly on areas of the shin that have been traumatized already.[15]

Ankle supports take the form of braces or even taping. There are various types of ankle braces, but most are either (1) soft ones made of cloth with added support straps or (2) hard ones made up of a very hard plastic shell lined with foam on the inside and two straps that go around to support the ankle joint.[3]

Taping, another way of protecting the ankle joint, can be done in many different ways, depending on what area is injured.

Pads may be used to protect the feet. They come in the form of arch supports for the longitudinal arch or the metatarsal arch and can either be bought over the counter or be custom fitted. Protecting the heel—from being bruised or because of pre-existing trauma—can be achieved by heel pads, heel spur pads, and heel cups, among others.

Socks can also be classified as part of protective equipment, simply because they help protect the foot and ankle from friction-type problems, preventing blisters.[1,3] Shoes are also important.

Ideally, the athlete's shoe should have a wide toe box and good heel counter support and cushioning. It should also provide firm support for the arches of the foot.[1,3] Depending on whether the athlete has a pre-existing injury, high-top, medium-cut, or low-top shoes can be worn.

TAPING AND WRAPPING

Taping and wrapping are a part of everyday life for athletic trainers. The skills are important because, when applied correctly,[2] tape can help prevent injury or support an injured area during rehabilitation or in competition.[3, 9] Athletic trainers have individual styles for taping, usually derived from what their predecessors taught them. There are general guidelines for taping. Areas that are going to be taped should be shaved to prevent hair loss and skin irritation. Some sort of tape adherent, whether Tuff-Skin or a quick-drying adherent, should be used, to ensure that the tape sticks and to protect the skin. Underwrap should be used in areas where the skin is very tender, to help decrease friction.[6,16] The problem with underwrap is that it does not increase, and may actually decrease, the stabilizing effect of the taping technique. In areas where prewrap is not enough, grease pads or some other sort of lubricant should be used to prevent blisters.[2,3] In learning to tape, technique is much more important than neatness. Neatness is usually learned after many hours of practice.

Foot and Ankle

ANKLE SPRAINS

When taping the ankle for support after an ankle sprain, three overlapping anchor strips should be placed at the musculotendinous junction of the Achilles tendon and the gastrocnemius muscle. Next, three stirrups and three Gibney straps should be placed in alternating fashion. These should be located posterior and inferior to the lateral malleolus, since this is the area where the soft tissue structures have been injured. Heel locks, one on each side, should be made, to lock the heel and ensure the stability of that region. Then a figure-of-eight should be taped, to prevent excessive plantar flexion, which can also cause a sprain. Strips of tape should be placed over each other to cover the stirrups and to help stabilize the ankle joint (Fig. 92–5).

ACHILLES TENDON INJURIES

The basic taping for an athlete with an Achilles tendon injury includes one anchor strip placed at the musculotendinous junction of the Achilles tendon and the gastrocnemius muscle. Anchor strips are also placed at the midportion of the foot. Foot placement is important, since taping should prevent overstretching of the tendon. Using two to three strips of elastic tape, the person taping places one end of the tape at the base of the foot and, with a slight pulling action, attaches the other end to the anchor strip of the calf (Fig. 92–6). The tape can also be split from the heel to the top of the musculotendinous junction, to provide two separate end pieces to wrap around the anterior portion of the shin. Several anchor strips should be placed over the calf as well as over the foot, to ensure proper attachment.[2,3,6,9]

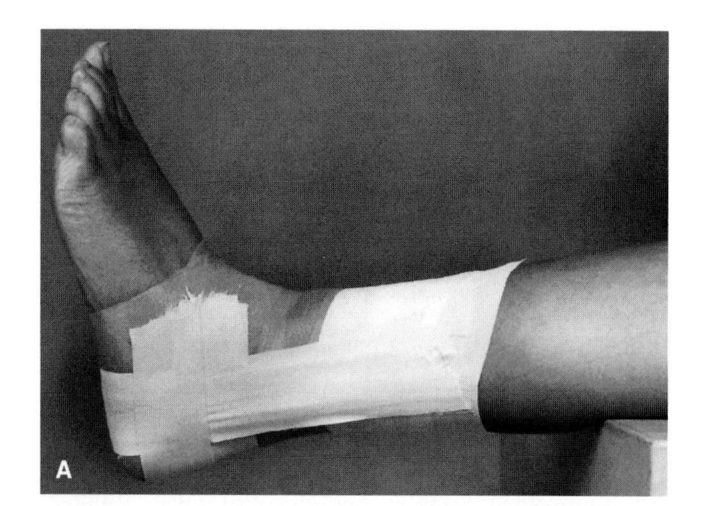

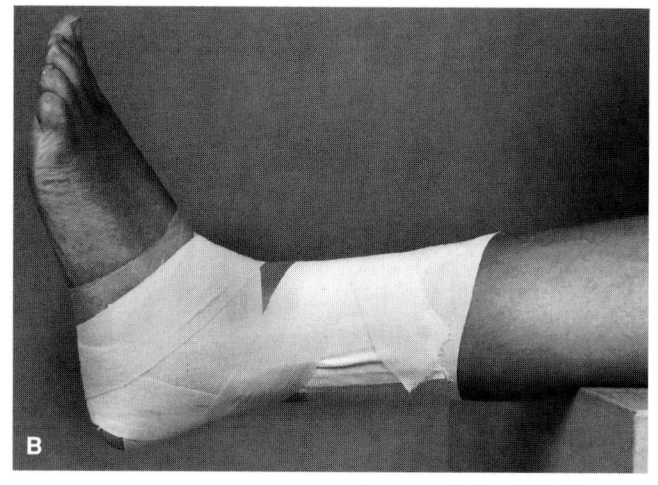

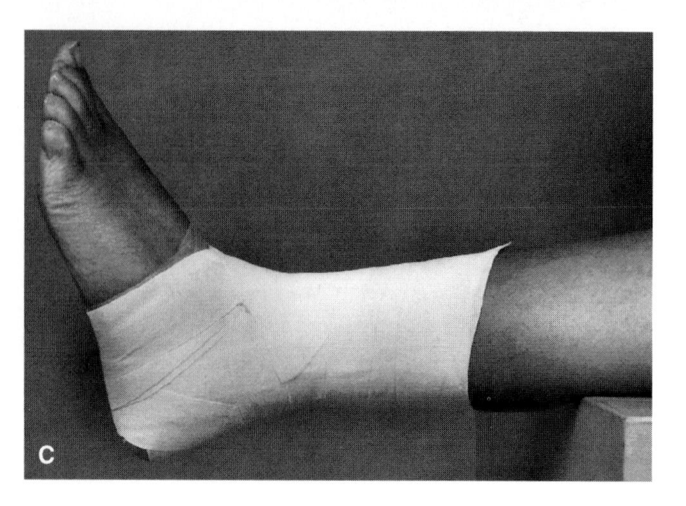

Fig. 92–5. Basic taping to support the ankle includes anchor strips at the musculotendinous junction of the Achilles tendon and gastrocnemius, followed by three stirrups and three Gibney straps *(A)*. After heel locks are added, a figure-of-eight should be applied, to prevent excessive plantar flexion *(B)*. Finally, strips of tape should be placed to cover the stirrups and to help stabilize the ankle joint *(C)*.

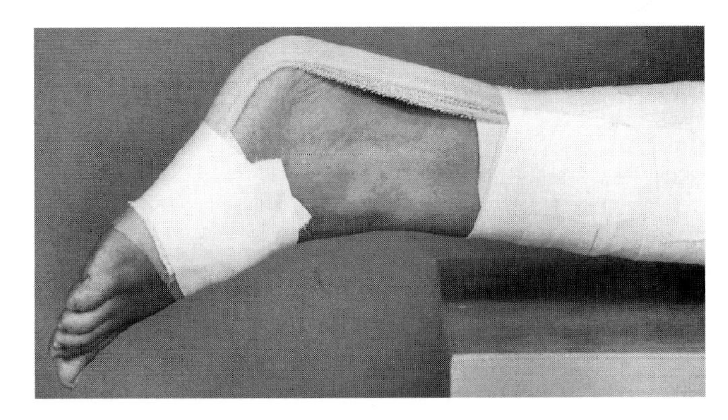

Fig. 92–6. Taping for a patient with an Achilles tendon injury should keep the foot positioned in plantar flexion, to prevent premature stretching of the tendon.

THE LONGITUDINAL ARCH

The anchor strip is placed around the distal portion of the foot. Alternating strips of tape are then started from the medial and lateral portions of the foot (usually six to eight strips) with the foot in a relaxed position. This is followed by several strips going lateral to medial along the plantar surface of the foot.[2,3,6,9]

TURF TOE

Anchor strips are placed around the forefoot and the great toe. Starting from the great toe, strips of tape should go all the way to the forefoot anchor strip. These strips should overlap each other until the toe is stabilized, to prevent hyperextension. Additional anchor strips should be placed around the great toe and around the forefoot as the final step (Fig. 92–7).[9]

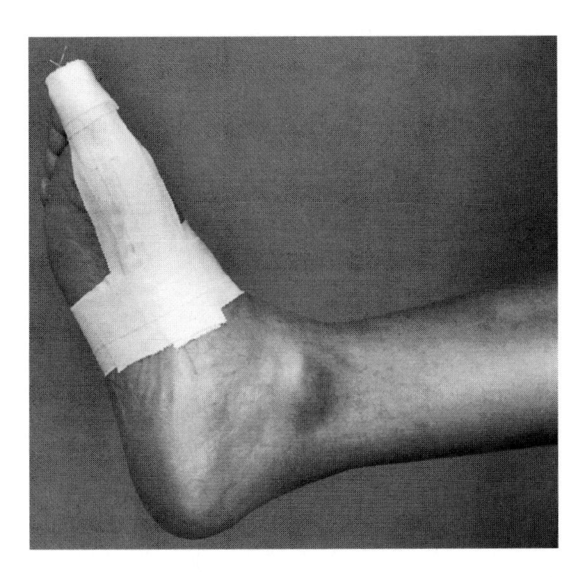

Fig. 92–7. For the athlete with turf toe, the taping should stabilize the great toe to prevent hyperextension.

Lower Leg

SHIN SPLINTS

Starting distally, strips of tape are placed overlapping each other, going from the lateral to the medial aspect, around the calf. Elastic tape is the tape of choice because it allows the muscles to expand.[3,6]

Knee

MEDIAL AND LATERAL SPRAINS

Several anchor strips are placed above and below the joint. Then, strips of tape alternating in an X fashion should be placed over the medial or lateral side, to help protect those structures from varus and valgus forces (Fig. 92–8). A rotation strip may be applied, if necessary. Finally, anchor strips are applied, once again, over the other strips to ensure their attachments.[2,3,6,9]

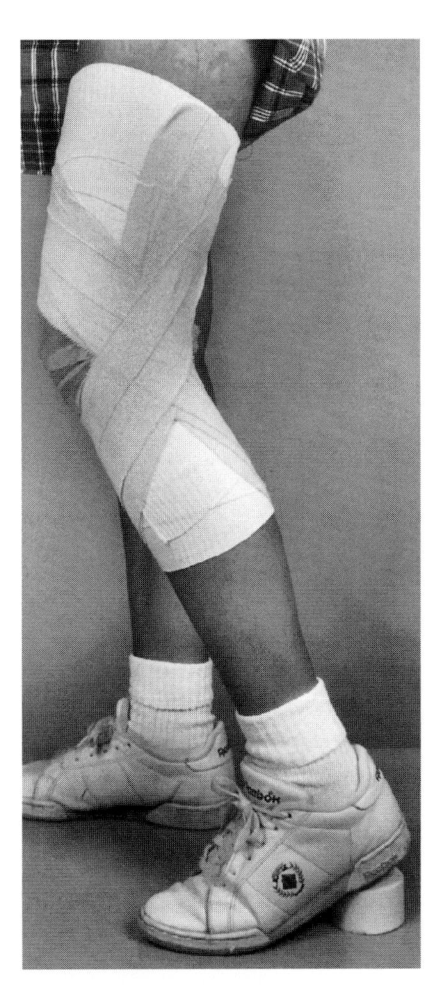

Fig. 92–8. Taping to stabilize the knee after a medial or lateral sprain should include several strips forming an X over the sides of the knee, to protect it from varus and valgus forces.

HYPEREXTENSION

To prevent hyperextension of the knee, anchor strips are placed above and below the joint. A patch should be placed in the popliteal area, to prevent friction and irritation. A sequence of alternating strips forming an X pattern is placed over the posterior portion of the knee joint, followed by anchor strips, once again, above and below the joint, to make sure their attachments are strong.(2,3,6)

Hip and Thigh

HAMSTRINGS AND QUADRICEPS STRAINS

Usually, protection is provided with a 6-inch Ace wrap. It is wrapped around the upper leg to control swelling and provide support.(2,3)

GROIN PULL

A 6-inch–wide elastic wrap should be used, starting at the distal portion of the thigh. Going from medial to lateral, the wrap should rotate upward. It should also be placed around the hip, to ensure proper support and prevent the wrap from slipping down the thigh.(2,3,6)

Shoulder

CLAVICLE FRACTURES

An Ace wrap is used to make an X, pulling the shoulders back to prevent the fractured clavicle from puncturing any arteries or veins in the traumatized area.(2)

ACROMIOCLAVICULAR JOINT SPRAINS

A series of overlapping strips should be placed along the clavicle and acromioclavicular joint, to help stabilize the joint. A pad should be placed over the nipple, to prevent irritating friction.

Elbow

HYPEREXTENSION

To protect the elbow from hyperextension, anchor strips are placed above and below the joint. The elbow is bent short of the position where pain begins. Two or three strips of tape, placed either directly on top of each other or in an X, should be placed on top of the anchor strips at both ends. Additional anchor strips should be placed over the overlapping strips, to help prevent the tape from detaching (Fig. 92–9).(2,3,6,9)

Wrist, Hand, and Fingers

Wrist support can be achieved by placing tape either around the wrist or in an X over the dorsal or plantar surface of the hand.(2,3,6,9)

Finger support is achieved by "buddy" taping—taping fingers together. The thumb can be stabilized with a figure-of-eight pattern, adding strips to prevent abduction and adduction.(2,3,9)

Custom Splinting

At some point during the athletic season, an athlete might need a customized pad. When making such pads,

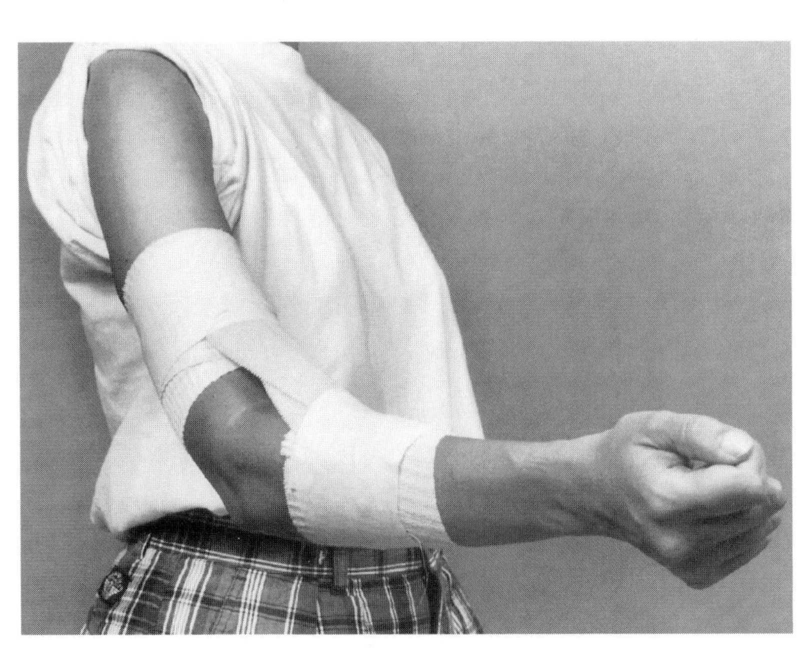

Fig. 92–9. Hyperextension of the elbow can be prevented by placing anchor straps on the upper arm and forearm and using several strips placed over the front of the elbow with the joint flexed to act as a checkrein.

the trainer, physician, or coach must ensure that they meet the rules and regulations of state high school associations or the NCAA.[7] Materials often used in the construction of specialized splints or pads are Orthoplast, 3M Scotch wrap, and silicone (RTV-11).[2,4,9] These materials can be used to make "bubble" pads for the acromioclavicular joint, and they help to stabilize joint injuries, particularly in the forearm, wrist, and hand. Scotch wrap and silicone are particularly helpful because they allow limited motion and are rubbery, and therefore unlikely to harm the athlete or an opponent.[2,3,6,9]

REFERENCES

1. McSorley, T.: Advanced Clinical Competencies Workshop; Seminar notes and handouts. Sport Physical Therapy Section, American Physical Therapy Association. Columbus, GA, 1987.
2. American Academy of Orthopaedic Surgeons: Athletic Training and Sports Medicine. 2nd Ed. Park Ridge, IL, The American Academy of Orthopaedic Surgeons, 1991.
3. Arnheim, D. D., and Prentice, W. E.: Principles of Athletic Training. 8th Ed. St. Louis, Mosby Year Book, 1993.
4. Gieck, J., and McCue, F. C. III: Fitting of protective football equipment. Am. J. Sports Med. *8*:192, 1980.
5. Mueller, F. O., and Ryan, A. J.: Prevention of Athletic Injuries: The Role of the Sports Medicine Team. Philadelphia, F. A. Davis, 1991.
6. Roy, S., and Irvin, R.: Sports Medicine—Prevention, Evaluation, Management, and Rehabilitation. Englewood Cliffs, NJ, Prentice-Hall, 1983.
7. NCAA Sports Medicine Handbook. 3rd ed. Overland Park, KS, NCAA, 1987.
8. Doberstin, S. T.: A procedure for fitting mouth-formed mouth guards. J. Athletic Training *25*:244, 1990.
9. Mellion, M. B., Walsh, W. M, and Shelton, G. L.: The Team Physician's Handbook. Philadelphia, Hanley & Belfus/Mosby Year Book, 1990.
10. Smith, C. R.: Mouth guards take a bite out of injuries. Physician Sportsmed. *20*(7):23, 1992.
11. Duda, M.: Which athletes should wear mouth guards. Physician Sportsmed. *15*(9):179, 1987.
12. Wilkinson, E. E., and Powers, J. M.: Properties of custom-made mouth protector materials. Physician Sportsmed. *14*(6):77, 1986.
13. Erie, J. C.: Eye injuries—prevention, evaluation, and treatment. Physician Sportsmed. *19*(11):108, 1991.
14. Pine D.: Preventing sports related eye injuries. Physician Sportsmed. *19*(2):129, 1991.
15. Steele, B. E.: Protective pads for athletes. Physician Sportsmed. *13*(3):179, 1985.
16. Shahady, E. J., and Petrizzi, M. J.: Sports Medicine for Coaches and Trainers. 2nd Ed. Chapel Hill, University of North Carolina Press, 1991.

V

SPORT-SPECIFIC PROBLEMS

93

Michael J. Axe and Sandra Gibney

Weight Lifting—A Brief Overview

This chapter is based on the assumption that most weight lifting injuries are preventable. In the senior author's 25 years of weight lifting experience, both as a participant and professionally, as the physician for the East Coast Gold Team of the United States Weight Lifting Federation, this contention has been supported again and again. Most of the recommendations for avoiding injury that we put forth in this chapter are informed by common sense. Unfortunately, as in all athletic activities, myths passed on from generation to generation of lifters have perpetuated environments and behaviors that are unsafe. The following information is offered to demonstrate to coaches, trainers, and sports physicians that weight training can be a safe and effective means of enhancing physical performance.

MAXIMAL LIFTS AND THE THREE PERCENT RULE

While overuse and repetitive trauma can lead to injury, most significant trauma results from a maximal single effort. The senior author has used a formula developed by Jeffrey Wright and implemented in 1983 by then University of Pittsburgh strength and conditioning coach, Charles "Buddy" Morris. It is invaluable in the design of safe and effective weight training programs. The 3% rule allows estimation of maximal lifts from known multiple repetition maxima. For the reader's convenience, the formulas were transformed into tabular form (Table 93–1); the values were rounded off to the nearest 5 pounds. MAX stands for the single repetition maximum; REPMAX, for the maximum weight used for two or more repetitions; and REPS, for the number of repetitions. The table allows a reasonable estimation of the athlete's single maximum effort, within 5 pounds.

These formulas and the data in the table are predicated on the assumption that the REPMAX is an exhaustive effort and that all repetitions are completed. The table guidelines are used for all major power lifts: bench press, military press, dead lift, and squat. The table allows adjustments in repetitions per set and conversion to the percentages of the maximum lift used by some strength and conditioning coaches and weight lifting programs. A 5-pound increase in single repetition maximum is expected for every 4 to 6 weeks of training, and the repetitions can be adjusted appropriately. Test maximum efforts are limited to only one, or at most two times, per year.[1] Using this approach, neither the University of Pittsburgh nor the All Sports Clinic of Delaware has seen injuries result from a maximal single effort lift.

ENVIRONMENTAL CONSIDERATIONS

Physical Plant

Weight rooms should be large and uncluttered, to avoid accidents. Most facilities have too much equipment and not enough space to allow all the pieces to be used simultaneously, as during a team "station cycle" work out. Moving from station to station, athletes trip over the weights or the racks. We suggest it is preferable to limit the amount of equipment rather than to crowd the weight room. Again, to avoid loss of balance and falling into equipment, the floor should be of a nonslippery material and should be padded. If the floors are not padded, dropped weights can break. Worse yet, an athlete may be injured if, because of poor lifting posture he loses balance and does not drop the weight for fear of drawing negative attention from the coach for the noise and distraction.

Supervision

Supervision is critical to the prevention of weight lifting injury, particularly if the weight lifting is done in the

Table 93-1 The Three Percent Rule

Lifts:
- Bench press
- Military press
- Squat
- Dead lift

MAX = Single repetition maximum

REP MAX = Maximum weight used for repetitions of two or more

REPS = Number of repetitions

MAX = (3% REP MAX × REPS) + REPMAX

$$\text{REP MAX} = \frac{\text{MAX}}{\text{3\% REPS} + 1}$$

Repetitions	*10*	*9*	*8*	*7*	*6*	*5*	*4*	*3*	*2*
MAX									
155	115	120	125	130	130	135	140	145	145
160	120	125	130	130	135	140	145	150	150
165	125	130	130	135	140	145	150	155	155
170	130	130	135	140	145	150	155	155	160
175	130	135	140	145	150	155	160	160	165
180	135	140	145	150	155	160	160	165	170
185	140	145	150	155	155	160	165	170	175
190	145	145	150	155	160	165	170	175	180
195	145	150	155	160	165	170	175	180	185
200	150	155	160	165	170	175	180	185	190
205	155	160	165	170	175	180	185	190	195
210	160	165	170	175	180	185	190	195	200
215	160	165	170	175	185	190	195	200	205
220	165	170	175	180	185	190	195	200	205
225	170	175	180	185	190	195	205	210	215
230	175	180	185	190	195	200	205	215	220
235	175	180	190	195	200	205	210	215	225
240	180	185	190	200	205	210	215	220	230
245	185	190	195	200	210	215	220	225	235
250	190	195	200	205	215	220	225	230	240
255	190	200	205	210	215	225	230	235	240
260	195	200	210	215	220	230	235	240	245
265	200	205	210	220	225	230	240	245	250
270	205	210	215	225	230	235	245	250	255
275	205	215	220	225	235	240	250	255	260
280	210	215	225	230	240	245	250	260	265
285	215	220	230	235	240	250	255	265	270
290	220	225	230	240	245	255	260	270	275
295	220	230	235	245	250	260	265	275	280
300	225	235	240	250	255	265	270	280	285
305	230	235	245	250	260	265	275	280	290
310	235	240	250	255	265	270	280	285	295
315	235	245	250	260	270	275	285	290	300
320	240	250	255	265	270	280	290	295	305
325	245	250	260	270	275	285	295	300	310
330	250	255	265	270	280	290	295	305	315
335	250	260	270	275	285	295	300	310	320
340	255	265	270	280	290	300	305	315	325
345	260	265	275	285	295	300	310	320	330
350	265	270	280	290	300	305	315	325	335
355	265	275	285	295	300	310	320	330	335
360	270	280	290	295	305	315	325	335	340
365	275	285	290	300	310	320	330	340	345
370	280	285	295	305	315	325	335	340	350
375	280	290	300	310	320	330	340	345	355
Percentage	75%	77.5%	80%	82.5%	85%	87.5%	90%	92.5%	95%

(Continued)

Table 93–1 The Three Percent Rule—*(Continued)*

Repetitions	*10*	*9*	*8*	*7*	*6*	*5*	*4*	*3*	*2*
MAX									
380	285	295	305	315	325	335	340	350	360
385	290	300	310	320	325	335	345	355	365
390	295	300	310	320	330	340	350	360	370
395	295	305	315	325	335	345	355	365	375
400	300	310	320	330	340	350	360	370	380
405	305	315	325	335	345	355	365	375	385
410	310	320	330	340	350	360	370	380	390
415	310	320	330	340	355	365	375	385	395
420	315	325	335	345	355	370	380	390	400
425	320	330	340	350	360	370	385	395	405
430	325	335	345	355	365	375	385	400	410
435	325	335	350	360	370	380	390	400	415
440	330	340	350	365	375	385	395	405	420
445	335	345	355	365	380	390	400	410	425
450	340	350	360	370	385	395	405	415	430
455	340	355	365	375	385	400	410	420	430
460	345	355	370	380	390	405	415	425	435
465	350	360	370	385	395	405	420	430	440
470	355	365	375	390	400	410	425	435	445
475	355	370	380	390	405	415	430	440	450
480	360	370	385	395	410	420	430	445	455
485	365	375	390	400	410	425	435	450	460
490	370	380	390	405	415	430	440	455	465
495	370	385	395	410	420	435	445	460	470
500	375	390	400	415	425	440	450	465	475
510	385	395	410	420	435	445	460	470	485
520	390	405	415	430	440	455	470	480	495
530	400	410	425	435	450	465	475	490	505
540	405	420	430	445	460	475	485	500	515
550	415	425	440	455	470	480	495	510	525
560	420	435	450	460	475	490	505	520	530
570	430	440	455	470	485	500	515	525	540
580	435	450	465	480	495	510	520	535	550
590	445	455	470	485	500	515	530	545	560
600	450	465	480	495	510	525	540	555	570
610	460	475	490	505	520	535	550	565	580
620	465	480	495	510	525	545	560	575	590
630	475	490	505	520	535	550	565	585	600
640	480	495	510	530	545	560	575	590	610
650	490	505	520	535	555	570	585	600	620
660	495	510	530	545	560	580	595	610	625
670	505	520	535	555	570	585	605	620	635
680	510	525	545	560	580	595	610	630	645
690	520	535	550	570	585	605	620	640	655
700	525	545	560	580	595	615	630	650	665
Percentage	75%	77.5%	80%	82.5%	85%	87.5%	90%	92.5%	95%

(Summer Conditioning Football Program, University of Pittsburgh, 1983.)

home. Weight lifters who lift without a spotter are obviously at risk, but so are children who are allowed to play in the weight room. Children between ages 2 and 4 years had 2270 visits to the emergency room in 1986 owing to injuries associated with a weight room;[2] those in the 5- to 14-year age group had 5940 visits. Most of these injuries occurred in an unsupervised weight room. One 4-year-old boy died after he fell from a weight training bench and struck his head on the floor.[2] A 9-year-old boy who had been playing with his older brother's set of weights, died from a ruptured right atrium after a 23-kg barbell fell 1 m onto his chest.[3] The equipment naturally attracts inquisitive young people's eyes and hands; thus, the area should be capable of being locked.

The importance of adequate supervision in all weight rooms cannot be overstated. Trained personnel should be available in sufficient numbers to ensure safe and appropriate use of available equipment.

Weight Belts

Traditional leather weight belts and newer, lighter-weight fabric belts or supports are often used to enhance lumbar spine stability during heavy lifting. Competitive power lifters, serious weight lifters, and even recreational lifters use abdominal weight belts to enhance spine stability and reduce lumbar stress. Studies have demonstrated that intra-abdominal pressure can reduce the compressive force on the lumbar spine by as much as 50%.[4] In addition to the beneficial effect on spinal forces and musculature, subjects have reported feeling more secure while wearing a weight belt.[5]

The choice of weight belt varies with the magnitude and intensity of the workouts. A light weight belt typically consists of a single layer of leather (approximately 7 mm) that tapers from a wide center (10 cm) to 7 cm at both ends. This type of belt is probably best for most recreational or noncompetitive lifters because it is less restrictive and allows for a somewhat tighter fit. Heavy belts usually are thicker (three layers of leather) and wide (10 cm) throughout their length. These are probably best suited for competitive lifters or those with a long trunk who can achieve proper belt tightening.[5]

Weight belts may have some disadvantages: Constant use of a belt may prevent or diminish the development of maximum strength in the abdominal and back muscles. Therefore, it may be valuable to perform less strenuous, lighter-weight lifts without using a belt, to help strengthen the abdominal and back muscles;[6] though those who have a history of back injury should use a weight belt for all levels of lifting activities. Increased intra-abdominal pressure from a tightened weight belt can decrease abdominal blood flow back to the heart. Loosening the belt between sets is recommended, to allow the lifter to breathe deeply and reduce intra-abdominal pressure.[7,8] Weight belts are *never* a substitute for proper exercise form and execution, which are crucial to avoiding injury.

PHYSICAL CONSIDERATIONS

Skeletal Immaturity

Preadolescent athletes who are mentally and emotionally mature enough to begin weight training can do so at any age, provided they adhere to the basic guidelines offered by the American Academy of Pediatrics' Committee on Sports Medicine (APCSM). We have developed the following "composite" guidelines based on theirs and on recommendations of other experts for skeletally immature weight lifters[9–13]:

Pediatric athletes should have a preparticipation physical examination.

A knowledgeable supervisor should be present during weight-lifting activity.

Athletes should wear clothing that cannot be inadvertently caught in the equipment. Shoes should have a firm toe box and nonskid soles.

Warm-up should include jogging, stretching, and calisthenics.

A 4- to 6-week period of body weight–type exercises, including pushups, pull-ups, and situps, should be used both for preparticipation and general conditioning, and to establish the child's commitment to a weight-lifting program. This is particularly true if a financial investment in equipment is anticipated.

Specific guidelines for skeletally immature athletes include these:

1. A routine of 20 to 30 minutes' duration.
2. A 12-week progressive cycle followed by a 6-week cycle of body weight exercises, including pushups, pull-ups, situps, and dips.
3. No more than 4 workouts per week and 1 day of no lifting between workouts.
4. Eight to fifteen repetitions per set, two to three sets per exercise, and one to two exercises per body part.
5. Weight progression no greater than 5 additional pounds per week.
6. Wrists should be supported with tape or wraps.
7. The dead lift, squat, military press, power clean, and dynamic lifts of the swatch and clean and jerk should be avoided until male and female athletes have reached Tanner Stage 5 in their development of secondary sexual characteristics (i.e., pubic hair is adult in quantity and type with extension onto the thighs, for males the genitalia are adult in size and shape, and for females the areola has recessed to the general contour of the breast).[14] At this point, the athlete will have passed through the period of maximal growth in height, during which the bony epiphyses appear to be more vulnerable to injury. This recommendation is designed to prevent injuries to the growth plates.

Female Athletes

The incidence of weight lifting injuries is much lower in women than in men. Though an overall smaller number of participants may account for this, other factors may contribute. Females attain skeletal maturity earlier than males, and they are therefore less susceptible to injuries described previously. In fact, approximately 2 years after the onset of regular menstruation, it is rare that female athletes have not reached skeletal maturity. It has been observed by Coach Morris and the authors that female athletes adhere more strictly to optimal lifting form and are less likely to allow their ego to place them at risk.

When women who engage in body building and power lifting fail to adhere to basic weight-lifting tenets, injuries occur as they would in men. In a study of shoulder instability as a result of training errors, 4 of the 20 athletes were women,[15] and Matthews and coworkers reported on a 27-year-old policewoman and body builder who developed degenerative arthritis of the acromioclavicular joint (osteolysis of the distal clavicle).[16]

TRAINING ERRORS

The Squat

The squat, an exercise that engages most of the body's muscle mass, is the most important exercise for improving power. Many health professionals and coaches are concerned about this controversial, and potentially "dangerous," lift.[17] It is not sound thinking to engage in this lift until an athlete has reached Tanner Stage 5. After reaching skeletal maturity, lifters who execute properly can expect to remain injury free and increase their lean body mass and improve lower body power and athletic performance. In 1991, the National Strength and Conditioning Association published a position paper on the squat (Table 93–2).[17] Recognized experts in that organization offered insights into common errors of technique:

Improper head position with the eyes directed toward the ceiling rather than straight ahead.
Improper foot position, with the feet not at shoulder width and turned slightly outward.
Uneven bar grip, causing a twisting movement when coming from the bottom position.
Malalignment of the spine with hyperkyphosis (round back).
Excessive forward leaning, allowing the knees to travel forward over the toes and the heels to come off the floor, compromising balance.
Bar racked too high on the neck, encouraging forward leaning.
Failure to reach parallel.
Descending too rapidly, causing loss of balance, leading to knee flexion well beyond parallel, which increases the likelihood of trapping the meniscus.

Squatting technique may be impaired by lack of flexibility in the lower back and pelvis or inherent weaknesses in the back and abdomen. Correction of these weak links may reduce the likelihood of injury.[18,19]

Upper Body

The athlete's philosophy of "more is better" is clearly reflected in weight lifters' attitudes toward chest and shoulder exercises. Multiple exercises per body part or excessive sets (four to ten) with repetitions from one to fifteen can lead to overuse problems from the shoulder to the fingers,[20] particularly in older and in preadolescent athletes.

Adequate recovery between workouts must be ensured, and the smaller stabilizing muscles of the rotator cuff must not be ignored while the lifter focuses on

Table 93–2. NSCA Position Paper: The Squat Exercise in Athletic Conditioning

Position Statement: The following nine points related to the use of the squat exercise constitute the Position Statement of the Association. They have been approved by the Research Committee of the Association.
Squats, when performed correctly and with appropriate supervision, are not only safe, but may be a significant deterrent to knee injuries.
The squat exercise can be an important component of a training program to improve the athlete's ability to forcefully extend the knees and hips, and can considerably enhance performance in many sports.
Excessive training, overuse injuries and fatigue-related problems do occur with squats. The likelihood of such injuries and problems is substantially diminished by adherence to established principles of exercise program design.
The squat exercise is not detrimental to knee joint stability when performed correctly.
Weight training, including the squat exercise, strengthens connective tissue, including muscles, bones, ligaments and tendons.
Proper form depends on the style of the squat and the muscles to be conditioned. Bouncing in the bottom position of a squat to help initiate ascent increases mechanical loads on the knee joint and is therefore contraindicated.
While squatting results in high forces on the back, injury potential is low with appropriate technique and supervision.
Conflicting reports exist as to the type, frequency and severity of weight-training injuries. Some reports of high injury rates may be based on biased samples. Others have attributed injuries to weight training, including the squat, which could have been caused by other factors.
Injuries attributed to the squat may result not from the exercise itself, but from improper technique, pre-existing structural abnormalities, other physical activities, fatigue or excessive training.

(Chandler, T. J., Stone, M.: The squat exercise in athletic conditioning: A position statement and review of literature. National Strength and Conditioning Journal. *13*(5):51, 1991.)

the deltoid, pectoral, and latissimus muscles. Imbalance can lead to injury of the rotator cuff and can thereby increase the strain on the ligaments of the shoulder girdle.[21] The University of Delaware's strength and conditioning coach, Anthony Decker, ATC, CSCS, suggests that athletes are at particular risk immediately following completion of a collision sport season, as they return to the progressive "building" weight-lifting programs rather than an in-season maintenance program. In the senior author's experience as a football player and team physician, this problem often occurs in late January and early February, week 6 of the winter 12-week cycle. Decker recommends weight program modifications for athletes with rotator cuff strain or contusion. Modifications with regard to the bench press include being cautious of excessively wide grips, and perhaps unloading the cuff with a reversed hand "chin-up" grip and using less weight. The rotator cuff exercises, using either dumbbells or Theraband, should be the final shoulder exercises for the weight-lifting workout.[22]

Gross and colleagues reported on 20 recreational weight lifters who became symptomatic when lifting with the shoulder abducted 90° and externally rotated (i.e., wide grip bench press, incline and supine flys, bent arm pullovers, latissimus pulldowns and the behind-the-neck military press).[15] Studies of the anterior ligaments of the shoulder demonstrate that the inferior and middle glenohumeral ligaments are in maximal strain in this position.[21,23,24] The anterior capsular ligaments can become stretched because of chronic strain or an acute event, and the athlete complains of pain when performing these "at-risk" lifts. Most acute injuries are associated with working without spotters and missing the standards when racking the weights.

The case files of the senior author contain two particularly severe examples. A varsity baseball player who missed the rack while performing behind-the-neck presses suffered an anteroinferior dislocation of his nonthrowing shoulder, and a 260-pound power lifter who, after a squat lift, was racking well over 700 pounds, missed the standards and was forced into a hyperflexed position, rupturing both quadriceps tendons. Adequate supervision and instruction should have prevented both injuries.

Elimination of behind-the-neck lifts with substitution exercises and modification of hand position to shoulder width can, on most occasions, allow an athlete to continue to lift with minimal symptoms once inflammation is controlled. Oral nonsteroidal anti-inflammatory medications have often been used successfully to treat this condition, and occasionally an intra-articular injection of a long-acting corticosteroid was needed. In our practice, we have found that, when symptoms of pain persist—or more commonly when the inability to increase in poundage of lifts persists—surgical repair of the strained capsular ligaments may be necessary.

Modification in exercises include shrugs, isolated dumbbell work for the middle and anterior heads of the deltoid, upright straight bar shoulder extensions for rear deltoids, and upright rows and sitting rows for the latissimus muscles. Another recommendation is that, within any given 12-week cycle, either flat *or* inclined bench be the major exercise for the pectoral muscle group, but not both.

OSTEOLYSIS AND OTHER PATHOLOGIC CONDITIONS

The senior author firmly believes that degenerative arthritis of the acromioclavicular joint—osteolysis of the clavicle—is an unavoidable liability of years of weight training. While many athletes with this condition have participated in collision sports, Scavenius and coworkers reported on 25 weight lifters who had no history of acute traumatic injury but developed clavicular osteolysis.[25] Cahill and Slawski have shown that, once the process becomes symptomatic, all measures short of surgery are merely temporizing,[26,27] and the senior author's experience bears out this observation. In the senior author's experience, pathologic changes in the glenohumeral joint and of the anterolateral acromion can be associated with osteolysis of the distal clavicle. Thus, diagnostic arthroscopy should include the glenohumeral joint and the subacromial space, rather than being limited to the acromioclavicular joint. Many weight lifters return to their 1 year preinjury level of lifting within 6 to 12 months after distal clavicle excision, though not all. The association of intra-articular lesions in the glenohumeral joint, including loose bodies, chondral defects of the glenoid and humeral head, attenuated glenohumeral ligaments, partial rotator cuff tears, and superior labrum, anterior and posterior (SLAP) lesions would be missed if only an open procedure were performed.

The impingement that many weight lifters experience is on the anterolateral aspect of the acromion, an area that is difficult to visualize and palpate in an open procedure without compromising the deltoid attachments. This impingement can be secondary to a bony hook on the acromion or to calcific deposits in the rotator cuff tendons as appreciated on preoperative radiographs. Other arthroscopic findings include a large, thickened subacromial bursa and, on occasion, a short tendon with a hypertrophic supraspinatus muscle. For this reason, coracoacromial ligament release and subacromial decompression, with particular attention to the anterolateral aspect of the acromion, has become the standard for the senior author.

Having required excision of both clavicles and repair of partial avulsions of both subscapularis tendons as a result of injuries from too rapid progression in press loads (Fig. 93–1), the senior author has gained keen awareness of osteolysis and associated lesions. Thus, the recommendation to address the glenohumeral joint and the anterolateral aspect of the acromion is also offered as a personal insight, as both a patient and a sports orthopedist.

Athletes must have reasonable expectations; for athletes to achieve the level of performance they enjoyed 1 year before an injury is a reasonable subjective goal that most can attain.

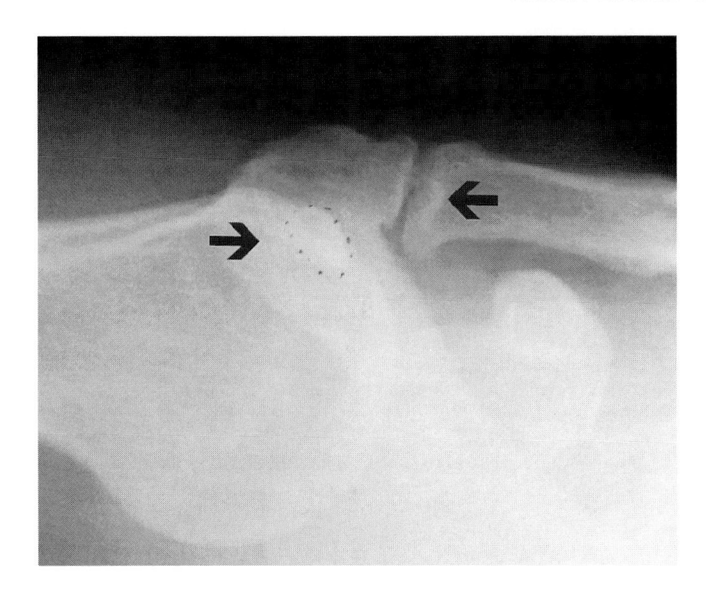

Fig. 93–1. 40-year-old sports orthopaedist with osteolysis of the clavicle *(left arrow)* and an avulsion fracture of the subscapularis *(right arrow).*

After surgery for osteolysis, the senior author has had success with the following modifications for weight lifting: For the first 12 weeks after surgery, no shoulder weight lifting exercises should be done, only stretching and range of motion exercises. In weeks 12 to 16 after surgery, upper extremity exercises, including pushups and sitting dips, are allowed, and the number is increased as tolerated. At 12 to 24 weeks after surgery, (1) the athlete should always get a lift off when doing bench exercises and get an assist setting the bar back after the lift; (2) no lifts should be performed above nipple level; (3) no more than two exercises should be done per body part; (4) repetitions should be no fewer than eight and no more than fifteen; and (5) all sets combined should total no more than 40 repetitions per body part. Weight lifters can expect inflammation to recur with the progression of the program. Occasionally, subacromial corticosteroid injections may be required during the first 6 months after surgery to control this inflammation. Weight lifters who are also throwing athletes may begin batting at 12 weeks, and some may be able to begin throwing programs at 16 weeks. After rehabilitation, weight lifters can expect to return to lifting the amount that they were able to lift 1 year before their symptoms began. Inclined bench and military press are strongly discouraged for the first 9 months after surgery.

Most acute injuries in weight lifting are associated with improper techniques, either in performing the lift or, as mentioned previously, when racking the bar. Tendon ruptures and avulsions—of the subscapularis, pectoralis major,[28–31] biceps proximally and distally,[32,33] triceps,[34,35] hamstrings and quadriceps tendons, patellar tendon,[36] and others—have been reported. Fractures that appear to be of acute onset, including ribs,[37] clavicle, and scaphoid, have been described, usually in case reports. There are also reports of nerves being stretched and trapped, including the long thoracic,[38] suprascapular,[39] and ulnar nerves.[34] Injuries, including costochondritis from bouncing the bar on the chest and toe fractures from dropping the weight on one's foot, are other acute processes that can be avoided with appropriate technique and care.

CONCLUSION

While weight lifting remains a safe and controlled activity, guidelines offered in this chapter, if followed, help athletes avoid injury. We suggest limiting maximum lifting effort to no more than twice per year and offer a way of estimating maximal lift poundage from multiple repetition maximums. Our focus was to offer useful guidelines for sports physicians, coaches, and trainers who care for the weight-lifting population.

REFERENCES

1. University of Pittsburgh: Summer Conditioning Football Program. Pittsburgh, University of Pittsburgh, 1983.
2. National Electronic Injury Surveillance System. 1986 Data Summary on Injuries Caused by Weightlifting. Washington, DC, U.S. Consumer Products Safety Commission, 1987.
3. George, D. H., Stakiw, K., and Wright, C. J.: Fatal accident with weight-lifting equipment: Implications for safety standards. Can. Med. Assoc. J. *140*:925, 1989.
4. Lander, J. E., Bates, B. T., and Devita, P.: Biomechanics of the squat exercise using a modified center of mass bar. Med. Sci. Sports Exerc. *18*:469, 1986.
5. Lander, J. E., Simonton, R. L., and Giacobbe, J. K. F.: The effectiveness of weight-belts during the squat exercise. Med. Sci. Sports Exerc. *22*:117, 1990.
6. Cholewicki, J., and McGill, S. M.: Lumbar posterior ligament involvement during extremely heavy lifts estimated from fluoroscopic measurements. J. Biomech. *25*:17, 1992.
7. Harman, E. A., Rosenstein, R. M., Frykman, P. N., and Nigro, G. A.: Effects of a belt on intra-abdominal pressure during weight lifting. Med. Sci. Sports Exerc. *21*:186, 1989.
8. Kumar, S., and Davis, P. R.: Spinal loading in static and dynamic postures; EMG and intra-abdominal pressure study. Ergonomics. *26*:913, 1983.
9. American Academy of Pediatrics Committee on Sports Medicine: Strength training, weight and power lifting, and body building by children and adolescents. Pediatrics. *86*:801, 1990.
10. Mazur, L. J., Yetman, R. J., and Risser, W. L.: Weight-training injuries: Common injuries and preventative methods. Sports Med. *16*:57, 1993.
11. Risser, W. L., Risser, J. M., and Preston, D.: Weight-training injuries in adolescents. Am. J. Dis. Children. *144*:1015, 1990.
12. Risser, W. L.: Musculoskeletal injuries caused by weight training: Guidelines for prevention. Clin. Pediatrics. *29*:305, 1990.
13. Risser, W. L.: Weight-training injuries in children and adolescents. Am. Family Physician. *44*:2104, 1991.
14. Tanner, J. M.: Growth at Adolescence. 2nd Ed. Oxford, Blackwell Scientific Publications, 1962.
15. Gross, M. L., Brenner, S. L., Esformes, I., and Sonzogni, J. T.: Anterior shoulder instability in weightlifters. Am. J. Sports Med. *21*:599, 1993.
16. Matthews, L. S., Simonson, B. G., and Wolock, B. S.: Osteolysis of the distal clavicle in a female body builder: A case report. Am. J. Sports Med. *21*:150, 1993.
17. Chandler, T. J., and Stone, M. H.: The squat exercise in athletic conditioning: A position statement and review of the literature. National Strength Conditioning Association Journal *13*(5):51, 1991.
18. Fairchild, D., Hill, B., Ritchie, M., and Sochor, D.: Common technique errors in the back squat (roundtable). National Strength Condition. Assoc. J. *13*(5):52, 1993.

19. Fry, A.: Coaching considerations for the barbell squat—part II. National Strength Condition. Assoc. J. *15*:28, 1993.
20. Kiefhaber, T. R., and Stern, P. J.: Upper extremity tendinitis and overuse syndromes in the athlete. Clin. Sports Med. *11*:39, 1992.
21. Matsen, F. A. III, Harryman, D. T. II, and Sidles, J. A.: Mechanics of glenohumeral instability. Clin. Sports Med. *10*:783, 1991.
22. Personal Communication, Anthony Decker, ATC, CSCS, Strength Coach, University of Delaware.
23. Cain, P. R., Mutschler, T. A., Fu, F. H., and Lee, S. K.: Anterior stability of the glenohumeral joint: A dynamic model. Am. J. Sports Med. *15*:144, 1987.
24. O'Connell, P. W., Nuber, G. W., Mileski, R. A., and Lautenschlager, E.: The contribution of the glenohumeral ligaments to anterior stability of the shoulder joint. Am. J. Sports Med. *18*:579, 1990.
25. Scavenius, M., and Iversen, B. F.: Nontraumatic clavicular osteolysis in weight lifters. Am. J. Sports Med. *20*:463, 1992.
26. Cahill, B. R.: Osteolysis of the distal part of the clavicle in male athletes. J. Bone Joint Surg. *64A*:1053, 1982.
27. Slawski, D. P., and Cahill, B. R.: Atraumatic osteolysis of the distal clavicle. Am. J. Sports Med. *22*:267, 1994.
28. Liu, J., et al.: Avulsion of the pectoralis major tendon. Am. J. Sports Med. *20*:366, 1992.
29. Reut, R. C., Bach, B. R., and Johnson, C.: Pectoralis major rupture: Diagnosing and treating a weight-training injury. Physician Sportsmed. *19*(3):89, 1991.
30. Rijnberg, W. J., and van Linge, B.: Rupture of the pectoralis major muscle in body-builders. Arch. Orthop. Trauma Surg. *112*:104, 1993.
31. Wolfe, S. W., Wickiewicz, T. L., and Cavanaugh, J. T.: Ruptures of the pectoralis major muscle: An anatomic and clinical analysis. Am. J. Sports Med. *20*:587, 1992.
32. Neviaser, T. J.: Weight lifting: Risk and injuries to the shoulder. Clin. Sports Med. *10*:615, 1991.
33. D'Alessandro, D. F., Shields, C. L., Jr., Tibone, J. E., and Chandler, R. W.: Repair of distal biceps tendon ruptures in athletes. Am. J. Sports Med. *21*:114, 1993.
34. Herrick, R. T., and Herrick, S.: Ruptured triceps in a powerlifter presenting as a cubital tunnel syndrome: A case report. Am. J. Sports Med. *15*:514, 1987.
35. Stannard, J. P., and Bucknell, A. L.: Ruptures of the triceps tendon associated with steroid injections. Am. J. Sports Med. *21*:482, 1993.
36. Glossbrenner, H.: Matt Dimel: His comeback story. Powerlifting USA *16*(7):9, 1993.
37. Goeser, C. D., and Aikenhead, J. A.: Rib fracture due to bench pressing. J. Manipulative Physiol. Therapeutics *13*:26, 1990.
38. Schultz, J. S., and Leonard, J. A., Jr.: Long thoracic neuropathy from athletic activity. Arch. Phys. Med. Rehabil. *73*:87, 1992.
39. Zeiss, J., Woldenberg, L. S., Saddemi, S. R., and Ebraheim, N. A.: MRI of suprascapular neuropathy in a weight lifter. J. Comput. Assisted Tomogr. *17*:303, 1993.

94 *Thomas K. Miller*

Triathlon

Although a variety of multisport events exist, most triathlons consist of three events contested consecutively, swimming, biking, and running. The best-known triathlon, the Hawaiian Iron Man, demands swimming 2.4 miles, cycling 112 miles, and running 26.2 miles (a marathon). More commonly, events are contested at the sprint (swim 0.5 mile, bike 13 miles, and run 3 miles) or the international (swim 1.5 km, bike 40 km, and run 10 km) distance with winning times for international distance events under 2 hours. The sport's World Championship has been held annually at this international distance since 1989, and triathlon has been included in the program for the 1994 Goodwill Games and the 1995 Pan-American Games.

Unlike many other athletes, participants in triathlon usually have a primary background in other endurance sports, the most common one being running. Though boredom with single-sport competition is often mentioned as a reason for investigating triathlon, athletes may take up the sport because of an injury in a primary sport. Interest in cross-training has been associated with the concept of multisport activities as a means of continued participation after injury. Though cross-training may not directly result in improvement in a primary sport (improvement in one sporting activity requires sport-specific training), it may allow improvement in muscle balance, and cross-training activities may allow the athlete to maintain fitness while recovering from injury in a primary sport. Participants in triathlon range from the age of 10 years (youngest age group in the Iron Kids series) to more than 70 years old. Unlike many sports, the World Championship of Triathlon is contested not only by professionals but by amateurs in these age groups. Given the broad age range and varied sporting backgrounds, participants bring with them not only primary sport expertise but also old injuries. Athletes of masters age often develop injuries more commonly seen in sporting novices as they take up new activities (e.g., swimmer's shoulder in a 50-year-old runner). As a result, the injuries seen are those of longterm overuse *and* those of a novice's training errors.

INJURIES

Injuries of triathletes often can be grouped by the "primary" sport from which they arise. In swimming, the most common problem is related to the shoulder—impingement and overuse. Cycling can produce both acute and chronic injuries. Acromioclavicular separations, clavicle fractures, and "road rash" are the most common acute injuries; knee problems (especially patellofemoral conditions) are an overuse phenomenon. The running component of triathlon is associated with knee injuries (both intra- and peri-articular), stress fractures, and Achilles tendon injuries. The pattern of injuries can also be evaluated by anatomic system.

Shoulder Injuries

The most common shoulder problems are overuse syndromes, usually secondary to swimming. With these injuries, prior history is especially important. "Retired" swimmers usually have a history of shoulder problems, and they complain of having in the past had "tendinitis" or "bursitis," which was quiescent until they resumed swimming. Novice swimmers usually experience the gradual onset of problems secondary to poor technique or training errors.

Rotator cuff irritation or impingement (swimmer's shoulder) is caused by repetitive abrasion of the rotator cuff against the coracoacromial arch. The principal function of the rotator cuff is to depress and center the humeral head, thus positioning the head on the glenoid for the remainder of the shoulder motion. Any factor that compromises the space between the rotator cuff and the coracoacromial arch results in abrasion and irritation of the cuff that causes shoulder pain. With swimmers, muscle imbalance between internal rotators (chest wall propulsion) and external rotators (rotator cuff) is common. Subsequently, there is progressive anterior displacement and proximal migration of the humeral head to an impingement position. While mere repetition of the swimmer's stroke does not necessarily imply that impingement or abrasion will occur, the progressive muscle imbalance that can be associated with training does lead to "shoulder pain at increased distances." Abnormal scapular mechanics, especially scapular winging, can cause anterior closure of the coracoacromial arch and lead to impingement. Abnormal acromial shape or spurring can decrease the space available to the rotator cuff during motion.

Impingement syndrome is diagnosed both by history and by examination. Athletes often complain of pain at the leading edge of the acromion or at the level of the bicipital groove. It is associated with specific strokes (butterfly or freestyle) and is distance- or intensity related. Essential in the evaluation of a swimmer with shoulder pain is both history and examination to rule out a proximal (neurologic) cause for the pain. Treatment relies on relief of rotator cuff irritation, restoration of normal glenohumeral flexibility, and restoration of rotator cuff balance. Short-term use of nonsteroidal anti-inflammatory drugs is appropriate. Training modifications include changing absolute distance and frequency or length of interval workouts. Careful evaluation of swimming technique may reveal extremes of internal rotation or thumb lead on water entry. Bilateral breathing decreases asymmetric cuff load. Establishment of a stable scapular platform and improvement of rotator cuff strength and relative rotator cuff balance are also essential.

In addition to the stress associated with swimming, cycling accidents may result in acromioclavicular separation, clavicle fracture, or contusions about the shoulder. Aside from the injury itself, muscle weakness and altered swim techniques are consequences of such an injury.

The use of triathlon aerodynamic handlebars also adds stress to the shoulders. These systems rely on a position of shoulder adduction, flexion, and internal rotation (impingement). Athletes riding in this position carry significant body load on the glenohumeral and humeroacromial articulations. Minimal impingement symptoms can be exacerbated by use of the bars. Modification of hand position and forearm rotation, stem length, elbow pad position, bar height, or the amount of time spent in the "aero" position may be necessary if shoulder problems develop when such devices are used.

Knee Injuries

Knee problems are related to both cycling and running; patellofemoral problems (quadriceps insertion tendinitis, chondromalacia, patellar tendon tendinitis) are the most common ones. Athletes present with tenderness at the quadriceps insertion, complaints of crepitation and pain of a true retropatellar nature, or tenderness at the origin of the patellar tendon. On occasion this may be associated with a knee effusion. For cyclists, this is usually an error in bike setup or training. "Pushing" large gears at a high load, slow cadence, or low saddle height contributes to irritation of the extensor mechanism. In runners, this is often secondary to prolonged downhill running or underlying patellofemoral malalignment. In either case, this can be addressed by training modification and appropriate rehabilitation.

Use of appropriate gearing during cycling, which allows riding at lower resistance and faster cadence (80 to 100 rpm) significantly decreases load on the extensor mechanism. In addition, elevating the saddle so that knee flexion is 20° to 25° at the bottom of each pedal stroke decreases patellofemoral contact pressure. Rehabilitation should consist of aggressive hamstrings flexibility exercises, quadriceps rehabilitation done with short arc and terminal extension exercises, and avoidance of eccentric load activities such as downhill running.

Medial shelf plica irritation is also commonly seen. With medial shelf irritation, the typical complaint is peripatellar irritation just above the joint line. Patients report an intermittent catch, pop, or snap. Effusion is an intermittent phenomenon. Examination often reveals specific point tenderness in the medial peripatellar area. Usually the hamstrings are extremely tight and the quadriceps relatively weak, particularly the vastus medialis obliquus (VMO). In cycling, this is often due to inappropriate cleat alignment with excessive *external* rotation, resulting in tension and repetitive abrasion of the medial shelf plica. In runners, this can be secondary to training on a steeply banked road, patellofemoral malalignment, or quadriceps—especially VMO—weakness. Rehabilitation consists of modification of cleat position or use of rotational freedom cleat systems in cycling, avoidance of cambered roads or repeated, unvaried track workouts in running, attention to hamstrings flexibility, and quadriceps rehabilitation with specific attention to the vastus medialis obliquus (including the use of a muscle stimulation unit).

Athletes with pes anserine tendinitis or bursitis present similarly with complaints and swelling just below the level of the joint line rather than around the patella. Its origin is similar to that of medial shelf plica syndrome, but excessive saddle height is a secondary cause. The treatment is similar to that for plica syndrome. Most important is attention to hamstrings flexibility. On occasion, the athlete may require iontophoresis to the pes insertion or selective corticosteroid injection.

Athletes with iliotibial band tendinitis complain of lateral knee discomfort, most often during the pedal stroke. They report a pop and catch over the lateral femoral condyle during knee extension. This is often associated with a zone of tenderness along the posterolateral femoral condyle and intermittent, nonspecific, posterolateral swelling. It is related to excessive saddle height, posterior saddle position, or excessive internal rotation during pedaling. It may be related to running on cambered roads (affecting the down-side leg), which places abnormal tension on the iliotibial band. Iliotibial band tendinitis is treated by modifying cleat position or using rotational freedom cleats, positioning the saddle farther forward, decreasing saddle height, aggressive flexibility exercises, and anti-inflammatory medications. Occasionally, injections about the iliotibial band may be useful, and for rare refractory cases, incision or resection of a portion of the iliotibial band is required.

Stress Fractures

Given the running component of the sport and the primary running background of most triathletes, stress fractures are not uncommon (though they may be more common in single-sport athletes). Stress fractures occur when stress applied repeatedly to bone over a long time exceeds the capacity of the bone to remodel in response to that stress. Patients present with some degree of discomfort, ranging from the occasional pain of shin splints to intractable pain during rest and activity. Hyperpronation may render an athlete more susceptible to medial tibial stress syndrome, including true tibial stress fractures. Any person involved in repetitive contact-load activities (e.g., running) who suddenly changes the duration or intensity of activity and who presents with nonspecific bone pain should be suspected of having a stress fracture. Plain films may not necessarily show a lesion in the initial phases, so bone scintigraphy may be necessary. Female endurance athletes are at particular risk for stress fractures because of the "female athlete triad" of eating disorders, amenorrhea, and osteoporosis. Treatment consists of curtailment of repetitive impact activities while continuing low-load and aerobic activities until the athlete is pain free. This is followed by gradual resumption of activities with increasing loads but with mandatory plateaus every 4 to 6 weeks. A note of caution: Any runner, especially a female runner, who reports a history of hip or groin pain must be assumed to have a femoral neck stress fracture until that can be ruled out.

One of the advantages for persons interested in multisport competition is that lower extremity problems secondary to one sport (typically running) may be addressed or rehabilitated by increasing training time in a nonload activity.

Heel Injuries

Discomfort about the heel in triathletes typically is secondary to Achilles tendinitis or plantar fasciitis, again, most often related to running. Affected athletes complain of pain, either in the body of the Achilles tendon or at its insertion. In plantar fasciitis, the discomfort is principally at the origin of the plantar fascia (volar medial aspect of the heel) and is described as a *stone bruise*. In both cases, this is usually related to repeated hill running or interval work. Examination reveals diffuse swelling or point tenderness about the Achilles tendon or the plantar fascia origin. Usually it is worst on arising in the morning but is relieved or at least diminishes with activity, only to return with rest. Hyperpronation or heel valgus posture somewhat increases the risk for these problems. Treatment requires restoration of heel cord and plantar fascia flexibility; orthotic devices that control direct pressure on the heel and extremes of pronation or hindfoot valgus often help. Fortunately, the motion of cycling often addresses these complaints in athletes whose primary sport is running. Injection of steroids into or about the Achilles tendon is contraindicated.

In summary, training errors and overuse are the principal causes of injuries in triathletes. As compared with "single-sport" competitive swimmers, decreasing training distance and load should enable triathlon swimmers to remain competitive even if they have a history of shoulder problems. Rotator cuff rehabilitation, posterior capsule flexibility exercises, and scapular stabilization are essential for those who have previous injuries and should be considered part of "pre-hab" for novice swimmers. Persons who have no background in swimming should consider early coaching to learn appropriate techniques and to avoid problems. For cyclists, proper bike fit is essential, with attention to saddle height and position and with special consideration of "rotational freedom" pedals, to avoid medial and lateral knee problems. "Spinning" at fast cadence and lower load helps avoid patellofemoral problems. Athletes who are primarily runners often benefit from decreased running distance secondary to inclusion of a new lower extremity sport (cycling). Injured triathletes accept alternative activities better than those concerned about participation in a single sport. Cycling in conjunction with the repetitive impact of running may improve overall lower extremity balance and flexibility.

95 *Angelo Galante*

Gymnastics

Gymnastics is one of the fastest growing sports in the world today. Current estimates place the number of participants at approximately 2,000,000 on club, school, and collegiate levels.[1] Gymnastics competitions have six events for men and four for women.[1] The men's events—the rings, pommel horse, parallel bars, horizontal bar, vault (long horse), and floor exercise—stress strength, agility, and grace. The women's events require grace, artistry, rhythm, and dance, as well as power, displayed on the balance beam, side horse vault, uneven parallel bars, and in the floor exercise. Because, today, participants begin the sport at younger and younger ages, they are vulnerable not only to musculoskeletal injuries but to mental and emotional stress. Physical development is not the gymnast's only concern.

INJURIES

Along with gymnastics' rise in popularity, the level of competition has risen; it demands from participants many long hours of practice. With more exposure time, injury rates have risen steadily.[2–4]

Because it is so demanding, gymnastics causes injury to all body parts. In descending order of frequency, the affected areas are the lower extremity (ankle and knee), the upper extremity (shoulder, elbow, and wrist), the trunk, and the spine. Many injuries result from overuse, and others from specific maneuvers such as dismounts, round-offs, and swings. Although injuries encompass a broad spectrum, only the more common ones are discussed here.

Ankle Injuries

In most surveys of gymnastic injuries, the ankle is the body part most commonly injured.[2,3] Overuse injuries such as plantar fasciitis and Achilles tendinitis are common. Repetitive stress coupled with ligamentous laxity can predispose the gymnast to ankle sprains.

High-energy dismounts cause a significant number of ankle problems in gymnasts. The athlete repeatedly lands in a nonplantigrade position, causing extreme dorsiflexion of the ankle joint. This can lead to dorsal impingement and ankle instability. The pathogenesis seems to be soft tissue hypertrophy in the anterolateral gutter, resulting in impingement. Rehabilitation of ankle sprains should be complete before the athlete is allowed to return to practice.

Elbow Injuries

Gymnasts frequently use their arms for weight bearing and also impart high-impact loads to their elbows. Hyperextension injuries can cause elbow dislocation, which results in injury to both the capsule and the posterior and medial ligaments. Although the incidence of elbow injuries is not high, they are very specific.[7] To prevent loss of flexion and extension, our suggested treatment for fractures and dislocations is a short period of immobilization followed by early motion. Aggressive rehabilitation and conditioning should restore full function within 3 months.

Conditions such as osteochondritis dissecans of the capitellum also affect gymnasts. See Chapters 50, 53, and 54 for further discussions of this entity. The key to limiting the extent of elbow injuries is early detection. Early diagnosis and treatment prevent disruption of normal growth in young gymnasts.[8]

Wrist Injuries

Because of the chronic overload of the wrist and the need for proper function, wrist pain is a leading cause of disability in gymnasts. One study of collegiate gymnasts indicates a 72% prevalence of wrist pain for males and 33% for females.[5] It is so prevalent that some gymnasts consider pain at the dorsal aspect of the wrist part of being a gymnast.

Most gymnasts with wrist pain complain of pain during compression and on impact with rotation or with forced dorsiflexion. Chronic overload of a non–weight-bearing joint during growth and development can change the normal structure of the wrist. It is theorized that because of this trauma to the distal radial physis the length of the ulna relative to the radius is increased.[5] The development of positive ulnar variance may confer increased risk for impingement, triangular fibrocartilage complex tears, ligamentous tears, and secondary chondromalacia of the different articulations of the wrist. Coaches should be educated about this condition and about the potential for inhibition of normal growth or for further injury. Young gymnasts with wrist pain should, during the healing phase, discontinue any activity that puts significant stress on the wrist.[6]

Stress fractures are also a significant problem because of increased load.

Spine Disorders

The demands on the lower back of a young gymnast are unparalleled in sports. Because of these excessive demands, a broad spectrum of problems can develop from acute and chronic injuries. The acute injuries usually occur from falls or poor technique and are the most devastating. Chronic injuries occur from repeated flexion, extension, and rotation of the spine. Common problems include damage to the pars interarticularis that results in spondylolysis and spondylolisthesis.[9] There has been some speculation that hereditary factors may predispose certain athletes to these injuries. The condition usually appears between age 10 and 13, and the chief complaint is back pain. Conditioning of the abdominal and paravertebral muscles is recommended to prevent hyperlordotic posture.[2]

Back problems in gymnasts are potentially serious and should never be ignored. Coaches and physicians who care for these athletes should look for warning signs such as low back pain. Pain lasting longer than 2 weeks is an indication for a complete evaluation, which includes a history and physical examination with radiographic studies. These injuries are seen more commonly in gymnasts, even though other injuries are also associated with the sport (Table 95–1).

Injury Prevention

The high rate of injury among gymnasts has prompted those who care for them to suggest the following measures to prevent injury: (1) maintenance of height charts for competitive gymnasts, (2) preseason examination that includes musculoskeletal screening and maturity assessment, (3) supervision by trained personnel (i.e., athletic trainers) of gymnasts identified as injured or at risk of injury in the preseason health examination, (4) ongoing supervision of injury rehabilitation and return to practice by trained personnel, and (5) reduced training loads for gymnasts experiencing a growth spurt indicated by height charts or maturity assessment information. When height measures or special periodic checkups show that any temporary physiologic imbalance related to the growth spurt has abated, normal training levels can be resumed.[10]

Table 95–1. Gymnastics Injuries

Ankle:	Sever's disease, osteochondritis dissecans, ligament instability
Knee:	Ligament injury, meniscal tears, fractures
Wrist:	Impingement, triangular fibrocartilage complex tears, ligament tears, chondromalacia
Forearm:	Fractures of both forearm bones (results from malfunction of leather dowel grips)
Elbow:	Fractures, dislocations, osteochondritis dissecans, loose bodies
Shoulder:	Impingement (common), rotator cuff injury, subluxations or dislocations, labrum tears
Spine:	Spondylolysis, spondylolisthesis

MEDICAL AND PSYCHOLOGICAL PROBLEMS

Although this demanding sport carries great risk for injury, good training, proper coaching, and good medical care can reduce the incidence and morbidity of musculoskeletal injuries. However, the stresses of gymnastics also create the potential for serious medical and psychological problems. These problems include issues of nutrition, endocrine imbalance, and psychological stress from intense competitiveness.

Endocrine

Menstrual dysfunction is common in female gymnasts. It occurs in as many as 50% of elite gymnasts.[11] The origin is multifactorial: little body fat, poor nutrition, high-intensity training, and high energy demands. Adding to the problem is the fact that most gymnasts start intensive training before puberty, which can delay the onset of menses by as long as 2 years. The longterm effects may include increased risk of premature osteoporosis, stress fractures, and pathologic fractures.

Psychological

Eating disorders are thought to be prevalent among gymnasts because of the great emphasis on body image and appearance. The societal image of Olga Korbut and Nadia Comaneci as ideal gymnasts has created this desire for a thin, lean look. Striving for leanness leads to calorie restriction, which can cause nutritional deficiencies (especially iron and calcium) and eating disorders (anorexia nervosa and bulimia). Because children are starting the sport younger, such undesirable consequences appear early. This can place increased stress on an already fragile self-esteem and can have longterm psychological effects.

The medical and psychological problems of the sport must be considered and dealt with as aggressively as are the orthopedic problems, not only because they affect performance but because they can have even greater impact on lifelong health. For all who are involved with the care of gymnasts, an awareness of the potential for these problems and the information to treat them can help circumvent longterm morbidity, and even mortality.

REFERENCES

1. Weiker, G. G.: Introduction and history of gymnastics. Clin. Sports Med. *4*:3, 1985.
2. Garrick, J. G., and Requa, R. K.: Epidemiology of women's gymnastics injuries. Am. J. Sports Med. *8*:261, 1980.
3. Snook, G. A.: Injuries in women's gymnastics. A five-year study. Am. J. Sports Med. *7*:242, 1979.
4. McAuley, E., Hudash E., Shields K., Albright J., et al.: Injuries in women's gymnastics—the state of the art. Am. J. Sports Med. *15*:558, 1987.
5. Mandelbaum, B. R., Bartolozzi A. R., Davis C. A., Teurlings L., and Bragonier, B.: Wrist pain syndrome in the gymnast: Pathogenetic, diagnostic, and therapeutic considerations. Am. J. Sports Med. *17*:305, 1989.
6. Roy, S., Caine, D., and Singer, K. M.: Stress changes of the distal radial epiphysis in young gymnasts. Am. J. Sports Med. *13*:301, 1985.
7. Meeusen, R., and Borms, J.: Gymnastics injuries. Sports Med. *13*:337, 1992.
8. Caine, D. J., and Lindner, K. T.: Overuse injuries of growing bones: The young female gymnast at risk? Physician Sportsmed. *13*(12):51, 1985.
9. Ciullo, J. V., and Jackson, D. W.: Pars interarticularis stress reaction spondylolysis, and spondylolisthesis in gymnasts. Clin. Sports Med. *4*:95, 1985.
10. Caine, D., Cochrane, B., Caine, C., and Zemper, E.: An epidemiologic investigation of injuries affecting young competitive female gymnasts. Am. J. Sports Med. *17*:811, 1989.
11. Calabrese, L. H.: Nutritional and medical aspects of gymnastics. Clin. Sports Med. *4*:23, 1985.

96

R. Todd Dombroski

Wrestling

INJURIES

More than a quarter of a million high school students participate in wrestling,[1] and many more in collegiate and local wrestling club teams. While much of the attention on sports-related injuries has focused on football, wrestling injury rates are a very close second. Approximately 30% of high school wrestlers sustain injuries that cause them to lose time from play.[2] Collegiate wrestlers average 1 to 2½ injuries per wrestler per season.[3] The absolute number of injuries is higher in practice than in competition; however, per minute of wrestling, the injury rate can be 40 times greater during a match.[4] Therefore, primary care physicians and orthopedists who work with wrestling teams should make sure that a physician is present at all matches, and, ideally, that he or she has an appreciation of the basic rules, biomechanics, and trauma associated with wrestling.

Risk factors for injury include time in the season (more injuries occur early in the season), level (junior varsity wrestlers have more injuries than varsity athletes), weight (lighter-weight wrestlers have more injuries), and the position of the wrestler with less control (i.e., during take down or while on the bottom).

The time allowed for a medical assessment is only 2 minutes in high school wrestling and 90 seconds in collegiate matches; this does not include bleeding injuries. The goal of a ringside physician is a directed examination to determine if an injury is serious enough to require the wrestler to forfeit the match. A more thorough examination and the follow-up plan can be completed later. The number of specific types of injury may vary, but generally the knee is the area more often injured, followed by the shoulder, ribs, and elbow.

Knee Injuries

Unlike football injuries, many wrestling knee injuries result from repetitive microtrauma. For example, the most common knee injury is prepatellar bursitis,[4] which is probably caused by repetitive rubbing rather than a traumatic blow. Prepatellar bursitis has a high recurrence rate. Aggressive treatment with a compressive dressing and immobilization (splinting) and wearing a donut dressing around the bursa during practice is recommended. The use of nonsteroidal anti-inflammatory medication and dicloxacillin is advised. Aspiration or use of a Penrose drain is controversial because this may introduce infection from skin bacteria and cause a fistula. Neoprene knee pads (not elastic) afford the best prevention for prepatellar bursitis.

The fact that the ratio of lateral meniscus injury to medial meniscus injury is nearly equal in wrestling is unique. Wrestling causes more varus stress to the knee and multiple episodes of microtrauma. Often there is no history of a traumatic event associated with lateral meniscal injury. Given the time constraints for injury assessment, if the wrestler has full range of motion, can hop on one leg, and can duck walk, the knee injury should not cause him to forfeit the match. To prevent more varus stress, wrestlers should be taught not to hook their ankle around the opponent's leg (Fig. 96–1). For collateral ligament sprains, the knee may be braced or taped, but the coach or trainer should remember that both knees should have something on them to avoid "marking" the injured knee for the opponent.

Shoulder Injuries

The most common shoulder injury among wrestlers is to the acromioclavicular (AC) joint. This usually occurs from direct trauma to the lateral shoulder, not to the AC joint itself. A palpable step-off, decreased range of motion, or upper extremity weakness is cause for forfeiture. Mild AC joint sprains may be padded, but padding has not been proven to prevent injury or to stay on during competition. Capsule sprains may require forfeiture,

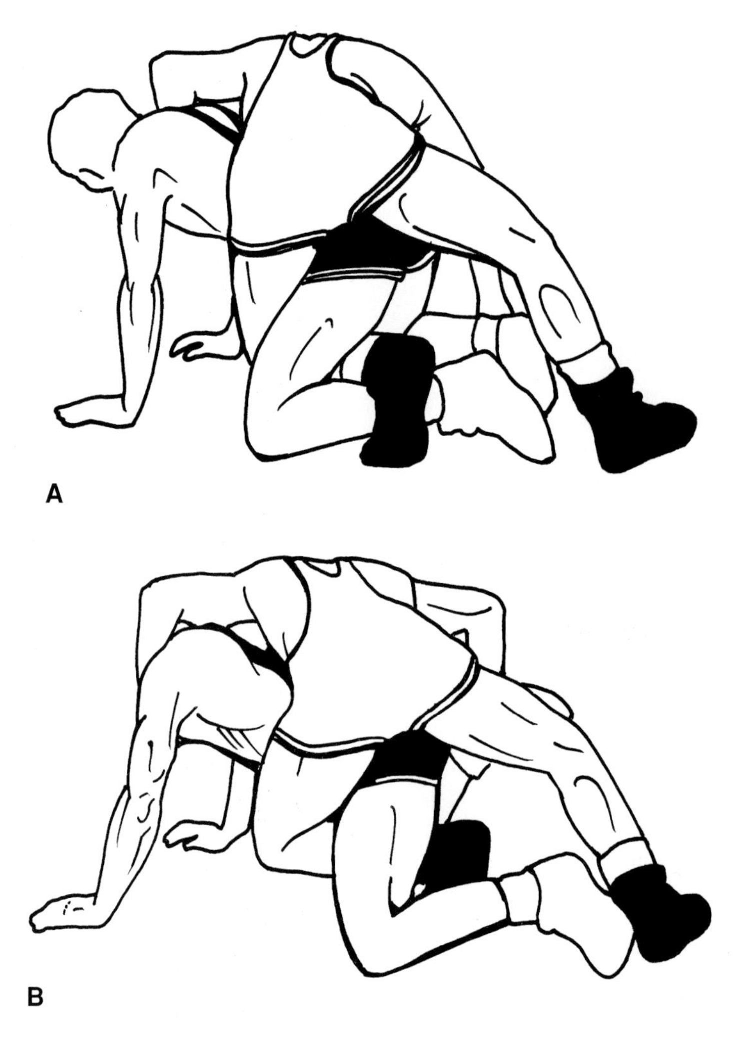

Fig. 96–1. *(A)* **Hooking the ankle around an opponent's leg can cause excessive varus stress to the knee.** *(B)* **The wrestler should be taught the correct position to avoid these stresses.**

but they usually do well with conservative treatment. Fortunately, shoulder subluxations and dislocations are rare.

Elbow Injuries

Elbow injuries commonly occur during a fall when the elbow is in full extension. This injury can result in hyperextension or fracture-dislocation. Wrestlers should be taught not to "lock" the elbow in full extension. Taping and bracing can be helpful for these injuries. Olecranon bursitis is also practically unique to wrestling and is treated like the aforementioned prepatellar bursitis.

Skin Diseases and Injuries

Skin diseases and injuries plague wrestlers. Many skin diseases can be prevented with twice daily disinfectant cleaning of the mats, careful use of personal towels and no sharing of towels among teammates. Herpes simplex virus type 1 causes herpes gladiatorum. Treatment includes oral acyclovir, 200 mg five times a day, for 5 days and application of acyclovir cream when the athlete is not wrestling. A clear plastic Tegaderm or Op-site (not gauze) should be applied over the lesions only during matches; and the athlete should be careful to avoid the mat during practices. Those with recurrent lesions may use oral acyclovir, 200 mg three times a day, during the season, but it is not recommended for use for longer than 12 months.[5] For the treatment of molluscum contagiosum and impetigo see Chapter 26.

Lacerations and nosebleeds are common wrestling injuries. Steri-strips can be a quick fix for lacerations. Nasal packing without epinephrine can help the athlete with a nosebleed through the match, but the evaluation after the match should include examination for septal hematoma.

Head and Neck Injuries

An auricular hematoma (cauliflower ear) is seen as a proud "war wound" by some athletes. Therefore, prompt evacuation of the hematoma and application of a collodion gauze pressure dressing may not be well accepted by the wrestler. Suturing cotton dental bolsters to both sides of the ear after evacuation may be less effective in preventing hematoma recurrence, but it enhances compliance.

Wrestling is second only to football in the incidence of catastrophic neck injuries.[1] Cervical strains are common and may lead to transient neurapraxia. Any athlete with a deficit in upper extremity motor strength should forfeit the match and be evaluated promptly with cervical spine radiographs.

Trunk Injuries

Injuries to the trunk include rib fractures, rib contusions, rib subluxations, costochondral sprains, and strains of the rectus abdominis and oblique muscles of the abdomen. All these injuries are painful and frustrating. Rest and nonsteroidal anti-inflammatory medication can ameliorate symptoms so the athlete can continue training.

Many other injuries that occur less commonly in wrestling are covered in other parts of this book. The problems of diet restriction and "cutting weight" are obviously a major concern in a sport based on weight classes. The chapters on nutrition and body composition discuss these in more detail.

Caring for wrestlers can be frustrating because of their high rate of noncompliance.[4] Earning trust as the "team physician" who is interested in initial aggressive treatment and prompt return to wrestling is the best asset. Also, early involvement of coaches, parents, and trainers should help to make the care of the "wrestling family" an enjoyable experience.

REFERENCES

1. Strauss, R. H., Lanese, R. R.: Injuries among wrestlers in high school and college tournaments. JAMA. *248*: 2016, 1982.
2. Estwanik, J., Bergfield, J., and Collins H.: Injuries in interscholastic wrestling. Physician Sportsmed. *8*(3):111, 1980.
3. Snook, G. A.: Injuries in intercollegiate wrestling. Am. J. Sports Med. *10*:142, 1982.
4. Wroble, R. R., Mysnyk, M. C., Foster, D. T., and Albright, J. P.: Patterns of knee injuries in wrestling: A six-year study. Am. J. Sports Med. *14*:55, 1986.
5. Becker, T. M., Kodsi, R., and Bailey, P., et al,: Grappling with herpes: Herpes gladiatorum. Am. J. Sports Med. *16*:665, 1988.

INDEX

Page numbers in *italics* indicate figures; those followed by "t" indicate tables.